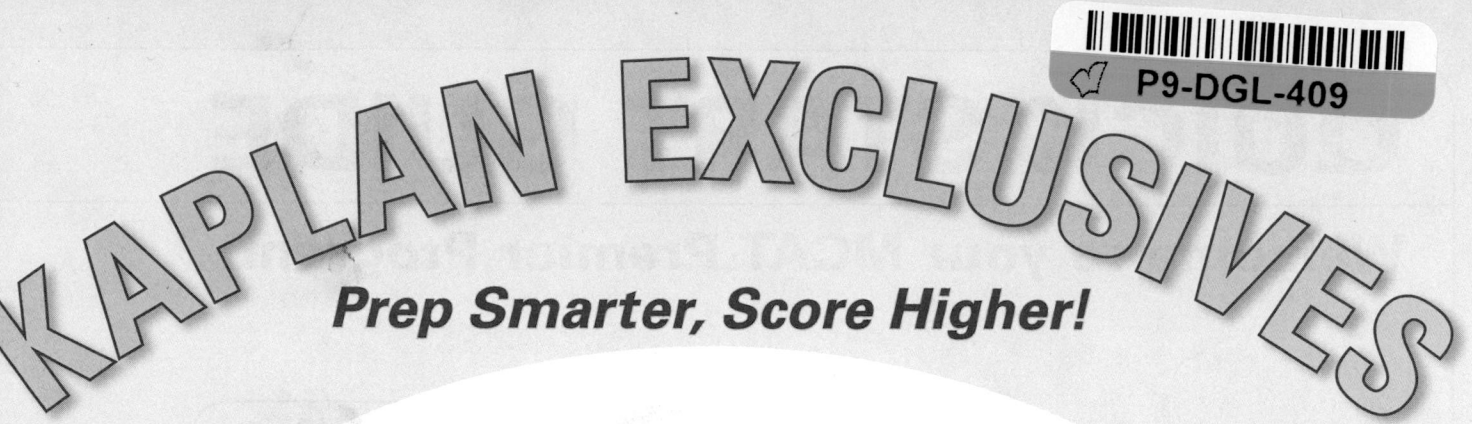

KAPLAN EXCLUSIVES

Prep Smarter, Score Higher!

Watch a Kaplan teacher explain key concepts from each section!

FAST FACT TEACHER VIDEOS

NEW QUIZZES EVERY MONTH

EXTENSIVE PRACTICE ONLINE

Take 3 total practice tests!

Come back each month for syllabus updates.

QUICK START GUIDE

Welcome to your MCAT Premier Program!

DOUBLE CHECK!

The serial number on the inside back cover of your book is your key to the online companion. *Enter it carefully and make sure all of the numbers and letters match exactly!*

1 REGISTER YOUR ONLINE COMPANION

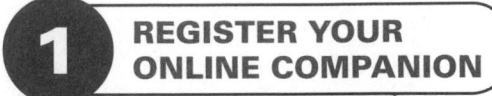
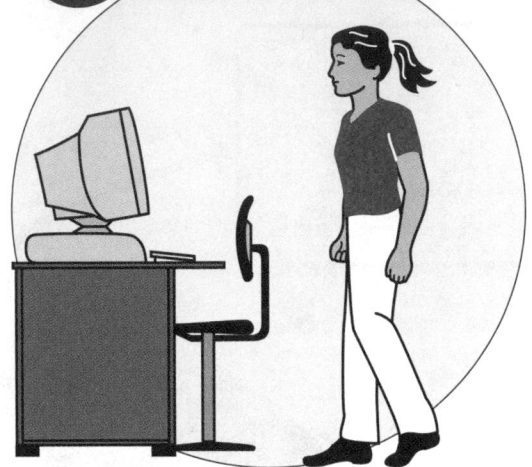

2 TAKE THE ONLINE DIAGNOSTIC QUIZ

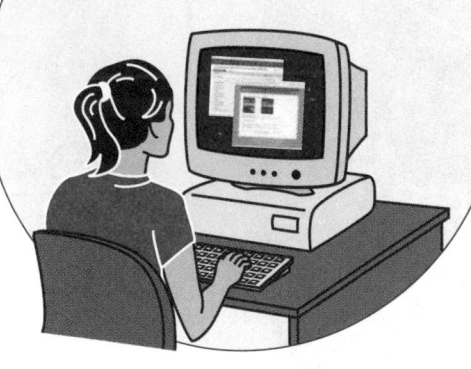

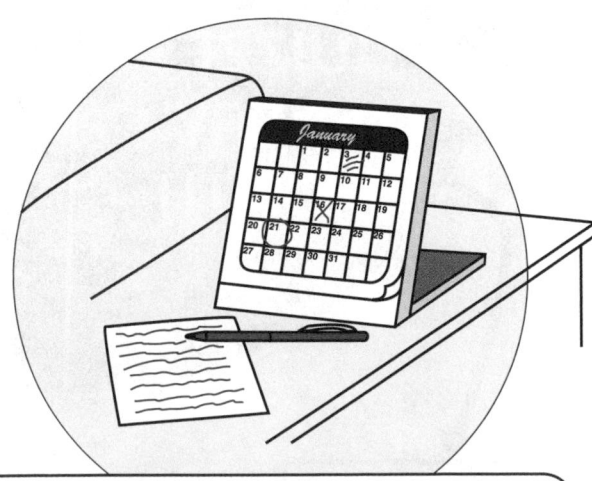

3 GET TO KNOW YOUR SYLLABUS AND THE MCAT FORMAT

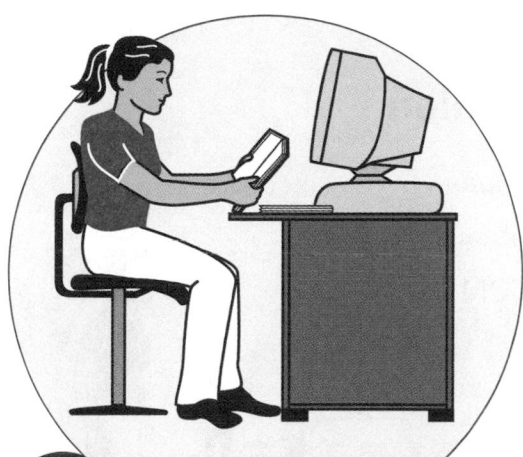

4 TAKE A NEW PRACTICE QUIZ EVERY MONTH!

☑ Register
☑ Diagnostic Test
☑ Practice Test
☐ Watch Lesson
☐ Online Content

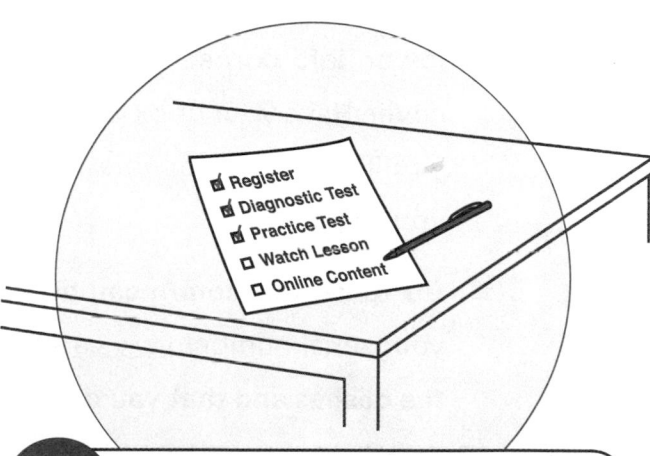

5 MONITOR YOUR PROGRESS WITH PRACTICE TESTS

6 WATCH A KAPLAN LESSON ONLINE

→ # THE FOLLOWING STEPS OF YOUR ONLINE PROGRAM WILL LEAD YOU ON THE PATH TO MCAT SUCCESS!

1 Register Your Online Companion

To begin your Kaplan MCAT test prep experience and access your course syllabus, you must first register your ONLINE COMPANION. Follow these simple steps:

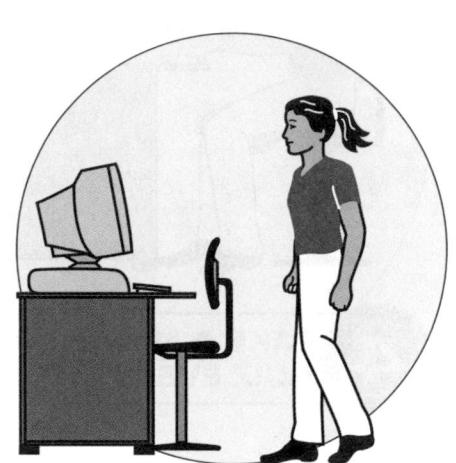

■ Locate the serial number in the book. You'll find the serial number on the lower left corner of the inside back cover. Have your book with you because you'll be asked for this number when you register.

■ **Go to kaptest.com/mcatbooksonline.** This is where it all begins! Insert your serial number <u>very carefully</u> to register. **Make sure you don't forget the dashes and that you don't enter any extra spaces!**

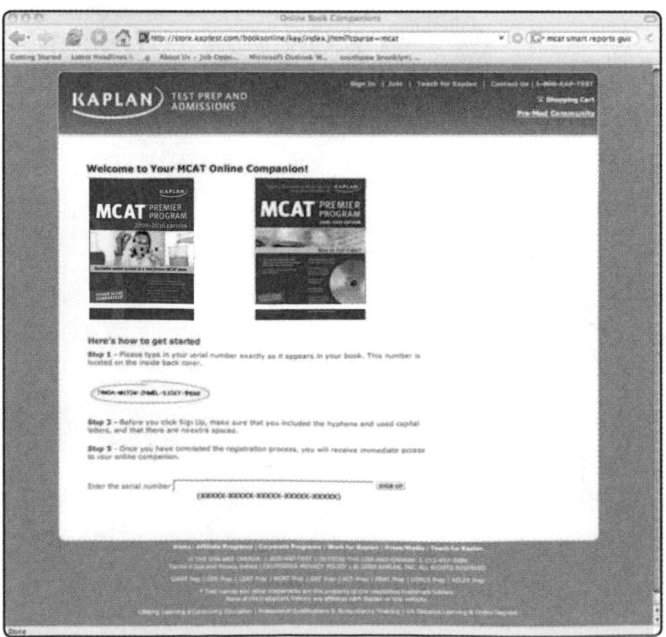

You can return to your Online Companion 24/7 through any Internet browser by going to **Kaptest.com** and selecting the "My Page" link.

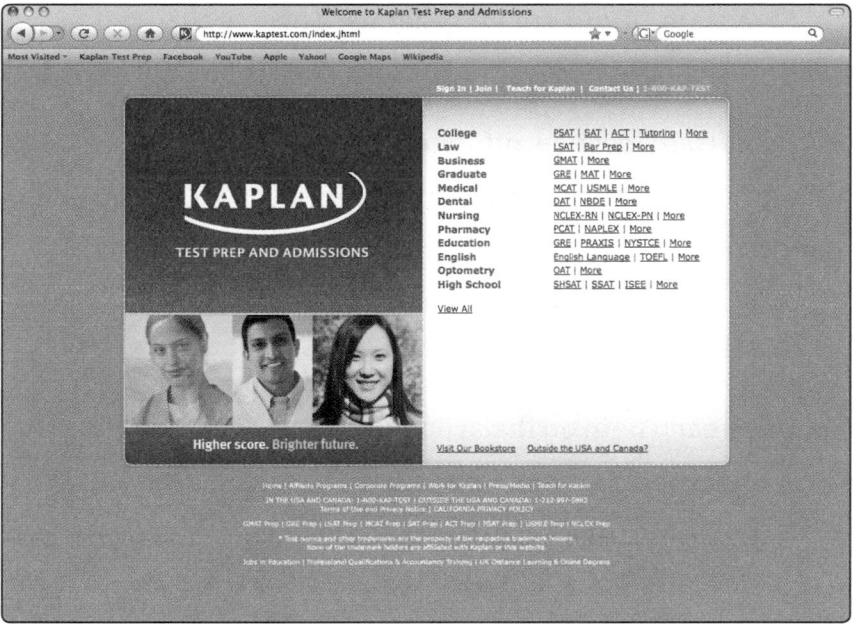

The Online Companion gives you access to MCAT Premier Program components that are not included between the covers of this book, including your Diagnostic Quiz, fresh new quizzes monthly, MCAT practice tests, and more!

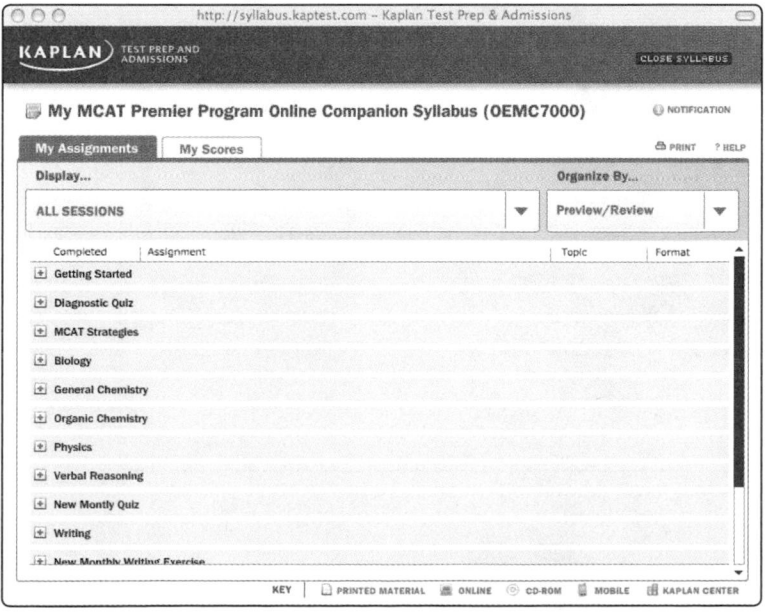

2 Take the Online Diagnostic Quiz

Once you have registered, begin by reviewing all of the items in the "Getting Started" section of the online syllabus. These items will assist you in using each of the course components to the fullest possible advantage.

The "Getting Started" section offers resources such as a direct link to the official MCAT registration website, an overview of MCAT question strategies, a scoring rubric that will assist you in evaluating your practice essays, and technical support.

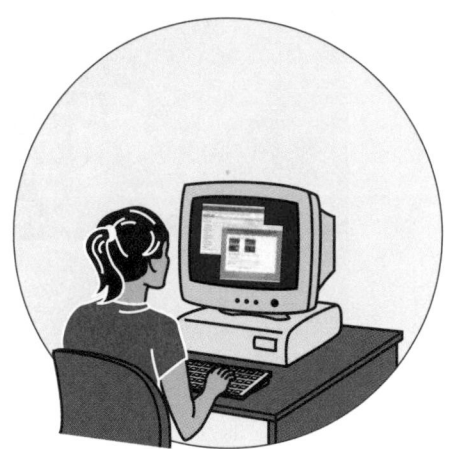

As you complete each item on the syllabus, remember to check it off so that you know which material you've already covered.

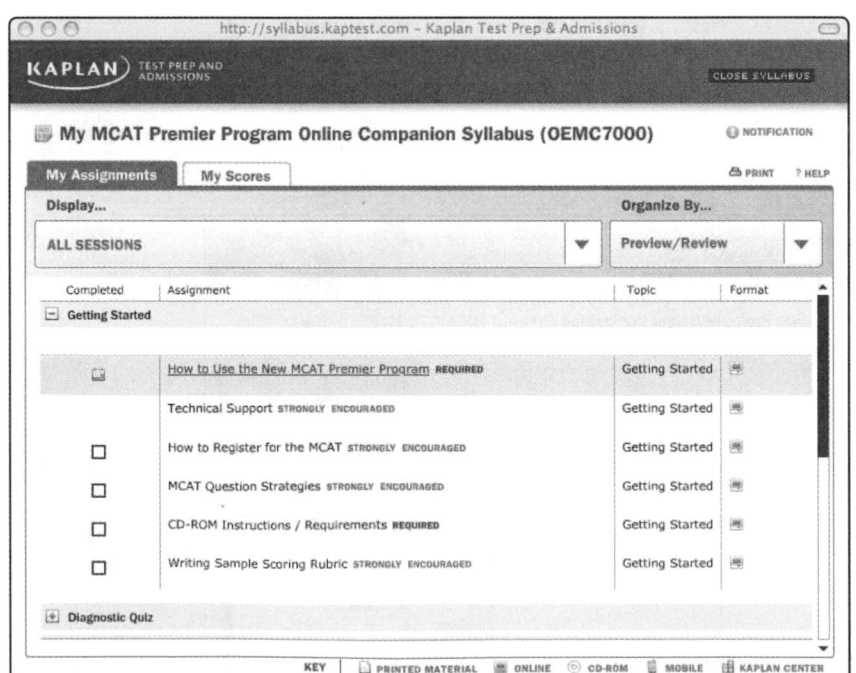

After you review the items in Getting Started, you are ready to take the online Diagnostic Quiz. The purpose of the Diagnostic Quiz is to help you gauge where you need to focus your review. The quiz will tell you if you are stronger or weaker in one of the sciences, or if you need more practice with Verbal Reasoning—that way, you'll know where to spend the majority of your time and energy reviewing.

Go to the "Diagnostic Quiz" session, and click on the "MCAT Diagnostic Quiz" link that appears. This will prompt a separate window to appear with the quiz.

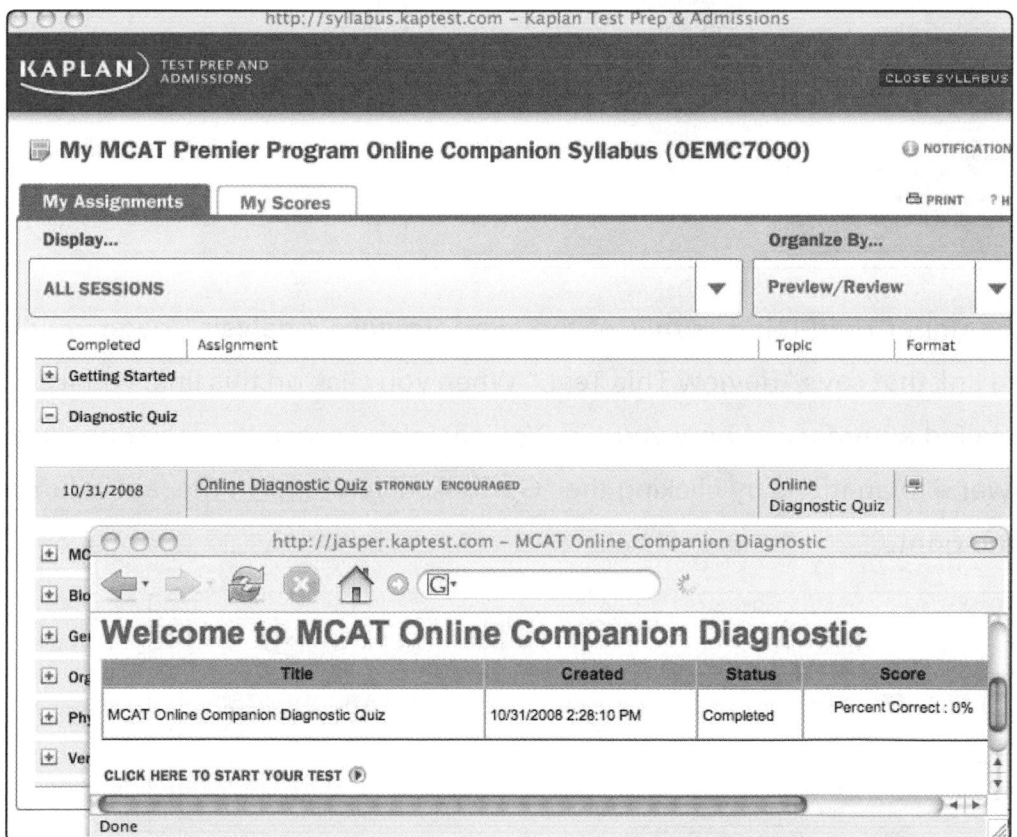

The MCAT Diagnostic Quiz is a sampling of what you will see on the real test. It includes samples of each question type found in the MCAT. When you complete the quiz and submit your answers, you will see a summary of your performance on the "Performance Analysis" page.

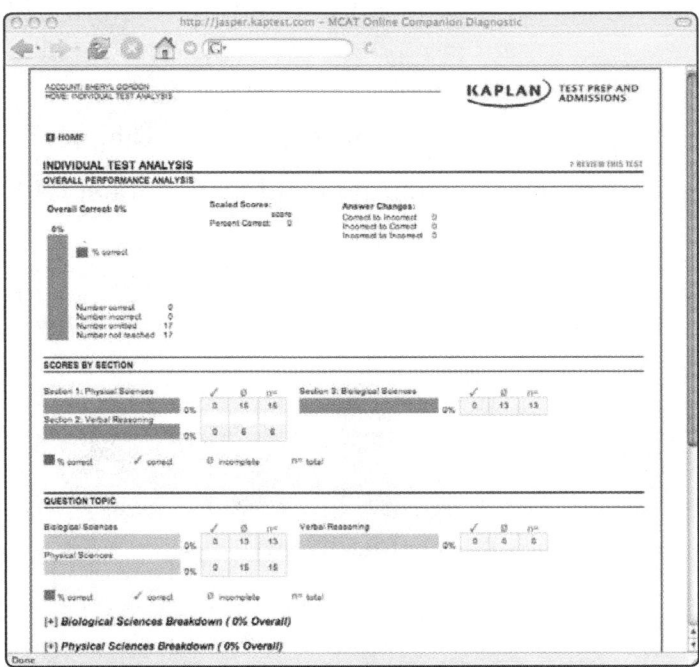

In the upper right-hand corner of the "Performance Analysis" page, you'll see a link that says "Review This Test." When you click on this link, you'll see a detailed summary of how you did. You can also access the questions and answer explanations by clicking the "Go To Analysis" link in the last column on the right.

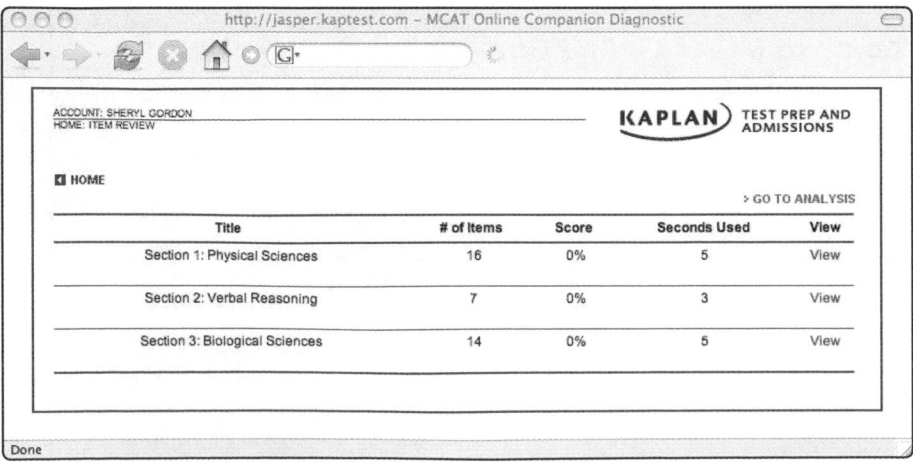

Title	# of Items	Score	Seconds Used	View
Section 1: Physical Sciences	16	0%	5	View
Section 2: Verbal Reasoning	7	0%	3	View
Section 3: Biological Sciences	14	0%	5	View

TWO EASY STEPS TO DIAGNOSING YOUR RESULTS

▶ ## STEP 1: Evaluate your general performance

Look at the summary of your performance on the "Performance Analysis" page to see what your scaled score would be, and to get a sense of:

- The number of questions you got right, wrong, skipped, or didn't answer by section.

- How long it took you to answer each question.

- How frequently you changed your mind.

▶ ## STEP 2: Identify your strengths and weaknesses

Now look at the detailed summary of your performance on each question in the "Review This Test" page, as well as the answer explanations. Make a list of your *personal* strengths and weaknesses by identifying whether or not:

- You know and understand the concepts being tested.

- You find certain question types especially challenging.

- You are answering questions quickly enough.

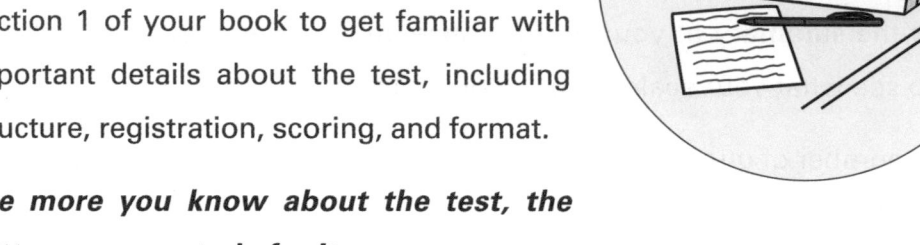

3 Get to Know Your Syllabus and the MCAT Format

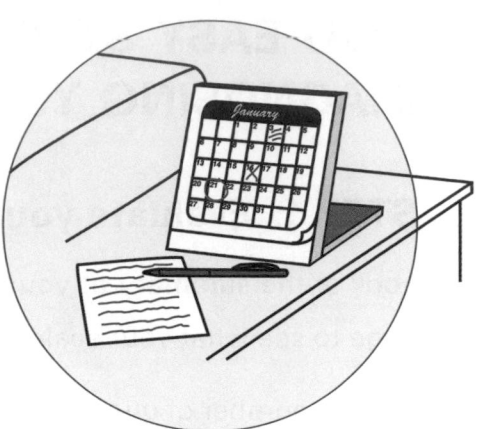

Before you dive into the many study sessions offered on your Online Companion, review Section 1 of your book to get familiar with important details about the test, including structure, registration, scoring, and format.

The more you know about the test, the better you can study for it.

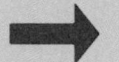

NAVIGATING AROUND YOUR SYLLABUS

Important components from your book, including Kaplan's comprehensive science, verbal reasoning, and writing review (Sections 2 through 7) make up the next part (and the bulk) of your syllabus.

- The strategies section offers test preparation advice and talks about MCAT question types, breaking them down into manageable parts and identifying methods for uncovering the correct answer.

- The comprehensive review section incorporates reading from your book as well as online workshops that delve into specific topics in greater depth.

You may wish to review all of these sections from start to finish, or you may choose to skip around or review only those areas where the Diagnostic Quiz indicated you needed additional review.

To start a workshop or online quiz

■ Choose the subject you want to practice.

■ When you roll your mouse over the name of the test or prompt, the name will turn into a hyperlink (it will change color and become underlined).

■ Click on the hyperlink. A separate window will appear.

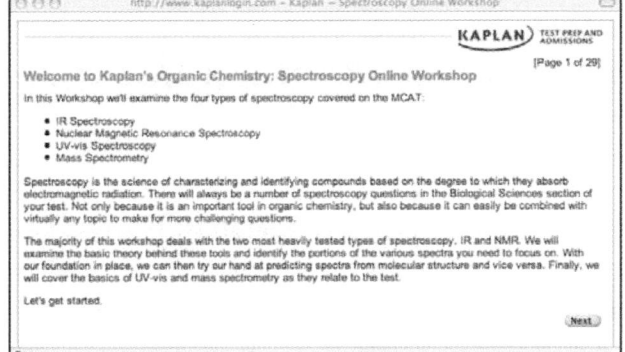

■ Read the explanation of the activity and click "Next" or "Click Here to Start..." to begin.

To suspend a quiz at any time

■ Click on the "Suspend" button at the bottom left side of the quiz window.

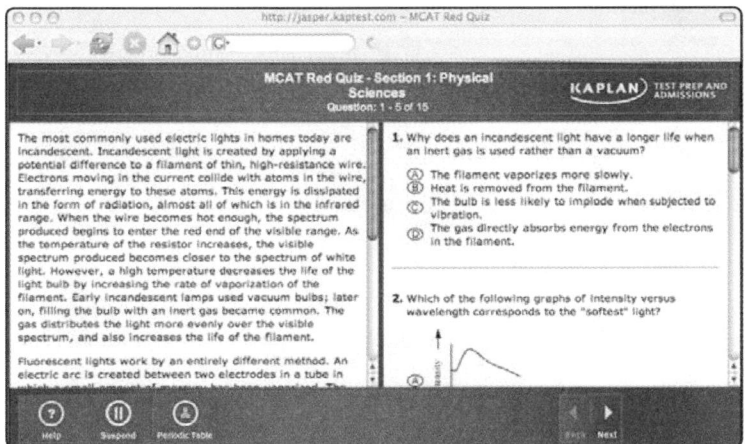

To resume a quiz

■ Select the quiz from the corresponding session.

■ A pop-up will appear with a table showing the status.

■ Click the "Resume" button in the right-hand column of the table.

To start a quiz over again

- Select the quiz from the corresponding session.

- A pop-up will appear with a table showing the status.

- Click the "Click Here to Start…" link.

To add completion dates for all activities

- Go to the corresponding session.

- Click on the box to the left of the task you completed.

- A pop-up will appear allowing you to select the date.

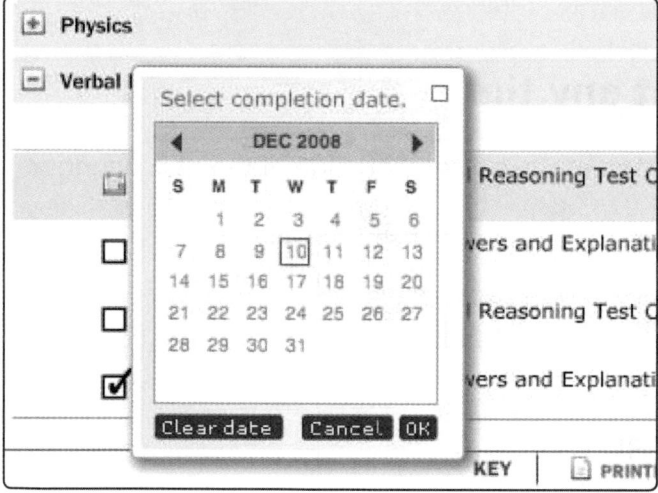

CUSTOMIZING THE ORGANIZATION OF YOUR ONLINE COMPANION

You can rearrange your home page syllabus to look however you like!

After logging in to your Online Companion, you will arrive at the default "My Assignments" page with the default "Preview/Review" category. This option presents all the assets for every session.

▶ To see all the assets of just one session:

■ Go to the "Display" pull-down menu.

■ Click on the "ALL SESSIONS" option.

■ Select the title of the session you want.

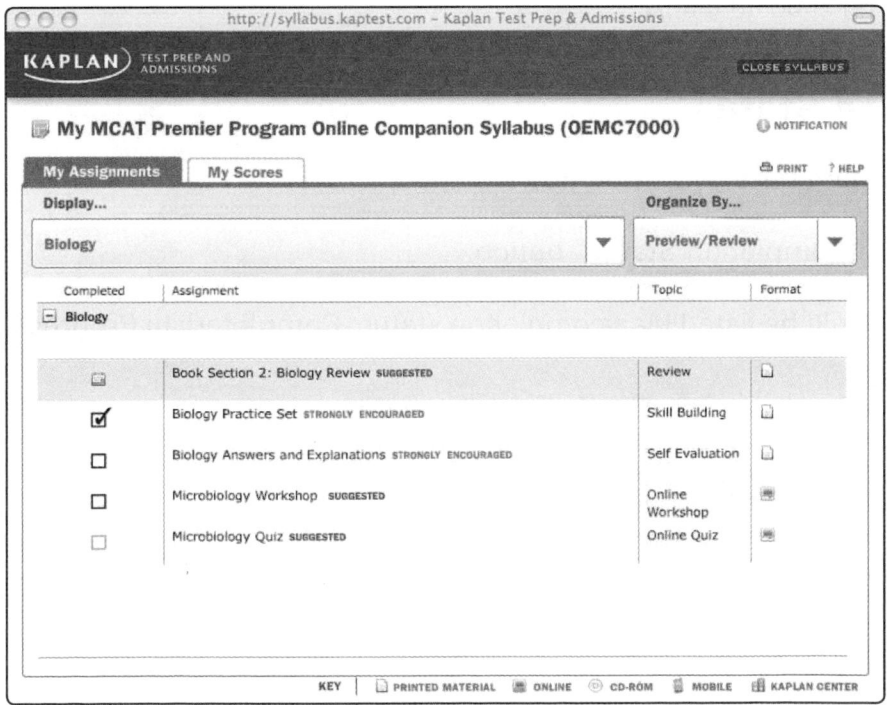

▶ ## Reorganize Your Syllabus by Category

There are six categories: Preview/Review, Requirement Level, Completion Status, Assignment Name, Topic, and Format.

Requirement Level

- Go to the "Organize by..." pull-down menu.

- Select the "Requirement Level" option.

- Each asset will be listed by a requirement level: Required (in red); Strongly Encouraged (in green); Suggested (in blue).

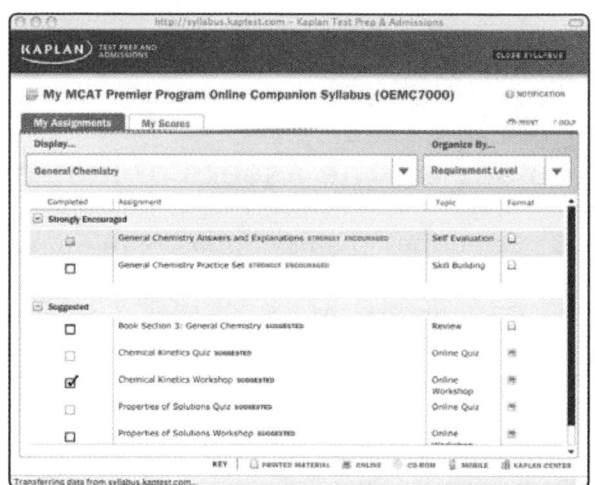

Completion Status

- Go to the "Organize by..." pull-down menu.

- Select the "Completion Status" option.

- Each asset will be listed by a completion status: Completed; In Progress; Incomplete.

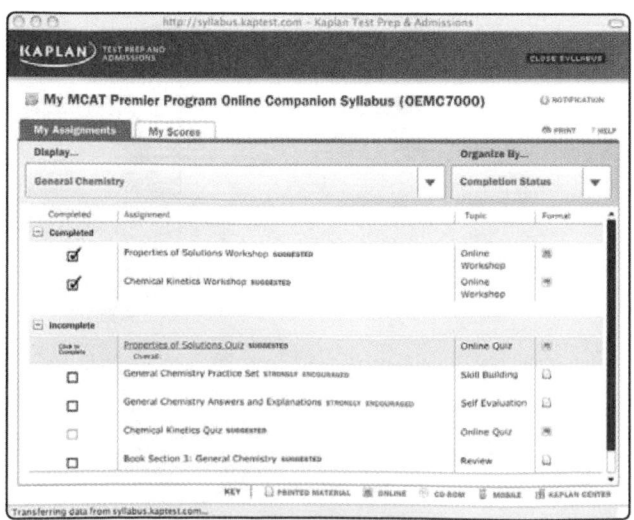

Assignment Name

■ Go to the "Organize by..." pull-down menu.

■ Select the "Assignment Name" option.

■ Each asset will be listed alphabetically (not by session).

Topic

■ Go to the "Organize by..." pull-down menu.

■ Select the "Topic" option.

■ Each asset will be listed by topic, such as "Review," "Skillbuilding, or "Practice Test."

Format

■ Go to the "Organize by..." pull-down menu.

■ Select the "Format" option.

■ Each asset will be listed by format (Online or Print).

4 Take a NEW Practice Quiz Every Month!

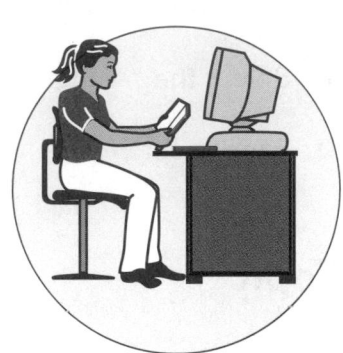

After the review sections and specific subject quizzes, you'll find online rotating quizzes and essay practice sessions that test your level of preparation and readiness for the full length exam. Under the section New Monthly Quiz, the quizzes refresh each month with new content so that you'll never run out of material to gauge your progress.

5 Monitor Your Progress with Practice Tests.

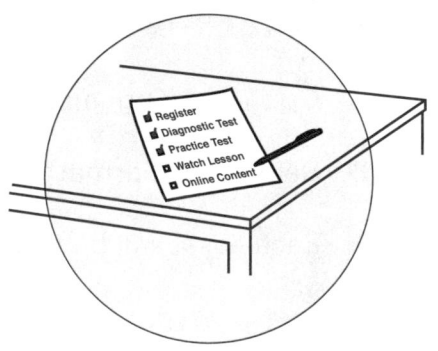

Once you feel comfortable that you've reviewed the necessary material and have demonstrated adequate proficiency on the quizzes and essay practice, you are ready to evaluate yourself by taking a practice tests.

The online component of your program offers **3 full-length practice tests**. Your book also offers a complete full-length practice test.

You may want to take some or all of these depending on your time frame, level of confidence, and overall readiness. We recommend that you set aside time to complete a full-length test under timed conditions, as it will prepare you for the rigor of the real exam.

View a Summary of Your Test and Quiz Scores in Your "My Scores" Page

■ Click on the "My Scores" tab next to the "My Assignments" tab.

■ The scores from the online assets will automatically appear here. Scores you fill in from other assets will appear here, too!

6 Watch a Kaplan Lesson Online

The MCAT Fast Fact videos feature a Kaplan instructor explaining the highest-yield concepts in more depth.

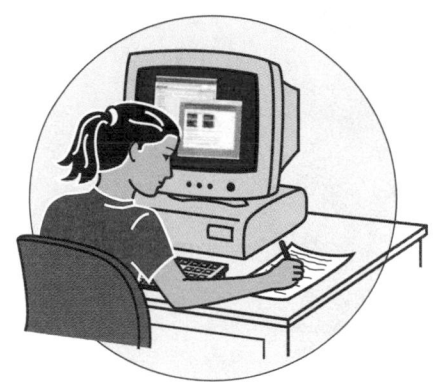

These videos bring the Kaplan Classroom experience into your own home!

Visit the "Fast Fact" section of your syllabus and click on the subject you would like to view. Each video is 3-5 minutes of in-depth MCAT analysis and explanation from a top-ranked Kaplan teacher.

HOW DID WE DO?

After you have completed the MCAT Premier Program and have taken the test, go back to the Online Companion and fill out the online survey. We want to know how you did on the exam—and how we did in helping you to prepare.

Good luck!

MCAT® PREMIER PROGRAM

2009–2010 EDITION

Other Kaplan Books Relating to Medical School Admissions

Get Into Medical School, Second Edition

MCAT® Practice Tests, Sixth Edition

MCAT® Advanced

MCAT in a Box, Second Edition

MCAT® PREMIER PROGRAM

2009–2010 EDITION

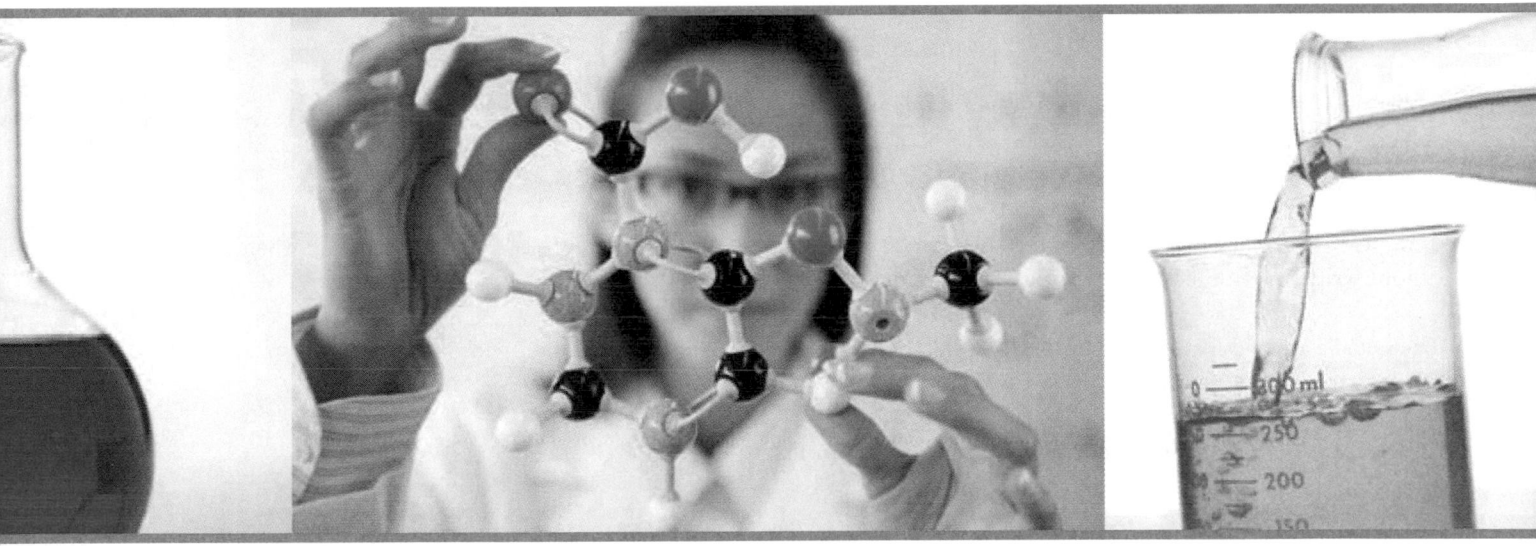

Rochelle Rothstein, M.D.

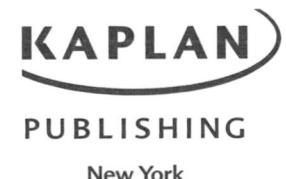

PUBLISHING

New York

© 2009 Kaplan , Inc.

Published by Kaplan Publishing, a division of Kaplan, Inc.
1 Liberty Plaza, 24th Floor
New York, NY 10006

"The Old-Fashioned Modernism of John Marin," by Helen Dudar, Smithsonian vol. 20, no. 11 (Feb 1990), pp. 20, 52–53, used by permission

Excerpt from *Community and Society in Roman Italy*, reprinted by permission of Stephen L. Dyson. © 1992. Johns Hopkins University Press.

Printed in the United States of America

April 2009
10 9 8 7 6 5 4 3 2

ISBN-13: 978-1-4195-5272-4

Kaplan Publishing books are available at special quantity discounts to use for sales promotions, employee premiums, or educational purposes. Please email our Special Sales Department to order or for more information at kaplanpublishing@kaplan.com, or write to Kaplan Publishing, 1 Liberty Plaza, 24th Floor, New York, NY 10006.

CONTENTS

Authors

Tessa Cigler
B.A. (Biochemistry), Harvard University
M.D. (in progress), Duke University

Richard Cohen, Ph.D.
B.S. (Physics), Brown University
Ph.D. (Physics), University of Maryland

William Dracos
B.A. (Biology), Duke University
M.B.A. (Health Services Management, in progress), Duke University

Sailesh Harwani, M.D., Ph.D.
B.S. (Biology), Loyola University
B.A. (Philosophy), Loyola University
M.D., Rush Medical College
Ph.D., Rush Medical College

Sharon Klotz
B.S. (Physics), Massachusetts Institute of Technology

Andy Koh, M.D.
B.A. (Biology), Harvard University
B.A. (English Literature), Oxford University
M.D., Harvard Medical School

Karl Lee, MA
B.A. (Chemistry), Amherst College
M.A. (Physical Chemistry), Harvard University

Alan Levine, MS
B.A. (Mathematics), Rice University
M.S. (Chemistry), University of Houston

Michael Manley, M.D.
B.S. (Psychobiology), University of California, Los Angeles
M.D., University of California, San Diego

Leslie Manley, Ph.D.
B.A. (Biochemistry & Cell Biology), University of California, San Diego
Ph.D. (Physiology & Pharmacology), University of California, San Diego

Stacie Orell
B.A. (Biology), University of Pennsylvania

Rochelle Rothstein, M.D.
B.A. (Biology), Princeton University
M.D., University of California, San Diego

Evan Skowronski, Ph.D.
B.S. (Chemistry), Duke University
Ph.D. (Microbiology), Loma Linda University

Andrew Taylor
B.A. (Biology), Boston University

Readers' Comments

"Well organized science review . . . very accurate test tips and pointers . . . great ideas on writing sample organization. The reading comprehension tests were amazingly close to the actual MCAT."
                    —Marcus Wilson, Mauldin, SC

"With Kaplan's help, I raised my score from a 25 to a 32 within the time frame of a single test administration . . . "
                    —Thomas E. Crosslin, Columbus, OH

"Excellent layout of topics, 'In a Nutshell,' and mnemonic tips . . . not as verbose as a college textbook."
                    —Christine C. Scavedra, Houston, TX

"[The] notes in the margins easily explained difficult portions."
                    —Emily Fox, Madison, SD

"Very easy to understand difficult topics . . . 'Clinical Correlates', mnemonics wonderful."
                    —Ashley Neils, Beloit, WI

"Concise presentation of information with examples. This book was very informative and the information presented closely correlated to that on the practice MCAT."
                    —Cody Starnes, Lindsay, TX

"Tips, mnemonics, practice sets, and more . . . "
                    —Rochelle Price, Coon Rapids, MN

PREFACE

If you're serious about going to medical school, you need to be serious about preparing for the MCAT. For all but a handful of medical schools, MCAT scores are vital admissions criteria. Your MCAT scores can make the difference in where you go to medical school and even *if* you go to medical school. You owe it to yourself to make sure that your performance on the MCAT accurately reflects your readiness to embark on a medical career.

The MCAT is a *prospective*, not a *retrospective* examination: It isn't designed to assess what you've learned in college. Instead, it attempts to predict whether you'll be successful in medical school. The emphasis is on applying concepts rather than on regurgitating information. In addition to covering a broad spectrum of content areas, the MCAT tests a wide range of "higher order" cognitive skills including reading comprehension, data analysis, critical reasoning, and writing ability. This means that the MCAT is not like your college examinations; it's probably unlike any exam you've ever taken. To do well, you'll need to make sure that you have a solid understanding of the content tested, can apply your knowledge in the setting of MCAT-style passages, and have the strategic know-how and confidence to finish the exam in the allotted time while under the stress of Test Day.

We have designed *MCAT Premier Program* to help you prepare for the many challenges presented by the MCAT. Throughout the program, you'll be exposed to Kaplan's proven methods and strategies. You'll learn to take control of the process. You can trust Kaplan. We've been preparing premeds for the MCAT for over 40 years in our comprehensive courses throughout North America. And in the past 15 years alone, we've helped over 400,000 students prepare for this important test and improve their chances of medical school admission.

We're confident that this guide can help you achieve your goals of MCAT success and admission into medical school.

Good luck!

Rochelle Rothstein, M.D.

MCAT
STRATEGIES

INTRODUCTION TO THE MCAT

The Medical College Admission Test, affectionately known as the MCAT, is different from any other test you've encountered in your academic career. It's not like the knowledge-based exams from high school and college, whose emphasis was on memorizing and regurgitating information. Medical schools can assess your academic prowess by looking at your transcript. The MCAT isn't even like other standardized tests you may have taken, where the focus was on proving your general skills.

Medical schools use MCAT scores to assess whether you possess the foundation upon which to build a successful medical career. Though you certainly need to know the content to do well, the stress is on thought process, because the MCAT is above all else a thinking test. That's why it emphasizes reasoning, critical and analytical thinking, reading comprehension, data analysis, writing, and problem-solving skills.

The MCAT's power comes from its use as an indicator of your abilities. Good scores can open doors. Your power comes from preparation and mindset, because the key to MCAT success is knowing what you're up against. And that's where this section of this book comes in. We'll explain the philosophy behind the test, review the sections one by one, show you sample questions, share some of Kaplan's proven methods, and clue you in to what the test makers are really after. You'll get a handle on the process, find a confident new perspective, and achieve your highest possible scores.

> **Test Tip**
>
> The MCAT places more weight on your thought process. However you must have a strong hold of the required core knowledge. The MCAT may not be a perfect gauge of your abilities, but it is a relatively objective way to compare you with students from different backgrounds and undergraduate institutions.

ABOUT THE MCAT

Information about the MCAT CBT is included below. For the latest information about the MCAT, visit www.kaptest.com/mcat.

MCAT CBT

Format	U.S. — All administrations on computer International — Most on computer with limited paper and pencil in a few isolated areas
Essay Grading	One human and one computer grader
Breaks	Optional break between each section
Length of MCAT Day	Approximately 5.5 hours
Test Dates	Multiple dates in January, March, April, May, June, July, August, and September Total of 24 administrations in 2009
Delivery of Results	Within 30 days in 2009 or if scores are delayed notification will be posted online at www.aamc.org/mcat Electronic and paper
Security	Government-issued ID Electronic thumbprint Electronic signature verification
Testing Centers	Small computer testing sites

PLANNING FOR THE TEST

As you look towards your preparation for the MCAT consider the following advice:

Complete your core course requirements as soon as possible. Take a strategic eye to your schedule and get core requirements out of the way now.

Take the MCAT once. The MCAT is a notoriously grueling standardized exam that requires extensive preparation. It is longer than the graduate admissions exams for business school (GMAT, $3\frac{1}{2}$ hours), law school (LSAT, $3\frac{1}{4}$ hours) and graduate school (GRE, $2\frac{1}{2}$ hours). You do not want to take it twice. Plan and prepare accordingly.

> **Kaplan Exclusive**
>
> Go online and sign up for a local Kaplan Pre-Med Edge event to get the latest information on the test.

THE ROLE OF THE MCAT IN ADMISSIONS

More and more people are applying to medical school and more and more people are taking the MCAT. It's important for you to recognize that while a high MCAT score is a critical component in getting admitted to top med schools, it's not the only factor. Medical school admissions officers weigh grades, interviews, MCAT scores, level of involvement in extracurricular activities, as well as personal essays.

In a Kaplan survey of 130 pre-med advisors, 84% called the interview a "very important" part of the admissions process, followed closely by college grades (83%) and MCAT scores (76%). Kaplan's college admissions consulting practice works with students on all these issues so they can position themselves as strongly as possible. In addition, the AAMC has made it clear that scores will continue to be valid for 3 years, and that the scoring of the computer-based MCAT will not differ from that of the paper and pencil version.

REGISTRATION

The only way to register for the MCAT is online. The registration site is: www.aamc.org/mcat.

You will be able to access the site approximately 6 months before your test date. Payment must be made by MasterCard or Visa.

Go to www.aamc.org/mcat/registration.htm and download *MCAT Essentials* for information about registration, fees, test administration, and preparation. For other questions, contact:

MCAT Care Team
Association of American Medical Colleges
Section for Applicant Assessment Services
2450 N. St., NW
Washington, DC 20037
www.aamc.org/mcat
Email: mcat@aamc.org

You will want to take the MCAT in the year prior to your planned start date. For example, if you want to start medical school in Fall 2010, you will need to take the MCAT and apply in 2009. Don't drag your feet gathering information. You'll need time not only to prepare and practice for the test, but also to get all your registration work done.

> **Go Online**
>
> Link directly to the AAMC website in the "Getting Started" section of your online syllabus.

ANATOMY OF THE MCAT

Before mastering strategies, you need to know exactly what you're dealing with on the MCAT. Let's start with the basics: The MCAT is, among other things, an endurance test.

If you can't approach it with confidence and stamina, you'll quickly lose your composure. That's why it's so important that you take control of the test.

The MCAT consists of four timed sections: Physical Sciences, Verbal Reasoning, Writing Sample, and Biological Sciences. Later in this section we'll take an in-depth look at each MCAT section, including sample question types and specific test-smart hints, but here's a general overview, reflecting the order of the test sections and number of questions in each.

> **Test Tip**
>
> The MCAT should be viewed just like any other part of your application: as an opportunity to show the medical schools who you are and what you can do. Take control of your MCAT experience.

Physical Sciences

Time	70 minutes
Format	• 52 multiple-choice questions: approximately 7–9 passages with 4–8 questions each • approximately 10 stand-alone questions (not passage-based)
What it tests	basic general chemistry concepts, basic physics concepts, analytical reasoning, data interpretation

Verbal Reasoning

Time	60 minutes
Format	• 40 multiple-choice questions: approximately 7 passages with 5–7 questions each
What it tests	critical reading

Writing Sample

Time	60 minutes
Format	• 2 essay questions (30 minutes per essay)
What it tests	critical thinking, intellectual organization, written communication skills

Biological Sciences

Time	70 minutes
Format	• 52 multiple-choice questions: approximately 7–9 passages with 4–8 questions each • approximately 10 stand-alone questions (not passage-based)
What it tests	basic biology concepts, basic organic chemistry concepts, analytical reasoning, data interpretation

Test Tip

There's no penalty for a wrong answer on the MCAT, so NEVER LEAVE ANY QUESTION BLANK, even if you have time only for a wild guess.

The sections of the test always appear in the same order:

Physical Sciences
[optional 10-minute break]
Verbal Reasoning
[optional 10-minute break]
Writing Sample
[optional 10-minute break]
Biological Sciences

SCORING

Each MCAT section receives its own score. Physical Sciences, Verbal Reasoning, and Biological Sciences are each scored on a scale ranging from 1–15, with 15 as the highest. The Writing Sample essays are scored alphabetically on a scale ranging from J to T, with T as the highest. The two essays are each evaluated by two official readers, so four critiques combine to make the alphabetical score.

Test Tip

The percentile figure tells you how many other test takers scored at or below your level. In other words, a percentile figure of 80 means that 80 percent did as well or worse than you did, and that only 20 percent did better.

The number of multiple-choice questions that you answer correctly per section is your "raw score." Your raw score will then be converted to yield the "scaled score"—the one that will fall somewhere in that 1–15 range. These scaled scores are what are reported to medical schools as your MCAT scores. All multiple-choice questions are worth the same amount—one raw point—and *there's no penalty for guessing*. That means that *you should always select an answer for every question, whether you get to that question or not!* This is an important piece of advice, so pay it heed. Never let time run out on any section without selecting an answer for every question.

Your score report will tell you—and your potential medical schools—not only your scaled scores, but also the national mean score for each section, standard deviation, national scoring profile for each section, and your percentile ranking.

WHAT'S A GOOD SCORE?

There's no such thing as a cut-and-dry "good score." Much depends on the strength of the rest of your application (if your transcript is first rate, the pressure to strut your stuff on the MCAT isn't as intense) and on where you want to go to school (different schools have different score expectations). Here are a few interesting statistics:

For each MCAT administration, the average scaled scores are approximately 8s for Physical Sciences, Verbal Reasoning, and Biological Sciences, and N for the Writing Sample. You need scores of at least 10–11s to be considered competitive by most medical schools, and if you're aiming for the top you've got to do even better, and score 12s and above.

You don't have to be perfect to do well. For instance, on the AAMC's Practice Test 5R, you could get as many as 10 questions wrong in Verbal Reasoning, 17 in Physical Sciences, and 16 in Biological Sciences and still score in the 80th percentile. To score in the 90th percentile, you could get as many as 7 wrong in Verbal Reasoning, 12 in Physical Sciences, and 12 in Biological Sciences. Even students who receive perfect scaled scores usually get a handful of questions wrong.

It's important to maximize your performance on every question. Just a few questions one way or the other can make a big difference in your scaled score. Here's a look at recent score profiles so you can get an idea of the shape of a typical score distribution.

Physical Sciences		
Scaled Score	Percent Achieving Score	Percentile Rank Range
15	0.1	99.9–99.9
14	1.2	98.7–99.8
13	2.5	96.2–98.6
12	5.1	91.1–96.1
11	7.2	83.9–91.0
10	12.1	71.8–83.8
9	12.9	58.9–71.1
8	16.5	42.4–58.5
7	16.7	25.7–42.3
6	13.0	12.7–25.6
5	7.9	04.8–12.6
4	3.3	01.5–04.7
3	1.3	00.2–01.4
2	0.1	00.1–00.1
1	0.0	00.0–00.0
Scaled Score Mean = 8.1 Standard Deviation = 2.32		

Verbal Reasoning		
Scaled Score	Percent Achieving Score	Percentile Rank Range
15	0.1	99.9–99.9
14	0.2	99.7–99.8
13	1.8	97.9–99.6
12	3.6	94.3–97.8
11	10.5	83.8–94.2
10	15.6	68.2–83.7
9	17.2	51.0–68.1
8	15.4	35.6–50.9
7	10.3	25.3–35.5
6	10.9	14.4–25.2
5	6.9	07.5–14.3
4	3.9	03.6–07.4
3	2.0	01.6–03.5
2	0.5	00.1–01.5
1	0.0	00.0–00.0
Scaled Score Mean = 8.0 Standard Deviation = 2.43		

Test Tip

The raw score of each administration is converted to a scaled score. The conversion varies with administrations. Hence, the same raw score will not always give you the same scaled score.

Writing Sample		
Scaled Score	Percent Achieving Score	Percentile Rank Range
T	0.5	99.9–99.9
S	2.8	94.7–99.8
R	7.2	96.0–99.3
Q	14.2	91.0–95.9
P	9.7	81.2–90.9
O	17.9	64.0–81.1
N	14.7	47.1–63.9
M	18.8	30.4–47.0
L	9.5	21.2–30.3
K	3.6	13.5–21.1
J	1.2	06.8–13.4
		02.9–06.7
		00.9–02.8
		00.2–00.8
		00.0–00.1

75th Percentile = Q
50th Percentile = O
25th Percentile = M

Biological Sciences		
Scaled Score	Percent Achieving Score	Percentile Rank Range
15	0.1	99.9–99.9
14	1.2	98.7–99.8
13	2.5	96.2–98.6
12	5.1	91.1–96.1
11	7.2	83.9–91.0
10	12.1	71.8–83.8
9	12.9	58.9–71.1
8	16.5	42.4–58.5
7	16.7	25.7–42.3
6	13.0	12.7–25.6
5	7.9	04.8–12.6
4	3.3	01.5–04.7
3	1.3	00.2–01.4
2	0.1	00.1–00.1
1	0.0	00.0–00.0

Scaled Score
Mean = 8.2
Standard Deviation = 2.39

WHAT THE MCAT REALLY TESTS

It's important to grasp not only the nuts and bolts of the MCAT, so you'll know *what* to do on test day, but also the underlying principles of the test so you'll know *why* you're doing what you're doing on test day. We'll cover the straightforward MCAT facts later. Now it's time to examine the heart and soul of the MCAT, to see what it's really about.

THE MYTH

Most people preparing for the MCAT fall prey to the myth that the MCAT is a straightforward science test. They think something like this:

> "It covers the four years of science I had to take in school: biology, chemistry, physics, and organic chemistry. It even has equations. OK, so it has Verbal Reasoning and Writing, but those sections are just to see if we're literate, right? The important stuff is the science. After all, we're going to be doctors."

Well, here's the little secret no one seems to want you to know: The MCAT is not just a science test; it's also a thinking test. This means that the test is designed to let you demonstrate your thought process, not only your thought content.

The implications are vast. Once you shift your test-taking paradigm to match the MCAT modus operandi, you'll find a new level of confidence and control over the test. You'll begin to work with the nature of the MCAT rather than against it. You'll be more efficient and insightful as you prepare for the test, and you'll be more relaxed on test day. In fact, you'll be able to see the MCAT for what it is rather than for what it's dressed up to be. We want your test day to feel like a visit with a familiar friend instead of an awkward blind date.

THE ZEN OF MCAT

Medical schools do not need to rely on the MCAT to see what you already know. Admission committees can measure your subject-area proficiency using your undergraduate coursework and grades. Schools are most interested in the potential of your mind.

In recent years, many medical schools have shifted pedagogic focus away from an information-heavy curriculum to a concept-based curriculum. There is currently more emphasis placed on problem solving, holistic thinking, and cross-disciplinary study. Be careful not to dismiss this important point, figuring you'll wait to worry about academic trends until you're actually in medical school. This trend affects you right now, because it's reflected in the MCAT. Every good tool matches its task. In this case the tool is the test, used to measure you and other candidates, and the task is to quantify how likely it is that you'll succeed in medical school.

Your intellectual potential—how skillfully you annex new territory into your mental boundaries, how quickly you build "thought highways" between ideas, how confidently and creatively you solve problems—is far more important to admission committees than your ability to recite Young's modulus for every material known to man. The schools assume they can expand your knowledge base. They choose applicants carefully because expansive knowledge is not enough to succeed in medical school or in the profession. There's something more. And it's this "something more" that the MCAT is trying to measure.

Every section on the MCAT tests essentially the same higher-order thinking skills: analytical reasoning, abstract thinking, and problem solving. Most test takers get trapped into thinking they are being tested strictly about biology, chemistry, etc. Thus, they approach each section with a new outlook on what's expected. This constant mental gear-shifting can be exhausting, not to mention counterproductive. Instead of perceiving the test as parsed into radically different sections, you need to maintain your focus on the underlying nature of the test: It's designed to test your thinking skills, not your information-recall skills. Each test section thus presents a variation on the same theme.

WHAT ABOUT THE SCIENCE?

With this perspective, you may be left asking these questions: "What about the science? What about the content? Don't I need to know the basics?" The answer is a resounding "Yes!" You must be fluent in the different languages of the test. You cannot do well on the MCAT if you don't know the basics of physics, general chemistry, biology, and organic chemistry. We recommend that you take one year each of biology, general chemistry, organic chemistry, and physics before taking the MCAT, and that you review the content in this book thoroughly. Knowing these basics is just the beginning of doing well on the MCAT. That's a shock to most test takers. They presume that once they recall or relearn their undergraduate science, they are ready to do battle against the MCAT. Wrong! They merely have directions to the battlefield. They lack what they need to beat the test: a copy of the test maker's battle plan!

You won't be drilled on facts and formulas on the MCAT. You'll need to demonstrate ability to reason based on ideas and concepts. The science questions are painted with a broad brush, testing your general understanding.

TAKE CONTROL: THE MCAT MINDSET

In addition to being a thinking test, as we've stressed, the MCAT is a standardized test. As such, it has its own consistent patterns and idiosyncrasies that can actually work in your favor. This is the key to why test preparation works. You have the opportunity to familiarize yourself with those consistent peculiarities, to adopt the proper test-taking mindset.

Test Tip

Don't think of the sections of the MCAT as unrelated timed pieces. Each is a variation on the same theme, since the underlying purpose of each section and of the test as a whole is to evaluate your thinking skills. Memorizing formulas won't boost your score. Understanding fundamental scientific principles will.

The following are some overriding principles of the MCAT Mindset that will be covered in depth in the chapters to come:

- Read actively and critically.
- Translate prose into your own words.
- Save the toughest questions for last.
- Know the test and its components inside and out.
- Do MCAT-style problems in each topic area after you've reviewed it.
- Allow your confidence to build on itself.
- Take full-length practice tests a week or two before the test to break down the mystique of the real experience.
- Learn from your mistakes—get the most out of your practice tests.
- Look at the MCAT as a challenge, the first step in your medical career, rather than as an arbitrary obstacle.

And that's what the MCAT Mindset boils down to: Taking control. Being proactive. Being on top of the testing experience so that you can get as many points as you can as quickly and as easily as possible. Keep this in mind as you read and work through the material in this book and, of course, as you face the challenge on test day.

Now that you have a better idea of what the MCAT is all about, let's take a tour of the individual test sections. Although the underlying skills being tested are similar, each MCAT section requires that you call into play a different domain of knowledge. So, though we encourage you to think of the MCAT as a holistic and unified test, we also recognize that the test is segmented by discipline and that there are characteristics unique to each section. In the overviews, we'll review sample questions and answers and discuss section-specific strategies. For each of the sections—Verbal Reasoning, Physical/Biological Sciences, and the Writing Sample—we'll present you with the following:

- **The Big Picture**
  You'll get a clear view of the section and familiarize yourself with what it's really evaluating.

- **A Closer Look**
  You'll explore the types of questions that will appear and master the strategies you'll need to deal with them successfully.

- **Highlights**
  The key approaches to each section are outlined, for reinforcement and quick review.

Test Tip

Those perfectionist tendencies that make you a good student and a good medical school candidate may work against you in MCAT Land. If you get stuck on a question or passage, move on. Perfectionism is for medical school—not the MCAT. And you don't need to understand every word of a passage before you go on to the questions—what's tripping you up may not even be relevant to what you'll be asked.

 Go Online

Find a one-page summary of key MCAT question strategies.

PHYSICAL AND BIOLOGICAL SCIENCES

THE BIG PICTURE

The two science sections on the MCAT, Physical and Biological, are similar in their format, though their content obviously differs. In each 70-minute section, you'll find about 7–9 passages, each followed by 4 to 8 multiple-choice questions, and approximately 10 stand-alone multiple-choice questions (also referred to as *discretes*)—not based on any passage. The Physical Sciences section is comprised of physics and general chemistry, approximately evenly divided in content though mixed throughout the section. The Biological Sciences section consists of biology and organic chemistry questions mixed throughout, with greater emphasis on biology (specifically, on DNA and genetics).

The passages, each 250–300 words in length, will describe experiments, situations, or ideas from which questions are drawn. The information may be presented in the guise of journal or textbook articles, experimental research, data analysis, or scientific-style editorials. When reading the science passages, you should think about extracting information—not meaning and structure as in Verbal Reasoning. Consider the passages to be data that you must interpret and understand to be able to apply them to the specific needs of the questions. The passage-and-question structure allows you to demonstrate many skills, among them:

- Understanding the science presented in the passage, no matter how obscure or foreign to you
- Confidently connecting elements of your scientific "repertoire" to new situations
- Quickly assessing the kinds of situations feasible given the information in the passage

Physical Sciences at a Glance

- 70 minutes
- 52 multiple-choice questions
- Approximately 7–9 passages with 4 to 8 questions each
- Approximately 10 stand-alone questions (not passage based)
- Tests basic science concepts, anaytical reasoning, data interpretation

The stand-alone questions will draw on your knowledge of particular concepts or themes in the respective sciences. They're "wild cards" in the sense that you cannot group them together in any formal way; in fact, they appear scattered throughout the sections. Ranging in scope from a quantitative problem to a conceptual thought experiment, they are the test maker's way of randomly tapping into your knowledge base.

THE MCAT ATTITUDE

It's important to approach both science sections with the same mindset: MCAT science is just a window into your mind. The test makers are trying to see how you reason, how you solve problems, and how well you command your knowledge. They are not after a data dump from your core memory. It's crucial that you demonstrate conceptual understanding of scientific material and show proficiency in applying scientific themes in new situations. This is the kind of mental flexibility that will get you a great MCAT score.

Abstract Thinking

Another way to describe flexibility is as a form of abstraction. To think abstractly is to lift ideas out of a specific context and place them in a new context. It's a skill that allows you passage into seemingly unfamiliar territory, and on the MCAT that could mean the question around the corner. In the science sections, this skill is tested repeatedly.

For example, passages may provide hypothetical scenarios or describe experiments you've never seen before. You'll need to take the unfamiliar and make it familiar, and that's where abstract thinking comes in. If you understand the basic framework of experimental design and scientific method, you won't be overwhelmed by a specific unfamiliar context. You'll be able to "rise above" the details rather than get tripped up by them.

What About Formulas and Math?

Contrary to what you may presume, the MCAT is not a math-intensive test. Despite the scientific language on the MCAT, there is nothing more mathematically complex than algebra, exponents, logs, and a little bit of trig. There is no calculus, differential equations, or matrix mechanics. You may need to recall sine and cosine for standard angles, though such values are often provided if necessary. That's it! No higher math.

Similarly, many of the scientific formulas necessary to work through problems and answer questions will be provided on the test. This is just an indicator of how negligible is the value of "straight memorization." You gain little by having every nitty-gritty formula easily accessible unless you also have a broad understanding of what the formulas mean, what they imply, what their units indicate, how they relate to one another, and how to navigate among them.

Biological Sciences at a Glance

- 70 minutes
- 52 multiple-choice questions
- Approximately 7–9 passages with 4 to 8 questions each
- Approximately 10 stand-alone questions (not passage based)
- Tests basic science concepts, anaytical reasoning, data interpretation

In light of our discussion of concept-based testing, it makes sense that the MCAT will not reward you merely for the "brute force" of memorization. There will rarely be an opportunity on the MCAT to algebraically crunch away on a formula. The information you're given won't fit neatly into formulas. If it did, the MCAT would be nothing but a memory-and-algebra test. And, as we've discussed, it is much more. Again, you should not be concerned with memorizing formulas. You should be concerned with *understanding* formulas. The key point is that once you understand the scientific concepts behind a formula, you hardly need the formula itself anymore. Though this applies mostly to physics and chemistry, the underlying theme is relevant for both science sections: Think, don't compute!

Test Tip

You don't need to memorize as many math and science formulas as you may think. Understanding them is more important than memorizing them.

 Go Online

Need a science vocabulary refresher? Use the Flashcards!

A CLOSER LOOK

What follows is a review of the content areas you can expect to find in the science sections of the MCAT. This is not to suggest that your MCAT will cover all of these topics; instead, use this list as a guideline of the content that could possibly show up. All these areas will be covered in detail in the content review sections of this book.

PHYSICAL SCIENCES

PHYSICS

- Basic Units/Kinematics
- Newtonian Mechanics
- Force and Inertia
- Thermodynamics
- Fluids/Solids
- Electrostatics
- Magnetism
- Circuits
- Periodic Motion, Waves, Sound
- Light and Optics
- Atomic Phenomena
- Nuclear Physics

GENERAL CHEMISTRY

- Quantum Numbers
- Hund's Rule/Electron Configuration
- Periodic Table
- Reaction Types
- Balancing Equations
- Bonding
- Formal Charge/VSEPR Theory
- Intermolecular Forces
- Chemical Kinetics/Equilibrium
- Thermodynamics/Entropy
- Ideal Gas Law
- Phases of Matter
- Solutions
- Acids and Bases
- Electrochemistry

BIOLOGICAL SCIENCES

BIOLOGY

- Eukaryotic and Prokaryotic Cells
- Membrane Traffic
- Cell Division—Mitosis and Meiosis
- Embryogenesis
- Enzymatic Activity
- Cellular Metabolism
- Muscular and Skeletal Systems
- Digestive System
- Respiratory and Circulatory Systems
- Lymphatic System
- Immune System
- Homeostasis
- Endocrine System
- Nervous System
- Molecular Genetics/Inheritance
- Viruses
- Evolution

ORGANIC CHEMISTRY

- Nomenclature
- Stereochemistry
- Mechanisms
- Carboxylic Acids
- Amines
- Spectroscopy
- Carbohydrates and Lipids
- Hydrolysis and Dehydration
- Amino Acids and Proteins
- Oxygen-containing Compounds
- Hydrocarbons
- Laboratory Techniques
- IR and NMR Spectroscopy

SAMPLE PASSAGE AND QUESTIONS

This is probably your first chance to see what the passages, passage-based questions, and stand-alone questions will look like in the science sections. An answer key is provided, but try to work through these samples without consulting it. We'll use the following passage and questions to highlight general strategies. You'll find more MCAT-style practice questions at the end of each content review subject area.

Passage

A physics class is attempting to measure the acceleration due to gravity, *g*, by throwing balls out of classroom windows. They performed the following two experiments:

Experiment 1

Two class members lean out of different windows at the same height, h = 5.2 m, above the ground and drop two different balls. One ball is made out of lead and has a mass of 5 kg. The other ball is made out of plastic and has a mass of 1 kg. The students measure the velocity of the lead ball just before impact with the ground and find it to be 10 m/s. They also find that when the plastic ball hits the ground it bounces, and its momentum changes by 18 kg × m/s.

Experiment 2

Instead of dropping the plastic ball, a student throws the ball out of a higher window and observes its projectile motion. The ball is thrown from a height of 10 m above the ground with a velocity of 4 m/s directed at an angle of 30° above the horizontal. (Note: Assume that the air resistance is negligible unless otherwise stated.)

Passage-Based Questions

1. The students did not account for air resistance in their measurement of g in Experiment 1. How does the value of g they obtained compare with the actual value of g ?

    A. The value of g obtained in Experiment 1 is greater than the actual value of g because air resistance increases the time it takes the balls to fall from the windows to the ground.
    B. The value of g obtained in Experiment 1 is greater than the actual value of g because air resistance decreases the kinetic energy of the balls just before impact.
    C. The value of g obtained in Experiment 1 is less than the actual value of g because air resistance decreases the velocity of the balls just before impact.
    D. The value of g obtained in Experiment 1 is less than the actual value of g because air resistance decreases the time it takes the balls to fall from the windows to the ground.

2. Which of the following would change the measured value of g in Experiment 1?

    I.   Increasing the mass of the earth
    II. Using balls having a different mass but the same volume
    III. Throwing the balls horizontally instead of dropping them vertically

    A. I only
    B. III only
    C. I and II only
    D. II and III only

3. In Experiment 1, the change in momentum that the plastic ball experiences when it bounces off the ground does NOT depend on: (Note: Assume that the collision is perfectly elastic.)

    A. the velocity of the ball just before impact.
    B. the mass of the ball.
    C. the mass of Earth.
    D. the volume of the ball.

4. In Experiment 2, what was the maximum height above the window reached by the plastic ball? (Note: The acceleration due to gravity is $g =$ 9.8 m/s^2, sin 30° = 0.50, and cos 30° = 0.866.)

    A. 10.2 cm
    B. 20.4 cm
    C. 30.6 cm
    D. 61.2 cm

5. In a third experiment, a student throws the lead ball out of the same window used in Experiment 1 with a velocity of 3 m/s in the horizontal direction. What is the ratio of the work done by gravity on the lead ball in the first experiment to the work done by gravity on the ball in the third experiment?

    A. 1:1
    B. 1:3
    C. 1:9
    D. 3:1

Stand-Alone Questions

6. In the figure below, the velocity vector of a particle is represented at successive times t. Which of the following best represents the acceleration vector?

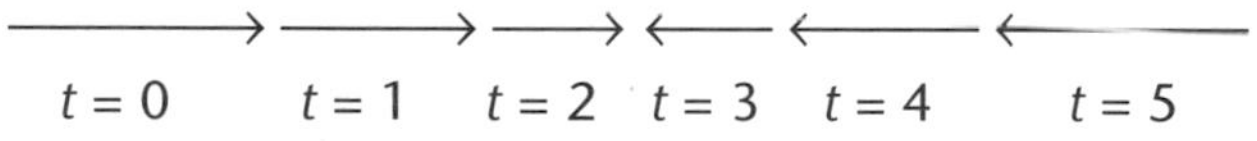

    A. ⟶
    B. ⟵
    C. The acceleration changes direction.
    D. The acceleration is zero.

7. All of the following statements are true of most transition elements EXCEPT:

    A. they have partially filled d subshells.
    B. they have extremely high ionization energies.
    C. they exhibit metallic character.
    D. they have multiple oxidation states.

8. A patient is taking a drug that has the side effect of being a sympathetic nervous system inhibitor. Which of the following would most likely be seen as a result of this drug?

    A. Decreased bowel motility
    B. Decreased heart rate
    C. Increased pupil diameter
    D. Decreased blood supply to skin

Were You Able to Think Abstractly?

Did you get bogged down in details, or were you able to rise above them? Were you able to come up with your own answers before looking at the choices? As you review the following answer explanations you'll be able to assess your performance and pick up important strategies.

ANSWER REVIEW

Passage

The passage describes a series of experiments performed by some students. As you read, you should be making notes in the margins or underlining important information (i.e., the height = 5.2 meters, mass = 5 kg, etc.). You might make a chart to list out the respective "given" data for each experiment:

Experiment 1	**Experiment 2**
2 balls	*height*
masses for each	*initial velocity*
height	*angle above horizon*
final velocity for lead ball	
plastic ball: change in momentum	

Passage-Based Questions

1. **C**

    This is a question you could answer without reference to the passage. It's really asking about how a measurement of *g* would change depending on whether or not air resistance is considered (with all other variables presumed constant). Because air resistance is a force working in the opposite direction from gravity, it's a force of resistance, like friction. Therefore, it slows down the motion of the ball, making it take longer to fall the same distance. Thus the velocity just before impact decreases when air resistance is considered. We know that air resistance opposes the motion of freefall so the object is unable to accelerate as much as it would have if that force was negligible (e.g. observed value is less than actual value). This allows us to cancel **Choices (A)** and **(B)**. **Choice (D)** has false logic as it states that air resistance decreases the time it takes for the object to fall. This is an opposite answer so **(D)** is out. We are left with **Choice (C)** which is correct because decreasing velocity means that it will take a longer time for the balls to free fall and this is due to the effects of the opposing force (air resistance).

Key Strategy: A chart helps you organize what you know from the passage, so you can access the information quickly while answering the questions. Remember, you're reading for data—not for meaning or structure. Be sure, however, that you understand the context of every piece of data you collect.

Key Strategy: Don't read more complexity into a question than is there. In some cases, passage-based questions will actually be testing in a stand-alone style, with little or no reference back to the passage.

> **Test Tip**
>
> Use your scratch paper to make notes or draw charts and diagrams.

2. **A**

This roman numeral–style question asks about what factors would change the measured value of *g* in the first experiment. Be careful to consider only the information from Experiment 1 when answering this question.

Let's consider the first statement. If it's wrong, then you can eliminate any answer choice that has it listed. If you decide it is true, then you must choose an answer that includes it in its list of numerals. In the first experiment, the students neglected air resistance, so we have only gravity to consider. The first statement requires that we think about how *g* is related to the mass of the earth. You should recall that the gravitational force between an object and the earth is $G = mM/R^2$, where G is the universal gravitational constant, *m* is the mass of the object, *M* is the mass of the earth, and *R* is the distance between. But remember also that the weight of an object = mg. We can equate these two forces ($GmM/R^2 = mg$) to solve for $g = GM/R^2$. Therefore, changing the mass of the earth would indeed change the value of *g*. So, Statement I is true, and you can eliminate **Choices (B)** and **(D)**. Now we need consider only Statement II to decide between **(A)** and **(C)**. Let's look at Statement II. It says that using balls with different mass but the same volume would change *g*. We know that in Experiment 1, the students ignored air resistance, so the volume of the balls is not relevant. What about the mass? Well, we saw above that *g* is independent of the object's mass. So, Statement II is not true and **Choice (A)** is correct.

> **Test Tip**
>
> Some passage-based questions can actually be answered without referring to the passage. Don't let unnecessary information confuse you.

If you were unsure about Statement I, though, you'd have to work through Statement III to decide which answer choice is correct. The key to the third statement is realizing that vertical trajectory will be unchanged by any initial horizontal velocity. The same vertical force—gravity—will be at work. So, Statement III is untrue, confirming **(A)** as the correct answer choice.

Key Strategy: Use the structure of a Roman numeral question to your advantage! Eliminate choices as soon as you find them to be inconsistent with the truth or falsehood of a statement in the stimulus. Similarly, consider only those choices that include a statement that you've already determined to be true.

Key Strategy: You don't have to consider the statements in order. Knowing about any one of them will get you off to a great start answering the question, so if you're unsure about the first statement, go on to the second or third.

3. **D**

This question asks about which variable is *not* a factor in determining the change in momentum for the plastic ball in Experiment 1. You'll be looking for the answer that does not play a role in the momentum shift. One of the first things to note is that you're given a hint about the collision between the ball and the ground—it is elastic, implying that both kinetic energy and momentum are conserved during the collision. The question stimulus tells you, then, that at the time of impact, the two surfaces act like solid, hard surfaces (like billiard balls) with no energy lost to the collision.

Because the mass of the ball doesn't change, its change in momentum is dependent on its change in velocity. So change in momentum = $mv_{final} - mv_{initial}$. In considering the answers, however, there is no need to painstakingly step through calculations. There is one choice that jumps out as inconsistent. **Choice (D)** mentions a variable—the volume of the ball—which has no bearing on the ball's change in momentum. All the other choices mention variables which are relevant in considering the change in momentum of the ball as it hits the earth.

Key Strategy: Don't do more work than you have to on the test. Work smart. The MCAT rewards test takers who can save time by seeing a creative strategy (i.e., looking for a variable that's not relevant rather than plodding through every choice, solving equations, and wasting time).

4. **B**

   Be careful to read the question. It asks for the maximum height above the window reached by the plastic ball in Experiment 2. Since we're looking for maximum height, we know the vertical velocity will be 0 (when the ball stops and turns around to fall back to the ground). From the passage, we know that the ball's initial velocity is 4 meters per second at an angle of 30°. The initial vertical velocity component is $4 \times$ sine 30, or $4 \times 1/2$, which is 2 meters per second. Using kinematics, we know that $v^2 - v_0^2 = 2ay$, where a is acceleration and y is distance. We know $v_0 = 2$ meters per second; we can estimate g to be 10 meters per second squared. Solving the equation, we see that y maximum = .2 meters or 20 centimeters. This is closest to **Choice (B)**, the correct answer. The height of the window doesn't even come into play. Notice that **Choice (D)** derives from using the cosine rather than sine of 30° to find the vertical component of velocity. **Choice (A)** results from a simple calculation error. **Choice (C)** is incorrect as well.

Go Online

The diagnostic test can help you decide where to focus your review.

Key Strategy: Estimate whenever you can to save time.

Key Strategy: Don't get flustered by unnecessary information. In this case, you had more information than you needed to solve the problem. Don't just plug in numbers and hope for a match. Think before you calculate!

5. **A**

   You're asked for a ratio. The implication is that some component of the problem is not solvable, so don't expect to work with actual numbers. In this case, you need to compare the work done in two different scenarios. We need to know that work is force through a distance, or $F \times d$. Since gravity works only along the vertical axis, we need to know the vertical distance traveled by both balls to compare the work done. In both cases, the ball drops 5.2 meters. The ball mentioned in the question has some horizontal velocity, but this has no bearing on the vertical dynamics. So, the distance traveled by the balls in the two different experiments is the same. Furthermore, because the mass is identical, the work done is the same. So, the ratio is 1:1—or **Choice (A)**.

Test Tip

You won't always be dealing with exact numerical factors or solutions. You may be working with ratios, or be required to estimate.

Key Strategy: In many cases with ratio questions, you will not be able to solve for actual numbers. You may have to work with relationships, fractions, and formulas to arrive at the solution.

Key Strategy: We reviewed these questions in order, but you don't have to do the questions in order. Start with the ones that seem most feasible and mark and return to the ones that seem difficult or time-intensive.

Stand-Alone Questions

6. B

This question is a great example of how the MCAT rewards the careful thinker. You're told that the vectors represent successive measurements of velocity for a particle. You're then asked which answer choice best represents the acceleration vector. Without having actual numbers to work with, you have to be able to construct a relationship between velocity and acceleration and "visualize" that relationship using vectors. The way to approach this question is to ask yourself, "What is the connection between velocity and acceleration?" Once you answer that, you can begin to home in on an appropriate answer choice. So, what *is* the relationship? Recall that, dimensionally, acceleration is velocity per unit time or displacement per time squared. Theoretically speaking, acceleration is the *rate of change of velocity through a period of time.*

So, the answer choice will be a vector that matches the general rate of change amongst the given velocity vectors. At $t = 0$, the velocity is positive and at a maximum. At $t = 1$, it is still positive but the magnitude has decreased, indicating a *deceleration*. At $t = 2$, the velocity is still positive but is diminished in magnitude even more. What the vectors are describing is a particle, mass, car, thing, object, or whatever is slowing down. At $t = 3$, something that looks a little tricky happens: the velocity becomes negative but with the same magnitude as $t = 2$. The object we're tracking has changed direction from "forward" to "reverse". The trend continues through $t = 4$ and $t = 5$; we see that the particle is going faster (greater magnitude) but in the opposite direction from its original orientation. Let's get a picture of what we've just figured out. A particle—suppose it's a car—is moving forward at some velocity. It slows down, stops at some point, and then reverses direction and speeds up.

OK, now that we understand the stimulus, we're ready to tackle the answer choices. Remember, we're looking for acceleration. We said earlier that acceleration is the rate of change in velocity. Even though the velocity vectors change direction, the acceleration vector maintains its negative direction throughout the time sampled. So, even though the car speeds up in the "negative" direction, its acceleration remains negative. It continually *decelerates* throughout its movement. The implication is that the force acting on the car is in a direction *opposing* the original direction of movement. Once this clicks, the correct answer—**Choice (B)**—leaps out as correct.

Let's step through the others. **Choice (A)** suggests that the particle keeps accelerating, but the velocity vectors get *smaller* in magnitude at first, not larger. So, even if you forgot that the "negative acceleration" for time markers 3, 4, and 5 has a negative direction, there's no way **Choice (A)** makes sense. **Choice (C)** replicates the behavior of the velocity vectors, and if you're not thinking carefully, you may fall for this choice because it *seems* to be consistent with the information you're given. **Choice (D)** presumes that you may visually "add up" all the vectors in the stimulus rather than apply them. If you do try to add them, you'll get a sum of 0. However, that sum is *not* the acceleration. In fact, it's the total *displacement*. The car essentially moves forward, slowing down to a stop, and then reverses, speeding up back to its original position.

Key Strategy: Understand the question clearly before you move to the answer choices. Otherwise, you'll be vulnerable to persuasive but incorrect choices.

Key Strategy: Use reason. Don't compute.

Test Tip

Before you go to the answer choices, make certain you understand the question.

7. **B**

    This question has the "all except" format, which means you're looking for the answer that is the *exception* (i.e., it's *not* true). The stimulus asks about transition elements. Before you rush to the answer choices, think about what you know of transition elements. They're in the middle of the periodic table and have partially filled *d* subshells. You might also recall that their electrons are loosely held by the nucleus and they are sometimes called *transition metals*.

    Choice (B)—they have high ionization energies—is the correct choice because its statement about transition elements is false. Transition elements are easy to ionize because their electrons are not strongly bound. **Choice (A)** can't be the correct choice because it says something *true* about transition elements. **Choice (C)** is also true—they do exhibit metallic properties because their electrons are mobile. **Choice (D)** is also true about transition elements; they can lose electrons from both s and d orbitals, resulting in multiple oxidation states.

Key Strategy: When answering a question in the "all/except" format, remember that you're looking for the choice that is *not* true.

Key Strategy: When answering a question in the "all/except" format, be sure to consider all the answer choices to be confident you've picked the most appropriate one.

8. **B**

This question is based on various functions of the different branches of the nervous system. Specifically, it requires knowledge of the pathways innervated by the sympathetic division of the autonomic nervous system. The autonomic nervous system is divided into two branches: the sympathetic and the parasympathetic. The sympathetic system mediates the "fight or flight" responses that ready the body for action. The parasympathetic system innervates those pathways that return the body to its normal state following fight or flight. The sympathetic system prepares the body by increasing heart rate, inhibiting digestion, causing vasoconstriction of blood vessels in the skin, and promoting pupil dilation.

From this list of functions, you can eliminate **Choices (A)**, **(C)**, and **(D)** since they're all functions of the sympathetic nervous system and would, therefore, not be likely responses to a drug that inhibits the activity of the sympathetic system. So by the process of elimination you see that **Choice (B)** is the correct answer. Since sympathetic innervation normally increases heart rate, of the four choices, an inhibitor of the system would most likely result in a *decrease* in heart rate.

<u>Key Strategy</u>: If you approach a stand-alone question that tests specific knowledge you do not possess, skim the choices carefully to see if you can glean any clues or information from them. If not, guess quickly, don't look back, and move on. You don't have time to waste.

HIGHLIGHTS

READING THE PASSAGES

- Passages may sound difficult or unfamiliar. Don't be daunted!
- Make notes on scratch paper or draw diagrams to help you summarize the information presented.

FACING THE QUESTIONS

- You can skip around. Tackle the easiest questions first, leaving the harder ones for later. The difficult questions are worth the same as the easy ones.
- Use numerical approximations when you can. Don't do any long calculations.
- Base your answers on the passage, not on your own knowledge.
- Use a process of elimination to get to the right answer or to increase your chances of guessing the right answer.
- If you don't know an answer, guess! Try to do so while you're still working on the passage, so you won't have to reread it later. There's no penalty for wrong answers. Leave no question unanswered!

3

VERBAL REASONING

THE BIG PICTURE

The Verbal Reasoning section is perhaps the most recognizable section of the MCAT, because it's similar to the reading comprehension sections of other standardized tests. It's 60 minutes long and consists of about 7 passages, with anywhere from 5 to 7 questions per passage. The passages, often complex, are drawn from the social sciences, philosophy, and other humanistic disciplines as well as from the natural sciences.

The Verbal Reasoning section tests your ability to:

- Read critically and actively
- "Possess" or truly comprehend written material
- Capture the essence of a passage by recognizing its main idea
- Intuit a writer's tone
- Draw inferences/conclusions

The passages you'll confront on test day probably won't be fun to read. Odds are, they'll be boring. If they're too engaging, check the cover. You may be taking the wrong test. As part of the challenge, you must be able to concentrate and glean meaning regardless of the nature of the text. This will involve working through your resistance to dry passages and overcoming any anxiety or frustration. The more control you can muster, the quicker you can move through each passage, through the questions, and to a higher score. Remember, Verbal Reasoning isn't there to entertain you or to provide relief from the science but to put you through a mental obstacle course.

> **Verbal Reasoning at a Glance**
>
> - 60 minutes
> - 40 multiple-choice questions
> - 7 passages with 5 to 7 questions each
> - Tests for critical reading

> **Test Tip**
>
> Don't be fooled by familiarity. Just because you've dealt with reading comprehension on other standardized tests doesn't mean you can get away with not preparing for the Verbal Reasoning section.

DO YOU NEED TO STUDY FOR VERBAL REASONING?

Don't make the mistake that so many MCAT participants make in underestimating the challenge of the Verbal Reasoning section. Sometimes it falls under the shadow cast by the looming science sections. Also, students figure that there isn't anything to "study" for this section. Be aware that the scoring gradient for Verbal Reasoning is very steep. It's hard to get a good score, so you can't afford to be cavalier. Some medical schools add all your MCAT scores together for a composite score—if you blow off Verbal Reasoning, you could kill your composite. Practice Verbal Reasoning as you would the other test sections, and challenge yourself to acquire the specialized reading skills required on the MCAT.

HOW TO READ ACTIVELY

Usually we read for entertainment or information. Rarely do we read critically, to understand how the writer organizes ideas and uses detail to support themes. MCAT Verbal Reasoning requires that you abandon standard reading habits and take on the role of a critical, or active, reader. This means that you create a mental model of the passage while you're reading, capturing each idea the author constructs and making it part of your vision of the passage.

This can happen only if you resist feeling overwhelmed by the themes in the passage. If you're too awed by the author or bored by the subject matter, you won't be able to take possession of the passage. This notion of "taking possession" is the key to active reading. It means that you keep a distance from the words and that you remain analytical rather than get emotional.

Your goals from the outset of the passage are to figure out what the author is saying and how the ideas are linked. Every passage contains one main idea. You can usually figure it out in the first few lines of the passage and redefine your sense of it as you move through the passage. When you're done reading, you should be able to state the main idea in your own words. Being an active reader implies that you constantly ask yourself what the author intends and how that intention is conveyed and supported. Successfully answering the questions depends on your ability to quickly glean the author's point, to map out the passage in your mind, and to assess the inferences.

Pay Attention to Structure

The structure of each passage can help you organize a mental map. You know, for example, that each paragraph will explore a new angle of the main idea or provide detail associated with a key idea. The MCAT Verbal Reasoning passages are, for the most part, very logical in their construction. They may contain complicated words or ideas, but their structure is very manageable, even predictable. Look for certain keywords (e.g., *consequently*) or phrases (e.g., *on the other hand*) that hold ideas together and can alert you as to what's ahead in the passage.

Some test takers feel more anchored as they read the passage if they've scoped out the questions first. As a rule, it won't save you time or effort to do so. Most of the questions will require that you demonstrate a general understanding of the passage's main idea and overall construction—neither of which can be derived from any particular section of the passage. You need to read for meaning and for organization whether or not you've reviewed the questions.

A CLOSER LOOK

Here's a chance to begin familiarizing yourself with Verbal Reasoning passages and questions, to learn how to approach them. You'll have more opportunities to practice this section in the content review section of this book; for now we want to open your eyes to structure and strategy.

SAMPLE PASSAGE AND QUESTIONS

As you read through the MCAT-style passage below, try to articulate the main idea to yourself. Read actively and critically. Consider what the author is trying to say and how the ideas are communicated. You might want to pause between paragraphs to digest what you've read and put the ideas into your own words.

In a real MCAT situation, you'll need to be time-conscious while you read. For now, just go at whatever pace feels comfortable to you. Keep in mind that the passages you'll see on the MCAT can come from history, philosophy, the arts, and other disciplines, and can vary in length and complexity.

> In 1948, *Look* magazine polled America's art critics and major artists, among them Edward Hopper, Stuart Davis, and Charles Burchfield, for a consensus on the creative spirit who could be pronounced the best of the age. It is a fair measure of the art
> 5 establishment's limited attention span that a generation after John Marin was crowned prince of painters by his peers, his name had begun to fade. New styles raced in to seize the interest of the gallery and museum worlds; fashion embraced Abstract Expressionism, then thrilled to the distancing imagery of Pop Art and later,

---

> **Test Tip**
>
> Remember, key words are signals.
>
> **contrast:**
>
> although, however, but, contrary, on the one hand
>
> **comparison:**
>
> likewise, similarly
>
> **continuing argument:**
>
> also, further, in addition, moreover
>
> **introducing examples:**
>
> for instance, consider the case of, one example of this is
>
> **conclusion:**
>
> then, therefore, finally, thus, in conclusion

10 for about five minutes, went gaga over a frail phenomenon labeled Op Art. To be sure, Marin's death in 1953 was the occasion for lavish obituary tributes. But mention him today to a reasonably literate American or a cultured, well traveled European and, likely as not, the response will be a puzzled stare.

15 That is not only odd but hard to understand. Marin's legacy embraces more than 3,000 works, many of them memorable. There are prime etchings, splendid, if demanding, oils and, in the main, watercolors—2,500 of them, amazing in color, design, and complexity. He seemed to have set down everything in a transport of

20 excitement, as if he were recording themes for a fevered gavotte. Indeed, he once wrote of the acts of drawing and painting as "a sort of mad wonder dancing."

Everything that came from Marin's loving hand radiated spontaneity. Here, it appeared, was a natural, creative spirit, a lucky

25 man who was freed, rather than constrained, by his magnanimous imagination. In truth, hardly anything Marin turned out was unrehearsed. The paintings which hinted at the impetuosity of an artist struggling to convey the "warring, pushing, pulling forces" of his surroundings were, as often as not, studio works. Even his letters,

30 with their blithe disregard for punctuation, were discovered to be the result of many drafts.

As a husband and father, Marin lived a life of singular regularity. He had one wife and, as far as anyone knows, no extramarital entanglements. When he put away his paints at the end of his working

35 day, Marin became a man of simple, harmless pleasures. Late pictures show a wiry-looking figure with a long, thin Yankee nose, the parched skin of a farmer, and a humorous mouth that often held a cigarette. No one ever saw him down more drink than was good for his speech or balance. His idea of fun was a good game of billiards.

40 The contrast between the art and the man who made it was extreme, fascinating, and a trifle baffling. Marin's pictures were daring, the work of a sophisticated eye, an unfailing imagination, a virtuoso hand; some of them verge on elegant abstraction, although he looked down on abstract art. He hated efforts to interpret his art—

45 or for that matter anyone else's. The attitude is not uncommon to artists, particularly American artists, but Marin's distrust of the critical and academic establishments verged on the fanatic. "Intellectuals," he once pronounced, "have in their makeup a form of Nazism."

1. The main point of the passage is to:
    A. explain why John Marin's work was virtually forgotten after his death.
    B. consider the contrast between Marin's artistic style and his personal life and habits.
    C. argue that the art establishment was unable to reach a consensus on the "best of the age" because of its limited attention span.
    D. suggest that Marin's vivacious watercolors were a reaction against Nazism in the art world.

2. Of the following, the author of the passage is most likely:
    A. a contemporary painter.
    B. a magazine art critic.
    C. an investigative reporter.
    D. a museum curator.

3. The author refers to Op Art (line 11) in order to:
    A. place Marin's art within a specific category or genre.
    B. identify the origins of Marin's artistic style.
    C. emphasize the fleeting popularity of artistic styles.
    D. compare Marin's stylistic simplicity with later psychedelic trends.

4. The author's attitude toward Marin may be described as one of:
    A. grudging approval.
    B. playful irreverence.
    C. flippant disrespect.
    D. reverent appreciation.

5. The passage discusses all of the following aspects of Marin's life EXCEPT his:
    A. political beliefs.
    B. physical appearance.
    C. artistic style.
    D. family life.

6. In saying that intellectuals "have in their makeup a form of Nazism," (line 48), Marin most probably means that:
    A. the academic establishment is clearly fascist in its structure.
    B. intellectuals often have leftist political and social leanings.
    C. critics often misread extremist political messages in the works of artists.
    D. the criticism and interpretation of art represents a sort of tyranny.

7. The author characterizes Marin's work as:
   A. fevered and energetic.
   B. simple and colorful.
   C. constrained and precise.
   D. tortured and impenetrable.

8. The author characterizes Marin's paintings as "studio works" in line 29 in order to make the point that:
   A. Marin's painting exhibit the influences of many studio artists.
   B. despite attempts at objectivity, Marin's works expressed the academic biases of his time.
   C. although Marin's work seemed spontaneous, it was the result of precise crafting.
   D. Marin's paintings never reflected his complexity and vivid imagination.

Did You Catch the Main Idea?

The author's intent was to contrast John Marin's flamboyant artistic style with his subdued personal life. We get the first hint of this theme in the second paragraph, where the author describes the ostensible mechanism by which Marin created his art ("mad wonder dancing"). The idea is further developed in the next paragraph, where we get the sense that the process through which Marin produced art was not as it seemed ("In truth, hardly anything Marin turned out was unrehearsed.") The fourth paragraph describes the subject's personal life, showing it to be as dull as his art was wild. The last paragraph begins with a clear statement of the passage's main idea; the rest of the paragraph solidifies the intent of the passage.

There's more to understanding the passage than just being able to figure out the main idea. You have to construct a mental outline of the structure of the passage so you'll be able to refer back to it while you answer the questions. The questions following a passage test your understanding of the passage, its structure, its implications, and its tone. It's important that you gather information about the passage as you read so you'll be able to answer the questions quickly and confidently.

ANSWER REVIEW

1. **B**

   Choice (B) has the proper scope to reflect the main idea. **Choice (A)** makes reference to a minor point in the first paragraph, **Choice (C)** distorts an idea from the passage and magnifies a detail, and **Choice (D)** connects two ideas presented separately.

2. **B**

The citation after the passage and the general tone of the writing suggest that "magazine art critic" is most fitting. Were the writer a painter, we would expect more information about the artwork. An investigative reporter would have a confrontational tone. Finally, we might expect that a museum curator would focus more on Marin's artwork and its effect on the public rather than on the relation between his art and his life.

3. **C**

Go back to the passage to find the reference. We find it in conjunction with the writer's implication that the art world has a short attention span. This is most consistent with **Choice (C)**. **Choices (A)** and **(B)** mistakenly connect Op Art to the work of Marin, a connection the author does not make in the passage. **Choice (D)** assumes a comparison also not drawn from the passage.

4. **D**

Only **Choice (D)** matches the overall tone of the passage. Most tone questions have adjectives and nouns in the answer choices. Remember that both must match the passage for the choice to be correct.

5. **A**

This type of question requires that you find an exception. **Choice (A)**—political beliefs—is the only aspect among the answer choices not discussed in the passage. If you misinterpreted Marin's "Nazi" quote as being political instead of philosophical, you might have had a hard time answering this question.

> **Test Tip**
>
> Certainly knowing a little about the topic discussed can be helpful. But remember to answer the questions based on what's in the passage, not based on your own outside knowledge.

6. **D**

Here, you must show that you interpreted the quote correctly. Marin used the phrase Nazism to describe a repressive, tyrannical system of criticism—not a political attitude. Only **Choice (D)** resonates with the metaphorical interpretation of the phrase.

7. **A**

The answer can't be found in a particular line from the passage. You must conclude the best answer based on the attitude and tone of the passage. **Choice (A)** accurately reflects the writer's characterizations of Marin's work. **Choice (B)** might be tempting because the writer *does* describe Marin as simple, but in his personal life, not in reference to his art. **Choice (C)** describes Marin's life as depicted by the author but has no connection to his art. Finally, **Choice (D)** conveys too much negativity to match the tone of the passage.

8. C

Refer to the line referenced in the question stem to see how the sentence functions in the passage. We see that the author was trying to suggest that despite their seeming spontaneity, Marin's paintings were actually quite "crafted." **Choice (C)** is thus consistent with the intent of the passage. **Choice (A)** is a tricky interpretation of the sentence. **Choice (B)** sounds erudite, but it has no relation to the passage whatsoever. Lastly, **Choice (D)** makes an illogical leap to conclude that Marin's paintings showed no imagination, but the passage never suggests this is the case.

SIX QUESTION TYPES

There are six Verbal Reasoning question styles you'll find on the MCAT: Main Idea, Detail, Inference, Application, Tone, and Logic. Familiarity with the question types helps you anticipate the kinds of answers you should be choosing. The ability to anticipate correct answers will speed up your testing time, give you extra confidence, and—ultimately—boost your score!

1. Main Idea

Description: Main Idea questions ask for a restatement of the author's main point, the primary idea, or the overall gist of the passage. Question 1 in the preceding sample is a Main Idea question, because it's asking you for the point of the Marin excerpt.

Strategy: Look for the answer that best matches the scope of the main theme. Wrong answers will be either too narrow or too broad in their restatement of the author's main point or will distort it in some way.

Strategy Applied: If you look for the "big idea" of the preceding sample passage as you read it, you see that your interpretation of the author's purpose matches only one answer, that there was a sharp contrast between Marin's artistic style and personal life.

2. Detail

Description: Detail questions require you to recall a specific point from the passage or to relocate it using information from the question stem. Correct answers will be those that approximate information directly from the passage. One type of Detail question—"Scattered Detail"—will ask you to consider many details from various places in the passage and may ask you to identify a detail as an exception among the answer choices. For example: "The author uses as evidence all the following except . . . ." Question 5 in the preceding sample is a Scattered Detail question because it requires that you recall or look back to the passage to determine a characteristic of Marin's life that is not mentioned.

> **Test Tip**
>
> Key phrases in the Main Idea question stem include:
>
> "The author's main purpose is . . . ."
>
> "The main idea of the passage is . . . ."
>
> "The general theme is . . . ."

> **Test Tip**
>
> Phrases that identify a question as a Detail question include:
>
> "According to the passage, ..."
>
> "Based on the information in the passage, ..."

Strategy: Refer to any notes you made on your scratch paper or to notes in your mental outline to identify the detail under consideration. If the question is in the "all except" format, you should be looking for the exception, for the choice that fits the stimulus. By all means, look back to the passage. You're not supposed to memorize details!

Strategy Applied: In the case of the sample, you're looking for the exception, so you should ask yourself, "Does this fit the stimulus?" for each answer choice. The answer is "no" for only one—the passage does not discuss Marin's political beliefs.

3. Inference

Description: Inference questions ask you to make a small logical leap from the passage to another idea that would be consistent with the main idea. Correct answers to Inference questions will have the proper degree of "distance" from the passage itself—not so close as to be a detail but not so far as to be illogical.

Strategy: Choose an answer that is consistent with the passage but is not a simple restatement of information already presented.

Strategy Applied: There wasn't an Inference question in the sample, but let's say that you were asked how Marin's work was affected by critical interpretation. Since you're told that Marin did not like interpretation of his or anyone else's art, you can infer that he would not adjust his art to suit the critics, that his work would be unaffected.

4. Application

Description: Application questions ask you to take an essential idea from the passage and relate it to a different context. These questions may set up analogies or metaphors; you'll need to figure out how they relate to one another and determine which one presents an idea that parallels the passage. Question 2 in the sample is an Application question because it asks you to use what you know about the passage to guess at the source of the passage.

Strategy: Pick an answer choice that effectively "translates" an idea from the passage into a new context or scenario.

Strategy Applied: Taking what you know about the sample passage (the author's point of view and tone) and applying this to a scenario outside the passage (the source of the piece), you can judge that the author was most likely a magazine art critic.

> **Test Tip**
>
> Inference questions can relate to details or to the general theme of the passage and are indicated by question-stem phrases such as:
>
> "It can be inferred from the passage that. . . ."
>
> "The author suggests that. . . ."

> **Test Tip**
>
> Here are some phrases to watch for in Application question stems:
>
> "The passage was probably written by a . . . ."
>
> "The example in paragraph 2 would be most similar to . . . ."

5. Tone

<u>Description</u>: Questions of Tone require you to identify the author's attitude or opinion about a passage's subject matter. Such questions may be focused on a detail or may refer to the tone of the whole passage. Question 4 from the sample passage is an example of a Tone question because it asks you to determine the author's attitude.

<u>Strategy</u>: Go with the answer choice that is consistent with your "gut feel" from the passage—positive, neutral, or negative.

<u>Strategy Applied</u>: Based on the first paragraph in the sample passage, you know that the author holds Marin in high esteem, so the correct answer about the author's tone will have to reflect a completely positive attitude. Only one choice does so.

6. Logic

<u>Description</u>: Logic questions require that you analyze the function of certain portions of the passage. You may be asked how a particular detail serves the purpose of the passage, or you may be asked about overall passage structure. A Logic question is derived from the overall plan and layout of the passage—not from the specifics contained within the passage. Question 8 in the sample is a Logic question because it asks you about the logical structure of the passage.

<u>Strategy</u>: Refer to your mental map and passage outline, the source of all logic questions. Choose an answer that maintains the integrity of your passage blueprint.

<u>Strategy Applied</u>: In the sample, you're asked to determine the meaning of the term *studio works*. To do so, you need to read a few sentences back from the term and figure out its context. You clearly see, then, that "studio works" refers to artistic pieces crafted out of a deliberate process.

HIGHLIGHTS

GETTING OFF ON THE RIGHT FOOT

- You usually won't save time by scanning the questions before reading the passage, as most of the questions are based on a holistic understanding of the passage. Besides, having the questions in mind can distract you from focusing on the passage.
- Read the opening lines of each paragraph slowly and carefully to "orient" yourself to the subject matter and its main point.
- Read for the Main Idea, often, but not always, expressed in the opening lines.

READING THE PASSAGES

- Read actively!
- Don't get emotional. Read with distance.
- Don't judge the passages. You'll need to overcome the hurdle of reading material that doesn't interest you.
- Create a mental map.
- Feel free to make notes on scratch paper.
- Don't try to memorize details. Know the purpose of the detail, not the detail itself.
- Look for structural keywords to help you anticipate new ideas in the passage.
- Check the citation at the end of the passage. It may give clues about tone or context.

Go Online

Rotating monthly quizzes will keep you on top of your game.

FACING THE QUESTIONS

- When you're finished reading, don't rush to the questions. Take a moment to rephrase the main idea to yourself.
- Remember that wrong answer choices will distort or reverse the author's main point, blow a detail out of proportion, confuse or misplace details, or be totally irrational. Use a process of elimination to increase your chances of getting to the right answer.
- You should look back at the passage to find or clarify details while you're answering the questions.
- Answer questions based on the passage—not based on outside knowledge.
- If you don't know an answer, guess! Try to do so while you're still working on the passage, so you won't have to reread it later. There's no penalty for wrong answers. Leave no question unanswered!

4

WRITING SAMPLE

THE BIG PICTURE

Medical schools want an assessment of your written communication skills, as these are a reflection of your ability to effectively convey information to your future patients, healthcare colleagues, and the public. This is where the Writing Sample section of the MCAT comes in.

You'll be writing two essays during the MCAT, each in response to a stimulus and each within a half-hour allotment. The Writing Sample is the only section that is not comprised of multiple-choice questions. Like the Verbal Reasoning section, this one tends to be underestimated by MCAT test takers. Most think they can just apply their everyday writing skills to the MCAT and do OK on the essays. This is a dangerous presumption. In every facet, the MCAT is a test of analytical reasoning—even in the Writing Sample.

THE STIMULUS

The statement you're to respond to will be in a format along the lines of: *True leadership leads by example rather than by command.* It may be an opinion, a widely shared belief, a philosophical dictum, or an assertion regarding general policy concerns in such areas as history, political science, business, ethics, or art. You can be sure that the statement will not concern scientific or technical subjects, your reasons for entering the medical profession, emotionally charged religious or social issues, or obscure social or political issues that may require specialized knowledge. In fact, you will not need any specialized knowledge to do well on this part of the MCAT.

Most test takers make the mistake of using the essay stimulus as a platform from which to emote, lecture, convince, or just babble. Instead, your goal should be to analyze the statement, present it from two perspectives, and explain how and when you might apply the statement. Your essays need to

---

Writing Sample at a Glance

- 60 minutes in two 30-minute time blocks
- 2 essays
- Tests critical thinking, intellectual organization, written communication skills

---

Test Tip

A stimulus, or statement, is the provided focus of your essay your jumping-off point.

be written with a critical mind, not an emotional one. This theme is in keeping with the overall goals and intentions of the MCAT—the test makers want to see how you think.

THE THREE-TASK ESSAY

Though worded slightly differently each time, the instructions that follow the statement will ask you to perform three tasks. When completed properly, the following tasks create a balanced essay.

Task One

Provide your interpretation or explanation of the statement. The degree to which you develop the statement in this first task dictates the depth and sophistication of your entire essay.

Task Two

Offer a concrete example that illustrates a point of view *directly opposite* to the one expressed in or implied by the statement. You must give an explicit counter example; it can be factual or hypothetical.

Task Three

Explain how the conflict between the viewpoint expressed in the statement and the viewpoint you described in the second task might be resolved. You'll be coming up with a kind of "test" or rule that you could apply in situations to see whether or not the statement holds true.

A CLOSER LOOK

Here's an opportunity to begin familiarizing yourself with the essay subjects and an actual essay. You should try your hand at addressing the three tasks (observing the 30-minute time limit, of course), compare your essay with the sample that's provided below, and review the strategies that follow. You'll have the opportunity to boost your essay-writing skills in the content review section of this book.

SAMPLE STIMULUS AND ESSAY

Stimulus

Consider this statement:

> *Heroes are people who place the needs of others above their own needs.*

Write a unified essay in which you perform the following tasks:

- Explain what you think the above statement means.
- Describe a specific situation in which a person could be heroic while placing his or her own needs above the needs of others.
- Discuss what you think determines whether or not people who put their own needs above the needs of others can be heroes.

> ### Test Tip
>
> It's essential that you keep the three tasks in mind as you write. The graders will look carefully to see if you fulfilled them.

Essay

The statement suggests that being heroic means subjugating one's own needs to external forces of need, relinquishing one's inner compass to be directed by the power of others in need. The classic hero, of course, is the firefighter who runs back into a burning building to save a child. The urgency of momentary crisis can compel people to forget their own safety, their own need for security, in order to guarantee the safety or security of others. In that a hero, by definition, is someone who is emulated and respected, the statement above carries with it the assumption that we respect people who sacrifice themselves to the needs of others.

In a more sophisticated sense, however, many of our historical and fictional heroes have been men and women who stood strong against a tide of negative judgment—people who did not indulge the needs of others but rather played out their own needs. Shakespeare's famous line is often quoted: "This above all: To thine own self be true and good will follow thee as night the day." We make heroes out of individualists who implement unique and personal vision. Ayn Rand is famous and well read in part because her characters—such as Howard Roark in *The Fountainhead*—refuse to place the needs of others above their own. Indeed, the more lyrical classic hero is the one who stands alone without the title of "hero" until long after the true heroism has passed—the heroism of maintaining a course consistent with one's principles regardless of outside pressure or persuasion. It is in the fuller circle of time that the person comes to be seen as heroic. These are the kinds of heroes who last through history—not just through tomorrow's news.

There are indeed times when sacrifice is heroic. No one would deny a soldier a Purple Heart earned in battle. However, we also see that there are circumstances in which self-actualization rather than self-denial is the heroic choice. Being a hero, then, seems to be more about courage and choice-making than about any particular outcome or event. Heroes of all kinds—those who put their own needs first (i.e., the "compassionate hero") and those who don't (i.e., the "principled hero")—are people who act according to a standard of "what is right." So, the thing that determines whether or not a sacrificial person can be a hero seems to be the gradient of courage he or she must climb on the way to action.

 Go Online

Rotating monthly essays and sample responses will refine your skills.

Did You Address All Three Tasks?

Don't be intimidated by this ideal essay. It's there for you to learn from, not for you to hold up as a standard that may be unrealistic considering the time limit. The sample completes all three tasks and does so with vivid examples and a strong organization. The statement is handled confidently, leading to an essay with interpretive depth, and the writing is crisp, focused, and easy to follow. On the whole the essay is well balanced, with strong counter examples and a strong resolution.

It begins by immediately defining the "classic hero" and developing an understanding of what is meant by the word *hero*. This gives the reader a context for the essay. When we get to the next paragraph—where we see a discussion of heroes who don't place others' needs above their own—the polarity emerges immediately. Through a series of examples, the essay becomes balanced in its discussion of heroism in relation to self-sacrifice. The stage is set for the resolution in the last paragraph.

As you familiarize yourself with the following seven-step approach to the Writing Sample, you'll see exactly how this particular essay follows each step.

SEVEN-STEP APPROACH TO THE WRITING SAMPLE

Your writing skills are directly linked to your ability to think analytically and logically. You might have a wonderful command of the English language, but if you can't get your thoughts organized and your ideas clear in your mind, your essay will be a jumbled mess.

Step 1: Read and Take Notes

<u>Purpose</u>: Clarify for yourself what the statement says and what the instructions require.

<u>Process</u>:
- Read the statement and instructions carefully.
- Write down any key words or phrases that are easy to miss but crucial to a good understanding, are ambiguous or confusing, or refer to vague or abstract concepts.
- Read the instructions, noting the tasks and jotting down any words that will help you remember exactly what it is you're supposed to do.

Application: Key words from the preceding sample statement, *heroes are people who place the needs of others above their own needs,* would be *hero, needs,* and *above.* These words form the seed of thought from which grows a personal interpretation of the statement.

Step 2: Prewrite the First Task

Purpose: On scratch paper, develop a clear interpretation of the statement.

Process:
- Think of one or more supporting examples.
- Clarify/define/interpret abstract, ambiguous, or confusing words.
- Ask yourself questions to get beyond the superficial meaning of the statement.

Test Tip

1. Read and take notes.
2. Prewrite the first task on paper.
3. Prewrite the second task on paper.
4. Prewrite the third task on paper.
5. Clarify the main idea and plan.
6. Write.
7. Proofread.

Application: For the preceding sample, you would want to expand the ideas in the statement by asking, "What is a hero? What are examples of self-sacrificial heroism and what makes those situations heroic?" Try to distill the implications of the statement. This is where the idea of the classic hero comes in as a context for understanding the statement.

Step 3: Prewrite the Second Task

Purpose: On scratch paper, further explore the meaning of the statement by examining a situation that represents an opposing point of view.

Process:
- Think up one or more specific situations that demonstrate a way in which the statement is not true (even if you agree with the statement).
- It's OK to discuss more than one example, but don't spread yourself too thin.

Test Tip

5 minutes—Steps 1–5
23 minutes—Step 6
2 minutes—Step 7

Application: Here's where, for the sample essay, you would consider opposing situations along the lines of, "When is a hero not sacrificial?" and "What are instances in which heroism has been defined by lack of self-sacrifice?" These extremes help balance and deepen the essay. Shakespeare's quote and Ayn Rand's characters help set up the duality of the essay by opposing the fireman example introduced earlier.

Step 4: Prewrite the Third Task

Purpose: On scratch paper, find a way to resolve the conflict between the statement given in the essay topic and the opposing situation(s) you conceived for the second task.

Process:
- Read the instructions for the third task carefully.
- Look back at the ideas you generated for the first and second tasks.
- Develop your response based on these ideas.
- You don't have to resolve the conflict in support of, or in opposition to, the statement. It's your reasoning that counts, not your stance on the conflict.

Application: Once the seeming dichotomy is set up, as in the hero essay, you need to find a way to resolve it. Sometimes a hero must act to save another. Sometimes saving oneself from moral inconsistency is the heroic act. Both must exist in the context of heroism, so there must be some "deciding" factor. Perhaps it's the difficulty of the act—the amount of courage it requires—or the degree of risk taken in order to achieve one's goal, selfless or otherwise.

Step 5: Clarify the Main Idea and Plan

Purpose: Do final organization and clarification of ideas; take a mental "breath" before beginning to write.

Process:
- Take a quick moment to look back over your notes in light of the ideas you have reached in prewriting the third task.
- Check to make sure your ideas are consistent with each other.
- Decide in what order your essay will address the three tasks.

Application: Take note of how solid organization provides a sense of unity in the sample essay.

Step 6: Write

Purpose: Type a straightforward essay that thoroughly presents your response to each of the three tasks.

Process:
- Use your prewriting notes for guidance.
- Stick to the tasks.
- Think about the quality of the essay, not the length.
- Try not to use clichés, slang expressions, redundant words or phrases (e.g., "refer back" instead of "refer"), and water-treading sentences (sentences that get you nowhere or serve only to restate the essay directions).
- Vary sentence length and structure, to give your essay a rhythm.
- Avoid making repeated references to yourself (e.g., "I feel.").

Application: You can see in the hero essay what a difference writing in a strong, confident voice makes.

Step 7: Proofread

<u>Purpose</u>: Quickly review your essay for blatant errors or significant omissions.

<u>Process</u>:
- You don't have time to revise your essay substantially.
- Look for problems in meaning (missing words, sentence fragments, illegible words, confusing punctuation, etc.) and problems in mechanics (misspelled words, capitalization, etc.).
- Learn the types of mistakes you tend to make and look for them.

<u>Application</u>: The sample essay would have made quite a different impression if words had been misspelled throughout. Reading through the essay carefully to see how it sounds is an important step.

YOUR ESSAY SCORE

Your essays will be graded on a six-tier scale, with Level 6 being the highest. Graders will be looking for an overall sense of your essay; they won't be assigning separate scores for specific elements like grammar or substance. They realize you're writing under time pressure and expect you to make a certain number of mistakes of this kind. A series of mistakes can mar your essay's overall impression, though, so work on any areas you're particularly weak in.

One reader reads your essay and assigns a score. Your essay is also graded by computer. The two scores are added together, and this combined score will then be converted into an alphabetical rating (ranging from J to T). Statistically speaking, there will be few Level 6 essays. An essay of 4 or 5 would place you at the upper range of those taking the exam.

Here's a quick look at what determines your score:

Score Level 6

- Fulfills all three tasks
- Develops the statement in depth
- Demonstrates careful thought
- Presents an organized structure
- Uses language in sophisticated manner

Score Level 5

- Fulfills all three tasks
- Interprets statement in some depth
- Demonstrates some in-depth thought
- Presents a fairly organized essay
- Shows good command of word choice and structure

Score Level 4

- Addresses all three tasks
- Considers the statement somewhat but not in depth
- Shows logical thought but nothing very complex
- Shows overall organization but may have digressions
- Demonstrates strong skills in word use

Score Level 3

- Overlooks or misses one or more of the tasks
- Offers a barely adequate consideration of the statement
- Contains ideas that lack depth
- Shows basic control of word choice and essay structure
- May have problems with clarity of meaning

Score Level 2

- Glaringly omits or misinterprets one or more tasks
- Offers an unacceptable consideration of the statement
- Shows lack of unity or is incoherent
- Exhibits errors in basic grammar, punctuation, or word use
- May be hard to follow or understand

Score Level 1

- Shows significant problems in basic writing construction
- Presents confusing or disjointed ideas
- May disregard or ignore the given assignment

You can see by this scoring outline that in order to receive higher than a Level 3 score you must successfully address all three tasks. Also note that to receive a top-level score you must develop the statement in depth and show sophisticated thought. Furthermore, for a great writing score, you need to demonstrate a strong and logical style, a confident tone, and an eloquent use of language.

HIGHLIGHTS

GETTING OFF ON THE RIGHT FOOT

- Spend about five minutes prewriting on scratch paper, outlining your thoughts before you start typing.
- If you can't come up with real-life examples, use literary examples or your imagination!

WRITING THE ESSAY

- Use a paragraph structure that matches the tasks, so your essay will be easy for readers to follow.
- Avoid clichés, slang expressions, junk phrases, redundant words or phrases, and water-treading sentences.
- Don't get emotional—graders don't care *what* you think, they care *how* you think and how many of the tasks you've fulfilled.

REVIEWING YOUR ESSAY

- Be strict with yourself so you have at least a few minutes left at the end to read over what you've written. Don't let yourself get cut off.
- Be sure you've addressed all three tasks. Your essay must be balanced.

5

TEST EXPERTISE

The first year of medical school is a frenzied experience for most students. In order to meet the requirements of a rigorous work schedule, s-tudents either learn to prioritize and budget their time or else fall hopelessly behind. It's no surprise, then, that the MCAT, the test specifically designed to predict success in the first year of medical school, is a high-speed, time-intensive test. It demands excellent time-management skills as well as that sine qua non of the successful physician—grace under pressure.

It's one thing to answer a Verbal Reasoning question correctly; it's quite another to answer several correctly in a limited time frame. And the same goes for Physical and Biological Sciences—it's a whole new ball game once you move from doing an individual passage at your leisure to handling a full section under actual timed conditions. You also need to budget your time for the Writing Sample, but this section isn't as time sensitive. But when it comes to the multiple-choice sections, time pressure is a factor that affects virtually every test taker.

So when you're comfortable with the content of the test, your next challenge will be to take it to the next level—test expertise—which will enable you to manage the all-important time element of the test.

> **Test Tip**
>
> For complete MCAT success, you've got to get as many correct answers as possible in the time you're allotted. Knowing the strategies is not enough. You have to perfect your time management skills so that you get a chance to use those strategies on as many questions as possible.

THE FIVE BASIC PRINCIPLES OF TEST EXPERTISE

On some tests, if a question seems particularly difficult you'll spend significantly more time on it, as you'll probably be given more points for correctly answering a hard question. Not so on the MCAT. Remember, every MCAT question, no matter how hard, is worth a single point. There's no partial credit or "A" for effort. And since there are so many questions to do in so little time, you'd be a fool to spend ten minutes getting a point for a hard question and then not have time to get a couple of quick points from three easy questions later in the section.

Given this combination—limited time, all questions equal in weight— you've got to develop a way of handling the test sections to make sure you get as many points as you can as quickly and easily as you can. Here are the principles that will help you do that:

1. FEEL FREE TO SKIP AROUND

One of the most valuable strategies to help you finish the sections in time is to learn to recognize and deal first with the questions that are easier and more familiar to you. That means you must temporarily skip those that promise to be difficult and time-consuming, if you feel comfortable doing so. You can always come back to these at the end, and if you run out of time, you're much better off not getting to questions you may have had difficulty with, rather than not getting to potentially feasible material. Of course, because there's no guessing penalty, always put an answer to every question on the test, whether you get to it or not. (It's not practical to skip passages, so do those in order.)

This strategy is difficult for most test takers; we're conditioned to do things in order. But give it a try when you practice. Remember, if you do the test in the exact order given, you're letting the test makers control you. But you control how you take this test. On the other hand, if skipping around goes against your moral fiber and makes you a nervous wreck—don't do it. Just be mindful of the clock, and don't get bogged down with the tough questions.

2. LEARN TO RECOGNIZE AND SEEK OUT QUESTIONS YOU CAN DO

Another thing to remember about managing the test sections is that MCAT questions and passages, unlike items on the SAT and other standardized tests, are not presented in order of difficulty. There's no rule that says you have to work through the sections in any particular order; in fact, the test makers scatter the easy and difficult questions throughout the section, in effect rewarding those who actually get to the end. Don't lose sight of what you're being tested for along with your reading and thinking skills: efficiency and cleverness.

Don't waste time on questions you can't do. We know that skipping a possibly tough question is easier said than done; we all have the natural instinct to plow through test sections in their given order. But it just doesn't pay off on the MCAT. The computer won't be impressed if you get the toughest question right. If you dig in your heels on a tough question, refusing to move on until you've cracked it, well, you're letting your ego get in the way of your test score. A test section (not to mention life itself) is too short to waste on lost causes.

3. USE A PROCESS OF ANSWER ELIMINATION

Using a process of elimination is another way to answer questions both quickly and effectively. There are two ways to get all the answers right on the MCAT. You either know all the right answers, or you know all the wrong answers. Since there are three times as many wrong answers, you should be able to eliminate some if not all of them. By doing so you either get to the correct response or increase your chances of guessing the correct response. You start out with a 25 percent chance of picking the right answer, and with each eliminated answer your odds go up. Eliminate one, and you'll have a 33 1/3 percent chance of picking the right one, eliminate two, and you'll have a 50 percent chance, and, of course, eliminate three, and you'll have a 100 percent chance. Increase your efficiency by actually crossing out the wrong choices on the screen using the strike-through feature. Remember to look for wrong-answer traps when you're eliminating. Some answers are designed to seduce you by distorting the correct answer.

4. REMAIN CALM

It's imperative that you remain calm and composed while working through a section. You can't allow yourself to become so rattled by one hard reading passage that it throws off your performance on the rest of the section. Expect to find at least one killer passage in every section, but remember, you won't be the only one to have trouble with it. The test is curved to take the tough material into account. Having trouble with a difficult question isn't going to ruin your score—but getting upset about it and letting it throw you off track will. When you understand that part of the test maker's goal is to reward those who keep their composure, you'll recognize the importance of not panicking when you run into challenging material.

5. KEEP TRACK OF TIME

Of course, the last thing you want to happen is to have time called on a particular section before you've gotten to half the questions. Therefore, it's essential that you pace yourself, keeping in mind the general guidelines for how long to spend on any individual question or passage. Have a sense of how long you have to do each question, so you know when you're exceeding the limit and should start to move faster.

So, when working on a section, always remember to keep track of time. Don't spend a wildly disproportionate amount of time on any one question or group of questions. Also, give yourself 30 seconds or so at the end of each section to fill in answers for any questions you haven't gotten to.

SECTION-SPECIFIC PACING

Let's now look at the section-specific timing requirements and some tips for meeting them. Keep in mind that the times per question or passage are only averages; there are bound to be some that take less time and some that take more. Try to stay balanced. Remember, too, that every question is of equal worth, so don't get hung up on any one. Think about it: If a question is so hard that it takes you a long time to answer it, chances are you may get it wrong anyway. In that case, you'd have nothing to show for your extra time but a lower score.

VERBAL REASONING

Allow yourself approximately eight to ten minutes per passage and respective questions. It may sound like a lot of time, but it goes quickly. Keep in mind that some passages are longer than others. On average, give yourself about three or four minutes to read and then four to six minutes for the questions.

PHYSICAL AND BIOLOGICAL SCIENCES

Averaging over each section, you'll have about one minute and 20 seconds per question. Some questions, of course, will take more time, some less. A science passage plus accompanying questions should take about eight to nine minutes, depending on how many questions there are. Stand-alone questions can take anywhere from a few seconds to a minute or more. Again, the rule is to do your best work first. Also, don't feel that you have to understand everything in a passage before you go on to the questions. You may not need that deep an understanding to answer questions, since a lot of information may be extraneous. You should overcome your perfectionism and use your time wisely.

WRITING SAMPLE

You have exactly 30 minutes for each essay. As mentioned in discussion of the 7-step approach to this section, you should allow approximately 5 minutes to prewrite the essay, 23 minutes to write the essay, and 2 minutes to proofread. It's important that you budget your time, so you don't get cut off.

Test Tip

For Verbal Reasoning, here are some of the important time techniques to remember:

- Spend eight to ten minutes per passage
- Allow about three to four minutes to read and four to six minutes for the questions

---

Test Tip

Some suggestions for maximizing your time on the science sections:

- Spend about eight to nine minutes per passage
- Maximize points by doing the questions you can do first
- Don't waste valuable time trying to understand extraneous material

---

COMPUTER-BASED TESTING STRATEGIES

ARRIVE AT THE TESTING CENTER EARLY
Get to the testing center early to jump-start your brain. However, if they allow you to begin your test early, decline.

USE THE MOUSE TO YOUR ADVANTAGE
If you are right-handed, practice using the mouse with your left hand for test day. This way, you'll increase speed by keeping the pencil in your right hand to write on your scratch paper. If you are left-handed, use your right hand for the mouse.

KNOW THE TUTORIAL BEFORE TEST DAY
You will save time on test day by knowing exactly how the test will work. Click through any tutorial pages and save time.

PRACTICE WITH SCRATCH PAPER
Going forward, always practice using scratch paper when solving questions because this is how you will do it on test day. Never write directly on a written test.

GET NEW SCRATCH PAPER
Between sections, get a new piece of scratch paper even if you only used part of the old one. This will maximize the available space for each section and minimize the likelihood of you running out of paper to write on.

REMEMBER YOU CAN ALWAYS GO BACK
Just because you finish a passage or move on, remember you can come back to questions about which you are uncertain. You have the "marking" option to your advantage. However, as a general rule minimize the amount of questions you mark or skip.

MARK INCOMPLETE WORK
If you need to go back to a question, clearly mark the work you've done on the scratch paper with the question number. This way, you will be able to find your work easily when you come back to tackle the question.

LOOK AWAY AT TIMES
Taking the test on computer leads to faster eye-muscle fatigue. Use the Kaplan strategy of looking at a distant object at regular intervals. This will keep you fresher at the end of the test.

PRACTICE ON THE COMPUTER

This is the most critical aspect of adapting to computer-based testing. Like anything else, in order to perform well on computer-based tests you must practice. Spend time reading passages and answering questions on the computer. You often will have to scroll when reading passages.

6

TEST MENTALITY

In this section, we first glanced at the content that makes up each specific section of the MCAT, focusing on the strategies and techniques you'll need to tackle individual questions and passages. Then we discussed the test expertise involved in moving from individual items to working through full-length sections. Now we're ready to turn our attention to the often overlooked attitudinal aspects of the test, to put the finishing touches on your comprehensive MCAT approach.

THE FOUR BASIC PRINCIPLES OF GOOD TEST MENTALITY

Knowing the test content arms you with the weapons you need to do well on the MCAT. But you must wield those weapons with the right frame of mind and in the right spirit. Otherwise, you could end up shooting yourself in the foot. This involves taking a certain stance toward the entire test. Here's what's involved:

> **Test Tip**
>
> The important elements of good test mentality are:
>
> - Test awareness
> - Stamina
> - Confidence
> - The right attitude

1. TEST AWARENESS

To do your best on the MCAT, you must always keep in mind that the test is like no other test you've taken before, both in terms of content and in terms of the scoring system. If you took a test in high school or college and got a number of the questions wrong, you wouldn't receive a perfect grade. But on the MCAT, you can get a handful of questions wrong and still get a "perfect" score. The test is geared so that only the very best test takers are able to finish every section. But even these people rarely get every question right.

What does this mean for you? Well, just as you shouldn't let one bad passage ruin an entire section, you shouldn't let what you consider to be a subpar performance on one section ruin your performance on the entire test. If you allow that subpar performance to rattle you, it can have a cumulative negative

Test Tip

Keep cool. Losing a few extra points here and there won't do serious damage to your score, but losing your head will. Keeping your composure is an important test-taking skill.

effect, setting in motion a downward spiral. It's that kind of thing that could potentially do serious damage to your score. Losing a few extra points won't do you in, but losing your cool will.

Remember, if you feel you've done poorly on a section, don't sweat it. Chances are it's just a difficult section, and that factor will already be figured into the scoring curve. The point is, remain calm and collected. Simply do your best on each section, and once a section is over, forget about it and move on.

2. STAMINA

You must work on your test-taking stamina. Overall, the MCAT is a fairly grueling experience, and some test takers simply run out of gas on the last section. To avoid this, you must prepare by taking a few full-length practice tests in the weeks before the test, so that on test day, three sections plus a writing sample will seem like a breeze. (Well, maybe not a breeze, but at least not a hurricane.)

Take the full-length practice test included in this book and the test offered in your online companion. You'll be able to review answer explanations and assess your performance. For additional practice material, contact the Association of American Medical Colleges to receive the MCAT Practice Tests it publishes:

AAMC
Membership and Publication Orders
2450 N Street, NW
Washington, DC 20037
http://www.aamc.org

The AAMC sells online access to four full-length practice tests. Test 3R is available on the AAMC website free of charge. Tests 4R, 5R, 6R, 7, 8, and 9 are available for purchase. Tests 5R and 6R are also available for purchase in paper format.

Your best option, if you have some time, would be to take the full Kaplan course. We'll give you access to all the released material plus loads of additional material (more than 1,000 MCAT-style passages in total), so you can really build up your MCAT stamina. You'll also have the benefit of our expert live instruction on every aspect of the MCAT. To go this route, call 1-800-KAP-TEST for a Kaplan center location near you.

Reading this chapter is a great start in your preparation for the test, but it won't get you your best score. That can only happen after lots of practice and skill-building. You've got to train your brain to be test smart! Kaplan has been helping people do that for over 65 years, so giving us a call would be a great way to move your test prep into high gear!

3. CONFIDENCE

Confidence feeds on itself, and unfortunately, so does the opposite of confidence—self-doubt. Confidence in your ability leads to quick, sure answers and a sense of well-being that translates into more points. If you lack confidence, you end up reading the sentences and answer choices two, three, or four times, until you confuse yourself and get off track. This leads to timing difficulties, which only perpetuate the downward spiral, causing anxiety and a tendency to rush in order to finish sections.

If you subscribe to the MCAT Mindset we've described, however, you'll gear all of your practice toward the major goal of taking control of the test. When you've achieved that goal—armed with the principles, techniques, strategies, and approaches set forth in this book—you'll be ready to face the MCAT with supreme confidence. And that's the one sure way to score your best on test day.

4. THE RIGHT ATTITUDE

Those who approach the MCAT as an obstacle, who rail against the necessity of taking it, who make light of its importance, who spend more time making fun of the AAMC than studying for the test, usually don't fare as well as those who see the MCAT as an opportunity to show off the reading and reasoning skills that the medical schools are looking for. Don't waste time making value judgments about the MCAT. It's not going to go away. Deal with it. Those who look forward to doing battle with the MCAT—or, at least, who enjoy the opportunity to distinguish themselves from the rest of the applicant pack—tend to score better than do those who resent or dread it.

It may sound a little dubious, but take our word for it: Attitude adjustment is a proven test-taking technique. Here are a few steps you can take to make sure you develop the right MCAT attitude:

- Look at the MCAT as a challenge, but try not to obsess over it; you certainly don't want to psyche yourself out of the game.
- Remember that, yes, the MCAT is obviously important, but, contrary to what some premeds think, this one test will not single-handedly determine the outcome of your life.

> **Test Tip**
>
> You wouldn't run a marathon without working on your stamina well in advance of the race, would you? The same goes for taking the MCAT.

Test Tip

Develop an MCATtitude. It sounds touchy-feely, we know, but your attitude toward the test rea-lly does affect your performance. We're not asking you to "think nice thoughts about the MCAT," but we are recommending that you change your mental stance toward the test.

- Try to have fun with the test. Learning how to match your wits against the test makers can be a very satisfying experience, and the reading and thinking skills you'll acquire will benefit you in medical school as well as in your future medical career.
- Remember that you're more prepared than most people. You've trained with Kaplan. You have the tools you need, plus the know-how to use those tools.

KAPLAN'S TOP TEN MCAT TIPS

1. **Relax!**

2. **Remember: It's primarily a thinking test.**
   Never forget the purpose of the MCAT: It's designed to test your powers of analytical reasoning. You need to know the content, as each section has its own particular "language," but the underlying MCAT intention is consistent throughout the test.

3. **Feel free to skip around within each section.**
   Attack each section confidently. You're in charge. Move around between questions if you feel comfortable doing so. Work your best areas first to maximize your opportunity for MCAT points. Don't be a passive victim of the test structure!

4. **For passage-based questions, choose an answer based on the information given.**
   Be careful not to be "too smart for your own good." Passages—especially those that describe experimental findings (an MCAT favorite, by the way)—often generate their own data. Your answer choices must be consistent with the information in the passage, even if that means an answer is inconsistent with the science of ideal theoretical situations.

5. **Avoid wrong-answer traps.**
   Try to anticipate answers before you read the answer choices. This helps boost your confidence and protects you from persuasive or tricky incorrect choices. Most wrong answer choices are logical twists on the correct choice.

6. **Think, think, think!**
   We said it before, but it's important enough to say again: Think. Don't compute.

7. **Don't look back.**

   Don't spend time worrying about questions you had to guess on. Keep moving forward. Don't let your spirit start to flag, or your attitude will slow you down. You can recheck answers within a section if you have time left, but don't worry about a section after time has been called.

8. **Practice for the MCAT on the computer.**

   The MCAT is a computer-based test and you will perform better on test day if you practice on the computer. Use your CD-ROM, which reflects the new CBT technology, and take the practice tests and quizzes online.

9. **Don't leave any questions unanswered.**

   There are no points taken off for wrong answers, so if you're not sure of an answer, **guess**. And guess quickly, so you'll have more time to work through other questions.

10. **Call us! We're here to help! 1-800-KAP-TEST.**

HOW TO USE THE REVIEW SECTION

The quantity of material you need to know for the MCAT is voluminous. MCAT Premier Program covers every subject in the Physical and Biological Sciences that you're likely to need for the test. We also give you numerous Verbal Reasoning practice passages and detailed advice on crafting your Writing Sample. In addition, our clear, concise margin notes give you key facts at a glance, identify "MCAT favorite" topics, and help you connect ideas among the different scientific disciplines.

Throughout this book, you'll see the following margin notes:

KAPLAN EXCLUSIVE:

These sidebars contain information that is exclusive to Kaplan. You will find important MCAT ideas or mnemonics here.

MCAT SYNOPSIS:

These synopses are found on pages where lots of important and complex information is presented. In the days right before the MCAT, make sure to review the Synopsis notes.

CLINICAL CORRELATE:

These illustrate how a concept discussed in the text relates to the practice of medicine. Because you are a premed (if not, you're reading the wrong book), we feel that these correlations will be of interest to you (if not, you're choosing the wrong profession) and will help solidify your understanding of some key concepts. Remember, the MCAT passages are often based on med school level content. You need to feel comfortable that if you know the basics, you can analyze anything a passage may throw your way. The clinical correlates will help you with this goal.

REAL-WORLD ANALOGY:

These sidebars provide "real world" examples of important scientific principles. Being able to relate a concept to something you are familiar with from day-to-day life should help you better understand and remember key information for Test Day.

MCAT FAVORITE:

This note highlights a concept that has traditionally been tested on the MCAT.

BRIDGE:

We use "Bridges" to alert you to the conceptual links that occur between disciplines. Bridges contain specific chapter references for the other subjects.

FLASHBACK:

Flashbacks refer to something you've seen earlier in the book.

PAVLOV'S DOG:

Pavlov conducted famous experiments where he conditioned a dog to salivate when a bell was rung. Our margin-note version presents the proposition that if you see a particular word/phrase/concept, you should undergo a cognitive salivation process and immediately think of a specific word/phrase/concept.

PREMIER PROGRAM:

These notes are distinguished by icons and refer you to specific online components of the premier program for additional practice or interactive review.

TEST TIP:

When you see this sidebar, you will find important information about the exam and ways you can strategize to perform your best on exam day.

BIOLOGY

1

THE CELL

The cell is the fundamental unit of all living things. Every function in biology involves a process that occurs within cells or at the interface between cells. Therefore, to understand biology, you need to appreciate the structure and function of the different parts of the cell (the organelles) as well as the properties that define the plasma membrane that surrounds the cell.

CELL THEORY

The cell was not discovered or studied in detail until the development of the microscope in the seventeenth century. Since then much more has been learned, and a unifying theory known as the **Cell Theory** has been proposed.

The Cell Theory may be summarized as follows:

- All living things are composed of cells.
- The cell is the basic functional unit of life.
- Cells arise only from pre-existing cells.
- Cells carry genetic information in the form of **DNA**. This genetic material is passed from parent cell to daughter cell.

METHODS AND TOOLS

There are many tools available to study the cell and its structures. Three primary methods are **microscopy, autoradiography,** and **centrifugation.**

A. MICROSCOPY

Of the many tools used by scientists to study cells, the microscope is the most basic. **Magnification** is the increase in apparent size of an object. **Resolution** is the differentiation of two closely situated objects.

1. **Compound Light Microscope**

   A compound light microscope uses two lenses or lens systems to magnify an object. The total magnification is equal to the product of the eyepiece magnification (usually 10×) and the magnification of the selected objective lens (usually 4×, 10×, 20×, or 100×). The chief components of the microscope are the **diaphragm,** the **coarse adjustment knob,** and the **fine adjustment knob** (see Figure 1.1).

   - The diaphragm controls the amount of light passing through the specimen.
   - The coarse adjustment knob roughly focuses the image.
   - The fine adjustment knob sharply focuses the image.

   In general, the compound light microscope is used in the observation of nonliving specimens. Light microscopy requires contrast between cells and cell structures; such contrast is obtained through staining techniques that result in cell death. Various stains and dyes may be used for light microscopy. For example, the dye hematoxylin reveals the distribution of **DNA** and **RNA** within a cell due to its affinity for negatively charged molecules.

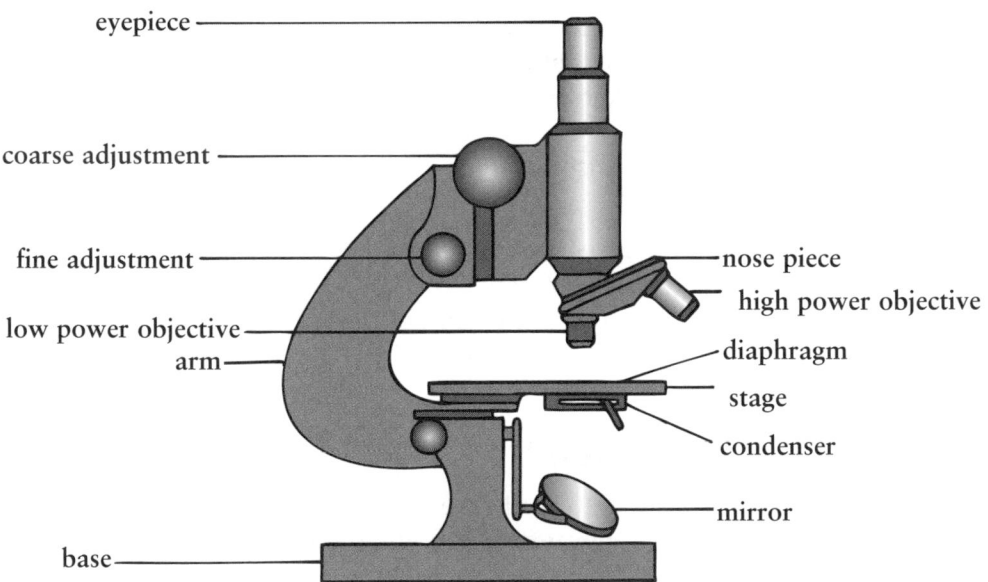

Figure 1.1. Compound Light Microscope

2. **Phase Contrast Microscope**

   A phase contrast microscope is a special type of light microscope that permits the study of living cells. Differences in refractive index are used to produce contrast between cellular structures. This technique does not kill the specimen.

3. **Electron Microscope**

An electron microscope uses a beam of electrons to allow a thousandfold higher magnification than is possible with light microscopy. Unfortunately, examination of living specimens is not possible because of the preparations necessary for electron microscopy; tissues must be fixed and sectioned and, sometimes, stained with solutions of heavy metals.

B. AUTORADIOGRAPHY

This technique uses radioactive molecules to trace and identify cell structures and biochemical activity. Cells are exposed to a radioactive compound for a brief, measured period of time (enough time for it to be incorporated into the cell). They are incubated, fixed at various intervals, and processed for microscopy. Each preparation is covered with a film of photographic emulsion. The preparations must be kept in the dark for several days while the radioactive compound decays. The emulsion is then developed; dark silver grains reveal the distribution of radioactivity within the specimen. Autoradiography can be used to study protein synthesis: Labeling amino acids with radioactive isotopes allows the pathways of protein synthesis to be examined. Similar techniques are used to study the mechanisms of DNA and RNA synthesis.

C. CENTRIFUGATION

Differential centrifugation can be used to separate cells or mixtures of cells without destroying them in the process. At lower speeds, cell mixtures separate into layers on the basis of cell type. Spinning fragmented cells at high speeds in the centrifuge will cause their components to sediment at different levels in the test tube on the basis of their respective densities. For example, centrifugation of a **eukaryotic** cell sediments high-density **ribosomes** at the bottom of the test tube, while low-density **mitochondria** and **lysosomes** remain at the top.

PROKARYOTES VS. EUKARYOTES

Cells can be structurally categorized into two distinct groups, **prokaryotic** and **eukaryotic**. **Viruses** occupy a unique category and are not technically considered cells since they are not capable of living independently.

 Go Online

Find an in-depth review of Microbiology topics in the Microbiology Workshop.

A. PROKARYOTES

Prokaryotes, which include **bacteria** and **cyanobacteria** (blue-green algae), are unicellular organisms with a simple cell structure. Prokaryotic cells have an outer cell membrane but do not contain any membrane-bound organelles. There is no true nucleus; the genetic material consists of a single circular molecule of DNA concentrated in an area of the cell called the **nucleoid** region. In addition, there may be smaller rings of DNA called **plasmids,** consisting of just a few genes. Plasmids replicate independently of the main chromosome, and often contain genes that allow the prokaryote to survive adverse conditions. Plasmids are one mechanism, for example, of imparting resistance to antibiotics.

Bacteria have a **cell wall**, a **cell membrane**, **cytoplasm**, ribosomes (somewhat different from those found in eukaryotes), and sometimes **flagella** (also different from those in eukaryotes) that are used for locomotion. Respiration occurs at the cell membrane (see Figure 1.2).

B. EUKARYOTES

All multicellular organisms and all nonbacteria unicellular organisms are composed of eukaryotic cells. A typical eukaryotic cell is bounded by a cell membrane and contains cytoplasm. Cytoplasm contains **organelles** suspended in a semifluid medium called the **cytosol**. The genetic material consists of linear strands of DNA organized into **chromosomes** and located within a membrane-enclosed organelle called the **nucleus**. Although both animal and plant cells are eukaryotic, they differ from each other. **Centrioles**, located in the centrosome area, are found in animal cells but not in plant cells (see Figure 1.3).

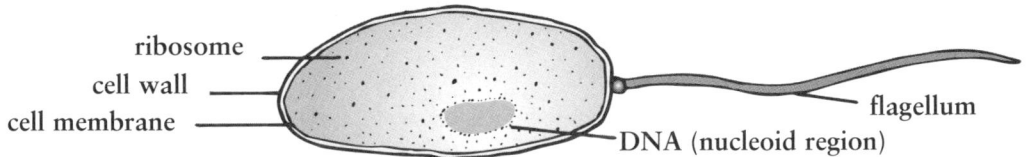

Figure 1.2. Prokaryotic Cell

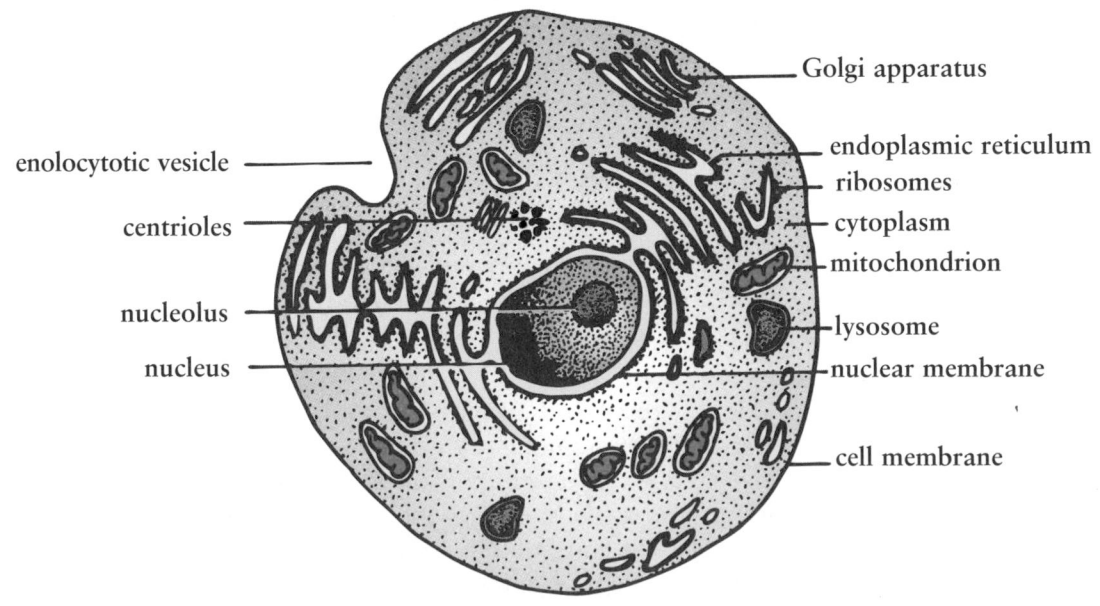

Figure 1.3. Eukaryotic Cell

EUKARYOTIC ORGANELLES

Cytosol is the fluid component of the cytoplasm and consists of an aqueous solution containing free proteins, nutrients, and other solutes. The **cytoskeleton**, which is composed of **microtubules, microfilaments, intermediate fibers**, and other accessory proteins, is also found in the cytosol. These proteinaceous filaments give the cell its shape and anchor the organelles. They also function in cell maintenance and aid in intracellular transport. The cell membrane surrounds the cell and regulates passage of materials in both directions.

The organelles are specialized structures of unique form and function. They include the nucleus, ribosomes, **endoplasmic reticulum**, **Golgi apparatus**, **vesicles, vacuoles**, lysosomes, **microbodies**, mitochondria, chloroplasts, and centrioles.

A. CELL MEMBRANE

The cell membrane (plasma membrane) encloses the cell and is composed of a **phospholipid bilayer**. Phospholipids have both a hydrophilic (polar) phosphoric acid and a hydrophobic (non-polar) fatty acid region. In a lipid bilayer, the hydrophilic regions are found on the exterior surfaces of the membrane whereas the hydrophobic regions are found on the interior of the membrane (see Figure 1.4).

This phospholipids bilayer structure allows the cell membrane to regulate the passage of material and molecules in and out of the cell and exhibits **selective permeability**. Selective permeability means that the cell membrane allows some compounds/molecules to pass through freely, where others are prohibited or regulated. Specifically, small non-polar (hydrophobic) molecules generally pass through freely (diffuse) across the cell membrane. In contrast, charged ions and large molecules such as proteins and complex carbohydrates do not diffuse freely. They may require carrier proteins to help carry them across the cell membrane.

According to the generally accepted fluid mosaic model, the cell membrane consists of a phospholipids bilayer with proteins embedded throughout. The lipids and many of the proteins can move freely within the membrane. Cholesterol molecules are often embedded in the hydrophobic interior and contribute to the cell membrane's fluidity. Proteins interspersed throughout the membrane may be partially or completely embedded in the bilayer; one or both ends of the protein may

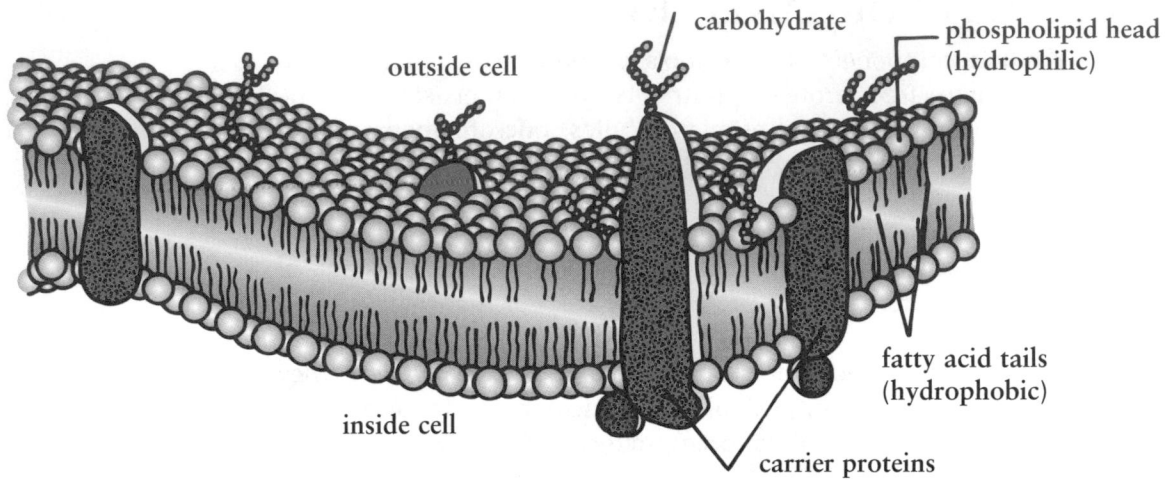

Figure 1.4. Fluid Mosaic Model

extend beyond the membrane on either side. Such proteins can play a role in cell adhesion by forming junctions with proteins on adjacent cells. Transport proteins are membrane-spanning proteins that allow certain ions and polar molecules to pass through the lipid bilayer. Cell adhesion molecules (CAMs) are proteins that contribute to cell recognition and adhesion, and are particularly important during development.

Receptors are complex proteins or glycoproteins generally embedded in the membrane with sites that bind to specific molecules in the cell's external environment. The receptor may carry the molecule into the cell via **pinocytosis** or it may signal across the membrane and into the cell via a second messenger (see chapter 11).

B. NUCLEUS

The nucleus controls the activities of the cell, including cell division. It is surrounded by a **nuclear membrane**, or **envelope**, which is a double membrane that maintains a nuclear environment distinct from that of the cytoplasm. Interspersed throughout the nuclear membrane are **nuclear pores** that allow selective two-way exchange of materials between the nucleus and the cytoplasm. The nucleus contains the DNA, which is complexed with structural proteins called **histones** to form chromosomes. The **nucleolus** is a dense structure in the nucleus where ribosomal RNA (rRNA) synthesis occurs.

C. RIBOSOMES

Ribosomes are the sites of protein production and are synthesized by the nucleolus (see chapter 14). Ribosomes consist of two subunits, one large and one small; each subunit is composed of rRNA and proteins. **Free**

> ### MCAT Favorite
>
> 1) Non-polar (hydrophobic) compounds pass through plasma membrane easily.
>
> 2) Polar (hydrophilic) compounds do NOT pass through plasma membrane easily. They may require the use of carrier proteins.

ribosomes are found in the cytoplasm, while **bound ribosomes** line the outer membrane of the endoplasmic reticulum.

D. ENDOPLASMIC RETICULUM

The endoplasmic reticulum (**ER**) is a network of membrane-enclosed spaces connected at points with the nuclear membrane. ER with ribosomes lining its outer surface is known as **rough ER (RER)** and ER without ribosomes is known as **smooth ER**.

In general, ER is involved in the transport of materials throughout the cell, especially those materials destined to be secreted from the cell. Smooth ER is involved in lipid synthesis and the detoxification of drugs and poisons, while rough ER is involved in protein synthesis. Proteins synthesized by the bound ribosomes cross into the cisternae of the RER, where they undergo chemical modification. The proteins then cross into smooth ER, where they are secreted into cytoplasmic vesicles and transported to the Golgi apparatus.

E. GOLGI APPARATUS

The Golgi apparatus consists of a stack of membrane-enclosed sacs. The Golgi receives vesicles and their contents from smooth ER, modifies them (e.g., glycosylation), repackages them into vesicles, and distributes them. The Golgi is particularly active in the distribution of newly synthesized materials to the cell surface. **Secretory vesicles**, produced by the Golgi, release their contents to the cell's exterior by the process of **exocytosis**.

F. VESICLES AND VACUOLES

Vesicles and vacuoles are membrane-bound sacs involved in the transport and storage of materials that are ingested, secreted, processed, or digested by the cell. Vacuoles are larger than vesicles and are more likely to be found in plant cells.

G. LYSOSOMES

Lysosomes are membrane-bound vesicles that contain hydrolytic enzymes involved in intracellular digestion. These enzymes are maximally effective at a pH of 5 and therefore need to be enclosed within the lysosome—an acidic environment distinct from the neutral pH of the cytosol. Lysosomes fuse with endocytotic vacuoles, thereby breaking down the material ingested by the cell. Lysosomes also aid in renewing a cell's own components by breaking down the old ones and releasing their molecular building blocks into the cytosol for reuse. A cell in an injured or dying tissue may "commit suicide" by rupturing the lysosome membrane and releasing its hydrolytic enzymes, which will digest cellular contents; this process is referred to as **autolysis**.

H. MICROBODIES

Microbodies are membrane-bound organelles specialized as containers for metabolic reactions. Two important types of microbodies are **peroxisomes** and **glyoxysomes**. Peroxisomes contain oxidative enzymes that catalyze a class of reactions in which hydrogen peroxide is produced by the transfer of hydrogen from a substrate to oxygen. Peroxisomes break fats down into smaller molecules that can be used for fuel, and are also used in the liver to detoxify compounds harmful to the body, such as alcohol. Glyoxysomes are usually found in fat tissue of germinating seedlings. They are used by the seedling to convert fats into sugars until the seedling is mature enough to produce its own supply of sugars by photosynthesis.

I. MITOCHONDRIA

Mitochondria are the sites of aerobic respiration within the cell and hence the suppliers of energy. Each mitochondrion is bound by an outer and an inner phospholipid bilayer membrane. The outer membrane is smooth and acts as a sieve, allowing molecules through on the basis of size. The area between the inner and outer membranes is known as the **intermembrane space**. The inner membrane has many convolutions called **cristae** and a high protein content that includes the proteins of the electron transport chain. The area bounded by the inner membrane is known as the mitochondrial **matrix** and is the site of many of the reactions in cell respiration (see chapter 3). Mitochondria are different from the other organelles in that they are **semiautonomous**; i.e., they contain their own DNA (which is circular) and ribosomes, which enable them to produce some of their own proteins and to self-replicate by **binary fission**. Mitochondria are believed by many to have been early prokaryotic cells that evolved a symbiotic relationship with the ancestors of eukaryotic cells.

J. CELL WALL

Many eukaryotic cells such as plant cells and fungi are surrounded by a tough outer cell wall that protects the cell from external stimuli and desiccation. Animal cells are **not** surrounded by a cell wall.

K. CENTRIOLES

Centrioles are a specialized type of microtubule (see below) involved in spindle organization during cell division and are **not** bound by a membrane. Animal cells usually have a pair of centrioles that are oriented at right angles to each other and lie in a region called the **centrosome**. Plant cells do **not** contain centrioles.

L. CYTOSKELETON

The cytoskeleton gives the cell mechanical support, maintains its shape, and functions in cell motility. It is composed of microtubules, microfilaments, and intermediate filaments.

Microtubules are hollow rods made up of polymerized **tubulins** that radiate throughout the cell and provide it with support. Microtubules provide a framework for organelle movement within the cell. Centrioles, which direct the separation of chromosomes during cell division, are composed of microtubules (see chapter 4). **Cilia** and flagella are specialized arrangements of microtubules that extend from certain cells and are involved in cell motility.

Microfilaments are solid rods of **actin**, involved in cell movement as well as support. Muscle contraction, for example, is based on the interaction of actin with **myosin** in muscle cells (see chapter 6). Microfilaments move materials across the plasma membrane, for instance, in the contraction phase of cell division, and in amoeboid movement.

Intermediate filaments are a collection of fibers involved in maintenance of cytoskeletal integrity. Their diameters fall between those of microtubules and microfilaments.

MOVEMENT ACROSS THE CELL MEMBRANE

Substances can move into and out of cells in various ways. Some methods occur passively, without energy, while others are active and require energy expenditure (ATP).

A. SIMPLE DIFFUSION

Simple diffusion is the net movement of dissolved particles down their concentration gradients—from a region of higher concentration to a region of lower concentration. This is a passive process (see Figure 1.5). **Osmosis** is the simple diffusion of water from a region of lower solute concentration to a region of higher solute concentration. If a membrane is impermeable to a particular solute, then water will flow across the membrane until the differences in the solute concentrations have been equilibrated. Differences in the concentration of substances to which the membrane is impermeable affect the direction of osmosis. When the cytoplasm of the cell has a lower solute concentration than the extracellular medium, the medium is said to be **hypertonic** to the cell and water will flow out, causing the cell to shrink. When the cytoplasm of a cell has a higher solute concentration than the extracellular medium, the medium is said to be **hypotonic** to the cell and water will flow in, causing the

MCAT Favorite

Gradients rule! Be on the lookout throughout biology for examples in which gradients drive physiological function:

- Oxygen-carbon dioxide exchange in tissues and lungs
- Urine formation in the kidneys
- Depolarization of neurons and conduction of the action potential
- Proton gradient in mitochondria
- Exchange of materials between the maternal and fetal blood across the placenta

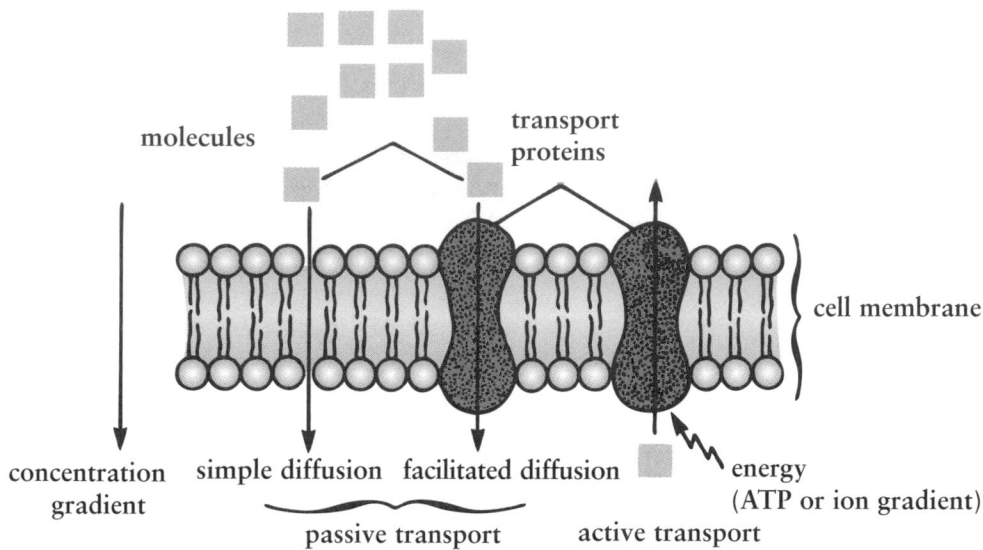

Figure 1.5. Movement Across Memberances

cell to swell; if too much water flows in, the cell may **lyse**. When the solute concentrations inside and outside the cell are equal, the cell and the medium are said to be **isotonic**, and there is no net flow of water in either direction (see Figure 1.6).

B. FACILITATED DIFFUSION

Facilitated diffusion (passive transport) is the net movement of dissolved particles down their concentration gradient with the help of carrier molecules. This process, like simple diffusion, does not require energy (see Figure 1.5).

C. ACTIVE TRANSPORT

Active transport is the net movement of dissolved particles against their concentration gradient with the help of transport proteins. Unlike diffusion, active transport requires energy (see Figure 1.5). Active transport is required to maintain membrane potentials in specialized cells such as neurons (see chapter 12).

D. ENDOCYTOSIS

Endocytosis is a process in which the cell membrane invaginates, forming a vesicle that contains extracellular medium (see Figure 1.7). Pinocytosis is the ingestion of fluids or small particles, and **phagocytosis** is the engulfing of large particles. Particles may first bind to receptors on the cell membrane before being engulfed.

Bridge

Diffusion is the biological version of a ball rolling down a hill—down its potential energy gradient. Active transport is the biological equivalent of pushing a ball up a hill; energy, in the form of ATP, must be expended and work is performed. See chapter 3 in the Physics section.

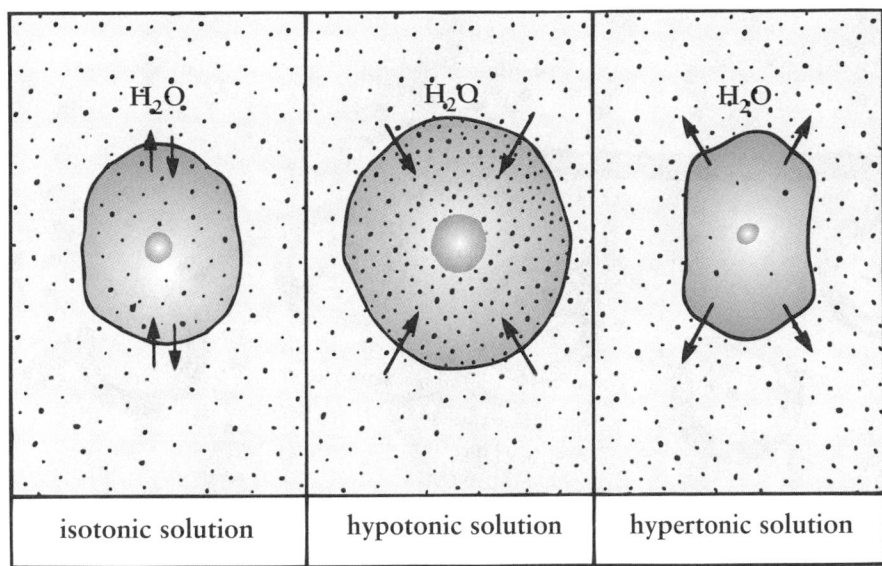

| isotonic solution | hypotonic solution | hypertonic solution |

Figure 1.6. Osmosis

E. EXOCYTOSIS

In exocytosis, a vesicle within the cell fuses with the cell membrane and releases its contents to the outside. Fusion of the vesicle with the cell membrane can play an important role in cell growth and intercellular signalling (see Figure 1.7). Note that in both endocytosis and exocytosis, the material never actually crosses through the cell membrane.

MCAT Synopsis

Types of transport:

Passive diffusion
• Down gradient
• No carrier
• No energy required

Facilitated diffusion
• Down gradient
• Carrier
• No energy required

Active transport
• Against gradient
• Carrier
• Energy required

Table 1.1: Movement Across the Cell Membrane

	Diffusion	Osmosis	Facilitated Transport	Active Transport
Concentration Gradient	High → Low	High → Low	High → Low	Low → High
Membrane Protein Required	No	No	Yes	Yes
Energy Required	NO – this is a PASSIVE process	NO – this is a PASSIVE process	NO – this is a PASSIVE process	YES – this is a ACTIVE process. Requires ATP
Type of Molecule/s Transported	Small non-polar (O_2, CO_2, etc...)	H_2O	Large non-polar (e.g glucose)	Polar molecules or ions (eg. Na^+, Cl^-, K^+ etc...)

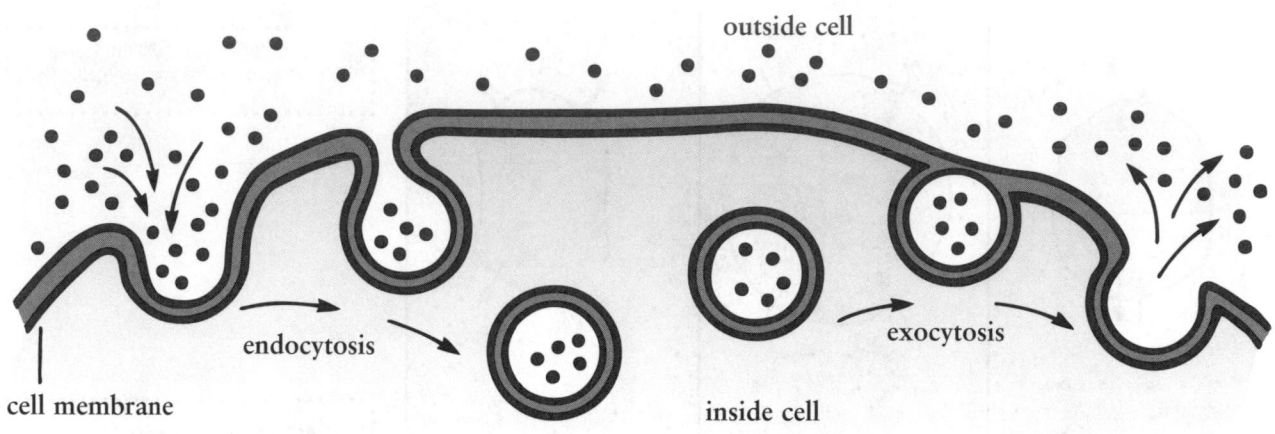

Figure 1.7. Endocytosis and Exocytosis

TISSUES

Tissues are groups of morphologically and functionally related cells. The four basic types of tissue found in the body are **epithelial**, **connective**, **nervous**, and **muscle**.

A. EPITHELIAL TISSUE

Epithelial tissue covers the surfaces of the body and lines the cavities, protecting them against injury, invasion, and desiccation. Epithelium is also involved in absorption, secretion, and sensation.

B. CONNECTIVE TISSUE

Connective tissue is involved in body support and other functions. Specialized connective tissues include bone, cartilage, tendons, ligaments, adipose tissue, and blood.

C. NERVOUS TISSUE

Nervous tissue is composed of specialized cells called neurons that are involved in the perception, processing, and storage of information concerning the internal and external environments (see chapter 12).

D. MUSCLE TISSUE

Muscle tissue has a great contractile capability and is involved in body movement. The three types of vertebrate muscle tissue are **skeletal** muscle, **cardiac** muscle, and **smooth** muscle (see chapter 6).

VIRUSES

Viruses are unique acellular structures composed of nucleic acid enclosed by a protein coat. Viruses range in size from 20–300 nm. In contrast, prokaryotes are 1–10 mm and eukaryotic cells are 10–100 mm. The nucleic acid can be either linear or circular, and has been found in four varieties: single-stranded DNA, double-stranded DNA, single-stranded RNA, and double-stranded RNA. The protein coat, or **capsid**, is composed of many protein subunits and may be enclosed by a membranous envelope.

Viruses are **obligate intracellular parasites**; i.e., they can express their genes and reproduce only within a living host cell, since they lack the structures necessary for independent activity and reproduction. A virus attaches itself to a host cell and injects its nucleic acid, taking control of protein synthesis within the cell. The viral genome replicates itself many times, produces new protein coats, and assembles new **virions** that leave the host cell in search of new hosts. Viruses that exclusively infect bacteria are called **bacteriophages**. The bacteriophage injects its nucleic acid into a bacterial cell; the phage capsid does not enter the cell (see chapter 14).

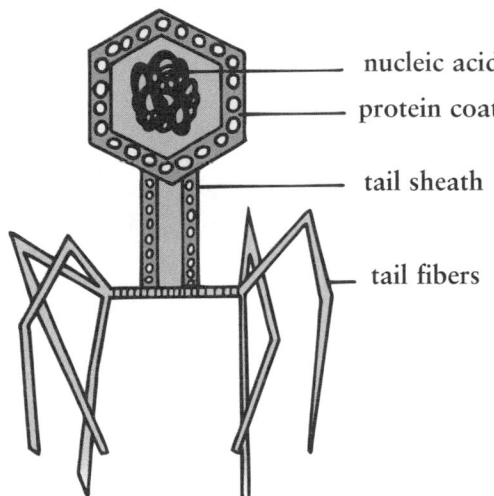

nucleic acid

protein coat

tail sheath

tail fibers

Figure 1.8. Bacteriophage

2

ENZYMES

Enzymes are protein catalysts that accelerate reactions, such as those in metabolic pathways, by reducing the initial energy **(activation energy)** necessary for them to proceed. The enzyme does not change the equilibrium point of a reaction; it changes only the rate at which it is attained. During the course of reactions, the enzymes themselves are neither consumed nor changed. Most enzyme reactions are reversible; the product synthesized by an enzyme can also be decomposed by the same enzyme. Figure 2.1 compares an uncatalyzed reaction with an enzymatically catalyzed reaction. The activation energy of the catalyzed reaction is lower, yet the overall **change in free energy** (ΔG) of the two reactions remains the same.

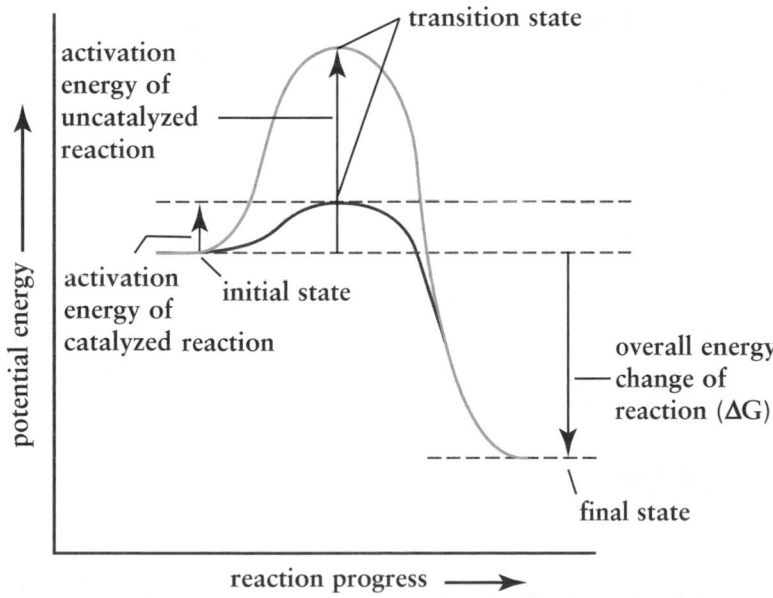

Figure 2.1. Reaction Coordinate

In a Nutshell

Enzymes:
- Lower activation energy of a reaction
- Increase the rate of the reaction
- Do not affect the overall ΔG of the reaction
- Are not changed or consumed in the course of the reaction

ENZYME SPECIFICITY

Enzymes are very selective; they may catalyze only one reaction or one specific class of closely related reactions. Urease, for example, selectively catalyzes the breakdown of urea. (Note that the suffix *ase* generally denotes an enzyme.) Chymotrypsin, on the other hand, selectively catalyzes the hydrolysis of specific types of peptide bonds, enabling it to catalyze the hydrolysis of more than one type of peptide (see chapter 7).

The molecule upon which an enzyme acts is called the **substrate**. There is an area on each enzyme to which the substrate bonds to form an **enzyme-substrate complex**. This area, the **active site**, has a three-dimensional shape into which the substrate fits and is held at a particular orientation. There are two models describing the formation of an enzyme-substrate complex: the **lock and key theory** and the **induced fit hypothesis**.

A. THE LOCK AND KEY THEORY

This theory holds that the spatial structure of an enzyme's active site (lock) is exactly complementary to the spatial structure of its substrate (key). Their 3-D configurations are such that the active site and the substrate fit together, forming an enzyme-substrate complex.

B. THE INDUCED FIT HYPOTHESIS

The induced fit hypothesis describes the active site of an enzyme as having some flexibility of shape. When the appropriate substrate comes in contact with the active site, the conformation of the active site changes such that it surrounds the substrate, creating a close fit (see Figure 2.2). A substrate of the wrong shape will not induce a conformational change in the enzyme's active site, thereby preventing the formation of an enzyme-substrate complex.

Studies suggest that the induced fit hypothesis is more plausible than the lock and key theory, and induced fit is currently more widely accepted.

Table 2.1. Activation Energy

1. LOWER the ACTIVATION ENERGY
2. INCREASE the RATE OF THE REACTION
3. DO NOT alter the equilibrium constant
4. ARE NOT CHANGED OR CONSUMED in the reaction. This means that they will appear in both the reactants and products.
5. Enzymes are pH and temperature sensitive, with optimal activity at specific pH ranges and temperatures.
6. DO NOT affect the overall ΔG of the reaction
7. Are SPECIFIC for a particular REACTION or CLASS of REACTIONS

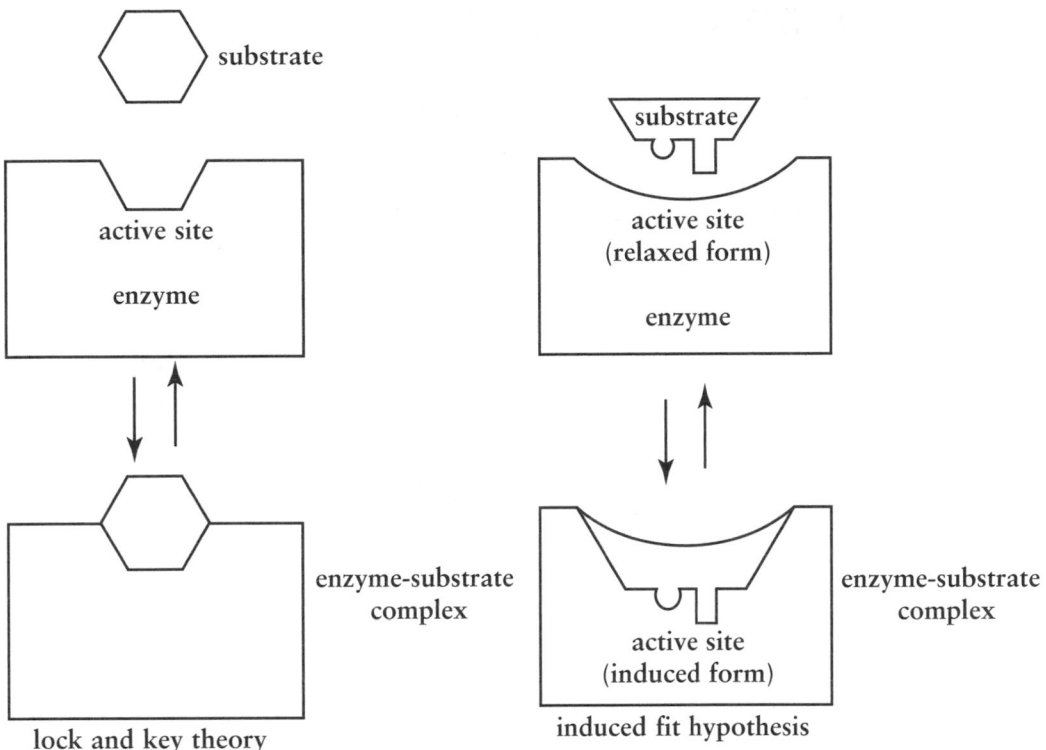

Figure 2.2. Models for Enzyme-Substrate Interactions

COFACTORS

Many enzymes require the incorporation of a nonprotein molecule to become catalytically active. These molecules, called **cofactors**, can aid in binding the substrate to the enzyme or in stabilizing the enzyme in an active conformation. An enzyme devoid of its necessary cofactor is called an **apoenzyme** and is catalytically inactive, while an enzyme containing its cofactor is called a **holoenzyme**. Cofactors can be bound to their enzymes by weak noncovalent interactions or by strong covalent bonds. Tightly bound cofactors are called **prosthetic groups**.

Two important types of cofactors are metal cations (e.g., Zn^{2+}, Fe^{2+}) and small organic groups (e.g., biotin). These latter organic cofactors are called **coenzymes**. Most coenzymes cannot be synthesized by the body and are obtained from the diet as vitamin derivatives. Lack of a particular vitamin can impair the action of its corresponding enzyme and lead to disease.

Clinical Correlate

Deficiencies in vitamin cofactors can result in devastating disease. Thiamin is an important cofactor for several enzymes involved in cellular metabolism and nerve conduction. Thiamin deficiency, often seen in alcoholics, results in a disease known as Wernicke-Korsokoff syndrome. In this disorder, patients suffer from a variety of neurological deficits, including delirium, balance problems, and in severe cases, the inability to form new memories.

ENZYME KINETICS

The rate of an enzyme-catalyzed reaction is related to a number of factors, including the concentrations of both the enzyme and the substrate, and environmental variables such as temperature and pH.

A. EFFECTS OF CONCENTRATION

The concentrations of substrate [S] and enzyme [E] during the course of a reaction greatly affect the reaction rate. When the concentration of the substrate is low compared to that of the enzyme, many of the active sites are unoccupied and the reaction rate is low. Initial increases in the substrate concentration (at constant enzyme concentration) lead to proportional increases in the rate of the reaction because unoccupied active sites on the enzyme readily bind to the additional substrate. However, once most of the active sites are occupied, the reaction rate levels off, regardless of further increases in substrate concentration. At high concentrations of substrate, the reaction rate approaches its **maximal velocity**, **Vmax**. At this point, increases in substrate concentration will no longer increase reaction rate (see Figure 2.3.)

According to the Michaelis-Menten model proposed in 1913, an enzyme-substrate complex, ES, is formed at rate k_1 from enzyme E and substrate S. The ES complex can either dissociate into E and S at rate k_2, or form product P at rate k_3. The relationship between the three rates is defined by the **Michaelis constant**, **K_m**, as $\dfrac{(k_2 + k_3)}{k_1}$, or the ratio of the breakdown of the ES complex to its formation.

$$E + S \underset{k_2}{\overset{k_1}{\rightleftharpoons}} ES_{\frac{1}{2}} \overset{k_3}{\longrightarrow} E + P$$

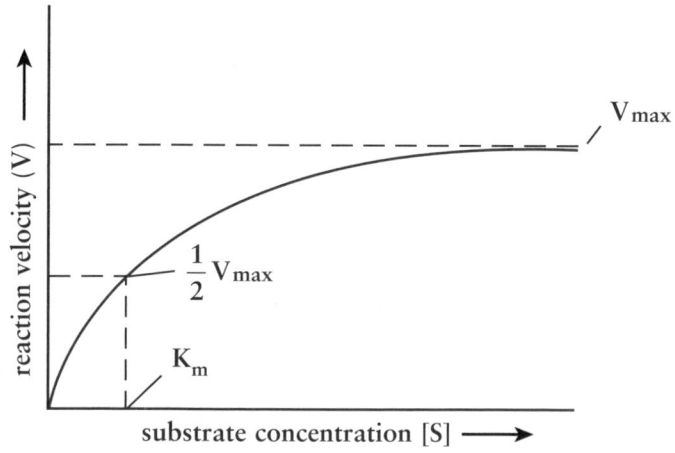

Figure 2.3. Michaelis-Menten Model

When the reaction rate is equal to $\frac{1}{2} V_{max}$, $K_m = [S]$ and can be understood as the point at which half of the enzyme's active sites are filled (see Figure 2.3). When [S] is less than K_m, changes in substrate concentration greatly affect the reaction rate. In contrast, at high concentrations of substrate, [S] is larger than K_m, and V approaches V_{max}.

B. EFFECTS OF TEMPERATURE

Rates of enzyme-catalyzed reactions tend to double for every 10°C increase in temperature until their optimal temperature is reached. For most enzymes operating in the human body, the optimal temperature is 37°C. At higher temperatures, enzymes become denatured: their 3-D structure is destroyed and the enzyme becomes nonfunctional. Enzymes that are partially denatured can sometimes regain their activity upon being cooled (see Figure 2.4).

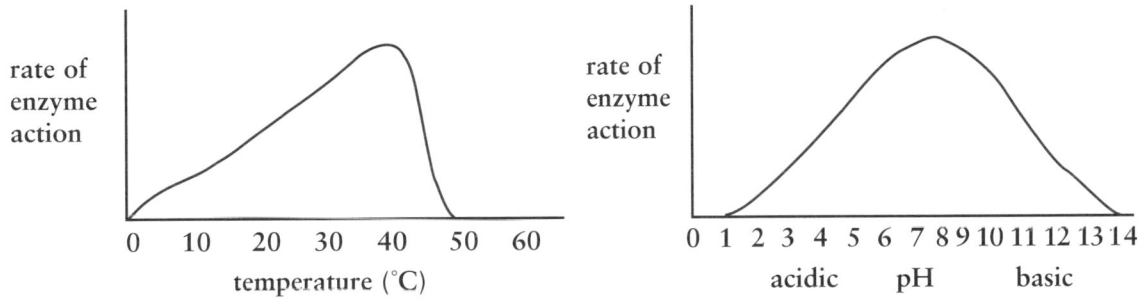

Figure 2.4. Effects of Temperature and pH on Enzyme Activity

C. EFFECTS OF pH

For each enzyme there is also an optimal pH above and below which enzymatic activity declines. Maximal activity of many human enzymes occurs around pH 7.4 (7.35–7.45), which is the pH of most body fluids and tissues. Plueral fluid is an exception and has a standard pH closer to 7.6. The other exceptions include pepsin, which works best in the highly acidic conditions of the stomach (pH = 2), and pancreatic enzymes, which work optimally in the alkaline conditions of the small intestine (pH = 8.5).

REGULATION OF ENZYMATIC ACTIVITY

The regulation of enzymatic activity is accomplished in a number of ways, most notably through allosteric effects and inhibitory interactions.

A. ALLOSTERIC EFFECTS

An **allosteric enzyme** has at least one active or catalytic site and at least one separate regulatory site. Often, these enzymes possess a quarternary structure. An allosteric enzyme oscillates between two configurations—an active state capable of catalyzing a reaction, and an inactive state that cannot. An interaction between an allosteric enzyme and a **regulator** (a molecule other than the substrate that binds to the enzyme) can stabilize either configuration, depending on the type of regulator involved. There are two types of regulators—**allosteric inhibitors** and **allosteric activators**. An inhibitor prevents an enzyme from binding to its substrate by stabilizing the inactive conformation, whereas an activator stabilizes the active configuration, promoting the formation of enzyme-substrate complexes.

Another allosteric effect involves increased affinity of an enzyme for its substrate. Sometimes the binding of a regulator at the allosteric site, or the binding of substrate at one of the enzyme's active sites, may stimulate the other active sites on the enzyme to bind more efficiently by increasing their affinity for the substrate. This type of cooperation is not unique to allosteric enzymes. Hemoglobin is composed of four subunits, each with its own oxygen-binding site; the binding of oxygen at one subunit increases the affinity for oxygen at the remaining three active sites (see chapter 9).

B. INHIBITION

An enzyme's activity may be regulated by one of the products of the reactions it catalyzes, or by a substance that binds to the enzyme and inhibits it from binding substrate. These interferences with enzymatic activity can be categorized as **feedback inhibition**, **competitive inhibition**, and **noncompetitive inhibition**.

1. Feedback Inhibition

Many biological reactions are regulated by feedback inhibition mechanisms, in which the end product of a sequence of enzymatic reactions becomes an allosteric modulator (in this case, an inhibitor) of one of the preceding enzymes in the sequence. In the following reaction sequence (Figure 2.5), product D is an inhibitory modulator for enzyme 1. Thus, when the concentration of D reaches some critical level, virtually all enzyme 1 molecules are inhibited and production of B (and thus of C and D) is halted. The process is sometimes reversible and can be instantaneous; as D levels decrease, enzyme 1 inhibition decreases, and A is again converted to B. This feedback process allows organisms to avoid overproduction of metabolites. (For an additional discussion of feedback inhibition see chapter 11.)

2. Competitive Inhibitors

Competitive inhibitors compete with the substrate directly by binding to the active site of the enzyme. The active site of an enzyme is

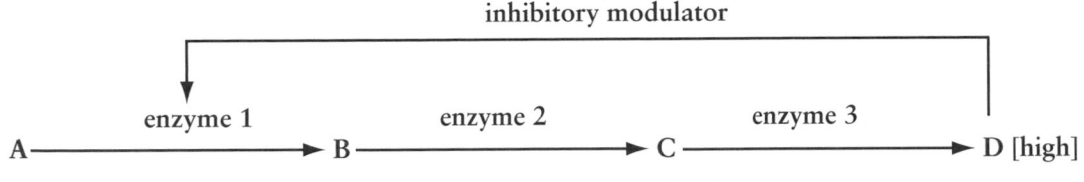

Figure 2.5. Negative Feedback

specific for a particular substrate or class of substrates. However, it is possible for molecules that are structurally similar to the substrate to bind to the active site of the enzyme. If this similar molecule is present in a concentration comparable to the concentration of the substrate, it will compete with the substrate for bonding sites on the enzyme and it will interfere with enzyme activity. This is known as competitive inhibition because the enzyme is inhibited by the inactive substrate, or competitor, so called because it *competes* with the substrate for the active site. Competitive inhibition is reversible with increased concentrations of substrate.

3. **Noncompetitive Inhibitors**

   A noncompetitive inhibitor is a substance that forms strong covalent bonds with an enzyme and consequently may not be displaced by the addition of excess substrate. Therefore, noncompetitive inhibition is irreversible. A noncompetitive inhibitor may be bonded at, near, or remote from the active site. This is an example of allosteric inhibition. Non-competitive inhibition can be overcome by increasing the concentration of the enzyme.

INACTIVE ENZYMES

A **zymogen** is an enzyme that is secreted in an inactive form. The zymogen is cleaved under certain physiological conditions to the active form of the enzyme. Important examples of zymogens include pepsinogen, trypsinogen, and chymotrypsinogen, which are cleaved in the digestive tract to yield the active enzymes pepsin, trypsin, and chymotrypsin, respectively (see chapter 7).

Clinical Correlate

The concept of competitive inhibition has relevance in the clinical setting. For example, methanol (wood alcohol), if ingested, is enzymatically converted to toxic metabolites that can cause blindness and even death. Administration of intravenous ethanol is the treatment of choice for a patient suffering from methanol poisoning. Ethanol works by competing with methanol for the active sites of the enzymes involved.

3

CELLULAR METABOLISM

Cellular metabolism is the sum total of all chemical reactions that take place in a cell. These reactions can be generally categorized as either **anabolic** or **catabolic**. Anabolic processes are energy-requiring, involving the biosynthesis of complex organic compounds from simpler molecules. Catabolic processes release energy as they break down complex organic compounds into smaller molecules. The metabolic reactions of cells are coupled so that energy released from catabolic reactions can be harnessed to fuel anabolic reactions.

TRANSFER OF ENERGY

A. THE FLOW OF ENERGY

The ultimate energy source for living organisms is the sun. **Autotrophic** organisms, such as green plants, convert sunlight into **bond energy** stored in the bonds of organic compounds (chiefly glucose) in the anabolic process of **photosynthesis**. Autotrophs do not need an exogenous supply of organic compounds. **Heterotrophic** organisms obtain their energy catabolically, via the breakdown of organic nutrients that must be ingested. Figure 3.1 is an energy flow diagram for biological systems; note that some energy is dissipated as heat at every stage.

Glucose plays an essential role in the energetics of cell metabolism. The production of glucose ($C_6H_{12}O_6$) by autotrophs involves the breaking of C–O and O–H bonds in CO_2 and H_2O, and the forming of C–H, C–O, C–C, and O–H bonds in glucose. The net reaction of photosynthesis:

$$6CO_2 + 6H_2O + Energy \longrightarrow C_6H_{12}O_6 + 6O_2$$
$$\text{glucose}$$

Heterotrophic organisms metabolize glucose and other organic molecules to release the stored bond energies. The net reaction of glucose catabolism, which is essentially the reversal of photosynthesis, is:

$$C_6H_{12}O_6 + 6O_2 \longrightarrow 6CO_2 + 6H_2O + \text{Energy}$$
glucose

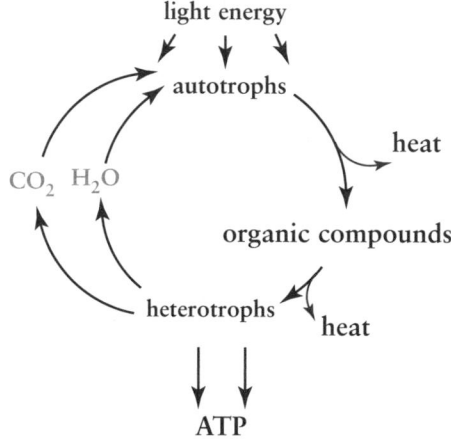

Figure 3.1. Energy Flow in Biological Systems

B. ENERGY CARRIERS

During metabolism, the cell uses various molecular carriers, such as **ATP** and the coenzymes **NAD⁺**, **NADP⁺**, and **FAD**, to shuttle energy between reactions.

1. ATP

ATP, or **adenosine triphosphate**, is the cell's main energy currency. Through its formation and degradation, cells have a quick way of releasing and storing energy. ATP is synthesized during glucose catabolism. ATP is composed of the nitrogenous base adenine, the sugar ribose, and three weakly linked phosphate groups. The energy of ATP is stored in the covalent bonds attaching these phosphate groups, often referred to as high-energy bonds.

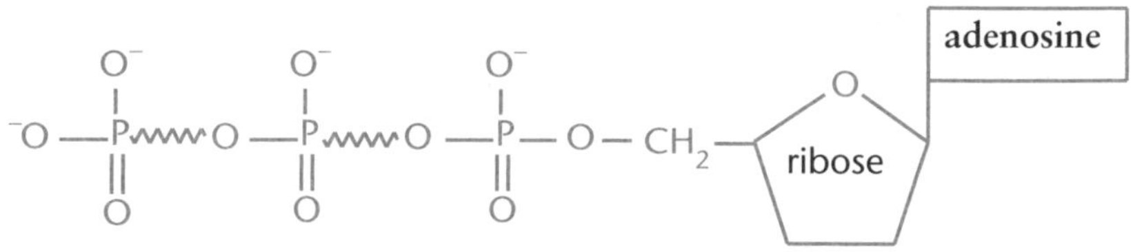

Figure 3.2. ATP

Hydrolysis of ATP to **ADP (adenosine diphosphate)** and P_i (**inorganic phosphate**) releases stored bond energy that the cell can use in metabolic processes. Approximately 7 kcal of energy are released per mole of ATP. This provides energy for **endergonic** (endothermic) reactions such as muscle contraction, motility, and the active transport of substances across plasma membranes. ATP may also be hydrolyzed into **AMP (adenosine monophosphate)** and PP_i (**pyrophosphate**):

$$ATP \longrightarrow ADP + P_i + 7 \text{ kcal/mole}$$

$$ATP \longrightarrow AMP + PP_i + 7 \text{ kcal/mole}$$

Alternatively, ADP and P_i combine to form ATP; in this way the cell regenerates its ATP supply. This process requires energy (supplied by the degradation of glucose):

$$ADP + P_i + 7 \text{ kcal/mole} \longrightarrow ATP$$

2. **NAD^+, $NADP^+$, and FAD**

A second mechanism by which the cell stores chemical energy is in the form of **high potential electrons**. Electrons are transferred as **hydride ions ($H:^-$)** or as pairs of hydrogen atoms. During glucose oxidation, hydrogen atoms are removed. Most of these are accepted by the carrier coenzymes **NAD^+ (nicotinamide adenine dinucleotide)**, **FAD (flavin adenine dinucleotide)**, and **$NADP^+$ (nicotinamide adenine dinucleotide phosphate)**. These molecules transport the high-energy electrons of the hydrogen atoms to a series of carrier molecules on the inner mitochondrical membrane that are collectively known as the **electron transport chain**.

Oxidation refers to the loss of an electron. NAD^+, $NADP^+$, and FAD are referred to as oxidizing agents because they cause other molecules to lose electrons and undergo oxidation. In the process, they themselves undergo **reduction**; that is, they gain electrons. For example, when NAD^+ accepts electrons in the form of a hydride ion it is reduced to **NADH**, while the donating molecule is oxidized. Likewise, when FAD accepts electrons in the form of hydrogen atoms, it is reduced to **$FADH_2$**. In their reduced forms, NADH, NADPH, and $FADH_2$ all behave as reducing agents. NADH transfers its electrons to another electron acceptor (e.g., the first carrier of the electron transport chain), thereby reducing it, and in the process NADH is oxidized back to NAD^+. NADPH is found in plant, not animal, cells. Thus, these coenzymes temporarily store and release energy in the form of electrons through their successive oxidations and reductions.

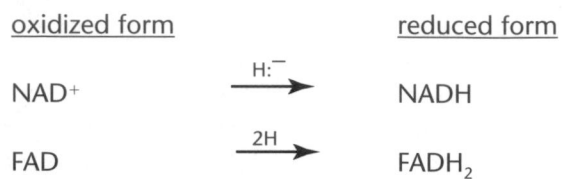

Figure 3.3. Reduction of NAD$^+$ and FAD

Bridge

Refer to chapter 14 in the Organic Chemistry notes for more on the structure of glucose and other carbohydrates.

GLUCOSE CATABOLISM

The degradative oxidation of glucose occurs in two stages, **glycolysis** and **cellular respiration**.

A. GLYCOLYSIS

The first stage of glucose catabolism is glycolysis. Glycolysis is a series of reactions that lead to the oxidative breakdown of glucose into two molecules of **pyruvate** (the ionized form of pyruvic acid), the production of ATP, and the reduction of NAD$^+$ into NADH. All of these reactions occur in the cytoplasm and are mediated by specific enzymes. The glycolytic pathway is outlined below in Figure 3.4.

Test Tip

You do *not* need to memorize the individual reactions of glycolysis for the MCAT. You will need to memorize them in medical school.

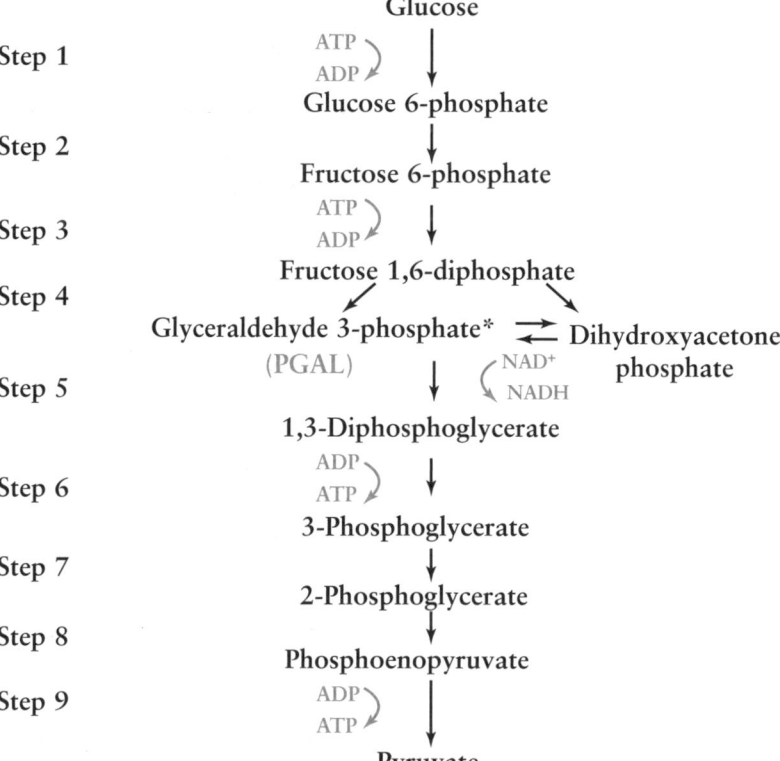

*NOTE: Steps 5–9 occur twice per molecule of glucose (see text).

Figure 3.4. Glycolysis

1. **Glycolytic Pathway**

   Note that at step 4, fructose 1,6-diphosphate is split into 2 three-carbon molecules: **dihydroxyacetone phosphate** and **glyceraldehyde 3-phosphate (PGAL)**. Dihydroxyacetone phosphate is isomerized into PGAL so that it can be used in subsequent reactions. Thus, 2 molecules of PGAL are formed per molecule of glucose, and all of the subsequent steps occur twice for each glucose molecule.

   From one molecule of glucose (a six-carbon molecule), 2 molecules of pyruvate (a three-carbon molecule) are obtained. During this sequence of reactions, 2 ATP are used (in steps 1 and 3) and 4 ATP are generated (2 in step 6, and 2 in step 9). Thus, there is a net production of 2 ATP per glucose molecule. This type of phosphorylation is called **substrate level phosphorylation**, since ATP synthesis is directly coupled with the degradation of glucose without the participation of an intermediate molecule such as NAD^+. One NADH is produced per PGAL, for a total of 2 NADH per glucose.

   The net reaction for glycolysis is:

   $$Glucose + 2ADP + 2P_i + 2NAD^+ \longrightarrow$$
   $$2Pyruvate + 2ATP + 2NADH + 2H^+ + 2H_2O$$

   This series of reactions occurs in both prokaryotic and eukaryotic cells. However, at this stage, much of the initial energy stored in the glucose molecule has not been released and is still present in the chemical bonds of pyruvate. Depending on the capabilities of the organism, pyruvate degradation can proceed in one of two directions. Under **anaerobic** conditions (in the absence of oxygen), pyruvate is reduced during the process of fermentation. Under **aerobic** conditions (in the presence of oxygen), pyruvate is further oxidized during cell respiration in the mitochondria.

B. CELLULAR RESPIRATION—ANAEROBIC

Cellular respiration can be described as aerobic or anaerobic.

2. **Fermentation**

   NAD^+ must be regenerated for glycolysis to continue in the absence of O_2. This is accomplished by reducing pyruvate into **ethanol** or **lactic acid**. Fermentation refers to all of the reactions involved in this process—glycolysis and the additional steps leading to the formation of ethanol or lactic acid. Fermentation produces only 2 ATP per glucose molecule.

> **Bridge**
>
> The conversion of acetaldehyde to ethanol is a typical reduction reaction of an aldehyde to an alcohol. See chapter 8 of the Organic Chemistry notes for more on this type of reaction.

a. Alcohol fermentation

Alcohol fermentation commonly occurs only in yeast and some bacteria. The pyruvate produced in glycolysis is decarboxylated to become acetaldehyde, which is then reduced by the NADH generated in step 5 of glycolysis to yield ethanol.

In this way, NAD$^+$ is regenerated and glycolysis can continue.

$$\text{Pyruvate (3C)} \xrightarrow{\quad\quad} \text{Acetaldhyde (2C)} \xrightarrow{\quad\quad} \text{Ethanol (2C)}$$

CO$_2$

NADH + H$^+$ NAD$^+$

b. Lactic acid fermentation

Lactic acid fermentation occurs in certain fungi and bacteria and in human muscle cells during strenuous activity. When the oxygen supply to muscle cells lags behind the rate of glucose catabolism, the pyruvate generated is reduced to lactic acid. As in alcohol fermentation, the NAD$^+$ used in step 5 of glycolysis is regenerated when pyruvate is reduced. In humans, lactic acid may accumulate in the muscles during exercise, causing a decrease in blood pH that leads to muscle fatigue. Once the oxygen supply has been replenished, the lactic acid is oxidized back to pyruvate and enters cellular respiration. The amount of oxygen needed for this conversion is known as **oxygen debt**.

$$\text{Pyruvate (3C)} \xrightarrow{\quad\quad} \text{Lactic acid (3C)}$$

NADH + H$^+$ NAD$^+$

C. CELLULAR RESPIRATION—ANAEROBIC

Cellular respiration is the most efficient catabolic pathway used by organisms to harvest the energy stored in glucose. Whereas glycolysis yields only 2 ATP per molecule of glucose, cellular respiration can yield 36–38 ATP. Cellular respiration is an aerobic process; oxygen acts as the final acceptor of electrons that are passed from carrier to carrier during the final stage of glucose oxidation. The metabolic reactions of cell respiration occur in the eukaryotic mitochondrion and are catalyzed by reaction-specific enzymes. Cellular respiration can be divided into three stages: **pyruvate decarboxylation**, the **citric acid cycle**, and the **electron transport chain**.

1. Pyruvate Decarboxylation

The pyruvate formed during glycolysis is transported from the cytoplasm into the mitochondrial matrix where it is decarboxylated; i.e., it loses a CO$_2$, and the acetyl group that remains is transferred to coenzyme A to form **acetyl CoA**. In the process, NAD$^+$ is reduced to NADH.

$$\text{NAD}^+ \qquad \text{NADH} + \text{H}^+$$

Pyruvate (3 C) + Coenzyme A $\longrightarrow$ Acetyl CoA (2C)

2. Citric Acid Cycle

The citric acid cycle is also known as the **Krebs cycle** or the **tricarboxylic acid cycle (TCA cycle)**. The cycle begins when the two-carbon acetyl group from acetyl CoA combines with **oxaloacetate**, a four-carbon molecule, to form the six-carbon **citrate**. Through a complicated series of reactions, 2 CO_2 are released, and oxaloacetate is regenerated for use in another turn of the cycle (Figure 3.5).

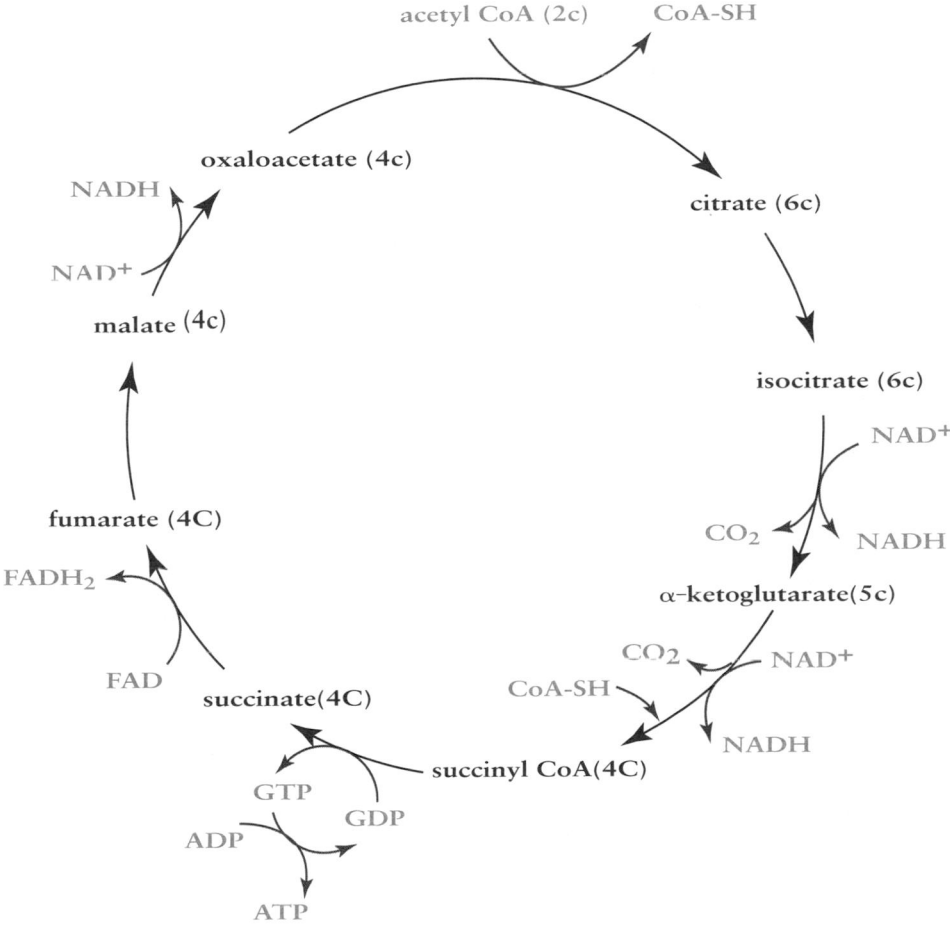

Figure 3.5. Citric Acid Cycle

For each turn of the citric acid cycle 1 ATP is produced by substrate level phosphorylation via a GTP intermediate. In addition, electrons are transferred to NAD^+ and FAD, generating NADH and $FADH_2$, respectively. These coenzymes then transport the electrons to the electron transport chain, where more ATP is produced via **oxidative phosphorylation**. Studying the cycle, we can do some bookkeeping; keep in mind that for each molecule of glucose, 2 pyruvates are decarboxylated and channeled into the citric acid cycle.

$$2 \times 3 \text{ NADH} \longrightarrow 6 \text{ NADH}$$
$$2 \times 1 \text{ FADH}_2 \longrightarrow 2 \text{ FADH}_2$$
$$2 \times 1 \text{ GTP (ATP)} \longrightarrow 2 \text{ ATP}$$

The net reaction of the citric acid cycle per glucose molecule is:

$$2\text{Acetyl CoA} + 6NAD^+ + 2FAD + 2ATP + 2P_i + 4H_2O \longrightarrow$$
$$4CO_2 + 6NADH + 2FADH_2 + 2ATP + 4H^+ + 2CoA$$

> ## MCAT Synopsis
>
> Energy checkpoint:
>
> | | |
> |---|---|
> | 2ATP | (from glycolysis) |
> | 2NADH | (from glycolysis) |
> | 2NADH | (from decarboxylation of pyruvate) |
> | 6NADH | (TCA cycle) |
> | 2FADH$_2$ | (TCA cycle) |
> | 2ATP | (TCA cycle) |

3. **Electron Transport Chain**
   a. **Electron transfer**

   The electron transport chain (**ETC**) is a complex carrier mechanism located on the inside of the inner mitochondrial membrane. During oxidative phosphorylation, ATP is produced when high energy potential electrons are transferred from NADH and $FADH_2$ to oxygen by a series of carrier molecules located in the inner mitochondrial membrane. As the electrons are transferred from carrier to carrier, free energy is released, which is then used to form ATP. Most of the molecules of the ETC are **cytochromes**, electron carriers that resemble hemoglobin in the structure of their active site. The functional unit contains a central iron atom, which is capable of undergoing a reversible redox reaction; that is, it can be alternatively reduced and oxidized.

   FMN (flavin mononucleotide) is the first molecule of the ETC. It is reduced when it accepts electrons from NADH, thereby oxidizing NADH to NAD^+. Sequential redox reactions continue to occur as the electrons are transferred from one carrier to the next; each carrier is reduced as it accepts an electron and is then oxidized when it passes it on to the next carrier.

   The last carrier of the ETC, **cytochrome a_3**, passes its electron to the final electron acceptor, O_2. In addition to the electrons, O_2 picks up a pair of hydrogen ions from the surrounding medium, forming water.

$$2H^+ + 2e^- + \frac{1}{2}O_2 \longrightarrow H_2O$$

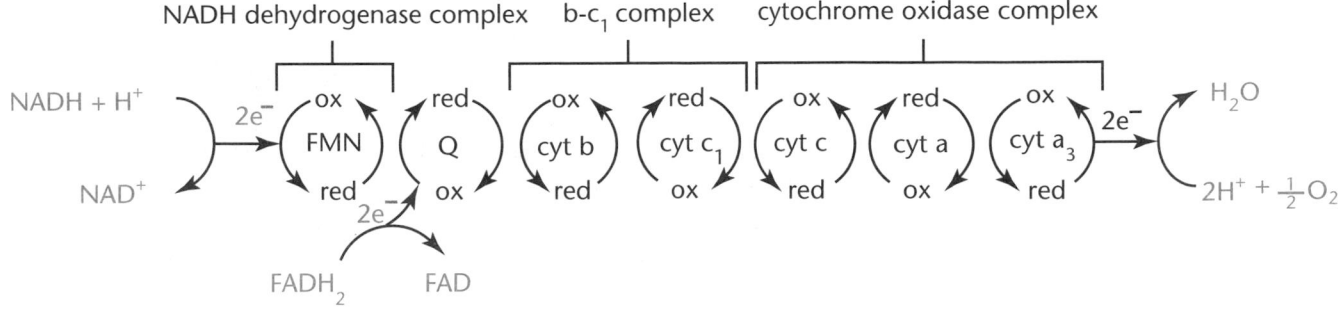

Figure 3.6. Electron Transport Chain

Without oxygen, the ETC becomes backlogged with electrons. As a result, NAD^+ cannot be regenerated and glycolysis cannot continue unless lactic acid fermentation occurs. Likewise, ATP synthesis comes to a halt if respiratory poisons such as **cyanide** or **dinitrophenol** enter the cell. Cyanide blocks the transfer of electrons from cytochrome a_3 to O_2. Dinitrophenol uncouples the electron transport chain from the proton gradient established across the inner mitochondrial membrane.

b. ATP generation and the proton pump

The electron carriers are categorized into three large protein complexes: **NADH dehydrogenase**, the **b-c_1 complex**, and **cytochrome oxidase**. There are energy losses as the electrons are transferred from one complex to the next; this energy is then used to synthesize 1 ATP per complex. Thus, an electron passing through the entire ETC supplies enough energy to generate 3 ATP. NADH delivers its electrons to NADH dehydrogenase complex, so that for each NADH, 3 ATP are produced. However, $FADH_2$ bypasses the NADH dehydrogenase complex and delivers its electrons directly to **carrier Q (ubiquinone)**, which lies between the NADH dehydrogenase and b-c_1 complexes. Therefore, for each $FADH_2$, there are only two energy drops, and only 2 ATP are produced.

The operating mechanism in this type of ATP production involves coupling the oxidation of NADH to the phosphorylation of ADP. The coupling agent for these two processes is a **proton gradient** across the inner mitochondrial membrane, maintained by the ETC. As NADH passes its electrons to the ETC, free hydrogen ions (H^+) are released and accumulate in the mitochondrial matrix. The ETC pumps these ions out of the matrix, across the inner mitochondrial membrane, and into the intermembrane space at each of the three protein complexes. The continuous translocation of H^+ creates a positively charged acidic environment in the intermembrane space. This electrochemical gradient generates a

proton-motive force, which drives H$^+$ back across the inner membrane and into the matrix. However, to pass through the membrane (which is impermeable to ions), the H$^+$ must flow through specialized channels provided by enzyme complexes called **ATP synthetases**. As the H$^+$ pass through the ATP synthetases, enough energy is released to allow for the phosphorylation of ADP to ATP. The coupling of the oxidation of NADH with the phosphorylation of ADP is called **oxidative phosphorylation.**

C. REVIEW OF GLUCOSE CATABOLISM

It is important to understand how all of the events described above are interrelated. Figure 3.7 is a eukaryotic cell with a mitochondrion magnified for detail.

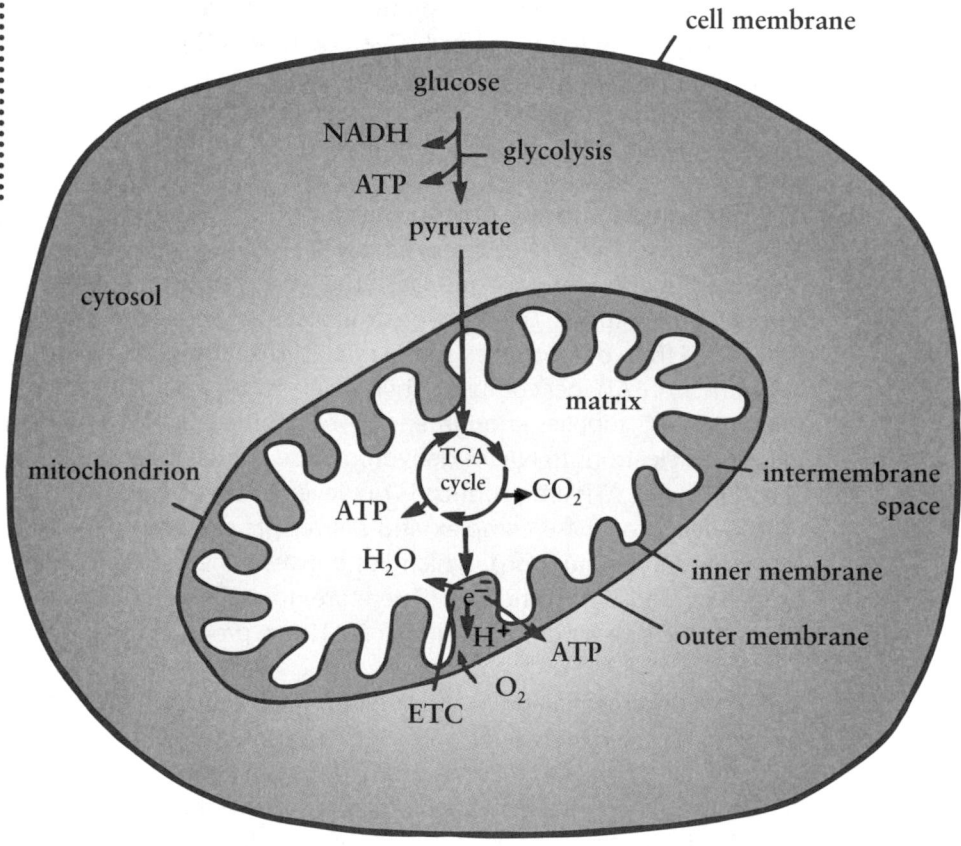

Figure 3.7. Schematic of Glucose Catabolism

To calculate the net amount of ATP produced per molecule of glucose we need to tally the number of ATP produced by substrate level phosphorylation and the number of ATP produced by oxidative phosphorylation.

1. **Substrate Level Phosphorylation**
   Degradation of one glucose molecule yields a net of 2 ATP from glycolysis and 1 ATP for each turn of the citric acid cycle. Thus, a total
   of 4 ATP are produced by substrate level phosphorylation.

2. **Oxidative Phosphorylation**
   Two pyruvate decarboxylations yield 1 NADH each for a total of 2
   NADH. Each turn of the citric acid cycle yields 3 NADH and 1 $FADH_2$,
   for a total of 6 NADH and 2 $FADH_2$ per glucose molecule. Each $FADH_2$
   generates 2 ATP, as previously discussed. Each NADH generates 3 ATP
   except for the 2 NADH that were reduced during glycolysis; these
   NADH cannot cross the inner mitochondrial membrane and must
   transfer their electrons to an intermediate carrier molecule, which
   delivers the electrons to the second carrier protein complex, Q.
   Therefore, these NADH generate only 2 ATP per glucose. So the 2
   NADH of glycolysis yield 4 ATP, the other 8 NADH yield 24 ATP, and
   the 2 $FADH_2$ produce 4 ATP, for a total of 32 ATP by oxidative phosphorylation.

   The total amount of ATP produced during eukaryotic glucose catabolism is therefore 4 via substrate level phosphorylation plus 32 via
   oxidative phosphorylation, for a total of 36 ATP. (For prokaryotes the
   yield is 38 ATP, because the 2 NADH of glycolysis don't have any
   mitochondrial membranes to cross and therefore don't lose energy.)
   See Table 3.1 for a summary of eukaryotic ATP production.

> **MCAT Synopsis**
>
> In an ANAEROBIC environment, eukaryotic cells can generate only 2 net ATP; in an AEROBIC environment, these cells can generate a net of 36 ATP!

Table 3.1. Eukaryotic ATP Production per Glucose Molecule

Glycolysis		
2 ATP invested (steps 1 and 3)	− 2	ATP
4 ATP generated (steps 6 and 9)	+ 4	ATP (substrate)
2 NADH × 2 ATP/NADH (step 5)	+ 4	ATP (oxidative)
Pyruvate Decarboxylation		
2 NADH × 3 ATP/NADH	+ 6	ATP (oxidative)
Citric Acid Cycle		
6 NADH × 3 ATP/NADH	+18	ATP (oxidative)
2 $FADH_2$ × 2 ATP/$FADH_2$	+ 4	ATP (oxidative)
2 GTP × 1 ATP/GTP	+ 2	ATP (substrate)
Total	**+36**	**ATP**

ALTERNATE ENERGY SOURCES

When glucose supplies run low, the body uses other energy sources. These sources are used by the body in the following preferential order: other carbohydrates, fats, and proteins. These substances are first converted to either glucose or glucose intermediates, which can then be degraded in the glycolytic pathway and TCA cycle.

A. CARBOHYDRATES

Disaccharides are hydrolyzed into monosaccharides, most of which can be converted into glucose or glycolytic intermediates. Glycogen stored in the liver can be converted, when needed, into glucose 6-phosphate, a glycolytic intermediate.

B. FATS

Fat molecules are stored in adipose tissue in the form of triglyceride. When needed, they are hydrolyzed by lipases to fatty acids and glycerol, and are carried by the blood to other tissues for oxidation. Glycerol can be converted into PGAL, a glycolytic intermediate. A fatty acid must first be "activated" in the cytoplasm; this process requires 2 ATP. Once activated, the fatty acid is transported into the mitochondrion and taken through a series of **beta-oxidation cycles** that convert it into two-carbon fragments, which are then converted into acetyl CoA. Acetyl CoA then enters the TCA cycle. With each round of β-oxidation of a saturated fatty acid, 1 NADH and 1 $FADH_2$ are generated.

Of all the high-energy compounds used in cellular respiration, fats yield the greatest number of ATP per gram. This makes them extremely efficient energy storage molecules. Thus, while the amount of glycogen stored in humans is enough to meet the short-term energy needs of about a day, the stored fat reserves can meet the long-term energy needs for about a month.

C. PROTEINS

The body degrades amino acids (the building blocks of proteins) only when there is not enough carbohydrate available. Most amino acids undergo a **transamination** reaction in which they lose an amino group to form an α-keto acid. The carbon atoms of most amino acids are converted into acetyl CoA, pyruvate, or one of the intermediates of the citric acid cycle. These intermediates enter their respective metabolic pathways, allowing cells to produce fatty acids, glucose, or energy in the form of ATP.

Clinical Correlate

Diabetic ketoacidosis (DKA) occurs when diabetics (primarily insulin dependent) fail to take their insulin. The blood glucose levels accumulate and the cells are, ironically, starved for glucose since there is no insulin. As a result, their bodies resort to the breakdown of fats, which produces β-ketoacids, eventually resulting in a coma, as they build up in the bloodstream.

METABOLIC MAP

Below is a diagram illustrating the relationship between fats, protein, and carbohydrate catabolism. Note where the products of fats and protein catabolism feed into the reactions of carbohydrate catabolism.

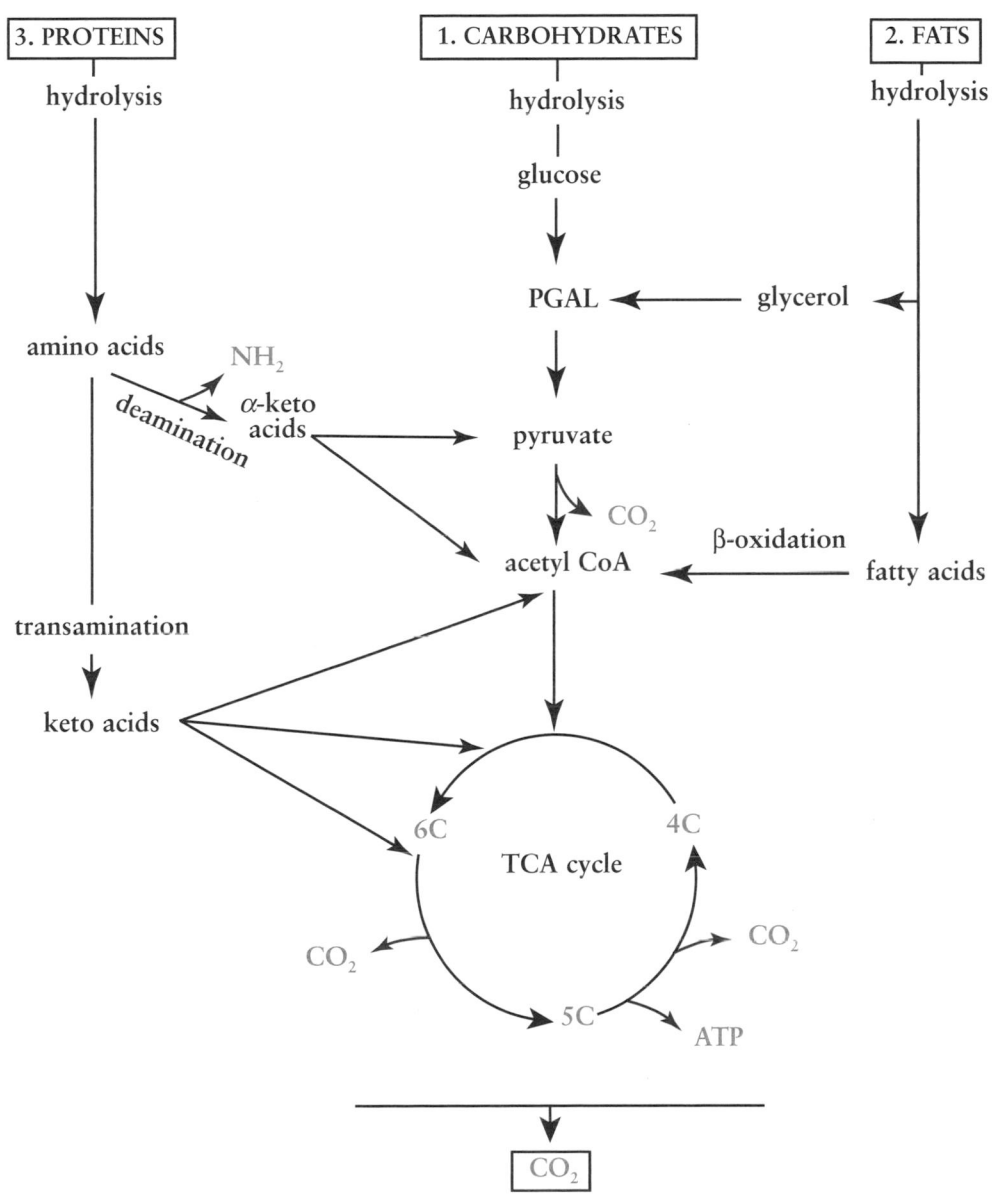

Figure 3.8. Nutrient Metabolism

4

REPRODUCTION

Reproduction is the process by which an organism perpetuates itself and its species, ensuring the precise duplication of genetic material and its representation in successive generations. Reproduction can be divided into three topics: **cell division, asexual reproduction**, and **sexual reproduction**.

CELL DIVISION

Cell division is the process by which a cell doubles its organelles and cytoplasm, replicates its DNA, and then divides in two. For unicellular organisms, cell division is a means of reproduction, while for multicellular organisms it is a method of growth, development, and replacement of worn-out cells. Prokaryotes and eukaryotes differ in their means of cell division.

Prokaryotes divide by a process called **binary fission** (a type of asexual reproduction). The single DNA molecule attaches to the plasma membrane during replication and duplicates, while the cell continues to grow in size. The cell membrane pinches inward, splitting the cell into two equal halves, with each daughter cell receiving a complete copy of the original chromosome.

Eukaryotic cell division is more complicated than binary fission because cells must duplicate and equally distribute chromosomes, organelles, and cytoplasm to both daughter cells. Eukaryotic **somatic**, or **autosomal**, cells contain the diploid number of chromosomes characteristic of its species, which is designated as **2N** (**N** is the number of chromosomes found in a **haploid** cell, or **gamete**). The diploid number for humans is 46, and the haploid number is 23; 23 chromosomes are inherited from each parent.

The life cycle of a eukaryotic cell can be broken down into four distinct stages collectively known as the **cell cycle.**

A. THE CELL CYCLE

The four stages of the cell cycle are designated as **G₁**, **S**, **G₂**, and **M**. The first three stages of the cell cycle are **interphase** stages, that is, they occur between cell divisions. The fourth stage, **mitosis**, includes the actual cell division.

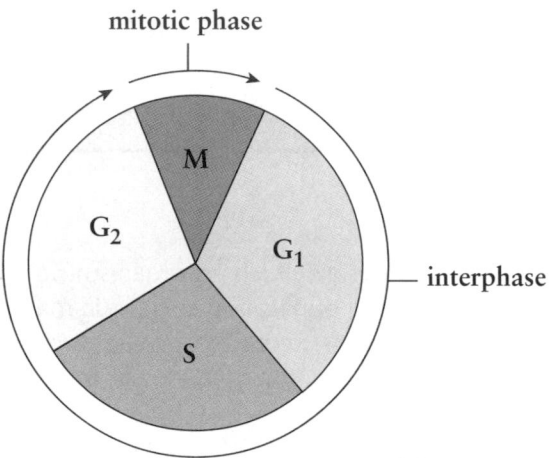

Figure 4.1. The Cell Cycle

1. **Interphase**
    This is by far the longest part of the cell cycle. A cell normally spends at least 90 percent of the cycle in interphase.

    a. **G₁ stage (presynthetic gap)**
        This stage is one of intense biochemical activity and growth. The cell doubles in size and new organelles such as mitochondria, ribosomes, endoplasmic reticulum, and centrioles are produced. A typical cell proceeds through the G₁ stage, passing a **restriction point**, after which it is committed to continue through the rest of the cell cycle and divide. However, some cells, including specialized skeletal muscle cells and nerve cells, never pass this point, instead entering a nondividing phase sometimes referred to as **G₀**.

    b. **S stage (synthesis)**
        In the synthetic stage each chromosome is replicated so that during division, a complete copy of the genome can be distributed to both daughter cells. After replication, the chromosomes, consist of two identical **sister chromatids** held together at a central region called the **centromere**. The ends of the chromosome are called the **telomeres**. Note that after DNA replication, the cell still contains the diploid number (2N) of chromosomes, but since each chromosome now consists of two chromatids, cells entering G₂ actually contain twice as much DNA as cells in G₁.

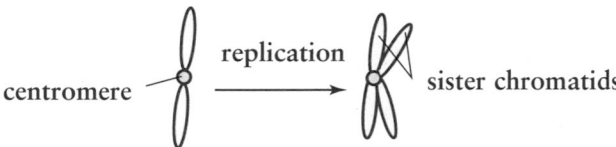

Figure 4.2. Chromosome Replication

c.   **G$_2$ stage (postsynthetic gap)**
The cell continues to grow in size, while assembly of new organelles and other cell structures continues.

2.   **M Stage (Mitotic Stage)**
This stage consists of mitosis and **cytokinesis.** Mitosis is the division and distribution of the cell's DNA to its two daughter cells such that each cell receives a complete copy of the original genome. Cytokinesis refers to the division of cytoplasm that follows.

a.   **Mitosis**
During interphase, the nucleus is membrane-bound and clearly visible, and one or more nucleoli may be observed. Individual chromosomes are not visible under a light microscope because they are active and uncoiled. The DNA appears granular and is called **chromatin.** As mitosis begins, the chromosomes coil up, condense, and become visible under high-power microscopy. This coiling facilitates their movement during the later stages of mitosis.

Chromosome movement is dependent on certain cytoplasmic organelles. The centrioles, which are typically found in pairs, are cylindrical organelles located outside of the interphase nucleus in an area referred to as the **centrosome.** During the first stage of mitosis, the centrioles, which have already replicated, migrate to opposite poles of the cell, and a system of **spindle fibers** composed of microtubules and associated proteins appears near each pair of centrioles. The spindle fibers radiate outward from the centrioles, forming structures called **asters.** The asters extend toward the center of the nucleus, forming the **spindle apparatus.** The movement of chromosomes toward opposite poles of the cell during the later stages of mitosis is caused by the shortening of the spindle apparatus.

Although mitosis is a continuous process, four stages are discernible: **prophase**, **metaphase**, **anaphase**, and **telophase**.

- **Prophase**

  The chromosomes condense, the centriole pairs separate and move toward opposite poles of the cell, and the spindle apparatus forms between them. The nuclear membrane dissolves, allowing spindle fibers to enter the nucleus, while the nucleoli become less distinct or disappear. **Kinetochores**, with attached **kinetochore fibers**, appear at the chromosome centromere.

- **Metaphase**

  The centriole pairs are now at opposite poles of the cell. The kinetochore fibers interact with the fibers of the spindle apparatus to align the chromosomes at the **metaphase plate** (equatorial plate), which is equidistant to the two poles of the spindle fibers.

- **Anaphase**

  The centromeres now split, so that each chromatid has its own distinct centromere, thus allowing the sister chromatids to separate. The telomeres are the last part of the chromatids to separate. The sister chromatids are pulled toward the opposite poles of the cell by the shortening of the kinetochore fibers.

- **Telophase**

  The spindle apparatus disappears. A nuclear membrane forms around each set of chromosomes and the nucleoli reappear. The chromosomes uncoil, resuming their interphase form. Each of the two new nuclei has received a complete copy of the genome identical to the original genome and to each other. Cytokinesis occurs.

  See Figure 4.3 for a summary of mitosis.

b. **Cytokinesis**

  Near the end of telophase, the cytoplasm divides into two daughter cells, each with a complete nucleus and its own set of organelles. In animal cells, a cleavage furrow forms; the cell membrane indents along the equator of the cell and finally pinches through the cell, separating the two nuclei.

  The life cycle of a cell is not an arbitrary series of events; cell division is a specified sequence of events dictated by the nucleus. For

---

KAPLAN) EXCLUSIVE

Mitosis = PMAT

Prophase:	chromosomes condense; spindles form
Metaphase:	chromosomes align
Anaphase:	sister chromatids separate
Telophase:	new nuclear membranes form

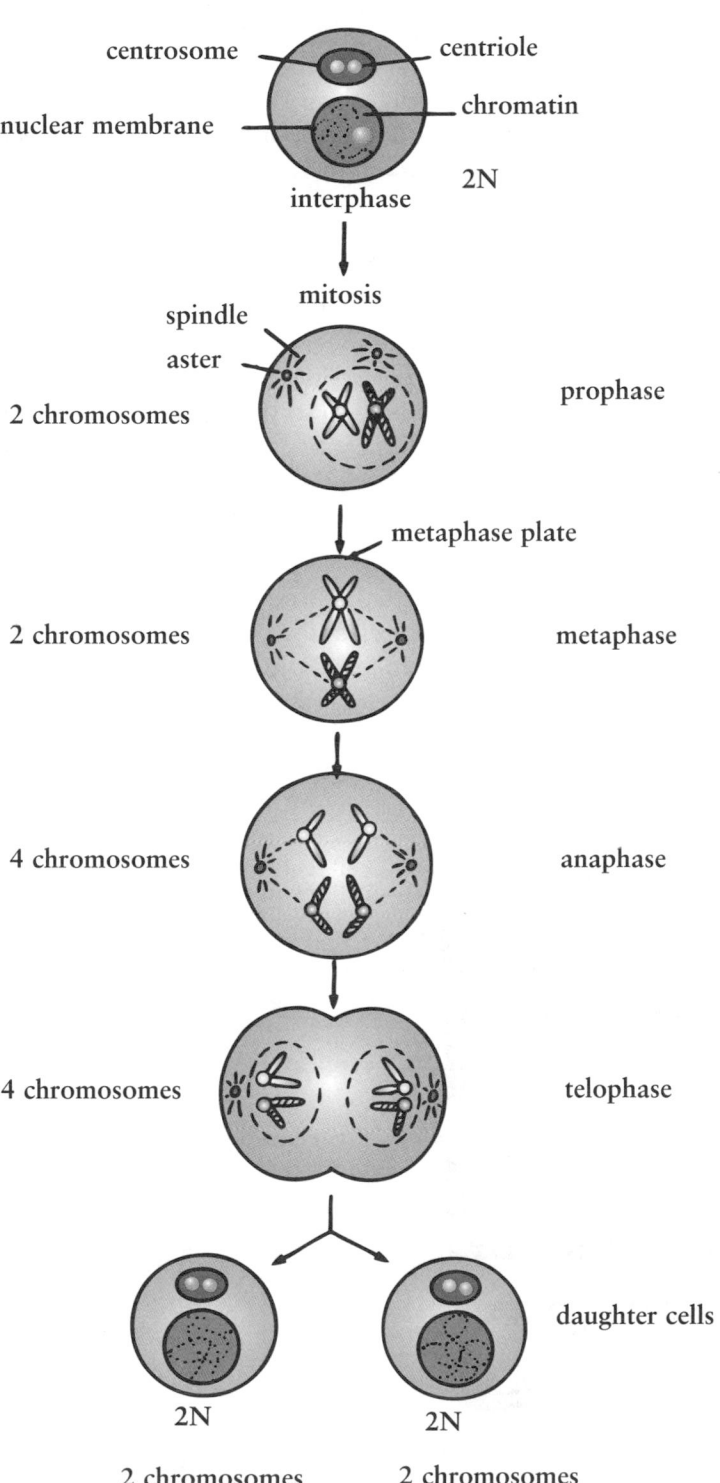

centrosome — centriole

nuclear membrane — chromatin

2N

interphase

mitosis

spindle
aster

2 chromosomes

prophase

metaphase plate

2 chromosomes

metaphase

4 chromosomes

anaphase

4 chromosomes

telophase

daughter cells

2N

2N

2 chromosomes   2 chromosomes

Figure 4.3. Mitosis

example, a typical somatic cell is programmed to divide between 20 and 50 times and then die. As mentioned earlier, some cells, such as muscle and nerve cells, never divide at all. Cancer cells can divide indefinitely; they do not respond to the control mechanisms that normally regulate cell division.

ASEXUAL REPRODUCTION

Asexual reproduction is the production of offspring without fertilization. New organisms are formed by division of a single parent cell. Offspring are essentially genetic carbon copies of their parent cells. Thus, except for random mutations, the offspring are genetically identical to the parent cells. The different types of asexual reproduction are **binary fission**, **budding**, **regeneration**, and **parthenogenesis.**

A. BINARY FISSION

Binary fission is a simple form of asexual reproduction seen in prokaryotes. The circular chromosome replicates and a new plasma membrane and cell wall grow inward along the midline of the cell, dividing it into two equally sized cells, each containing a duplicate of the parent chromosome. A very similar process occurs in some primitive eukaryotic cells.

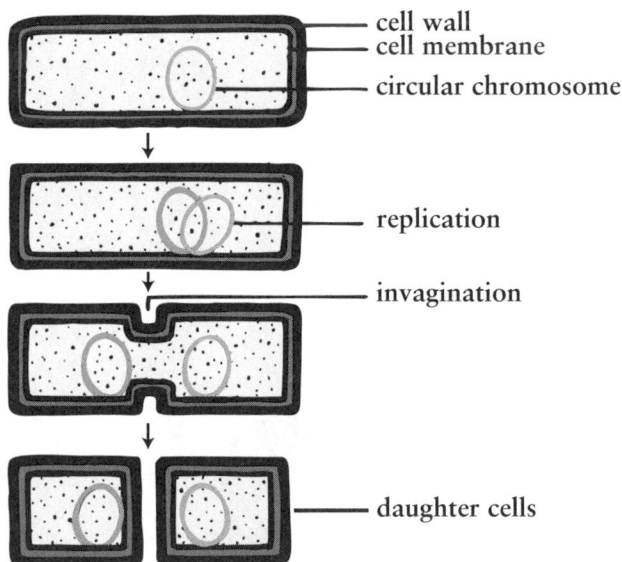

Figure 4.4. Binary Fission

B. BUDDING

Budding is the replication of the nucleus followed by unequal cytokinesis. The cell membrane pinches inward to form a new cell that is smaller in size but genetically identical to the parent cell and which subsequent-

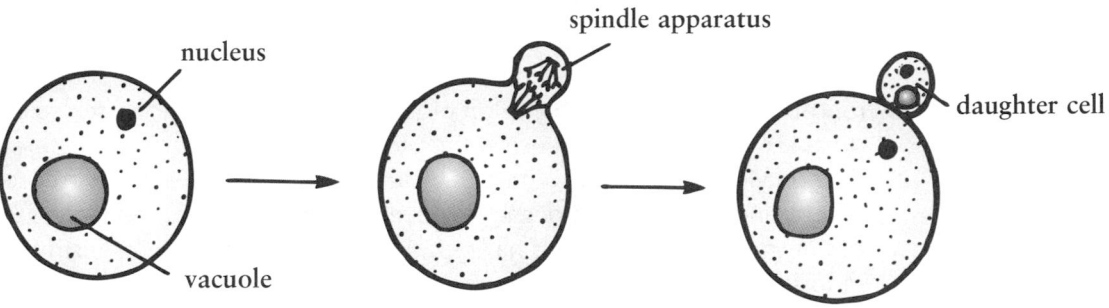

Figure 4.5. Budding

ly grows to adult size. The new cell may separate immediately from the parent or it may remain attached to it, develop as an outgrowth, and separate at a later stage. Budding occurs in hydra and yeast.

C. REGENERATION

Regeneration is the regrowth of a lost or injured body part. Replacement of cells occurs by mitosis. Some lower animals such as hydra and starfish have extensive regenerative capabilities. If a starfish loses an arm, it can regenerate a new one; the severed arm may even be able to regenerate an entire body, as long as the arm contains a piece of an area called the central disk. Salamanders and tadpoles can generate new limbs. The extent of regeneration depends on the nerve damage to the severed body part. In adult birds and mammals, regeneration is usually limited to the healing of tissues, although some internal organs, such as the liver, have considerable regenerative capabilities as long as part of the organ remains viable.

D. PARTHENOGENESIS

Parthenogenesis is the development of an unfertilized egg into an adult organism. This process occurs naturally in certain lower organisms. For example, in most species of bees and ants, the males develop from unfertilized eggs, and several species of all-female, parthenogenetic salamander exist. The eggs of some higher organisms can be induced to develop parthenogenetically (although the process does not occur naturally), with the resulting embryos surviving for variable lengths of time. Frog eggs have been induced to develop into tadpoles, and unfertilized rabbit eggs have been stimulated to develop into adult rabbits. Since the organism develops from a haploid cell, all of its cells will be haploid.

SEXUAL REPRODUCTION

Sexual reproduction differs from asexual reproduction in that there are two parents involved, and the end result is genetically unique offspring. Sexual reproduction occurs via the fusion of two gametes—specialized sex cells produced by each parent. **Meiosis** is the process whereby these sex cells are produced. Meiosis is similar to mitosis in that a cell duplicates its chromosomes before undergoing the process. However, mitosis preserves the diploid number of the cell, while meiosis halves it, resulting in haploid cells. Furthermore, mitosis comprises one division resulting in two diploid cells, while meiosis comprises two divisions resulting in four haploid gametes. Somatic cells undergo mitosis, while specialized cells called **gametocytes** undergo meiosis. During fertilization, two haploid gametes fuse, restoring the diploid number.

MCAT Favorite

Remember that MITOSIS occurs in all of the cells of the body that divide. MEIOSIS occurs only in the sex cells (a.k.a., "germ cells" or gametocytes) found in the reproductive system (the testes and ovaries).

A. MEIOSIS

As in mitosis, the gametocyte's chromosomes are replicated during the S phase of the cell cycle and the centrioles replicate at some point during interphase. The first round of division (meiosis I) produces two intermediate daughter cells. The second round of division (meiosis II), similar to mitosis, involves the separation of the sister chromatids, resulting in four genetically distinct haploid gametes. Each meiotic division has the same four stages as mitosis.

1. **Meiosis I**
   a. **Prophase I**

   The chromatin condenses into chromosomes, the spindle apparatus forms, and the nucleoli and nuclear membrane disappear. **Homologous chromosomes** (chromosomes that code for the same traits, one inherited from each parent), come together and intertwine in a process called **synapsis.** Since at this stage each chromosome consists of two sister chromatids, each synaptic pair of homologous chromosomes contains four chromatids and is, therefore, often called a **tetrad.** Sometimes chromatids of homologous chromosomes break at corresponding points and exchange equivalent pieces of DNA; this process is called **crossing over.** Note that crossing over occurs between homologous chromosomes and not between sister chromatids of the same chromosome. (The latter are identical, so crossing over would not produce any change.) Those chromatids involved are left with an altered but structurally complete set of genes. The chromosomes remain joined at points called **chiasmata** where the crossing over occurred. Such **genetic recombination** can "unlink" **linked genes** (see chapter 13), thereby increasing the variety of genetic combinations that can be produced via gametogenesis. Recombination among chromosomes results in

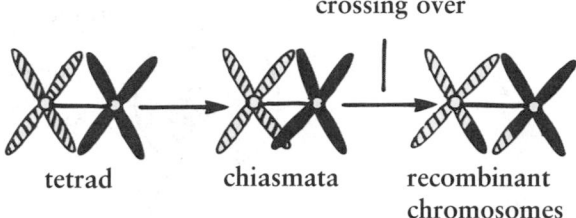

crossing over

tetrad   chiasmata   recombinant chromosomes

Figure 4.6. Synapsis

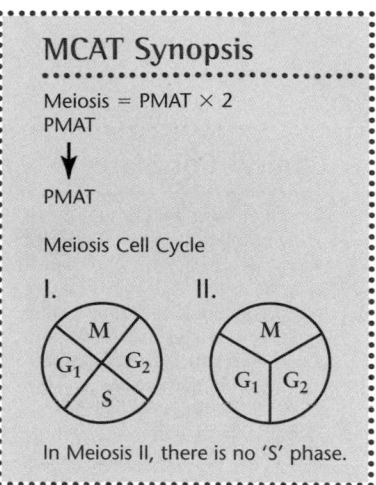

MCAT Synopsis

Meiosis = PMAT × 2
PMAT

↓

PMAT

Meiosis Cell Cycle

I.   II.

In Meiosis II, there is no 'S' phase.

increased genetic diversity within a species. Note that sister chromatids are no longer identical after recombination has occurred (see Figure 4.6).

b. Metaphase I

Homologous pairs (tetrads) align at the equatorial plane, and each pair attaches to a separate spindle fiber by its kinetochore.

c. Anaphase I

The homologous pairs separate and are pulled to opposite poles of the cell. This process is called **disjunction**, and it accounts for a fundamental **Mendelian law** (see chapter 13). During disjunction, each chromosome of paternal origin separates (or disjoins) from its homologue of maternal origin, and either chromosome can end up in either daughter cell. Thus, the distribution of homologous chromosomes to the two intermediate daughter cells is random with respect to parental origin. Each daughter cell will have a unique pool of **alleles** (genes coding for alternative forms of a given trait; e.g., yellow flowers or purple flowers) from a random mixture of maternal and paternal origin.

d. Telophase I

A nuclear membrane forms around each new nucleus. At this point each chromosome still consists of sister chromatids joined at the centromere. The cell divides (by cytokinesis) into two daughter cells, each of which receives a nucleus containing the haploid number of chromosomes. Between cell divisions there may be a short rest period, or **interkinesis**, during which the chromosomes partially uncoil.

2. Meiosis II

This second division is very similar to mitosis, except that meiosis II is not preceded by chromosomal replication.

a. Prophase II

The centrioles migrate to opposite poles and the spindle apparatus forms.

Clinical Correlate

If, during anaphase I or II of meiosis, homologous chromosomes (anaphase I) or sister chromatids (anaphase II) fail to separate (nondisjunction), then one of the resulting gametes will have two copies of a particular chromosome and the other gamete will have no copies. Subsequently, during fertilization, the resulting zygote may have one too many or one too few copies of the chromosome. Note that nondisjunction can affect both the autosomal chromosomes (e.g., trisomy 21; Down's syndrome) and the sex chromosomes (Klinefelter's; Turner's).

MCAT Synopsis

1) Sex cells
2) Diploid ⟶ Haploid
   2N ⟶ 1N
3) 4 daughter cells in males (except in females; there is only 1 daughter cell)

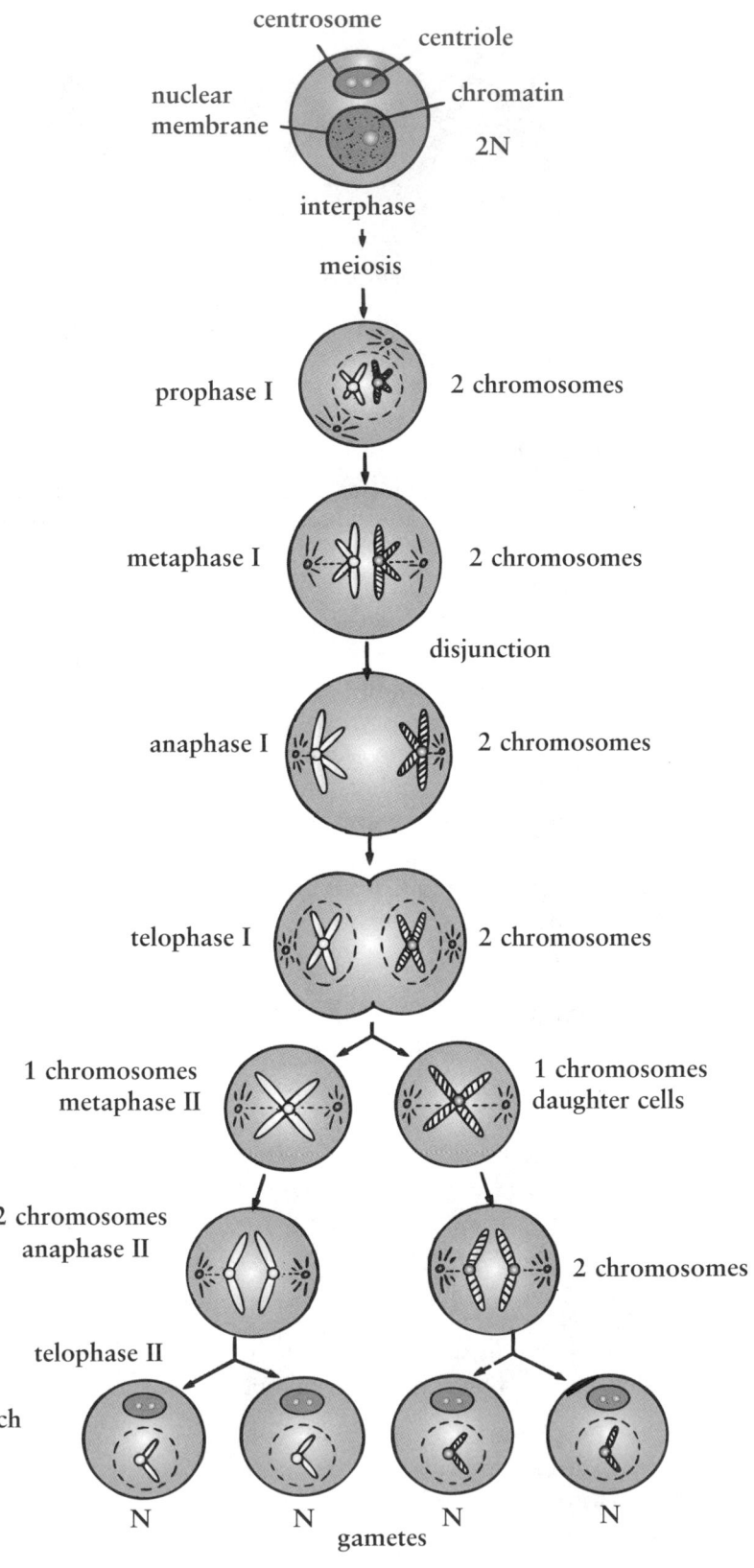

Figure 4.7. Meiosis

b. **Metaphase II**

The chromosomes line up along the equatorial plane. The centromeres divide, separating the chromosomes into pairs of sister chromatids.

c. **Anaphase II**

The sister chromatids are pulled to opposite poles by the spindle fibers.

d. **Telophase II**

A nuclear membrane forms around each new (haploid) nucleus. Cytokinesis follows and two daughter cells are formed. Thus, by the completion of meiosis II, four haploid daughter cells are produced per gametocyte. (In women, only one of these becomes a functional gamete.)

The random distribution of chromosomes in meiosis, coupled with crossing over in prophase I, enables an individual to produce gametes with many different genetic combinations. Thus, as opposed to asexual reproduction, which produces identical offspring, sexual reproduction produces genetic variability in offspring. The possibility of so many different genetic combinations is believed to increase the capability of a species to evolve and adapt to a changing environment.

B. HUMAN SEXUAL REPRODUCTION

Human reproduction is a highly complex process involving not only sexual intercourse between male and female but also interactions between the reproductive and endocrine systems within the body. Children are the product of fertilization—the fusion of **sperm** and **egg** (the gametes) in the female reproductive tract. The gametes are produced in the primary reproductive organs, or **gonads.**

1. **Male Reproductive Anatomy**

The male gonads, called the **testes,** contain two functional components: the **seminiferous tubules** and the **interstitial cells (cells of Leydig).** Sperm are produced in the highly coiled seminiferous tubules, where they are nourished by **Sertoli cells.** The interstitial cells, located between the seminiferous tubules, secrete **testosterone** and other **androgens** (male sex hormones) (see chapter 11). The testes are located in an external pouch called the **scrotum,** which maintains testes temperature 2–4°C lower than body temperature, a condition essential for sperm survival. Sperm pass from the seminiferous tubules into the coiled tubules of the **epididymis.** Here they

---

MCAT Synopsis

Mitosis	Meiosis
2N → 2N	2N → N
Occurs in all dividing cells	Occurs in sex cells only
Homologous chromosomes don't pair up	Homologous chromosomes pair up at metaphase plate forming tetrads
No crossing over	Crossing over can occur

MCAT Synopsis

To remember the pathway of sperm, think SEVEN UP.

Seminiferous tubules
Epididymus
Vas deferens
Ejaculatory duct
(Nothing)
Urethra
Penis

acquire motility, mature, and are stored until **ejaculation**. During ejaculation they travel through the **vas deferens** to the ejaculatory duct and then to the **urethra**. The urethra passes through the **penis** and opens to the outside at its tip. In males, the urethra is a common passageway for both the reproductive and excretory systems.

Sperm is mixed with **seminal fluid** as it moves along the reproductive tract; seminal fluid is produced by three glands: the **seminal vesicles**, the **prostate gland**, and the **bulbourethral glands.** The paired seminal vesicles secrete a fructose-rich fluid that serves as an energy source for the highly active sperm. The prostate gland releases an alkaline milky fluid that protects the sperm from the acidic environment of the female reproductive tract. Finally, the bulbourethral glands secrete a small amount of viscous fluid prior to ejaculation; the function of this secretion is not known. Seminal fluid aids in sperm transport by lubricating the passageways through which the sperm will travel. Sperm plus seminal fluid is known as **semen.**

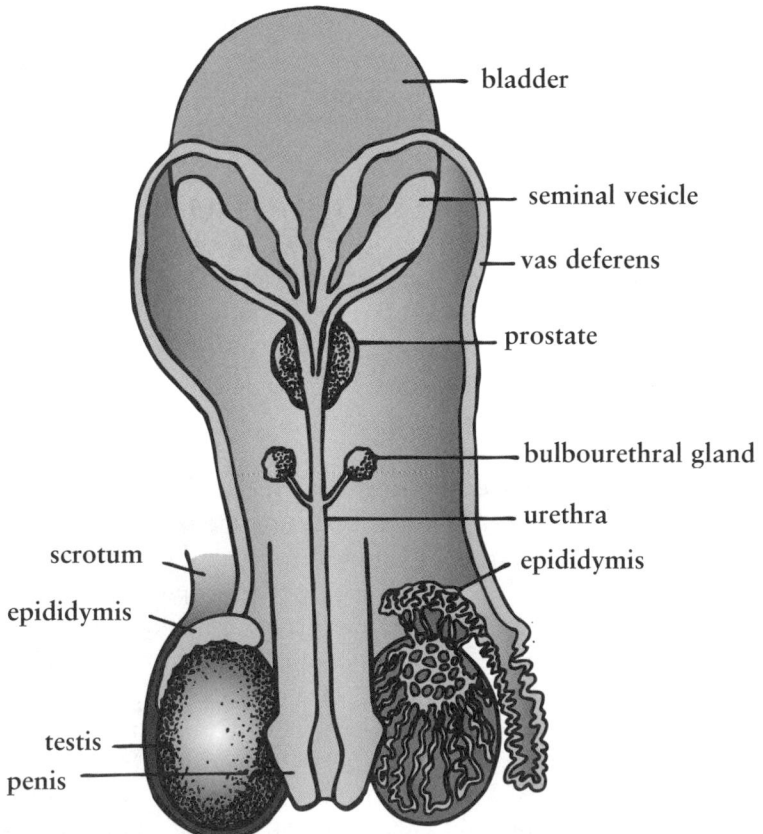

Figure 4.8. Male Reproductive Tract

2. Spermatogenesis

Spermatogenesis, or sperm production, occurs in the seminiferous tubules. Diploid cells called **spermatogonia** differentiate into diploid cells called **primary spermatocytes,** which undergo the first meiotic division to yield two haploid **secondary spermatocytes** of equal size; the second meiotic division produces four haploid **spermatids** of equal size. Following meiosis, the spermatids undergo a series of changes leading to the production of mature sperm, or **spermatozoa,** which are specialized for transporting the sperm nucleus to the egg, or **ovum.** The mature sperm is an elongated cell with a head, neck, body, and tail. The head consists almost entirely of the nucleus. The tail (flagellum) propels the sperm, while mitochondria in the neck and body provide energy for locomotion. A caplike structure called the **acrosome,** derived from the Golgi apparatus, develops over the anterior half of the head. The acrosome contains enzymes needed to penetrate the tough outer covering of the ovum. After a male has reached sexual maturity, approximately three million primary spermatocytes begin to undergo spermatogenesis per day, the maturation process taking a total of 65–75 days.

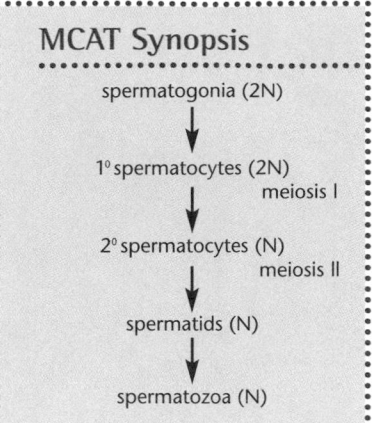

MCAT Synopsis

spermatogonia (2N)

↓

1° spermatocytes (2N)

meiosis I

↓

2° spermatocytes (N)

meiosis II

↓

spermatids (N)

↓

spermatozoa (N)

3. Female Reproductive Anatomy

The female gonads, called the **ovaries,** produce eggs (**ova**), and secrete the hormones estrogen and progesterone (see chapter 11). The ovaries are found in the abdominal cavity, below the digestive system. The ovaries consist of thousands of **follicles;** a follicle is a multilayered sac of cells that contains, nourishes, and protects an immature ovum. It is actually the follicle cells that produce estrogen. Once a month, an immature ovum is released from the ovary into the abdominal cavity and drawn into the nearby **fallopian tube.** The inner surface of the fallopian tube is lined with cilia that create currents that move the ovum

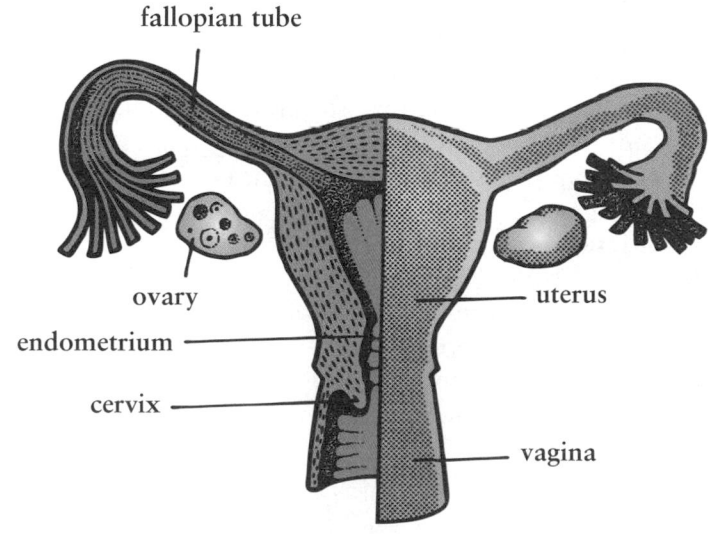

Figure 4.9. Female Reproductive Tract

into and along the tube. Each fallopian tube opens into the upper end of a muscular chamber called the **uterus,** which is the site of fetal development. The lower, narrow end of the uterus is called the **cervix.** The cervix connects with the **vaginal canal,** which is the site of sperm deposition during intercourse and is also the passageway through which a baby is expelled during childbirth. The external female genitalia is referred to as the **vulva.** Note that in the mammalian (placental) female, the reproductive and excretory systems are distinct from one another; i.e., the urethra and the vagina are not connected.

4. **Oogenesis**

Oogenesis, which is the production of female gametes, occurs in the ovarian follicles. At birth, all of the immature ova, known as **primary oocytes,** that a female will produce during her lifetime are already in her ovaries. Primary oocytes are diploid cells that form by mitosis in the ovary. After menarche (the first time a female gets her period), one primary oocyte per month completes meiosis I, yielding two daughter cells of unequal size—a **secondary oocyte** and a small cell known as a **polar body.** The secondary oocyte is expelled from the follicle during ovulation. Meiosis II does not occur until fertilization. The oocyte cell membrane is surrounded by two layers of cells; the inner layer is the **zona pellucida,** the outer layer is the **corona radiata.** Meiosis II is triggered when these layers are penetrated by a sperm cell, yielding two haploid cells—a mature ovum and another polar body. (The first polar body may also undergo meiosis II; eventually, the polar bodies die.) The mature ovum is a large cell containing a lot of cytoplasm, RNA, organelles, and nutrients needed by a developing embryo.

Women ovulate approximately once every four weeks (except during pregnancy and, usually, lactation) until menopause, which typically occurs between the ages of 45 and 50. During menopause, the ovaries become less sensitive to the hormones that stimulate follicle development (FSH and LH), and eventually they atrophy. The remaining follicles disappear, estrogen and progesterone levels greatly decline, and ovulation stops. The profound changes in hormone levels are often accompanied by physiological and psychological changes that persist until a new balance is reached.

5. **Fertilization**

An egg can be fertilized during the 12–24 hours following ovulation. Fertilization occurs in the lateral, widest portion of the fallopian tube. Sperm must travel through the vaginal canal, cervix, uterus, and into the fallopian tubes to reach the ovum. Sperm remain viable and capable of fertilization for one to two days following intercourse.

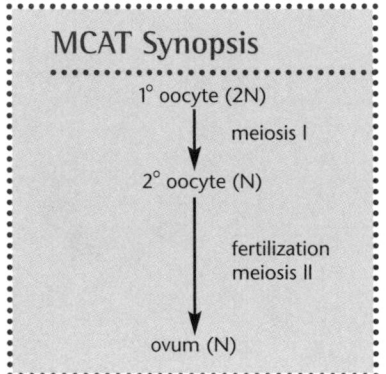

MCAT Synopsis

1° oocyte (2N)

meiosis I

2° oocyte (N)

fertilization
meiosis II

ovum (N)

The first barrier that the sperm must penetrate is the corona radiata. Enzymes secreted by the sperm aid in penetration of the corona radiata. The acrosome is responsible for penetrating the zona pellucida; it releases enzymes that digest this layer, thereby allowing the sperm to come into direct contact with the ovum cell membrane. Once in contact with the membrane, the sperm forms a tubelike structure called the **acrosomal process,** which extends to the cell membrane and penetrates it, fusing the sperm cell membrane with that of the ovum. The sperm nucleus now enters the ovum's cytoplasm. It is at this stage of fertilization that the ovum completes meiosis II.

The acrosomal reaction triggers a **cortical reaction** in the ovum, causing calcium ions to be released into the cytoplasm; this, in turn, initiates a series of reactions that result in the formation of the **fertilization membrane.** The fertilization membrane is a hard layer that surrounds the ovum cell membrane and prevents multiple fertilizations. The release of Ca^{2+} also stimulates metabolic changes within the ovum, greatly increasing its metabolic rate. This is followed by the fusion of the sperm nucleus with the ovum nucleus to form a diploid zygote. The first mitotic division of the zygote soon follows (see chapter 5).

6. **Multiple Births**
   a. **Monozygotic (identical) twins**
      Monozygotic twins result when a single zygote splits into two embryos. If the splitting occurs at the two-cell stage of development, the embryos will have separate chorions and separate placentas; if it occurs at the blastula stage, then the embryos will have only one chorionic sac and will therefore share a placenta and possibly an amnion (see chapter 5). Occasionally the division is incomplete, resulting in the birth of "Siamese" twins, which are attached at some point on the body, often sharing limbs and/or organs. Monozygotic twins are genetically identical, since they develop from the same zygote. Monozygotic twins are therefore of the same sex, blood type, and so on.

   b. **Dizygotic (fraternal) twins**
      Dizygotic twins result when two ova are released in one ovarian cycle and are fertilized by two different sperm. The two embryos implant in the uterine wall individually, and each develops its own placenta, amnion, and chorion (although the placentas may fuse if the embryos implant very close to each other). Fraternal twins share no more characteristics than any other siblings, since they develop from two distinct zygotes.

5

EMBRYOLOGY

Embryology is the study of the development of a unicellular zygote into a complete multicellular organism. In the course of nine months, a unicellular human zygote undergoes cell division, cellular differentiation, and morphogenesis in preparation for life outside the uterus. Much of what is known about mammalian development stems from the study of less complex organisms such as sea urchins and frogs.

EARLY DEVELOPMENTAL STAGES

A. CLEAVAGE

Early embryonic development is characterized by a series of rapid mitotic divisions known as **cleavage.** These divisions lead to an increase in cell number without a corresponding growth in cell protoplasm, i.e., the total volume of cytoplasm remains constant. Thus, cleavage results in progressively smaller cells, with an increasing ratio of nuclear-to-cytoplasmic material. Cleavage also increases the surface-to-volume ratio of each cell, thereby improving gas and nutrient exchange. An **indeterminate cleavage** is one that results in cells that maintain the ability to develop into a complete organism. Identical twins are the result of an indeterminate cleavage (see chapter 4). A **determinate cleavage** results in cells whose future **differentiation** pathways are determined at an early developmental stage. Differentiation is the specialization of cells that occurs during development.

The first complete cleavage of the zygote occurs approximately 32 hours after fertilization. The second cleavage occurs after 60 hours, and the third cleavage after approximately 72 hours, at which point the 8-celled embryo reaches the uterus. As cell division continues, a solid ball of embryonic cells, known as the **morula,** is formed. **Blastulation** begins when the morula develops a fluid-filled cavity called the **blastocoel,** which by the fourth day becomes a hollow sphere of cells called the **blastula.** The mammalian blastula is called a **blastocyst** (see Figure 5.1) and consists of two cell groups: the **inner cell mass,** which protrudes into the blastocoel, and the **trophoblast,** which surrounds the blastocoel and later gives rise to the chorion.

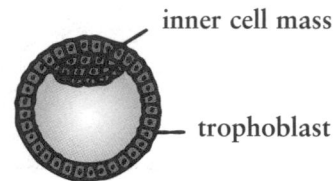

inner cell mass

trophoblast

Figure 5.1. Mammalian Blastocyst

B. IMPLANTATION

The embryo implants in the uterine wall during blastulation, approximately five to eight days after fertilization. The uterus is prepared for implantation by the hormone progesterone (see chapter 11), which causes glandular proliferation in the **endometrium**—the mucosal lining of the uterus. The embryonic cells secrete proteolytic enzymes that enable the embryo to digest tissue and implant itself in the endometrium. Eventually, maternal and fetal blood exchange materials at this site, later to be the location of the placenta.

C. GASTRULATION

Once implanted, cell migrations transform the single cell layer of the blastula into a three-layered structure called a **gastrula.** In the sea urchin, gastrulation begins with the appearance of a small invagination on the surface of the blastula. An inpocketing forms as cells continue to move toward the invagination, eventually eliminating the blastocoel. The result is a two-layered cup, with a differentiation between an outer cellular layer—the **ectoderm,** and an inner cellular layer—the **endoderm.** The newly formed cavity of the two-layered gastrula is called the **archenteron,** and later develops into the gut. The opening of the archenteron is called the **blastopore.** (In organisms classified as **deuterostomes,** such as humans, the blastopore is the site of the future anus, whereas in organisms classified as **protostomes,** the blastopore is the site of the future mouth.) Proliferation and migration of cells into the space between the ectoderm and the endoderm gives rise to a third cell layer, called the **mesoderm.** These three **primary germ layers** are responsible for the differential development of the tissues, organs, and systems of the body at later stages of growth.

- **Ectoderm**—integument (including the epidermis, hair, nails, and epithelium of the nose, mouth, and anal canal), the lens of the eye, and the nervous system.

- **Endoderm**—epithelial linings of the digestive and respiratory tracts (including the lungs), and parts of the liver, pancreas, thyroid, and bladder.

- **Mesoderm**—musculoskeletal system, circulatory system, excretory system, gonads, connective tissue throughout the body, and portions of digestive and respiratory organs.

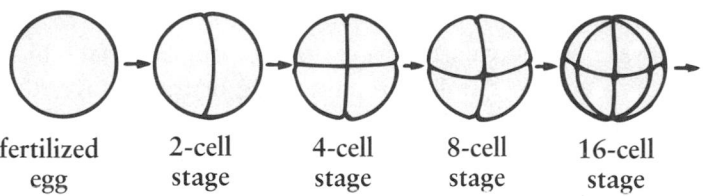

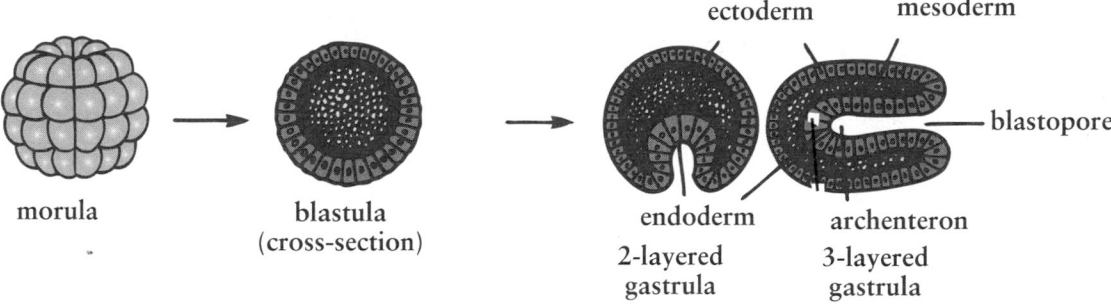

Figure 5.2. Amphibian Cleavage and Gastrulation

Despite the fact that all embryonic cells are derived from a single zygote and therefore have the same DNA, cells and tissues differentiate to perform unique and specialized functions. Most of this differentiation is accomplished through selective transcription of the genome. As the embryo develops, different tissue types express different genes. Most of the genetic information within any given cell is never expressed.

Induction is the influence of a specific group of cells (sometimes known as the **organizer**) on the differentiation of another group of cells. Induction is most often mediated by chemical substances (**inducers**) passed from the organizer to adjacent cells. In development of the eyes, lateral outpocketings from the brain (optic vesicles) grow out and touch the overlying ectoderm. The optic vesicle induces the ectoderm to thicken and form the lens placode. The lens placode then induces the optic vesicle to flatten and invaginate inward, forming the optic cup. The optic cup then induces the lens placode to invaginate and form the cornea and lens. Experiments with frog embryos show that if this ectoderm is transplanted to the trunk (after the optic vesicles have grown out), a lens will develop in the trunk. If, however, the ectoderm is transplanted before the outgrowth of the optic vesicles, it will not form a lens.

D. NEURULATION

By the end of gastrulation, regions of the germ layers begin to develop into a rudimentary nervous system; this process is known as **neurulation.** A rod of mesodermal cells, called the **notochord,** develops along the long-itudinal axis just under the dorsal layer of ectoderm. The notochord has an inductive effect on the overlying ectoderm, causing it to bend inward and form a groove along the dorsal surface of the embryo. The dorsal ectoderm folds on either side of the groove; these **neural folds** grow upward and finally fuse, forming a closed tube. This is the **neural tube,** which gives rise to the brain and spinal cord (**central nervous system**). Once the neural tube is formed, it detaches from the surface ectoderm. The cells at the tip of each neural fold are called the **neural crest** cells. These cells migrate laterally and give rise to many components of the **peripheral nervous system,** including the sensory ganglia, autonomic ganglia, adrenal medulla, and Schwann cells (see chapter 12).

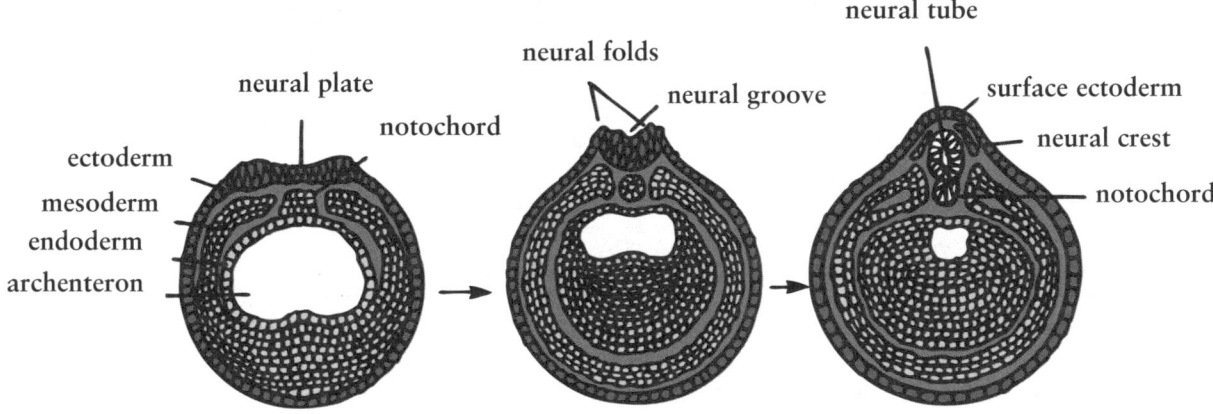

Figure 5.3. Neurulation

FETAL RESPIRATION

The growing **fetus** (the embryo is referred to as a fetus after eight weeks of **gestation**) receives oxygen directly from its mother through a specialized circulatory system. This system not only supplies oxygen and nutrients to the fetus, but removes carbon dioxide and metabolic wastes as well. The two components of this system are the **placenta** and the **umbilical cord,** which both develop in the first few weeks following fertilization.

The placenta and the umbilical cord are outgrowths of the four extra-embryonic membranes formed during development: the **amnion, chorion, allantois,** and **yolk sac.** The amnion is a thin, tough membrane containing a watery fluid called **amniotic fluid.** Amniotic fluid acts as a shock absorber of external and localized pressure from uterine contractions during **labor.** Placenta formation begins with the chorion, a membrane that completely surrounds the amnion. About two weeks after fertilization the chorion extends villi into the uterine wall. These **chorionic villi** become closely associated with endometrial cells, developing into the spongy tissue of the placenta. A third membrane, the allantois, develops as an outpocketing of the gut. The blood vessels of the allantoic wall enlarge and become the **umbilical vessels,** which will connect the fetus to the developing placenta. The yolk sac, the site of early development of blood vessels, becomes associated with the umbilical vessels. At some point the allantois and yolk sac are enveloped by the amnion, forming the primitive **umbilical cord,** which is the initial connection between the fetus and the placenta. The mature umbilical cord consists of the umbilical vessels, which developed from the allantoic vessels, surrounded by a jellylike matrix. As the embryo grows, it remains attached to the placenta by the umbilical cord, which permits it to float freely in the amniotic fluid.

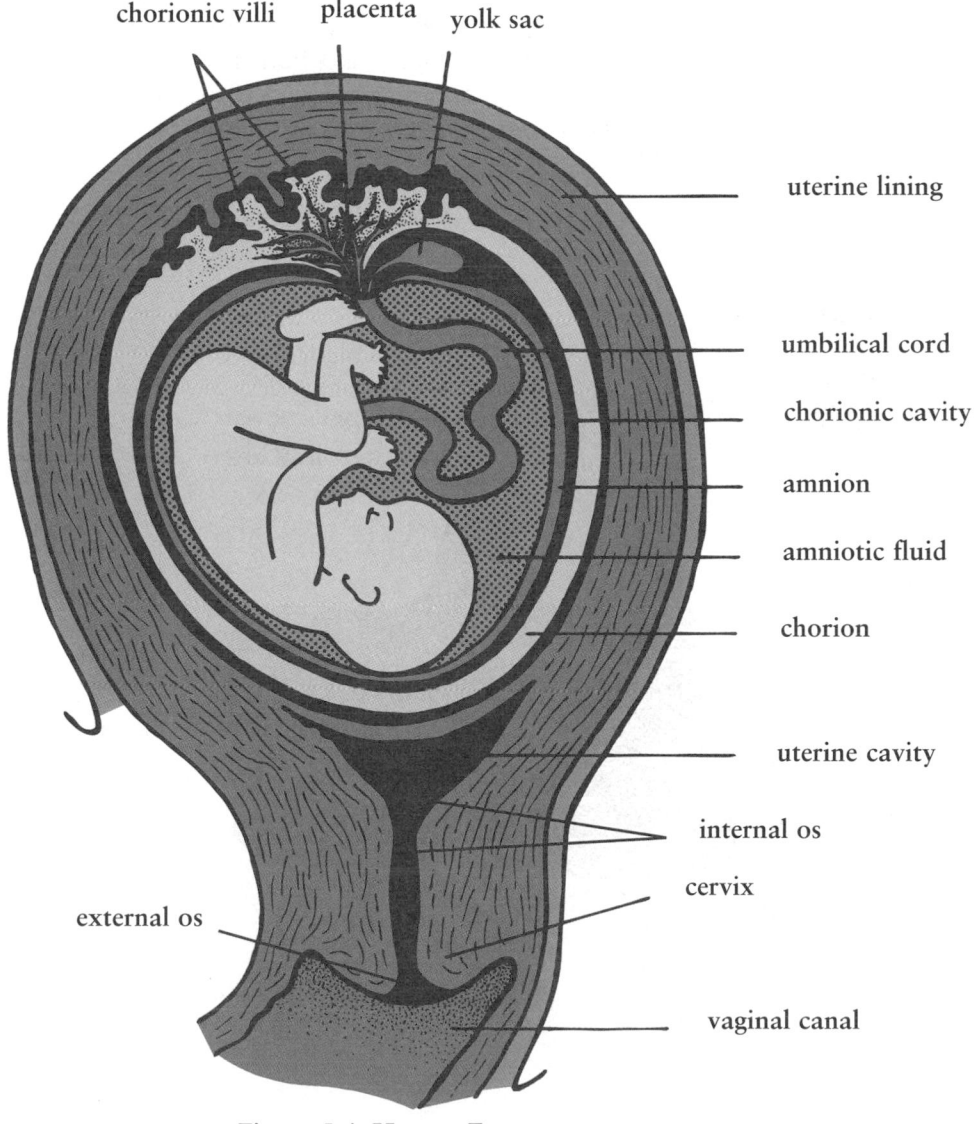

chorionic villi   placenta   yolk sac

uterine lining

umbilical cord

chorionic cavity

amnion

amniotic fluid

chorion

uterine cavity

internal os

cervix

external os

vaginal canal

Figure 5.4. Human Fetus

The placenta is the site of nutrition, respiration, and waste disposal for the fetus. Water, glucose, amino acids, vitamins, and inorganic salts diffuse across maternal capillaries into fetal blood. **Fetal hemoglobin (Hb-F)** has a greater affinity for oxygen than does adult hemoglobin **(Hb-A)**; consequently, oxygen preferentially diffuses into fetal blood. Concurrently, metabolic wastes and carbon dioxide diffuse in the opposite direction—from fetal blood into maternal blood. Note that the circulatory systems of the mother and the fetus are not directly connected, so maternal and fetal blood do not mix. As can be seen in Figure 5.5, all exchange of material between maternal and fetal blood vessels occurs in the placenta via diffusion.

In addition to nutritive and respiratory functions, the placenta offers the fetus some immunological protection by preventing the diffusion of foreign matter (e.g., bacteria) into fetal blood. However, the placenta is permeable to viruses, alcohol, and many drugs and toxins, all of which can adversely affect fetal development. The placenta also functions as an endocrine gland, producing the hormones progesterone, estrogen, and human chorionic gonadotropin (HCG)—all of which are essential for maintaining a pregnancy (see chapter 11). The presence of HCG in urine is the simplest test for pregnancy.

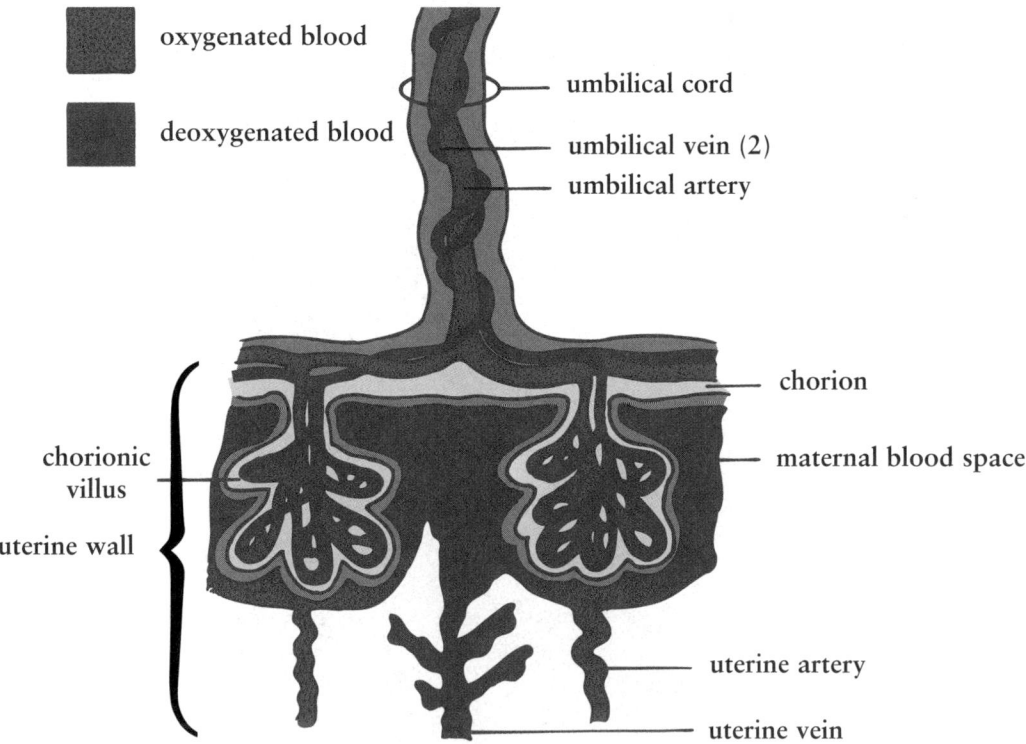

Figure 5.5. Placenta

FETAL CIRCULATION

Fetal circulation differs from adult circulation in several important ways. The major difference is that in fetal circulation, blood is oxygenated in the placenta (because fetal lungs are nonfunctional prior to birth), while in adult circulation, blood is oxygenated in the lungs. In addition, the fetal circulatory route contains three shunts that divert blood flow away from the developing fetal liver and lungs. The **umbilical vein** carries oxygenated blood from the placenta to the fetus. The blood bypasses the fetal liver by way of a shunt called the **ductus venosus**, before converging with the inferior vena cava. The inferior and superior venae cavae return deoxygenated blood to the right atrium. Since the oxygenated blood from the umbilical vein mixes with the deoxygenated blood of the venae cavae, the blood entering the right atrium is only partially oxygenated. Most of this blood bypasses the pulmonary circulation and enters the left atrium directly from the right atrium by way of the **foramen ovale,** a shunt that diverts blood away from the pulmonary arteries. The remaining blood in the right atrium empties into the right ventricle and is pumped into the pulmonary artery. Most of this blood is shunted directly from the pulmonary artery to the aorta via the **ductus arteriosus**, diverting even more blood away from the lungs. This means that in the fetus, the pulmonary arteries carry partially oxygenated blood to the lungs. The blood that does reach the lungs is further deoxygenated as the blood unloads its oxygen to the developing lungs. Remember, gas exchange does not occur in the fetal lungs—it occurs in the placenta. The deoxygenated blood then returns to the left atrium via the pulmonary veins. Despite the fact that this blood mixes with the partially oxygenated blood that crossed over from the right atrium (via the foramen ovale) before being pumped into the systemic circulation by the left ventricle, the blood delivered via the aorta has an even lower partial pressure of oxygen than the blood that was delivered to the lungs. This deoxygenated blood is returned to the placenta via the **umbilical arteries.**

In contrast, in adult circulation, deoxygenated blood enters the right atrium, the right ventricle pumps this blood to the lungs via the pulmonary arteries (those same arteries that carried partially oxygenated blood in the fetus), and gas exchange occurs in the lungs. Oxygenated blood is returned to the left atrium via the pulmonary veins (those same veins that carried deoxygenated blood in the fetus), and the left ventricle pumps the blood into circulation via the aorta. (For a more complete discussion of adult circulation, see chapter 9.)

> **MCAT Synopsis**
>
> A small amount of blood must reach the pulmonary circulation in order to nourish the developing fetal lungs.

> **MCAT Synopsis**
>
> Fetal circulation can be considered the opposite of adult circulation.
>
> Umbilical vein = oxygenated blood
>
> Umbilical arteries = deoxygenated blood
>
> Three shunts shift fetal blood from the right-sided circulation to the left-sided circulation:
>
> 1) Ductus venosus (shunts blood from the fetal liver)
> 2) Ductus arteriorsus (shunts blood from the lungs)
> 3) Foramen ovale (shunts blood from the lungs)

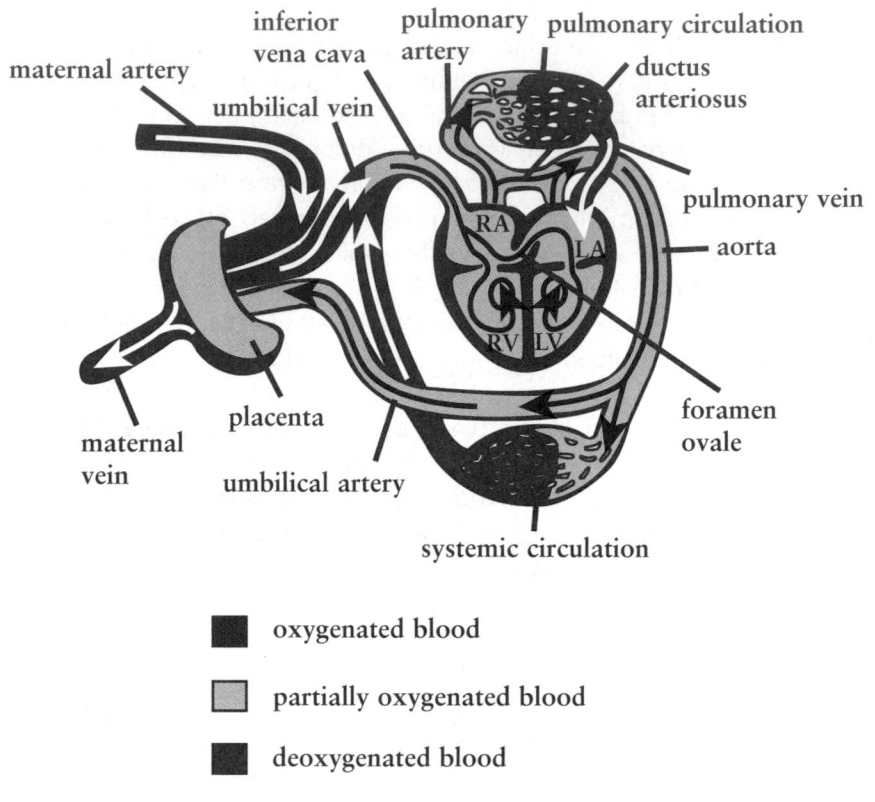

oxygenated blood

partially oxygenated blood

deoxygenated blood

Figure 5.6. Fetal Circulation

After birth, a number of changes occur in the circulatory system as the fetus adjusts to breathing on its own. The lungs expand with air and rhythmic breathing begins. Resistance in the pulmonary blood vessels decreases, causing an increase in blood flow through the lungs. When umbilical blood flow stops, blood pressure in the inferior vena cava decreases, causing a decrease in pressure in the right atrium. In contrast, left atrial pressure increases due to increased blood flow from the lungs. Increased left atrial pressure coupled with decreased right atrial pressure causes the foramen ovale to close. In addition, the ductus arteriosus constricts and later closes permanently. The ductus venosus degenerates over a period of time, completely closing in most infants three months after birth. The infant begins to produce adult hemoglobin, and by the end of the first year of life little fetal hemoglobin can be detected in the blood.

GESTATION

Human pregnancy, or gestation, is approximately 9 months (266 days), and can be subdivided into 3 **trimesters.** The primary developments that occur during each trimester are described below.

A. FIRST TRIMESTER

During the first weeks, the major organs begin to develop. The heart begins to beat at approximately 22 days, and soon afterward, the eyes, gonads, limbs, and liver start to form. By 5 weeks the embryo is 10 mm in length; by 6 weeks the embryo has grown to 15 mm. The cartilaginous skeleton begins to turn into bone by the seventh week (see chapter 6). By the end of 8 weeks, most of the organs have formed, the brain is fairly developed, and the embryo is referred to as a fetus. At the end of the third month, the fetus is about 9 cm long.

B. SECOND TRIMESTER

During the second trimester, the fetus does a tremendous amount of growing. It begins to move around in the amniotic fluid, its face appears human, and its toes and fingers elongate. By the end of the sixth month, the fetus is 30–36 cm long.

C. THIRD TRIMESTER

The seventh and eighth months are characterized by continued rapid growth and further brain development. During the ninth month, antibodies are transported by highly selective active transport from the mother to the fetus for protection against foreign matter. The growth rate slows and the fetus becomes less active, as it has less room to move about.

BIRTH

Childbirth is accomplished by labor, a series of strong uterine contractions. Labor can be divided into three distinct stages. In the first stage, the cervix thins out and dilates, and the amniotic sac ruptures, releasing its fluids. During this time contractions are relatively mild. The second stage is characterized by rapid contractions, resulting in the birth of the baby, followed by the cutting of the umbilical cord. During the final stage, the uterus contracts, expelling the placenta and the umbilical cord.

6

MUSCULOSKELETAL SYSTEM

The musculoskeletal system forms the basic internal framework of the vertebrate body. Muscles and bones work in close coordination to produce voluntary movement. In addition, bone and muscle perform a number of other independent functions.

SKELETAL SYSTEM

The skeleton functions primarily as the physical support of an organism. In contrast to the external skeleton (**exoskeleton**) of arthropods, vertebrates have an internal skeleton, or **endoskeleton.** The mammalian skeleton is divided into the **axial** and **appendicular** skeletons. The axial skeleton is the basic framework of the body, consisting of the skull, the vertebral column, and the rib cage. The appendicular skeleton consists of the limb bones and the pelvic and pectoral girdles. In addition to providing the lever upon which skeletal muscles act during locomotion, the skeleton surrounds and protects delicate organs such as the brain and the spinal cord. Furthermore, skeletal bone marrow houses much of the body's blood-forming elements.

The two major components of the skeleton are **cartilage** and **bone**.

CARTILAGE

Cartilage is a type of connective tissue that is softer and more flexible than bone. It is made of a firm but elastic matrix called **chondrin,** which is secreted by specialized cells called **chondrocytes.** Cartilage is the principal component of embryonic skeletons in higher animals. During mammalian development, however, much of it hardens and calcifies into bone. Cartilage is retained in adults in places where firmness and flexibility are needed. For example, in humans, the external ear, the nose, the walls of the larynx and trachea, and the skeletal joints contain cartilage. Most cartilage is avascular (i.e., contains no blood or lymph vessels) and is devoid of nerves; it receives nourishment from capillaries located in nearby connective tissue and bone via diffusion through the surrounding fluid.

BONE

Bone is a specialized type of mineralized connective tissue that has the ability to withstand physical stress. Ideally designed for body support, bone tissue is hard and strong, while at the same time, somewhat elastic and lightweight.

A. MACROSCOPIC BONE STRUCTURE

There are two basic types of bone: **compact bone** and **spongy bone**. Compact bone is dense bone that does not appear to have any cavities when observed with the naked eye. Spongy bone, also called **cancellous bone**, is much less dense, and consists of an interconnecting lattice of bony spicules (trabeculae); the cavities in between the spicules are filled with **yellow** and/or **red bone marrow**. Yellow marrow is inactive and infiltrated by adipose tissue; red marrow is involved in blood cell formation (see chapter 9).

The bones of the appendages, the **long bones**, are characterized by a cylindrical shaft called a **diaphysis** and dilated ends called **epiphyses**. The diaphysis is primarily compact bone surrounding a cavity containing bone marrow. The epiphyses are spongy bone surrounded by a thin layer of compact bone. The **epiphyseal plate** is a disk of cartilaginous cells separating the diaphysis from the epiphysis and is the site of longitudinal growth. A fibrous sheath called the **periosteum** surrounds the long bone and is the site of attachment to muscle tissue. Some periosteum cells differentiate into bone-forming cells.

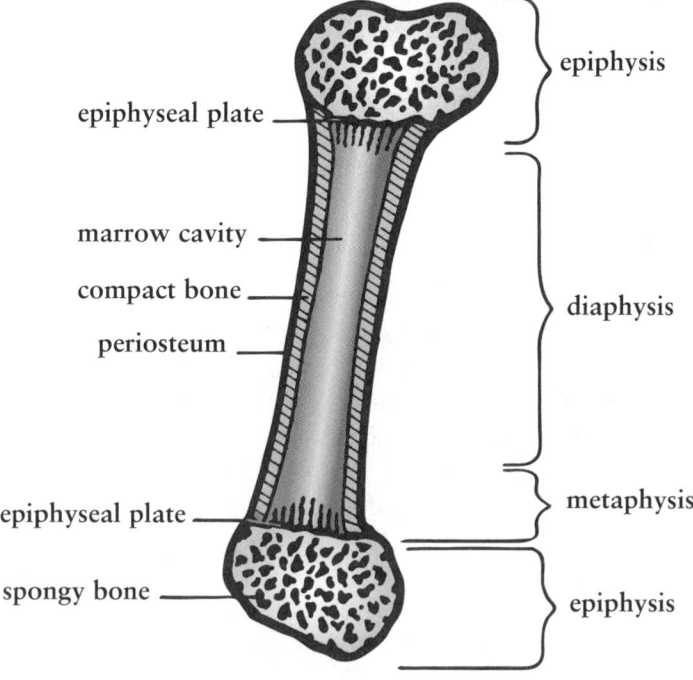

Figure 6.1. Long Bone

B. MICROSCOPIC BONE STRUCTURE

Compact bone is a dense, hardened **bone matrix**, which contains both organic and inorganic components. The organic components include proteins (principally collagen fibers and glycoproteins), while the inorganic components include calcium, phosphate, and hydroxide (which combine and harden to form **hydroxyapatite crystals**), as well as sodium, potassium, and magnesium ions. The association of hydroxyapatite crystals with collagen fibers gives bone its characteristic strength.

The bony matrix is deposited in structural units called **osteons (Haversian systems)**. Each osteon consists of a central microscopic channel called a **Haversian canal**, surrounded by a number of concentric circles of bony matrix called **lamellae**. There are blood vessels, nerve fibers, and lymph in the Haversian canals, vascularizing and innervating bone tissue. Interspersed within the matrix are spaces called **lacunae**, which house mature bone cells called **osteocytes**. Osteocytes are involved in bone maintenance. Radiating from each lacuna are a number of minute canals called **canaliculi**. The canaliculi interconnect with each other and with the Haversian canals, allowing for exchange of nutrients and wastes (see Figure 6.2).

> ### MCAT Synopsis
>
> Don't forget that bone is much more dynamic than you might think. Bone is both vascular and innervated. The bone's blood supply can become infected after an injury (a disease known as osteomyelitis) and if you break a bone, it will hurt (a lot). In addition, remember that bone is in a dynamic equilibrium between being broken down (by osteoCLASTS) and being built up (by osteoBLASTS.) This is known as bone remodeling.

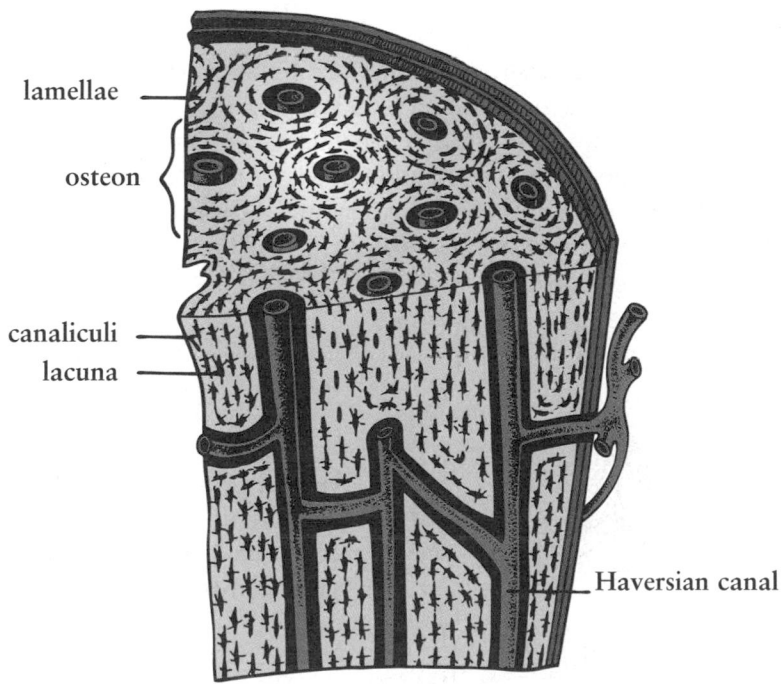

Figure 6.2. Microscopic Bone Structure

Two other types of cells found in bone tissue are **osteoblasts** and **osteoclasts.** Osteoblasts synthesize and secrete the organic constituents of the bone matrix; once they have become surrounded by their matrix, they mature into osteocytes. Osteoclasts are large, multinucleated cells involved in **bone resorption.**

C. BONE FORMATION (OSSIFICATION)

Bone formation occurs by either **endochondral ossification** or by **intramembranous ossification.** In endochondral ossification, existing cartilage is replaced by bone. Long bones arise primarily through endochondral ossification. In intramembranous ossification, **mesenchymal** (embryonic, undifferentiated) connective tissue is transformed into, and replaced by, bone.

D. BONE REMODELING

Bone matrix is dynamic; i.e., it is continuously and simultaneously degraded and reformed. During **bone reformation,** inorganic ions (e.g., calcium and phosphate) are absorbed from the blood for use in bone formation; in the process of **bone resorption** (degradation), these ions are released into the blood. These two processes are collectively known as **bone remodeling.** Vitamin D and hormones such as parathyroid hormone and calcitonin are all involved in the regulation of bone remodeling (see chapter 11). Bone use and stress during exercise are also factors in bone remodeling.

JOINTS

Joints are connective tissue structures that join bones together. Bones that do not move relative to each other, such as skull bones, are held in place by **immovable joints.** Bones that do move relative to one another are held together by **movable joints** and are additionally supported and strengthened by **ligaments.** Movable joints consist of a **synovial capsule,** which encloses a **joint cavity (articular cavity).** Movement is facilitated by **synovial fluid,**

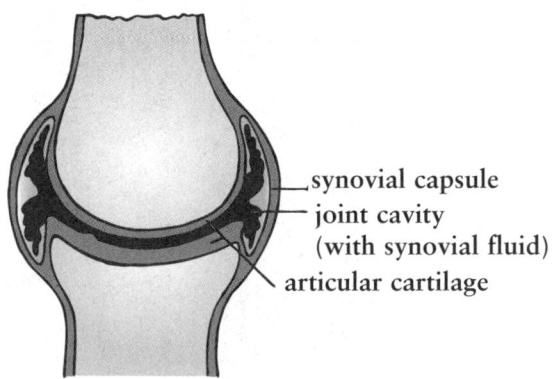

synovial capsule
joint cavity
(with synovial fluid)
articular cartilage

Figure 6.3. Movable Joint

which lubricates the joint, and by **articular cartilage** on the opposing bone surfaces, which is smooth and reduces tension during movement (see Figure 6.3).

MUSCULAR SYSTEM

Muscle tissue consists of bundles of specialized contractile fibers held together by connective tissue. There are three morphologically and functionally distinct types of muscle in mammals: **skeletal muscle, smooth muscle,** and **cardiac muscle.**

Table 6.1. Skeletal Muscle

Smooth Muscle	Cardiac Muscle	Skeletal Muscle
• Non-striated	• Striated	• Striated
• One nucleus per cell	• 1-2 Nuclei per cell	• Multinucleated cells
• Involuntary/Autonomic Nervous System	• Involuntary/Autonomic Nervous System	• Voluntary/Somatic Nervous System
• Smooth continuous contractions	• Strong Forceful Contractions	• Strong Forceful Contractions

SKELETAL MUSCLE

Skeletal muscle is responsible for voluntary movements and is innervated by the **somatic nervous system** (see chapter 12). A muscle is a bundle of parallel fibers. Each fiber is a multinucleated cell created by the fusion of several mononucleate embryonic cells. The nuclei are usually found at the periphery of the cell. Embedded in the fibers are filaments called **myofibrils,** which are further divided into contractile units called **sarcomeres.** The myofibrils are enveloped by a modified endoplasmic reticulum that stores calcium ions and is called the **sarcoplasmic reticulum.** The cytoplasm of a muscle fiber is called **sarcoplasm,** and the cell membrane is called the **sarcolemma.** The sarcolemma is capable of propagating an action potential (see chapter 12), and is connected to a system of **transverse tubules (T system)** oriented perpendicularly to the myofibrils. The T system provides channels for ion flow throughout the muscle fibers, and can also propagate an action potential (see Figure 6.4).

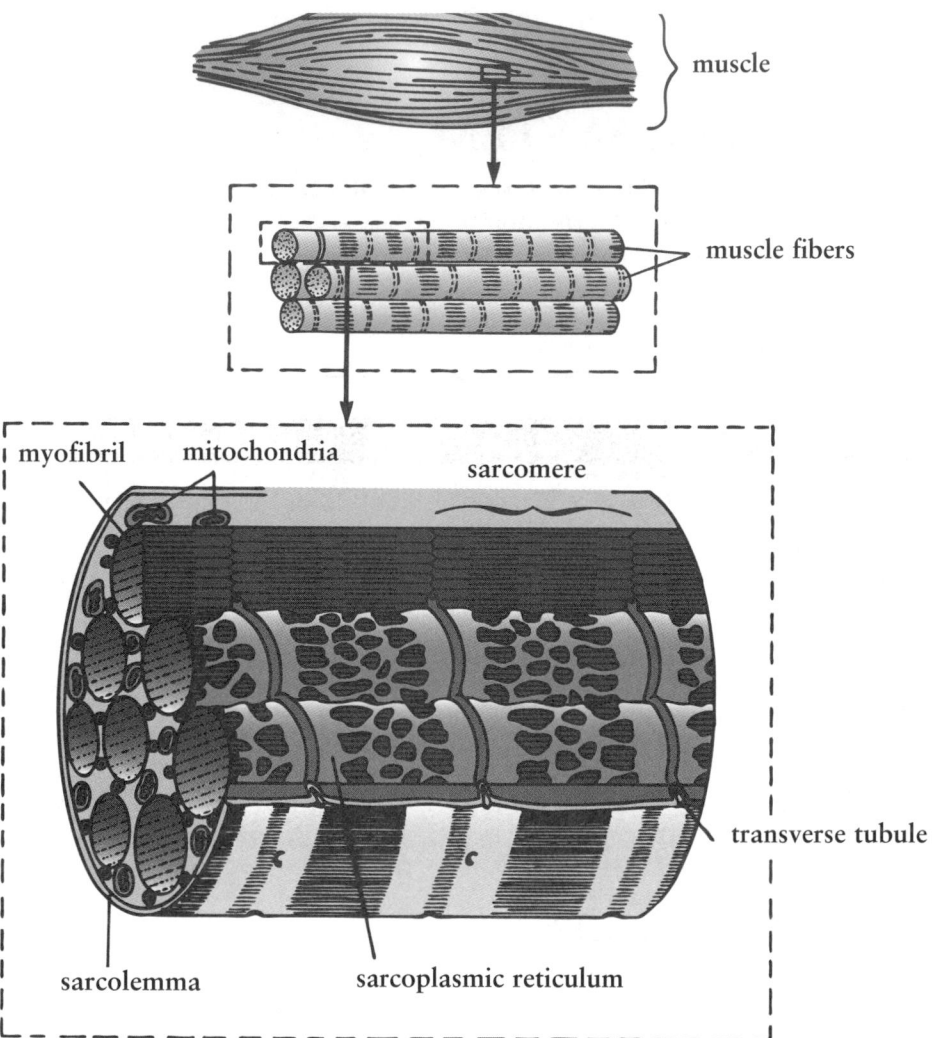

Figure 6.4. Skeletal Muscle

Skeletal muscle has striations of light and dark bands, and is therefore also referred to as **striated** muscle. Skeletal muscle fibers can be characterized as either red or white. **Red fibers** (slow-twitch fibers) have a high **myoglobin** content (a protein resembling hemoglobin) and many mitochondria. They derive their energy primarily from aerobic respiration and are capable of sustained and vigorous activity. **White fibers** (fast-twitch fibers) are anaerobic and therefore contain less myoglobin and fewer mitochondria than red fibers. White fibers have a greater rate of contraction than red fibers; however, white fibers fatigue more easily.

THE SARCOMERE

A. STRUCTURE

The sarcomere is composed of **thin** and **thick filaments**. The thin filaments are chains of globular **actin** molecules associated with two other proteins, **troponin** and **tropomyosin**. The thick filaments are composed of organized bundles of **myosin** molecules; each myosin molecule has a head region and a tail region.

Electron microscopy reveals that the sarcomere is organized as follows: **Z lines** define the boundaries of a single sarcomere and anchor the thin filaments. The **M line** runs down the center of the sarcomere. The **I band** is the region containing thin filaments only. The **H zone** is the region containing thick filaments only. The **A band** spans the entire length of the thick filaments and any overlapping portions of the thin filaments. Note that during contraction, the A band is not reduced in size, while the H zone and I band are.

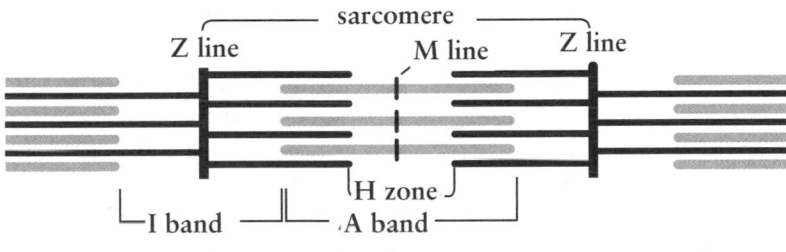

Figure 6.5. Sarcomere

B. CONTRACTION

1. Initiation

Muscle contraction is stimulated by a message from the somatic nervous system sent via a **motor neuron**. The link between the **nerve terminal (synaptic bouton)** and the sarcolemma of the muscle fiber is called the **neuromuscular junction**. The space between the two is known as the **synapse**, or **synaptic cleft**. Depolarization of the motor neuron results in the release of **neurotransmitters** (e.g., acetylcholine) from the nerve terminal. The neurotransmitter diffuses across the synaptic cleft and binds to special receptor sites on the sarcolemma. If enough of these receptors are stimulated, the permeability of the sarcolemma is altered and an **action potential** is generated (see chapter 12). The action potential then quickly spreads through the transverse tubules to sequentially contract the entire muscle with spontaneous synchronization.

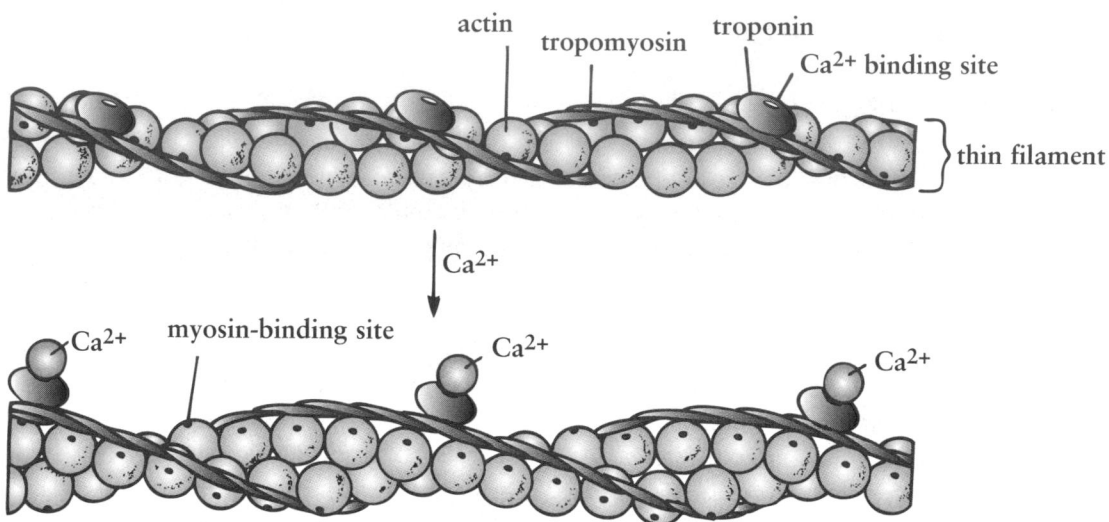

Figure 6.6. Thin Filament

2. Shortening of the Sarcomere

Once an action potential is generated, it is conducted along the sarcolemma and the T system, and into the interior of the muscle fiber. This causes the sarcoplasmic reticulum to release Ca^{2+} into the sarcoplasm. The Ca^{2+} binds to the troponin molecules, causing the tropomyosin strands to shift, thereby exposing the **myosin-binding sites** on the actin filaments (see Figure 6.6).

The free globular heads of the myosin molecules move toward and then bind to the exposed binding sites on the actin molecules, forming actin-myosin cross-bridges. In creating these cross-bridges, the myosin pulls on the actin molecules, drawing the thin filaments toward the center of the H zone and shortening the sarcomere (see Figure 6.7). ATPase activity in the myosin head provides the

> **MCAT Favorite**
>
> When the muscle contracts—the 'H' and 'I' bands are eliminated.

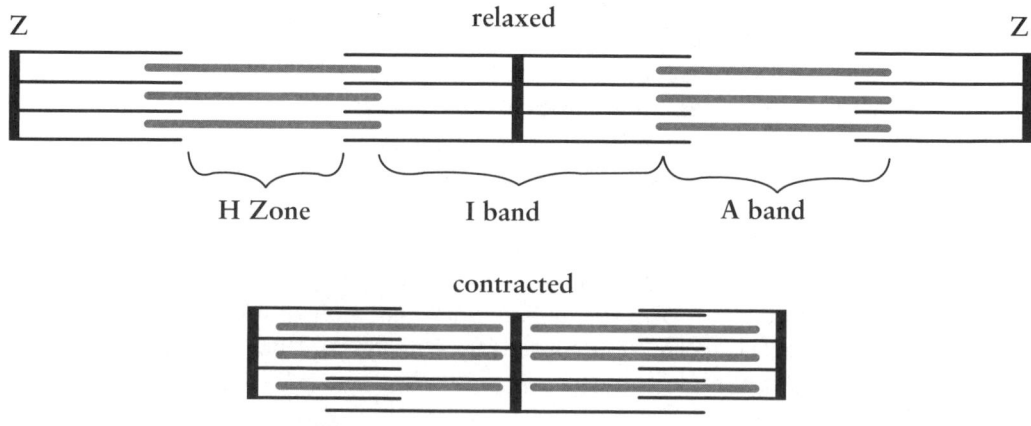

Figure 6.7. Contraction

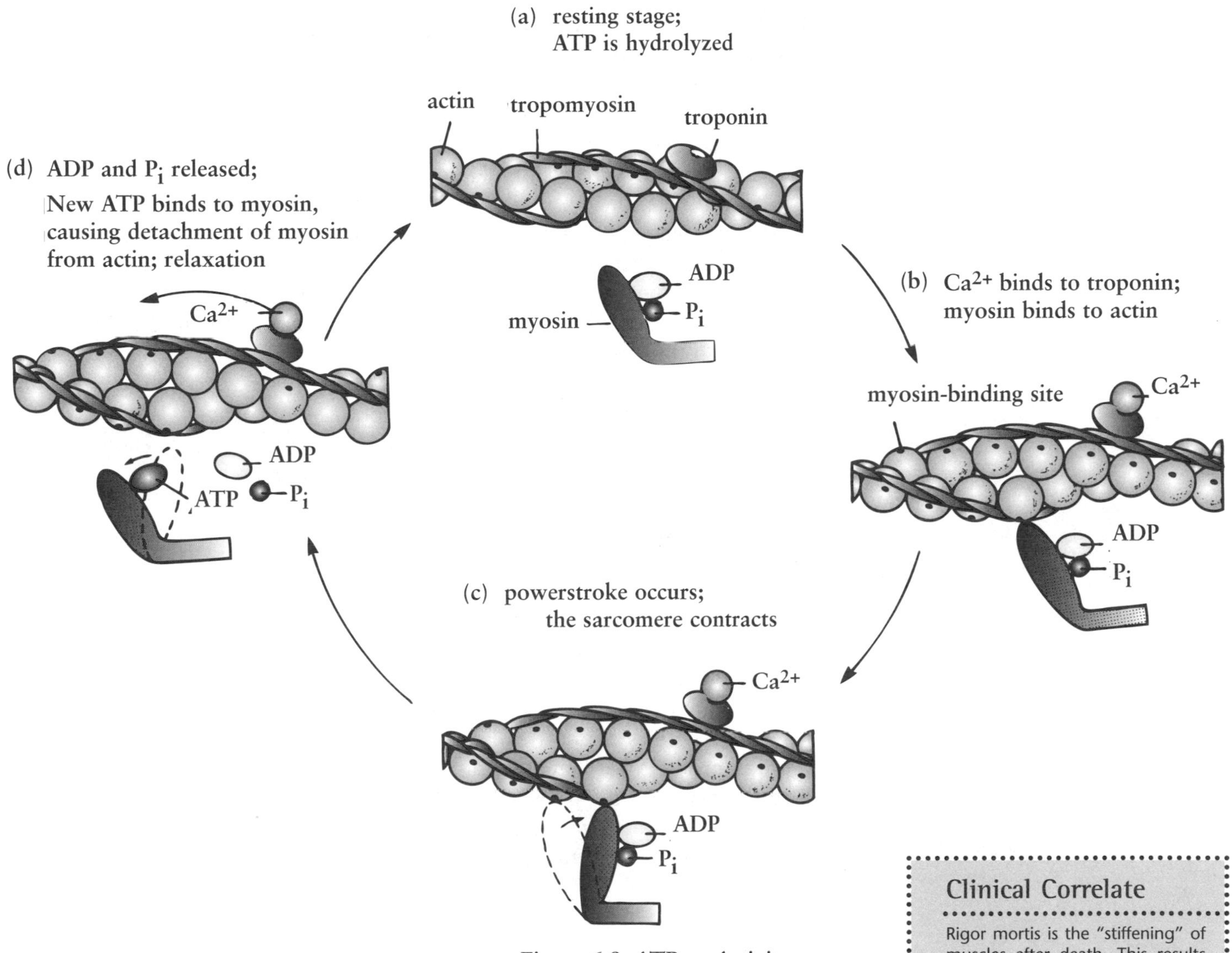

(a) resting stage;
ATP is hydrolyzed

actin   tropomyosin   troponin

(d) ADP and P_i released;
New ATP binds to myosin,
causing detachment of myosin
from actin; relaxation

ADP

myosin — P_i

Ca^{2+}

(b) Ca^{2+} binds to troponin;
myosin binds to actin

myosin-binding site Ca^{2+}

Ca^{2+}

ADP

ATP — P_i

ADP

P_i

(c) powerstroke occurs;
the sarcomere contracts

Ca^{2+}

ADP

P_i

Figure 6.8. ATPase Activity

energy for the powerstroke that results in the dissociation of the myosin head from the actin. (An ATPase is an enzyme that hydrolyzes ATP.) The myosin returns to its original position and is now free to bind to another actin molecule and repeat the process, thus further pulling the thin filaments towards the center of the H zone.

3. **Relaxation**
When the sarcolemmic receptors are no longer stimulated, the Ca^{2+} is pumped back into the sarcoplasmic reticulum. The products of ATP hydrolysis are released from the myosin head, a new ATP binds to the head, resulting in the dissociation of the myosin from the thin filament, and the sarcomere returns to its original width.

C. STIMULUS AND MUSCLE RESPONSE

1. Stimulus Intensity

Individual muscle fibers generally exhibit an **all-or-none response**; only a stimulus above a minimal value called the **threshold value** can elicit contraction. The strength of the contraction of a single muscle fiber cannot be increased, regardless of the strength of the stimulus. Whole muscle, on the other hand, does not exhibit an all-or-none response. Although there is a minimal threshold value needed to elicit a muscle contraction, the strength of the contraction can increase as stimulus strength is increased by involving more fibers. A maximal response is reached when all of the fibers have reached the threshold value and the muscle contracts as a whole.

Tonus refers to the continual low-grade contractions of muscle, which are essential for both voluntary and involuntary muscle contraction. Even at rest, muscles are in a continuous state of tonus.

2. Simple Twitch

A simple twitch is the response of a single muscle fiber to a brief stimulus at or above the threshold stimulus and consists of a **latent period**, a **contraction period**, and a **relaxation period.** The latent period is the time between stimulation and the onset of contraction. During this time lag, the action potential spreads along the sarcolemma and Ca^{2+} ions are released. Following the contraction period, there is a brief relaxation period in which the muscle is unresponsive to a stimulus; this period is known as the **absolute refractory period.** This is followed by a **relative refractory period,** during which a greater-than-normal stimulus is needed to elicit a contraction (see Figure 6.9).

simple twitch (single fiber)   summation and tetanus (whole muscle)

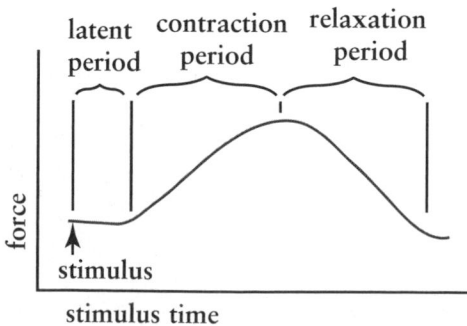
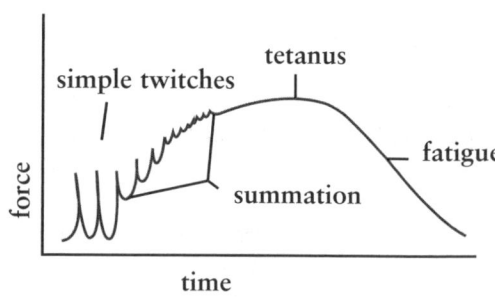

Figure 6.9. Simple Twitch and Summation/Tetanus

3. **Summation and Tetanus**

When the fibers of a muscle are exposed to very frequent stimuli, the muscle cannot fully relax. The contractions begin to combine, becoming stronger and more prolonged. This is known as **frequency summation.** The contractions become continuous when the stimuli are so frequent that the muscle cannot relax. This type of contraction is known as **tetanus** and is stronger than a simple twitch of a single fiber. If tetanization is prolonged, the muscle will begin to fatigue (see Figure 6.9).

SMOOTH MUSCLE

Smooth muscle is responsible for involuntary actions and is innervated by the **autonomic nervous system** (see chapter 12). Smooth muscle is found in the digestive tract, bladder, uterus, and blood vessel walls, among other places. Smooth muscle cells possess one centrally located nucleus. While smooth muscle cells also contain actin and myosin filaments, these filaments lack the organization of skeletal sarcomeres; consequently, smooth muscles lack the striations of skeletal muscle.

As in skeletal muscle, smooth muscle contractions result from the sliding of actin and myosin over one another and are regulated by an influx of calcium ions. However, smooth muscle contractions are slower and are capable of being sustained longer than skeletal muscle contractions. Smooth muscle typically has both inhibitory and excitatory synapses that regulate contraction via the nervous system. Smooth muscle also has the property of reflexively contracting without nervous stimulation; this is called **myogenic** activity.

CARDIAC MUSCLE

The muscle tissue of the heart is composed of cardiac muscle fibers. These fibers possess characteristics of both skeletal and smooth muscle fibers. As in skeletal muscle, actin and myosin filaments are arranged in sarcomeres, giving cardiac muscle a striated appearance. However, cardiac muscle cells generally have only one or two centrally located nuclei. Cardiac muscle is innervated by the autonomic nervous system, which serves only to modulate its inherent beat, since cardiac muscle, like smooth muscle, is myogenic (see chapter 9).

MCAT Synopsis

Skeletal Muscle
- Striated
- Voluntary
- Somatic innervation
- Many nuclei per cell
- Ca^{2+} required for contraction

Cardiac Muscle
- Striated
- Involuntary
- Autonomic innervation
- One to two nuclei per cell
- Ca^{2+} required for contraction

Smooth Muscle
- Non-striated
- Involuntary
- Autonomic innervation
- One nucleus per cell
- Ca^{2+} required for contraction

ENERGY RESERVES

A. CREATINE PHOSPHATE

High-energy compounds, such as fatty acids, glycogen, and glucose, can be degraded in muscle cells to produce ATP. In addition, energy can be temporarily stored in a high-energy compound called **creatine phosphate**. During resting periods, creatine phosphate is produced via a reaction that transfers a high-energy phosphate group from ATP to creatine. During exercise, the reaction proceeds in reverse, resynthesizing ATP from creatine phosphate and ADP, thus replenishing the ATP supply without the need for additional oxygen.

$$\text{creatine + ATP} \rightleftharpoons \text{creatine phosphate + ADP}$$

B. MYOGLOBIN

Myoglobin is a hemoglobin-like protein found in muscle tissue. Myoglobin has a high O_2-affinity; it binds to O_2 from the bloodstream and holds onto it. During strenuous exercise, when muscle cells rapidly run out of available O_2, myoglobin releases its O_2. In this way, myoglobin acts as an additional oxygen reserve for active muscle. However, during strenuous exercise, the oxygen supply to muscles may be insufficient to meet its energy demands, despite the extra O_2 supplied by myoglobin. During this period the muscle obtains additional energy via anaerobic respiration, resulting in the build-up of lactic acid (see chapter 3).

Flashback

Remember, in the absence of oxygen, pyruvate is reduced to lactic acid in the cytoplasm, and the TCA cycle and electron transport chain do not come into play. Lactic acid build-up is responsible for the "feel the burn" stage of vigorous exercise. See chapter 3.

CONNECTIVE TISSUE

The major function of connective tissue is to bind and support other tissue. Connective tissue is a sparsely scattered population of cells contained in an amorphous ground substance which may be liquid, jellylike, or solid. **Loose connective tissue** is found throughout the body. It binds epithelium to underlying tissues and is the packing material that holds organs in place. It contains proteinaceous fibers of three types: **collagenous fibers,** which are composed of collagen and have great tensile strength; **elastic fibers,** which are composed of elastin and endow connective tissue with resilience; and **reticular fibers,** which are branched, tightly woven fibers that join connective tissue to adjoining tissue. There are two major cell types in loose connective tissue: **fibroblasts,** which secrete substances that are components of extracellular fibers, and **macrophages,** which engulf bacteria and dead cells via phagocytosis.

Dense connective tissue is connective tissue with a very high proportion of collagenous fibers. The fibers are organized into parallel bundles that give the fibers great tensile strength. Dense connective tissue forms **tendons,** which attach muscle to bone, and **ligaments,** which hold bones together at the joints.

MUSCLE-BONE INTERACTIONS

Locomotion is dependent on interactions between the skeletal and muscular systems. If a given muscle (including associated joints) is attached to two bones, contraction of the muscle will cause only one of the two bones to move. The end of the muscle attached to the stationary bone is called the **origin;** in limb muscles it corresponds to the **proximal end.** The end of the muscle attached to the bone that moves during contraction is called the **insertion;** in limb muscles, the insertion corresponds to the **distal end.**

Often muscles work in antagonistic pairs; one relaxes while the other contracts. Such is the case in the arm, where the biceps and triceps work antagonistically. When you move your hand toward your shoulder, the biceps contract and the triceps relax; when you move your hand down again, the biceps relax and the triceps contract (see Figure 6.10). There are also **synergistic muscles,** which assist the principal muscles during movement.

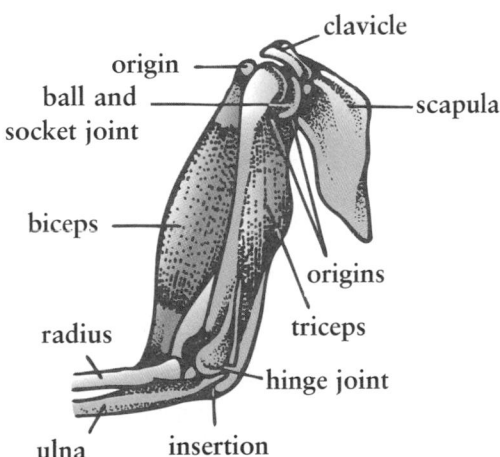

Figure 6.10. Muscles of the Upper Arm

A **flexor** muscle will contract to decrease the angle of a joint, whereas an **extensor muscle** will contract to straighten the joint. An **abductor** moves a part of the body away from the body's midline; an **adductor** moves a part of the body toward the midline.

7

DIGESTION

Digestion consists of the degradation of large molecules into smaller molecules that can be absorbed into the bloodstream and used directly by cells. **Intracellular digestion** occurs within the cell, usually in membrane-bound vesicles. **Extracellular digestion** refers to a digestive process that occurs outside of the cell, within a lumen or tract. Mammals have a one-way digestive tract known as the **alimentary canal.** Mammalian digestive tracts tend to be complex and are organized into regions specialized for the digestion and absorption of specific nutrients.

The human digestive tract begins with the **oral cavity** and continues with the **pharynx,** the **esophagus,** the **stomach,** the **small intestine,** and the **large intestine** (see Figure 7.1). Accessory organs, such as the **salivary glands,** the **pancreas,** the **liver,** and the **gall bladder,** also play essential roles in the digestive process.

Most body surfaces (e.g., the skin and lungs, and the linings of the nose, mouth, esophagus, stomach, and intestines) are covered or lined by continuous sheets of epithelial cells. Epithelial cells are joined tightly together, facilitating their ability to act as a barrier against mechanical injury, invading organisms, and fluid loss. The free surface of epithelium is exposed to air or liquid and may be ciliated. The inner surface is attached to underlying connective tissue by a **basement membrane.**

THE ORAL CAVITY

The oral cavity (the mouth) is where mechanical and chemical digestion of food begins. Mechanical digestion is the breakdown of large food particles into smaller particles through the biting and chewing action of teeth (mastication). While mechanical digestion does not lead to changes in the molecular composition of food, the total surface area of the food is increased, allowing for faster and more efficient enzymatic action. **Chemical digestion** refers to the enzymatic breakdown of macromolecules into smaller molecules and begins in the

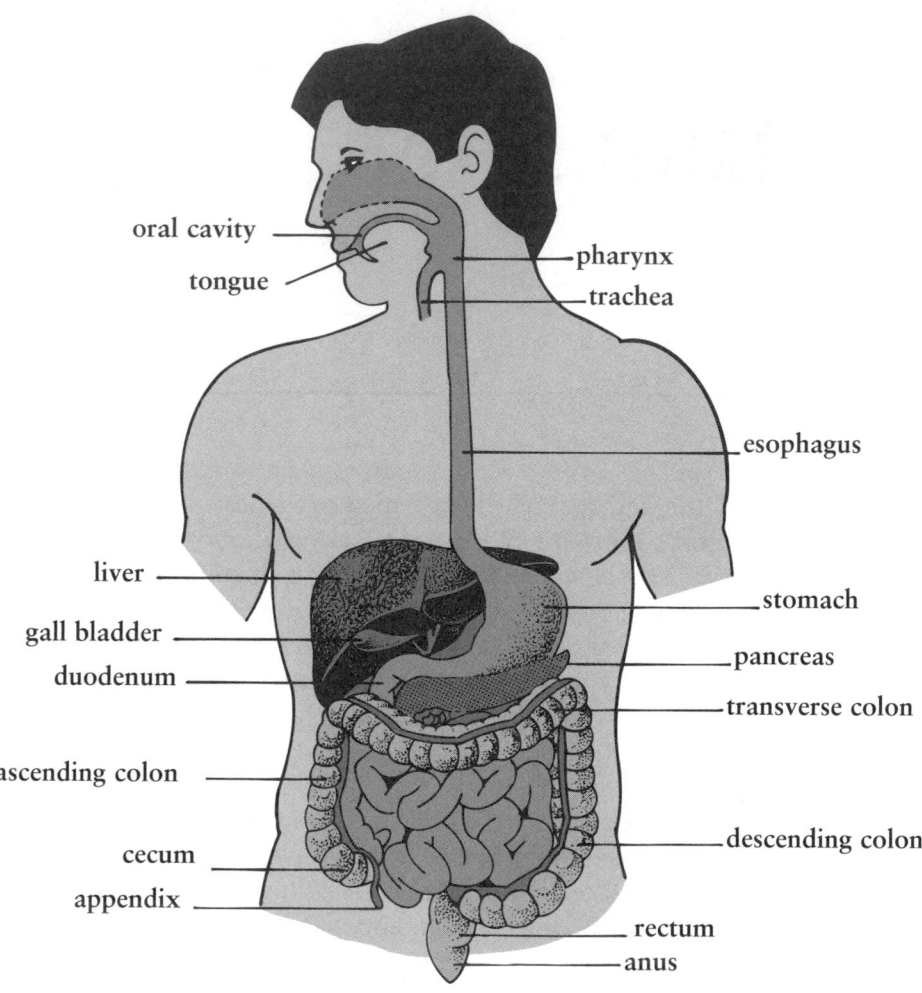

Figure 7.1. Human Digestive Tract

mouth when the salivary glands secrete saliva. Saliva lubricates food to facilitate swallowing and provides a solvent for food particles. Saliva is secreted in response to a nervous reflex triggered by the presence of food in the oral cavity. Saliva contains the enzyme salivary amylase (ptyalin), which hydrolyzes starch into simple sugars. However, since food does not remain in the mouth for long, only a small portion of starch is hydrolyzed there. The muscular tongue, containing the taste buds, manipulates the food, rolls it into a ball called a bolus, and pushes the bolus into the pharynx.

THE PHARYNX

The pharynx is the cavity that leads food from the mouth into the esophagus. The pharynx also functions in respiration as the passageway through which air enters the trachea. During swallowing, the opening of the trachea is covered by a flap called the **epiglottis,** thereby preventing food particles from being aspirated into the lungs.

THE ESOPHAGUS

The esophagus is the muscular tube leading from the pharynx to the stomach. Food is moved down the esophagus by rhythmic waves of involuntary muscular contractions called **peristalsis.** When a wave of peristalsis spreads down the esophagus, a specialized ring of muscle in the lower esophagus opens, allowing food to enter the stomach. Following the peristaltic wave, this muscle, called the **lower esophageal sphincter** or **cardiac sphincter,** returns to its normal closed state, thus preventing the regurgitation of stomach contents into the esophagus.

THE STOMACH

The stomach, a large, muscular organ located in the upper abdomen, stores and partially digests food. The walls of the stomach are lined by the thick gastric mucosa, which contains the **gastric glands** and **pyloric glands.** The gastric glands are stimulated by nervous impulses from the brain, which responds to the sight, taste, and/or smell of food. The gastric glands are composed of three types of secretory cells: **mucous cells, chief cells,** and **parietal cells.** Mucous cells secrete mucus, which protects the stomach lining from the harshly acidic juices (pH = 2) present in the stomach. **Gastric juice** is composed of the secretions of the chief cells and the parietal cells. Chief cells secrete **pepsinogen,** the zymogen of the protein-hydrolyzing enzyme **pepsin.** The chief cells also secrete intrinsic factor which plays a role in the absorption of vitamin B12. Parietal cells secrete **hydrochloric acid (HCl).** HCl kills bacteria, dissolves the intercellular "glue" holding food tissues together, and facilitates the conversion of pepsinogen to pepsin. Pepsin hydrolyzes specific peptide bonds to yield polypeptide fragments. The pyloric glands secrete the hormone **gastrin** in response to the presence of certain substances in food. Gastrin stimulates the gastric glands to secrete more HCl and also stimulates muscular contractions of the stomach, which churn food. This churning produces an acidic, semifluid mixture of partially digested food known as **chyme.**

At the junction of the stomach and the small intestine is the muscular **pyloric sphincter,** which regulates the passage of chyme from the stomach into the small intestine via alternating contractions and relaxations. Although nutrient absorption occurs in the small intestine, alcohol and certain drugs (e.g., aspirin) can be directly absorbed into the systemic circulation through capillaries in the stomach wall.

THE SMALL INTESTINE

Chemical digestion is completed in the small intestine. The small intestine is divided into three sections: the **duodenum,** the **jejunum,** and the **ileum.** In order to maximize the surface area available for digestion and absorption, the intestine is extremely long (greater than six meters in length) and highly coiled. In addition, numerous fingerlike projections called **villi** extend out of the intestinal submucosa, and tiny cytoplasmic projections called **microvilli** project from the surface of the individual cells lining the villi (see Figure 7.2). The total surface area of the small intestine is approximately 300 m^2.

A. DIGESTIVE FUNCTIONS

Most digestion in the small intestine occurs in the duodenum, where the secretions of the intestinal glands, pancreas, liver, and gall bladder mix together with the acidic chyme entering from the stomach. The presence of chyme triggers hormonal release, which in turn stimulates and regulates the secretions of the small intestine and its accessory organs.

The intestinal mucosa secretes enzymes that hydrolyze carbohydrates into monosaccharides, such as **maltase, lactase**, and **sucrase**, and **peptidases**, which hydrolyze dipeptides and oligo peptides. The hormone **secretin** is

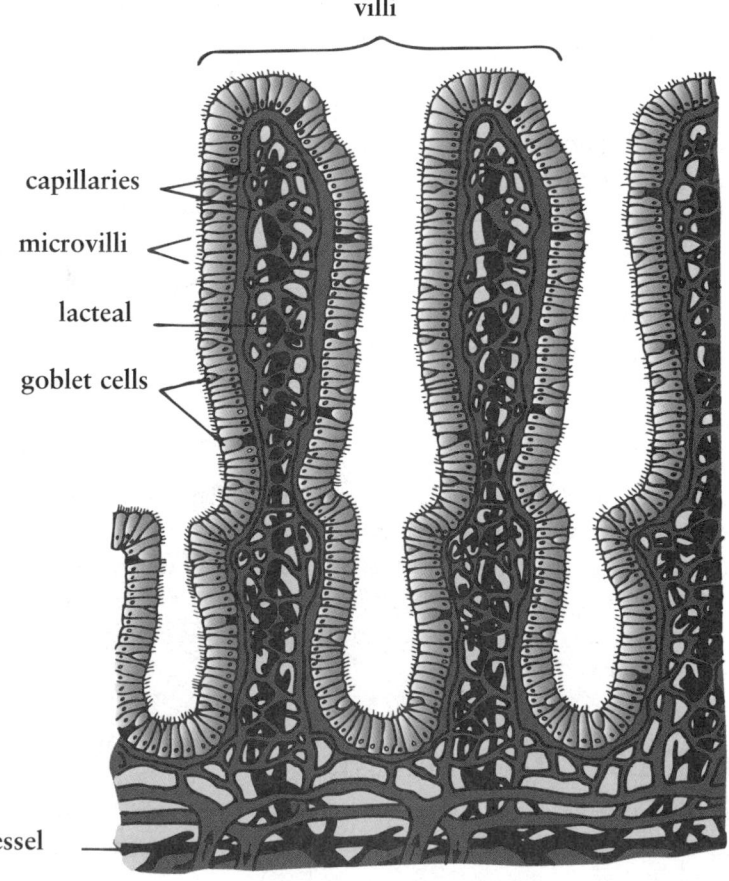

Figure 7.2. Intestinal Villi

villi

capillaries

microvilli

lacteal

goblet cells

lymphatic vessel

released by the duodenum in response to the acidity of chyme, stimulating the pancreas to secrete **pancreatic juice.** The enzymes of the small intestine function optimally at a slightly basic pH and are denatured by acid; pancreatic juice is an alkaline fluid (due to a high concentration of bicarbonate) that helps neutralize the acidity of chyme and contains enzymes that digest carbohydrates, proteins, and lipids. **Trypsinogen** is a proteolytic zymogen secreted by the pancreas and is converted to its active form, **trypsin,** by an enzyme called **enterokinase** (secreted by the intestinal glands). Trypsin then converts another pancreatic zymogen, **chymotrypsinogen,** to its active form, **chymotrypsin.** Each of these enzymes cleaves specific peptide bonds within proteins, producing polypeptide fragments. The pancreas also secretes **carboxypeptidase** (also secreted as a zymogen and activated by trypsin). Proteolytic enzymes in the pancreatic juice break down proteins into dipeptides and oligopeptides. Then, similar to the hydrolysis of carbohydrates, the intestinal mucosa breaks these compounds into amino acids by secreting amino peptidase.

The hormone **CCK (cholecystokinin)** is secreted into the bloodstream by the duodenum in response to the presence of chyme. CCK stimulates the secretion of pancreatic enzymes and the release of **bile.** Bile is an alkaline fluid synthesized and secreted by the liver, stored and concentrated in the gall bladder, and released into the duodenum. Bile is composed of bile salts, bile pigments, and cholesterol. Bile salts are molecules with a water-soluble region on one end and a fat-soluble region on the other. This structure, similar to that of detergents, allows bile salts to emulsify, i.e. dissolve, fat globules and to surround and maintain these particles in finely dispersed complexes called **micelles,** which are soluble in aqueous media. This process is called the **emulsification** of fat and exposes more of the lipids' surface area to the actions of **lipases,** which hydrolyze molecules of fat into glycerol and fatty acids. The amount of bile released is proportional to the amount of fat ingested. If the chyme is particularly fatty, the duodenum releases the hormone **enterogastrone,** which inhibits stomach peristalsis, thus slowing down the release of chyme into the small intestine (fats take a longer time to digest than the other macromolecules).

In addition to hormonal regulation, the digestive processes are also stimulated by the **parasympathetic nervous system** and inhibited by the **sympathetic nervous system** (See chapter 12).

B. ABSORPTIVE FUNCTIONS

The majority of nutrient absorption occurs across the walls of the jejunum and the ileum (a small amount of absorption occurs in the duodenum). Monosaccharides are absorbed via active transport and facilitated diffusion into the epithelial cells lining the villi; amino acids are absorbed into the

> **Clinical Correlate**
>
> Lactose intolerance results from the absence of lactase. Hence, lactose passes to the colon undigested. This results in the symptoms experienced by those with this deficiency.

> **MCAT Synopsis**
>
> We've now reviewed two important "good" functions of cholesterol: contributor to the fluidity of cell membranes (chapter 1) and key component of bile. More to come...

epithelium via active transport. Monosaccharides, amino acids, and small fatty acids diffuse directly into the intestinal capillaries and enter portal circulation via the **hepatic portal vein.** Larger fatty acids, glycerol, and cholesterol diffuse into the mucosal cells; the fatty acids and glycerol recombine to form triglycerides, which, along with phosphoglycerides and cholesterol, are packaged into protein-coated droplets called **chylomicrons.** The chylomicrons are secreted into tiny lymph vessels within the villi called **lacteals,** which lead into the lymphatic system; the lymphatic system converges with venous blood at the thoracic duct located in the neck. The chylomicrons are processed in the bloodstream and delivered to the liver. They are repackaged there and released into the bloodstream as LDLs, VLDLs, and HDLs (lipoproteins or proteins complexed with lipids).

Vitamins and minerals are also absorbed in the small intestine. The fat-soluble vitamins (A, D, E, and K) are absorbed along with fats, and most water-soluble vitamins (e.g., the vitamin B complexes and vitamin C) are absorbed via simple diffusion into the circulatory system. Approximately seven liters of fluid enter the small intestine every day; the majority of it is absorbed through the walls of the small intestine.

THE LARGE INTESTINE

The large intestine is approximately 1.5 m long and consists of six parts: the **cecum,** the **ascending colon, transverse colon, descending colon, sismoid colon,** and the **rectum.** The cecum is a blind outpocketing at the junction of the small and large intestines. At the tip of the cecum is a small, fingerlike projection called the **appendix.** The appendix is a **vestigial structure** (see chapter 15) containing lymphoid tissue that is often surgically removed if it becomes infected. The colon functions in the absorption of salts and the absorption of any water not already absorbed by the small intestine. If digested matter moves through the colon too quickly, too little water is absorbed, causing diarrhea and dehydration. Alternatively, if movement through the bowels is too slow, too much water is absorbed, causing constipation. The rectum stores **feces,** which consist of bacteria (particularly **E. coli**), water, undigested food, and unabsorbed digestive secretions (e.g., enzymes and bile). The **anus** is the opening through which wastes are eliminated and is separated from the rectum by two sphincters that regulate elimination.

Table 7.1. Digestive Enzymes

Nutrient	Enzyme	Site of Production	Site of Function	Function
Carbohydrates	Salivary amylase (Ptyalin)	Salivary glands	Mouth	Hydrolyzes starch to maltose
	Pancreatic amylase	Pancreas	Small intestine	Hydrolyzes starch to maltose
	Maltase	Intestinal glands	Small intestine	Hydrolyzes maltose to two glucose molecules
	Sucrase	Intestinal glands	Small intestine	Hydrolyzes sucrose to glucose and fructose
	Lactase	Intestinal glands	Small intestine	Hydrolyzes lactose to glucose and galactose
Proteins	Pepsin (secreted as pepsinogen)	Gastric glands	Stomach	Hydrolyzes specific peptide bonds
	Trypsin (secreted as trypsinogen)	Pancreas	Small intestine	Hydrolyzes specific peptide bonds Converts chymotrypsinogen to chymotrypsin
	Chymotrypsin (secreted as chymotrypsinogen)	Pancreas	Small intestine	Hydrolyzes specific peptide bonds
	Carboxypeptidase	Pancreas	Small intestine	Hydrolyzes terminal peptide bond at carboxyl end
	Aminopeptidase	Intestinal glands	Small intestine	Hydrolyzes terminal peptide bond at amino end
	Dipeptidases	Intestinal glands	Small intestine	Hydrolyzes pairs of amino acids
	Enterokinase	Intestinal glands	Small intestine	Converts trypsinogen to trypsin
Lipids	Bile*	Liver	Small intestine	Emulsifies fat
	Lipase	Pancreas	Small intestine	Hydrolyzes lipids

* Note that bile is NOT an enzyme.

ACCESSORY ORGANS

A. LIVER

The liver has many functions such as storage of glycogen, gluconeogenesis, conversion of ammonia to urea, lipid metabolism, synthesis of the majority of proteins in the human blood stream, detoxification of drugs and their metabolites in the blood stream, and production and secretion of bile into the gastrointestinal tract to emulsify fats.

B. GALLBLADDER

The gall bladder is primarily responsible for the storage and secretion of excess bile.

C. PANCREAS

The pancreas has both exocrine and endocrine function. The endocrine function of the pancreas arises from its production of insulin and glucagons, and somatostatin primarily relates to glucose metabolism. In contrast, the exocrine function of the pancreas refers to its secretions of bicarbonate and digestive enzymes such as trypsin, chymotrypsin, enterokinase, amylase, and lipase into the small intestine for digestion.

SUMMARY OF DIGESTION

Digestion begins in different parts of the digestive tract for each of the three classes of macromolecules. Carbohydrate digestion begins in the mouth; protein digestion begins in the stomach; and lipid digestion begins in the small intestine. Table 7.1 is a summary of the digestive enzymes.

8

RESPIRATION

Respiration is a broad term referring to the exchange of gases between an organism and its external environment, the transport of these gases within the organism, and the diffusion of gases into and out of cells. (Cellular respiration, discussed in chapter 3, refers to the role that these gases play in generating energy at the cellular level.) Aerobic organisms exchange CO_2 generated during cellular respiration for O_2 obtained from the external environment. Higher vertebrates have developed respiratory systems whereby gas exchange occurs at a single **respiratory surface**, the **lungs**.

ANATOMY

In the human respiratory system, air enters the lungs after traveling through a series of respiratory airways, as outlined in Figure 8.1. Air enters the respiratory tract through the **external nares** (nostrils) and then travels through the nasal cavities, where it is filtered by mucous and nasal hairs. It then passes through the pharynx and into a second chamber called the **larynx.** Ingested food also passes through the pharynx en route to the esophagus. To ensure that food does not accidentally enter the larynx and induce choking, a piece of tissue called the epiglottis covers the glottis (the opening to the larynx) during swallowing, thereby channeling food into the esophagus (see chapter 7). Air passes from the larynx into the cartilaginous **trachea,** which divides into two bronchi, one entering the right lung, the other entering the left. Both the trachea and bronchi are lined by ciliated epithelial cells, which filter and trap particles inhaled along with the air. The bronchi repeatedly branch into smaller bronchi, the terminal branches of which are called **bronchioles.** Each bronchiole is surrounded by clusters of small air sacs called **alveoli.** Gas exchange between the lungs and the circulatory system occurs across the very thin walls of the alveoli. Each alveolus is coated with a thin layer of liquid containing **surfactant** and is surrounded by an extensive network of capillaries. Surfactant lowers the surface tension of the alveoli and facilitates gas exchange across the membranes. Three hundred million alveoli provide approximately 100 m^2 of moist respiratory surface for gas exchange.

Following gas exchange, air rushes back through the respiratory pathway and is exhaled.

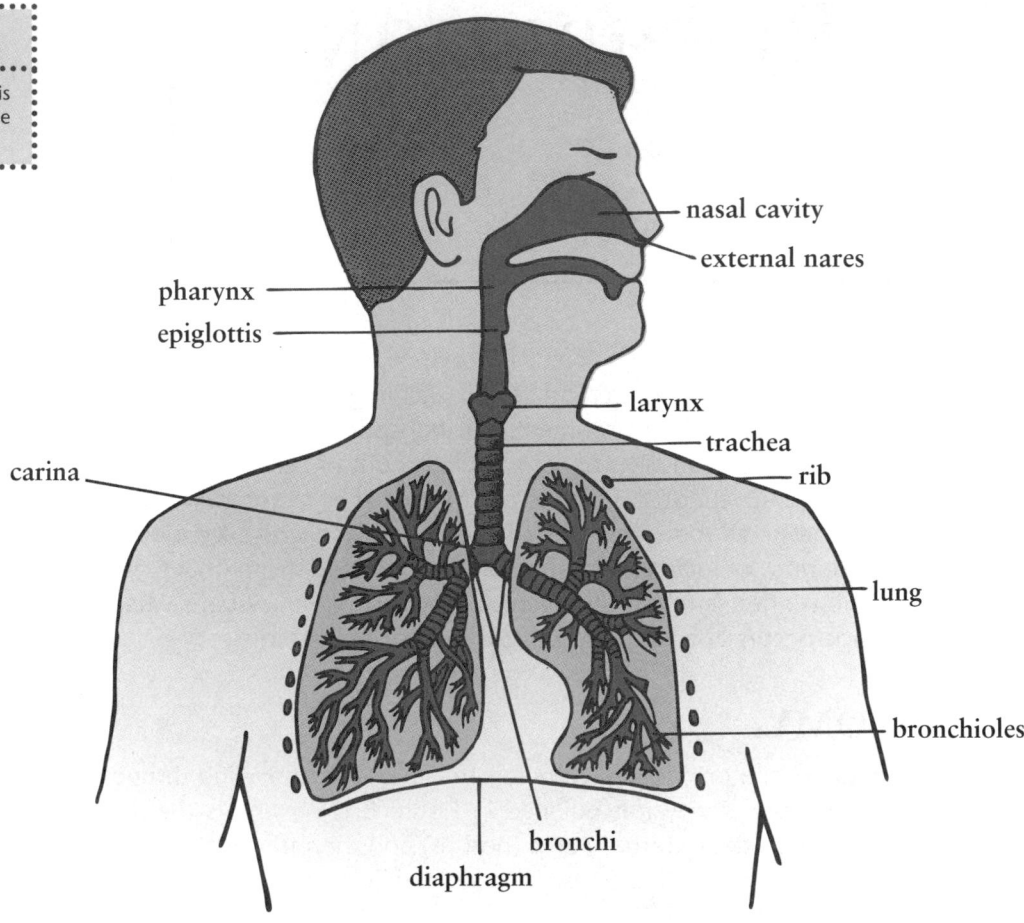

Figure 8.1. Respiratory System

VENTILATION

Ventilation of the lungs (breathing) is the process by which air is inhaled and exhaled. The purpose of ventilation is to take in oxygen from the atmosphere and eliminate carbon dioxide from the body. The ventilating mechanism is dependent upon pressure changes in the **thoracic cavity,** the body cavity that contains the heart and lungs. The thoracic cavity is separated from the abdominal cavity by a muscle known as the **diaphragm** and is bounded on the sides by the chest wall. The lungs are surrounded by membranes called the **visceral pleura** and the **parietal pleura**. The space between the two pleura, the **intrapleural space,** contains a thin layer of fluid (see Figure 8.2). The pressure differential between the intrapleural space and the lungs (which is essentially atmospheric pressure) prevents the lungs from collapsing.

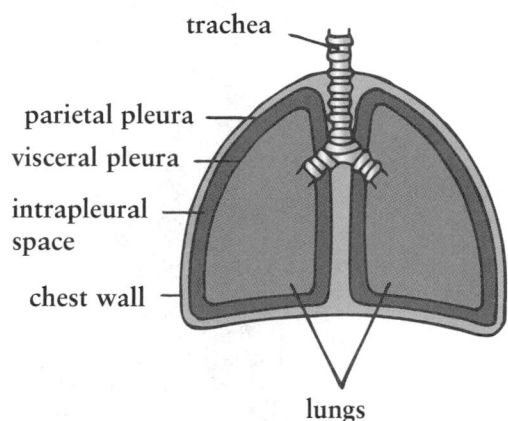

trachea

parietal pleura

visceral pleura

intrapleural space

chest wall

lungs

Figure 8.2. Thoracic Cavity (neutral position)

A. STAGES OF VENTILATION

1. Inhalation

During inhalation, the diaphragm contracts and flattens, and the **external intercostal muscles** contract, pushing the rib cage and chest wall up and out. This causes the thoracic cavity to increase in volume. This volume increase, in turn, reduces the intrapleural pressure, causing the lungs to expand and fill with air. This is referred to as **negative-pressure breathing** because air is drawn in by a vacuum.

2. Exhalation

Exhalation is generally a passive process. The lungs and chest wall are highly elastic and tend to recoil to their original positions following inhalation. The diaphragm and external intercostal muscles relax and the chest wall pushes inward. The consequent decrease in thoracic cavity volume causes the air pressure in the intrapleural space to increase. This causes the lungs to deflate, forcing air out of the alveoli. During forced exhalation, the **internal intercostal muscles** contract, pulling the rib cage down. Surfactant reduces the high surface tension of the fluid lining the alveoli, preventing alveolar collapse during exhalation.

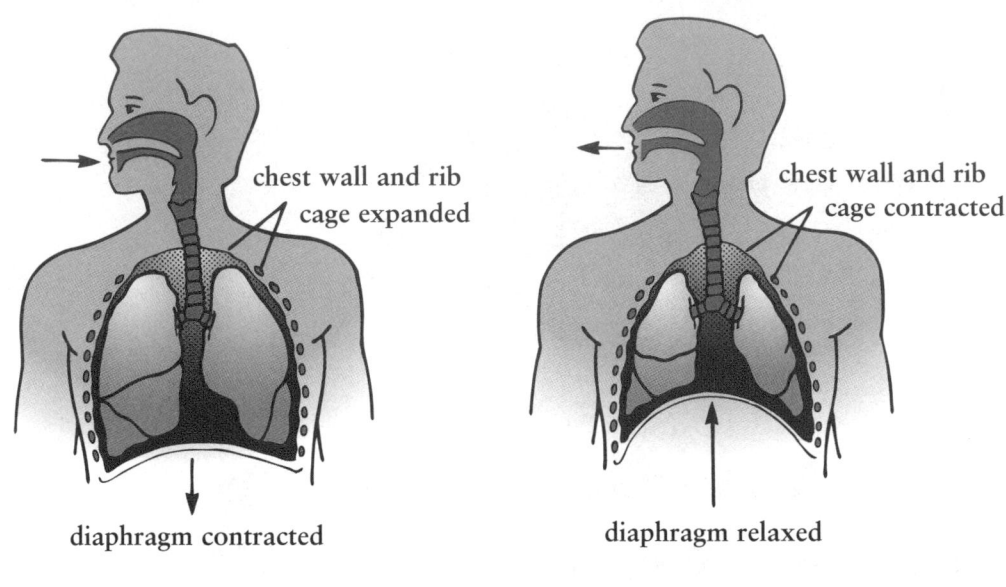

chest wall and rib cage expanded

chest wall and rib cage contracted

diaphragm contracted

diaphragm relaxed

inhalation

exhalation

Figure 8.3. Ventilation

B. CONTROL OF VENTILATION

Ventilation is regulated by neurons (referred to as **respiratory centers**) located in the **medulla oblongata,** whose rhythmic discharges stimulate the intercostal muscles and/or the diaphragm to contract. These neural signals can be modified by **chemoreceptors** (e.g., in the aorta), which respond to changes in the pH and the partial pressure of CO_2 in the blood. For example, when the partial pressure of CO_2 rises, the medulla oblongata stimulates an increase in the rate of ventilation.

To a limited extent, ventilation can be consciously controlled by the cerebrum. However, if a person tries to hold his breath indefinitely, the high concentration of CO_2 in the blood will stimulate the medulla oblongata to "override" this conscious attempt and stimulate inhalation. Hyperventilation (deep, rapid breathing) lowers the partial pressure of CO_2 in the blood below normal; chemoreceptors sense this and send signals to the respiratory center, which temporarily inhibits breathing.

LUNG CAPACITIES AND VOLUMES

An instrument called a **spirometer** measures the amount of air normally present in the respiratory system and the rate at which ventilation occurs. The maximum amount of air that can be forcibly inhaled and exhaled from the lungs is called the **vital capacity.** The amount of air normally inhaled and exhaled with each breath is called the **tidal volume.** The residual volume is the air that always remains in the lungs, preventing the alveoli from collapsing. The **expiratory reserve volume** is the volume of air that can still be forcibly exhaled following a normal exhalation (see Figure 8.4). **Total lung capacity** is equal to the vital capacity plus the residual volume.

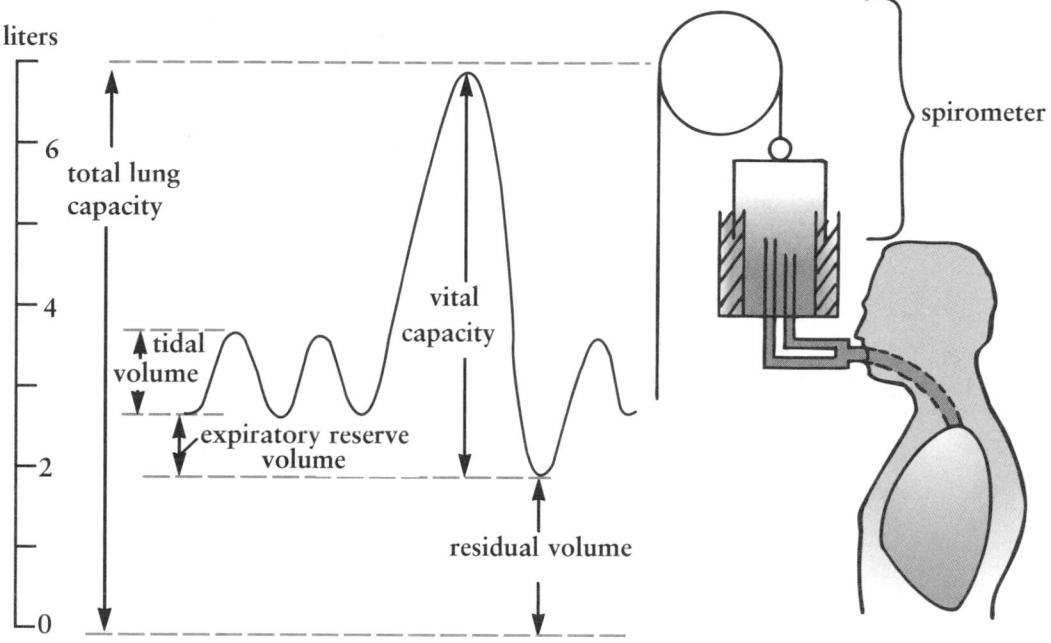

Figure 8.4. Spirometer

GAS EXCHANGE

A dense network of minute blood vessels called the pulmonary capillaries surrounds the alveoli. Gas exchange occurs by diffusion across these capillary walls and those of the alveoli; gases move from regions of higher partial pressure to regions of lower partial pressure. Blood enters the pulmonary capillaries in a deoxygenated state and thus has a lower partial pressure of O_2 than does the inhaled air in the alveoli. Hence, O_2 diffuses down its gradient into the capillaries where it binds with hemoglobin and returns to the heart via the pulmonary veins. In contrast, the partial pressure of CO_2 in the capillaries is greater than that of the inhaled alveolar air; thus CO_2 diffuses from the capillaries into the alveoli, where it is subsequently released into the external environment during exhalation (see Figure 8.5).

> **MCAT Synopsis**
>
> O_2 in the alveoli flows down its partial pressure gradient from the alveoli into the pulmonary capillaries where it can bind to hemoglobin for transport. Meanwhile, CO_2 flows down its partial pressure gradient from the capillaries into the alveoli for expiration.

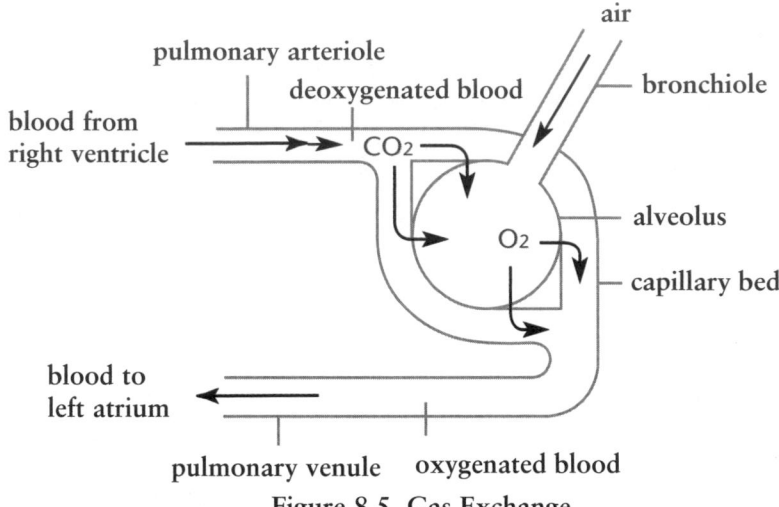

Figure 8.5. Gas Exchange

At high altitudes, the partial pressure of O_2 in the atmosphere declines, making it more difficult to get sufficient oxygen to diffuse into the capillaries. The body can compensate for these conditions in a variety of ways, such as by increasing the rate of ventilation (hyperventilation) and by increasing the production of red blood cells to carry more oxygen (polycythemia). In addition, the affinity of hemoglobin for oxygen decreases to facilitate unloading of oxygen in tissues, and there is greater vascularization of the peripheral tissues.

9

CIRCULATION

Higher organisms rely on a complex **cardiovascular system** to transport respiratory gases, nutrients, and wastes to and from cells. A secondary circulatory system, the **lymphatic system,** collects excess body fluids and returns them to the cardiovascular circulation.

THE CARDIOVASCULAR SYSTEM

The human cardiovascular system is composed of a muscular four-chambered **heart**, a network of **blood vessels,** and the **blood** itself. The right side of the heart pumps deoxygenated blood into the lungs via the pulmonary arteries. Oxygenated blood returns from the lungs to the left side of the heart via the pulmonary veins. It is then pumped into the **aorta,** which branches into a series of arteries. The arteries branch into arterioles, and then into microscopic capillaries. Exchange of gases, nutrients, and cellular waste products occurs via diffusion across capillary walls. The capillaries then converge into venules, and eventually into veins, leading deoxygenated blood back toward the right side of the heart. Blood returning from the lower body and extremities enters the heart via the **inferior vena cava,** while deoxygenated blood from the upper head and neck region flows through the **jugular vein** and into the **superior vena cava,** which also leads into the right atrium of the heart. The blood then flows to the right ventricle through the tricuspid valve. From the right ventricle, the blood goes to the pulmonary artery and is pumped to the lungs to be oxygenated (see chapter 8). The blood then returns from the lungs to the left atrium via the pulmonary veins. The left atrium then pumps the blood to the left ventricle through the mitral valve. Finally, the blood enters systemic circulation as it enters the aorta from the left ventricle. Oxygenated blood is supplied to heart muscle by the **coronary arteries.** The first branches off the aorta; **the coronary veins** and **coronary sinus** return deoxygenated blood to the right side of the heart.

In systemic circulation there are three special circulatory routes, referred to as **portal systems,** in which blood travels through *two* capillary beds before returning to the heart. There is a portal system in the liver (hepatic portal circulation), in the kidneys (see chapter 10), and in the brain (hypophyseal portal circulation; see chapter 11).

A. THE HEART

The heart is the driving force of the circulatory system. The right and left halves can be viewed as two separate pumps: The right side of the heart pumps deoxygenated blood into pulmonary circulation (toward the lungs), while the left side pumps oxygenated blood into systemic circulation (throughout the body). The two upper chambers are called **atria** and the two lower chambers are called ventricles. The atria are thin-walled,

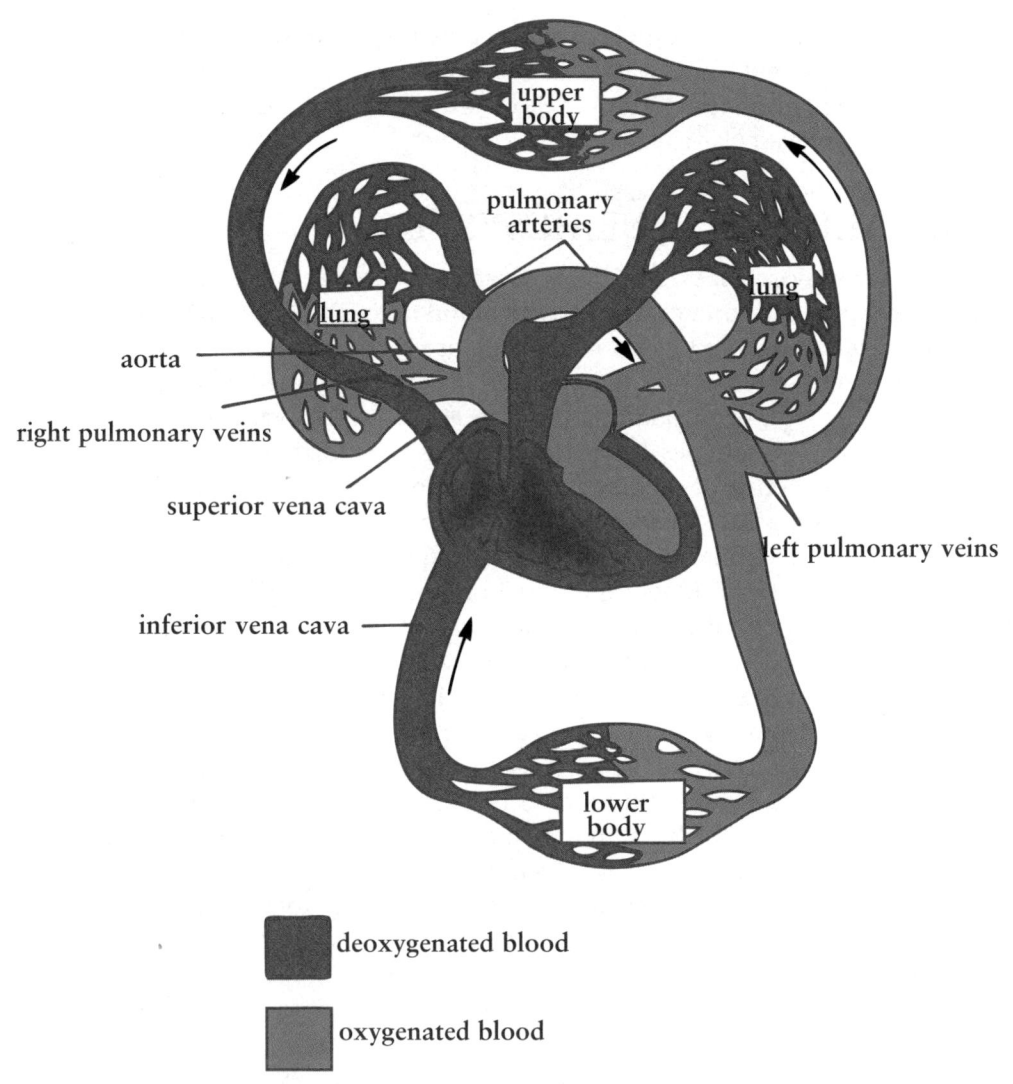

Figure 9.1. Circulation

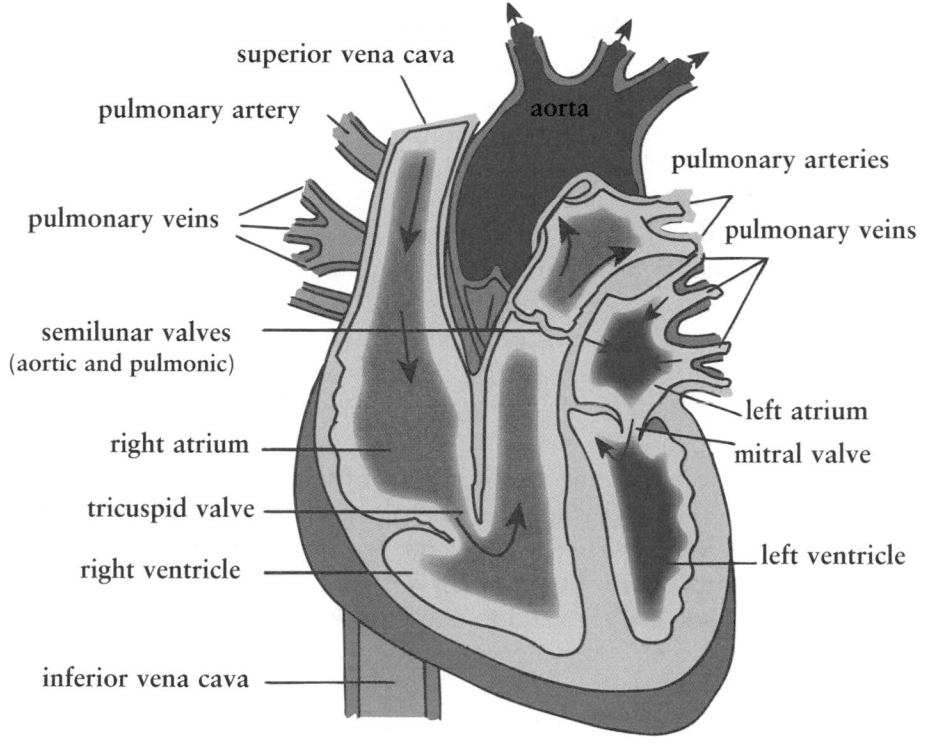

superior vena cava

pulmonary artery

aorta

pulmonary arteries

pulmonary veins

pulmonary veins

semilunar valves
(aortic and pulmonic)

left atrium

right atrium

mitral valve

tricuspid valve

right ventricle

left ventricle

inferior vena cava

Figure 9.2. Human Heart

MCAT Synopsis

Blood Flow

Superior and inferior vena cavae
↓
Right atrium
↓
Right ventricle
↓
Pulmonary artery
↓
Lungs
↓
Pulmonary veins
↓
Left atrium
↓
Left ventricle
↓
Aorta

while the **ventricles** are extremely muscular. The left ventricle is more muscular than the right ventricle because it is responsible for generating the force that propels systemic circulation and because it pumps against a higher resistance.

1. **Valves**

   The **atrioventricular valves**, located between the atria and ventricles on both sides of the heart, prevent backflow of blood into the atria. The valve on the right side of the heart has three cusps and is called the **tricuspid valve.** The valve on the left side of the heart has two cusps and is called the **mitral valve.** The **semilunar valves** have three cusps and are located between the left ventricle and the aorta (the aortic valve) and between the right ventricle and the pulmonary artery (the pulmonic valve).

2. **Contraction**

   a. **Phases**

   The heart's pumping cycle is divided into two alternating phases, **systole** and **diastole,** which together make up the **heartbeat.** Systole is the period during which the ventricles contract. Diastole is the period of cardiac muscle relaxation during which blood drains into all four chambers. **Cardiac output** is defined as

Clinical Correlate

The "lub dubs" you hear when you listen to someone's heart with a stethoscope are referred to as the heart sounds. The first heart sound, S1, is produced when the two atrioventricular valves close at the start of systole. (Those valves must close so that the blood flows out of the heart instead of back up into the atria). The second heart sound, S2, is produced when the two semilunar valves close at the conclusion of systole. (If they didn't close at that point, blood would flow back into the ventricles.)

the total volume of blood the left ventricle pumps out per minute. Cardiac output = **heart rate** (number of heartbeats per minute) × **stroke volume** (volume of blood pumped out of the left ventricle per contraction).

b. **Mechanism and control**

Cardiac muscle (see chapter 6) contracts rhythmically without stimulation from the nervous system, producing impulses that spread through its internal conducting system. An ordinary cardiac contraction originates in, and is regulated by, the **sinoatrial (SA) node** (the **pacemaker**), a small mass of specialized tissue located in the wall of the right atrium. The SA node spreads impulses through both atria, stimulating them to contract simultaneously. The impulse arrives at the **atrioventricular (AV) node,** which conducts slowly, allowing enough time for atrial contraction and for the ventricles to fill with blood. The impulse is then carried by the **bundle of His (AV bundle),** which branches into the right and left bundle branches and through the **Purkinje fibers** in the walls of both ventricles, generating a strong contraction.

The **autonomic nervous system** (see chapter 12) modifies the rate of heart contraction. The parasympathetic system innervates the heart via the **vagus nerve** and causes a decrease in the heart rate. The sympathetic system innervates the heart via the cervical and upper thoracic ganglia and causes an increase in the heart rate.

Clinical Correlate

The heart's electrical impulses can be detected on the body's surface by placing electrodes on the skin on opposite sides of the heart. A recording of these currents is called an electrocardiogram (a.k.a., ECG or EKG). Electrocardiograms are incredibly powerful tools for assessing the status of a patient's heart. A normal EKG is shown below.

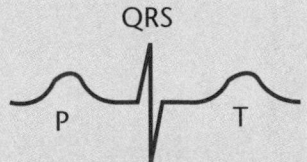

Since depolarization will precede cardiac muscle contraction, the electrical spokes of the EKG occur just before a cardiac contractile event. The P wave occurs immediately before the atria contract and the QRS complex occurs just before the ventricles contract. The T wave represents ventricular repolarization.

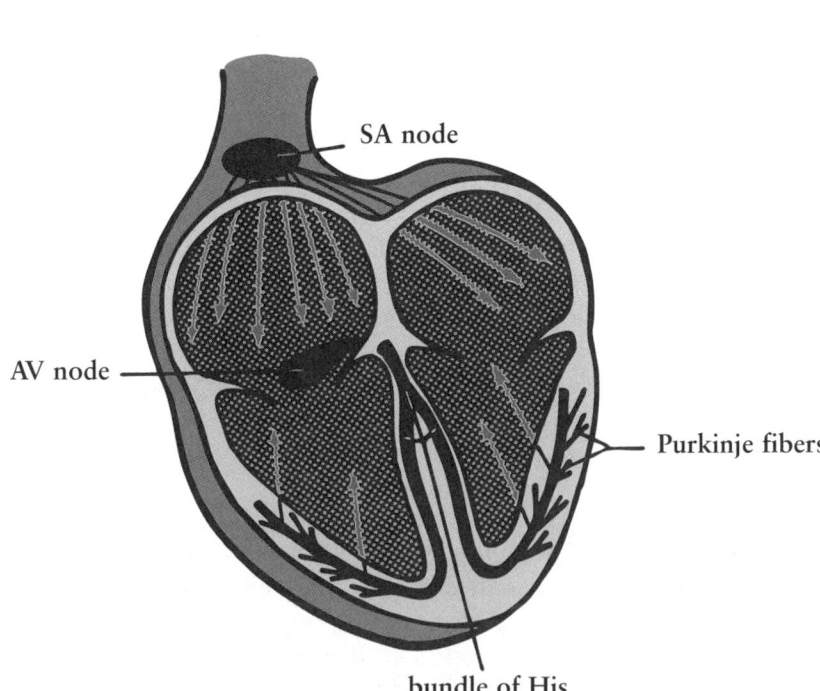

Figure 9.3. Contraction

The adrenal medulla exerts hormonal control via epinephrine (adrenaline) secretion, which causes an increase in heart rate (see chapter 11).

B. BLOOD VESSELS

The three types of blood vessels are arteries, veins, and capillaries. **Arteries** are thickly-walled, muscular, elastic vessels that transport oxygenated blood away from the heart—except for the pulmonary arteries, which transport deoxygenated blood from the heart to the lungs. **Veins** are relatively thinly walled, inelastic vessels that conduct deoxygenated blood towards the heart—except for the pulmonary veins, which carry oxygenated blood from the lungs to the heart. Much of the blood flow in veins depends on their compression by skeletal muscles during movement, rather than on the pumping of the heart. Venous circulation is often at odds with gravity; thus larger veins, especially those in the legs, have valves that prevent backflow. **Capillaries** have very thin walls composed of a single layer of endothelial cells across which respiratory gases, nutrients, enzymes, hormones, and wastes can readily diffuse. Capillaries have the smallest diameter of all three types of vessels; red blood cells must often travel through them single file.

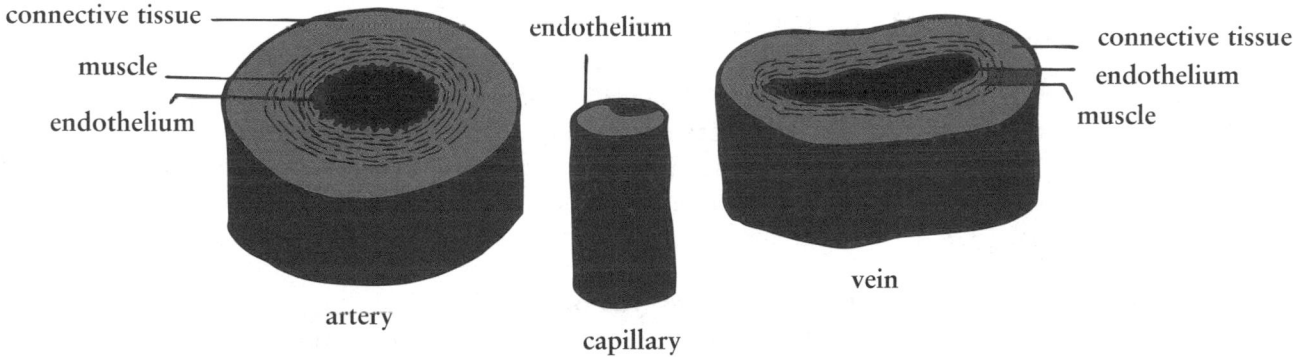

connective tissue
muscle
endothelium

endothelium

connective tissue
endothelium
muscle

artery

capillary

vein

Figure 9.4. Blood Vessels

C. BLOOD PRESSURE

Blood pressure is the force per area that blood exerts on the walls of the blood vessels. Blood pressure is measured by an instrument called a **sphygmomanometer** (a.k.a., "blood pressure cuff") and is expressed as systolic pressure/diastolic pressure. As blood flows through the circulatory system from artery to capillary, blood pressure gradually drops, due to friction between blood and the walls of the vessels, and to the increase in cross-sectional area afforded by the numerous capillary beds (see Figure 9.5).

> **Bridge**
>
> In chapter 5 (Fluids and Solids) of the Physics section, pressure is defined as force/area. This holds true for blood pressure as well.

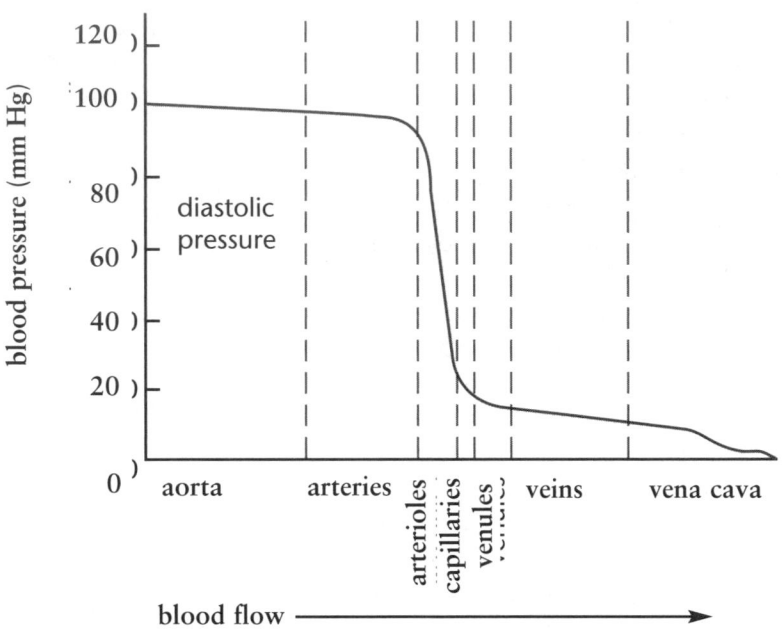

Figure 9.5. Blood Pressure

BLOOD

A. COMPOSITION

On the average, the human body contains 4–6 liters of blood. Blood has both liquid (55 percent) and cellular components (45 percent; formed elements). **Plasma** is the liquid portion of the blood. It is an aqueous mixture of nutrients, salts, respiratory gases, wastes, hormones, and blood proteins (e.g., immunoglobulins, albumin, and fibrinogen). The cellular components of the blood are **erythrocytes, leukocytes,** and **platelets.**

1. **Erythrocytes (red blood cells)**

    Erythrocytes are the oxygen-carrying components of blood. An erythrocyte contains approximately 250 million molecules of **hemoglobin,** each of which can bind up to four molecules of oxygen. Adult hemoglobin consists of 2β chains and 2α chains. Erythrocytes have a distinct biconcave, disklike shape, which gives them both increased surface area for gas exchange and greater flexibility for movement through those tiny capillaries. Erythrocytes are formed from stem cells in the bone marrow, where they lose their nuclei, mitochondria, and membranous organelles. Since erythrocytes lack mitochondria, they are anaerobic and obtain their ATP via glycolysis alone. Once mature, erythrocytes circulate in the blood for about 120 days, after which they are phagocytized by special cells in the spleen and liver. There are about 5 million erythrocytes per one mm³ of blood.

2. **Leukocytes (white blood cells)**

   Leukocytes arise from stem cells in the marrow of long bones. Leukocytes are larger than erythrocytes and have protective functions. The number of leukocytes in the blood varies widely; there are normally 5,000–10,000 leukocytes per one mm^3 of blood, but this number substantially increases when the body is battling an infection. There are three types of leukocytes: **granular leukocytes, lymphocytes,** and **monocytes.**

   Granular leukocytes are non-specific and attack general invading pathogens, such as bacteria or parasites. Granular leukocytes (**neutrophils, basophils,** and **eosinophils**) play key roles in inflammation, allergic reactions, pus formation, and the destruction of invading bacteria and parasites. Neutrophiles predominantly fight bacterial infections, where eosmophiles are associated with parasitic infections. Basophiles are responsible for allergies and allergic reactions through the release of histamine.

   Lymphocytes play an important role in the **immune response;** they are produced in the lymph nodes, tonsils, spleen, appendix, thymus, and bone marrow and are involved in the production of **antibodies.** As a result, lymphocytes are involved in the specific immune response against a specific invading pathogen. For example, if you have antibodies against influenza virus, you can still be infected with another strain. The two types of lymphocytes are **B lymphocytes** and **T lymphocytes.** Monocytes are involved in the nonspecific immune response. They phagocytize foreign matter and organisms such as bacteria. Some monocytes migrate from the blood to tissue, where they mature into stationary cells called **macrophages.** Macrophages have greater phagocytic capability than monocytes.

3. **Platelets**

   Platelets are cell fragments approximately 2–3 μm in diameter and are also formed in the bone marrow. Platelets lack nuclei and function in clot formation. There are about 250,000–500,000 platelets per one mm^3 of blood.

> **Clinical Correlate**
>
> Anasarca is a condition of generalized edema in the tissues. It is caused by very low albumin concentration in the blood, i.e. low osmotic pressure in the capillary at the venule end

B. BLOOD ANTIGENS

Erythrocytes have characteristic cell-surface proteins (**antigens**). Antigens are macromolecules that are foreign to the host organism and trigger an immune response. The two major groups of red blood cell antigens are the **ABO group** and the **Rh factor.**

1. **ABO Group**

   There are four ABO blood groups, **A**, **B**, **AB**, and **O**; see Table 9.1.

Table 9.1.

Blood Type	Antigen on Red Blood Cell	Antibodies Produced
A	A	anti-B
B	B	anti-A
AB (universal recipient)	A and B	none
O (universal donor)	none	anti-A and anti-B

It is extremely important during blood transfusions that donor and recipient blood types be appropriately matched. The aim is to avoid transfusion of red blood cells that will be clumped ("rejected") by antibodies (proteins in the immune system that bind specifically to antigens) present in the recipient's plasma. The rule of blood matching is as follows: If the donor's antigens are already in the recipient's blood, no clumping occurs. Type AB blood is termed the "**universal recipient**," as it has neither anti-A nor anti-B antibodies. Type O blood is considered to be the "**universal donor;**" it will not elicit a response from the recipient's immune system since it does not possess any surface antigens (see chapter 13 for further discussion of ABO blood groups).

2. **Rh Factor**

   The Rh factor is another antigen that may be present on the surface of red blood cells. Individuals may be Rh$^+$, possessing the Rh antigen, or Rh$^-$, lacking the Rh antigen. Consideration of the Rh factor is particularly important during pregnancy. An Rh$^-$ woman can be sensitized by an Rh$^+$ fetus if fetal red blood cells (which will have the Rh factor) enter maternal circulation during birth. If this woman subsequently carries another Rh$^+$ fetus, the anti-Rh antibodies she produced when sensitized by the first birth may cross the placenta and destroy fetal red blood cells. This results in a severe anemia for the fetus, known as **erythroblastosis fetalis**. Erythroblastosis is not caused by ABO blood-type mismatches between mother and fetus, since anti-A and anti-B antibodies cannot cross the placenta.

FUNCTIONS OF THE CIRCULATORY SYSTEM

Blood transports nutrients and O_2 to tissue, and wastes and CO_2 from tissue. Platelets are involved in injury repair. Leukocytes are the main component of the immune system.

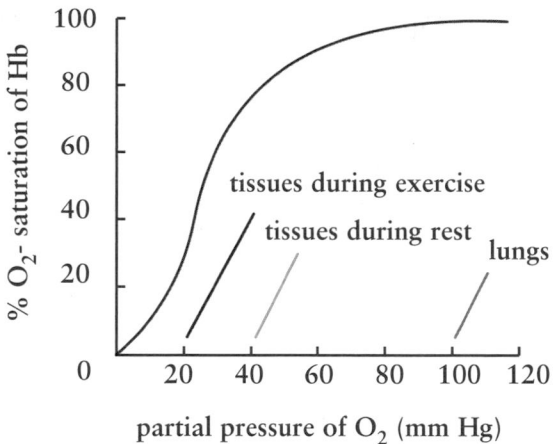

Figure 9.6. Hemoglobin Dissociation Curve

A. TRANSPORT OF GASES

Erythrocytes transport O_2 throughout the circulatory system. Actually, it is the hemoglobin molecules in erythrocytes that bind to O_2. A hemoglobin molecule is composed of four polypeptide chains, each containing a prosthetic heme group. Each heme group is capable of binding to one molecule of oxygen. Thus, each hemoglobin molecule is capable of binding to four molecules of O_2. The binding of O_2 at the first heme group induces a conformational change that facilitates the binding of O_2 at the other three heme groups. Similarly, the unloading of O_2 at one heme group facilitates the unloading of O_2 at the other three heme groups. This cooperation between the heme groups is an allosteric effect (see chapter 2); this is reflected in hemoglobin's S-shaped **dissociation curve** (see Figure 9.6).

Hemoglobin also binds to CO_2. Carbon dioxide diffuses from tissue into erythrocytes, where it combines with H_2O to form carbonic acid (H_2CO_3). Carbonic acid then dissociates into a bicarbonate ion (HCO_3^-) and a hydrogen ion (H^+). The H^+ binds to the hemoglobin molecule, while HCO_3^- diffuses into the plasma. There is an allosteric relationship between the concentrations of CO_2, H^+, and O_2, known as the **Bohr effect**. According to the Bohr effect, increasing concentrations of H^+ (a decrease in pH) and CO_2 (an increase in HCO_3^-) in the blood decrease hemoglobin's O_2 affinity. Thus, the presence of high concentrations of H^+ and CO_2 in metabolically active tissue, such as muscle, enhances the release of O_2 to this tissue. Conversely, a high concentration of O_2, as in the alveolar capillaries, promotes O_2 uptake and CO_2 release from hemoglobin. In the lungs, HCO_3^- and H^+ reassociate to form CO_2 and H_2O, which are expelled during exhalation (see chapter 8). Both formation and dissociation of carbonic acid are catalyzed by the enzyme **carbonic anhydrase**.

> **MCAT Synopsis**
>
> Only a small percentage of carbon dioxide is actually bound directly to hemoglobin to form carboxyhemoglobin; most of the CO_2 is dissolved in plasma and lives as HCO_3^-.

$$CO_2 + H_2O \xrightleftharpoons[\text{anhydrase}]{\text{carbonic}} H_2CO_3 \rightleftharpoons H^+ + HCO_3^-$$

B. TRANSPORT OF NUTRIENTS AND WASTES

Amino acids and simple sugars are absorbed into the bloodstream at the intestinal capillaries and transported to the liver via the hepatic portal vein. After processing, they are transported throughout the body. Fats enter the lymphatic system through lymph capillaries in the small intestine and drain into the bloodstream at the large veins of the neck, thereby bypassing the liver. Throughout the body, metabolic waste products (e.g., water, urea, and carbon dioxide) diffuse into capillaries from surrounding cells; these wastes are then delivered to the appropriate excretory organs (see chapter 10).

The exchange of materials is greatly influenced by the balance between the **hydrostatic pressure** and the **osmotic pressure** of the blood and tissue fluids. The hydrostatic pressure at the arteriole end of the capillaries is greater than the hydrostatic pressure of the surrounding tissue fluids (interstitial fluid). This causes fluid to move out of the capillaries at the arteriole end. However, because blood has a higher solute concentration than the tissue fluid, osmotic pressure causes fluid to move back into the capillaries at the venule end. Proteins, such as albumin, are primarily responsible for the majority of this osmotic pressure.

As shown in Figure 9.7, the hydrostatic pressure at the arteriole end of the capillary bed is approximately 36 mm Hg, while the opposing osmotic pressure is approximately 25 mm Hg. This 11 mm Hg difference favors the

MCAT Synopsis

Think of it this way—hydrostatic pressure pushes fluid out of vessels while osmotic pressure pulls fluid back into the vessels. Hydrostatic pressure is dependent on the blood pressure driven by the heart; osmotic pressure is dependent on the number of particles dissolved in the plasma.

Clinical Correlate

Anasarca is a condition of generalized edema in the tissues. It is caused by very low albumin concentration in the blood, i.e., low osmotic pressure in the capillary at the venule end.

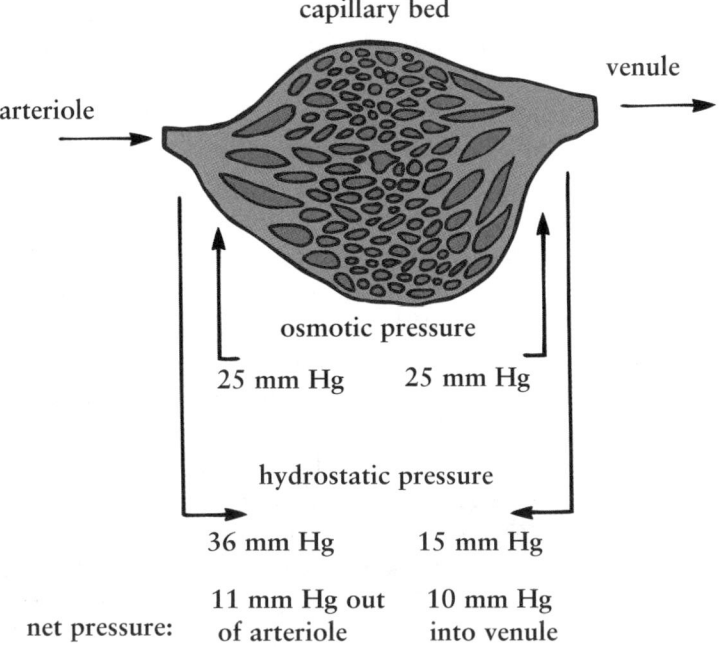

Figure 9.7. Net Fluid Flow at Capillary Bed

hydrostatic pressure, and so there is a net flow of fluid out of the capillaries. At the venule end of the capillary bed, the osmotic pressure across the wall is greater than the hydrostatic pressure, which has dropped to 15 mm Hg. This difference tends to draw fluid into the capillaries. Hence, most of the fluid is forced out of the capillaries at the arteriole end and is reabsorbed by the capillaries at the venule end. The remaining fluid is transported back into the blood via the lymphatic system.

C. CLOTTING

When platelets come into contact with the exposed collagen of a damaged vessel, they release a chemical that causes neighboring platelets to adhere to one another, forming a platelet plug. Subsequently, both the platelets and the damaged tissue release the clotting factor **thromboplastin.** Thromboplastin, with the aid of its cofactors calcium and vitamin K, converts the inactive plasma protein **prothrombin** to its active form, **thrombin.** Thrombin then converts **fibrinogen** (another plasma protein) into **fibrin.** Threads of fibrin coat the damaged area and trap blood cells to form a **clot.** Clots prevent extensive blood loss while the damaged vessel heals itself. People suffering from the genetic disease **hemophilia** lack one of the agents involved in clot formation and bleed excessively, even from minor cuts and bruises (see chapter 13).

D. IMMUNOLOGICAL REACTIONS

The body has the ability to distinguish between "self" and "nonself," and to "remember" nonself entities (antigens) that it has previously encountered. These defense mechanisms are an integral part of the **immune system.** The immune system is composed of two **specific defense mechanisms: humoral immunity,** which involves the production of antibodies; and **cell-mediated immunity,** which involves cells that combat fungal and viral infection. Lymphocytes are responsible for both of these immune mechanisms. The body also has a number of nonspecific defense mechanisms.

1. Humoral Immunity

One of the body's defense mechanisms is the production of antibodies. Humoral immunity is responsible for the proliferation of antibodies following exposure to antigens. Antibodies, also called **immunoglobulins** (Igs), are complex proteins that recognize and bind to specific antigens and trigger the immune system to remove them. Antibodies either attract other cells (such as leukocytes) to phagocytize the antigen, or cause the antigens to clump together (agglutinate) and form large insoluble complexes, facilitating their removal by phagocytic cells. An antibody molecule consists of four polypeptide chains—two identical **heavy chains** and two identical **light chains**—held together by disulfide linkages and noncovalent bonds. Certain regions on the chains (called **variable regions**) serve as antigen-binding sites; these sites are structured so as to bind to one specific antigen. The remaining part of the chains (the **constant regions**) aid in the process by which foreign antigens are destroyed (see Figure 9.8). There are five types of constant regions—M, A, D, G, and E—defining five classes of immunoglobulins: **IgM, IgA, IgD, IgG,** and **IgE.**

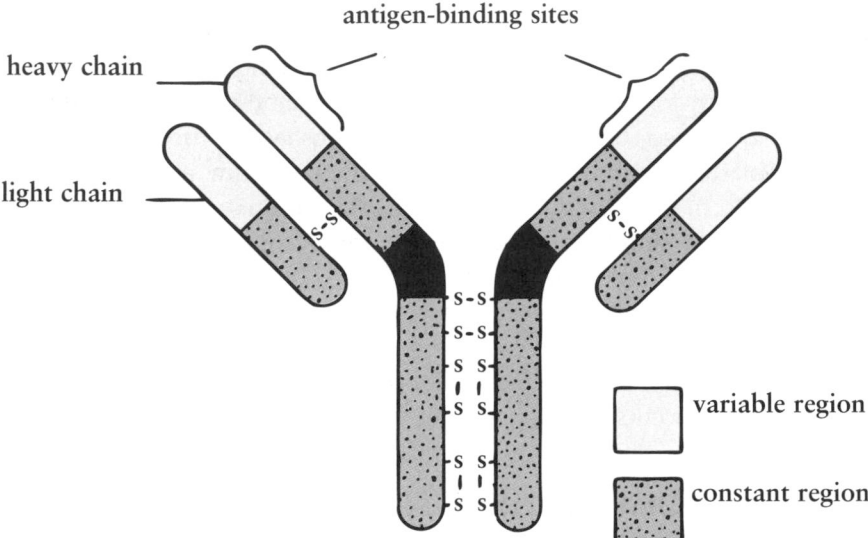

Figure 9.8. Antibody Structure

The lymphocytes involved in the humoral response are the B lymphocytes, or **B cells**, which originate in the bone marrow and differentiate in the spleen, lymph nodes, and other lymphatic organs. When exposed to a specific antigen, B lymphocytes specific for that antigen proliferate. Some of the daughter cells become **memory cells**, and others become **plasma cells (effector cells)**; this is known as the **primary response.** Plasma cells produce and release antibodies specific for the antigen. It generally takes 7–10 days for the plasma cells to generate a sufficient amount of antibody. Memory cells "remember" the antigen and are long-lived in the bloodstream, sometimes remaining there permanently. Memory cells are able to elicit a more immediate response upon subsequent exposure to the same antigen; this is referred to as the **secondary response.**

Active immunity refers to the production of antibodies during an immune response. Active immunity can be conferred by vaccination; an individual is injected with a weakened, inactive, or related form of a particular antigen, that stimulates the immune system to produce specific antibodies against it. Active immunity may require weeks to build up. **Passive immunity** involves the transfer of antibodies produced by another individual or organism. Passive immunity is acquired either passively or by injection. For example, during pregnancy, some maternal antibodies cross the placenta and enter fetal circulation, conferring passive immunity upon the fetus. Although passive immunity is acquired immediately, it is very short-lived, lasting only as long as the antibodies circulate in the blood system.

2. **Cell-Mediated Immunity**

The lymphocytes involved in cell-mediated immunity are T lymphocytes, or **T cells,** which develop in bone marrow and mature and proliferate in the thymus. T cells act primarily against the body's own cells that are infected by a fungus or virus. T cells differentiate into effector cells: **cytotoxic T cells** destroy antigens directly; **helper T cells** activate other B and T cells, as well as nonlymphocyte cells such as macrophages, through the secretion of **lymphokines** (e.g., interleukins); **suppressor T cells** regulate other B and T cells to decrease their activity against antigens. Some T cells differentiate into memory cells. These events constitute the primary components of a cell-mediated response. During a secondary response, these memory cells proliferate vigorously and produce a large number of cytotoxic T cells to combat the invader.

T cells play important roles in allergic reactions and in the rejection of organ transplants. Sometimes pollen or certain foods can act as antigens, stimulating the release of substances (e.g., **histamine**) responsible for allergic symptoms, such as hives and mucous membrane inflammation. Cell-mediated immunity plays an important role in transplant rejection; i.e., tissue from a donor is recognized by the recipient as foreign because the recipient's body does not recognize the antigens on the transplanted cells, and in response, cytotoxic T cells are sent out to destroy the foreign cells. In certain diseases, the body mistakenly identifies its own cells as foreign and elicits an **autoimmune** response, destroying its own cells.

3. **Nonspecific Defense Mechanisms**

The body employs a number of nonspecific defenses against foreign material: *1* Skin is a physical barrier against bacterial invasion. In addition, pores on the skin's surface secrete sweat, which contains an enzyme that attacks bacterial cell walls. *2* Passages (e.g., the respiratory tract) are lined with ciliated mucous-coated epithelia, which filter and trap foreign particles. *3* Macrophages engulf and destroy foreign particles. *4* The **inflammatory response** is initiated by the body in response to physical damage: injured cells release histamine, which causes blood vessels to dilate, thereby increasing

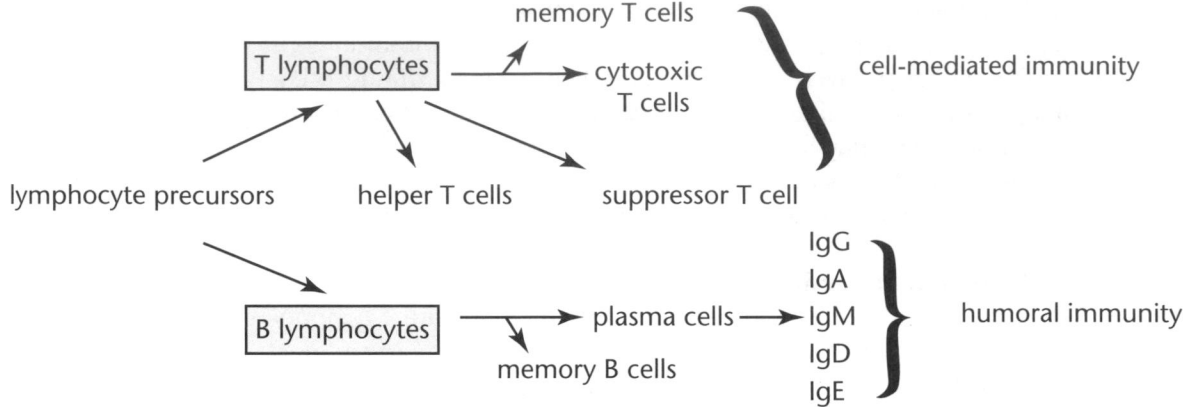

Figure 9.9. Lymphocyte Differentiation

blood flow to the damaged region. Granulocytes attracted to the injury site phagocytize antigenic material. An inflammatory response is often accompanied by a fever. *5* Proteins called **interferons** are produced by cells under viral attack. Interferons diffuse to other cells, where they help prevent the spread of the virus.

THE LYMPHATIC SYSTEM

The lymphatic system is a secondary circulatory system distinct from cardiovascular circulation. Its vessels transport excess interstitial fluid, called **lymph,** to the cardiovascular system, thereby keeping fluid levels in the body constant. **Lymph capillaries** (lacteals) collect fats by absorbing chylomicrons in the small intestine and transporting them to cardiovascular circulation (see chapter 7). Lymph capillaries are closed at one end and lead into other lymph vessels that have valves to prevent the backflow of lymph. These lymph vessels then converge in the region of the upper chest and neck, where they drain into the large veins of the cardiovascular system. Lymph flow is regulated by contraction of neighboring skeletal muscles and rhythmic contractions of the lymphatic vessels themselves. **Lymph nodes** are swellings along lymph vessels containing phagocytic cells (leukocytes) that filter the lymph, removing and destroying foreign particles.

10

HOMEOSTASIS

Homeostasis is the process by which a stable internal environment within an organism is maintained. Some important homeostatic mechanisms include the maintenance of a water and solute balance (**osmoregulation**), the removal of metabolic waste products (**excretion**), the regulation of blood glucose levels, and the maintenance of a constant internal body temperature (**thermoregulation**). In mammals, the primary homeostatic organs are the **kidneys**, the **liver**, the **large intestine**, and the **skin**.

THE KIDNEYS: OSMOREGULATION

The kidneys regulate the concentration of salt and water in the blood through the formation and excretion of urine. The kidneys are bean-shaped and are located behind the stomach and liver. Each kidney is composed of approximately one million units called **nephrons**.

A. STRUCTURE

The kidney is divided into three regions: the **cortex**, the **medulla,** and the **pelvis.** Blood enters the kidney through the **renal artery,** which divides into many **afferent arterioles** that run through the medulla and into the cortex (see Figure 10.1). Each afferent arteriole branches into a convoluted network of capillaries called a **glomerulus** (see Figure 10.2). Rather than converging directly into a vein, the capillaries converge into an **efferent arteriole,** which divides into a fine capillary network known as the **vasa recta.** The vasa recta enmeshes the nephron tubule and then converges into the **renal vein.** This arrangement of tandem capillary beds is a portal system (see chapter 9).

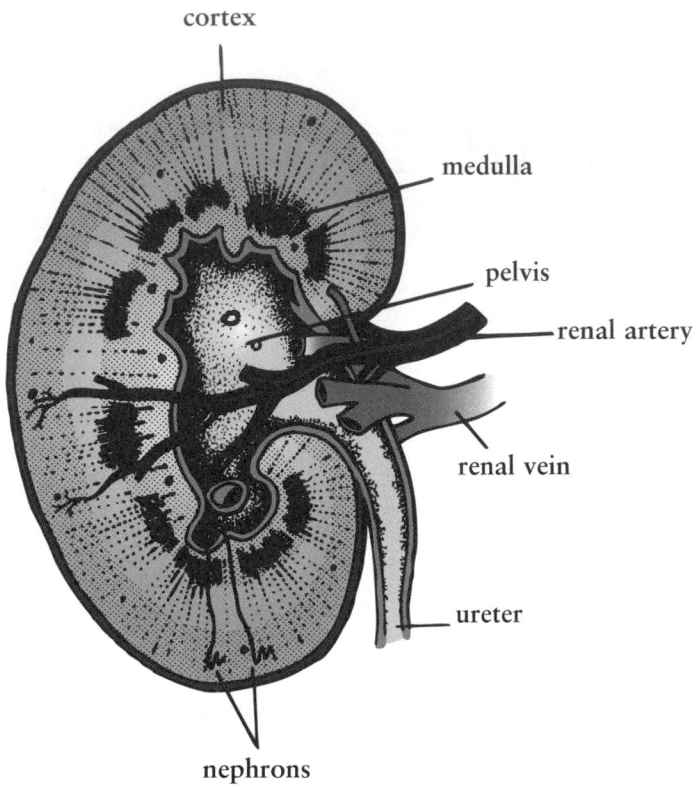

Figure 10.1. Kidney

A nephron consists of a bulb called **Bowman's capsule,** which embraces a glomerulus and leads into a long coiled tubule that is divided into five units: the **proximal convoluted tubule,** the **descending limb** of the **loop of Henle,** the **ascending limb** of the **loop of Henle,** the **distal convoluted tubule,** and the **collecting duct.** The nephron is positioned such that the loop of Henle runs through the medulla, while the convoluted tubules and Bowman's capsule are in the cortex (see Figure 10.2).

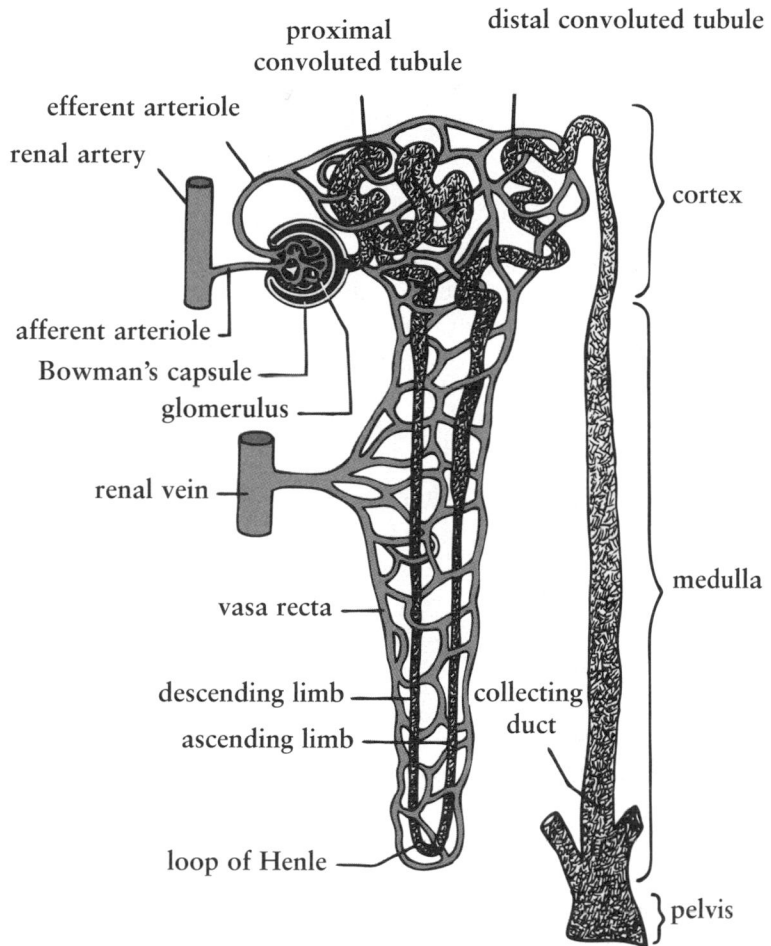

Figure 10.2. Nephron

B. FUNCTION

1. Overview

Filtration, secretion, and **reabsorption** are the three processes that regulate salt and water balance in the blood.

a. Filtration

Blood pressure forces 20 percent of the blood plasma entering the glomerulus into the surrounding Bowman's capsule. The fluid and small solutes entering the nephron are called the **filtrate.** The filtrate is isotonic with blood plasma. Molecules too large to filter through the glomerulus, such as blood cells and albumin, remain in the circulatory system.

> ### MCAT Synopsis
>
> Imagine that the glomerulus is like a sieve or collander. Small molecules dissolved in the fluid will pass through the glomerulus (e.g., glucose that is later reabsorbed), while large molecules such as proteins and blood cells will not. If blood cells or protein are found in the urine, this indicates a problem at the level of the glomerulus.

b. **Secretion**

The nephron secretes substances such as acids, bases, and ions from the interstitial fluid into the filtrate by both passive and active transport. Secretion maintains blood pH, potassium concentration in the blood, and nitrogenous waste concentration in the filtrate.

c. **Reabsorption**

Essential substances (glucose, salts, and amino acids) and water are reabsorbed from the filtrate and returned to the blood. This results in the formation of concentrated urine, which is hypertonic to the blood.

2. **Nephron Function**

Through the selective permeability of its walls and the maintenance of an osmolarity gradient, the nephron reabsorbs nutrients, salts, and water from the filtrate and returns them to the body, thus maintaining the bloodstream's solute concentration.

a. **Selective permeability**

The walls of the proximal tubule and the descending limb of the loop of Henle are permeable to water. The walls of the lower ascending limb are permeable only to salt. In the presence of ADH, the walls of the collecting duct are permeable to water and urea but only slightly permeable to salt.

b. **Osmolarity gradient**

The selective permeability of the tubules establishes an **osmolarity gradient** in the surrounding interstitial fluid. By exiting and then reentering at different segments of the nephron, solutes create an osmolarity gradient, with tissue osmolarity increasing from cortex to inner medulla. The solutes that contribute to the maintenance of the gradient are urea and salt (Na^+ and Cl^-). Urea diffuses out of the collecting duct; it eventually reenters the nephron by diffusing into the ascending limb. Salt is cycled between the two limbs of the loop of Henle. Na^+ and Cl^- diffuse out of the lower half of the ascending limb, while the upper half actively pumps out Na^+ (Cl^- passively follows). This combination of passive diffusion and active transport of solutes maximizes water conservation and the excretion of urine hypertonic to the blood (see Figure 10.3).

> **Clinical Correlate**
>
> In certain conditions (e.g., congestive heart failure), the body tends to accumulate excess water in the form of fluid in the lungs or in peripheral tissues. The judicious use of a diuretic drug can help the body get rid of excess fluids. Diuretics typically inhibit the reabsorption of sodium in one or more regions of the nephron, thereby increasing sodium excretion. The increased sodium excretion, in turn, results in an increased excretion of water, thereby relieving the body of some of its excess fluid.

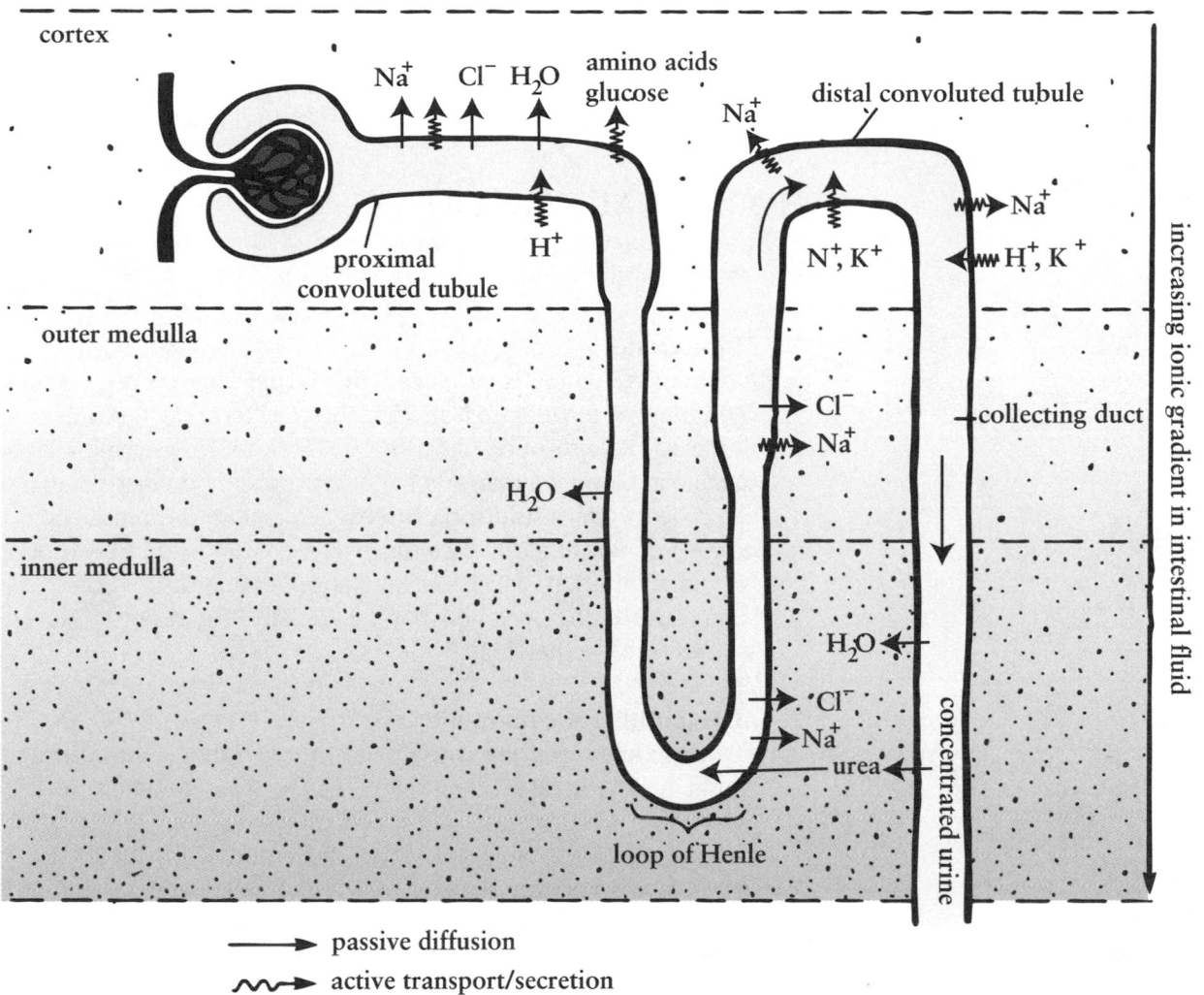

passive diffusion

active transport/secretion

Figure 10.3. Selective Permeability and Osmolarity Gradient
in the Nephron

c. **Flow of filtrate**

Filtrate enters Bowman's capsule and flows into the proximal
convoluted tubule, where virtually all glucose, amino acids, and
other important organic molecules are reabsorbed via active
transport. In addition, 60–70 percent of the Na⁺ in the filtrate is
reabsorbed (by both active and passive mechanisms); water and
Cl⁻ passively follow. The filtrate then flows down the descending
limb into the renal medulla, where there is an increasing ionic
concentration in the interstitial fluid, causing more water to diffuse out of the nephron. The filtrate flows through the ascending
limb, which is impermeable to water, and then into the distal

convoluted tubule. The filtrate continues through the collecting duct, where water reabsorption is under hormonal (ADH) control. The remaining filtrate, urine, is hypertonic to the blood and highly concentrated in urea and other solutes.

C. HORMONAL REGULATION

Hormonal regulation plays a key role in urine formation. Two hormones that regulate water reabsorption are **aldosterone** and **ADH.**

1. Aldosterone

Aldosterone, which is produced by the adrenal cortex, stimulates both the reabsorption of Na+ from the collecting duct and the secretion of K+. Reabsorption of Na+ increases water reabsorption, leading to a rise in blood volume, and hence a rise in blood pressure. In a person suffering from **Addison's disease,** aldosterone is produced insufficiently or not at all. This causes overexcretion of urine with a high Na+ concentration, which causes a considerable drop in blood pressure. Aldosterone secretion is regulated by the **renin-angiotensin system** (see chapter 11).

2. ADH (antidiuretic hormone)

ADH, also known as **vasopressin,** is formed in the hypothalamus and stored in the posterior pituitary. As an "antidiuretic," it causes increased water reabsorption. It acts directly on the collecting duct, increasing its permeability to water. The amount of ADH produced is dependent on plasma osmolarity. A high solute concentration in the blood causes increased ADH secretion, while a low solute concentration in the blood reduces ADH secretion. Alcohol and caffeine inhibit ADH secretion, causing excess excretion of dilute urine and dehydration (see chapter 11).

D. EXCRETION

By the time filtrate exits the nephron, most of the water has been reabsorbed. The remaining fluid, composed of urea, uric acid, and other wastes, leaves the collecting tubule and exits the kidney via the **ureter,** a duct leading to the bladder. Urine is stored there until it is excreted from the body through the **urethra** (see Figure 10.4).

In a healthy individual, the nephron reabsorbs all of the glucose entering it, producing glucose-free urine. The urine of a diabetic, however, is not glucose-free. The high blood glucose concentration in a diabetic overwhelms the nephron's active transport system, leading to the excretion of glucose in the urine (see chapter 11).

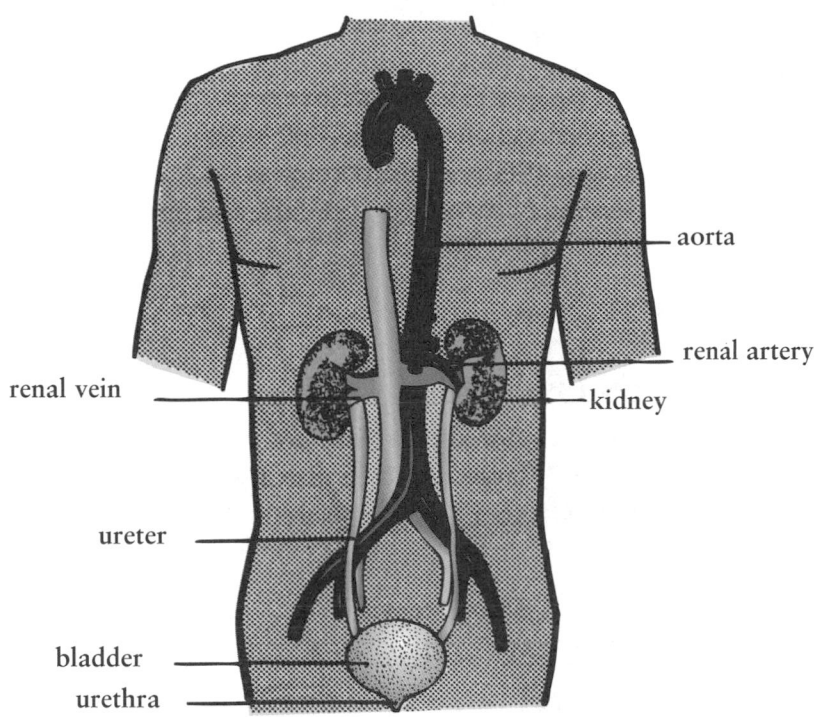

Figure 10.4. Human Excretory System

THE LIVER

The liver helps regulate blood glucose levels and produces urea. Glucose and other monosaccharides absorbed during digestion are delivered to the liver via the **hepatic portal vein** (see chapter 7). Glucose-rich blood is processed by the liver, which converts excess glucose to glycogen for storage. If the blood has a low glucose concentration, the liver converts glycogen into glucose and releases it into the blood, restoring blood glucose levels to normal. In addition, the liver synthesizes glucose from noncarbohydrate precursors via the process of **gluconeogenesis**. Glycogen metabolism is under both hormonal and nervous control (see chapter 11).

The liver is also responsible for the processing of nitrogenous wastes. Excess amino acids are absorbed in the small intestine and transported to the liver via the hepatic portal vein. There the amino acids undergo a process called **deamination,** in which the amino group is removed from the amino acid and converted into ammonia, a highly toxic compound. In a complex biochemical process, the liver combines ammonia with carbon dioxide to form urea, a relatively nontoxic compound, which is released into the blood and eventually excreted by the kidneys.

The liver is also responsible for:
- Detoxification of toxins
- Storage of iron and vitamin B$_{12}$
- Destruction of old erythrocytes
- Synthesis of bile
- Synthesis of various blood proteins
- Defense against various antigens
- Beta-oxidation of fatty acids to ketones
- Interconversion of carbohydrates, fats, and amino acids

THE LARGE INTESTINE

The large intestine absorbs water and sodium not previously absorbed in the small intestine (see chapter 7). However, the large intestine also functions as an excretory organ for excess salts. Excess calcium, iron, and other salts are excreted into the colon and then eliminated with the feces.

THE SKIN: OSMOREGULATION AND THERMOREGULATION

A. STRUCTURE

The skin is the largest organ of the body, comprising an average of 16 percent of total body weight. The two major layers of the skin are the **epidermis** and the **dermis,** beneath which lies subcutaneous tissues, sometimes called the **hypodermis.**

The epidermis is the outermost epithelial layer and is composed of five cellular layers: the **stratum basalis (or stratum germinativum),** the **stratum spinosum,** the **stratum granulosum,** the **stratum lucidum,** and the **stratum corneum.** The deepest layer, the stratum basalis, continuously proliferates, pushing older epidermal cells outward. As the older cells reach the outermost layer (stratum corneum), they die, lose their nuclei, and transform into squames (scales) of keratin. The keratinized cells of the stratum corneum are tightly packed, serving as a protective barrier against microbial attack. Hair projects above the surface of the epithelium; sweat pores open to the surface.

The dermis can be subdivided into a layer of loose connective tissue known as the **papillary layer** and a layer of dense connective tissue known as the **reticular layer.** Within the dermis are the sweat glands, the sense organs, blood vessels, and the bulbs of hair follicles.

The **hypodermis,** composed of loose connective tissue, is abundant in fat cells and binds the outer skin layers to the body (see Figure 10.5).

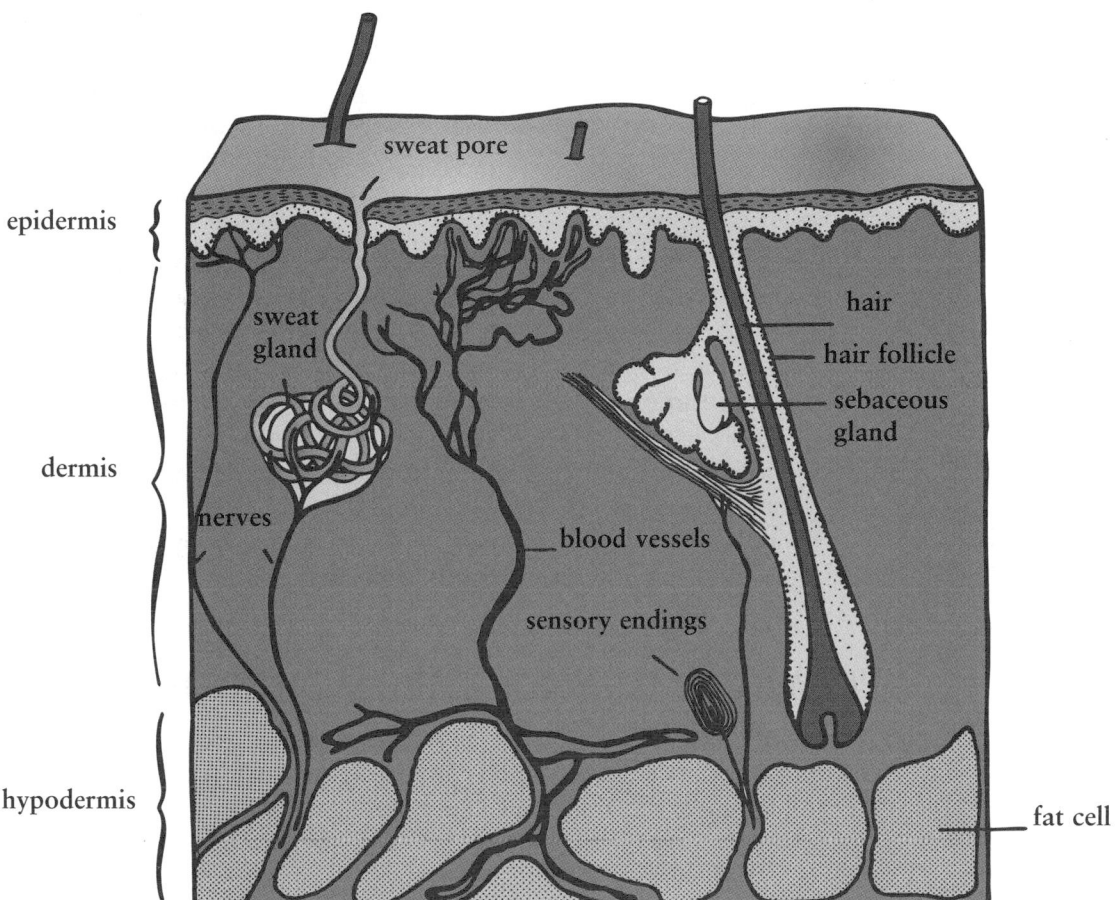

Figure 10.5. Human Skin

B. FUNCTION

The skin protects the body from microbial invasion and from environmental stresses, such as dry weather and wind. Specialized epidermal cells called **melanocytes** synthesize the pigment **melanin**, which protects the body from ultraviolet light. The skin is a receptor of stimuli, such as pressure and temperature. The skin is also an excretory organ (removing excess water and salts from the body) and a thermoregulatory organ (helping control both the conservation and release of heat).

Sweat glands secrete a mixture of water, dissolved salts, and urea via sweat pores. As sweat evaporates, the skin is cooled. Thus, sweating has both an excretory and a thermoregulatory function. Sweating is under nervous control.

Subcutaneous fat in the hypodermis insulates the body. Hair entraps and retains warm air at the skin's surface. Hormones such as epinephrine can increase the metabolic rate, thereby increasing heat production. In addition, muscles can generate heat by contracting rapidly (shivering). Heat loss can be inhibited through the constriction of blood vessels in the dermis. Likewise, dilation of these same blood vessels dissipates heat.

Alternative mechanisms are used by some mammals to regulate their body temperature. For example, **panting** is a cooling mechanism that evaporates water from the respiratory passages. Most mammals have a layer of fur; fur traps and conserves heat. Some mammals exhibit varying states of **torpor** in the winter months in order to conserve energy; their metabolism, heart rate, and respiration rate greatly decrease during these months. **Hibernation** is a type of torpor during which the animal remains dormant over a period of weeks or months with body temperature maintained below normal. Animals with a constant body temperature are referred to as **homeotherms (endotherms).**

THYROID GLAND: THERMOREGULATION

The basal metabolic rate of the human body contributes a great deal to the warmth or coolness of the body. The thyroid hormones, primarily thyroxine, control the basal metabolic rate (see chapter 11). When there is overproduction of these hormones (hyperthyroidism), the person will feel excessively warm. When there is a decrease in the level of these hormones (hypothyroidism), the person will feel cold.

> **MCAT Synopsis**
>
> While this chapter focused on the homeostatic roles played by the kidney, liver, and skin, you should be aware that homeostasis is not limited to those organs; all the organs of the body are involved in one way or another in preserving physiologic equilibrium.

11

ENDOCRINE SYSTEM

The endocrine system acts as a means of internal communication, coordinating the activities of the organ systems. **Endocrine glands** (see Figure 11.1) synthesize and secrete chemical substances called **hormones** directly into the circulatory system. (In contrast, **exocrine glands,** such as the gall bladder, secrete substances that are transported by ducts.) Hormones regulate the function of **target organs** or tissues.

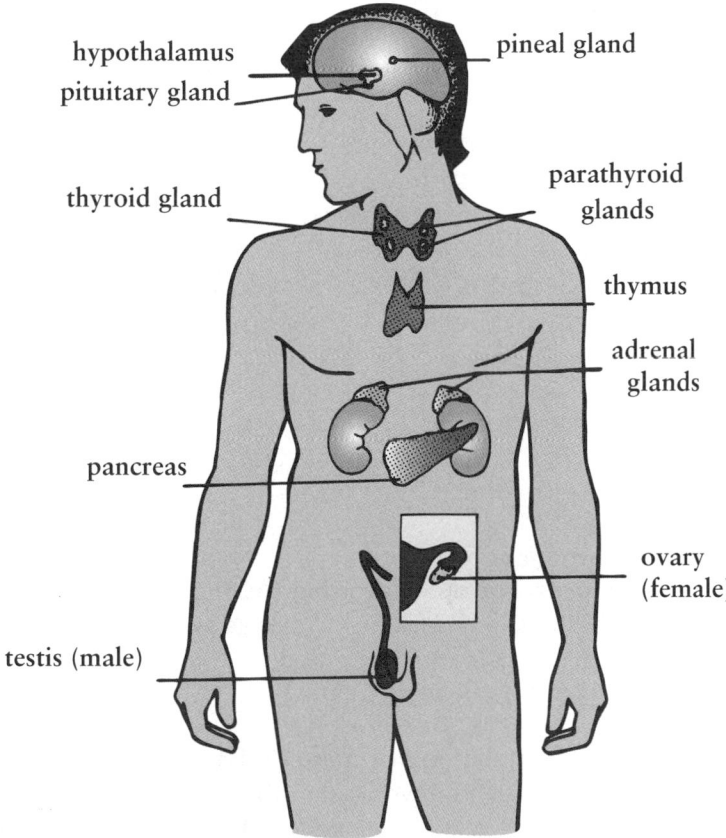

Figure 11.1. Human Endocrine System

ENDOCRINE GLANDS

Glands that synthesize and/or secrete hormones include the **pituitary, hypothalamus, thyroid, parathyroids, adrenals, pancreas, testes, ovaries, pineal, kidneys, gastrointestinal glands, heart,** and **thymus.** Some hormones regulate a single type of cell or organ, while others have more widespread actions. The specificity of hormonal action is determined by the presence of specific receptors on or in the target cells.

A. PITUITARY GLAND

The pituitary (**hypophysis**) is a small, trilobed gland lying at the base of the brain. The two main lobes, **anterior** and **posterior,** are functionally distinct. (In humans, the third lobe, the intermediate lobe, is rudimentary.)

1. Anterior Pituitary

The anterior pituitary synthesizes both direct hormones, which directly stimulate their target organs, and tropic hormones, which stimulate other endocrine glands to release hormones. The hormonal secretions of the anterior pituitary are regulated by hypothalamic secretions called **releasing/inhibiting hormones** or factors.

a. Direct hormones
- **Growth hormone (GH, somatotropin)**
  GH promotes bone and muscle growth, inhibits the uptake of glucose by certain cells, and stimulates the breakdown of **fatty acid,** thus conserving glucose. GH secretion is stimulated by the hypothalamic releasing hormone **GHRH** and inhibited by somatostatin. Secretion is also under neural and metabolic control. In children, a GH deficiency can lead to stunted growth (**dwarfism**), while overproduction of GH results in **gigantism**. Overproduction of GH in adults causes **acromegaly,** a disorder characterized by a disproportionate overgrowth of bone, localized especially in the skull, jaw, feet, and hands.

- **Prolactin**
  Prolactin stimulates milk production and secretion in female **mammary glands.**

b. Tropic hormones
- **Adrenocorticotropic hormone (ACTH)**
  ACTH stimulates the adrenal cortex to synthesize and secrete glucocorticoids and is regulated by the releasing hormone **corticotropin releasing factor (CRF).**

- **Thyroid-stimulating hormone (TSH)**
  TSH stimulates the thyroid gland to absorb iodine and then synthesize and release thyroid hormone. TSH is regulated by the releasing hormone **TRH.**

- **Luteinizing hormone (LH)**
  In females, LH stimulates ovulation and formation of the corpus luteum. In males, LH stimulates the interstitial cells of the testes to synthesize **testosterone.** LH is regulated by **estrogen, progesterone,** and **gonadotropin releasing hormone (GnRH).**

- **Follicle-stimulating hormone (FSH)**
  In females, FSH causes maturation of ovarian follicles; in males, FSH stimulates maturation of the seminiferous tubules and sperm production. FSH is regulated by estrogen and by GnRH.

2. **Posterior Pituitary**
   The posterior pituitary does not synthesize hormones; it stores and releases the hormones **oxytocin** and **ADH,** which are produced by the neurosecretory cells of the hypothalamus. Hormone secretion is stimulated by action potentials descending from the hypothalamus.

   a. **Oxytocin**
      Oxytocin, which is secreted during childbirth, increases the strength and frequency of uterine muscle contractions. Oxytocin secretion is also induced by suckling; oxytocin stimulates milk secretion in the mammary glands.

   b. **Antidiuretic Hormone (ADH, vasopressin)**
      ADH increases the permeability of the nephron's collecting duct to water, thereby promoting water reabsorption and increasing blood volume (see chapter 10). ADH is secreted when plasma osmolarity increases, as sensed by **osmoreceptors** in the hypothalamus, or when blood volume decreases, as sensed by **baroreceptors** in the circulatory system.

B. HYPOTHALAMUS

The hypothalamus is part of the forebrain and is located directly above the pituitary gland. The hypothalamus receives neural transmissions from other parts of the brain and from peripheral nerves that trigger specific responses from its neurosecretory cells. The neurosecretory cells regulate pituitary gland secretions via negative feedback mechanisms and through the actions of inhibiting and releasing hormones.

1. **Interactions with Anterior Pituitary**
   Hypothalamic releasing hormones are hormones that stimulate or inhibit the secretions of the anterior pituitary. For example, GnRH stimulates the anterior pituitary to secrete FSH and LH. Releasing hormones are secreted into the **hypothalamic–hypophyseal portal system** (see Figure 11.2). In this circulatory pathway, blood from the capillary bed in the hypothalamus flows through a portal vein into the anterior

KAPLAN) EXCLUSIVE

To remember the six hormones of the anterior pituitary, think FLAT PiG:

_F_SH
_L_H
_A_CTH
_T_SH

_P_rolactin
_i_(gnore)
_G_H

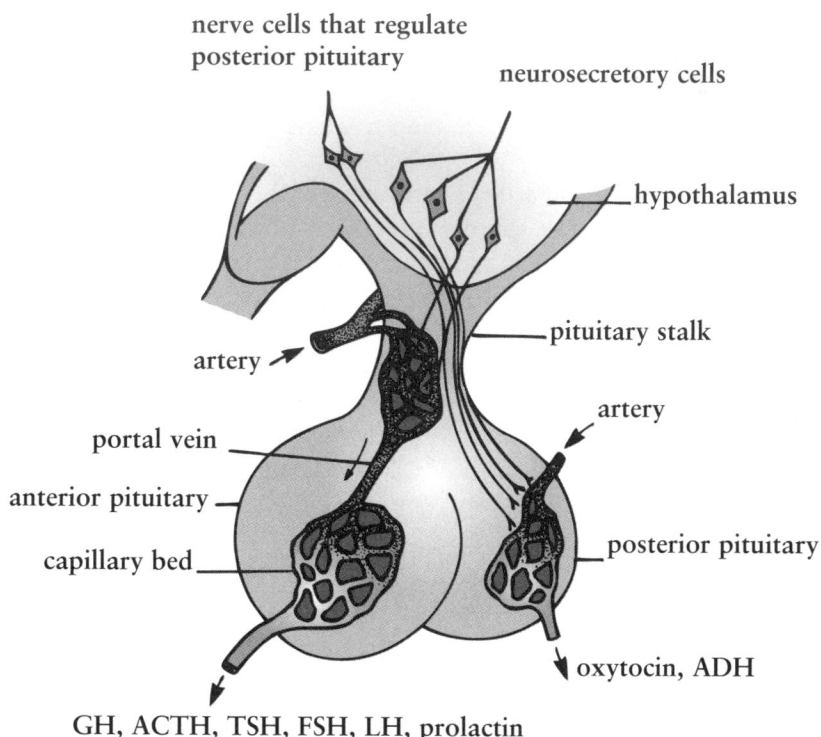

Figure 11.2. Hypothalamus and Pituitary Gland

pituitary, where it diverges into a second capillary network. In this way, releasing hormones can immediately reach the anterior pituitary.

Oversecretion of hormones is potentially harmful to an organism and so a preventive mechanism, called **negative feedback**, has evolved (see chapter 2). A high hormone level inhibits further production of that hormone. For example, when plasma levels of adrenal cortical hormones reach a critical level, the hormones themselves exert an inhibitory effect on the pituitary and on the hypothalamus, inhibiting CRF and ACTH release. In the absence of CRF, the anterior pituitary stops ACTH secretion, and the adrenal cortex stops secreting adrenal cortical hormones. When adrenal hormone levels are too low, the hypothalamus is stimulated to release CRF. This stimulates the anterior pituitary to secrete ACTH, which, in turn, stimulates the adrenal cortex to release adrenal cortical hormones (see Figure 11.3).

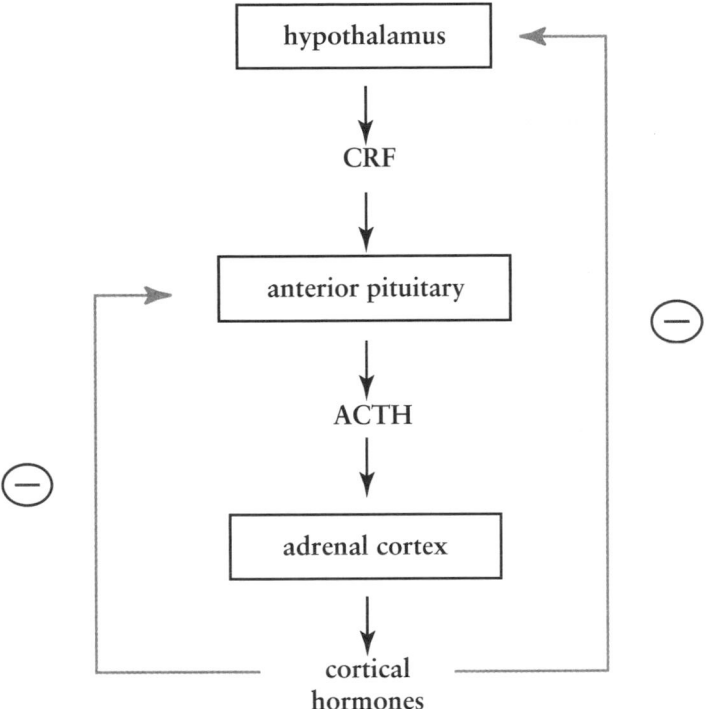

Figure 11.3. Negative Feedback Mechanism

2. Interactions with Posterior Pituitary

Neurosecretory cells in the hypothalamus synthesize both oxytocin and ADH and transport them via their axons into the posterior pituitary for storage and secretion.

C. THYROID GLAND

The thyroid gland is a bilobed structure located on the ventral surface of the trachea. It produces and secretes **thyroxine, triiodothyronine (the thyroid hormones),** and **calcitonin.**

1. Thyroid Hormones (Thyroxine and Triiodothyronine)

Thyroxine (T_4) and triiodothyronine (T_3) are derived from the iodination of the amino acid tyrosine. Thyroid hormones are necessary for growth and neurological development in children. They increase the rate of cellular respiration and the rate of protein and fatty acid synthesis and degradation in many tissues. High plasma levels of thyroid hormones inhibit TRH and TSH secretion, thereby returning plasma levels to normal.

Inflammation of the thyroid or iodine deficiency causes **hypothyroidism,** in which thyroid hormones are undersecreted or not secreted at all. Common symptoms of hypothyroidism include a slowed heart rate and respiratory rate, fatigue, cold intolerance, and weight gain. Hypothyroidism in newborn infants, called **cretinism**, is characterized by mental retardation and short stature. In **hyperthyroidism**, the thyroid is overstimulated, resulting in the oversecretion of thyroid hormones. Symptoms often include increased metabolic rate, feelings of excessive warmth, profuse sweating, palpitations, weight loss, and protruding eyes. In both disorders, the thyroid often enlarges, forming a bulge in the neck called a **goiter.**

2. **Calcitonin**
   Calcitonin decreases plasma Ca^{2+} concentration by inhibiting the release of Ca^{2+} from bone. Calcitonin secretion is regulated by plasma Ca^{2+} levels.

D. PARATHYROID GLANDS

The parathyroid glands are four small pea-shaped structures embedded in the posterior surface of the thyroid. These glands synthesize and secrete **parathyroid hormone (PTH)**, which, together with calcitonin and vitamin D, regulates plasma Ca^{2+} concentration. In turn, the plasma Ca^{2+} concentration regulates PTH secretion by means of a negative feedback mechanism. PTH raises the Ca^{2+} concentration in the blood by stimulating Ca^{2+} release from bone and decreasing Ca^{2+} excretion in the kidneys. In addition, PTH converts vitamin D into its active form, which stimulates intestinal calcium absorption.

E. ADRENAL GLANDS

The adrenal glands are situated on top of the kidneys and consist of the **adrenal cortex** and the **adrenal medulla.**

1. **Adrenal Cortex**
   In response to stress, ACTH stimulates the adrenal cortex to synthesize and secrete the steroid hormones, which are collectively known as **corticosteroids.** The corticosteroids, derived from cholesterol, include **glucocorticoids, mineralocorticoids,** and **cortical sex hormones.**

   a. **Glucocorticoids**
      Glucocorticoids, such as **cortisol** and **cortisone,** are involved in glucose regulation and protein metabolism. Glucocorticoids raise blood glucose levels by promoting gluconeogenesis and decrease protein synthesis. They also reduce the body's immunological and inflammatory responses. Cortisol secretion is governed by a negative feedback mechanism.

b. **Mineralocorticoids**

Mineralocorticoids, particularly **aldosterone,** regulate plasma levels of sodium and potassium and, consequently, the total extracellular water volume. Aldosterone causes active reabsorption of sodium and passive reabsorption of water in the nephron (see chapter 10). This results in a rise in both blood volume and blood pressure. Aldosterone also stimulates the secretion of potassium ion and hydrogen ion into the nephron and their subsequent excretion in urine.

Aldosterone secretion is regulated by the **renin-angiotensin** system. When blood volume falls, the juxtaglomerular cells of the kidney produce **renin**—an enzyme that converts the plasma protein **angiotensinogen** to **angiotensin I.** Angiotensin I is converted to **angiotensin II,** which stimulates the adrenal cortex to secrete aldosterone. Aldosterone helps to restore blood volume by increasing sodium reabsorption at the kidney, leading to an increase in water reabsorption. This removes the initial stimulus for renin production.

c. **Cortical sex hormones**

The adrenal cortex secretes small quantities of **androgens** (male sex hormones) in both males and females. Since, in males, most of the androgens are produced by the testes, the physiologic effect of the adrenal androgens is quite small. In females, however, overproduction of the adrenal androgens may have masculinizing effects, such as excessive facial hair.

2. **Adrenal Medulla**

The secretory cells of the adrenal medulla can be viewed as specialized sympathetic nerve cells that secrete hormones into the circulatory system. The adrenal medulla produces **epinephrine (adrenaline)** and **norepinephrine (noradrenaline),** both of which belong to a class of amino acid-derived compounds called **catecholamines.**

Epinephrine increases the conversion of glycogen to glucose in liver and muscle tissue, causing a rise in blood glucose levels and an increase in the basal metabolic rate. Both epinephrine and norepinephrine increase the rate and strength of the heartbeat and dilate and constrict blood vessels in such a way as to increase the blood supply to skeletal muscle, the heart, and the brain, while decreasing the blood supply to the kidneys, skin, and digestive tract. These effects are known as the "**fight or flight response,**" and are elicited by sympathetic nervous stimulation in response to stress. Both of these hormones are also neurotransmitters (see chapter 12).

> **Flashback**
>
> The secretions of the exocrine pancreas (see chapter 7) are components of the pancreatic juice that enters into the duodenum:
>
> - Amylase (carbohydrate digestion)
> - Lipase (lipid digestion)
> - Trypsin, chymotrypsin and carboxypeptidase (protein digestion)

F. PANCREAS

The pancreas is both an exocrine organ and an endocrine organ. The exocrine function is performed by the cells that secrete digestive enzymes into the small intestine via a series of ducts. The endocrine function is performed by small glandular structures called the **islets of Langerhans**, which are composed of **alpha, beta,** and **delta cells.** Alpha cells produce and secrete **glucagon;** beta cells produce and secrete **insulin;** delta cells produce and secrete **somatostatin.**

1. Glucagon

Glucagon stimulates protein and fat degradation, the conversion of glycogen to glucose, and gluconeogenesis, all of which serve to increase blood glucose levels. Glucagon secretion is stimulated by a decrease in blood glucose and by gastrointestinal hormones (e.g., CCK and gastrin) and is inhibited by high plasma glucose levels. Glucagon's actions are largely antagonistic to those of insulin.

2. Insulin

Insulin is a protein hormone secreted in response to a high blood glucose concentration. It stimulates the uptake of glucose by muscle and adipose cells and the storage of glucose as glycogen in muscle and liver cells, thus lowering blood glucose levels (see Figure 11.4). It also stimulates the synthesis of fats from glucose and the uptake of amino acids. Insulin's actions are antagonistic to those of glucagon and the glucocorticoids. Insulin secretion is regulated by blood glucose levels. Overproduction of insulin causes **hypoglycemia** (low blood glucose levels). Underproduction of insulin, or an insensitivity to insulin, leads to **diabetes mellitus,** which is characterized by **hyperglycemia** (high blood glucose levels). High blood glucose levels lead to excretion of glucose and water loss. In addition, diabetes is associated with weakness and fatigue, and may lead to **ketoacidosis,** which is a dangerous lowering of blood pH due to excess keto acids and fatty acids in the plasma.

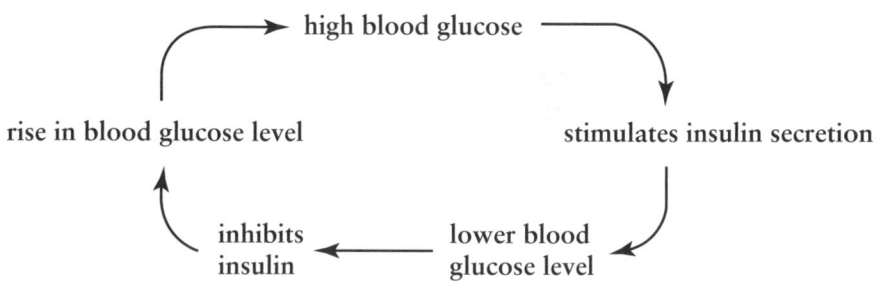

Figure 11.4. Regulation of Insulin Secretion

3. **Somatostatin**
Pancreatic somatostatin secretion is increased by high blood glucose or high amino acid levels, leading to both decreased insulin and glucagon secretion. Somatostatin is also regulated by CCK and GH levels.

G. TESTES

The interstitial cells of the testes produce and secrete androgens, e.g., testosterone (see chapter 4). Testosterone induces embryonic sexual differentiation and male sexual development at puberty and maintains secondary sex characteristics. Testosterone secretion is controlled by a negative feedback mechanism involving FSH and LH. Insensitivity to testosterone results in a syndrome called **testicular feminization**, in which a genetic male (XY) has female secondary sexual characteristics.

H. OVARIES

The ovaries synthesize and secrete estrogens and progesterone. The secretion of both estrogens and progesterone is regulated by LH and FSH, which, in turn, are regulated by GnRH.

1. **Hormones**
   a. **Estrogens**
   Estrogens are steroid hormones necessary for normal female maturation. They stimulate the development of the female reproductive tract and contribute to the development of secondary sexual characteristics and sex drive. Estrogens are also responsible for the thickening of the **endometrium** (uterine wall). Estrogens are secreted by the ovarian follicles and the **corpus luteum.**

   b. **Progesterone**
   Progesterone is a steroid hormone secreted by the corpus luteum during the luteal phase of the menstrual cycle. Progesterone stimulates the development and maintenance of the endometrial walls in preparation for implantation.

2. **The Menstrual Cycle**
   The hormonal secretions of the ovaries, the hypothalamus, and the pituitary play important roles in the female reproductive cycle. From **puberty** through **menopause**, interactions between these hormones result in a monthly cyclical pattern known as the **menstrual cycle.** The menstrual cycle may be divided into the **follicular phase, ovulation**, the **luteal phase**, and **menstruation** (see Figure 11.5).

MCAT Synopsis

- Follicles mature during the follicular phase (FSH, LH).
- LH surge at midcycle triggers ovulation.
- Ruptured follicle becomes corpus luteum and secretes estrogen and progesterone to build up uterine lining in preparation for implantation; LH and FSH inhibited.
- If fertilization doesn't occur, corpus luteum atrophies, progesterone and estrogen levels decrease, menses occurs, and LH and FSH levels begin to rise again.

a. **Follicular phase**

The follicular phase begins with the cessation of the **menstrual flow** from the previous cycle. During this phase, FSH and LH act together to promote the development of several ovarian follicles, which grow and begin secreting estrogen. Rising levels of estrogen in the latter half of this phase stimulate GnRH secretion, which in turn further stimulates LH secretion.

b. **Ovulation**

Midway through the cycle **ovulation** occurs—a mature ovarian follicle bursts and releases an **ovum.** Ovulation is caused by a surge in LH which is preceded by and, in part, caused by a peak in estrogen levels.

c. **Luteal phase**

Following ovulation, LH induces the ruptured follicle to develop into the corpus luteum, which secretes estrogen and progesterone. Progesterone causes the glands of the endometrium to mature and produce secretions that prepare it for the implantation of an embryo. Progesterone and estrogen are essential for the maintenance of the endometrium. Progesterone and estrogen together inhibit secretion of GnRH, thereby inhibiting LH and FSH secretion. This prevents the maturation of additional follicles during the remainder of the cycle.

d. **Menstruation**

If the ovum is not fertilized, the corpus luteum atrophies. The resulting drop in progesterone and estrogen levels causes the endometrium (with its superficial blood vessels) to slough off, giving rise to the menstrual flow (**menses**). Progesterone and estrogen levels decline and GnRH is no longer inhibited. GnRH restimulates LH and FSH secretion, and so the cycle begins anew. However, if the ovum is fertilized, menstruation ceases for the duration of the pregnancy.

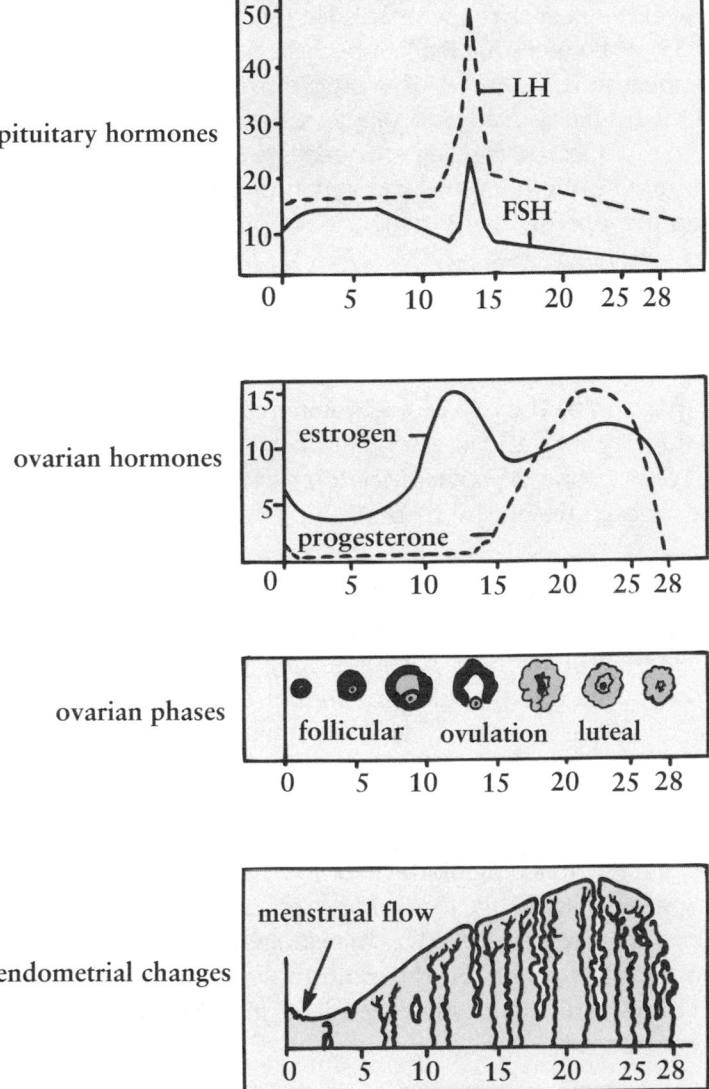

Figure 11.5. The Menstrual Cycle

3. **Pregnancy**

During the first trimester of pregnancy, the corpus luteum is preserved by **human chorionic gonadotropin (HCG)**, a hormone produced by the blastocyst and the developing placenta. Hence, progesterone and estrogen secretion by the corpus luteum is maintained during the first trimester. During the second trimester, HCG levels decline, but progesterone and estrogen levels rise, since they are now secreted by the placenta itself. High levels of progesterone and estrogen inhibit GnRH secretion, thus preventing FSH and LH secretion and the onset of a new menstrual cycle.

4. Menopause

Menopause is the period in a woman's life (usually between the ages of 45 and 55) when menstruation first becomes irregular and eventually stops. Menopause is the result of a progressive decline in the functioning of the ovaries with advancing age; some follicles fail to rupture, ovulation does not occur, and less estrogen is produced by the ovaries, thereby disrupting the hormonal regulation of other glands. Women undergoing menopause may experience symptoms such as bloating, hot flashes, and headaches.

I. PINEAL GLAND

The pineal gland is a tiny structure at the base of the brain that secretes the hormone **melatonin.** The role of melatonin in humans is unclear, but it is believed to play a role in the regulation of **circadian rhythms**— physiological cycles lasting 24 hours. Melatonin secretion is regulated by light and dark cycles in the environment.

J. OTHER ENDOCRINE ORGANS

Glandular tissue is found throughout the mucosa of the stomach and intestines. The primary stimulus for gastrointestinal hormone release is the presence of food in the gut, though neural input and exposure to other hormones also affect their release. Over 20 gastrointestinal peptides have been isolated; important examples are gastrin, secretin, and CCK (see chapter 7).

Clinical Correlate

Patients with chronic kidney disease can become anemic due to impaired erythropoietin production, causing inadequate red cell production from the bone marrow. Recently, genetically engineered erythropoietin has been employed to stimulate the bone marrow to produce more red blood cells in such patients.

Although the primary function of the kidneys is urine formation (see chapter 10), special cells within the kidneys have important endocrine functions. **Renin,** an enzyme secreted by the kidney, is involved in the regulation of aldosterone secretion. **Erythropoietin** is secreted by the kidney in response to decreased renal oxygen levels and stimulates bone marrow to produce red blood cells.

It has also been discovered that the heart and brain are endocrine organs; they release **atrial natriuretic hormone (ANH) and brain natriuretic peptide (BNP),** respectively. ANH and BNP are involved in the regulation of salt and water balance.

The thymus gland is located in the front neck region and secretes hormones such as **thymosin** during childhood. Thymosin stimulates T lymphocyte development and differentiation (see chapter 9). The thymus atrophies by adulthood, after the immune system has fully developed. See Table 11.1 for a listing of the principal hormones.

Table 11.1. Principal Hormones in Humans

Hormone	Source	Action
Growth hormone	Anterior pituitary	Stimulates bone and muscle growth
Prolactin	Anterior pituitary	Stimulates milk production and secretion
Adrenocorticotropic hormone (ACTH)	Anterior pituitary	Stimulates the adrenal cortex to synthesize and secrete glucocorticoids
Thyroid-stimulating hormone (TSH)	Anterior pituitary	Stimulates the thyroid to produce thyroid hormones
Luteinizing hormone (LH)	Anterior pituitary	Stimulates ovulation in females; testosterone synthesis in males
Follicle-stimulating hormone (FSH)	Anterior pituitary	Stimulates follicle maturation in females; spermatogenesis in males
Oxytocin	Hypothalamus; stored in posterior pituitary	Stimulates uterine contractions during labor, and milk secretion during lactation
Vasopressin (ADH)	Hypothalamus; stored in posterior pituitary	Stimulates water reabsorption in kidneys
Thyroid hormone	Thyroid	Stimulates metabolic activity
Calcitonin	Thyroid	Decreases the blood calcium level
Parathyroid hormone	Parathyroid	Increases the blood calcium level
Glucocorticoids	Adrenal cortex	Increase blood glucose level and decreases protein synthesis
Mineralocorticoids	Adrenal cortex	Increase water reabsorption in the kidneys
Epinephrine and Norepinephrine	Adrenal medulla	Increase blood glucose level and heart rate
Glucagon	Pancreas	Stimulates conversion of glycogen to glucose in the liver; increases blood glucose
Insulin	Pancreas	Lowers blood glucose and increases storage of glycogen
Somatostatin	Pancreas	Suppresses secretion of glucagon and insulin
Testosterone	Testis	Maintains male secondary sexual characteristics
Estrogen	Ovary/placenta	Maintains female secondary sexual characteristics
Progesterone	Ovary/placenta	Promotes growth/maintenance of endometrium
Melatonin	Pineal	Unclear in humans
Atrial natriuretic hormone	Heart	Involved in osmoregulation
Thymosin	Thymus	Stimulates T lymphocyte development

MECHANISMS OF HORMONE ACTION

Hormones are classified on the basis of their chemical structure into three major groups: **peptide hormones, steroid hormones,** and **amino acid-derived hormones.** There are two ways in which hormones affect the activities of their target cells: via extracellular receptors or intracellular receptors.

A. PEPTIDES: SECONDARY MESSENGER

Peptide hormones range from simple short peptides (amino acid chains) such as ADH, to complex polypeptides such as insulin. Synthesis of peptide hormones begins with the synthesis of a large polypeptide (see chapter 14). The polypeptide is then cleaved into smaller protein units and transported to the Golgi apparatus, where it is further modified into the active hormone. The hormone is packaged into secretory vesicles and stored until it is released by the cell via exocytosis.

Peptide hormones act as **first messengers.** Their binding to specific receptors on the surface of their target cells triggers a series of enzymatic reactions within each cell, the first of which may be the conversion of ATP to **cyclic adenosine monophosphate (cAMP);** this reaction is catalyzed by the membrane-bound enzyme **adenylate cyclase.** Cyclic AMP acts as a **second messenger,** relaying messages from the extracellular peptide hormone to cytoplasmic enzymes and initiating a series of successive reactions in the cell. This is an example of a **cascade effect;** with each step, the hormone's effects are amplified. Cyclic AMP activity is inactivated by the cytoplasmic enzyme **phosphodiesterase.**

B. STEROIDS: PRIMARY MESSENGER

Steroid hormones, such as estrogen and aldosterone, belong to a class of lipid-derived molecules with a characteristic ring structure. They are produced by the testes, ovaries, placenta, and adrenal cortex. In the synthesis of steroid molecules, precursors already present in the cell (such as cholesterol) undergo enzymatic reactions that convert them into active hormones. Steroid hormones pass through the cell membrane with ease because they are lipid-soluble. Steroid hormones are not stored, but are secreted at a rate determined by their rate of synthesis.

Steroid hormones enter their target cells directly and bind to specific receptor proteins in the cytoplasm. This receptor-hormone complex enters the nucleus and directly activates the expression of specific genes by binding to receptors on the chromatin. This induces a change in mRNA transcription and protein synthesis.

MCAT Synopsis

Peptide hormones:

- Surface receptors
- Generally act as first messengers

Steroid hormones:

- Intracellular receptors
- Hormone/receptor binding to DNA promotes transcription of specific genes

---

C. AMINO ACID DERIVATIVES

Amino acid derivatives are hormones composed of one or two modified amino acids. They are synthesized in the cytoplasm of glandular cells. Some are further modified and stored in granules until the cell is stimulated to release them, while others are initially synthesized as component parts of larger molecules and stored.

Some amino acid–derived hormones, such as epinephrine, activate their target cells as peptide hormones do; i.e., via second messengers. Others, such as thyroxine, act in the same manner as steroid hormones, entering the nucleus of their target cells and regulating gene expression.

12

NERVOUS SYSTEM

The nervous system enables organisms to receive and respond to **stimuli** from their external and internal environments. **Neurons** are the functional units of the nervous system. A neuron converts stimuli into electrochemical signals that are conducted through the nervous system.

NEURONS

A. STRUCTURE

The neuron is an elongated cell consisting of **dendrites,** a **cell body,** and an **axon.** Dendrites are cytoplasmic extensions that receive information and transmit it toward the cell body. The cell body **(soma)** contains the nucleus and controls the metabolic activity of the neuron. The **axon hillock** connects the cell body to the axon (nerve fiber), which is a long cellular process that transmits impulses away from the cell body. Most mammalian axons are ensheathed by an insulating substance known as **myelin,** which allows axons to conduct impulses faster. Myelin is produced by cells known as **glial cells. (Oligodendrocytes** produce myelin in the central nervous system, and **Schwann cells** produce myelin in the peripheral nervous system.) The gaps between segments of myelin are called **nodes of Ranvier.** Ultimately, the axons end as swellings known as **synaptic terminals** (sometimes also called synaptic boutons or knobs) (see Figure 12.1). Neurotransmitters are released from these terminals into the **synapse** (or **synaptic cleft**), which is the gap between the axon terminals of one cell and the dendrites of the next cell.

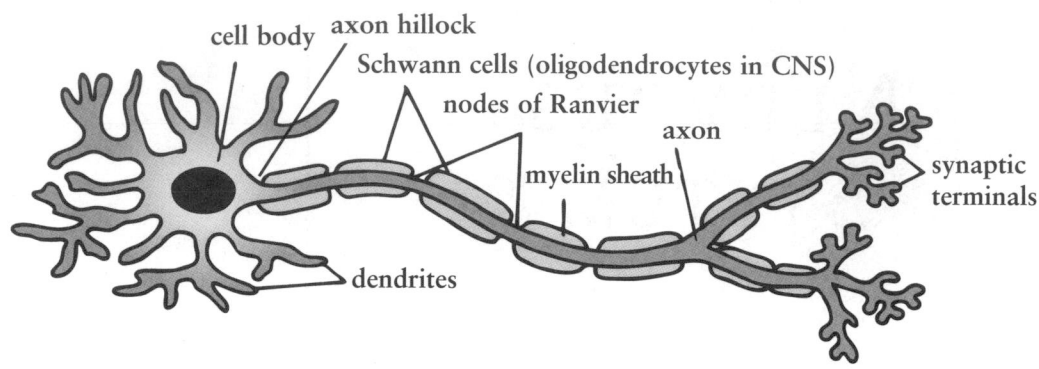

Figure 12.1. Peripheral Nerve

B. FUNCTION

Neurons are specialized to receive signals from sensory receptors or from other neurons in the body and transfer this information along the length of the axon. Impulses, known as **action potentials**, travel the length of the axon and invade the nerve terminal, thereby causing the release of neurotransmitter into the synapse. When a neuron is at rest, the potential difference between the extracellular space and the intracellular space is called the **resting potential.**

1. Resting Potential

Even at rest, a neuron is polarized. This potential difference is the result of an unequal distribution of ions between the inside and out-side of the cell. A typical resting membrane potential is −70 millivolts (mV), which means that the inside of the neuron is more negative than the outside. This difference is due to selective ionic permeability of the neuronal cell membrane and is maintained by the **Na⁺/K⁺ pump** (also called the Na⁺/K⁺ ATPase).

The concentration of K⁺ is higher inside the neuron than outside; the concentration of Na⁺ is higher outside than inside. Additionally, neg-atively charged proteins are trapped inside of the cell. The resting potential is created because the neuron is selectively permeable to K⁺, so K⁺ diffuses down its concentration gradient, leaving a net negative charge inside. (Neurons do not allow much Na⁺ to enter the cell under resting conditions, so the cell remains polarized.)

Because the transmission of action potentials leads to the disruption of the ionic gradients (see next section), the gradients must be restored by the Na⁺/K⁺ pump. This pump, using ATP energy, transports 3 Na⁺ out for every 2 K⁺ it transports into the cell (see Figure 12.2).

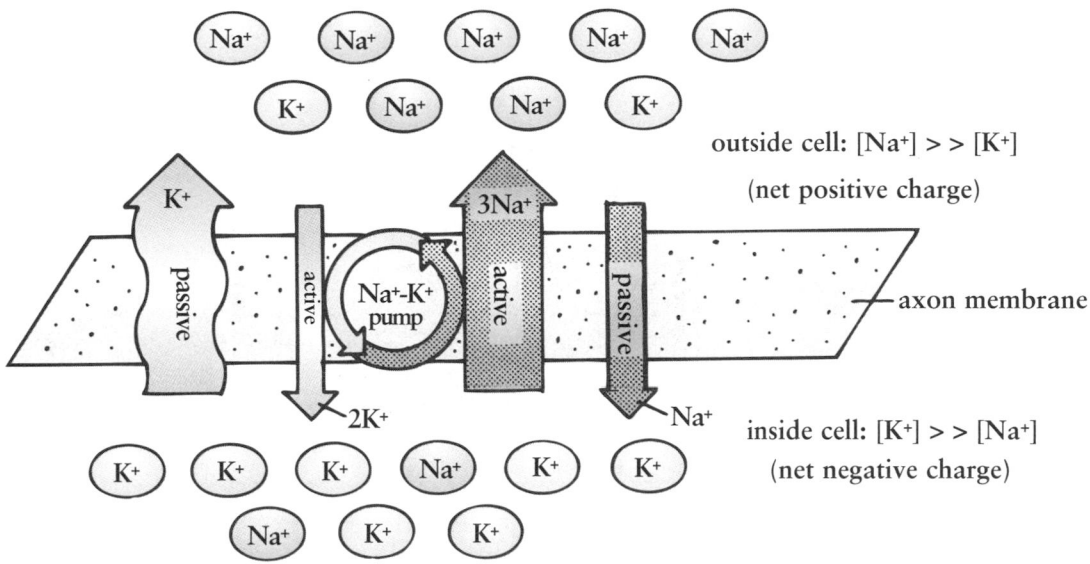

outside cell: [Na⁺] >> [K⁺]

(net positive charge)

— axon membrane

inside cell: [K⁺] >> [Na⁺]

(net negative charge)

Figure 12.2. Resting Potential of a Neuron

2. Action Potential

The nerve cell body receives both excitatory and inhibitory impulses from other cells. If the cell becomes sufficiently excited or **depolarized** (i.e., the inside of the cell becomes less negative), an action potential is generated. The minimum **threshold membrane potential** (usually around –50 mV) is the level at which an action potential is initiated.

Ion channels located in the nerve cell membrane open in response to these changes in voltage and are therefore called **voltage-gated ion channels.** An action potential begins when **voltage-gated Na⁺ channels** open in response to depolarization, allowing Na⁺ to rush down its **electrochemical gradient** into the cell, causing a rapid depolarization of that segment of the cell. The voltage-gated Na⁺ channels then close, and **voltage-gated K⁺ channels** open, allowing K⁺ to rush out down its electrochemical gradient. This returns the cell to a more negative potential, a process known as **repolarization**. In fact, the neuron may shoot past the resting potential and become even more negative inside than normal; this is called **hyperpolarization** (see Figure 12.3). Immediately following an action potential, it may be very difficult or impossible to initiate another action potential; this period of time is called the **refractory period**.

MCAT Synopsis

Na⁺ wants to go into the cell because it is more negative inside (electrical gradient) and because there is less Na⁺ inside (chemical gradient).

Clinical Correlate

There is a poison called tetrodotoxin (TTX) which is found in the puffer fish, a delicacy in Japan. TTX blocks the voltage-gated Na⁺ channels, thereby blocking neuronal transmission, and can rapidly cause death. For this reason, chefs that prepare puffer fish must be specially trained and licensed. If the fish is prepared correctly, you should only experience a slight numbing of your oral cavity.

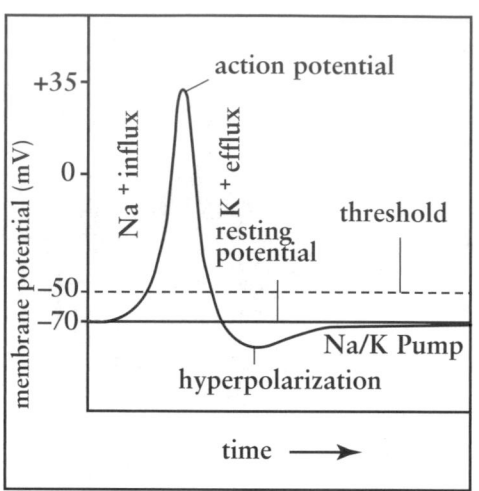

Figure 12.3. Action Potential

The action potential is often described as an **all-or-none response**. This means that whenever the threshold membrane potential is reached, an action potential with a consistent size and duration is produced. Neuronal information is coded by the frequency and number of action potentials rather than the size of the action potential. (In other words, the harder you hit your thumb with a hammer, the more action potentials will travel up your pain fibers, but the size and duration of each individual action potential will remain the same.)

3. **Impulse Propagation**

    If there is an adequate stimulus, the action potential will first be initiated at the axon hillock. Na^+ rushes into the neuron and diffuses to adjacent parts of the axon, causing nearby voltage-gated Na^+ channels to open. This occurs as previous segments are repolarizing. This chain of events (depolarization followed by a subsequent repolarization) continues along the length of the axon (see Figure 12.4). Although axons can theoretically propagate action potentials bidirectionally, information transfer will occur only in one direction: from dendrite to synaptic terminal. (This is because synapses operate only in one direction and because refractory periods make the backward travel of action potentials impossible.) Different axons can propagate action potentials at different speeds. The greater the diameter of the axon and the more heavily it is myelinated, the faster the impulses will travel. Myelin increases the conduction velocity by insulating segments of the axon, so that the membrane is permeable to ions only in the nodes of Ranvier. In this way, the action potential "jumps" from node to node; this process is called **saltatory conduction**.

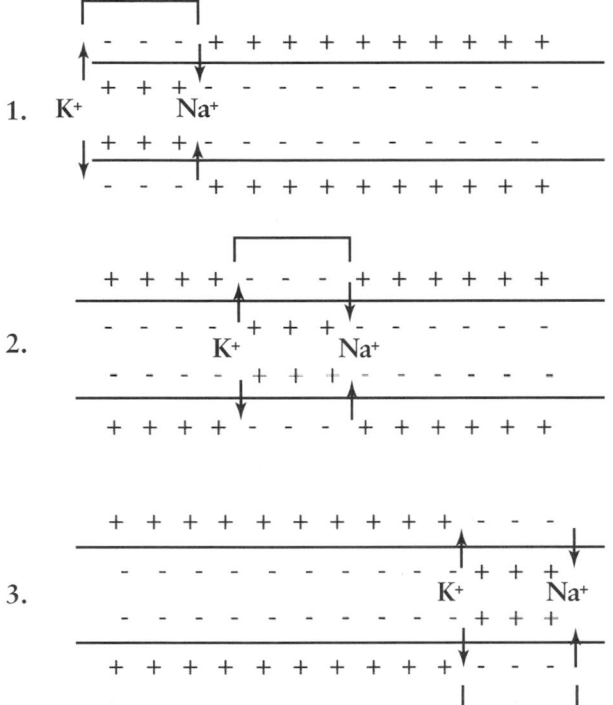

Figure 12.4. Propagation of an Action Potential

SYNAPSE

The synapse is the gap between the axon terminal of one neuron (called the **presynaptic neuron** because it is before the synapse) and the dendrites of another neuron **(postsynaptic neuron).** Neurons may also communicate with postsynaptic cells other than neurons, such as cells in muscles or glands; these are called **effector cells.** The vast majority of synapses in the human are **chemical synapses.** In chemical synapses, the nerve terminal contains thousands of membrane-bound vesicles full of chemical messengers known as **neurotransmitters.** When the action potential arrives at the nerve terminal and depolarizes it, the synaptic vesicles fuse with the presynaptic membrane and release neurotransmitter into the synapse via a calcium-dependent process of exocytosis. The neurotransmitter diffuses across the synapse and acts on receptor proteins embedded in the postsynaptic membrane (see Figure 12.5). Depending on the nature of the receptor, the neurotransmitter may have an excitatory or an inhibitory effect on the postsynaptic cell. Neurotransmitter is removed from the synapse in a variety of ways: it may be taken back up into the nerve terminal (via a protein known as an **uptake carrier**) where it may be reused or degraded; it may be degraded by enzymes located in the synapse (e.g., **acetylcholinesterase** inactivates the neurotransmitter acetylcholine); it may simply diffuse out of the synapse.

Clinical Correlate

Many common drugs (either in clinical use or street drugs) modify processes that occur in the synapse. For instance, cocaine acts by blocking neuronal uptake carriers, thus prolonging the action of neurotransmitters in the synapse by preventing neurotransmitter re-entry into the nerve terminal. There are clinically useful drugs (e.g., drugs used to treat glaucoma) that inhibit acetylcholinesterase, thereby elevating synaptic levels of acetylcholine. Nerve gases are extremely potent acetylcho-linesterase inhibitors which have been used in war and in recent terrorist activities. Nerve gas causes rapid death by preventing the action of skeletal muscle (most importantly, the diaphragm)—leading to respiratory arrest.

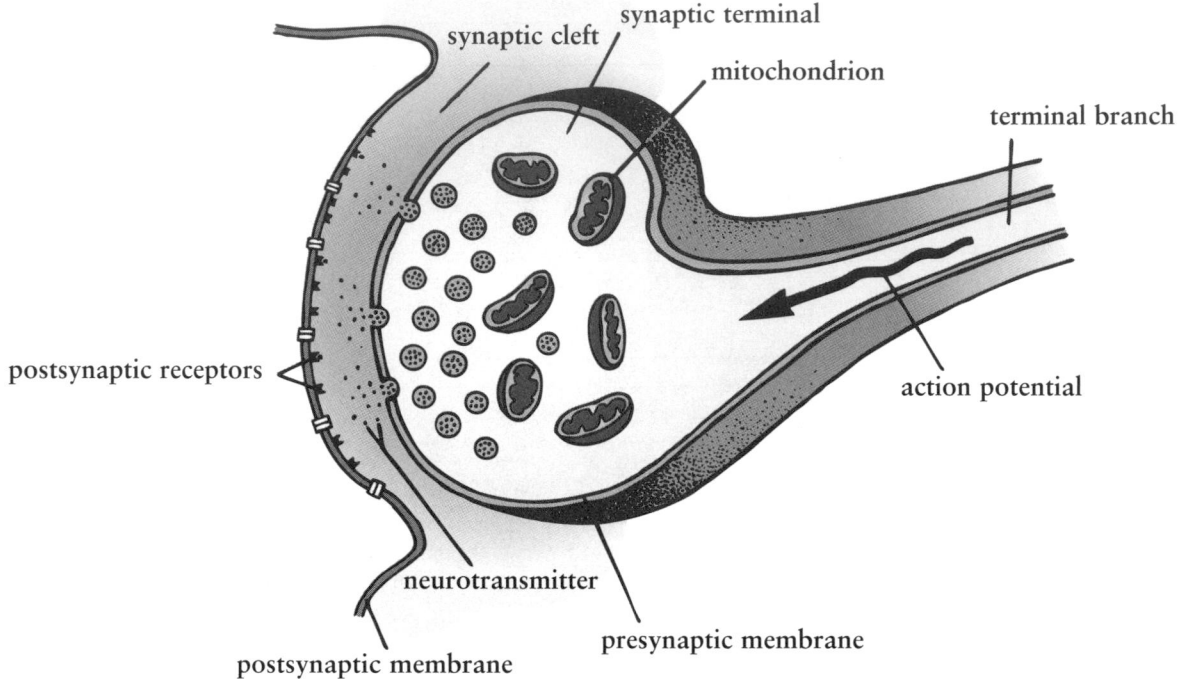

Figure 12.5. The Synapse

ORGANIZATION OF THE VERTEBRATE NERVOUS SYSTEM

There are many different kinds of neurons in the vertebrate nervous system. Neurons that carry information about the external or internal environment to the brain or spinal cord are called **afferent neurons**. Neurons that carry commands from the brain or spinal cord to various parts of the body (e.g., muscles or glands) are called **efferent neurons**. Some neurons (**interneurons**) participate only in local circuits; their cell bodies and their nerve terminals are in the same location.

Nerves are essentially bundles of axons covered with connective tissue. A nerve may carry only sensory fibers (a **sensory nerve**), only motor fibers (a **motor nerve**), or a mixture of the two (a **mixed nerve**). Neuronal cell bodies often cluster together; such clusters are called **ganglia** in the periphery; in the central nervous system, they are called **nuclei**. The nervous system itself is divided into two major systems, the **central nervous system** and the **peripheral nervous system** (see Figure 12.6).

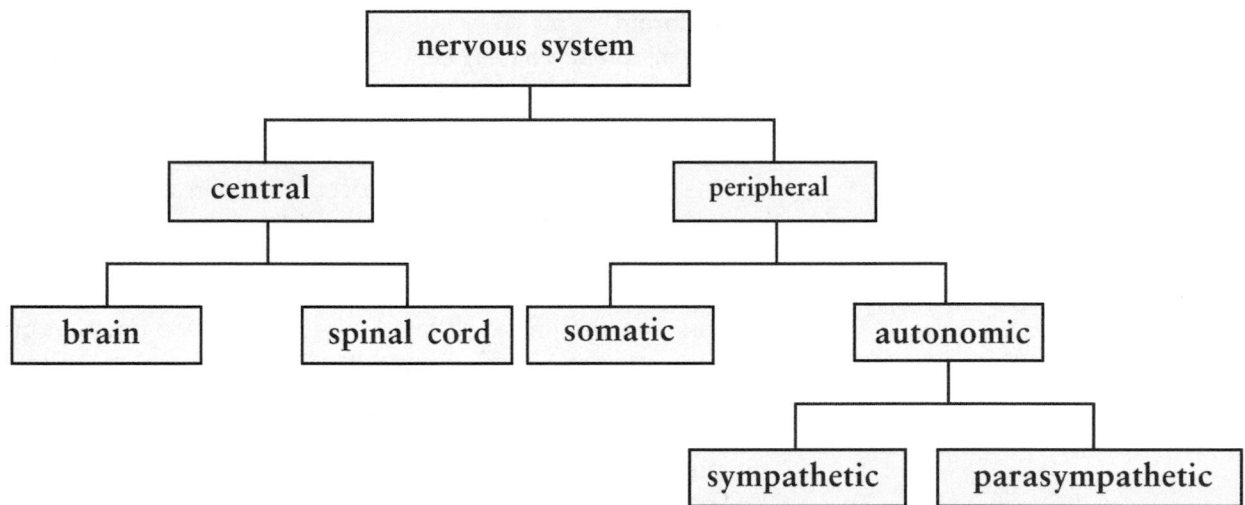

Figure 12.6. Organization of the Vertebrate Nervous System

A. CENTRAL NERVOUS SYSTEM

The central nervous system (CNS) consists of the **brain** and the **spinal cord.**

1. **Brain**

   The brain is a jellylike mass of neurons that resides in the skull. Its functions include interpreting sensory information, forming motor plans, and cognitive function (thinking). The brain consists of **gray matter** (cell bodies) and **white matter** (myelinated axons). The brain can be divided into the **forebrain, midbrain,** and **hindbrain.**

   a. **Forebrain**

      The forebrain consists of the **telencephalon** and the **diencephalon.** The telencephalon consists of right and left hemispheres; each hemisphere can be divided into four different lobes: **frontal, parietal, temporal,** and **occipital.** A major component of the telencephalon is the **cerebral cortex,** which is the highly convoluted gray matter that can be seen on the surface of the brain. The cortex processes and integrates sensory input and motor responses and is important for memory and creative thought. Right and left cerebral cortices communicate with each other through the **corpus callosum.**

      The diencephalon contains the **thalamus** and **hypothalamus.** The thalamus is a relay and integration center for the spinal cord and cerebral cortex. The hypothalamus controls visceral functions such as hunger, thirst, sex drive, water balance, blood pressure, and temperature regulation. It also plays an important role in the control of the endocrine system (see chapter 11).

b. **Midbrain**

The midbrain is a relay center for visual and auditory impulses. It also plays an important role in motor control.

c. **Hindbrain**

The hindbrain is the posterior part of the brain and consists of the **cerebellum**, the **pons**, and the **medulla**. The cerebellum helps to modulate motor impulses initiated by the motor cortex and is important in the maintenance of balance, hand-eye coordination, and the timing of rapid movements. One function of the pons is to act as a relay center to allow the cortex to communicate with the cerebellum. The medulla (also called the medulla oblongata) controls many vital functions such as breathing, heart rate, and gastrointestinal activity. Together, the midbrain, pons, and medulla constitute the **brainstem**.

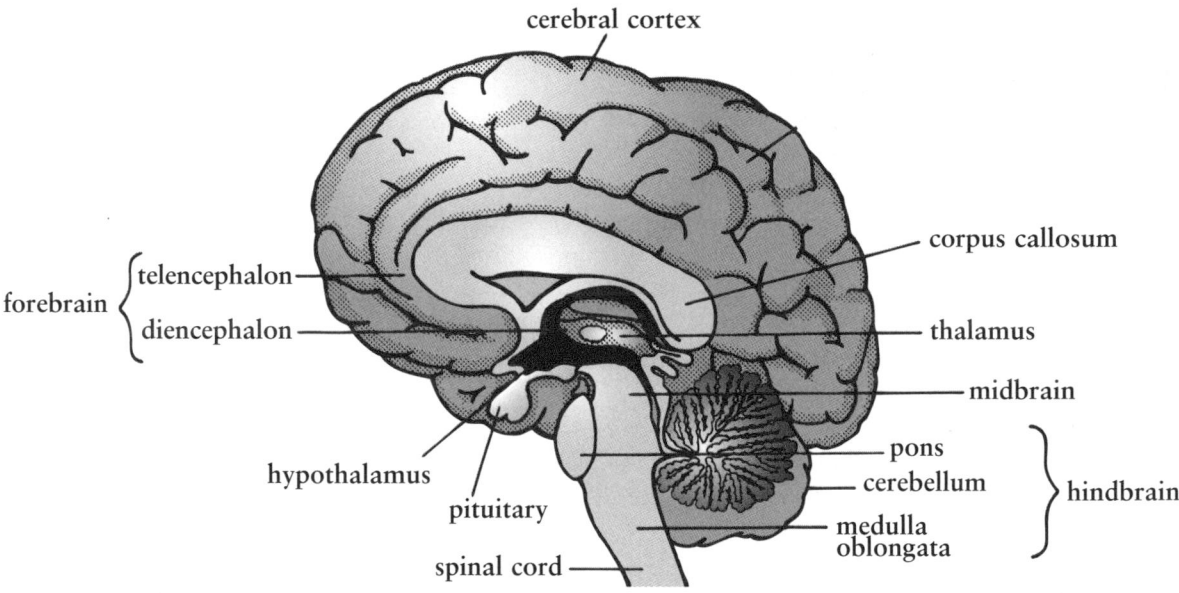

Figure 12.7. Human Brain

2. **Spinal Cord**

The spinal cord is an elongated structure, continuous with the brainstem, that extends down the dorsal side of vertebrates. Nearly all nerves that innervate the viscera or muscles below the head pass through the spinal cord, and nearly all sensory information from below the head passes through the spinal cord on the way to the brain. The spinal cord can also integrate simple motor responses (e.g., reflexes) by itself. A cross-section of the spinal cord reveals an outer white matter area containing motor and sensory axons and an inner gray matter area containing nerve cell bodies. Sensory information enters the spinal cord dorsally; the cell bodies of these sensory neurons are located in the **dorsal root ganglia**. All motor information exits the spinal cord ventrally. Nerves branches entering and leaving the cord are called **roots** (see Figure 12.8). The spinal cord is divided into four regions (going in order from the brainstem to the tail): **cervical, thoracic, lumbar,** and **sacral.**

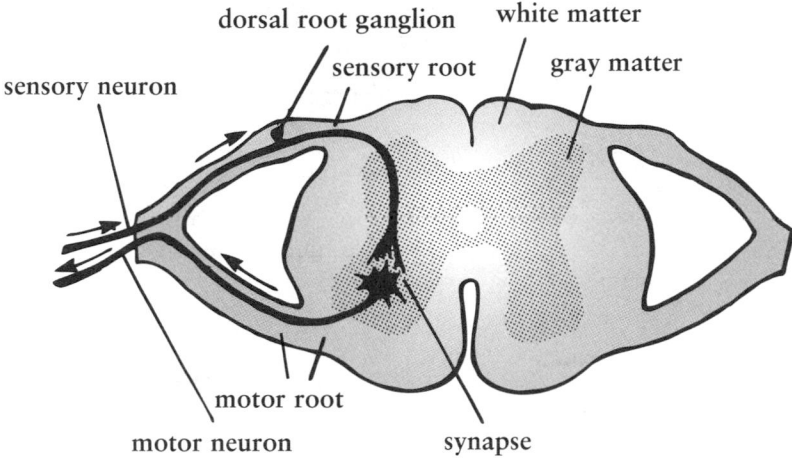

Figure 12.8. Spinal Cord

B. PERIPHERAL NERVOUS SYSTEM

The peripheral nervous system (PNS) consists of 12 pairs of cranial nerves, which primarily innervate the head and shoulders, and 31 pairs of spinal nerves, which innervate the rest of the body. Cranial nerves exit from the brainstem and spinal nerves exit from the spinal cord. The PNS has two primary divisions: the somatic and the autonomic nervous systems, each of which has both motor and sensory components.

1. Somatic Nervous System

The somatic nervous system (SNS) innervates skeletal muscles and is responsible for voluntary movement. Motor neurons release the neurotransmitter acetylcholine (ACh) onto ACh receptors located on skeletal muscle. This causes depolarization of the skeletal muscle, leading to muscle contraction. In addition to voluntary movement, the somatic nervous system is also important for reflex action. There are both **monosynaptic** and **polysynaptic** reflexes.

• Monosynaptic reflex pathways have only one synapse between the sensory neuron and the motor neuron. The classic example is the **knee-jerk reflex**. When the tendon covering the patella (kneecap) is hit, stretch receptors sense this and action potentials are sent up the sensory neuron and into the spinal cord. The sensory neuron synapses with a motor neuron in the spinal cord, which in turn, stimulates the quadriceps muscle to contract, causing the lower leg to kick forward (see Figures 12.8 and 12.9).

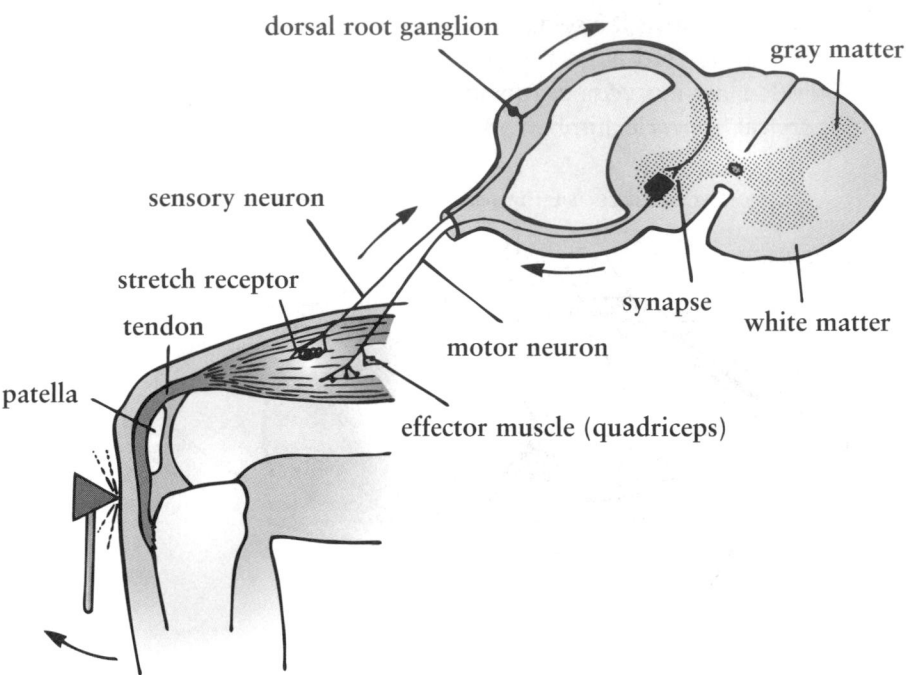

Figure 12.9. Reflex Arc for Knee-Jerk

- In polysynaptic reflexes, sensory neurons synapse with more than one neuron. A classic example of this is the **withdrawal reflex**. When a person steps on a nail, the injured leg withdraws in pain, while the other leg extends to retain balance.

2. **Autonomic Nervous System**

The autonomic nervous system **(ANS)** is sometimes also called the involuntary nervous system because it regulates the body's internal environment without the aid of conscious control. Whereas the somatic nervous system innervates skeletal muscle, the ANS innervates cardiac and smooth muscle. Smooth muscle is located in areas such as blood vessels, the digestive tract, the bladder, and bronchi, so it isn't surprising that the ANS is important in blood pressure control, gastrointestinal motility, excretory processes, respiration, and reproductive processes. ANS pathways are characterized by a two-neuron system. The first neuron (preganglionic neuron) has a cell body located within the CNS and its axon synapses in peripheral ganglia. The second neuron (postganglionic neuron) has its cell body in the ganglia and then synapses on cardiac or smooth muscle. The ANS is comprised of two subdivisions, the **sympathetic** and the **parasympathetic nervous systems**, which generally act in opposition to one another.

a. **Sympathetic nervous system**

The sympathetic division is responsible for the "flight or fight" responses that ready the body for action. It basically does everything you would want it to do in an emergency situation. It increases blood pressure and heart rate; it increases blood flow to skeletal muscles and it decreases gut motility. The preganglionic neurons emerge from the thoracic and lumbar regions of the spinal cord and use acetylcholine as their neurotransmitter; the postganglionic neurons typically release norepinephrine. The action of preganglionic sympathetic neurons also causes the adrenal medulla to release adrenaline (epinephrine) into the bloodstream.

b. **Parasympathetic nervous system**

The parasympathetic division acts to conserve energy and restore the body to resting activity levels following exertion ("rest and digest"). It acts to lower heart rate and to increase gut motility. One very important parasympathetic nerve that innervates many of the thoracic and abdominal viscera is called the **vagus nerve**. Parasympathetic neurons originate in the brainstem (cranial nerves) and the sacral part of the spinal cord. Both the preganglionic and postganglionic neurons release acetycholine.

SPECIAL SENSES

The body has three types of sensory receptors to monitor its internal and external environment: **interoceptors**, **proprioceptors**, and **exteroceptors**. Interoceptors monitor aspects of the internal environment such as blood pressure, the partial pressure of CO_2 in the blood, and blood pH. Proprioceptors transmit information regarding the position of the body in space. These receptors are located in muscles and tendons to tell the brain where the limbs are in space and are also located in the inner ear to tell the brain where the head is in space. Exteroceptors sense things in the external environment such as light, sound, taste, pain, touch, and temperature.

1. **The Eye**

The eye detects light energy (as photons) and transmits information about intensity, color, and shape to the brain. The eyeball is covered by a thick, opaque layer known as the **sclera**, which is also known as the white of the eye. Beneath the sclera is the **choroid** layer, which helps to supply the retina with blood. The innermost layer of the eye is the **retina**, which contains the photoreceptors that sense the light. The transparent **cornea** at the front of the eye bends and focuses light rays. The rays then travel through an opening called the **pupil**, whose diameter is controlled by the pigmented, muscular **iris**. The iris responds to the intensity of light in the surroundings (light makes the pupil constrict). The light continues through the lens, which is suspended behind the pupil. The lens, the shape of which is controlled by the **ciliary muscles**, focuses the image onto the retina. In the retina are photoreceptors that **transduce** light into action potentials. There are two main types of photoreceptors: **cones** and **rods**. Cones respond to high-intensity illumination and are sensitive to color, while rods detect low-intensity illumination and are important in night vision. The cones and rods contain various pigments that absorb specific wavelengths of light. The cones contain three different pigments that absorb red, green, and blue wavelengths; the rod pigment, **rhodopsin**, absorbs one wavelength. The photoreceptor cells synapse onto **bipolar cells**, which in turn synapse onto **ganglion cells**. Axons of the ganglion cells bundle to form the right and left **optic nerves**, which conduct visual information to the brain. The point at which the optic nerve exits the eye is called the **blind spot** because photoreceptors are not present there. There is also a small area of the retina called the **fovea**, which is densely packed with cones and is important for high acuity vision (see Figure 12.10).

The eye also has its own circulation system. Near the base of the iris, the eye secretes aqueous humor, which travels to the anterior chamber of the eye from which it exits and eventually joins venous blood.

Bridge

The lens in the eye is a converging (convex) lens. A convex lens with a smaller radius of curvature (i.e., thicker) has more refractive power and a shorter focal length (good for near vision). A lens with a larger radius of curvature (i.e., flatter) has less refractive power and a longer focal length (good for far vision). A convex lens forms an inverted and reversed image on the focal plane (i.e., the retina); it is up to the brain to sort that out.

Clinical Correlate

Some people develop a plumbing problem in the eye and cannot adequately drain aqueous humor. This disease is called glaucoma. Because of the draining problem, pressure builds in the anterior chamber and is transmitted to the vitreous humor, leading to increased pressure on the optic nerve. If the pressure is not relieved, this condition can permanently damage the optic nerve and lead to blindness.

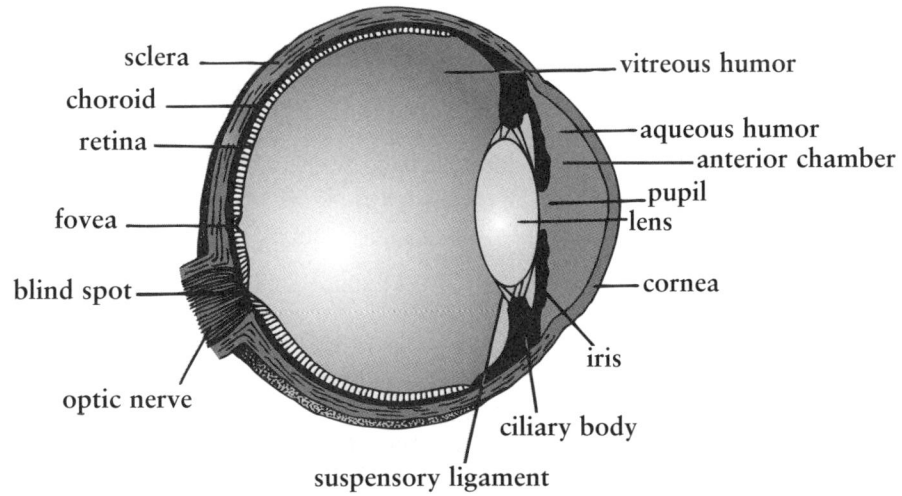

Figure 12.10. Human Eye

2. The Ear

The ear transduces sound energy (pressure waves) into impulses perceived by the brain as sound. The ear is also responsible for maintaining equilibrium (balance) in the body.

Sound waves pass through three regions as they enter the ear. First, they enter the **outer ear,** which consists of the **auricle** (pinna) and the **auditory canal.** At the end of the auditory canal is the **tympanic membrane (eardrum)** of the **middle ear,** which vibrates at the same frequency as the incoming sound. Next, the three bones, or **ossicles (malleus, incus,** and **stapes),** amplify the stimulus and transmit it through the **oval window,** which leads to the fluid-filled **inner ear.** The inner ear consists of the **cochlea** and the **semicircular canals.** The cochlea contains the **organ of Corti,** which has specialized sensory cells called hair cells. Vibration of the ossicles exerts pressure on the fluid in the cochlea, stimulating the hair cells to transduce the pressure into action potentials, which travel via the **auditory (cochlear) nerve** to the brain for processing (see Figure 12.11).

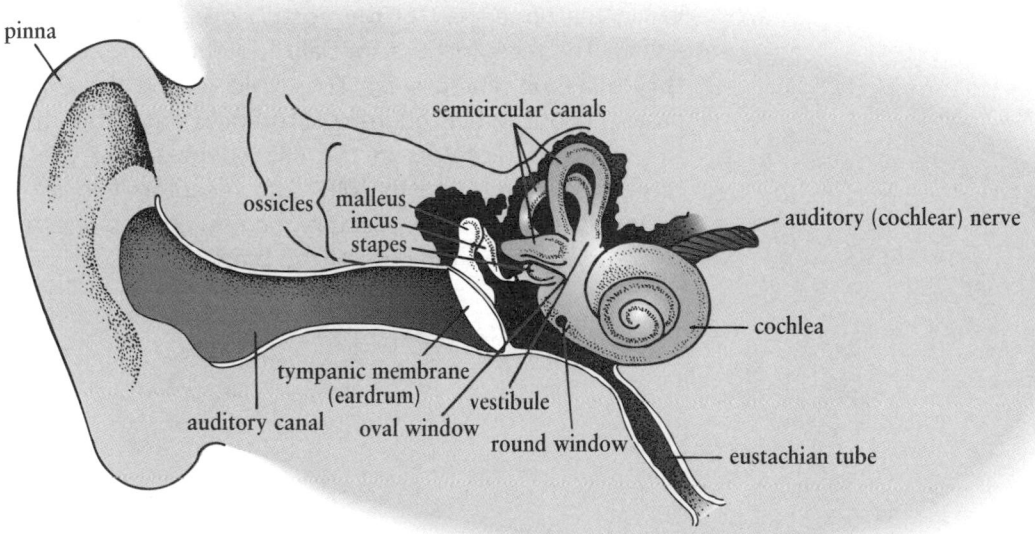

Figure 12.11. Human Ear

The three semicircular canals are each perpendicular to the other two and filled with a fluid called **endolymph.** At the base of each canal is a chamber with sensory hair cells; rotation of the head displaces endolymph in one of the canals, putting pressure on the hair cells in it. This changes the nature of impulses sent by the vestibular nerve to the brain. The brain interprets this information to determine the position of the head.

3. **The Chemical Senses**

The chemical senses are taste and smell. These senses transduce chemical changes in the environment, specifically in the mouth and nose, into **gustatory** and **olfactory** sensory impulses, which are interpreted by the nervous system.

a. **Taste**

Taste receptors, or **taste buds,** are located on the tongue, the soft palate, and the epiglottis. Taste buds are composed of approximately 40 epithelial cells. The outer surface of a taste bud contains a **taste pore**, from which microvilli, or **taste hairs,** protrude. The receptor surfaces for taste are on the taste hairs. Interwoven around the taste buds is a network of nerve fibers that are stimulated by the taste buds. These neurons transmit gustatory information to the brainstem via three cranial nerves. There are four kinds of taste sensations: sour, salty, sweet, and bitter. Although most taste buds will respond to all four stimuli, they respond preferentially; i.e., at a lower threshold, to one or two of them.

b. **Smell**

Olfactory receptors are found in the olfactory membrane, which lies in the upper part of the nostrils over a total area of about 5 cm^2. The receptors are specialized neurons from which **olfactory hairs,** or **cilia,** project. These cilia form a dense mat in the nasal mucosa. When odorous substances enter the nasal cavity, they bind to receptors in the cilia, depolarizing the olfactory receptors. Axons from the olfactory receptors join to form the **olfactory nerves.** The olfactory nerves project directly to the **olfactory bulbs** in the base of the brain.

13

GENETICS

Genetics is the study of how traits are inherited from one generation to the next. The basic unit of heredity is the **gene.** Genes are composed of DNA and are located on chromosomes. When a gene exists in more than one form, the alternate forms are called **alleles.** The genetic makeup of an individual is the individual's **genotype;** the physical manifestation of the genetic makeup is the individual's **phenotype.** Some phenotypes correspond to a single genotype, while other phenotypes correspond to several different genotypes.

MENDELIAN GENETICS

In the 1860s, Gregor Mendel developed the basic principles of genetics through his experiments with the garden pea. Mendel studied the inheritance of individual pea traits by performing genetic crosses: He took **true-breeding** individuals (which, if self-crossed, produce progeny only with the parental phenotype) with different traits, mated them, and statistically analyzed the inheritance of the traits in the progeny.

A. MENDEL'S FIRST LAW: LAW OF SEGREGATION

Mendel postulated four principles of inheritance:

- Genes exist in alternate forms (now referred to as alleles).
- An organism has two alleles for each inherited trait, one inherited from each parent.
- The two alleles segregate during meiosis, resulting in gametes that carry only one allele for any given inherited trait.
- If two alleles in an individual organism are different, only one will be fully expressed and the other will be silent. The expressed allele is said to be **dominant,** the silent allele, **recessive.** In genetics problems, dominant alleles are typically assigned capital letters, and recessive alleles are assigned lower case letters. Organisms that contain two copies of the same allele are **homozygous** for that trait; organisms that carry two different alleles are **heterozygous.**

1. **Monohybrid Cross**

   The principles of Mendelian inheritance can be illustrated in a cross between two true-breeding pea plants, one with purple flowers and the other with white flowers. Since only one trait is being studied in this particular mating, it is referred to as a **monohybrid cross**. The individuals being crossed are the **Parental** or **P generation**; the progeny generations are the **Filial** or **F generations**, with each generation numbered sequentially (e.g., F_1, F_2, etc.).

   The purple flower parent has the genotype PP (i.e., it has two P alleles) and is homozygous dominant. The white flower parent has the genotype pp and is homozygous recessive. When these individuals are crossed, they produce F_1 plants that are 100 percent heterozygous (genotype = Pp). Since purple is dominant to white, all the F_1 progeny have the purple flower phenotype.

2. **Punnett Square**

   One way of predicting the genotypes expected from a cross is by drawing a **Punnett square** diagram. The parental genotypes are arranged around a grid, as shown in Figure 13.1. Since the genotype of each progeny will be the sum of the alleles donated by the parental gametes, their genotypes can be determined by looking at the intersections on the grid. A Punnett square indicates all the potential progeny genotypes, and the relative frequencies of the different genotypes and phenotypes can be easily calculated (see Figure 13.1).

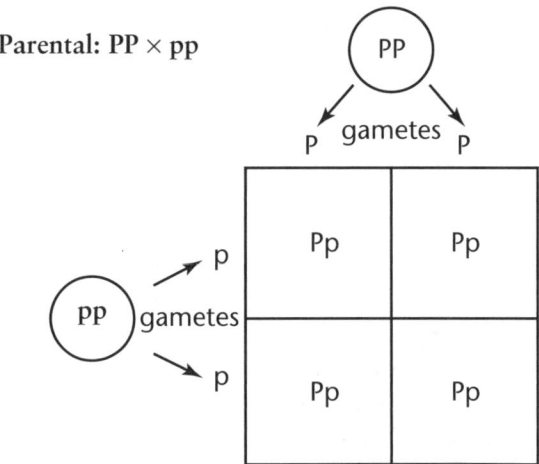

Parental: PP × pp

F_1 genotypes: 100% Pp (heterozygous)

F_1 phenotypes: 100% purple flowers

Figure 13.1. Monohybrid Cross

When the F_1 generation from our monohybrid cross is **self-crossed**, i.e., Pp × Pp, the F_2 progeny are more genotypically and phenotypically diverse than their parents. Since the F_1 plants are heterozygous, they will donate a P allele to half of their descendants and a p allele to the other half. One-fourth of the F_2 plants will have the genotype PP; 50 percent will have the genotype Pp; and 25 percent will have the genotype pp. Since the homozygous dominant and heterozygous genotypes both produce the dominant phenotype, purple flowers, 75 percent of the F_2 plants will have purple flowers, and 25 percent will have white flowers (see Figure 13.2).

This is a standard pattern of Mendelian inheritance. Its hallmarks are the disappearance of the silent (recessive) phenotype in the F_1 generation and its subsequent reappearance in 25 percent of the individuals in the F_2 generation.

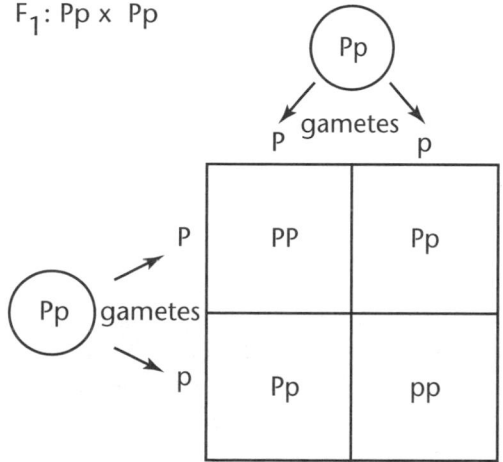

F_1: Pp × Pp

F_2 genotypes: 1:2:1; 1PP: 2Pp:1pp

F_2 phenotypes: 3:1; 3 purple:1 white

Figure 13.2. Self-Cross of F_1 Generation

3. **Testcross**

Only with a recessive phenotype can genotype be predicted with 100 percent accuracy. If the dominant phenotype is expressed, the genotype can be either homozygous dominant or heterozygous. Thus, homozygous recessive organisms always breed true. This fact can be used to determine the unknown genotype of an organism with a dominant phenotype. In a procedure known as a

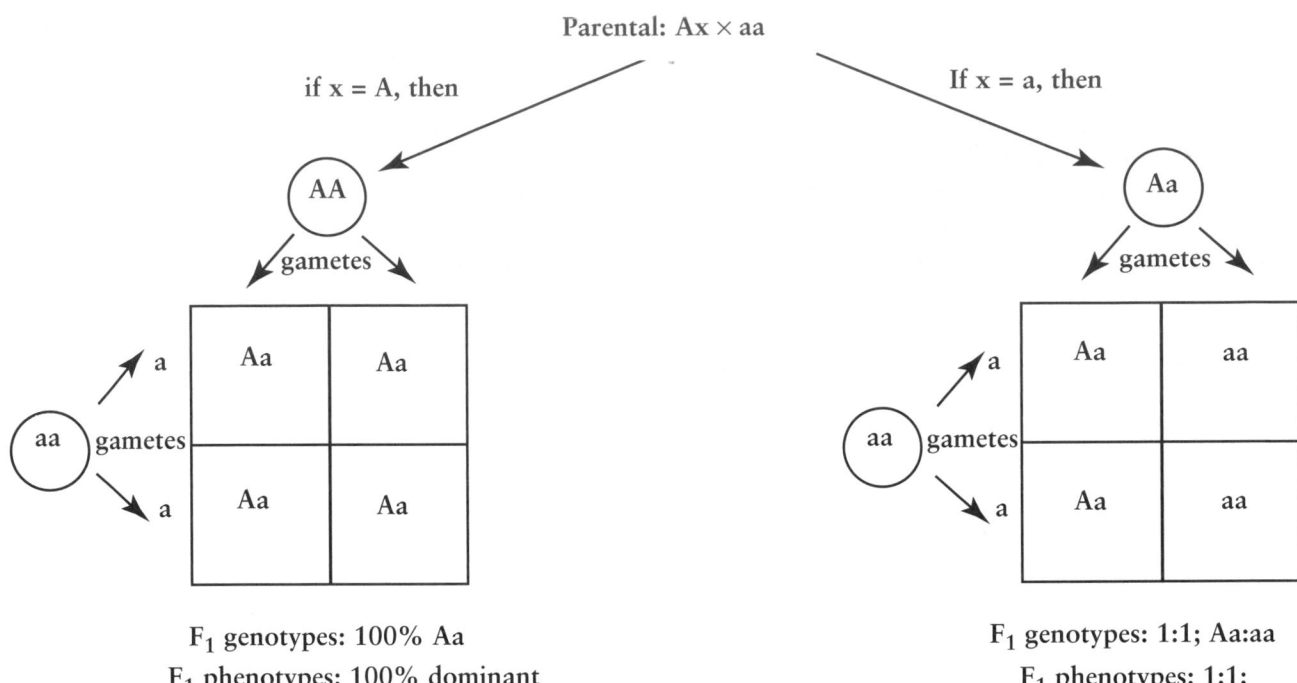

F₁ genotypes: 100% Aa
F₁ phenotypes: 100% dominant

F₁ genotypes: 1:1; Aa:aa
F₁ phenotypes: 1:1;
    dominant:recessive

Figure 13.3. Testcross

testcross or **backcross,** an organism with a dominant phenotype of unknown genotype (Ax) is crossed with a phenotypically recessive organism (genotype aa). Since the recessive parent is homozygous, it can donate only the recessive allele, a, to the progeny. If the dominant parent's genotype is AA, all of its gametes will carry an A, and thus all of the progeny will have genotype Aa. If the dominant parent's genotype is Aa, half of the progeny will be Aa and express the dominant phenotype, and half will be aa and express the recessive phenotype. In a testcross, the appearance of the recessive phenotype in the progeny indicates that the phenotypically dominant parent is genotypically heterozygous (see Figure 13.3).

B. MENDEL'S SECOND LAW: LAW OF INDEPENDENT ASSORTMENT

1. Dihybrid Cross

The principles of the monohybrid cross can be extended to a dihybrid cross in which the parents differ in two traits, as long as each trait assorts independently; i.e., the alleles of unlinked genes assort independently during meiosis. This is known as Mendel's **law of independent assortment.**

In the following example, a purple-flowered tall pea plant is crossed with a white-flowered dwarf pea plant; both plants are doubly homozygous (tall is dominant to dwarf, T = tall allele, t = dwarf allele; purple is dominant to white, P = purple allele, p = white allele). The purple parent's genotype is TTPP, and it thus produces only TP gametes; the white parent's genotype is ttpp and produces only tp gametes. The F_1 progeny will all have the genotype TtPp and will be phenotypically dominant for both traits.

When the F_1 generation is self-crossed (TtPp × TtPp), it produces 4 different phenotypes: tall purple, tall white, dwarf purple, and dwarf white, in the ratio 9:3:3:1, respectively. This is the typical pattern for Mendelian inheritance in a dihybrid cross between heterozygotes with independently assorting traits (see Figure 13.4).

> ## MCAT Synopsis
>
> Note that each trait assorts individually in a 3:1 ratio, as in a monohybrid cross. There are 9 purple tall and 3 purple dwarf, for a total of 12 purple; and there are 3 white tall and 1 white dwarf, for a total of 4 white. Hence, the purple:white ratio is 12:4 = 3:1. Likewise, the tall:dwarf ratio is 3:1.

Parental: TTPP × ttpp

F_1 genotypes: 100%   TtPp

(self-cross) F_1 × F_1: TtPp × TtPp

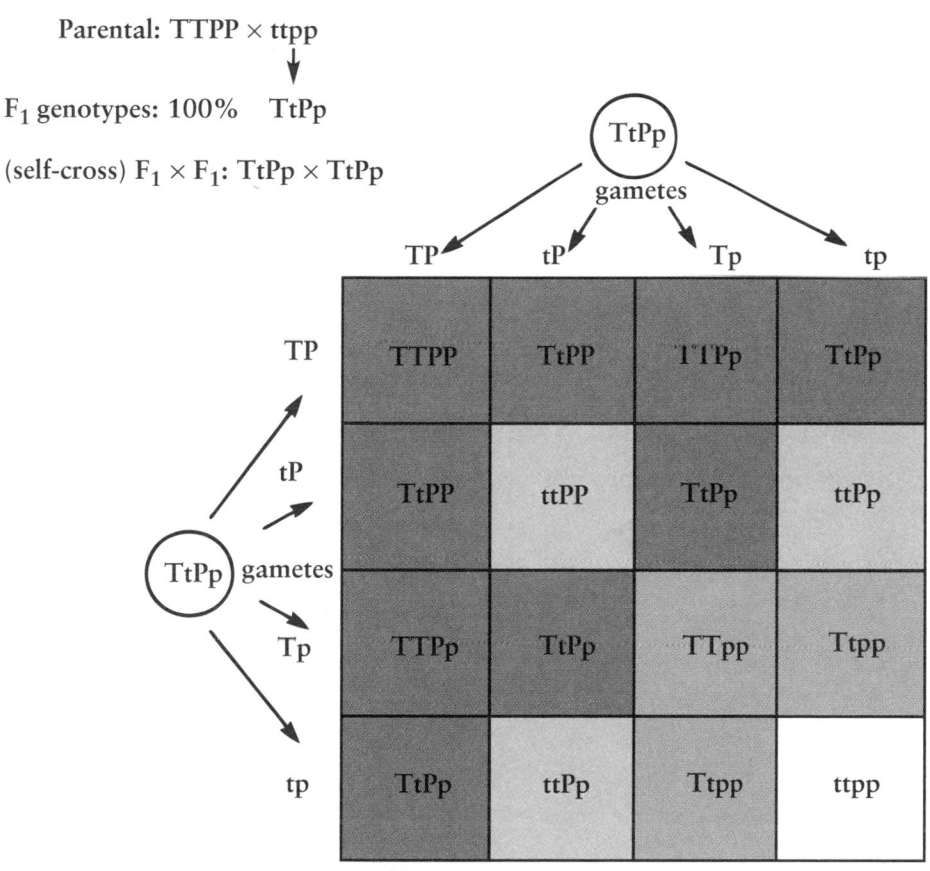

F_2 phenotypes: 9:3:3:1

9 tall purple:3 tall white:3 dwarf purple:1 dwarf white

Figure 13.4. Dihybrid Cross

2. **Statistical Calculations**

Each F_1 parent in the dihybrid cross can produce four possible gametes: TP, Tp, tP, and tp. The probability of a particular genotype appearing in the F_2 progeny can be determined by calculating the number of different gamete combinations that will produce this genotype. For example, the genotype TTPP can be produced in only o n e way, by the fusion of two TP gametes. Since $\frac{1}{4}$ of each parent's gametes will be TP, $\frac{1}{4}$ of the other parent's gametes will also be TP, $\frac{1}{4} \times \frac{1}{4}$ or $\frac{1}{16}$ of the total progeny will be TTPP. In statistical terms, the probability that one parent will donate a particular gamete ($\frac{1}{4}$ in this case) is independent of the probability that the other parent will donate a particular gamete (also $\frac{1}{4}$). Consequently, the probability of producing a genotype that requires the occurrence of both these independent events is equal to the *product* of the individual probabilities that these events will occur ($\frac{1}{16}$).

In contrast, the genotype TtPp can be produced by four different gamete combinations, TP + tp; Tp + tP; tP + Tp; and tp + TP. The probability of any one of these combinations is $\frac{1}{4} \times \frac{1}{4}$ or $\frac{1}{16}$ (e.g., $\frac{1}{4}$ of one parent's gametes will be TP, and $\frac{1}{4}$ of the other parent's gametes will be TP; the probability of these gametes fusing is the product of the individual probabilities). Since there are four ways to produce a TtPp genotype, the frequency of the TtPp genotype in the F_2 generation is $\frac{1}{16} + \frac{1}{16} + \frac{1}{16} + \frac{1}{16} = \frac{4}{16} = \frac{1}{4}$. In statistical terms, the probability of producing a genotype that can be the result of more than one event is equal to the *sum* of the individual probabilities that these events will occur. (Note that statistical calculations are most accurate with a large sample size.)

3. **Problem Solving**

In solving problems involving two independently assorted traits, it generally helps to consider each trait individually. For example, consider the cross between a purple tall plant of unknown genotype and a white tall plant, also of unknown genotype. The F_1 generation consists of 62 tall plants with purple flowers, 59 tall plants with white flowers, 20 dwarf plants with purple flowers, and 21 dwarf plants with white flowers. What are the genotypes of the parental generation?

Since both parents are tall, but the F_1 generation contains dwarf plants, both parents must be heterozygous for tallness and hence of genotype Tt. If so, then tall plants should outnumber dwarf plants in the F_1 generation by a ratio of 3 to 1. In fact, the ratio of tall plants (62 + 59 = 121) to dwarf plants (20 + 21 = 41) is 121:41 or approximately 3:1.

In addition, one parent is white; it must therefore be homozygous pp. But since the F_1 generation contained white-flowered plants, the purple parent must also have the allele for white flowers. If we now look at the segregation of purple and white alone, we find that the ratio of purple (62 + 20 = 82) to white (59 + 21 = 80) is almost 1:1. This is the ratio expected in a cross between a heterozygous dominant individual (Pp) and a homozygous recessive (pp). Thus, the genotype of the purple tall parent must be TtPp, and the genotype of the white tall parent must be Ttpp.

THE CHROMOSOMAL THEORY OF INHERITANCE

The principles of Mendelian genetics reflect the linear arrangement of genes on chromosomes. **Diploid** species have chromosome pairs (**homologues**). In diploids, the alleles for a given trait are segregated; one allele is located on one chromosome, and the other allele is found on its homologue.

A. SEGREGATION AND INDEPENDENT ASSORTMENT

Mendelian segregation and independent assortment are the consequences of chromosomal behavior during meiosis. Prior to meiosis, each chromosome is replicated, but the daughter copy remains attached to the parental chromosome via the centromere, forming sister chromatids. The sister chromatids pair with their homologues and align at the equatorial plate during metaphase I. During the first meiotic division, the homologous pairs separate, and following cytokinesis, the number of chromosomes per cell is reduced from 2N to N. This is the step in meiosis during which segregation and independent assortment occur. In the second meiotic division, the sister chromatids separate. Each gamete receives the haploid (N) complement of chromosomes; i.e., one sister

Flashback

Now may be an opportune time to review meiosis. See chapter 4.

chromatid from every homologous pair. The fusion of two gametes during fertilization restores the diploid number, 2N.

B. NONINDEPENDENT ASSORTMENT: GENETIC LINKAGE

Not all traits assort independently in a dihybrid cross. In the sweet pea plant, the allele for purple-colored pollen (A) is dominant to the allele for red pollen (a); the allele for long pollen (B) is dominant to the allele for round pollen (b). In a cross between two purple long dihybrids (AaBb $\times$ AaBb), if the two traits assort independently, then the expected phenotypic ratio is 9 purple long:3 purple round:3 red long:1 red round. The purple long F_1 progeny have the **parental phenotype**, purple long; the other phenotypes are **recombinant phenotypes**, since they recombine the parental traits. However, in this dihybrid cross, the F_1 genotypic ratio is 4 AABB:8 AaBb:4 aabb, or 1:2:1. The F_1 phenotypic ratio is 12 purple long:4 red round, or 3:1; the parental phenotype is overly represented in the progeny. In fact, the segregation pattern for these two traits in a dihybrid cross is like that of a single trait in a monohybrid cross. This is because genes A and B are **linked**; they are located on the same chromosome and are usually inherited together. This means that the parent AaBb does not produce four different types of gametes (AB, Ab, aB, ab). Instead, only two different gametes are produced; in this case, AB and ab. (If the two types of gametes were Ab and aB, then the genotypic ratio would have been 1 AAbb:2 AaBb:1 aaBB.)

Genetic linkage is a direct result of the organization of genes along chromosomes: linked genes are located on the same chromosome. Recall that during meiosis I, homologous chromosomes segregate into different cells. If two genes are located on the same chromosome, they tend to segregate together. The degree of genetic linkage can be tight and complete, with no recombinant phenotypes. Linkage can also be weak, as when the number of recombinants in the F_1 progeny approaches the number expected from independent assortment. Tightly linked genes recombine at a frequency close to 0 percent; weakly linked genes recombine at frequencies approaching 50 percent.

C. RECOMBINATION FREQUENCIES: GENETIC MAPPING

Linked genes can recombine at frequencies between 0 and 50 percent to produce recombinants. The recombinant chromosomes arise through the physical exchange of DNA between homologous chromosomes

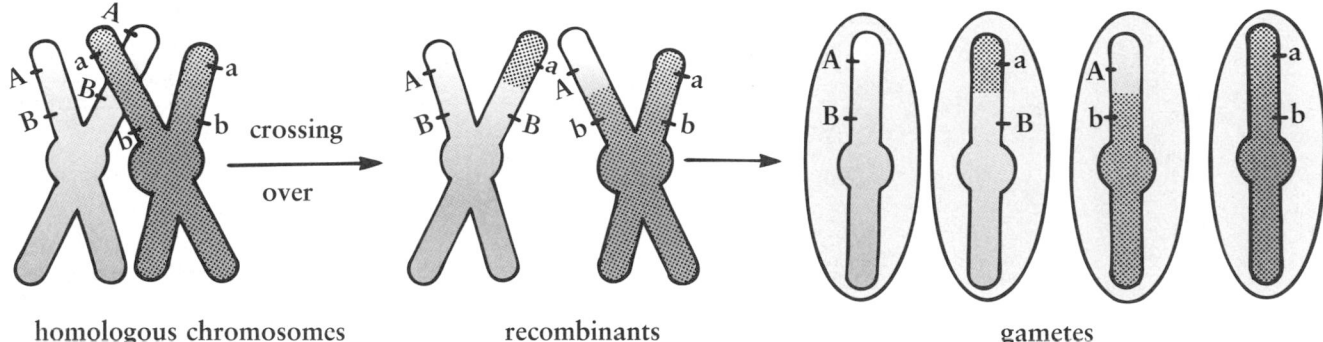

homologous chromosomes   recombinants   gametes

Figure 13.5. Crossing Over

paired during meiosis. This process is called **crossing over** or **genetic recombination** (see chapter 4). Crossing over can unlink linked genes (see Figure 13.5).

The degree of genetic linkage is a measure of how far apart two genes are on the same chromosome. The probability of a crossover and exchange occurring between two points is generally directly proportional to the distance between the points. For example, pairs of genes that are far apart from each other on a chromosome have a higher probability of being separated during crossing over than pairs of genes that are located close to each other. Thus, the frequency of genetic recombination between two genes is related to the distance between them.

Recombination frequencies can be used to construct a **genetic map**. One **map unit** is defined as a 1 percent **recombinant frequency**. Recombination frequencies are roughly additive. If genes are found on a map in the order XYZ, then the recombination frequency between X and Y plus the recombination frequency between Y and Z will be roughly equal to the recombination frequency between X and Z. Likewise, if you are given the recombinant frequencies for X and Y, X and Z, and Y and Z (which can be determined by dividing the number of recombinant offspring by the total number of offspring), then you can determine the relative positions of these genes on the chromosome. In Figure 13.6, we are given that X and Y have a recombination frequency of 8 percent; i.e., they are 8 map units apart. If X and Z recombine 12 percent of the time, then they are 12 map units apart. Depending on where you draw Z in relation to X on your map, Y and Z are either 20 map units apart, or 4 map units apart. Since we are also given that Y and Z recombine with a frequency of 4 percent, the genes are in the order XYZ (or ZYX) on the chromosome.

> **Flashback**
>
> Recall in Chapter 4 that crossing over occurs when the homologous chromosomes pair up into tetrads during prophase I.

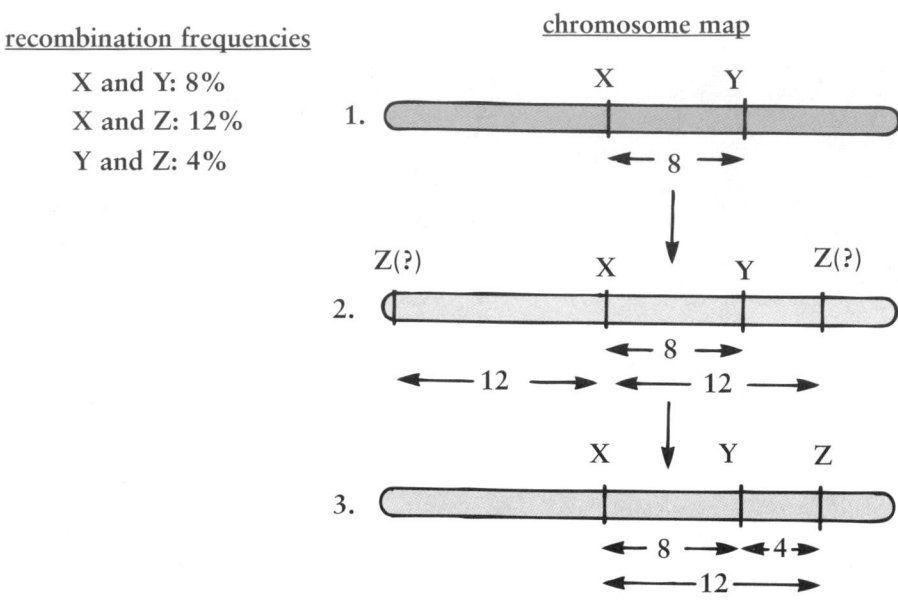

Figure 13.6. Chromosome Mapping

VARIATIONS ON MENDELIAN GENETICS

In real life, inheritance patterns are often more complicated than Mendel would have hoped. One major source of complication is in the relationship between phenotype and genotype. In theory, 100 percent of individuals with the recessive phenotype have a homozygous recessive genotype, and 100 percent of individuals with the dominant phenotype have either homozygous or heterozygous genotypes. Such clean concordance between genotype and phenotype is not always the case.

A. INCOMPLETE DOMINANCE

Some progeny phenotypes are apparently blends of the parental phenotypes. The classic example is flower color in snapdragons: homozygous dominant red snapdragons when crossed with homozygous recessive white snapdragons produce 100 percent pink progeny in the F_1 generation. When F_1 progeny are self-crossed, they produce red, pink, and white progeny in the ratio of 1:2:1, respectively (see Figure 13.7). The pink color is the result of the combined effects of the red and white genes in heterozygotes. An allele is **incompletely dominant** if the phenotype of the heterozygote is an intermediate of the phenotypes of the homozygotes.

snapdragons
R = allele for red flowers
r = allele for white flowers
Parental: RR × rr (red × white)

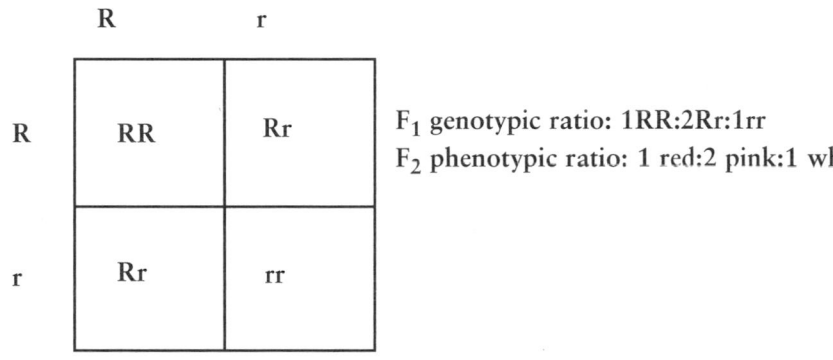

F_1 genotypic ratio: 100% Rr
F_1 phenotypic ratio: 100% pink

F_1: Rr × Rr (pink × pink)

F_1 genotypic ratio: 1RR:2Rr:1rr
F_2 phenotypic ratio: 1 red:2 pink:1 white

Figure 13.7. Incomplete Dominance

B. CODOMINANCE

Codominance occurs when multiple alleles exist for a given gene and more than one of them is dominant. Each dominant allele is fully dominant when combined with a recessive allele, but when two dominant alleles are present, the phenotype is the result of the expression of both dominant alleles simultaneously.

The classic example of codominance and multiple alleles is the inheritance of ABO blood groups in humans. Blood type is determined by three different alleles, I^A, I^B, and i. Only two alleles are present in any single individual, but the population contains all three alleles. I^A and I^B are both dominant to i. Individuals who are homozygous I^A or heterozygous I^Ai have blood type A; individuals who are homozygous I^B or heterozygous I^Bi have blood type B; and individuals who are homozygous ii have blood type O. However, I^A and I^B are codominant; individuals who are heterozygous $I^A I^B$ have a distinct blood type, AB, which combines characteristics of both the A and B blood groups.

C. PENETRANCE AND EXPRESSIVITY

A dominant allele is not necessarily expressed to the same degree in all individuals who carry it; phenotype is a combination of genetics and environment. The **penetrance** of a genotype is the percentage of individuals in the population carrying the allele who actually express the phenotype associated with it. The **expressivity** of a genotype is the degree to which the phenotype associated with the genotype is expressed in individuals who carry the allele. Both penetrance and expressivity can be affected by environment; e.g., in the fruitfly *Drosophila melanogaster*, the dominant gene curly (C^Y) gives rise to adult flies with abnormal wings that curl up if the pupae are kept at 25°C, but remain uncurled if the pupae are kept at 19°C. At 25°C, C^Y is 100 percent penetrant, whereas at 19°C, C^Y is 0 percent penetrant. The expressivity is the degree of curliness of the wings.

D. INHERITED DISORDERS

1. Recessive

Recessively inherited disorders are caused by recessive alleles that are inherited as simple recessive traits. Individuals homozygous for the recessive allele exhibit the disorder, while heterozygotes are **carriers** of the disorder, and are capable of passing the allele on to their offspring. Individuals afflicted with such disorders are usually the result of a mating between two carriers. As in a typical dominant/recessive monohybrid cross, one-fourth of the offspring of such a mating are predicted to have the disorder. The disorders can be mild, like albinism, a lack of skin pigmentation; or **lethal,** like Tay-Sachs disease, which results from a malfunctioning enzyme that causes lipids to accumulate in the brain, causing death in early childhood. Since these alleles are recessive and do not typically affect carriers, the allele remains in the gene pool, "hidden" in carriers who are not selected against by natural selection. Most lethal genes are **early acting,** i.e., they program an early death for homozygotes, typically during embryonic development. Sometimes, lethal genes impart an advantage to heterozygous individuals, as in the case of sickle-cell anemia. Heterozygous individuals are resistant to malaria, while homozygous individuals have abnormal hemoglobin, which causes the painful and often fatal anemia.

2. Dominant

Lethal alleles can also be dominant. These are **late-acting** genes; the classic example is the gene for Huntington's chorea in humans.

Huntington's chorea is 100 percent penetrant and fully dominant; all individuals carrying the allele succumb to the disease. Since the Huntington's chorea gene isn't expressed until middle age, most of its victims have already had children by the time of diagnosis; assuming the other parent is normal, 50 percent of the children are predicted to inherit the Huntington's chorea gene.

E. SEX DETERMINATION

Different species vary in their systems of sex determination. In sexually differentiated species, most chromosomes exist as pairs of homologues called **autosomes** but sex is determined by a pair of **sex chromosomes**. All humans have 22 pairs of autosomes; additionally, females have a pair of homologous **X chromosomes**, and males have a pair of heterologous chromosomes, an **X** and a **Y** chromosome. The sex chromosomes pair during meiosis and segregate during the first meiotic division. Since females can produce only gametes containing the X chromosome, the gender of a zygote is determined by the genetic contribution of the male gamete. If the sperm carries a Y chromosome, the zygote will be male; if it carries an X chromosome, the zygote will be female. For every mating there is a 50 percent chance that the zygote will be male and a 50 percent chance that it will be female.

> ### MCAT Synopsis
>
> The odds of a child being a boy or a girl are 50 percent. That means that regardless of how many sons or daughters a couple might have, the odds of having a boy or girl the next time around remains 50 percent. Each fertilization is an independent event!

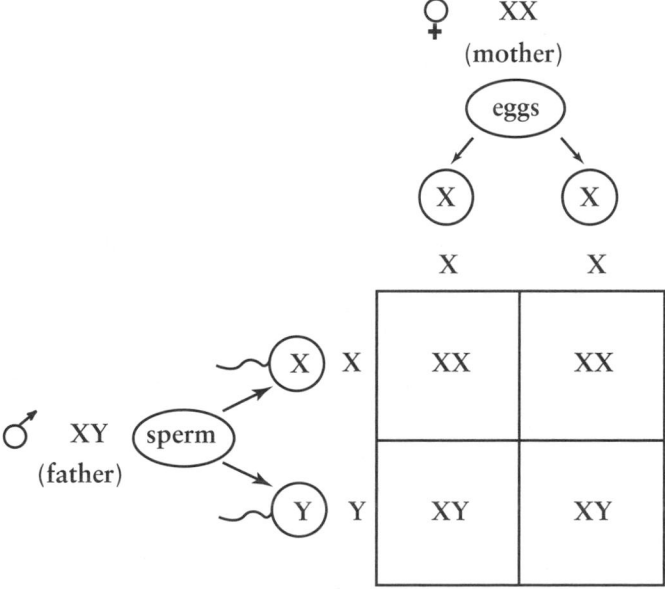

offspring: 50% XX = 50% female
50% XY = 50% male

Figure 13.8. Sex Determination in Humans

Genes that are located on the X or Y chromosome are called **sex-linked.** In humans, most sex-linked genes are located on the X chromosome, though some Y-linked traits have been found (e.g., hair on the outer ears).

F. SEX LINKAGE

In humans, females have two X chromosomes, and males have only one. As a result, recessive genes that are carried on the X chromosome will produce the recessive phenotypes whenever they occur in males, since no dominant allele is present to mask them. The recessive phenotype will thus be much more frequently found in males. Examples of sex-linked recessives in humans are the genes for hemophilia and for color blindness.

The pattern of inheritance for a sex-linked recessive is somewhat complicated. Since the gene is carried on the X chromosome, and males pass the X chromosome only to their daughters, affected males *cannot* pass the trait to their male offspring. Affected males will pass the gene to *all* of their daughters. However, unless the daughter also receives the gene from her mother, she will be a phenotypically normal carrier of the trait. Since all of the daughter's male children will receive their only X chromosome from her, half of her sons will receive the recessive sex-linked allele (see Figure 13.9). Thus, sex-linked recessives generally affect only males; they cannot be passed from father to son, but can be passed from father to grandson via a daughter who is a carrier, thereby skipping a generation.

a. Cross between a carrier female (X^hX) and a normal male (XY):

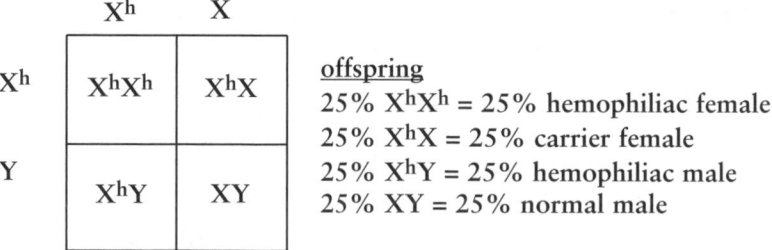

	X^h	X
X	X^hX	XX
Y	X^hY	XY

offspring
25% X^hX = 25% carrier female
25% XX = 25% normal female
25% X^hY = 25% hemophiliac male
25% XY = 25% normal male

b. Cross between a carrier female ($X^h X$) and a hemophiliac male (X^hY)

	X^h	X
X^h	X^hX^h	X^hX
Y	X^hY	XY

offspring
25% X^hX^h = 25% hemophiliac female
25% X^hX = 25% carrier female
25% X^hY = 25% hemophiliac male
25% XY = 25% normal male

Figure 13.9. Inheritance of Hemophilia Gene

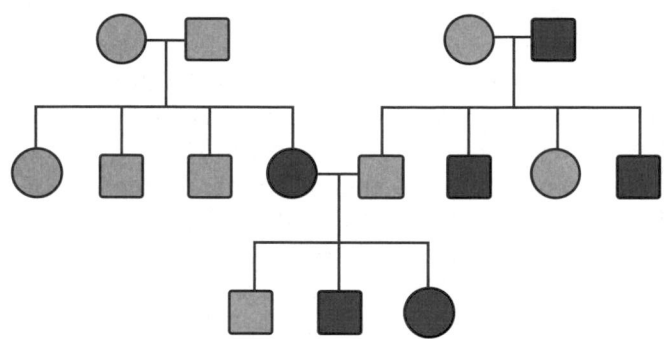

Figure 13.10a. Autosomal Recessive

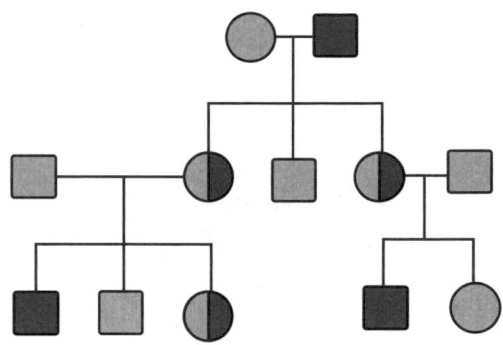

Figure 13.10b. Sex-linked Recessive

PEDIGREE ANALYSIS

Ethical constraints forbid geneticists from performing testcrosses on human populations. Instead, they must rely on examining matings that have already occurred. A **pedigree** is a family tree depicting the inheritance of a particular genetic trait over several generations. By convention, males are indicated by squares and females by circles. Matings are indicated by horizontal lines, and descendants are listed below. Individuals affected by the trait are generally shaded, and unaffected individuals are unshaded. When carriers of sex-linked traits have been identified (typically, female heterozygotes), they are usually half shaded in family trees.

A human pedigree for a recessive autosomal trait, such as albinism, is shown in Figure 13.10a (an affected child born to parents that are normal) and, for a sex-linked trait, such as hemophilia, in Figure 13.10b (the key here is more affected males than females). In analyzing pedigrees, look for individuals with the recessive phenotype. Such individuals have only one possible genotype: homozygous recessive. Matings between them and the dominant phenotype behave as testcrosses; the ratio of phenotypes among the offspring allows deduction of the dominant genotype.

MCAT Favorite

When analyzing a pedigree, look for the recessive phenotype (you'll know the genotype) and work from there. If only males are affected, suspect sex linkage.

CHROMOSOMAL ABERRATIONS

Chromosome number and structure can be altered by abnormal cell division during meiosis or by mutagenic agents.

A. NONDISJUNCTION

Nondisjunction is either the failure of homologous chromosomes to separate properly during meiosis I, or the failure of sister chromatids to separate properly during meiosis II (usually in a secondary spermatocyte or secondary oocyte). In the case of a secondary spermatocyte, it results in one gamete with two copies of the chromosome (polyploid), two normal haploid gametes, and one gamete with no copies of the chromosome (aneuploid). The resulting zygote may have either three copies of that chromosome, called **trisomy** (somatic cells will have **2N + 1** chromosomes) or a single copy of that chromosome, called **monosomy** (somatic cells will have **2N–1** chromosomes). A classic case of trisomy is the birth defect **Down's syndrome**, which is caused by trisomy of **chromosome 21.** Victims of Down's syndrome are of short stature, have characteristic facial features, and are mentally retarded. They are also usually sexually underdeveloped and have shorter-than-normal lifespans. Most monosomies and trisomies are lethal, causing the embryo to spontaneously abort early in the pregnancy.

Nondisjunction of the sex chromosomes may also occur, resulting in individuals with extra or missing copies of the X and/or Y chromosomes. **XXY** individuals are afflicted with **Klinefelter's syndrome;** they are sterile males with abnormally small testes. **XO** females have only one sex chromosome and suffer from **Turner's syndrome;** they fail to develop secondary sexual characteristics and are sterile and of short stature. **XXX** females are referred to as **metafemales** and are usually mentally retarded and sometimes infertile. **XYY** males are normal males, though they tend to be taller than average and, according to some studies, may be more violent.

B. CHROMOSOMAL BREAKAGE

Chromosomal breakage may occur spontaneously or be induced by environmental factors, such as mutagenic agents and X rays. The chromosome that loses a fragment is said to have a deficiency. The fragment may join with its homologous chromosome, resulting in a **duplication,** or it may join with a nonhomologous chromosome, an event termed a **translocation.** The fragment may also rejoin its original chromosome but in the reverse position; this is known as an **inversion.** For example, Down's syndrome can also be caused by the translocation of a chromosome 21 fragment.

14

MOLECULAR GENETICS

Genes are composed of **DNA (deoxyribonucleic acid)**, which contains information coded in the sequence of its base pairs, providing the cell with a blueprint for protein synthesis. Furthermore, DNA has the ability to self-replicate, which is crucial for cell division, and hence for organismal reproduction. DNA is the basis of heredity; self-replication ensures that its coded sequence will be passed on to successive generations. This is the central dogma of molecular genetics and it is summarized in Figure 14.1.

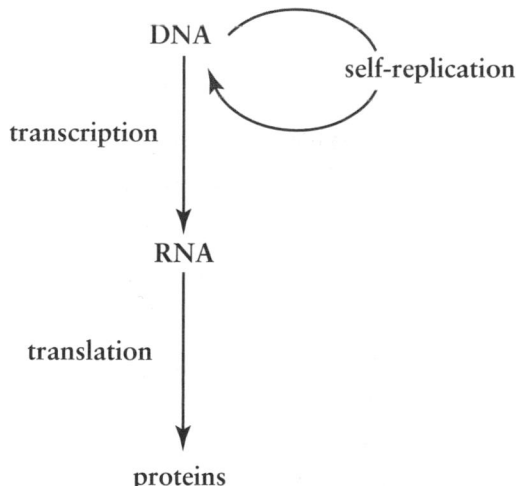

Figure 14.1. Central Dogma of Molecular Genetics

DNA

A. STRUCTURE

The basic unit of DNA is the **nucleotide**, which is composed of **deoxyribose** (a sugar) bonded to both a **phosphate group** and a **nitrogenous base**. There are two types of bases: the double-ringed **purines** and the single-ringed **pyrimidines**. The purines in DNA are **adenine (A)** and guanine (**G**), and the pyrimidines are **cytosine (C)** and **thymine (T)** (see Figure 14.2).

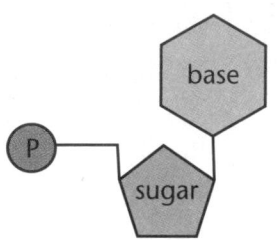

Figure 14.2. Nucleotide

Nucleotides bond together to form polynucleotides. The 3' hydroxyl group of the sugar on one nucleotide is joined to the 5' hydroxyl group of the adjacent sugar by a phosphodiester bond. The phosphate and sugar form a chain with the bases arranged as side groups off the chain.

A DNA molecule is a **double-stranded helix** with the sugar-phosphate chains on the outside of the helix and the bases on the inside. T always forms **two** hydrogen bonds with A; G always forms **three** hydrogen bonds with C. This **base-pairing** forms "rungs" on the interior of the double helix that link the two polynucleotide chains together (see Figure 14.3).

MCAT Synopsis

Due to complementary base pairing in DNA, the amount of A will equal the amount of T and G will equal C. Also, because G is triple bonded to C, the higher the G/C content of DNA, the more tightly bound the two strands will be.

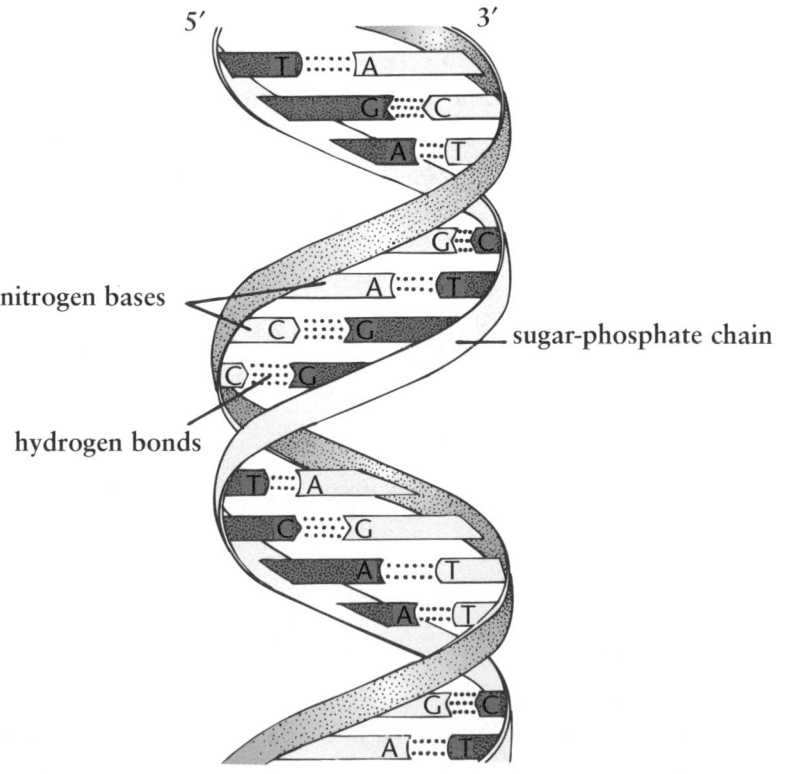

Figure 14.3. DNA Molecule

The strands are positioned **antiparallel** to each other, i.e., one strand has a **5′ → 3′ polarity**, and its complementary strand has a **3′ → 5′ polarity**. The 5′ end is designated as the end with a free hydroxyl group (or phosphate group) bonded to the 5′ carbon of the terminal sugar; the 3′ end is designated as the one with a free hydroxyl group attached to the 3′ carbon of the terminal sugar. This is known as the **Watson-Crick** model of DNA (see Figure 14.4).

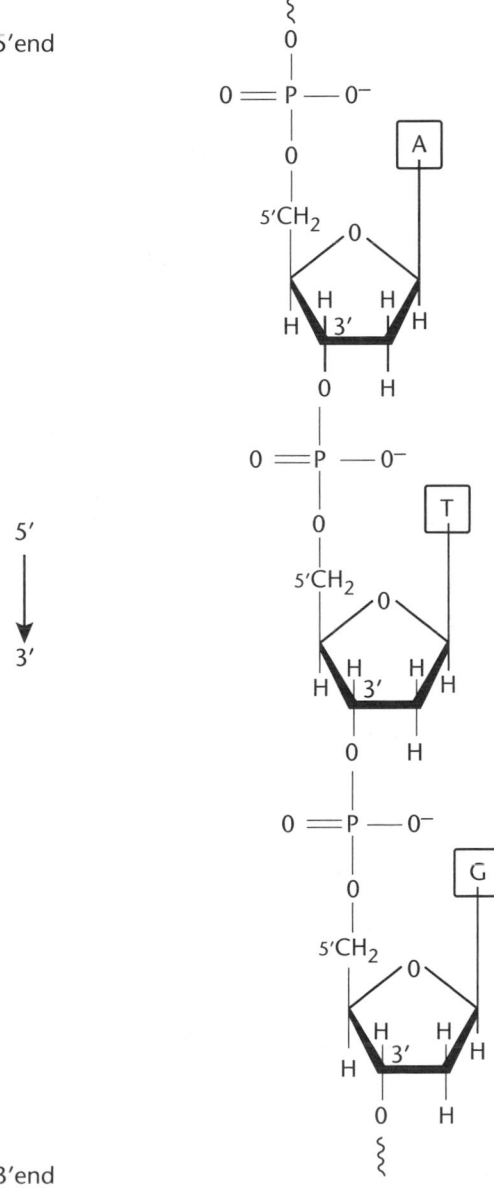

Figure 14.4. Single-Stranded DNA

B. DNA REPLICATION (EUKARYOTIC)

1. **Semiconservative Replication**

   During replication, the helix unwinds and each strand acts as a template for complementary base-pairing in the synthesis of two new daughter helices. Each new daughter helix contains an intact strand from the parent helix and a newly synthesized strand; thus DNA replication is **semiconservative**. The daughter DNA helices are identical in composition to each other and to the parent DNA (see Figure 14.5).

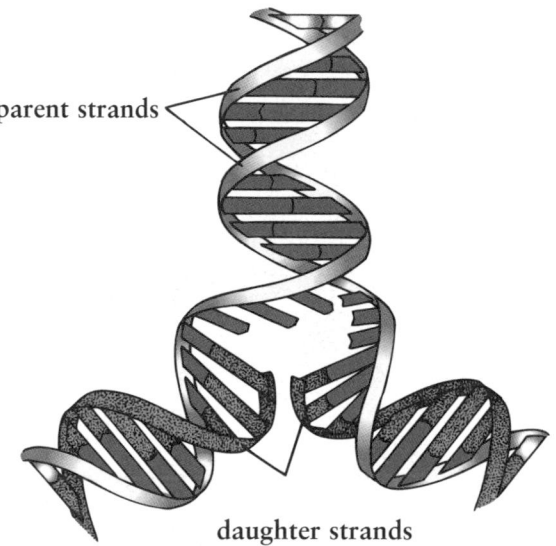

parent strands

daughter strands

Figure 14.5. Semiconservative Replication

2. **Origin of Replication**

   As the helix unwinds, both strands are simultaneously copied with the aid of more than a dozen enzymes, at the rate of about 50 nucleotide additions per second (in mammals). Replication begins at specific sites along the DNA called **origins of replication** and proceeds in both directions simultaneously. As replication proceeds in a given direction, a **replication fork** forms (see Figure 14.6).

3. **Unwinding and Initiation**

   The enzyme **helicase** unwinds the helix, while **single-strand binding** protein (SSB) binds to the single strands and stabilizes them, preventing them from recoiling and reforming a double helix. **DNA gyrase** is a type of *topoisomerase* that enhances the action of helicase by the introduction of negative supercoils into the DNA molecule.

   A **primer** chain, usually several nucleotides long and composed of RNA, is necessary for the initiation of DNA synthesis. An RNA polymerase, **primase**, synthesizes the primer, which binds to a segment of

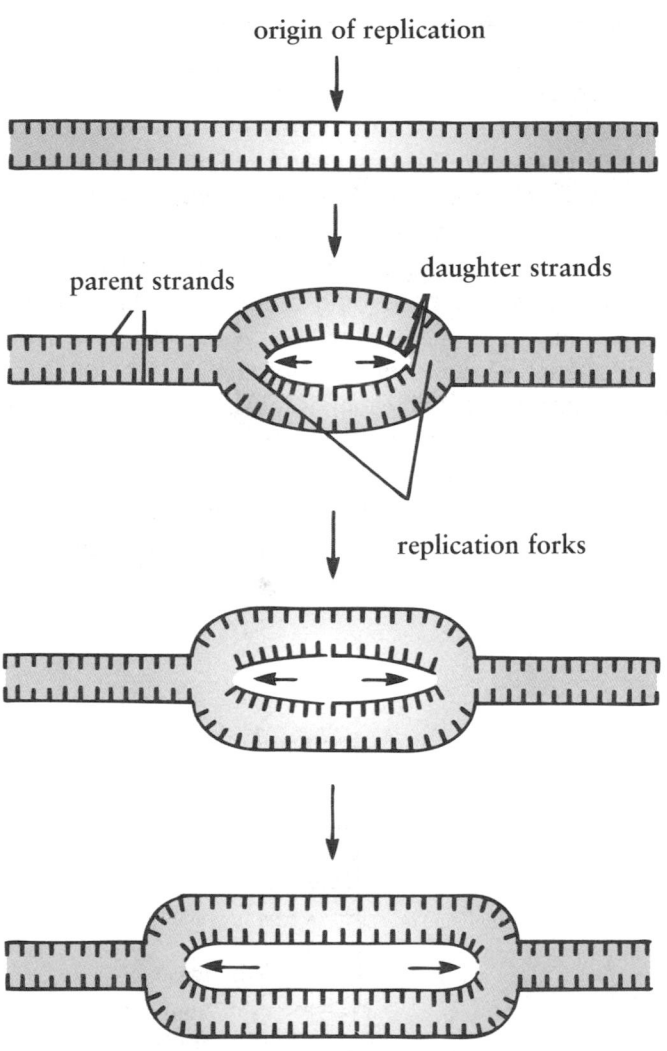

origin of replication

parent strands   daughter strands

replication forks

Figure 14.6. Origin of Replication

DNA to which it is complementary and serves as the site for nucleotide addition. The first nucleotide binds to the 3' end of the primer chain.

4. **Synthesis**

DNA synthesis proceeds in the 5' → 3' direction and is catalyzed by a group of enzymes collectively known as **DNA polymerases**. The double-stranded DNA ahead of the DNA polymerase is unwound by a helicase, and SSB again keeps the unwound DNA in a single-stranded form so that both strands can serve as templates. DNA gyrase concurrently introduces negative supercoils to relieve the tension created during unwinding. As the helix unwinds, free nucleotides (attached to pyrophosphate groups [PPi]) are aligned opposite the parent strands. The nucleotides form phosphodiester linkages, releasing the pyrophosphate, and the bases form H-bonds with their complements.

One daughter strand is the **leading strand** and the other daughter strand is the **lagging strand**. The leading strand is continuously synthesized by DNA polymerase in the $5' \rightarrow 3'$ direction. The lagging strand is synthesized discontinuously in the $5' \rightarrow 3'$ direction (since DNA polymerase synthesizes only in that direction) as a series of short segments known as **Okazaki fragments**; however, overall growth of the lagging strand occurs in the $3' \rightarrow 5'$ direction (see Figure 14.7). The lagging strand loops through DNA polymerase in the same direction as the leading strand. The looped segment of the lagging strand is primed with RNA, and DNA polymerase adds a short sequence of nucleotides (approximately 1,000). The lagging strand is released and a new loop is formed. Primase again synthesizes a short stretch of primer to initiate the formation of another Okazaki fragment. The RNA primers are removed and replaced by DNA. The gaps between the Okazaki fragments are also filled in with DNA. Finally, the fragments are covalently linked by the enzyme **DNA ligase** (see Figure 14.7).

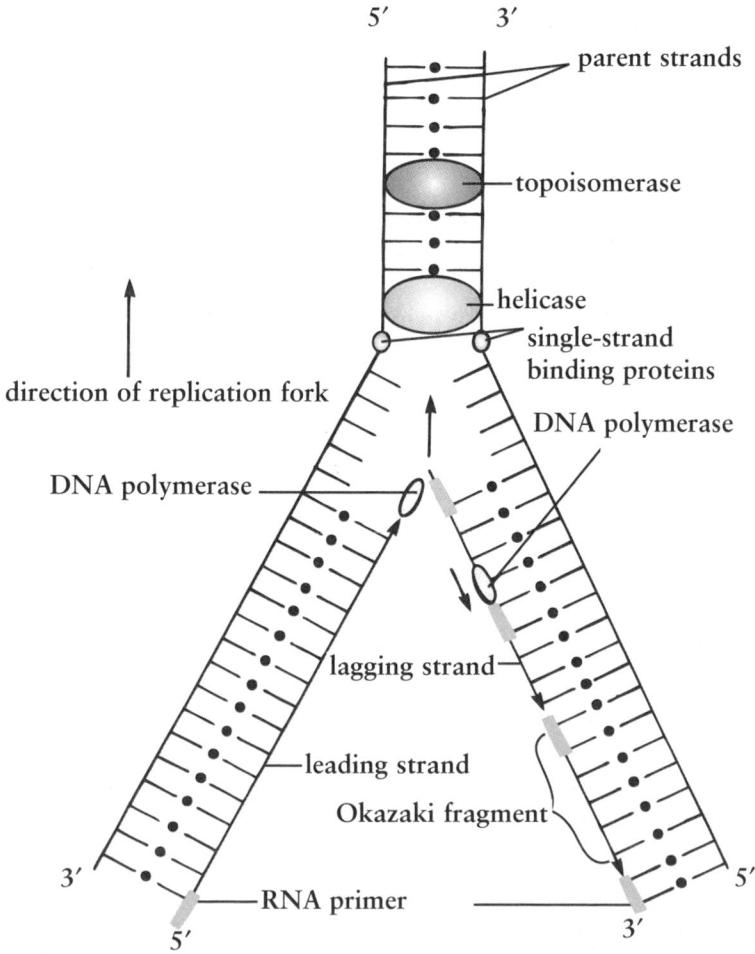

Figure 14.7. DNA Replication

RNA

RNA, ribonucleic acid, is a polynucleotide structurally similar to DNA except that its sugar is ribose, it contains uracil (U) instead of thymine, and it is usually **single-stranded**. RNA can be found in both the nucleus and the cytoplasm. There are several types of RNA, all of which are involved in some aspect of protein synthesis: **mRNA, tRNA, rRNA,** and **hnRNA**.

A. MESSENGER RNA (mRNA)

mRNA carries the complement of a DNA sequence and transports it from the nucleus to the ribosomes, where protein synthesis occurs. mRNA is **monocistronic**; i.e., one mRNA strand codes for one polypeptide.

B. TRANSFER RNA (tRNA)

tRNA is found in the cytoplasm and aids in the translation of mRNA's nucleotide code into a sequence of amino acids. tRNA brings amino acids to the ribosomes during protein synthesis. There is at least one type of tRNA for each amino acid, and approximately 40 known types of tRNA.

C. RIBOSOMAL RNA (rRNA)

rRNA is a structural component of ribosomes and is the most abundant of all RNA types. rRNA is synthesized in the nucleolus.

D. HETEROGENEOUS NUCLEAR RNA (hnRNA)

hnRNA is a large ribonucleoprotein complex that is the precursor of mRNA.

PROTEIN SYNTHESIS (EUKARYOTIC)

A. TRANSCRIPTION

Transcription is the process whereby information coded in the base sequence of DNA is transcribed into a strand of mRNA. The strand of mRNA is synthesized from a DNA template in a process similar to DNA replication. The DNA helix unwinds at the point of transcription, and synthesis occurs in the 5' → 3' direction, using only one DNA strand (the **antisense strand**) as a template. The base-pairing rules are the same as for DNA, with U replacing T (G bonds with C; A bonds with U). mRNA is synthesized by the enzyme **RNA polymerase**, which must bind to sites on the DNA called **promoters** to begin RNA synthesis. Synthesis continues until the polymerase encounters a **termination sequence**, which signals RNA polymerase to stop transcription, thus allowing the DNA helix to reform. The mRNA strand is then processed and leaves the nucleus through nuclear pores.

MCAT Synopsis

DNA:
- Double-stranded
- Sugar = deoxyribose
- Base pariing: A/T, G/C
- Found in nucleus only

RNA:
- Single-stranded
- Sugar = ribose
- Base pairing: A/U, G/C
- Found in nucleus and cytoplasm

KAPLAN EXCLUSIVE

INtrons are cut OUT!
Exons are expressed.

B. POST-TRANSCRIPTIONAL RNA PROCESSING

Most eukaryotic DNA does not code for proteins; noncoding or "garbage" sequences are found between coding sequences. A typical gene consists of several coding sequences, **exons**, interrupted by noncoding sequences, **introns**. The RNA initially transcribed is a precursor molecule, hnRNA, which contains both introns and exons. During hnRNA processing, the introns are cleaved and removed, while the exons are spliced to form a mRNA molecule coding for a single polypeptide. Processing occurs within the nucleus, and is also necessary for tRNA and rRNA production (see Figure 14.8).

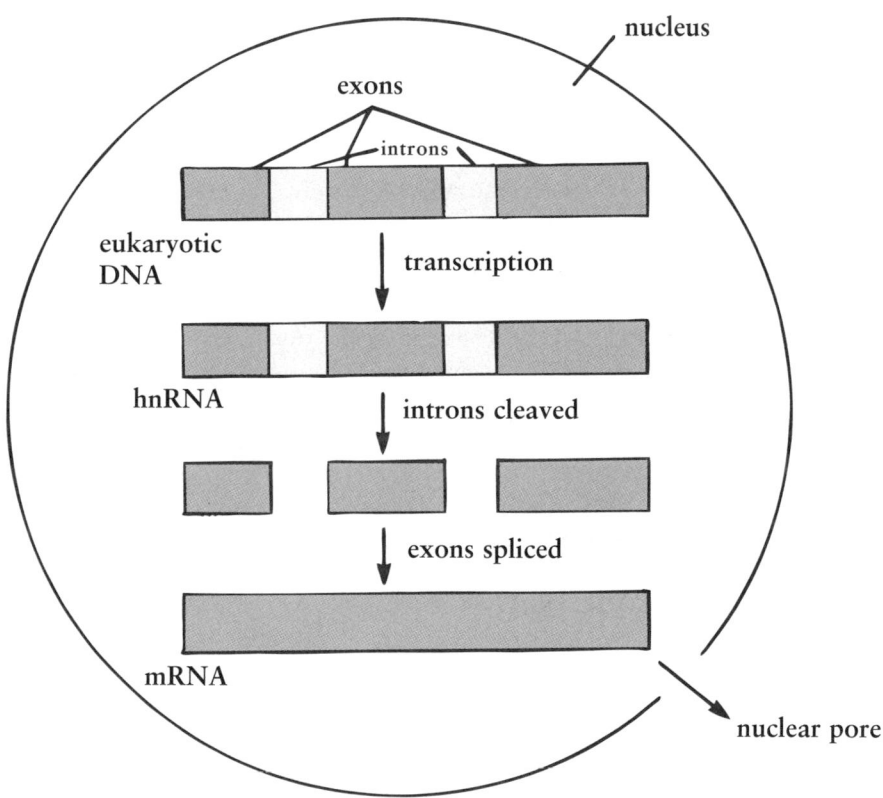

Figure 14.8. mRNA Processing

C. THE GENETIC CODE

The language of DNA consists of four "letters": A, T, C, and G. The language of proteins consists of 20 "words": the 20 amino acids. The DNA language must be translated by mRNA in such a way as to produce the 20 words in the amino acid language; hence, the **triplet code**. (A 2-letter [doublet] code would not suffice; with only 4 letters in the DNA alphabet, there would be only $4^2 = 16$ words possible—not enough to code for all 20 amino acids.) The base sequence of mRNA is translated as a series of triplets, otherwise known as **codons**. A sequence of three consecutive bases codes for a particular amino acid; e.g., the codon GGC specifies glycine, and the codon GUG specifies valine. The genetic code is universal for almost all organisms. (The exceptions are found in single-celled eukaryotes called ciliated protozoa, in mycoplasma, and in the mitochondria of several species.)

Given that there are 4^3, or 64, different codons possible based on the triplet code, and there are only 20 amino acids that need to be coded, the code must contain synonyms. Most amino acids have more than one codon specifying them. This property is referred to as the **degeneracy** or **redundancy** of the genetic code (see Table 14.1).

> **MCAT Synopsis**
>
> Each codon represents only one amino acid, but most amino acids are represented by more than one codon.

Table 14.1. The Genetic Code

		Second Base					
		U	**C**	**A**	**G**		
First Base (5')	**U**	UUU } Phe UUC UUA } Leu UUG	UCU UCC } Ser UCA UCG	UAU } Tyr UAC UAA } *Stop* UAG	UGU } Cys UGC UGA } *Stop* UGG } Trp	U C A G	Third Base (3')
	C	CUU CUC } Leu CUA CUG	CCU CCC } Pro CCA CCG	CAU } His CAC CAA } Gln CAG	CGU CGC } Arg CGA CGG	U C A G	
	A	AUU } Ile AUC AUA AUG } Start or Met	ACU ACC } Thr ACA ACG	AAU } Asn AAC AAA } Lys AAG	AGU } Ser AGC AGA } Arg AGG	U C A G	
	G	GUU GUC } Val GUA GUG	GGU GGC } Ala GGA GGG	GAU } Asp GAC GAA } Glu GAG	GGU GGC } Gly GGA GGG	U C A G	

D. TRANSLATION

Translation is the process whereby mRNA codons are translated into a sequence of amino acids. Translation occurs in the cytoplasm and involves tRNA, ribosomes, mRNA, amino acids, enzymes, and other proteins.

1. **tRNA**

   tRNA brings amino acids to the ribosomes in the correct sequence for polypeptide synthesis; tRNA "recognizes" both the amino acid and the mRNA codon. This dual function is reflected in its three-dimensional structure: one end contains a three-nucleotide sequence, the **anticodon**, which is complementary to one of the mRNA codons; the other end is the site of amino acid attachment and consists of a CCA sequence for all tRNA. Each amino acid has its own **aminoacyl-tRNA synthetase**, which has an active site that binds to both the amino acid and its corresponding tRNA, catalyzing their attachment to form an **aminoacyl-tRNA complex**. (This is an energy-requiring process.)

2. **Ribosomes**

   Ribosomes are composed of two subunits (consisting of proteins and rRNA), one large and one small, that bind together only during protein synthesis. Ribosomes have three binding sites: one for mRNA, and two for tRNA: the **P site** (peptidyl-tRNA binding site) and the **A site** (aminoacyl-tRNA complex binding site). The P site binds to the tRNA attached to the growing polypeptide chain, while the A site binds to the incoming aminoacyl-tRNA complex.

3. **Polypeptide Synthesis**

   Polypeptide synthesis can be divided into three distinct stages: **initiation**, **elongation**, and **termination**. All three stages are energy-requiring and are mediated by enzymes.

   a. **Initiation**

      Synthesis begins when the small ribosomal subunit binds to the mRNA near its 5′ end in the presence of proteins called **initiation factors**. The ribosome scans the mRNA until it binds to a start codon (AUG). The initiator aminoacyl-tRNA complex, **methionine-tRNA** (with the anticodon 3′-UAC-5′), base pairs with the start codon. The large ribosomal unit then binds to the small one, creating a complete ribosome with the met-tRNA complex sitting in the P site.

   b. **Elongation**

      Hydrogen bonds form between the mRNA codon in the A site and its complementary anticodon on the incoming aminoacyl-tRNA complex. The enzyme **peptidyl transferase** catalyzes the formation of a peptide bond between the amino acid attached to the tRNA in the A site and the met attached to the tRNA in the P site. Following peptide bond formation, a ribosome carries uncharged tRNA in the P site and peptidyl-tRNA in the A site. The cycle is completed by **translocation**, in which the ribosome advances 3 nucleotides along the mRNA in the 5′ → 3′ direction. In a concurrent action, the uncharged tRNA from the P site is expelled and the peptidyl-tRNA from the A site moves into the P site. The ribosome then has an empty A site ready for entry of the aminoacyl-tRNA corresponding to the next codon (see Figure 14.9).

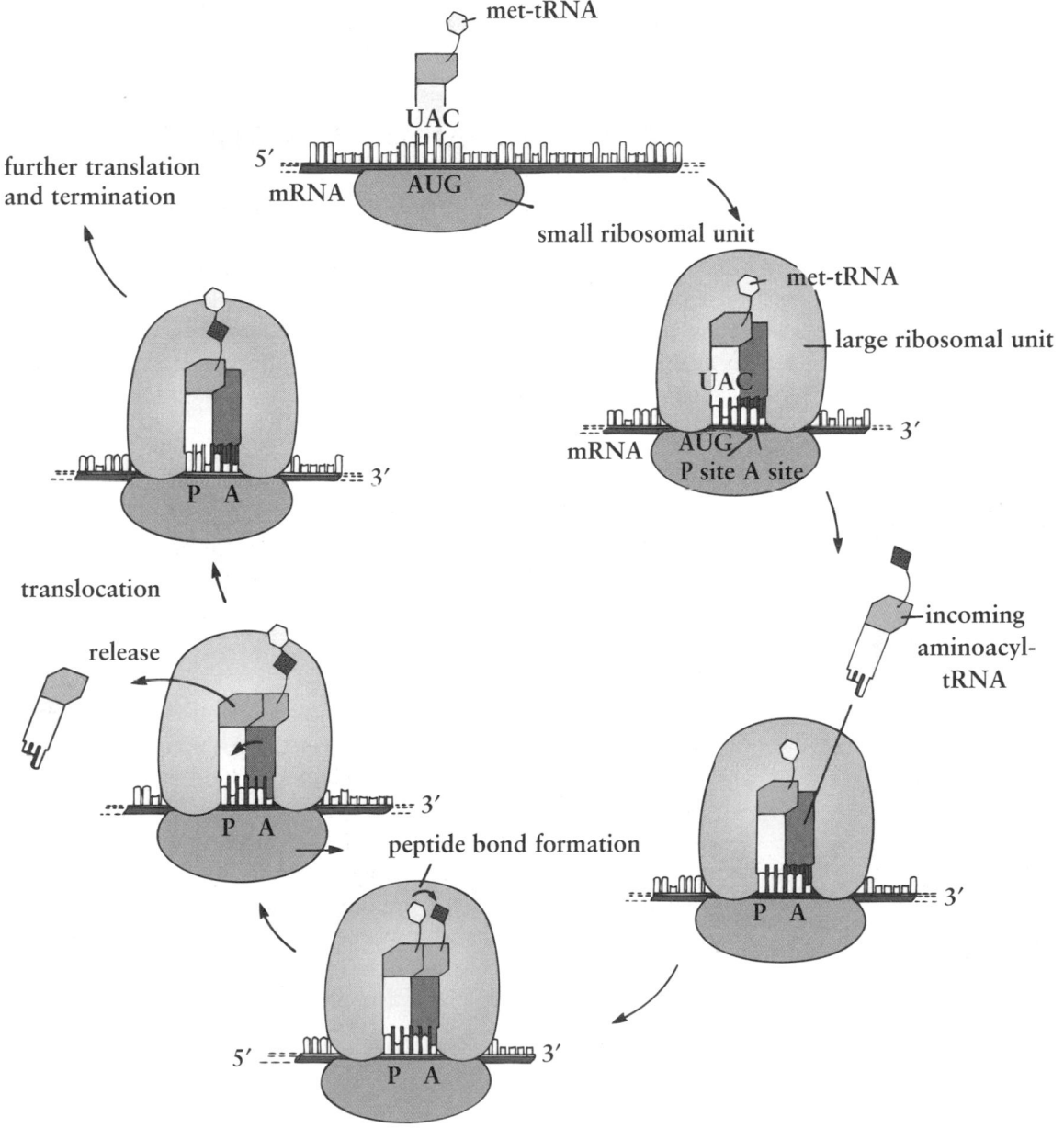

Figure 14.9. Initiation and Elongation

c. **Termination**

Polypeptide synthesis terminates when one of three special mRNA **termination codons** (UAA, UAG, or UGA) arrives in the A site. These codons signal the ribosome to terminate translation; they do not code for amino acids. Instead of another aminoacyl-tRNA complex coming into the A site and binding to the codon, a protein called **release factor** binds to the termination codon, causing a water molecule to be added to the polypeptide chain. This reaction precipitates the release of the polypeptide chain from the tRNA and the ribosome itself; the ribosome then dissociates into its two subunits. Frequently, many ribosomes simultaneously translate a single mRNA molecule, forming a structure known as a **polyribosome**.

E. POST-TRANSLATIONAL MODIFICATIONS

During and after its release, the polypeptide assumes the characteristic conformation determined by the primary sequence of amino acids. Disulfide bonds can form within or between polypeptide chains. There are often other post-translational modifications made to the polypeptide before it becomes a functional protein. For example, there might be cleavages and/or additions at the terminal ends of the chain; certain amino acids within the chain might be phosphorylated, carboxylated, methylated, or glycosylated.

F. MUTATIONS

A mutation is a change in the base sequence of DNA that may be inherited by offspring. The common types of mutations are **base-pair substitutions**, **base-pair insertions**, and **base-pair deletions**.

1. **Types of Mutations**

   a. **Point mutations**

   A point mutation occurs when a single nucleotide base is substituted by another. If the substitution occurs in a noncoding region, or if the substitution is transcribed into a codon that codes for the same amino acid, there will be no change in the amino acid sequence (a "silent" mutation). If the substitution changes the sequence, the result can range from insignificant to lethal, depending on the effect the substitution has on the protein. Sickle-cell anemia most commonly results from a single base-pair substitution; sickle-cell hemoglobin has a valine (codon GUG) where normal hemoglobin has a glutamic acid (codon GAG).

b. **Frame shift mutations**

Base-pair insertions and deletions involve the addition or loss of nucleotides, respectively. Such mutations usually have more serious effects on the coded protein, since nucleotides are read as a series of triplets. The addition or loss of a nucleotide(s) (except in multiples of three) will change the **reading frame** of the mRNA and is known as a **frameshift mutation**. The protein, if synthesized at all, will most likely be nonfunctional.

2. **Mutagenesis**

Mutagenesis is the creation of mutations; it can be caused by internal genetic "mistakes" or by external cancer-causing agents called **mutagens**. Internal mistakes can occur during DNA replication, resulting in gene mutations and dysfunctional proteins. Physical mutagens, such as X rays and ultraviolet radiation, and chemical mutagens, such as base analogs, all result in mutations. Furthermore, DNA itself can act as a mutagen; mobile pieces of DNA called **transposon**s can insert themselves in genes and cause mutation.

> **MCAT Favorite**
>
> Remember, a mutation will only be inherited if it occurs in the germ (sex) cell line. Mutations limited to somatic cells will not be passed on to the next generation. They may, however, play an important role in the development of tumors.

VIRAL GENETICS

The viral genome contains anywhere from several to several hundred genes and has either double-stranded **or** single-stranded DNA **or** RNA. Viruses are highly specific with respect to host selection and can be generally grouped into plant viruses, animal viruses, and bacteriophages (DNA viruses that infect bacteria).

A. INFECTION OF HOST CELL

A virus can only infect a host cell that has a surface receptor for the virus' capsid (protein coat). Viruses enter their host cells by a variety of mechanisms. Some viruses introduce only their nucleic acid into the host cell's cytoplasm, while others enter the host cell entirely (their nucleic acid is liberated from its capsid intracellularly).

B. GENOME REPLICATION AND TRANSCRIPTION

1. **DNA-Containing Viruses**

Viral DNA is replicated and viral mRNA is transcribed inside the host cell's nucleus (or nuclear region), using the host's DNA polymerases, RNA polymerases, and nucleotide pool. A few DNA viruses replicate and transcribe in the cytoplasm; these viruses must bring their own DNA and RNA polymerases with them.

2. RNA-Containing Viruses

Viral RNA is replicated and is transcribed in the host cell's cytoplasm. An enzyme called **RNA replicase** transcribes new RNA from an RNA template. Some viruses bring RNA replicase with them into the host; otherwise a portion of viral RNA functions as mRNA, which is translated to RNA replicase immediately after entering the host cell. **Retroviruses** are a special group of RNA viruses that use their genome as a template for DNA synthesis rather than for RNA synthesis. DNA is synthesized by the enzyme **reverse transcriptase**. The retroviral DNA becomes integrated into the host DNA. When viral DNA becomes integrated into host DNA it is called a **provirus** (animal viruses) or **prophage** (bacteriophages). The proviral DNA is later transcribed into mRNA that is needed for prophage assembly.

C. TRANSLATION AND PROGENY ASSEMBLY

The mRNA transcribed from viral nucleic acid is translated into the polypeptide chains that compose the viral protein coats with the aid of the host cell's tRNA, amino acids, ribosomes, and enzymes. Viral progeny self-assemble; the protein-nucleic acid configuration forms either spontaneously or with the aid of viral enzymes. A single virus is capable of producing hundreds of progeny.

D. PROGENY RELEASE

Once assembled, viral progeny may be released either by lysis of the host cell or by **extrusion**, a process similar to budding. In extrusion, the progeny are enclosed in vesicles derived from the host cell membrane; this permits viral replication without killing the host cell. The process of viral replication and extrusion in animal viruses is called a **productive cycle** (see Figure 14.10).

host cell membrane

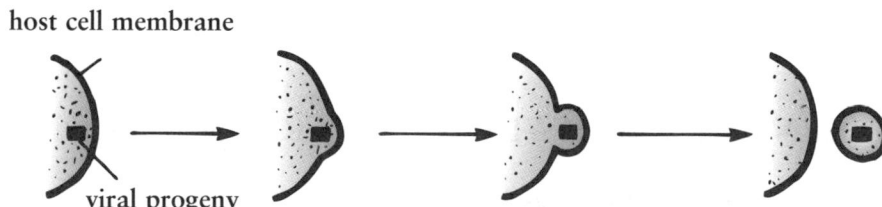

viral progeny

Figure 14.10. Extrusion

E. BACTERIOPHAGE

A bacteriophage infects its host bacterium by attaching to it, boring a hole through the bacterial cell wall, and injecting its DNA, while its protein coat remains attached to the cell wall. Once inside its host, the bacteriophage enters either a **lytic cycle** or a **lysogenic cycle**.

1. **Lytic Cycle**

   The phage DNA takes control of the bacterium's genetic machinery and manufactures numerous progeny. The bacterial cell then bursts (lyses), releasing new virions, each capable of infecting other bacteria. Bacteriophages that replicate by the lytic cycle, killing their host cells, are called **virulent**.

2. **Lysogenic Cycle**

   If the bacteriophage does not lyse its host cell, it becomes integrated into the bacterial genome in a harmless form (prophage or probacteriophage), lying dormant for one or more generations. The virus may stay integrated indefinitely, replicating along with the bacterial genome. However, either spontaneously or as a result of environmental circumstances (e.g., radiation, ultraviolet light, or chemicals), the prophage can reemerge and enter a lytic cycle (see Figure 14.11). Bacteria containing prophages are normally resistant to further infection ("superinfection") by similar phages.

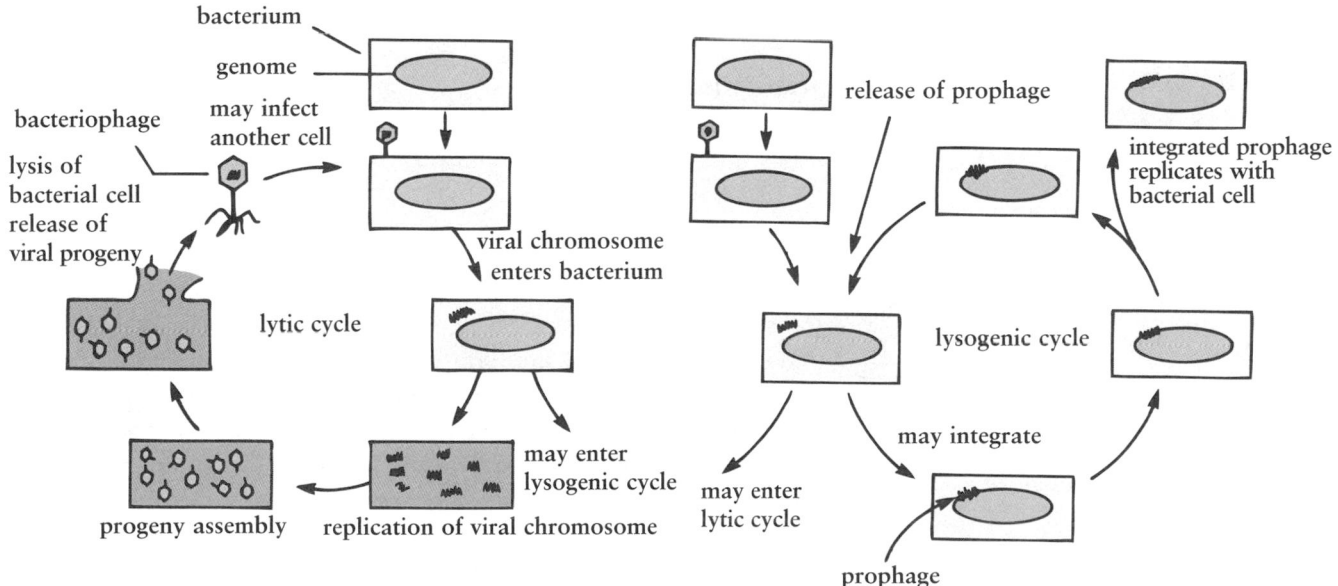

Figure 14.11. Bacteriophage Lifecycle

BACTERIAL GENETICS

A. BACTERIAL GENOME

The bacterial genome consists of a single circular chromosome located in the nucleoid region of the cell (see chapter 1). Many bacteria also contain smaller circular rings of DNA called **plasmids**, which contain accessory genes. **Episomes** are plasmids that are capable of integration into the bacterial genome. Since the bacterial chromosome is not separated from the cytoplasm by a nuclear membrane, transcription and translation occur almost simultaneously. As soon as a small portion of newly synthesized mRNA separates from its DNA template, translation begins. A strand of prokaryotic mRNA may be **polycistronic**, i.e., coding for more than one polypeptide (usually a group of related proteins).

B. REPLICATION

Replication of the bacterial chromosome begins at a unique origin of replication and proceeds in both directions simultaneously. DNA is synthesized in the 5′ → 3′ direction. Replication occurs at the rate of approximately 500 nucleotide additions per second.

C. GENETIC VARIANCE

Bacterial cells reproduce by binary fission and proliferate very rapidly under favorable conditions. Although binary fission is an asexual process, bacteria have three mechanisms for increasing the genetic variance of a population: **transformation**, **conjugation**, and **transduction**.

1. Transformation

Transformation is the process by which a foreign chromosome fragment (plasmid) is incorporated into the bacterial chromosome via recombination, creating new inheritable genetic combinations.

2. Conjugation

Conjugation can be described as sexual mating in bacteria; it is the transfer of genetic material between two bacteria that are temporarily joined. A cytoplasmic **conjugation bridge** is formed between the two cells and genetic material is transferred from the **donor male (+) type** to the **recipient female (−) type**. The bridge is formed from appendages called **sex pili**, which are found on the donor male. Only bacteria containing plasmids called **sex factors** are capable of forming pili and conjugating. The best studied sex factor is the **F factor** in *Escherichia coli*. Bacteria possessing this plasmid are termed **F+ cells**, those without it are called **F− cells**. During conjugation between an F+ and an F− cell, the F+ cell replicates its F factor and donates the copy to the recipient, converting it to an F+ cell (see Figure 14.12). Plasmids that do not induce pili formation may transfer into the recipient cell along with the sex factor.

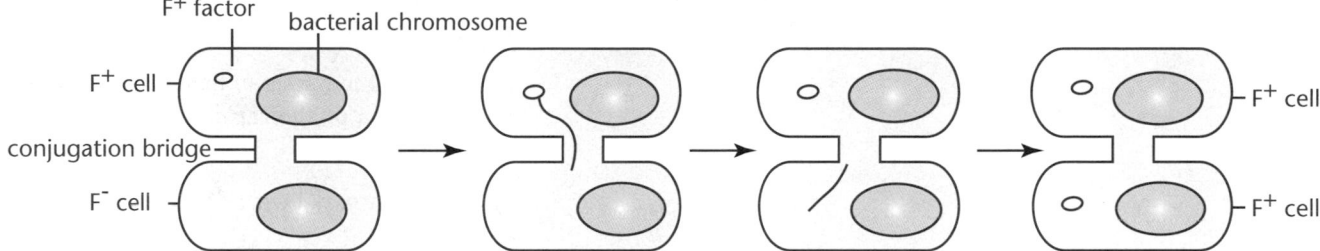

Figure 14.12. Conjugation

Sometimes the sex factor becomes integrated into the bacterial genome. During conjugation the entire bacterial chromosome replicates and begins to move from the donor cell into the recipient cell. The conjugation bridge usually breaks before the entire chromosome is transferred, but the bacterial genes that enter the recipient cell can easily recombine with the bacterial genes already present to form novel genetic combinations. These bacteria are called **Hfr cells**, meaning that they have a high frequency of recombination.

3. **Transduction**
Transduction is when fragments of the bacterial chromosome accidentally become packaged into viral progeny produced during a viral infection. These virions may infect other bacteria and introduce new genetic arrangements through recombination with the new host cell's DNA (see Figure 14.13). This process is similar to conjugation and may reflect an evolutionary relationship between viruses and plasmids.

D. GENE REGULATION
The regulation of gene expression (transcription) enables prokaryotes to control their metabolism. Regulation of transcription is based on the accessibility of RNA polymerase to the genes being transcribed and is directed by an **operon**, which consists of **structural genes**, an **operator gene**, and a **promoter gene**. Structural genes contain sequences of DNA that code for proteins. The operator gene is the sequence of nontranscribable DNA that is the repressor binding site. The promoter gene is the noncoding sequence of DNA that serves as the initial binding site for RNA polymerase. There is also a **regulator gene**, which codes for the synthesis of a repressor molecule that binds to the operator and blocks RNA polymerase from transcribing the structural genes.

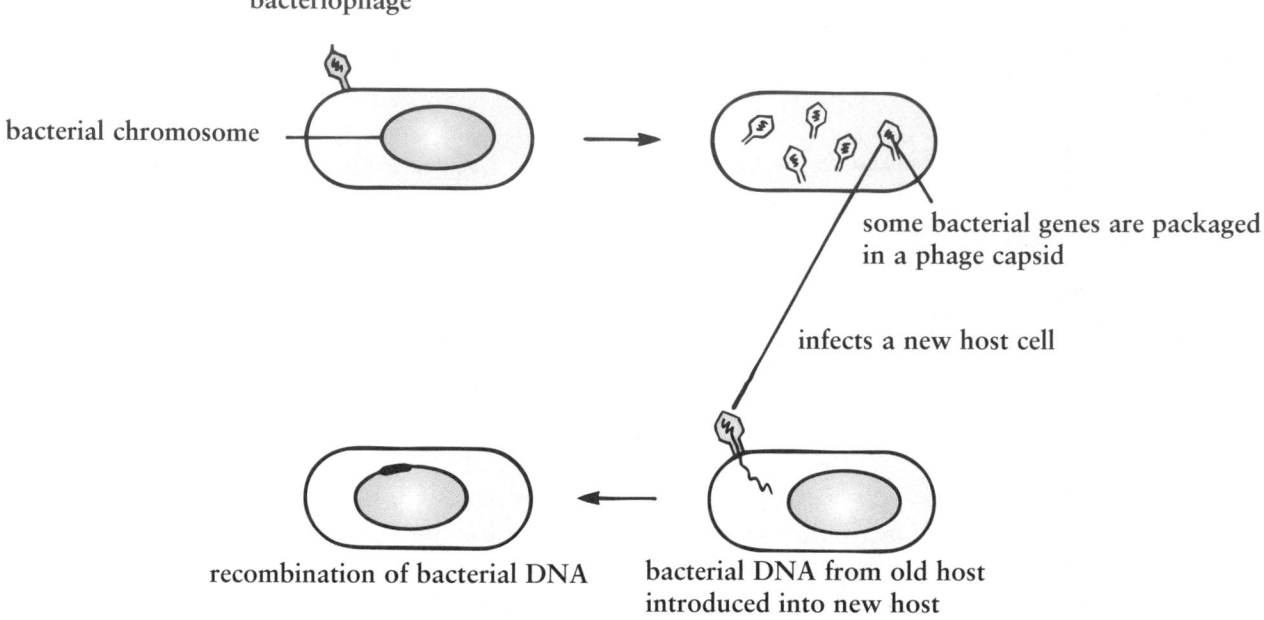

bacteriophage

bacterial chromosome

some bacterial genes are packaged in a phage capsid

infects a new host cell

recombination of bacterial DNA

bacterial DNA from old host introduced into new host

Figure 14.13. Transduction

Regulation may be via **inducible systems** or **repressible systems**. Inducible systems are those that require the presence of a substance, called an **inducer**, for transcription to occur. Repressible systems are in a constant state of transcription unless a **corepressor** is present to inhibit transcription.

1. **Inducible Systems**

   In an inducible system, the repressor binds to the operator, forming a barrier that prevents RNA polymerase from transcribing the structural genes. The repressor is active until it binds to the inducer. For transcription to occur, an inducer must bind to the repressor, forming an **inducer-repressor complex**. This complex cannot bind to the operator, thus permitting transcription. The proteins synthesized are thus said to be inducible. The structural genes typically code for an enzyme, and the inducer is usually the substrate, or a derivative of the substrate, upon which the enzyme normally acts. When the substrate (inducer) is present, enzymes are synthesized; when it is absent, enzyme synthesis is negligible. In this manner, enzymes are transcribed only when they are actually needed. An example of an inducible system is the ***lac* operon** (see Figure 14.14).

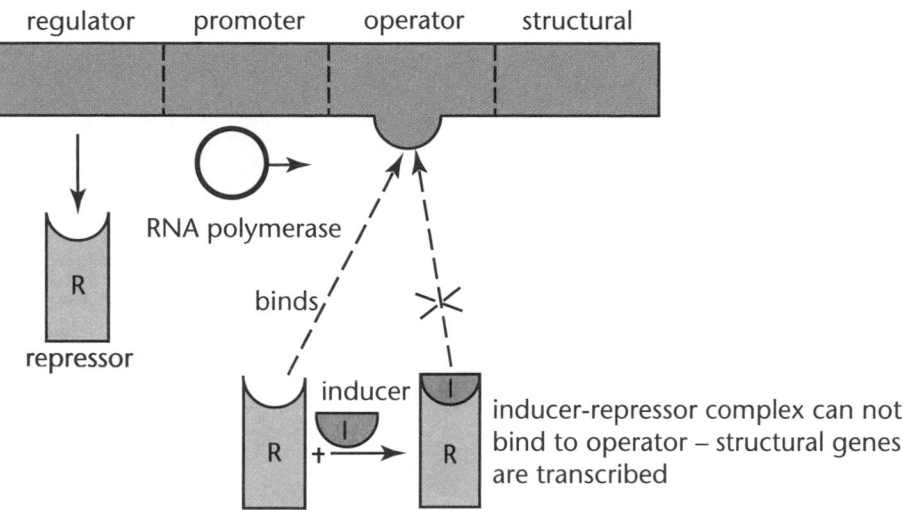

Figure 14.14. Inducible System

2. Repressible Systems

In a repressible system, the repressor is inactive until it combines with the corepressor. The repressor can bind to the operator and prevent transcription only when it has formed a **repressor-corepressor complex.** Corepressors are often the end-products of the biosynthetic pathways they control. The proteins produced (usually enzymes) are said to be repressible since they are normally being synthesized; transcription and translation occur until the corepressor is synthesized. An example of a repressible system is the ***trp* operon** (see Figure 14.15)

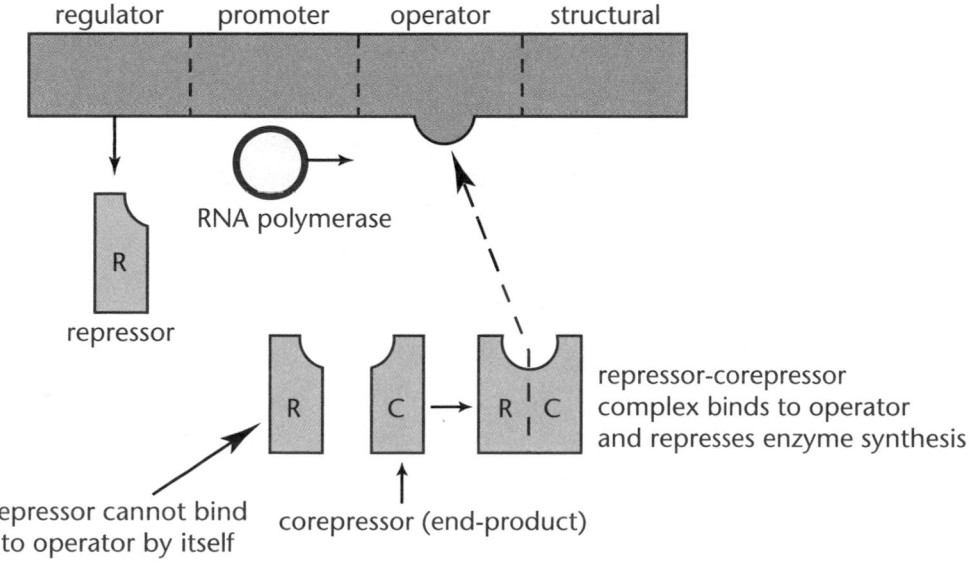

Figure 14.15. Repressible System

15

EVOLUTION

Evolution is a process of change and adaptation leading to the development of new life forms and genetic diversity.

THEORIES OF EVOLUTION

A. LAMARCK

Jean Baptiste Lamarck was an early evolution theorist. He formulated the concept of **use and disuse:** organs that are used extensively develop, while organs that are not used atrophy. Lamark theorized that newer, more complex species arise from older and simpler species through the accumulation and modification of **acquired characteristics**. Although it is now known that characteristics are inherited rather than acquired through use, Lamarck's work was the first systematic approach to understanding evolutionary processes.

> **Pavlov's Dog**
>
> If you see any hint of the buzz phrases "use and disuse" or "inheritance of acquired characteristics," think Lamarck. And don't forget—Lamarck was wrong!

B. DARWIN

Charles Darwin developed a theory of evolution in *The Origin of Species*, published in 1859. In it, Darwin outlined a number of basic agents leading to evolutionary change:

1. Organisms produce offspring, very few of which survive to reproductive maturity.

2. There are chance variations between individuals in any given population, some of which are inheritable. Variations that give the organism a slight advantage in the struggle for existence are called favorable variations.

3. Individuals who have inherited favorable variations are likely to live longer and produce more offspring than others; thus favorable variations become more common from generation to generation. This process is known as **natural selection.** Gradually, natural selection leads to variations that differentiate organisms into groups and ultimately

into distinct species. **Fitness** is measured in terms of reproductive success and the relative genetic contribution of an individual to the future of the population. Natural selection is the driving force of evolution.

C. NEO-DARWINISM (THE MODERN SYNTHESIS)

Most of Darwin's ideas persist in the current view of evolution, termed neo-Darwinism, or the modern synthesis. The science of genetics revealed that the ultimate source of hereditary variation lies in the processes of mutation and genetic recombination. Some gene combinations increase chances for survival and reproduction, while others decrease them. This leads to **differential reproduction;** i.e., individuals with favorable genes produce more offspring. As a result, after many generations, these favorable genes will have become pervasive in the **gene pool;** the gene pool consists of all of the genes in all individuals in a population at a given time.

D. PUNCTUATED EQUILIBRIUM

One remarkable aspect of the fossil record is that many organisms do not demonstrate gradual changes; instead there seem to be short periods of rapid change with long static periods between them. To explain this phenomenon, Eldredge and Gould (1972) proposed the model of **punctuated** equilibrium. They contend that evolution is characterized by long periods of stasis "punctuated" by evolutionary changes occurring in spurts. This is in contrast to Darwin's model, which proposes that evolutionary changes accumulate gradually and evenly over time.

EVIDENCE OF EVOLUTION

Evidence supporting modern evolutionary theory is drawn from many disciplines, including **paleontology, biogeography, comparative anatomy, comparative embryology,** and **molecular biology**.

A. PALEONTOLOGY

Paleontology, which is the study of the fossil record, is of particular significance to the study of evolution. With the use of radioactive dating techniques, paleontologists are able to determine the age of fossils, thus allowing them to determine the chronological succession of species in the fossil record.

B. BIOGEOGRAPHY

Biogeography refers to the distribution of life forms throughout the globe. Darwin observed that many species found on one of the Galapagos Islands seemed more closely related to species inhabiting the neighboring mainland than to species inhabiting the other Galapagos Islands. The biogeography of the Galapagos suggests that species migrated from the mainland to neighboring islands, where they adapted to the different island environments in isolation from each other.

C. COMPARATIVE ANATOMY

Homologous structures are similar in structure and share a common evolutionary origin. A classic example of homologous structures is found in the forelimbs of mammals: bat wings, whale flippers, horse forelegs, and human arms are all modifications of a common anatomical theme. In contrast, **analogous structures** share a functional similarity but arose from different evolutionary origins. The wings of insects and birds are both adaptations for flight but evolved from separate lines of descent. **Vestigial structures** are remnants of organs that have lost their ancestral functions, and thus are evidence of evolutionary forces at work. Examples include vestiges of limb bones in the adult python and the appendix and vestiges of the tail bone (coccyx) in man.

D. COMPARATIVE EMBRYOLOGY

The stages of embryonic development in closely related organisms resemble each other, indicating common evolutionary origins. The earliest stages tend to be the most similar. For example, all chordates exhibit certain features as embryos, such as gills.

E. MOLECULAR BIOLOGY

Through comparative DNA studies, biologists have been able to detect similarities in the DNA composition of related species. Taxonomically close species have a greater percentage of similar DNA than taxonomically distant species.

GENETIC BASIS OF EVOLUTION

Genetic variation functions as the raw material for natural selection. Sources of genetic variation include inheritable mutations and recombination. Mutations are random changes in the nucleotide sequence of DNA. Recombination refers to novel genetic combinations resulting from sexual reproduction and crossing over.

A. THE HARDY-WEINBERG EQUILIBRIUM

Evolution can be viewed as a result of changing **gene frequencies** within a population. Gene frequency is the relative frequency of a particular allele. When the gene frequencies of a population are not changing, the gene pool is stable, and the population is not evolving. However, this is true only in ideal situations in which the following conditions are met:

1. The population is very large.
2. There are no mutations that affect the gene pool.
3. Mating between individuals in the population is random.
4. There is no net migration of individuals into or out of the population.
5. The genes in the population are all equally successful at reproducing.

> **Flashback**
>
> If you didn't get it the first time out, it's time to revisit the concepts of recombination and mutation. See chapters 4 and 14.

Under these idealized conditions, a certain equilibrium will exist between all of the genes in a gene pool, which is described by the **Hardy-Weinberg equation.**

For a gene locus with only two alleles, T and t, **p** = the frequency of allele T and **q** = the frequency of allele t. By definition, for a given gene locus, **p + q = 1,** since the combined frequencies of the alleles must total 100 percent. Thus $(p + q)^2 = (1)^2$ and

$$p^2 + 2pq + q^2 = 1$$

where $\quad p^2 \;=\;$ frequency of TT (dominant homozygotes)
$2pq \;=\;$ frequency of Tt (heterozygotes)
$q^2 \;=\;$ frequency of tt (recessive homozygotes)

The Hardy-Weinberg equation may be used to determine gene frequencies in a large population in the absence of microevolutionary change (defined by the five conditions given above). For example, individuals from a nonevolving population can be randomly crossed to demonstrate that the gene frequencies remain constant from generation to generation. Assume that in the original gene pool the gene frequency of the dominant gene for tallness, T, is .80, and the gene frequency of the recessive gene for shortness, t, is .20. Thus, p = .80 and q = .20. In a cross between two heterozygotes, the resulting F_1 genotype frequencies are: 64 percent TT, 16 percent + 16 percent = 32 percent Tt, and 4 percent tt (see the Punnett square below).

	p = .80 (T)	q = .20 (t)
p = .80 (T)	$(p^2 = .64)$ TT = 64%	$(pq = .16)$ Tt = 16%
q = .20 (t)	$(pq = .16)$ Tt = 16%	$(q^2 = .04)$ tt = 4%

The gene frequencies of the F_1 generation can be calculated as follows:

64% TT	=	64% T allele	+	0% t allele
32% Tt	=	16% T allele	+	16% t allele
4% tt	=	0% T allele	+	4% t allele

Gene frequencies = 80% T allele + 20% t allele

Thus, p = .80 and q = .20. These frequencies are the same as those in the parent generation, thus demonstrating Hardy-Weinberg equilibrium in a nonevolving population.

B. MICROEVOLUTION

No population can be represented indefinitely by the Hardy-Weinberg equilibrium because such idealized conditions do not exist in nature. Real populations have unstable gene pools and migrating populations. The agents of microevolutionary change—**natural selection**, **mutation**, **assortive mating, genetic drift**, and **gene flow**—are all deviations from the five conditions of a Hardy-Weinberg population.

1. **Natural Selection**
   Genotypes with favorable variations are selected through natural selection, and the frequency of favorable genes increases within the gene pool.

2. **Mutation**
   Gene mutations change allelle frequencies in a population, shifting gene equilibria.

3. **Assortive Mating**
   If mates are not randomly chosen, but rather selected according to criteria such as phenotype and proximity, the relative genotype ratios will be affected, and will depart from the predictions of the Hardy-Weinberg equilibrium. On the average, the allele frequencies in the gene pool remain unchanged.

4. **Genetic Drift**
   Genetic drift refers to changes in the composition of the gene pool due to chance. Genetic drift tends to be more pronounced in small populations, where it is sometimes called the **founder effect.**

5. **Gene Flow**
   Migration of individuals between populations will result in a loss or gain of genes, and thus change the composition of a population's gene pool.

MODES OF NATURAL SELECTION

Natural selection is the only evolutionary process that assembles and maintains particular gene combinations over extended periods of time. Three different modes of natural selection are discussed below: **stabilizing selection, directional selection,** and **disruptive selection** (see Figure 15.1).

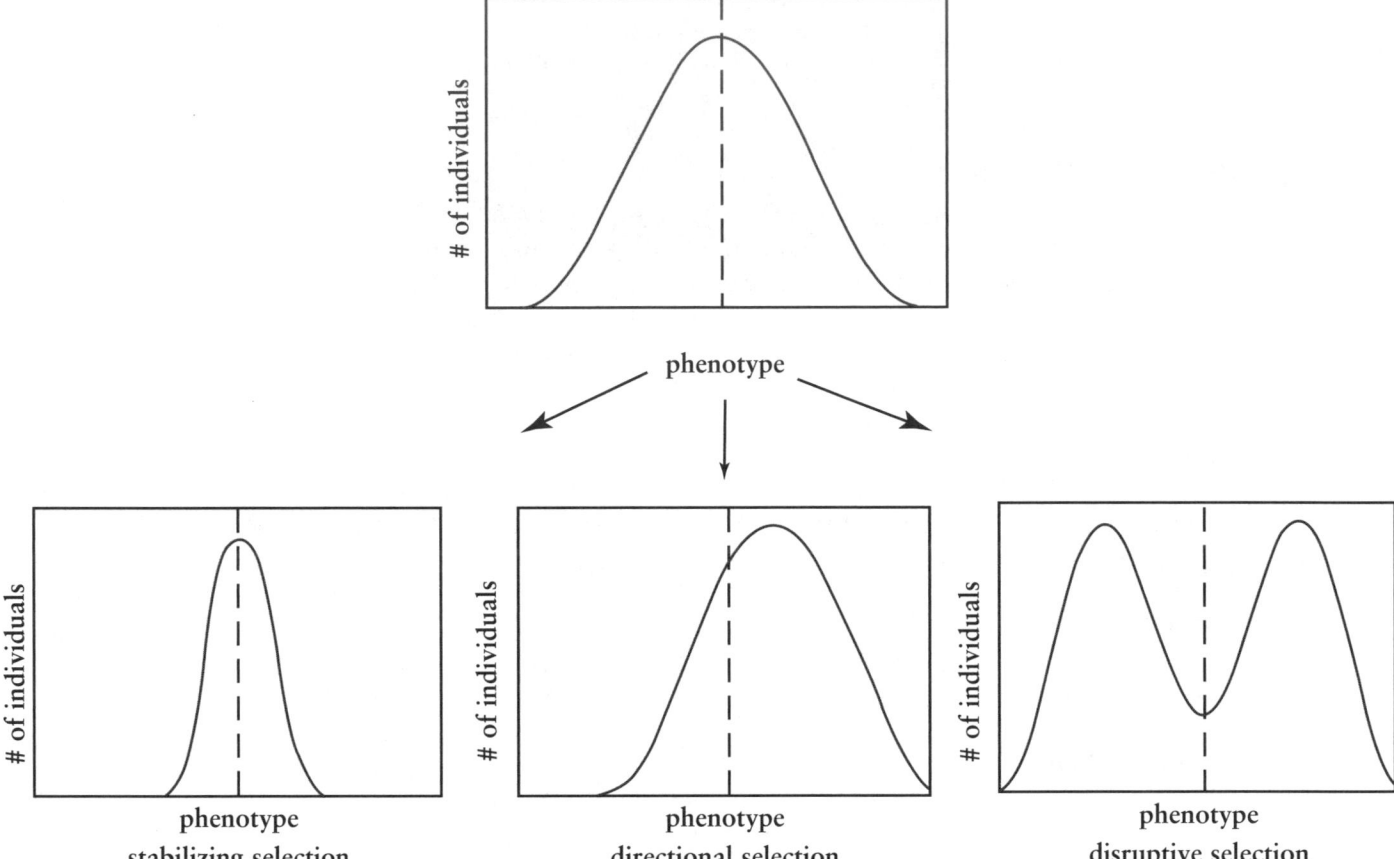

Figure 15.1. Modes of Natural Selection

A. STABILIZING SELECTION

Stabilizing selection maintains a well-adapted uniform character in a population by eliminating deviations from the norm. This process reduces the frequency of extreme phenotypes, thereby reducing variation. For example, stabilizing selection maintains human birth weights within a very narrow range.

B. DIRECTIONAL SELECTION

Directional selection produces an adaptive change over time, with an increase in the proportion of individuals with an extreme phenotype. Directional selection occurs when organisms must adapt to a changing environment. A familiar example of directional selection is the emergence of the DDT-resistant mosquito. The introduction of DDT produced a selectional advantage for those mosquitoes possessing the mutant gene for DDT resistance. After a period of time, the population of mosquitoes all possessed the gene for DDT resistance.

C. DISRUPTIVE SELECTION

Disruptive selection favors variants of both phenotypic extremes over the intermediates, leading to the existence of two or more phenotypic forms within a population (**polymorphism**).

ALTRUISTIC BEHAVIOR

Altruistic behavior is behavior that benefits one individual at the expense of another. An example is bee societies in which worker bees are sterile but labor for the benefit of the hive. Explaining the existence of such behavior in terms of natural selection has been a challenge to Darwinian theory. **Group selection** is the now-discredited hypothesis that certain individuals in a population inherit a gene for not reproducing, thus controlling population size at an advantageous level. This hypothesis is flawed because such a gene could not be passed on by its nonreproducing carriers. However, it led to the development of **kin selection** theory, which holds that natural selection can lead to behavior that does not improve the survival of an individual but does improve the survival of his near kin. Since increasing the survival and reproductive success of near kin, who share alleles, will often increase the survival of the individual's alleles, such behavior is consistent with neo-Darwinism. Since worker bees are the genetic sisters of the queen bee, their labor ensures the survival of their own alleles. **Inclusive fitness** describes fitness as the number of an individual's alleles that are inherited by the next generation.

ADAPTIVE RADIATION

Adaptive radiation is the emergence of a number of lineages from a single ancestral species. A single species may diverge into a number of distinct species; the differences between them are those adaptive to a distinct lifestyle, or **niche**. A classic example is Darwin's finches of the Galapagos Island chain. Over a comparatively short period of time, a single species of finch underwent adaptive radiation, resulting in 13 separate species of finches, some of them on the same island. Such adaptations minimized the competition among the birds, enabling each emerging species to become firmly established in its own environmental niche.

PATTERNS OF EVOLUTION

When examining apparent similarities in form or function between two species, it is important to determine whether the similarities are the result of a close evolutionary relationship or the result of similar adaptations to similar environments. Patterns of evolution are described in terms of **convergent evolution, divergent evolution,** and **parallel evolution** (see Figure 15.2).

A. CONVERGENT EVOLUTION

Convergent evolution refers to the independent development of similar characteristics in two or more lineages **not** sharing a recent common ancestor. For example, fish and dolphins have come to resemble one another physically, although they belong to different classes of vertebrates. They evolved certain similar features in adapting to the conditions of aquatic life.

B. DIVERGENT EVOLUTION

Divergent evolution refers to the independent development of dissimilar characteristics in two or more lineages sharing common ancestry. For example, seals and cats are both mammals belonging to the order Carnivora, yet differ markedly in general appearance. These two species live in very different environments, and adapted to different selection pressures while evolving.

C. PARALLEL EVOLUTION

Parallel evolution refers to the process whereby related species evolve in similar ways for a long period of time in response to analogous environmental selection pressures.

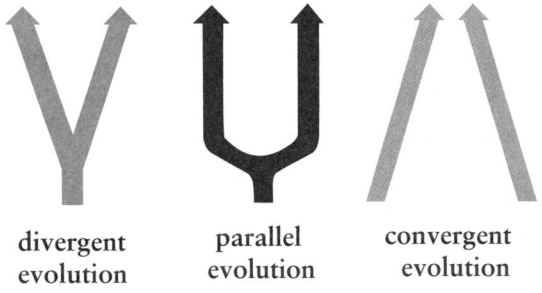

divergent evolution   parallel evolution   convergent evolution

Figure 15.2. Evolutionary Patterns

ORIGIN OF LIFE

The earliest evidence of primitive prokaryotic life is found in stromatolites, which are fossilized bands of sediment that contain microorganisms approximately 3.5 billion years old. It is not clear how life on Earth originated, but a hypothesis has been developed based on a theory proposed independently by both Oparin and Haldane in the 1920s and tested for the first time in the 1950s by Stanley Miller.

A. FORMATION OF ORGANIC MOLECULES

Oparin and Haldane proposed that conditions during the early years of Earth's existence favored the abiotic synthesis of organic molecules. Carbon, hydrogen, nitrogen, and small amounts of oxygen present in the atmosphere and seas bonded together in various ways and accumulated, forming a "**primordial soup**" of organic precursor molecules. The energy for the formation of these bonds was supplied by a number of sources, including the sun, lightning, radioactive decay, and volcanic activity.

Miller tested this hypothesis in a laboratory by simulating the conditions believed to have existed on primitive Earth. A mixture of gases was circulated past a source of electrical discharge (simulating lightning), and after one week, the reaction apparatus was found to contain a variety of organic compounds, including simple amino acids. During numerous modified replications of this experiment, all twenty amino acids, many lipids, and the five nitrogenous bases of DNA and RNA have all been generated. It is postulated that organic monomers were abiotically synthesized in a similar way on primitive Earth, and as they accumulated, were brought into close proximity, allowing them to react and form polymers.

B. FORMATION OF PROTOBIONTS

In laboratory experiments, abiotically produced polymers in an aqueous solution can spontaneously assemble into tiny proteinaceous droplets called **microspheres**. These microspheres have a selectively permeable membrane that separates them from their surroundings and maintains an independent internal chemical environment. Colloidal droplets called **coacervates** had been formed in Oparin's laboratory from a solution of polypeptides, nucleic acids, and polysaccharides. These coacervates are capable of carrying out enzymatic activity within their membrane if enzymes and substrate are present. Although microspheres and coacervates have some properties characteristic of life, they are not living cells. The molecular aggregates of organic polymers that are believed to have been the primitive ancestors of living cells are called **protobionts.**

C. FORMATION OF GENETIC MATERIAL

These hypothetical protobionts had the ability to grow in size and divide, but did not have a way of transmitting information to their next generation. The evolution of genetic material is difficult to map out, but it is believed that short strands of RNA were the first molecules capable of self-replication and of storing and transmitting information from one generation to the next. Experiments in the laboratory have shown that free bases can align with their complementary bases on a pre-existing short RNA sequence and bind together, creating a new short RNA chain. Natural selection may have favored RNA sequences whose three-dimensional conformations were more stable and could replicate faster. The next evolutionary step might have involved the association of specific amino acids with specific RNA bases. Thus, an RNA sequence could bring a number of amino acids together in a particular sequence and facilitate their bonding together to form a particular peptide. Natural selection could have selected for the synthesis of those peptides that enhanced the replication and/or the further activity of the RNA. Once this hereditary mechanism developed, proto-bionts would have been able to grow, split, and transmit important genetic information to their progeny. Self-replicating molecules eventually evolved to code for many of the molecules needed by primitive cells. Evolutionary trends led to the eventual establishment of DNA, which is a more stable molecule than RNA, as the primary warehouse of genetic information.

Biology Practice Set

Use this practice set to evaluate your mastery of the biology section of the test.

Read the explanations to all the practice problems, and revisit the chapters that relate to weak areas.

Good luck!

Biology Practice Set

Passage I (Questions 1–6)

The development of the nervous system is characterized by an initial overproduction of neurons, followed by the subsequent elimination of excess nerve cells through cell death. This system appears to provide an efficient way of establishing proper nerve pathways through synaptic connections: A given synapse is more likely to form when many neurons, rather than only a few, grow toward a target neuron. Once the appropriate synapse is produced, the superfluous neurons degenerate.

Scientists have long been intrigued by the mechanisms that regulate the growth and elimination of these superfluous neurons. Experiments have shown that *nerve growth factor* (NGF) causes the axons of sympathetic neurons to grow in great abundance along chemical tracks left by the diffusion of NGF. NGF is one of several proteins known as neurotrophic agents that appear to promote neuron growth. Another trophic agent currently under study is *ciliary neurotroph factor* (CNTF), which is believed to increase the growth of ciliary neurons and spinal motor neurons. The following assays were performed to test this hypothesis and the results are shown in Table 1 below.

Assay 1
In vivo treatment of developing chick embryos with CNTF*, in which test solution was injected into the embryos.

Assay 2
In vitro treatment of separate cultures of embryonic ciliary neurons and embryonic spinal motor neurons with CNTF*, in which test solution was administered to the cultures.

*Control assays were treated with an equal volume of the solution used to dilute CNTF.

Table 1

Assay	% of neurons in which growth was induced	
	In vivo	*In vitro*
Ciliary neurons + CNTF	0	25
Ciliary neurons + dilution fluid	0	0
Spinal motor neurons + CNTF	30	30
Spinal motor neurons + dilution fluid	0	0

1. From the information in the passage, it can be inferred that synapse formation:

   A. is a preprogrammed process with fully predictable results.
   B. is a completely random event.
   C. is a process that would occur much less efficiently without neurotrophic agents.
   D. is not absolutely essential for the formation of complex nervous pathways.

2. The experimental data shown in the table supports which of the following conclusions?

   A. *In vivo* growth of ciliary neurons is dependent on CNTF.
   B. Both *in vivo* and *in vitro* growth of ciliary neurons are dependent on CNTF.
   C. *In vivo* growth of spinal motor neurons is not dependent on CNTF.
   D. Neither *in vivo* nor *in vitro* growth of spinal motor neurons is dependent on dilution fluid.

3. According to the passage, NGF enhances the growth of sympathetic neurons. Based on this, which of the following physiological responses would most likely be compromised in an adult chicken if an NGF inhibitor were administered to the developing chick embryo?

   A. Inhibition of heart rate
   B. Stimulation of digestion
   C. Vasoconstriction of blood vessels in skeletal muscl
   D. Pupil dilation

4. Which of the following assays produced an unexpected result?

   A *In vivo* treatment of ciliary neurons with CNTF
   B. *In vitro* treatment of ciliary neurons with CNTF
   C. *In vivo* treatment of spinal motor neurons with CNTF
   D. *In vitro* treatment of spinal motor neurons with CNTF

5. The process by which a developing neuron contacts a target neuron and forms a synapse is most analogous to which of the following biological processes?

   A. Migration of chromosomes during cell division
   B. Packaging and exocytosis of a secretory protein
   C. Binding of a hormone to its cell surface receptors
   D. Fertilization of an ovum by a spermatozoan

6. If the assays described in the passage were performed on adult chickens and no neuron growth was observed, which of the following would best explain the results?

   A. Ciliary and spinal motor neurons degenerate during maturation.
   B. Adult chickens can form new synapses.
   C. CNTF can induce neuron growth only during a critical period early in embryonic development.
   D. CNTF cannot induce neuron growth of embryonic ciliary neurons in vivo.

Passage II (Questions 7–11)

Several methods of gene therapy have been developed to insert foreign genes into cells with genetic defects. Microinjection of a gene into a target cell with a fine glass pipette has been successful in some cases, but is very time-consuming and requires a high level of expertise. Another approach is electroporation, in which DNA is stimulated to enter cells by exposure to electric shock; however, this procedure is traumatic to the cells. To date, the most effective method of introducing foreign genes into cells is through a viral vector. With this method, foreign genes enter the cell via a normal viral infection mechanism.

The genome of a virus may consist of DNA or RNA, and may be either single- or double-stranded. When certain DNA viruses infect a cell, their DNA is inserted into the host's genome. Once integrated, viral genes can be transcribed into mRNA, which is then translated into protein. By contrast, the genomes of simple RNA viruses are translated directly into mRNA by the enzyme RNA replicase; DNA never enters the process. In retroviruses, the RNA genome is transcribed by the enzyme reverse transcriptase into DNA, which is then inserted into the host's genome. The viral genes can then be expressed, directing the synthesis of viral RNA and proteins. Retroviruses consist of an outer protein envelope surrounding a protein core that contains viral RNA and reverse transcriptase. The retroviral RNA contains the three coding regions *gag, pol,* and *env*, which code for the viral core proteins, reverse transcriptase, and the coat protein, respectively.

So far, retroviruses seem a more promising tool for gene therapy than either DNA viruses or simple RNA viruses. A retrovirus containing a gene of interest enters a cell via receptor-mediated endocytosis, and its RNA is then transcribed into DNA. This DNA randomly integrates into the cellular DNA, forming a provirus that is copied along with the chromosomal DNA during cell division. Retroviral vectors are constructed such that the therapeutic gene takes the place of *gag, pol,* or *env.* Problems associated with this form of gene therapy include the possibility that random integration could lead to activation of an oncogene, the fact that integration can occur only in cells that can divide, and the limitation that gene expression cannot be precisely controlled due to the randomness of integration.

7. Simple RNA viruses make poor gene-therapy vectors because:

    A. their genomes are not large enough to accommodate a therapeutic gene.
    B. a therapeutic gene inserted in the form of RNA cannot be copied and passed on to daughter cells.
    C. they can infect only specific cell types.
    D. insertion of a therapeutic gene into an RNA genome renders it too unstable to be used as a vector.

8. *In vitro* experiments have shown that a retroviral delivery system for gene therapy is preferable to physical methods of delivering DNA into cells, such as microinjection or electroporation. Which of the following is the most likely explanation for this observation?

    A. Retroviral delivery permits greater control over the site of integration.
    B. Retroviral delivery produces a greater proportion of cells that successfully integrate the therapeutic gene.
    C. Retroviral delivery is less labor-intensive and less destructive to the cells.
    D. Retroviral delivery allows therapeutic genes to be inserted into all cell types.

9. Which of the following cells would NOT be good targets for gene therapy involving a retroviral vector?

    A. Liver cells, because they divide continually, so the effects of the therapeutic gene would be diluted.
    B. Skin cells, because they are continually sloughed off the surface of the skin, so the therapeutic gene would be lost.
    C. Mature neuronal cells, because they are not capable of division, so the therapeutic gene would not be able to integrate.
    D. Bone marrow cells, because they cannot be removed from the body.

10. Which of the following events must occur for a retrovirus carrying a therapeutic gene to successfully infect its target cell and integrate into the cell's genome?

    A. The target cell's surface receptors must bind the retroviral protein envelope.

    B. New virions must be produced.

    C. The retroviral genome must be translated by reverse transcriptase.

    D. The retroviral proteins encoded by *gag, pol,* and *env* must be synthesized by the vector virus after integration has occurred.

11. Once a therapeutic gene has been integrated into a target cell's DNA, the retroviral DNA will most likely

    A. cause a nondisjunction event that corrects the genetic defect.

    B. be recognized as "foreign" by the host's immune system and degraded.

    C. replicate and form infectious virions.

    D. persist in the cell in a noninfectious form.

Questions 12 through 16 are NOT based on a descriptive passage.

12. The smallpox vaccine contains *vaccinia* virus, which has proven effective in providing active immunity to smallpox. The graph below plots the serum level of smallpox antibodies in a patient administered a smallpox vaccine on Days 1 and 50. The increase in serum level of smallpox antibody following the second vaccination can most likely be attributed to:

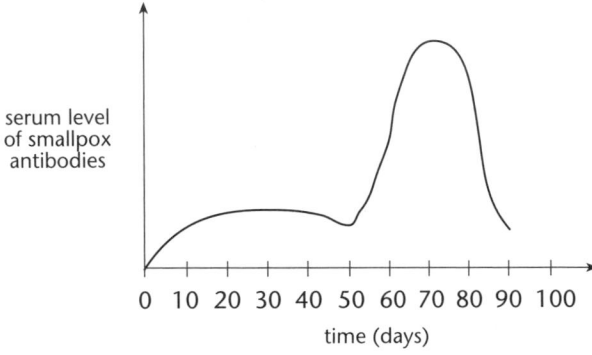

    A. the smallpox infection caused by *vaccinia* virus.

    B. the proliferation of B-lymphocytes exposed to *vaccinia* during the first vaccination.

    C. the synthesis of smallpox antibodies by *vaccinia* virus and by the recipient's B-lymphocytes.

    D. the fact that most vaccines require a minimum of 45 days for active immunity to be conferred on the vaccine recipient.

13. In patients with *myasthenia gravis*, a severe autoimmune disease of neuromuscular junctions, the body produces antibodies against the acetylcholine receptors of the muscle membrane (the sarcolemma), triggering their removal via phagocytosis. Based on this information, which of the following processes would be directly impaired by this condition?

    A. Sarcomere shortening during muscle contraction
    B. Calcium release by the sarcoplasmic reticulum
    C. Action potential conduction across the sarcolemma
    D. Acetylcholine synthesis

14. Which of the following factors would most likely cause an increase in left ventricle musculature (hypertrophy)?

    A. High systemic blood pressure
    B. Low systemic blood pressure
    C. High pulmonary blood pressure
    D. Low pulmonary blood pressure

15. What would be the most likely effect of infusing a concentrated solution of sodium chloride directly into the renal tubules of a healthy person?

    A. Decreased urine volume, due to increased filtrate osmolarity
    B. Increased urine volume, due to increased filtrate osmolarity
    C. Decreased urine volume, due to decreased filtrate osmolarity
    D. Increased urine volume, due to decreased filtrate osmolarity

16. A man with type AB blood marries a woman with type O blood. Which of the following are blood types that their children might inherit?

    A. Type A and type B
    B. Type O and type AB
    C. Type B and type O
    D. Type A and type AB

Passage III (Questions 17–21)

The human menstrual cycle is regulated by a group of hormones that interact with one another via a complex system of positive and negative biofeedback mechanisms. The cyclic changes governed by these hormones result in the monthly preparation of the female reproductive system for fertilization and pregnancy. For example, prior to ovulation, the uterine endometrium proliferates and the uterine glands increase in size; following ovulation, the ovarian follicle atrophies into the corpus luteum, which maintains the endometrium through its secretion of estrogens and progesterone. If fertilization occurs, the embryo implants in the endometrium and the menstrual cycle ceases until at least six weeks after delivery, longer if the mother breastfeeds. If the ovum is not fertilized, menstruation occurs. During this process, the endometrium sloughs off and is expelled from the uterus along with the unfertilized ovum. Menstruation averages 5 days, and the entire cycle averages 28 days.

Plasma concentrations of 4 of the hormones that regulate the menstrual cycle—progesterone, 17 β-estradiol (one of the estrogens), luteinizing hormone (LH), and follicle-stimulating hormone (FSH)—were assayed in 100 female volunteers with 28-day menstrual cycles, each at an equivalent point in their cycle. The data for Assays A – G were averaged and appear below in Table 1.

Table 1

Hormones	Assay						
	A	B	C	D	E	F	G
	Day 1	Day 5	Day 10	Day 15	Day 19	Day 25	Day 27
Progesterone $\left(\dfrac{ng}{mL}\right)$	0.11	0.11	0.11	0.20	0.43	1.81	0.20
17-β-estradiol $\left(\dfrac{pg}{mL}\right)$	40.4	49.0	240.2	198.1	65.0	140.2	30.0
LH $\left(\dfrac{IRP - hMG}{mL}\right)$	8.5	10.5	20.3	50.2	14.0	10.0	8.0
FSH $\left(\dfrac{IRP - hMG}{mL}\right)$	10.0	12.0	10.0	23.1	8.0	7.0	8.0

Figure 1 represents the in vivo biosynthesis of progesterone from its precursor, pregnenalone:

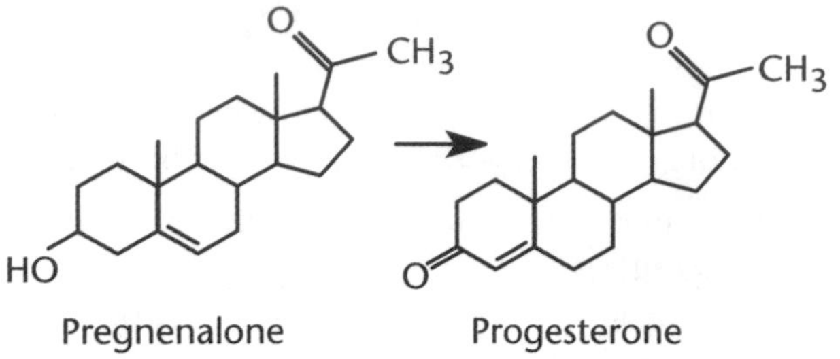

Pregnenalone   Progesterone

Figure 1

17. When 17 β-estradiol (a steroid hormone) contacts one of its target cells, it binds to an intracellular receptor and migrates to the nucleus; insulin (a peptide hormone) binds to extracellular receptors on the plasma membrane of its target cells. What is the most likely reason for this difference in mode of action?

 A. 17 β-estradiol is hydrophobic, and is therefore stable in cytoplasmic surroundings.
 B. 17 β-estradiol is lipid-soluble, and therefore easily traverses the plasma membrane.
 C. 17 β-estradiol is too small to bind to extracellular plasma membrane receptors.
 D. Insulin is too large to interact with DNA.

18. Based on the data in Table 1, what effect does the rising 17 β-estradiol plasma concentration appear to have on FSH secretion during the time interval between Assay B and Assay C?

 A. Positive biofeedback
 B. Competitive inhibition
 C. Negative biofeedback
 D. Allosteric activation

19. According to the passage, breast-feeding typically results in *secondary amenorrhea* (absence of menstrual periods). Given that breast-feeding is known to stimulate secretion of the hormone prolactin, which of the following explanations would best account for this effect?

    A. Prolactin inhibits ovulation, causing estrogen and progesterone secretion to decrease.

    B. Prolactin inhibits ovulation, causing estrogen and progesterone secretion to increase.

    C. Prolactin stimulates ovulation, causing estrogen and progesterone secretion to decrease.

    D. Prolactin stimulates ovulation, causing estrogen and progesterone secretion to increase.

20. Which of the following is the most likely explanation for the increase in progesterone and 17 β-estradiol plasma concentrations during the interval between Assay E and Assay F?

    A. The surge in LH secretion between Days 10 and 15 triggers the conversion of the ruptured ovarian follicle into the corpus luteum.

    B. 3-β-hydroxysteroid dehydrogenase, the enzyme that catalyzes the conversion of pregnenalone to progesterone, is inhibited by FSH.

    C. At Day 19, the uterine glands begin to secrete progesterone and 17 β-estradiol in anticipation of implantation.

    D. The surge in LH secretion between Days 15 and 19 increases 17 β-estradiol and progesterone production.

21. According to Figure 1, the biosynthesis of progesterone from pregnenalone results from which of the following?

    A. Reduction of a carbon-carbon single bond

    B. Oxidation of a carbon-carbon double bond

    C. Reduction of a hydroxy group

    D. Oxidation of hydroxy group

Passage IV (Questions 22–28)

DNA sequencing determines the precise base sequence of a given fragment of DNA. One such sequencing technique is the Maxam-Gilbert method, which separates DNA fragments that differ by only one nucleotide.

In the Maxam-Gilbert method, a sample containing multiple copies of a DNA fragment is radio-labeled with [^{32}P]. The DNA sample is divided into four equal portions, and each is subjected to a different chemical treatment. One cleaves the fragment before guanine (G) only; another before either purine, adenine (A) or guanine; a third before cytosine (C) only; and a fourth before either pyrimidine, thymine (T) or cytosine. If carried to completion, these reactions would cleave the fragment every time its particular base(s) appeared. However, limiting the reagent concentration and the duration of the reactions allows each fragment to be cleaved only once (on average). The procedure for cleaving guanines, for instance, produces a series of fragments of different lengths, each ending before a different guanine in the original molecule. Thus, all of the positions where a particular residue is found are represented in the series of fragments. The unlabeled fragments are ignored.

The products of the reactions are separated and their lengths identified by standard biochemical means. The four reaction mixtures are loaded onto four lanes of a polyacrylamide gel and subjected to electrophoresis. Larger residues migrate more slowly downward through the gel and the fragments spread out in a series of invisible bands. The positions of the fragments are then visualized using autoradiography: when the gel is held up to a photographic film, the radioactive phosphates expose the film, and the bands appear on the developed negative. DNA sequences up to 200 bases long can be analyzed in one set of experiments. Since molecular DNA is composed of two complementary strands, the first base in any chain can be identified by sequencing and identifying the final base of its complement.

Figure 1 shows the autoradiograph produced from Maxam-Gilbert sequencing of a short fragment of DNA. The band that appears at the top of the gel in all four lanes is the unreacted DNA fragment.

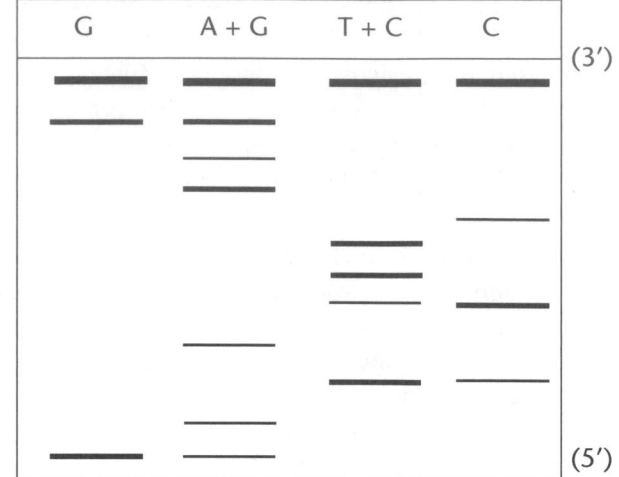

Figure 1

22. Why is the DNA fragment radio-labeled with [^{32}P] at the beginning of the Maxam-Gilbert sequencing procedure?

   A. To cleave the fragment before specific bases
   B. To divide the sample into four equal portions
   C. To limit the duration of the cleavage reactions
   D. To identify the polarity of the DNA fragment

23. If a fragment of DNA was found to have the sequence 5′ -AGACCTATG-3′, which of the following RNA fragments would form a DNA-RNA hybrid with it?

   A. 5′ -AGACCTATG-3′
   B. 5′ -CATAGGTCT-3′
   C. 5′ -CAUAGGUCU-3′
   D. 5′ -UCUGGAUAC-3′

24. After applying the Maxam-Gilbert method to a DNA fragment of unknown sequence, a researcher would identify a base as a guanine if a band appeared in:

   A. the G lane only.
   B. the A + G lane only.
   C. both the G lane and the A + G lane.
   D. neither the G lane nor the A + G lane.

25. What is the base sequence of the DNA fragment depicted in Figure 1?

   A. 5′ -GGACTTCAGA-3′
   B. 5′ -GACACTTCAAG-3′
   C 5′ -GAACTCACAG-3′
   D. 5′ -GATATCTAAG-3′

26. Which of the following is NOT a basic premise underlying the Maxam-Gilbert sequencing method?

   A. Each of the four chemical treatments cleaves the DNA fragment before only one nitrogen base.
   B. DNA contains the nitrogen bases adenine, guanine, thymine, and cytosine.
   C. The lengths of small DNA fragments can be compared by standard biochemical means.
   D. A single chemical treatment can produce labeled fragments of varying lengths.

27. According to the information in the passage, if the adenine + guanine cleavage reaction were allowed to continue to completion, how would this affect the appearance of the developed autoradiogram of the gel electrophoresis?

   A A greater number of distinct bands would appear in the A + G lane.
   B. A smaller number of distinct bands would appear in the A + G lane.
   C. A smaller number of distinct bands would appear in the A lane.
   D. The number of unlabeled fragments in the A + G lane would decrease.

28. If the [^{32}P]-radio-labeled DNA fragment 5'-[^{32}P]ACTATG-3' were subjected to the Maxam-Gilbert method, which of the following fragments would produce visible bands in either the C lane or the T + C lane?

   I.   [^{32}P]A
   II. [^{32}P]AC
   III. [^{32}P]ACT
   IV. [^{32}P]ACTA
   A. I and II only
   B. II and IV only
   C. I, II, and IV only
   D. I, II, III, and IV only

Questions 29 through 30 are NOT based on a descriptive passage.

29. Which of the following processes is NOT ATP-dependent?

   A. Exocytosis of synaptic vesicles at a nerve terminal
   B. Movement of urea across a cell membrane
   C. Movement of Ca^{2+} into a muscle cell
   D. Export of Na^+ from a neuron

30. In the diagram below, the reaction coordinate shows the progress of an enzyme-catalyzed reaction. If an inhibitor of the enzyme were added to the reaction vessel, how would the reaction most likely be affected?

   A. The free energy of the reactants would decrease.
   B. The free energy of the products would increase.
   C. The activation energy would increase.
   D. There would be no change.

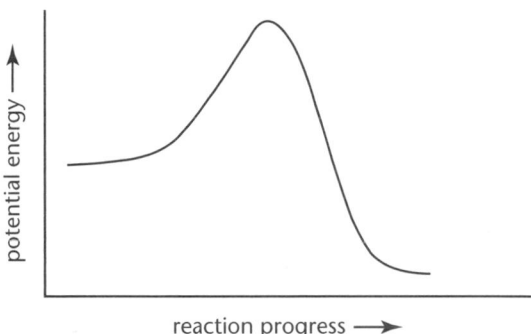

Passage V (Questions 31–35)

A researcher performed the following set of experiments in order to investigate the metabolism of two different strains of bacteria, Strain 1 and Strain 2.

Experiment 1

Strains 1 and 2 were incubated in separate broth cultures for 24 hours at 37.0°C. A sample of each culture was streaked onto three different plates—A, B, and C—each containing a different starch-agar medium; the plates were then incubated for another 48 hours at 37.0°C. The plates were then examined for surface colony growth and stained with iodine solution to determine the extent of starch digestion.

Table 1

	Surface colony growth			Starch digestion		
	A	B	C	A	B	C
Strain 1	+	+	+	–	–	–
Strain 2	+	+	–	+	+	–

Key: + = growth; – = no growth

Experiment 2

The two strains were incubated in the same manner as in Experiment 1. Two 100-mL portions of agar were poured into two beakers, which were maintained at 43.0°C. Next, 0.2 mL of broth culture from Strain 1 was pipetted into the first beaker, and 0.2 mL of broth culture from Strain 2 was pipetted into the second beaker. The agar was swirled around to distribute the bacteria evenly through the media and then poured onto plates. These plates were incubated for 48 hours at 37.0°C and then examined for colony growth both on the agar surface and lower down within the oxygen-poor agar layer.

Table 2

	Surface colony growth	Deep-agar colony growth
Strain 1	+	–
Strain 2	+	+

Key: + = growth; – = no growth

31. All of the following structures are found in both Strain 1 bacteria and Strain 2 bacteria EXCEPT:
    - A. circular DNA.
    - B. mitochondria.
    - C. cell walls.
    - D. ribosomes.

32. Based on the results of Experiment 2, Strain 2 bacteria would most likely be classified as:
    - A. obligate anaerobes.
    - B. obligate aerobes.
    - C. facultative anaerobes.
    - D. chemoautotrophs.

33. Which of the following statements best accounts for the experimental observations obtained for Strain 1 bacteria in Experiment 1?
    - A. Strain 1 bacteria do not possess the enzymes necessary to digest starch.
    - B. Strain 1 bacteria do not use starch for their first 48 hours of growth.
    - C. Strain 1 bacteria grow best under oxygenated conditions.
    - D. Strain 1 bacteria cannot grow on starch-agar medium C.

34. The researcher decided to incubate the plates from Experiment 1 for three more days; the results obtained were identical to those from Experiment 1 EXCEPT that starch digestion was observed for Strain 1 on all three starch-agar media. Which of the following conclusions might be drawn from these observations?

    I. Strain 1 requires longer incubation times to digest starch.
    II. Strain 2 requires oxygen for its early stages of growth.
    III. Strain 2 cannot digest the starch in starch-agar medium C.

    - A. I only
    - B. III only
    - C. I and III only
    - D. I, II, and III

35. Suppose that the researcher repeats Experiments 1 and 2, and this time, starch digestion is observed for Strain 2 in all of the starch media. These results can most likely be explained by the occurrence of which of the following processes?

    A. Mutation
    B. Transduction
    C. Nondisjunction
    D. Meiosis

Questions 36 through 38 are NOT based on a descriptive passage.

36. Animal studies have shown that certain lesions to the mesodermal embryonic primary germ layer may simulate the development of a rare human condition known as spina bifida, a congenital fissure in the lower vertebrae. Besides the spinal column, what other structures would most likely be affected by such lesions?

    I. Muscles
    II. Blood vessels
    III. Skin and hair
    IV. Intestinal epithelium

    A. I only
    B. I and II only
    C. II and III only
    D. III and IV only

37. Curve C on the graph below represents the normal hemoglobin dissociation curve at 38.0°C and physiological pH (7.4). Which curve most likely corresponds to the hemoglobin dissociation curve for a patient suffering from acidosis (low blood pH)?

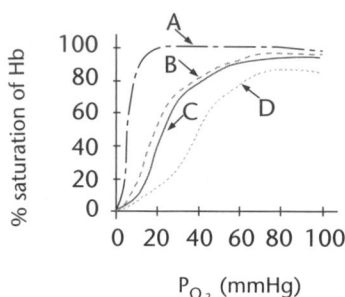

A.   Curve A
B.   Curve B
C.   Curve C
D.   Curve D

38. Which of the following graphs best represents the optimal pH for pepsin (a protease) activity?

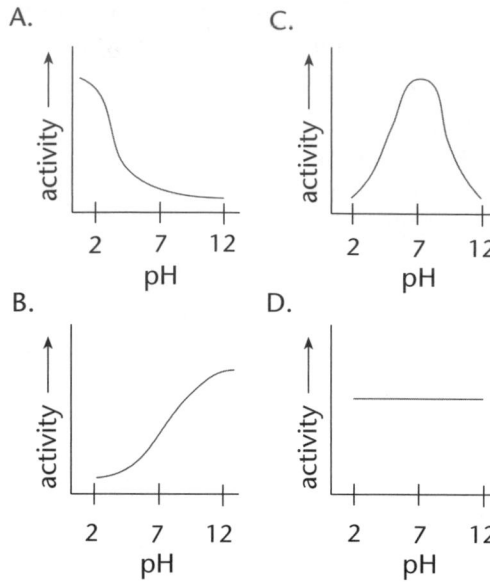

Biology Practice Set: Answers and Explanations

ANSWER KEY

1. C	11. D	21. D	31. B
2. D	12. B	22. D	32. C
3. D	13. C	23. C	33. B
4. A	14. A	24. C	34. C
5. D	15. B	25. B	35. A
6. C	16. A	26. A	36. B
7. B	17. B	27. B	37. D
8. C	18. C	28. C	38. A
9. C	19. A	29. B	
10. A	20. A	30. C	

EXPLANATIONS

Passage I (Questions 1–6)

1. C   The main concept in this passage is that the formation of synaptic connections in the nervous system is a complex procedure, somewhat comparable to shooting in the dark. Since neurons have no way of sensing each other, the probability that a single neuron growing towards a target neuron will form a synaptic connection is quite low. To compensate for this, the developing nervous system has evolved the following mechanism: it initially produces an abundance of neurons that grow toward a single target neuron. Once the proper synapse has formed, the superfluous neurons degenerate. Compare this to someone trying to shoot an arrow at a bullseye. The chances that one arrow will hit the center are much greater if many arrows are shot. The arrows that don't hit the target merely fall by the wayside. This analogy is appropriate because, as you're told in the passage, the growth of the neurons toward the target is not completely random; it is aimed, to some degree, by the neurotrophic agents that control neuron growth. This implies that without neurotrophic agents, synapse formation would occur much less efficiently; thus, choice (C) is right. Choice (A) is incorrect because, as just explained, the process of

synapse formation certainly does NOT have predictable results. Choice (B) is incorrect because we also know that the process of synapse formation isn't completely random; it's under the influence of neurotrophic agents. Choice (D) is incorrect because the passage states that proper nerve pathways are established trough synaptic connections. This means that synapse formation IS absolutely essential for the formation of complex nervous pathways.

2. D   The assays were performed in order to determine whether CNTF increases the growth of ciliary neurons and spinal motor neurons both in vivo and in vitro. As a control, both types of neurons were also treated with the fluid used to dilute CNTF in the experiment—again, under both in vivo and in vitro conditions. The dilution fluid was *not* expected to increase neuron growth; that's why it was used as the control. Anytime CNTF promoted neuron growth, it provided support for the hypothesis behind the assays. Turning now to the answer choices, since growth was *not* induced in vivo ciliary neurons treated with CNTF, then choice (A) cannot be concluded and must therefore be wrong. And although it might be concluded that *in vitro* growth of ciliary neurons is dependent on CNTF, since 25 percent of the neurons in that assay experienced growth, as just discussed this is NOT true for in *vivo* ciliary neurons. Therefore, choice (B) is also incorrect. Since 30 percent of spinal motor neurons treated in vivo with CNTF experienced growth, one would conclude that this growth was dependent on CNTF; thus choice (C) is also wrong. Choice (D), however, is supported by the data because NONE of the control assays were expected to cause neuron growth, and none of them did. Therefore, it can be concluded that neither in vivo nor in vitro growth of spinal motor neurons, or for that matter of ciliary neurons, is dependent on the dilution fluid used in the preparation of CNTF.

3. D This question takes a tiny little piece of information from the second paragraph and uses it as a springboard. To answer it, you have to know the differences between the parasympathetic and sympathetic divisions of the autonomic nervous system. These two divisions often elicit antagonistic responses when they innervate the same organ. In general, the parasympathetic division elicits physiological responses that conserve and gain energy, such as slowing down heart rate, vasoconstriction blood vessels in skeletal muscle, constricting pupils, and decreasing metabolic rate; the sympathetic division, on the other hand, stimulates responses that expend energy and prepare an organism for action, such as inhibiting digestive processes, increasing heart rate, vasodilating blood vessels in skeletal muscle, dilating pupils, and increasing metabolic rate. These responses are commonly known as the "flight-or-fight" responses. Based on this, it can be inferred that if a developing chick embryo were given an NGF inhibitor, then the axons of sympathetic neurons would not grow in abundance, and the proper synaptic connections would not be formed. And this means that some of the nervous pathways leading to the physiological responses associated with sympathetic innervation might very well be compromised in an adult chicken. Choice (D), pupil dilation, is the only sympathetic response among the four choices; therefore, it's the only one that might be compromised, and is the correct answer.

4. A In this experiment, it was expected that anywhere that ciliary neurotrophic growth factor was introduced, neuron growth would be induced. Thus, it's logical that anywhere CNTF was omitted, as in the four control experiments with dilution fluid, growth should not have been induced. However, in the in vivo assay of ciliary neurons plus CNTF, you notice that even though growth factor was introduced, no neuron growth occurred. This is an unexpected result, especially since growth was induced both in vivo and in vitro for the spinal motor neurons, and in vitro for the ciliary neurons. Therefore, choice (A) is the correct answer. There are many possible explanations for this result; one is that the experimental conditions may simply have gone awry. Another is that perhaps CNTF simply does not work this way within the body— that is, CNTFs in vitro neurotrophic effects may not

be due to the same mechanism that normally causes ciliary neurons to grow in vivo, so that even though it may serve as a neurotrophic agent for embryonic ciliary neurons in vitro, it doesn't in vivo. None of the remaining answer choices are correct, because they're all expected results.

5. D The process by which a target neuron forms a synapse with a developing neuron is largely determined by the probability that a neuron growing toward a target neuron actually synapses with it. The chances of this occurring would be quite low were it not for neurotrophic agents, which increase the number of neurons growing toward a single target. So during development, a large number of neurons are overproduced so as to ensure that at least one of them forms the proper synapse. Once the synapse has formed, the remaining neurons, which are no longer needed, will degenerate. Of the four answer choices, this process is most analogous to the fertilization of an ovum by a spermatozoan.

Sperm swimming through the female reproductive tract towards the egg are somewhat directed by chemical signals, just as neurotrophic agents direct neurons in their growth. Yet there is still the possibility that the ovum won't be fertilized, just as there's a chance that a single developing neuron won't synapse with its target neuron. To increase this probability, nature has dictated that millions of spermatozoa simultaneously attempt to fertilize the same egg, much like the initial overproduction of neurons increases the probability that the proper synapse will form. Thus, choice (D) is correct. Choice (A) is incorrect because there is no question of probability in the migration of chromosomes during cell division. This process is precisely controlled; the chromosomes are guided towards their objective—the cell poles—by spindle fibers that are attached to their centrioles. Choice (B) is incorrect because the packaging and exocytosis of a secretory protein is not in any way similar to the development of a neural pathway. It's not as if a thousand molecules of the same protein are synthesized in the hope that one of them makes it into a secretory vesicle and out of the cell. Finally, choice (C) is also incorrect because hormones are released into the circulatory system in minute quantities and then travel to their target cells, where they bind with surface receptors specific for them.

Hormones are *not* produced in excess, nor is there only a single cell with a single receptor that is receptive to the hormones' effects.

6. C According to information in the question stem, when the same exact procedures that had been performed on ciliary neurons and spinal neurons of embryonic chicks were performed on adult chickens instead, CNTF failed to induce any growth. The only difference between this set of experiments and the ones described in the passage is the age of the chickens. All four answer choices deal with this age discrepancy, so it makes sense to evaluate each of them to determine which best explains the experimental results. Choice (A) says that ciliary and spinal motor neurons degenerate during maturation. Not only is this false, but there's absolutely no evidence for it in the passage. What the passage *does* tell you is that the superfluous neurons produced by the developing embryonic nervous system degenerate after a synapse has properly formed. Thus, choice (A) is incorrect. If choice (B), which says that adult chickens can form new synapse, were actually true, then you would expect that CNTF would have induced neuron growth in the chickens. Since this did not occur, and since it's not clear from the passage whether adult chickens can or can't form new synapses, choice (B) must also be wrong. Choice (C), however, does provide a plausible explanation for the lack of CNTF-induced neuron growth in the adult chickens: Neuron growth can only be induced during a critical period of embryonic development. In other words, there is a limited period of time during which CNTF can induce the growth of ciliary and spinal motor neurons, and this period occurs during embryonic growth. After this critical period has passed, ciliary and spinal motor neurons are no longer sensitive to the effects of CNTF. So, choice (C) is correct. As for choice (D): While the claim that CNTF can't induce growth of embryonic ciliary neurons in vivo *is* supported by the results of the experiments described in the passage, this does not account for the lack of ciliary neuron growth and spinal motor neuron growth in adult chickens treated with CNTF; therefore, choice (D) is wrong.

Passage II (Questions 7–11)

7. B The key to this question is the fact that whereas simple RNA viruses are poor vectors for gene therapy, retroviruses are good ones. So the factor that makes simple RNA viruses bad vectors must be something that is not true of retroviruses. The major difference between the two is that retroviral genomes get reverse transcribed into DNA. Remember, the passage tells you that the genome of a simple RNA virus is directly transcribed into messenger RNA. If a simple RNA virus were used as the vector for a therapeutic gene, then the gene would not be replicated and passed on to daughter cells, because an RNA gene cannot become integrated into the cell's DNA genome. Integration is a necessary step of gene therapy and can only occur if the gene is in the form of DNA. Since integration cannot occur, the viral RNA is rapidly degraded by the cell. Choice (A) is wrong because there is no evidence in the passage that RNA viruses have smaller genomes than either DNA viruses of retroviruses, or that they might therefore not be able to accommodate a therapeutic gene. Choice (C) is also incorrect, because although it's true that certain viruses can infect only specific cell types, this is true for all viruses, not just simple RNA viruses, so it would not be a factor that would distinguish simple RNA viruses in particular. And, in any case, the problem of cell type specificity on the part of the virus is not even discussed in the passage, so there's no evidence to support this choice. Choice (D) is incorrect since there is also no evidence in the passage to support the statement that incorporation of a therapeutic gene into an RNA genome would render it too unstable to be used as a vector. Instead, the passage implies that it is possible to produce vectors carrying therapeutic genes from all kinds of viruses, but that retroviruses make the best vectors for some other reason—which is the reason described by correct choice (B).

8. C The passage described microinjection as a time-consuming technique requiring a high level of expertise, and electroporation as a technique that is traumatic for the cells. Neither of these criticisms is applied to retroviral delivery, which is described instead as occurring via a "normal" infection mechanism. Normal retroviral infection does not require any technique more complicated than adding the virus to the cells to be infected, and it does not harm the cells during the actual infection process, since the virus enters a lysogenic cycle. Thus, choice (C) is correct. Choice (A), which states that the site of gene integration can be more precisely controlled using a retroviral delivery system than by using physical methods, is wrong because the passage states that the retroviral DNA integrates into the cellular DNA at a random location—that is, not precisely at all! Choice (B) is also incorrect, since there is no evidence in the passage to suggest that a retroviral delivery system allows a greater proportion of its target cells to integrate the therapeutic gene than does electroporation or microinjection. And although you are not expected to know this, microinjection is probably the most efficient method of gene therapy in terms of the proportion of treated cells that are infected with the therapeutic gene. Finally, choice (D) is a wrong answer since the passage states that provirus integration occurs during RNA replication, thus, only cells that can divide are amenable to retroviral gene therapy.

9. C As you're told in the passage, a retrovirus integrates its DNA into cellular DNA during DNA replication, mainly during cell division, so it can only integrate into the chromosomes of cells that are capable of dividing. Of the four cell types listed as answer choices, only neuronal cells cannot divide. Choices (A) and (B) are both wrong, and for similar reasons. Liver cells would actually be *good* targets for retroviral gene therapy because they divide continuously. Continuous division means that the therapeutic gene would be replicated along with the cellular DNA and inherited by the daughter cells, thus ensuring a *continuous* supply of the therapeutic gene product; thus, choice (A) is wrong. Likewise, though dead skin cells are continually sloughed from the surface of the skin, they are replaced by living ones through cell division. The retrovirus could only successfully infect live cells, and once it had infected these cells, the therapeutic gene would not be lost, but rather inherited by the daughter skin cells. Choice (D) is incorrect because bone marrow cells are good targets for gene therapy involving a retroviral vector, for the very reason that they can be successfully removed from the body, infected, and then replaced. Moreover, bone marrow cells do divide and eventually produce important blood cell types, which makes them particularly fruitful subjects for gene replacement therapy. As you may be aware, bone marrow replacement has been used in recent years to treat lymphomas.

10. A For a retrovirus carrying a therapeutic gene to successfully infect and integrate into its target cell's genome, several events must occur. The first stage of infection is the binding of the retrovirus' protein envelope to receptors on the surface of the target cell. This facilitates the entry of the retrovirus into the cell, which consists of RNA, which is first transcribed into DNA by the enzyme reverse transcriptase. You might therefore have been tricked by choice (C), which actually says that the retroviral genome must be translated by reverse transcriptase; however, translation is a different process. The stage of protein synthesis during which a strand of messenger RNA transcribed from the genome is used to produce a strand of amino acids is translation. Thus, choice (C) is also wrong. Choice (D) would not occur during successful gene therapy; the retroviral proteins encoded by the genes *gag*, *pol*, and *env* are not synthesized after integration has already occurred. *Gag* and *env*, which code for the retroviral core proteins and protein envelope, respectively, would be synthesized after infection only if the retrovirus entered a lytic cycle. And although the *pol* region codes for reverse transcriptase, which is necessary for integration, reverse transcriptase is synthesized before integration occurs; so choice (D) is incorrect.

11. D This one can easily be answered by the process of elimination. Choice (A) is just plain ridiculous. Nondisjunction is either the failure of sister chromatids to properly separate during mitosis, or the failure of homologous chromosomes to properly separate during meiosis—the net result being that some daughter cells inherit multiple copies of one chromosome, while others lack the chromosome entirely. In any case, nondisjunction is not at all desirable and is in fact typically lethal. Therefore it is improbable that a therapeutic gene integrated into its target cell's DNA would normally

cause a nondisjunction event; this would not be expected to correct a genetic defect, and if a nondisjunction event did somehow occur, it would not be therapeutic; thus, choice (A) is wrong. Choice (B) is wrong because the host's immune system would have no opportunity to come into contact with and recognize the retroviral DNA as foreign since the viral DNA integrated along with the therapeutic gene into the host cell's DNA. Choice (C) is wrong because in order for replication of the retroviral DNA and formation of infectious virions to occur, the virus would have had to enter a lytic cycle, which does not occur in successful gene therapy. Remember, if the retrovirus was lytic, then the host cell would be killed, and this is clearly not the goal of retroviral gene therapy. The *goal* is to introduce a healthy gene into a genetically defective cell and produce its protein product without causing an infection, which necessarily implies that the retroviral DNA persists in the host DNA in an noninfectious form.

Discrete Questions

12. B Vaccines consist of attenuated—that is, weakened or inactive—bacterial or viral forms. Vaccines are specifically designed to "fool" the body into synthesizing antigens against a particular pathogen, without actually causing the disease typically associated with that pathogen. Therefore, choice (A) is wrong, because a smallpox vaccine containing *vaccinia* virus does not cause smallpox. The reason *vaccinia* is used in the smallpox vaccine is that its protein coat contains antigens similar enough to those found on the smallpox virus that they stimulate the proliferation of B lymphocytes that will then produce antibodies specific for both *vaccinia* virus and smallpox virus. The vaccine recipient is thus protected against a future smallpox infection. This type of acquired immunity is known as active immunity. Active immunity has two phases: First, the B lymphocytes differentiate into either plasma cells or memory cells. The plasma cells immediately start to synthesize antibodies; the memory cells remain inactive but retain surface receptors specific for the vaccine's antigens. This is known as the primary response. Upon subsequent exposure to the same antigen, such as a second vaccination or an exposure to the infectious agent, these same memory cells elicit a greater and more immediate proliferation of B lymphocytes, and this is known as the secondary response. On the graph, the curve following the first smallpox vaccination corresponds to the primary response, and the curve following the second smallpox vaccination corresponds to the secondary response. Thus, choice (B) is correct. As for choice (C), although the increase in the serum level of smallpox antibody can be attributed to the synthesis of smallpox antibodies, they are synthesized by the recipient's B lymphocytes, not by *vaccinia* virus. Being a virus, *vaccinia* can't synthesize anything but the proteins and nucleic acid it needs to replicate itself, and it can only do that with the use of a host cell's genetic machinery; it certainly can't synthesize antibodies, which are only produced by multicellular organisms. And there's no evidence in the question stem to support the claim that the smallpox vaccine or any other vaccine requires a minimum of 45 days to confer active immunity, choice (D).

13. C A neuromuscular junction is composed of the presynaptic membrane of a neuron and the postsynaptic membrane of a muscle fiber (which is called the sarcolemma). The two are separated by a synapse. In response to an incoming action potential, the presynaptic membrane of a neuromuscular junction releases the neurotransmitter acetylcholine into the synapse. Acetylcholine diffuses across the synapse and binds to acetylcholine receptors on the sarcolemma, causing the membrane to depolarize and generating an action potential. The action potential causes the sarcoplasmic reticulum to release large amounts of calcium ions into the sarcoplasm, which is the cytoplasm of a muscle fiber. This in turn leads to the shortening of the muscle fiber's sarcomeres, which contracts the muscle. According to the question stem, myasthenia gravis causes the body to produce antibodies that trigger the removal of the acetylcholine receptors found on muscle fibers. Without these receptors, acetylcholine can't bind to the membrane and trigger its depolarization. And if this doesn't occur, then neither can any of the events that normally follow it. So, of the four choices, the one that would be directly impaired by myasthenia gravis would be the conduction of an action potential across the sarcolemma: therefore, choice (C) is correct. Choices (A) and (B) are wrong, because although they too are impaired by myasthenia gravis, they're dependent on the conduction of an action potential, so it can't really be said that they are directly impaired. Choice (D), acetylcholine synthesis, is wrong because it's not at all affected by myasthenia gravis; acetylcholine is synthesized by the neuron itself, and this process is independent of whether or not acetylcholine receptors are present on the postsynaptic membrane.

14. A Muscular hypertrophy is an increase in muscle mass, which is due to an enlargement of its constituent cells. The most likely cause of hypertrophy in any muscle is an increased workload. Therefore, the most likely cause of hypertrophy of the left ventricle would be an increase in workload for the left ventricle. The left ventricle is responsible for pumping blood into the aorta and supplying the force necessary to propel it through the rest of the systemic circulation. Therefore, an increase in systemic blood pressure would increase the resistance of systemic circulation and force the left ventricle to work harder to overcome it; and as a result, the left ventricle would gradually hypertrophy. Thus, choice (A) is right and choice (B) is wrong. Choices (C) and (D) are wrong because pulmonary circulation is propelled by the *right* ventricle, and so any changes in pulmonary blood pressure would primarily affect the right ventricle.

15. B Water reabsorption in the kidneys is directly proportional to the osmolarity of the interstitial tissue, relative to the osmolarity of the filtrate. When the osmolarity of the filtrate is lower than the osmolarity of the kidney tissue, the tendency is for water to diffuse *out* of the nephron; when the osmolarity of the filtrate is higher, the tendency is for water to diffuse *into* the nephron. Infusing the nephron of a healthy person with a concentrated sodium chloride solution increases the filtrate osmolarity; thus, water will diffuse into the nephron to try and compensate for this change. So, you can rule out choices C and D. And since the volume of urine excreted is inversely proportional to the amount of water reabsorption, there will be a concomitant increase in urine volume. Therefore, choice (A) is wrong and choice (B) is correct.

16. A To answer this question correctly, you need to understand the genetics of the ABC blood system; that is, you need to know that the A and B alleles are codominant to the O allele. Thus, a person with the genotype AA or AO has a type A blood; a person with the genotype BB or BO has type B blood; a person with the genotype OO has type O blood. A man with type AB blood has the genotype AB and can therefore produce with either the A allele or with the B allele. A woman with type O blood has two O alleles and therefore only produce gametes of the O allele. So if this couple has children, the only two genotypes their children can possible inherit with respect to the blood groups are AO and BO, which correspond to the phenotypes type A blood and type B blood, respectively.

Passage III (Questions 17–21)

17. B   The main difference between the mechanisms of action of steroid hormones and peptide hormones is that steroids work intracellularly and peptide hormones work extracellularly. The barrier separating the intracellular environment from the extracellular environment is the lipid bilayer know as the plasma membrane. Peptide hormones must exert their effects extracelluarly, because they are not lipid-soluble and therefore can't easily cross the plasma membrane and enter a cell. Instead, peptide hormones bind to extracellular receptors on the plasma membranes of their target cells; and this binding then triggers a series of enzymatic reactions within the cells. Steroid hormones, on the other hand, are small hormones related to and synthesized from cholesterol, which is a component of eukaryotic plasma membranes. Thus, steroids are lipid-soluble and can easily traverse the plasma membrane, so they can and do act inside their target cells. Once inside a cell, a steroid hormone binds to a cytoplasmic receptor protein. The receptor-steroid complex enters the nucleus, where it induces protein synthesis by binding to the DNA and derepressing specific genes. Thus, choice (B) is the correct answer. Choice (A) doesn't hang together logically, and even if it did, it would not explain the differences between he modes of action of the two types of hormones. It's true that 17-β-estradiol is hydrophobic; however, this property doesn't make it stable in the cytoplasm, which is aqueous. Hydrophobic proteins, in fact, tend to be unstable in the cytoplasm, because their tertiary structure tends to be disturbed by a polar environment. However, a small steroid hormone like 17-β-estradiol has no tertiary structure to lose, so its stability won't be affected one way or the other by the cytoplasmic surroundings. Moreover, if it were true that this molecule is particularly stable in the cytoplasm, this would be a property that it shares with peptide hormones, so it wouldn't explain the differences in modes of action. Choice (C) is wrong because it's simply untrue. There is no need for estradiol to bind to extracellular plasma membrane receptors because it's lipid-soluble and therefore acts intracellularly. Finally, choice (D) can be eliminated for a number of reasons. First, the passage doesn't give you any information about the size of insulin versus the size of 17-β-estradiol; and although it's true (and you may have known) that proteins are generally larger than steroids, it's not the size of the hormones that dictates their mode of action but their solubility in the plasma membrane. In fact, as proteins go, insulin is fairly small, and enzymes much larger than insulin normally act in the nucleus, interacting with DNA during DNA replication and protein synthesis; so its size certainly wouldn't preclude insulin from interacting with DNA.

18. C   To answer this question, you first have to figure out what kind of influence increasing estradiol levels has on FSH secretion between Assay B and Assay C, which corresponds to the time interval between Days 5 and 10. During this interval, the estradiol plasma concentration rose from 49 to 240.2, while the plasma concentration of FSH decreased from 12 to 10. The question stem implies that this FSH decrease is a direct result of the estradiol increase; thus, it appears that this effect is one of negative biofeedback, choice (C). In biological systems there are many modes of regulation, one of which is negative biofeedback. Often, the concentration of a product or intermediate in a metabolic pathway inhibits the pathway that led to its formation. And although this is not exactly the case here, there is a negative relationship between estradiol and FSH; when the concentration of estradiol rises sharply prior to ovulation, it makes sense that FSH secretions should be inhibited, because FSH stimulates the maturation of an ovarian follicle, and it would be metabolically wasteful for a second follicle to mature before the first one is even mature, let alone ovulated. So, choice (C) is the correct answer. Choice (A), positive biofeedback, is another biological regulatory mechanism, in which the increased secretion of one product stimulates the increased secretion of a second product, which is not the effect that estradiol has on FSH production over the time period in question. Choice (B), competitive inhibition, might have sounded like a good choice, since FSH secretion does indeed appear to be inhibited by estradiol, but this inhibition is in no way competitive. Competitive inhibition is a regulatory mechanism in which molecules that are structurally similar compete with one another for substrate binding sites. The passage gives you no evidence at all about the mechanism whereby 17-β-estradiol affects FSH secretion, and certainly gives you no reason to believe that competitive inhibition is occurring; thus, choice (B) is wrong. Finally, choice (D), allosteric activation, is another regulatory mechanism. Allosteric effects occur in molecules with multiple active sites: The binding of substrate at one active site affects the properties of the others. Thus, allosteric activation is when substrate binding increases the reactivity of other active sites. Obviously, this is not occurring here, so choice (D) is wrong.

19. A Ovulation is followed by the conversion of the ruptured follicle to the corpus luteum, which maintains the uterine endometrium through its secretions of estrogens and progesterone. Therefore, it can be said that ovulation is indirectly responsible for the increases in estrogen concentration and progesterone concentration that follow it. So, if breast feeding stimulates secretion of the hormone prolactin, one of the results being the absence of menstrual periods, then this means that prolactin must inhibit ovulation. Thus, choices (C) and (D) can be eliminated. Since prolactin inhibits ovulation, then it must also inhibit progesterone and estrogen secretion; and you might also have known that estrogen stimulates LH and therefore helps bring on ovulation, which means that ovulation will tend to be inhibited by decreased, not increased, estrogen levels; therefore, choice (B) is wrong and choice (A) is correct.

20. A Answering this question requires a little bit of outside knowledge of the menstrual cycle and its hormonal regulation. Looking at Table 1, you should have either known outright that ovulation occurs midway through the cycle, around Day 14; or, if you recalled that ovulation is preceded by a surge in estrogen and LH secretion, you could have reasoned this out based on the table. The peak in estrogen concentration at Day 10 triggers the rise in LH concentration between Days 10 and 15, and it's this surge of LH secretion that triggers ovulation. Following ovulation, the ruptured ovarian follicle forms a yellowish mass of cells called the corpus luteum; as mentioned in the passage, this begins to secrete progesterone and estrogens, evoking the increase in progesterone and 17-β-estradiol secretion that takes place between Assay E and Assay F.

So, choice (A) is the correct answer. Even if you didn't know this, you might have been able to eliminate the other three choices. Choice (B) can be eliminated based on logic: It claims that FSH-induced inhibition of the enzyme that catalyzes the formation of progesterone from its precursor, pregnenalone, is responsible for the rise in progesterone and 17-β-estradiol secretion. Besides the fact that there's no evidence for any such mechanism in the passage, if this were in fact true, then you'd expect the progesterone concentration to decrease following the surge in FSH secretion on Day 15. You might also expect a significant decrease in FSH concentration around Day 23, when the progesterone level surges. Since neither of these is observed, choice (B) can be ruled out. On the other hand, if choice (C) were correct, it would explain the data in Table 1; however, it's untrue that the uterine glands secrete progesterone and 17-β-estradiol in anticipation of implantation. As discussed earlier, it's the corpus luteum that secretes these two hormones. As a matter of fact, although you might not have known this, the only glands that secret estrogens and progesterone in the uterus are those of the placenta, but this only happens if pregnancy occurs. As for choice (D), although LH does have a biofeedback relationship with estrogen and progesterone, which at times is one of negative biofeedback, and at other times positive biofeedback, you should have immediately ruled out this choice on a technicality: if you look at Table 1, you'll see that LH secretion decreases between Days 15 and 19.

21. D Pregnenalone is converted into progesterone; the question asks you to describe the change that occurs during this conversion. To answer this, you need to look at the structural differences between the two compounds, and also remember that a loss of hydrogen atoms is known as oxidation, while the opposite process, a gain of hydrogen atoms, is known as reduction. We can see that there are only two major changes from one structure to the other: The double bond in the second ring of pregnenalone is shifted into the first ring, and the -OH, or hydroxy group, in pregnenalone becomes a double-bond-O, or carbonyl group, in progesterone. The conversion of a hydroxy group into a carbonyl group is brought about by removal of hydrogen atoms, or oxidation. Therefore, choice (D), oxidation of a hydroxy group, is correct, and choice (C) is incorrect. Choice (A), reduction of a carbon-carbon single bond, is incorrect because the only reduction occurs at the carbon-carbon double bond in the second ring of pregnenalone. Here, hydrogen atoms are added to the double bond, making it a single carbon-carbon bond as the double bond shifts over to the first ring. In fact, a carbon-carbon single bond can't be reduced. Choice (B), oxidation of a double bond, is incorrect because what gets oxidized is a carbon-carbon single bond; and as we said, the double bond got reduced, not oxidized. Oxidation of a double bond would result in the removal of more hydrogen atoms and give a triple bond. Since there's no triple bond in progesterone, choice (B) is clearly incorrect.

Passage IV (Questions 22–28)

22. D The DNA fragment is labeled with radioactive phosphorus-32 to identify the polarity of the DNA fragment—that is, which is the 5′ end and which is the 3′ end. The radioactive phosphorus is inserted into phosphate which is then incorporated into DNA during replication since phosphate makes up the backbone of the double helix. According to the passage, the DNA is radiolabeled in such a way that the radioactive phosphate occurs only at the 5′ end. Therefore, when fragments of DNA are subjected to autoradiography following polyacrylamide gel electrophoresis, the 5′ end, which is labeled, can be distinguished from the unlabeled 3′ end which the passage says is ignored. So, choice (D) is correct. Even if you didn't see this, you could get the correct answer by a process of elimination, based on the descriptions of the procedure. According to the passage. the DNA is first radiolabeled, then divided into four parts, and then each part is subjected to a different chemical treatment. Thus, choice (A), which suggests that the radiolabeling causes the cleavage, is incorrect. And so is choice (B), which suggests that the radiolabeling itself functions to divide the sample into the four equal parts. Choice (C) is incorrect since radiolabeling merely replaces a nonradioactive phosphorus atom with a radioactive phosphorus atom; this does not change the reactivity of the molecule and therefore does not have any effect on the duration of the cleavage reaction. The duration presumably depends only on the amount of time the DNA sample is exposed to the reagent that causes cleavage.

23. C If a DNA–RNA hybrid were to be formed with a DNA fragment having the sequence AGACCTATG in the 5′ to 3′ direction, then the sequence of the RNA fragment would have to be complementary to the sequence of the DNA. There are two things you have to keep in mind: First, in RNA, uracil takes the place of thymine; that is, adenine binds with uracil. Second, in double-stranded nucleic acid, such as in a DNA helix or a DNA–RNA hybrid, the two strands run antiparallel; that is, the 5′ end of the DNA binds with the 3′ end of the RNA. Therefore, the sequence of the RNA fragment complementary to the DNA fragment would be CAUAGGUCU in the 5′ to 3′ direction, which means that choice (C) is the right answer. You

should have ruled out choices A and B immediately, since they both contain thymine, and RNA does not have thymine. Choice (D) is wrong because its polarity is wrong: Its sequence is backwards.

24. C If a band appeared at the same position in both the G lane and the A + G lane, then the base would be identified as guanine. One of the chemical reactions cleaves before either purine—that is, before adenine or before guanine. Therefore, for every adenine and every guanine a band will appear in the A + G lane. However, this band alone is not enough to distinguish between the two purines. One of the other chemical reactions cleaves the fragment only before guanines, and so for every guanine, a band will also appear in the G lane. Logically, therefore, if there is a band at the same position in both the G lane and the A + G lane, then the base can be conclusively identified as a guanine. Thus, choice (C) is correct and choice (D) is wrong. Choice (B) is also wrong, because by the same reasoning, a band that appears only in the A + G lane would be identified as an adenine. Finally, choice (A), the G lane only, is incorrect, since for every guanine, a band will appear in the G lane and in the A + G lane. In fact, you would never see a band in only the G lane, unless there was some sort of error in your procedure.

25. B The DNA fragment in Figure 1 has the sequence 5′-GACACTCAAG-3′. There are some clues to help you determine the proper sequence. First of all, the passage tells you that the band appearing in all four lanes at the top of the gel is unreacted DNA fragment. Second, the polarity of the gel is conveniently labeled for you: the 5′ end is at the bottom of the lane, and the 3′ end is at the top. So to read the sequence in the 5′ to 3′ direction, which you want to do since all the answer choices have this polarity, you have to work from the bottom up. Bands appearing in the G lane represent cleavage before a guanine; bands appearing in the C lane represent cleavage before a cytosine; bands appearing in the A + G lane represent cleavage before either a guanine or an adenine; and bands appearing in the T + C lane represent cleavage before either a thymine or a cytosine. If a band in the T + C lane has a corresponding band—that is, in the same position—in the C lane, then the cleavage was before a cytosine; if not, then the cleavage was before a thymine. If a band in the A + G lane has a corresponding band in the G lane, then the cleavage was before a guanine; if not, then the cleavage was before an adenine. Thus, reading from the bottom of the lanes to the top, the sequence of the DNA fragment in the 5' to 3' direction is GACACTCAAG, and choice (B) is correct.

26. A Two of the four chemical treatments used in the Maxam-Gilbert method cleave a DNA fragment before *two* different bases—in one case, before either adenine or guanine, and in the other, before either thymine or cytosine. Therefore choice (A), that each of the treatments cleaves the DNA before only one nitrogenous base, is false and thus is not a basic premise underlying the method. So, choice (A) is the right answer. Choices B, C, and D are all incorrect choices since they *are* basic premises underlying the procedure. Choice (B), that DNA contains four nitrogenous bases—adenine, guanine, thymine and cytosine—is a very basic fact about DNA that is a basis for this procedure, since these are the known points at which the fragment of DNA is cleaved by the four chemical treatments. Choice (C), that the lengths of small fragments of DNA must be comparable by standard biochemical means, is also true: Size comparison of the fragments in each of the four samples, which is effected by the gel electrophoresis step, is also necessary for determining the base sequence. So choice (C) is also a basic premise. Finally, choice (D) states that a single chemical procedure can produce labeled fragments of varying lengths. The passage tells us that the single chemical procedure for cleaving guanine produces a series of fragments of different lengths, each ending before a different guanine in the original molecule. This allows one to determine all of the positions occupied by a particular base along the DNA molecule. So this is also a basic premise of the Maxam-Gilbert method, and choice (D) is also wrong.

27. B According to the passage, if the A + G chemical treatment were carried to completion, the DNA fragment would be cleaved at every adenine and guanine present. This means that on average the original fragment would be cleaved many times, not just once. These DNA fragments would therefore have small molecular weights more similar to one another than the weights of

the two fragments produced by a single cleavage of the DNA. Since gel electrophoresis separates the DNA fragments into distinct bands on the basis of molecular weight, a series of fragments with similar molecular weights would produce a "fuzzy" band, as opposed to the more distinct band produced by the single cleavage DNA fragments. Therefore, choice (B) is correct and choice (A) is wrong. If you weren't quite clear on the concept behind this question, you might have looked at choices C and D first, since they can be easily eliminated. Choice (C) is wrong on a technicality, since there is no "A" lane present on the gel; while choice (D) is incorrect because unlabeled fragments do not show up on the developed autoradiogram of the gel electrophoresis, since they contain no radioactive phosphorus to expose the film.

28. C If the DNA fragment given in the question stem were subjected to the Maxam-Gilbert procedure, it would produce all five of the fragments listed. However, you're interested only in those fragments that would produce bands in the C lane or the T + C lane of the gel electrophoresis. Between them, the two chemical treatments that produce bands in the C lane and the T + C lane cleave before cytosine residues and thymine residues. Cleavage before cytosine residues would produce only one fragment, $^{32}P–A$; while cleavage before thymine residues would produce two fragments, $^{32}P–AC$ and $^{32}P–ACTA$. This corresponds to fragments I, II, and IV, and so choice (C) is correct.

Discrete Questions

29. B This is another knowledge-based question, requiring you to distinguish between biological processes that require ATP and those that don't. Exocytosis of synaptic vesicles containing neurotransmitters at a nerve terminal is an ATP-dependent process that is triggered by the transmission of an action potential along the length of a neuron; so choice (A) is wrong. Urea, a byproduct of amino acid metabolism, is a small uncharged molecule and, therefore, can cross the cell membrane by simple diffusion, which is a passive process. Therefore, choice (B) is independent of ATP and is thus the correct answer. The movement of calcium ions into muscle cells, choice (C), goes against the concentration gradient; therefore, calcium ions enter cells by active transport and ATP is therefore required. Choice (D), the export of sodium ions from a neuron, occurs in conjunction with the import of potassium ions; this is known as the sodium-potassium-ATPase pump, an ATP-dependent process necessary for the maintenance of a potential across the neuron membrane. Therefore, choice (D) is wrong.

30. C   This question is concerned with the kinetics of an enzyme catalyzed reaction. Enzymes speed up the rates of reactions that would eventually occur on their own in due time, by decreasing the activation energy without being consumed by the reaction. The activation energy is the amount of energy that the reactants must absorb from their surroundings to reach the transition state. In an exothermic reaction, such as the one depicted in the figure, the free energy of the reactants is greater than the free energy of the product. The initial free energy of the reactants and the final free energy of the products are independent of enzyme catalysis. Therefore, if the enzyme in question were blocked by an inhibitor, the free energy of the reactants and the products would remain the same—which means that choices (A) and (B) are wrong—but the activation energy would increase. This means that choice (D) is clearly wrong and choice (C) is the correct answer. You might have realized that the graph is superfluous in terms of answering this question.

Passage V (Questions 31–35)

31. B Identify which of the choices is not found in *any* bacteria. Bacteria are prokaryotes, and that the main characteristics of prokaryotes are that they have circular DNA, they don't have *any* membrane-bound organelles, they have ribosomes (which are structurally different from eukaryotic ribosomes), and they have cell walls composed of complex macromolecules of amino acids and amino sugars. Thus, choices (A), (C), and (D) are structures found in all bacteria, and thus can be eliminated. Choice (B), mitochondria, are the membrane-bound organelles that supply eukaryotic cells with ATP, and so choice (B) is the correct answer.

32. C Choice (D) is the odd man out, so it's worth checking quickly to see if it's correct or not. In fact, chemoautotrophs are organisms that derive their energy from the oxidation of inorganic chemical compounds rather than organic compounds and require carbon dioxide for growth; there's no reason to believe that this describes Strain 2; in fact, you have reason to believe that it doesn't, since Strain 2 can digest some starches, which are organic molecules. So choice (D) is incorrect. As for the other three: According to the results of Experiment 2, Strain 2 exhibited colony growth both on the surface of the agar, which is exposed to oxygen, and within the agar itself, which according to the passage, is oxygen-poor. To figure out whether this fits choice (A), (B), or (C), you have to know or figure out what these terms mean. An obligate anaerobe is an organism that obtains its energy via anaerobic processes such as fermentation. Since oxygen is a highly reactive compound, and since anaerobes don't consume oxygen in metabolism, oxygen tends to be toxic to anaerobic organisms. Thus, an obligate anaerobe would not be expected to grow on the surface of an agar plate. Since Strain 2 did exhibit growth under these conditions, choice (A) is incorrect. Obligate aerobes, choice (B), are organisms that require oxygen for metabolism, this implies that such an organism would not exhibit growth within an oxygen-poor environment such as the inside of the agar layer in Experiment 2. Thus, choice (B) is also incorrect. This leaves choice (C), facultative anaerobes. A facultative anaerobe is an organism that normally derives its energy aerobically, but also has metabolic pathways that allow it to exist under anaerobic conditions, such as with-

in the layer of agar. Since this definition corresponds to the results of Experiment 2, Strain 2 bacteria would most likely be classified as facultative anaerobes, and so choice (C) is correct.

33. B The results of Experiment 1 for Strain 1 indicate that Strain 1 is capable of growing on all three of the starch-agar plates used in the protocol, though iodine staining revealed that, at least for the first 48 hours of growth, Strain 1 does not digest Starch A, B, or C. In other words, although starch digestion is absent during the first 48 hours, colony growth occurs. This implies that Strain 1 bacteria must not use starch for its first 48 hours of growth, and so choice (B) must be correct. Choice (A), which says that Strain 1 bacteria do not possess the enzymes necessary for starch digestion, is tempting, since you know that starch digestion doesn't occur in the course of the experiment. However, metabolic pathways are not necessarily active at all times, and it's quite common for a bacterium to use one nutrient source preferentially over another and only to switch to a second source, and the pathways required to utilize it, after the first, more attractive nutrient has been exhausted. So, although it might be the case that the strain doesn't possess a starch digestion pathway, as a researcher, you would not be justified in drawing this conclusion after only 48 hours of incubation time. It could just be that the starch pathway is there but just isn't activated within 48 hours because there are enough other nutrients present to keep the cells alive for that time. In order to conclusively demonstrate that Strain 1 lacks the enzymatic machinery to digest starch, you would want to repeat Experiment 1 with a longer incubation time. Choice (C) says that Strain 1 bacteria grow best in an oxygenated environment. Although this claim was actually substantiated by the results of Experiment 2, this conclusion can't be drawn from Experiment 1 because plates A, B, and C are only examined for growth on the agar surface, not within the agar layer. Finally, choice (D) is incorrect because not only is it false that Strain 1 bacteria can't grow on starch-agar medium C—because they do—but even if it were true, this alone would not be enough to account for the discrepancy between starch digestion and colony growth, which is the issue that this question is actually addressing.

34. C This question investigates the mystery of how Strain 1 bacteria can grow on starch-agar media for 48 hours without actually digesting any of the starch. You're told that when the researcher repeated Experiment 1, the results were identical to those described in the passage, except that Strain 1 bacteria now exhibited starch digestion on all three of the starch-agar plates. So, you're asked to decide what conclusions might be drawn from this new data. Statement I says that Strain 1 bacteria require longer incubation times to digest starch. Based on the data, this conclusion does follow: With an incubation period of 120 hours, not only did Strain 1 grow on all three media—which we'd already seen from the original experiment 1—but it also digested all three types of starch. Statement I is correct, so choice (B), III only, can be eliminated. Statement II says Strain 2 needs oxygen for its early stages of development. This is clearly incorrect, because Experiment 1 did not address the oxygen metabolism of the bacterial strains—this was only tested in Experiment II. According to Table 2, Strain 2 grows in the oxygen-poor environment below the agar surface, so it doesn't need oxygen to grow. Thus, Statement II is false, and so choice (D) can also be ruled out. Finally, Statement III says that Strain 2 cannot grow on starch-agar medium C. Based on this, it is fairly safe to assume that if Strain 2 has not started to grow after this length of time, then it won't grow at all. Thus, Statement III is a valid conclusion, which means that choice (A) is wrong and choice (C) is the right answer.

35. A In this version of the experiments, Strain 2 exhibited starch digestion on all three of the starch-agar media, whereas in the first run of the experiments, Strain 2 digested only two out of the three different starches—it didn't digest Starch C. This means that between the first and second trials, something happened to some of the bacteria in Strain 2 that now allowed them to digest Starch C. Mutation, choice (A), is a change in DNA sequence; though most mutations are deleterious to an organism, mutations sometimes have beneficial results. An example of this would be if a mutation made Strain 2 able to digest Starch C in the second trial of Experiment 1, since this ability would increase the bacteria's survival ability. A mutation that resulted in the synthesis of an enzyme capable of digesting Starch C could plausibly explain the observed results. Thus, choice (A) is the correct answer. Transduction, choice (B), is

the transfer of bacterial DNA between two bacteria via a bacteriophage, which is a type of virus that infects only bacteria. Though transformation could account for Strain 2's newfound ability to digest Starch C, since the introduction of new DNA might provide the bacteria with some enzymes of metabolic pathways that it previously lacked, this is not the most likely explanation in this case, because there's no evidence of bacteriophage infection in the bacterial strains. Further, there's no bacterial strain around that can digest Starch C from which the capacity could be transformed. So, choice (B) is wrong. Choice (C), nondisjunction, is the failure of paired chromosomes or chromatids to properly separate during mitosis or meiosis, resulting in daughter cells that either lack a chromosome or have triplicate copies of one. Since bacteria don't have separate chromosomes but just one piece of circular DNA, nondisjunction can't possibly occur during bacterial DNA replication. And, even if the chromosome failed to replicate correctly, this wouldn't produce any new DNA, so it couldn't possibly give the bacteria a new metabolic pathway, and choice (C) is wrong. Finally, choice (D) is wrong because meiosis is the eukaryotic process by which gametes are formed. Prokaryotic organisms do not undergo meiosis at any stage of their existence; they replicate via binary fission, which is basically mitosis.

Discrete Questions

36. B You're required to know what structures and systems each of the three embryonic germ layers gives rise to. Spina bifida is a bone abnormality. Since bone arises from the mesodermal embryonic germ layer, a lesion to the mesoderm that simulates this disease would most likely also affect the development of other structures based on different types of connective tissue (such as blood, blood vessels, and muscles) and diffuse connective tissue of various organs. Thus, this lesion would affect the development of both muscles and blood vessels, Roman Numerals I and II. So choice (A) is wrong and choice (B) is correct. Skin and hair, along with the nervous system, originate from ectoderm, whereas intestine develops from endoderm. Therefore, Roman Numerals III and IV are wrong, and thus choices (C) and (D) are also wrong.

37. D Oxygen and hydrogen ions are in an allosteric relationship with respect to hemoglobin. An increase in the concentration of hydrogen ions decreases hemoglobin's affinity for oxygen; that is, the binding of hydrogen ions to a molecule of oxyhemoglobin enhances the release of oxygen. This interaction is known as the Bohr effect. According to the question, a patient suffering from acidosis has a decreased blood pH, which means that the concentration of hydrogen ions in the blood is higher than normal. And, as just discussed, a high concentration of hydrogen ions means that hemoglobin will release oxygen more readily than it does under normal conditions. With reference to the hemoglobin dissociation curve, this means that at a given partial pressure of oxygen in the blood, the percent saturation of hemoglobin with oxygen in a patient with acidosis will be lower than it would be at physiological pH. In terms of the graph, the hemoglobin dissociation curve corresponding to an acidotic patient would be shifted to the right of the curve for normal pH, and so curve D, choice (D), is correct.

38. A Pepsin is an enzyme secreted by the chief cells of the stomach's gastric glands; it digests proteins by hydrolyzing specific peptide bonds. In addition to pepsin, the gastric glands secrete hydrochloric acid, which give the stomach a pH of about 2. Thus, since the stomach is very acidic, and since pepsin functions in that environment, it follows that its pH optimum will be around 2; in other words, a graph of its activity as a function of pH would peak at a pH of 2 and slope downward as pH increases. Thus, choice (A) is correct. The reason pepsin works best in such an acidic environment is because the low pH of gastric juice denatures the proteins found in food, thereby exposing their peptide bonds to the enzyme's actions.

GENERAL CHEMISTRY

1

ATOMIC STRUCTURE

Chemistry is the study of the nature and behavior of matter. The **atom** is the basic building block of matter, representing the smallest unit of a chemical element. An atom in turn is composed of subatomic particles called **protons, neutrons,** and **electrons.** The protons and neutrons in an atom form the **nucleus,** the core of the atom. The electrons exist outside the nucleus in characteristic regions of space called **orbitals.** All atoms of an **element** show similar chemical properties and cannot be further broken down by chemical means.

SUBATOMIC PARTICLES

A. PROTONS

Protons carry a single positive charge and have a mass of approximately one **atomic mass unit** or amu (see below). The **atomic number** (Z) of an element equals the number of protons found in an atom of that element. All atoms of a given element have the same atomic number.

B. NEUTRONS

Neutrons carry no charge and have a mass only slightly larger than that of protons. Different **isotopes** of one element have different numbers of neutrons but the same number of protons. The **mass number** of an atom is equal to the total number of protons and neutrons. The convention $^A_Z X$ is used to show both the atomic number and mass number of an X atom, where Z is the atomic number and A is the mass number.

C. ELECTRONS

Electrons carry a charge equal in magnitude but opposite in sign to that of protons. An electron has a very small mass, approximately 1/1,837th the mass of a proton or neutron, which is negligible for most purposes. The electrons farthest from the nucleus are known as **valence electrons.** The farther the valence electrons are from the nucleus, the weaker the attractive force of the positively charged nucleus and the more likely the valence electrons are to be influenced by other atoms. Generally, the valence electrons and their activity determine the reactivity of an atom. In a neutral atom, the number of electrons is equal to the number of protons. A positive or negative charge on an atom is due to a loss or gain of electrons; the result is called an **ion.**

Some basic features of the three subatomic particles are shown in the table below.

Table 1.1

Subatomic Particle	Symbol	Relative Mass	Charge	Location
Proton	$_1^1H$	1	+1	Nucleus
Neutron	$_0^1n$	1	0	Nucleus
Electron	e^-	0	−1	Electron Orbitals

Example: Determine the number of protons, neutrons, and electrons in a Nickel-58 atom and in a Nickel-60 2+ cation.

Solution: ^{58}Ni has an atomic number of 28 and a mass number of 58. Therefore, ^{58}Ni will have 28 protons, 28 electrons, and 58 − 28, or 30, neutrons.

In the $^{60}Ni^{2+}$ species, the number of protons is the same as in the neutral ^{58}Ni atom. However, $^{60}Ni^{2+}$ has a positive charge because it has lost two electrons and thus, Ni^{2+} will have 26 electrons. Also the mass number is 2 units higher than for the ^{58}Ni atom, and this difference in mass must be due to 2 extra neutrons, thus it has a total of 32 neutrons.

MCAT Synopsis

- Atomic number = number of protons
- Mass number = number of protons and number of neutrons
- In a neutral atom, number of protons = number of electrons

ATOMIC WEIGHTS AND ISOTOPES

A. ATOMIC WEIGHTS

The atomic mass of an atom is the relative mass of that atom compared with the mass of a carbon-12 atom, which is used as a standard with an assigned mass of 12.000. Atomic masses are expressed in terms of atomic mass units (amu), with one amu defined as exactly one-twelfth the mass of the carbon-12 atom, approximately 1.66×10^{-24} grams (g). A more common convention used to define the mass of an atom is **atomic weight.** The atomic weight is the weight in grams of one mole (mol) of a given element and is expressed in terms of g/mol. A mole is a unit used to count particles and is represented by **Avogadro's number,** 6.022×10^{23} particles. For example, the atomic weight of carbon is 12.0 g/mol, which means that 6.022×10^{23} carbon atoms weigh 12.0 g (see chapter 4, Compounds and Stoichiometry).

B. ISOTOPES

For a given element, multiple species of atoms with the same number of protons (same atomic number) but different numbers of neutrons (different mass numbers) exist; these are called **isotopes** of the element. Isotopes are referred to either by the convention described above or, more commonly, by the name of the element followed by the mass number. For example, carbon-12 ($^{12}_{6}C$) is a carbon atom with 6 protons and 6 neutrons, while carbon-14 ($^{14}_{6}C$) is a carbon atom with 6 protons and 8 neutrons. Since isotopes have the same number of protons and electrons, they generally exhibit the same chemical properties.

In nature, almost all elements exist as a collection of two or more isotopes, and these isotopes are usually present in the same proportions in any sample of a naturally occurring element. The presence of these isotopes accounts for the fact that the accepted atomic weight for most elements is not a whole number. The masses listed in the periodic table are weighted averages that account for the relative abundance of various isotopes.

Example: Element Q consists of three different isotopes, A, B, and C. Isotope A has an atomic mass of 40.00 amu and accounts for 60.00 percent of naturally occurring Q. The atomic mass of isotope B is 44.00 amu and accounts for 25.00 percent of Q. Finally, isotope C has an atomic mass of 41.00 amu and a natural abundance of 15.00 percent. What is the atomic weight of element Q?

Solution: 0.60(40 amu) + 0.25(44 amu) + 0.15(41 amu)
= 24.00 amu + 11.00 amu + 6.15 amu = 41.15 amu

The atomic weight of element Q is 41.15 g/mol.

BOHR'S MODEL OF THE HYDROGEN ATOM

In 1911, Ernest Rutherford provided experimental evidence that an atom has a dense, positively charged nucleus that accounts for only a small portion of the volume of the atom. In 1900, Max Planck developed the first **quantum theory,** proposing that energy emitted as electromagnetic radiation from matter comes in discrete bundles called **quanta.** The energy value of a quantum is given by the equation $E = hf$ where h is a proportionality constant known as **Planck's constant,** equal to 6.626×10^{-34} J·s, and f (sometimes designated v) is the **frequency** of the radiation.

A. THE BOHR MODEL

In 1913, Niels Bohr used the work of Rutherford and Planck to develop his model of the electronic structure of the hydrogen atom. Starting from Rutherford's findings, Bohr assumed that the hydrogen atom consisted of a central proton around which an electron travelled in a circular orbit, and that the centripetal force acting on the electron as it revolved around the nucleus was the electrical force between the positively charged proton and the negatively charged electron.

> **Bridge**
>
> For more detail on Bohr's model of the atom, see chapter 11 in the Physics section.

Bohr's model used the quantum theory of Planck in conjunction with concepts from classical physics. In classical mechanics, an object, such as an electron, revolving in a circle may assume an infinite number of values for its radius and velocity. Therefore, the angular momentum ($L = mvr$) and kinetic energy ($KE = mv^2/2$) can take on any value. However, by incorporating Planck's quantum theory into his model, Bohr placed conditions on the value of the angular momentum. Like Planck's energy, the angular momentum of an electron is quantized according to the following equation:

$$\text{angular momentum} = nh/2\pi$$

where h is Planck's constant and n is a quantum number that can be any positive integer. As h, 2, and are constants, the angular momentum changes only in discrete amounts with respect to the quantum number, n. Bohr then equated the allowed values of the angular momentum to the energy of the electron. He obtained the following equation:

$$E = -R_H/n^2$$

where R_H is an experimentally determined constant (known as the Rydberg constant) equal to 2.18×10^{-18} J/electron. Therefore, like angular momentum, the energy of the electron changes in discrete amounts with respect to the quantum number.

A value of zero energy was assigned to the state in which the proton and electron were separated completely, meaning that there was no attractive force between them. Therefore, the electron in any of its quantized states in the atom would have a negative energy as a result of the attractive forces between the electron and proton. This explains the negative sign in the above equation for energy.

B. APPLICATIONS OF THE BOHR MODEL

In his model of the structure of hydrogen, Bohr postulated that an electron can exist only in certain fixed energy states. In terms of quantum theory, the energy of an electron is **quantized.** Using this model, certain generalizations concerning the characteristics of electrons can be made.

The energy of the electron is related to its orbital radius: the smaller the radius, the lower the energy state of the electron. The smallest orbit (radius) an electron can have corresponds to $n = 1$, which is the ground state of the hydrogen electron. At the **ground state** level, the electron is in its lowest energy state. The Bohr model is also used to explain the atomic emission spectrum and atomic absorption spectrum of hydrogen, and is helpful in interpretation of the spectra of other atoms.

1. **Atomic Emission Spectra**

   At room temperature, the majority of atoms in a sample are in the ground state. However, electrons can be excited to higher energy levels, by heat or other energy, to yield the excited state of the atom. Because the lifetime of the excited state is brief, the electrons will return rapidly to the ground state, emitting energy in the form of photons. The electromagnetic energy of these photons may be determined using the following equation:

   $$E = hc/\lambda$$

   where h is Planck's constant, c is the velocity of light (3.00×10^8 m/s), and λ is the wavelength of the radiation.

   The different electrons in an atom will be excited to different energy levels. When these electrons return to their ground states, each will emit a photon with a wavelength characteristic of the specific transition it undergoes. The quantized energies of light emitted under these conditions do not produce a continuous spectrum (as expected from classical physics). Rather, the spectrum is composed of light at specific frequencies and is thus known as a line spectrum, where each line on the emission spectrum corresponds to a specific electronic transition. Because each element can have its electrons excited to different distinct energy levels, each one possesses a unique **atomic emission spectrum,** which can be used as a fingerprint for the element. One particular application of atomic emissions spectroscopy is in the analysis of stars; while a physical sample cannot be taken, the light from a star can be resolved into its component wavelengths, which are then matched to the known line spectra of the elements.

   The Bohr model of the hydrogen atom explained the atomic emission spectrum of hydrogen, which is the simplest emission spectrum among all the elements. The group of hydrogen emission lines corresponding to transitions from upper levels $n > 2$ to $n = 2$ is known as the **Balmer series** (4 wavelengths in the visible region), while the group corresponding to transitions between upper levels $n > 1$ to $n = 1$ is known as the **Lyman series** (higher energy transitions, occur in the UV region).

MCAT Synopsis

Note that all systems tend toward minimal energy, thus atoms of any element will generally exist in the ground state unless subjected to extremely high temperatures or irradiation.

Bridge

E = hf for photons in physics. This also holds true here since we know that C = fλ. This is based on the formula V = fλ for photons.

MCAT favorite

Emission gives rise to fluorescence.

When the energy of each frequency of light observed in the emission spectrum of hydrogen was calculated according to Planck's quantum theory, the values obtained closely matched those expected from energy level transitions in the Bohr model. That is, the energy associated with a change in the quantum number from an initial value n_i to a final value n_f is equal to the energy of Planck's emitted photon. Thus:

$$E = hc/\lambda = -R_H[1/(n_i)^2 - 1/(n_f)^2]$$

and the energy of the emitted photon corresponds to the precise difference in energy between the higher-energy initial state and the lower-energy final state.

2. Atomic Absorption Spectra

When an electron is excited to a higher energy level, it must absorb energy. The energy absorbed as an electron jumps from an orbital of low energy to one of higher energy is characteristic of that transition. This means that the excitation of electrons in a particular element results in energy absorptions at specific wavelengths. Thus, in addition to an emission spectrum, every element possesses a characteristic **absorption spectrum**. Not surprisingly, the wavelengths of absorption correspond directly to the wavelengths of emission since the energy difference between levels remains unchanged. Absorption spectra can thus be used in the identification of elements present in a gas phase sample.

> **MCAT Favorite**
>
> Absorption is the basis for color of compounds

QUANTUM MECHANICAL MODEL OF ATOMS

While the concepts put forth by Bohr offered a reasonable explanation for the structure of the hydrogen atom and ions containing only one electron (such as He^{1+} and Li^{2+}), they did not explain the structures of atoms containing more than one electron. This is because Bohr's model does not take into consideration the repulsion between multiple electrons surrounding one nucleus. Modern quantum mechanics has led to a more rigorous and generalized study of the electronic structure of atoms. The most important difference between the Bohr model and modern quantum mechanical models is that Bohr's assumption that electrons follow a circular orbit at a fixed distance from the nucleus is no longer considered valid. Rather, electrons are described as being in a state of rapid motion within regions of space around the nucleus, called **orbitals.** An orbital is a representation of the probability of finding an electron within a given region. In the current quantum mechanical description of electrons, pinpointing the exact location of an electron at any given point in time is impossible. This idea is best

> **MCAT Synopsis**
>
> Note that the magnitude of ΔE is the same for absorption or emission between any two energy levels. The sign of ΔE indicates whether the energy goes in or out.

described by the **Heisenberg uncertainty principle,** which states that it is impossible to determine, with perfect accuracy, the momentum and the position of an electron simultaneously. This means that if the momentum of the electron is being measured accurately, its position will change, and vice versa.

A. QUANTUM NUMBERS

Modern atomic theory states that any electron in an atom can be completely described by four **quantum numbers:** n, ℓ, m_ℓ, and m_s. Further, according to the **Pauli exclusion principle,** no two electrons in a given atom can possess the same set of four quantum numbers. The position and energy of an electron described by its quantum numbers is known as its **energy state.** The value of n limits the values of ℓ, which in turn limits the values of m_ℓ. The values of the quantum numbers qualitatively give information about the orbitals: n about the size, ℓ about the shape, and m_ℓ about the orientation of the orbital. All four quantum numbers are discussed below.

1. **Principal Quantum Number**

   The first quantum number is commonly known as the **principal quantum number** and is denoted by the letter n. This is the quantum number used in Bohr's model that can theoretically take on any positive integer value. The larger the integer value of n, the higher the energy level and radius of the electron's orbit. The maximum number of electrons in energy level n (electron shell n) is $2n^2$. The difference in energy between adjacent shells decreases as the distance from the nucleus increases, since it is related to the expression $1/n_2^2 - 1/n_1^2$. For example, the energy difference between the third and fourth shells, $n = 3$ to $n = 4$, is less than that between the second and third shells, $n = 2$ to $n = 3$.

2. **Azimuthal Quantum Number**

   The second quantum number is called the **azimuthal (angular momentum) quantum number** and is designated by the letter ℓ. The second quantum number refers to the **subshells** or **sublevels** that occur within each principal energy level. For any given n, the value of ℓ can be any integer in the range of 0 to $n - 1$. The four subshells corresponding to $\ell = 0$, 1, 2, and 3 are known as the s, p, d, and f subshells, respectively. The maximum number of electrons that can exist within a subshell is given by the equation $4\ell + 2$. The greater the value of ℓ, the greater the energy of the subshell. However, the energies of subshells from different principal energy levels may overlap. For example, the 4s subshell will have a lower energy than the 3d subshell because its average distance from the nucleus is smaller (see Figure 1.1).

MCAT Synopsis

For any principal quantum number n, there will be n possible values for ℓ.

3. **Magnetic Quantum Number**
    The third quantum number is the **magnetic quantum number** and is designated m_ℓ. An orbital is a specific region within a subshell that may contain no more than two electrons. The magnetic quantum number specifies the particular orbital within a subshell where an electron is highly likely to be found at a given point in time. The possible values of m_ℓ are all integers from ℓ to $-\ell$, including 0. Therefore, the s subshell, where there is one possible value of m_ℓ (0), will contain 1 orbital; likewise, the p subshell will contain 3 orbitals, the d subshell will contain 5 orbitals, and the f subshell will contain 7 orbitals. The shape and energy of each orbital are dependent upon the subshell in which the orbital is found. For example, a p subshell has three possible m_ℓ values (–1, 0, +1). The three dumbbell-shaped orbitals are oriented in space around the nucleus along the x, y, and z axes and are often referred to as p_x, p_y, and p_z.

4. **Spin Quantum Number**

    The fourth quantum number is also called the **spin quantum number** and is denoted by ms. The spin of a particle is its intrinsic angular momentum and is a characteristic of a particle, like its charge. In classical mechanics an object spinning about its axis has an angular momentum; however, this does not apply to the electron. Classical analogies often are inapplicable in the quantum world. In any case, the two spin orientations are designated $+\frac{1}{2}$ and $-\frac{1}{2}$. Whenever two electrons are in the same orbital, they must have opposite spins. Electrons in different orbitals with the same ms values are said to have **parallel** spins.

    The quantum numbers for the orbitals in the second principal energy level, with their maximum number of electrons noted in parentheses, are shown in Table 1.2. Electrons with opposite spins in the same orbital are often referred to as paired.

Table 1.2

n	2(8)			
ℓ	0(2)		1(6)	
m_ℓ	0(2)	+1(2)	0(2)	−1(2)
m_s	$+\frac{1}{2}, -\frac{1}{2}$	$+\frac{1}{2}, -\frac{1}{2}$	$+\frac{1}{2}, -\frac{1}{2}$	$+\frac{1}{2}, -\frac{1}{2}$

B. ELECTRON CONFIGURATION AND ORBITAL FILLING

For a given atom or ion, the pattern by which subshells are filled and the number of electrons within each principal level and subshell are designated by an **electron configuration**. In electron configuration notation, the first number denotes the principal energy level, the letter designates the subshell, and the superscript gives the number of electrons in that subshell. For example, $2p^4$ indicates that there are four electrons in the second (p) subshell of the second principal energy level.

When writing the electron configuration of an atom, it is necessary to remember the order in which subshells are filled. Subshells are filled from lowest to highest energy, and each subshell will fill completely before electrons begin to enter the next one. The $(n + \ell)$ rule is used to rank subshells by increasing energy. This rule states that the lower the values of the first and second quantum numbers, the lower the energy of the subshell. If two subshells possess the same $(n + \ell)$ value, the subshell with the lower n value has a lower energy and will fill first. The order in which the subshells fill is shown in the following chart.

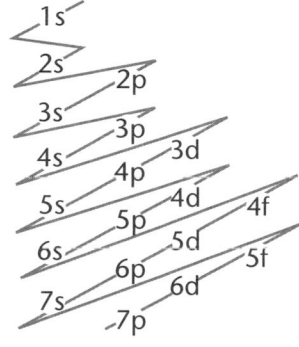

Figure 1.1

Example: Which will fill first, the 3d subshell or the 4s subshell?

Solution: For 3d, $n = 3$ and $\ell = 2$, so $(n + \ell) = 5$. For 4s, $n = 4$ and $\ell = 0$, so $(n + \ell) = 4$. Therefore, the 4s subshell has lower energy and will fill first. This can also be determined from the chart by examination.

To determine which subshells are filled, you must know the number of electrons in the atom. In the case of uncharged atoms, the number of electrons equals the atomic number. If the atom is charged, the number of electrons is equal to the atomic number plus the extra electrons if the atom is negative, or the atomic number minus the electrons if the atom is positive.

In subshells that contain more than one orbital, such as the 2p subshell with its 3 orbitals, the orbitals will fill according to **Hund's rule.** Hund's rule states that within a given subshell, orbitals are filled such that there are a maximum number of half-filled orbitals with parallel spins. Electrons "prefer" empty orbitals to half-filled ones because a pairing energy must be overcome for two electrons carrying repulsive negative charges to exist in the same orbital.

Example: What are the written electron configurations for nitrogen (N) and iron (Fe) according to Hund's rule?

Solution: Nitrogen has an atomic number of 7, thus its electron configuration is $1s^2\ 2s^2\ 2p^3$. According to Hund's rule, the two s orbitals will fill completely, while the three p orbitals will each contain one electron, all with parallel spins.

$$\underset{1s^2}{\uparrow\downarrow} \qquad \underset{2s^2}{\uparrow\downarrow} \qquad \underset{2p^3}{\uparrow\ \uparrow\ \uparrow}$$

Iron has an atomic number of 26, and its 4s subshell fills before the 3d. Using Hund's rule, the electron configuraton will be:

$$\underset{1s^2}{\uparrow\downarrow} \qquad \underset{2s^2}{\uparrow\downarrow}\quad \underset{2p^6}{\uparrow\downarrow\ \uparrow\downarrow\ \uparrow\downarrow}\quad \underset{3s^2}{\uparrow\downarrow}\quad \underset{3p^6}{\uparrow\downarrow\ \uparrow\downarrow\ \uparrow\downarrow}\quad \underset{3d^6}{\uparrow\downarrow\ \uparrow\ \uparrow\ \uparrow\ \uparrow}\quad \underset{4s^2}{\uparrow\downarrow}$$

Iron's electron configuration is written as $1s^2\ 2s^2\ 2p^6\ 3s^2\ 3p^6\ 3d^6\ 4s^2$. Subshells may be listed either in the order in which they fill (e.g., 4s before 3d) or with subshells of the same principal quantum number grouped together, as shown here. Both methods are correct.

The presence of paired or unpaired electrons affects the chemical and magnetic properties of an atom or molecule. If the material has unpaired electrons, a magnetic field will align the spins of these electrons and weakly attract the atom. These materials are said to be **paramagnetic.** Materials that have no unpaired electrons and are slightly repelled by a magnetic field are said to be **diamagnetic.**

C. VALENCE ELECTRONS

The valence electrons of an atom are those electrons that are in its outer energy shell *or* that are available for bonding. For elements in Groups IA and IIA, only the outermost s electrons are valence electrons. For elements in Groups IIIA through VIIIA, the outermost s and p electrons in the highest energy shell are valence electrons. For transition elements, the valence electrons are those in the outermost s subshell and in the d subshell of the next-to-outermost energy shell. For the inner transition elements, the valence electrons are those in the s subshell of the outermost energy shell, the d subshell of the next-to-outermost energy shell, and the f subshell of the energy shell two levels below the outermost shell.

IIIA–VIIA elements beyond Period II might, under some circumstances, accept electrons into their empty d subshell, which gives them more than 8 valence electrons (see Exceptions to the Octet Rule in chapter 3).

Example: Which are the valence electrons of elemental iron, elemental selenium, and the sulfur atom in a sulfate ion?

Solution: Iron has 8 valence electrons: 2 in its 4s subshell and 6 in its 3d subshell.

Selenium has 6 valence electrons: 2 in its 4s subshell and 4 in its 4p subshell. Selenium's 3d electrons are not part of its valence shell.

Sulfur in a sulfate ion has 12 valence electrons: its original 6 plus 6 more from the oxygens to which it is bonded. Sulfur's 3s and 3p subshells can contain only 8 of these 12 electrons; the other 4 electrons have entered the sulfur atom's 3d subshell, which in elemental sulfur is empty (see Figure 3.1).

PERIODIC TABLE OF THE ELEMENTS

Period	1 IA 1A	2 IIA 2A	3 IIIB 3B	4 IVB 4B	5 VB 5B	6 VIB 6B	7 VIIB 7B	8 -------	9 VIII --	10 -----	11 IB 1B	12 IIB 2B	13 IIIA 3A	14 IVA 4A	15 VA 5A	16 VIA 6A	17 VIIA 7A	18 vIIIA 8A
1	1 H 1.008																	2 He 4.003
2	3 Li 6.941	4 Be 9.012											5 B 10.81	6 C 12.01	7 N 14.01	8 O 16.00	9 F 19.00	10 Ne 20.18
3	11 Na 22.99	12 Mg 24.31						-------8-------					13 Al 26.98	14 Si 28.09	15 P 30.97	16 S 32.07	17 Cl 35.45	18 Ar 39.95
4	19 K 39.10	20 Ca 40.08	21 Sc 44.96	22 Ti 47.88	23 V 50.94	24 Cr 52.00	25 Mn 54.94	26 Fe 55.85	27 Co 58.47	28 Ni 58.69	29 Cu 63.55	30 Zn 65.39	31 Ga 69.72	32 Ge 72.59	33 As 74.92	34 Se 78.96	35 Br 79.90	36 Kr 83.80
5	37 Rb 85.47	38 Sr 87.62	39 Y 88.91	40 Zr 91.22	41 Nb 92.91	42 Mo 95.94	43 Tc (98)	44 Ru 101.1	45 Rh 102.9	46 Pd 106.4	47 Ag 107.9	48 Cd 112.4	49 In 114.8	50 Sn 118.7	51 Sb 121.8	52 Te 127.6	53 I 126.9	54 Xe 131.3
6	55 Cs 132.9	56 Ba 137.3	57 La* 138.9	72 Hf 178.5	73 Ta 180.9	74 W 183.9	75 Re 186.2	76 Os 190.2	77 Ir 190.2	78 Pt 195.1	79 Au 197.0	80 Hg 200.5	81 Tl 204.4	82 Pb 207.2	83 Bi 209.0	84 Po (210)	85 At (210)	86 Rn (222)
7	87 Fr (223)	88 Ra (226)	89 Ac~ (227)	104 Rf (257)	105 Db (260)	106 Sg (263)	107 Bh (262)	108 Hs (265)	109 Mt (266)	110 --- ()	111 --- ()	112 --- ()	114 --- ()		116 --- ()			118 --- ()

Lanthanide Series*	58 Ce 140.1	59 Pr 140.9	60 Nd 144.2	61 Pm (147)	62 Sm 150.4	63 Eu 152.0	64 Gd 157.3	65 Tb 158.9	66 Dy 162.5	67 Ho 164.9	68 Er 167.3	69 Tm 168.9	70 Yb 173.0	71 Lu 175.0
Actinide Series~	90 Th 232.0	91 Pa (231)	92 U (238)	93 Np (237)	94 Pu (242)	95 Am (243)	96 Cm (247)	97 Bk (247)	98 Cf (249)	99 Es (254)	100 Fm (253)	101 Md (256)	102 No (254)	103 Lr (257)

2

THE PERIODIC TABLE

In 1869, the Russian chemist Dmitri Mendeleev published the first version of his periodic table, in which he showed that ordering the elements according to atomic weight produced a pattern in which similar properties periodically recurred. This table was later revised, using the work of the physicist Henry Moseley, to organize the elements on the basis of increasing atomic number. Using this revised table, the properties of certain elements that had not yet been discovered were predicted: A number of these predictions were later borne out by experimentation. The substance of this work is summarized in the **periodic law,** which states that the chemical properties of the elements are dependent, in a systematic way, upon their atomic numbers.

In the periodic table used today, the elements are arranged in **periods** (rows) and **groups** (columns). There are seven periods, representing the principal quantum numbers $n = 1$ to $n = 7$, and each period is filled sequentially. Groups represent elements that have the same electronic configuration in their **valence,** or outermost shell, and share similar chemical properties. The electrons in the outermost shell are called **valence electrons.** They are involved in chemical bonding and determine the chemical reactivity and properties of the element. The Roman numeral above each group represents the number of valence electrons. There are two sets of groups, designated A and B. The A elements are the **representative elements,** which have either s or p sublevels as their outermost orbitals. The B elements are the **nonrepresentative elements,** including the **transition elements,** which have partly filled d sublevels, and the **lanthanide** and **actinide series,** which have partly filled f sublevels. The electron configuration for the valence electrons is given by the Roman numeral and letter designations. For example, an element in Group VA will have a valence electron configuration of s^2p^3 ($2 + 3 = 5$ valence electrons).

PERIODIC PROPERTIES OF THE ELEMENTS

The properties of the elements exhibit certain trends, which can be explained in terms of the position of the element in the periodic table, or in terms of the electron configuration of the element. All elements seek to gain or lose valence electrons so as to achieve the stable octet formation possessed by the **inert** or **noble gases** of Group VIII. Two other important trends exist within the periodic table. First, as one goes from left to right across a period, electrons are added one at a time; the electrons of the outermost shell experience an increasing amount of nuclear attraction, becoming closer and more tightly bound to the nucleus. Second, as one goes down a given column, the outermost electrons become less tightly bound to the nucleus. This is because the number of filled principal energy levels (which shield the outermost electrons from attraction by the nucleus) increases downward within each group. These trends help explain elemental properties such as atomic radius, ionization potential, electron affinity, and electronegativity.

A. ATOMIC RADII

The **atomic radius** of an element is equal to one-half the distance between the centers of two atoms of that element that are just touching each other. In general, the atomic radius decreases across a period from left to right and increases down a given group; The atoms with the largest atomic radii will be located at the bottom of groups, and in Group I.

As one moves from left to right across a period, electrons are added one at a time to the outer energy shell. Electrons within a shell cannot shield one another from the attractive pull of protons. Therefore, since the number of protons is also increasing, producing a greater positive charge attracting the valence electrons, the effective nuclear charge increases steadily across a period. This causes the atomic radius to decrease.

As one moves down a group of the periodic table, the number of electrons and filled electron shells will increase, but the number of valence electrons will remain the same. Thus, the outermost electrons in a given group will feel the same amount of effective nuclear charge, but electrons will be found farther from the nucleus as the number of filled energy shells increases. Thus, the atomic radii will increase.

B. IONIZATION ENERGY

The **ionization energy** (IE), or **ionization potential,** is the energy required to completely remove an electron from a gaseous atom or ion. Removing an electron from an atom always requires an input of energy (is endothermic; see chapter 6, Thermodynamics). The closer and more tightly bound an electron is to the nucleus, the more difficult it will be to remove, and the higher the ionization energy will be. The **first ionization energy** is the energy required to remove one valence electron from the parent atom, the **second ionization energy** is the energy needed to remove a second valence electron from the univalent ion to form the divalent ion, and so on. Successive ionization energies grow increasingly large; i.e., the second ionization energy is always greater than the first ionization energy. For example:

$$Mg\ (g) \longrightarrow Mg^+\ (g) \quad + e- \quad \text{First Ionization Energy} \quad + \quad 7.646\ eV$$
$$Mg^+\ (g) \longrightarrow Mg^{2+}\ (g) \quad + e- \quad \text{Second Ionization Energy} \quad + \quad 15.035\ eV$$

Ionization energy increases from left to right across a period as the atomic radius decreases. Moving down a group, the ionization energy decreases as the atomic radius increases. Group I elements have low ionization energies because the loss of an electron results in the formation of a stable octet.

C. ELECTRON AFFINITY

Electron affinity is the energy change that occurs when an electron is added to a gaseous atom, and it represents the ease with which the atom can accept an electron. The stronger the attractive pull of the nucleus for electrons (**effective nuclear charge**, or Z_{eff}), the greater the electron affinity will be. In discussing electron affinities, two sign conventions are used. The more common one states that a positive electron affinity value represents energy release when an electron is added to an atom; the other states that a negative electron affinity represents a release of energy. In this discussion, the first convention will be used.

Generalizations can be made about the electron affinities of particular groups in the periodic table. For example, the Group IIA elements, or **alkaline earths,** have low electron affinity values. These elements are relatively stable because their s subshell is filled. Group VIIA elements, or **halogens,** have high electron affinities because the addition of an electron to the atom results in a completely filled shell, which represents a stable electron configuration. Achieving the stable octet involves a release of energy, and the strong attraction of the nucleus for the electron leads to a high energy change. The Group VIII elements, or **noble gases,** have electron affinities on the order of zero, since they already possess a stable octet and cannot readily accept an electron. Elements of other groups generally have low values of electron affinity.

D. ELECTRONEGATIVITY

Electronegativity is a measure of the attraction an atom has for electrons in a chemical bond. The greater the electronegativity of an atom, the greater its attraction for bonding electrons. Electronegativity values are

MCAT Synopsis

To recall the various trends, remember this: Cesium, Cs, is the largest, most metallic, and least electronegative of all naturally occurring elements. It also has the smallest ionization energy and the least exothermic electron affinity.

MCAT Synopsis

L → R   Atomic Radius ↓
              Ionization Energy ↑
              Electronegativity ↑

Top → Bottom
              Atomic Radius ↑
              Ionization Energy ↓
              Electronegativity ↓

MCAT Synopsis

Electronegativity might better be called "nuclear positivity." It is a result of the nucleus' attraction for electrons, that is, the Z_{eff} perceived by the electrons in a bond.

not determined directly. The most common electronegativity scale is the Pauling electronegativity scale, with values ranging from 0.7 for the most electropositive elements, like cesium, to 4.0 for the most electronegative element fluorine. Electronegativities are related to ionization energies: Elements with low ionization energies will have low electronegativities because their nuclei do not attract electrons strongly, while elements with high ionization energies will have high electronegativities because of the strong pull their nuclei have on electrons. Therefore, electronegativity increases from left to right across periods. In any group, the electronegativity decreases as the atomic number increases, as a result of the increased distance between the valence electrons and the nucleus, i.e., greater atomic radius.

TYPES OF ELEMENTS

The elements of the periodic table may be classified into three categories: **metals,** located on the left side and in the middle of the periodic table; **nonmetals,** located on the right side of the table; and **metalloids (semimetals),** found along a diagonal line between the other two.

A. METALS

Metals are shiny solids (except for mercury) at room temperature, and generally have high melting points and densities. Metals have the characteristic ability to be deformed without breaking. The ability of a metal to be hammered into shapes is called **malleability** and the ability to be drawn into wires is called **ductility.** Many of the characteristic properties of metals, such as large atomic radius, low ionization energy, and low electronegativity, are due to the fact that the few electrons in the valence shell of a metal atom can easily be removed. Because the valence electrons can move freely, metals are good conductors of heat and electricity. Group IA and IIA represent the most reactive metals and will be discussed below. The transition elements, also discussed later, are metals which have partially filled d orbitals.

B. NONMETALS

Nonmetals are generally brittle in the solid state and show little or no metallic luster. They have high ionization energies and electronegativities, and are usually poor conductors of heat and electricity. Most nonmetals share the ability to gain electrons easily, but otherwise they display a wide range of chemical behaviors and reactivities. The nonmetals are located on the upper right side of the periodic table; they are separated from the metals by a line cutting diagonally through the region of the periodic table containing elements with partially filled p orbitals.

C. METALLOIDS

The metalloids or semimetals are found along the line between the metals and nonmetals in the periodic table, and their properties vary considerably. Their densities, boiling points, and melting points fluctuate widely. The electronegativities and ionization energies of metalloids lie between those of metals and nonmetals; therefore, these elements possess characteristics of both those classes. For example, silicon has a metallic luster, yet it is brittle and is not an efficient conductor. The reactivity of metalloids is dependent upon the element with which they are reacting. For example, boron (B) behaves as a nonmetal when reacting with sodium (Na) and as a metal when reacting with fluorine (F). The elements classified as metalloids are boron, silicon, germanium, arsenic, antimony, and tellurium.

THE CHEMISTRY OF GROUPS

A. ALKALI METALS

The **alkali metals** are the elements of Group IA. They possess most of the physical properties common to metals, yet their densities are lower than those of other metals. The alkali metals have only one loosely bound electron in their outermost shell, giving them the largest atomic radii of all the elements in their respective periods. Their metallic properties and high reactivity are determined by the fact that they have low ionization energies; thus they easily lose their valence electron to form univalent cations. Alkali metals have low electronegativities and react very readily with nonmetals, especially halogens.

B. ALKALINE EARTHS

The **alkaline earths** are the elements of Group IIA, which also possess many characteristically metallic properties. Like the alkali metals, these properties are dependent upon the ease with which they lose electrons. The alkaline earths have two electrons in their outer shell and thus have smaller atomic radii than the alkali metals. However, the two valence electrons are not held very tightly by the nucleus, so they can be removed to form divalent cations. Alkaline earths have low electronegativities and low electron affinities.

C. HALOGENS

The **halogens**, Group VIIA, are highly reactive nonmetals with seven valence electrons (one short of the favored octet configuration). Halogens are highly variable in their physical properties. For instance, the halogens range from gaseous (F_2 and Cl_2) to liquid (Br_2) to solid (I_2) at room temperature. Their chemical properties are more uniform: The electronegativities of halogens are very high, and they are particularly reactive towards alkali metals and alkaline earths, which "want" to donate electrons to the halogens to form stable ionic crystals. Fluorine (F) has the highest electronegativity of all the elements.

D. NOBLE GASES

The **noble gases,** also called the **inert gases,** are found in Group VIII (also called Group 0). They are fairly nonreactive because they have a complete valence shell, which is an energetically favored arrangement. This gives them little or no tendency to gain or lose electrons, high ionization energies, and no real electronegativities. They possess low boiling points and are all gases at room temperature.

E. TRANSITION ELEMENTS

The **transition elements,** Groups IB to VIIIB, are all considered metals; hence, they are also called the **transition metals.** These elements are very hard and have high melting points and boiling points. As one moves across a period, the five d orbitals become progressively more filled. The d electrons are held only loosely by the nucleus and are relatively mobile, contributing to the malleability and high electrical conductivity of these elements. Chemically, transition elements have low ionization energies and may exist in a variety of positively charged forms or **oxidation states.** This is because transition elements are capable of losing various numbers of electrons from the s and d orbitals of their valence shell. Theoretically, the transition metals in Group VIIIB could have eight different oxidation states, from +1 to +8; however, they typically do not exhibit so many. For instance, copper (Cu), in group IB, can exist in either the +1 or the +2 oxidation state, and manganese (Mn), in Group VIIB, occurs in the +2, +3, +4, +6, or +7 state. Because of this ability to attain positive oxidation states, transition metals form many different ionic and partially ionic compounds. The dissolved ions can form **complex ions** either with molecules of water (**hydration complexes**) or with nonmetals, forming highly colored solutions and compounds (e.g., $CuSO_4 \cdot 5H_2O$), and this complexation may enhance the relatively low solubility of certain compounds (e.g., $AgCl$ is insoluble in water, but quite soluble in aqueous ammonia due to the formation of the complex ion $[Ag(NH_3)_2]^+$). The formation of complexes causes the d orbitals to be split into two energy sublevels. This enables many of the complexes to absorb certain frequencies of light—those containing the precise amount of energy required to raise electrons from the lower to the higher d sublevel. The frequencies not absorbed—known as the subtraction frequencies—give the complexes their characteristic colors.

3

BONDING AND CHEMICAL INTERACTIONS

The atoms of many elements can combine to form **molecules.** The atoms in most molecules are held together by strong attractive forces called **chemical bonds.** These bonds are formed via the interaction of the valence electrons of the combining atoms. The chemical and physical properties of the resulting molecules are often very different than their constituent elements. In addition to the very strong forces within a molecule, there are weaker intermolecular forces between molecules. These **intermolecular forces,** although weaker than the intramolecular chemical bonds, are of considerable importance in understanding the physical properties of many substances.

BONDING

Many molecules contain atoms bonded according to the **Octet Rule,** which states that an atom tends to bond with other atoms until it has eight electrons in its outermost shell, thereby forming a stable electron configuration similar to that of the Group VIII (noble gas) elements. **Exceptions** to this rule are as follows: **hydrogen,** which can have only two valence electrons (the configuration of He); lithium and beryllium, which bond to attain two and four valence electrons, respectively; boron which bonds to attain six; and elements beyond the second row, such as phosphorus and sulfur, which can expand their octets to include more than eight electrons by incorporating d orbitals.

When classifying chemical bonds, it is helpful to introduce two distinct types: **ionic bonds** and **covalent bonds.** In ionic bonding, an electron(s) from an atom with a smaller ionization energy is transferred to an atom with a greater electron affinity. This results in a positive and negative ion. These resulting ions are held together by electrostatic forces. In covalent bonding, an electron pair is shared between two atoms. In many cases, the bond is partially covalent and partially ionic; we call such bonds polar covalent bonds.

IONIC BONDS

When two atoms with large differences in electronegativity react, there is a complete transfer of electrons from the less electronegative atom to the more electronegative atom. The atom that loses electrons becomes a positively charged ion, or **cation,** and the atom that gains electrons becomes a negatively charged ion, or **anion.** For this transfer to occur, the difference in electronegativity must be greater than 1.7. In general, the elements of Groups I and II (low electronegativities) bond ionically to elements of Group VII (high electronegativities). Hence, ionic bonds occur between metals and non-metals. Elements of Groups I and II give up their electrons to achieve a noble gas configuration, while Group VII elements gain an electron to achieve the noble gas configuration. For example, Na + Cl $\longrightarrow$ Na$^+$ Cl$^-$ (sodium chloride). The electrostatic force of attraction between the charged ions is called an **ionic** or **electrovalent bond.**

Ionic compounds have characteristic physical properties. They have high melting and boiling points due to the strong electrostatic forces between the ions. They can conduct electricity in the liquid and aqueous states, though not in the solid state. Ionic solids form crystal lattices consisting of infinite arrays of positive and negative ions in which the attractive forces between ions of opposite charge are maximized, while the repulsive forces between ions of like charge are minimized.

COVALENT BONDS

When two or more atoms with similar electronegativities interact, the energy required to form ions is greater than the energy that would be released upon the formation of an ionic bond (i.e., the process is not energetically favorable). However, since a complete transfer of electrons cannot occur, such atoms achieve a noble gas electron configuration by **sharing** electrons in a covalent bond. The binding force between the two atoms results from the attraction that each electron of the shared pair has for the two positive nuclei.

Covalent compounds contain discrete molecular units with weak intermolecular forces. Consequently, they are low-melting solids, and do not conduct electricity in the liquid or aqueous states.

A. PROPERTIES OF COVALENT BONDS

Atoms can share more than one pair of electrons. Two atoms sharing one, two, or three electron pairs are said to be joined by a **single, double,** or **triple covalent bond,** respectively. The number of shared electron pairs between two atoms is called the **bond order;** hence a single bond has a bond order of one, a double bond has a bond order of two, and a triple bond has a bond order of three.

A covalent bond can be characterized by two features: **bond length** and **bond energy.**

1. **Bond Length**

    Bond length is the average distance between the two nuclei of the atoms involved in the bond. As the number of shared electron pairs increases, the two atoms are pulled closer together, leading to a decrease in bond length. Thus, for a given pair of atoms, a triple bond is shorter than a double bond, which is shorter than a single bond.

2. **Bond Energy**

    Bond energy is the energy required to separate two bonded atoms. For a given pair of atoms, the strength of a bond (and therefore the bond energy) increases as the number of shared electron pairs increases. (Bond energy is further discussed in chapter 6, Thermodynamics.)

> **Bridge**
>
> | | Bond length | Bond strength |
> |---|---|---|
> | C—C | longest | weakest |
> | C=C | medium | medium |
> | C≡C | shortest | strongest |

B. COVALENT BOND NOTATION

The shared valence electrons of a covalent bond are called the **bonding electrons.** The valence electrons not involved in the covalent bond are called **nonbonding electrons.** The unshared electron pairs can also be called **lone electron pairs.** A convenient notation, called a **Lewis structure,** is used to represent the bonding and nonbonding electrons in a molecule, facilitating chemical "bookkeeping." The number of valence electrons attributed to a particular atom in the Lewis structure of a molecule is not necessarily the same as the number would be in the isolated atom, and the difference accounts for what is referred to as the **formal charge** of that atom. Often, more than one Lewis structure can be drawn for a molecule; this phenomenon is called **resonance.** Lewis structures, formal charge, and resonance are discussed in detail below.

1. **Lewis Structures**

    A Lewis structure, or **Lewis dot symbol,** is the chemical symbol of an element surrounded by dots, each representing one of the s and/or p valence electrons of the atom. The Lewis symbols of the elements found in the second period of the periodic table are shown below.

Table 3.1

·Li	Lithium	·N̈·	Nitrogen
·Be·	Beryllium	·Ö:	Oxygen
·B̈·	Boron	·F̈:	Fluorine
·C̈·	Carbon	:N̈e:	Neon

Just as a Lewis symbol is used to represent the distribution of valence electrons in an atom, it can also be used to represent the distribution of valence electrons in a molecule. For example, the Lewis symbol of an F ion is : $\ddot{\text{F}}$:; the Lewis structure of an F_2 molecule is : $\ddot{\text{F}}$ —— $\ddot{\text{F}}$:.

Certain steps must be followed in assigning a Lewis structure to a molecule. These steps are outlined below, using HCN as an example.

- Write the skeletal structure of the compound (i.e., the arrangement of atoms). In general, the least electronegative atom is the central atom. Hydrogen (always) and the halogens F, Cl, Br, and I (usually) occupy the end position.

  In HCN, H must occupy an end position. Of the remaining two atoms, C is the least electronegative, and therefore occupies the central position. The skeletal structure is as follows:

$$\text{H} - \text{C} - \text{N}$$

- Count all the valence electrons of the atoms. The number of valence electrons of the molecule is the sum of the valence electrons of all atoms present:

  > H has 1 valence electron;
  > C has 4 valence electrons;
  > N has 5 valence electrons; therefore,
  > HCN has a total of 10 valence electrons.

- Draw single bonds between the central atom and the atoms surrounding it. Place an electron pair in each bond (bonding electron pair).

$$\text{H} : \text{C} : \text{N}$$

Each bond has 2 electrons, so $10 - 4 = 6$ valence electrons remain.

- Complete the octets (8 valence electrons) of all atoms bonded to the central atom, using the remaining valence electrons still to be assigned. (Recall that H is an exception to the Octet Rule since it can have only 2 valence electrons.) In this example H already has 2 valence electrons in its bond with C.

$$: \text{H} : \text{C} : \ddot{\text{N}} :$$

- Place any extra electrons on the central atom. If the central atom has less than an octet, try to write double or triple bonds between the central and surrounding atoms using the nonbonding, unshared lone electron pairs.

The HCN structure above does not satisfy the Octet Rule for C because C possesses only 4 valence electrons. Therefore, 2 lone electron pairs from the N atom must be moved to form 2 more bonds with C, creating a triple bond between C and N. Finally, bonds are drawn as lines rather than pairs of dots.

$$H - C \equiv N :$$

Now the Octet Rule is satisfied for all three atoms, since C and N have 8 valence electrons and H has 2 valence electrons.

2. **Formal Charges**

The number of electrons officially assigned to an atom in a Lewis structure does not always equal the number of valence electrons of the free atom. The difference between these two numbers is the **formal charge** of the atom. Formal charge can be calculated using the following formula:

$$\text{Formal charge} = V - \frac{1}{2}N_{bonding} - N_{nonbonding}$$

where V is the number of valence electrons in the free atom, $N_{bonding}$ is the number of bonding electrons, and $N_{nonbonding}$ is the number of nonbonding electrons.

The formal charge of an ion or molecule equals the sum of the formal charges of the individual atoms comprising the ion or molecule.

Formal charge also contributes to stability. The lower the overall formal charge of the molecule, the more stable the molecule.

Example: Calculate the formal charge on the central N atom of $[NH_4]^+$.

Solution: The Lewis structure of $[NH_4]^+$ is

$$\left[\begin{array}{c} H \\ | \\ H - N - H \\ | \\ H \end{array} \right]$$

Nitrogen is in group VA; thus it has 5 valence electrons. In $[NH_4]^+$,

N has 4 bonds (i.e., 8 bonding electrons and no nonbonding electrons).

So, $V = 5$; $N_{bonding} = 8$; $N_{nonbonding} = 0$

$$\text{Formal charge} = 5 - \frac{1}{2}(8) - 0 = +1$$

Thus, the formal charge on the N atom in $[NH_4]^+$ is +1.

3. **Resonance**

For some molecules, two or more nonidentical Lewis structures can be drawn; these are called **resonance structures.** The molecule doesn't actually exist as either one of the resonance structures, but is rather a composite, or hybrid, of the two. For example, SO_2 has three resonance structures, two of which are minor: $O = S - O$ and $O - S = O$. The actual molecule is a hybrid of these three structures (spectral data indicate that the two S-O bonds are identically equivalent). This phenomenon is known as resonance, and the actual structure of the molecule is called the **resonance hybrid.** Resonance structures are expressed with a double-headed arrow between them; thus,

$$\ddot{O}\!=\!\ddot{S}\!=\!\ddot{O} \longleftrightarrow \ddot{O}\!=\!\ddot{S}\!-\!\ddot{O}\!: \longleftrightarrow :\!\ddot{O}\!-\!\ddot{S}\!=\!\ddot{O}$$

represents the resonance structures of SO_2.

The last two resonance structures of sulfur dioxide shown above have equivalent energy or stability. Often, nonequivalent resonance structures may be written for a molecule. In these cases, the more stable the structure, the more that structure contributes to the character of the resonance hybrid. Conversely, the less stable the resonance structure, the less that structure contributes to the resonance hybrid. It is the structure on the left of the diagram that is the most stable. Formal charges are often useful for qualitatively assessing the stability of a particular resonance structure; the following guidelines are used:

a. A Lewis structure with small or no formal charges is preferred over a Lewis structure with large formal charges.

b. A Lewis structure in which negative formal charges are placed on more electronegative atoms is more stable than one in which the formal charges are placed on less electronegative atoms.

Example: Write the resonance structures for $[NCO]^-$.

Solution: 1. C is the least electronegative of the three given atoms, N, C, and O. Therefore the C atom occupies the central position in the skeletal structure of $[NCO]^-$.

N C O

2. N has 5 valence electrons;
C has 4 valence electrons;
O has 6 valence electrons;
and the species itself has one negative charge.
Total valence electrons $= 5 + 4 + 6 + 1 = 16$

3. Draw single bonds between the central C atom and the surrounding atoms, N and O. Place a pair of electrons in each bond.

$$N : C : O$$

4. Complete the octets of N and O with the remaining $16 - 4 = 12$ electrons.

$$:\ddot{\underset{..}{N}}:C:\ddot{\underset{..}{O}}:$$

5. The C octet is incomplete. There are three ways in which double and triple bonds can be formed to complete the C octet: 2 lone pairs from the O atom can be used to form a triple bond between the C and O atoms;

$$:\underset{..}{\ddot{N}}—C\equiv O:$$

or 1 lone electron pair can be taken from both the O and the N atoms to form two double bonds, one between N and C, and the other between O and C;

$$:\ddot{N}=C=\ddot{O}:$$

or 2 lone electron pairs can be taken from the N atom to form a triple bond between the C and N atoms.

$$:N\equiv C—\ddot{\underset{..}{O}}:$$

These three are all resonance structures of [NCO]⁻.

6. Assign formal charges to each atom of each resonance structure.

The most stable structure is:

$$:N\equiv C—\ddot{\underset{..}{O}}:$$

since the negative formal charge is on the most electronegative atom, O.

4. **Exceptions to the Octet Rule**

Atoms found in or beyond the third period can have more than eight valence electrons, since some of the valence electrons may occupy *d* orbitals. These atoms can be assigned more than four bonds in Lewis structures. When drawing the Lewis structure of the sulfate ion, giving the sulfur 12 valence electrons permits 3 of the 5 atoms to be assigned a formal charge of zero. The

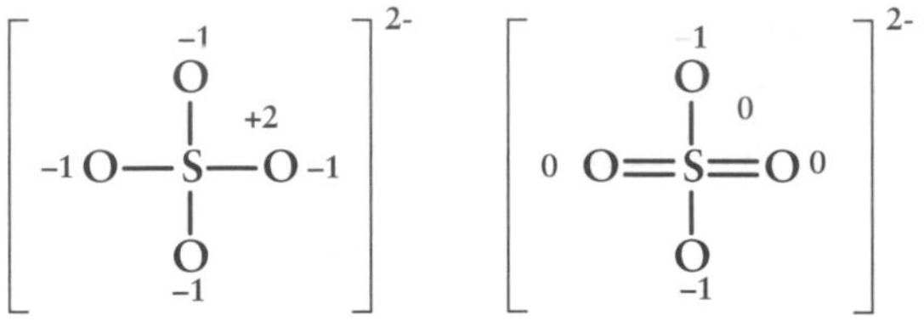

Figure 3.1

sulfate ion can be drawn in six resonance forms, each with the two double bonds attached to a different combination of oxygen atoms.

C. TYPES OF COVALENT BONDING

The nature of a covalent bond depends on the relative electronegativities of the atoms sharing the electron pairs. Covalent bonds are considered to be **polar** or **nonpolar** depending on the difference in electronegativities between the atoms.

> **Note**
>
> The Octet "Rule" is really not much of a rule. It always applies to neutral atoms and anions of C, N, O, and F only. It often (not always!) applies to the halogens and other representative elements, but never applies to H, He, Li, Be, or neutral B and Al. Nor does it apply to elements beyond period 3 since these elements have d orbitals.

1. Polar Covalent Bond

Polar covalent bonding occurs between atoms with small differences in electronegativity, generally in the range of 0.4 to 1.7 Pauling units. The bonding electron pair is not shared equally but pulled more toward the element with the higher electronegativity. As a result, the more electronegative atom acquires a partial negative charge, δ^-, and the less electronegative atom acquires a partial positive charge, δ^+, giving the molecule partially ionic character. For instance, the covalent bond in HCl is polar because the two atoms have a small difference in electronegativity (approximately 0.9). Chlorine, the more electronegative atom, attains a partial negative charge and hydrogen attains a partial positive charge. This difference in charge between the atoms is indicated by an arrow crossed (like a plus sign) at the positive end pointing to the negative end, as shown below:

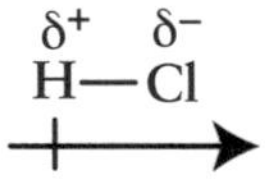

Figure 3.2

A molecule that has such a separation of positive and negative charges is called a polar molecule. The **dipole moment** itself is a vector quantity μ, defined as the product of the charge magnitude (q) and the distance between the two partial charges (r):

$$\mu = qr$$

The dipole moment is denoted by an arrow pointing from the positive to the negative charge, and is measured in Debye units (coulomb-meters).

2. **Nonpolar Covalent Bond**

   Nonpolar covalent bonding occurs between atoms that have the same electronegativities. The bonding electron pair is shared equally, with no separation of charge across the bond. Not surprisingly, nonpolar covalent bonds occur in diatomic molecules such as H_2, Cl_2, O_2, and N_2.

3. **Coordinate Covalent Bond**

   In a coordinate covalent bond, the shared electron pair comes from the lone pair of one of the atoms in the molecule. Once such a bond forms, it is indistinguishable from any other covalent bond. Distinguishing such a bond is useful only in keeping track of the valence electrons and formal charges. Coordinate bonds are typically found in Lewis acid-base compounds (see chapter 10, Acids and Bases). A **Lewis acid** is a compound that can accept an electron pair to form a covalent bond; a **Lewis base** is a compound that can donate an electron pair to form a covalent bond. For example, in the reaction between borontrifluoride (BF_3) and ammonia (NH_3):

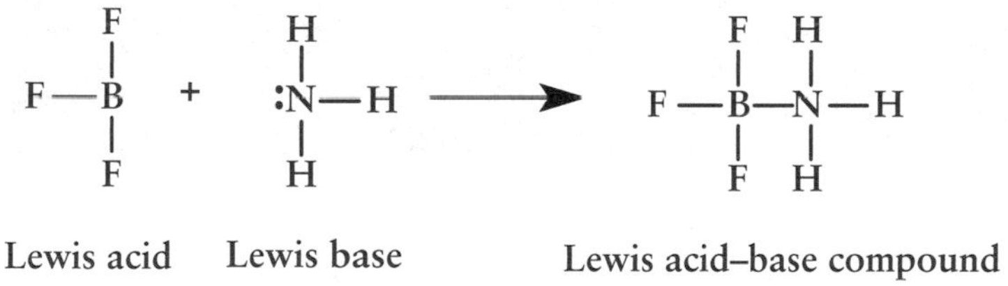

Lewis acid   Lewis base   Lewis acid–base compound

Figure 3.3

   NH_3 donates a pair of electrons to form a coordinate covalent bond; thus, it acts as a Lewis base. BF_3 accepts this pair of electrons to form the coordinate covalent bond; thus, it acts as a Lewis acid.

D. GEOMETRY AND POLARITY OF COVALENT MOLECULES

1. **The Valence Shell Electron-Pair Repulsion Theory**

   The valence shell electron-pair repulsion (VSEPR) theory uses Lewis structures to predict the molecular geometry of covalently bonded molecules. It states that the three-dimensional arrangement of atoms surrounding a central atom is determined by the repulsions between the bonding and the nonbonding electron pairs in the valence shell of the central atom. These electron pairs arrange themselves as far apart as possible, thereby minimizing repulsion.

The following steps are used to predict the geometrical structure of a molecule using the VSEPR theory.

- Draw the Lewis structure of the molecule.

- Count the total number of bonding and nonbonding electron pairs in the valence shell of the central atom.

- Arrange the electron pairs around the central atom so that they are as far apart from each other as possible. For example, the compound AX_2 has the Lewis structure, X : A : X. A has two bonding electron pairs in its valence shell. To make these electron pairs as far apart as possible, their geometric structure should be linear,

$$X - A - X$$

Valence electron arrangements are summarized in Table 3.2.

Table 3.2

Regions of Electron Density	Example	Geometric Arrangement of Electron Pairs Around the Central Atom	Shape	Angle between Electron Pairs
2	$BeCl_2$	X—A—X	linear	180.0°
3	BH_3		trigonal planar	120.0°
4	CH_4		tetrahedral	109.05°
5	PCl_5		trigonal bipyramidal	90.0°, 120°, 180°
6	SF_6		octahedral	90.0°, 180.0°

Example: Predict the geometry of NH_3.

Solution: 1.   The Lewis structure of NH_3 is:

$$\overset{\displaystyle H}{\underset{\displaystyle \ddot{}}{\overset{\displaystyle |}{H-N-H}}}$$

2.   The central atom, N, has 3 bonding electron pairs and 1 nonbonding electron pair, for a total of 4 electron pairs.

3.   The 4 electron pairs will be farthest apart when they occupy the corners of a tetrahedron. As one of the four electron pairs is a lone pair, the observed geometry is trigonal pyramidal.

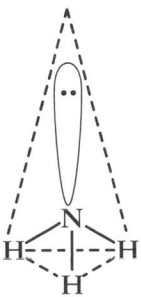

Figure 3.4

In describing the shape of a molecule, only the arrangement of atoms (not electrons) is considered. Even though the electron pairs are arranged tetrahedrally, the shape of NH_3 is pyramidal. It is not trigonal planar because the lone pair repels the 3 bonding electron pairs, causing them to move as far away as possible.

Example: Predict the geometry of CO_2.

Solution: The Lewis structure of CO_2 is $\ddot{O}::C::\ddot{O}$.

The double bond behaves just like a single bond for purposes of predicting molecular shape. This compound has two groups of electrons around the carbon. According to the VSEPR theory, the two sets of electrons will orient themselves 180° apart, on opposite sides of the carbon atom, minimizing electron repulsion. Therefore, the molecular structure of CO_2 is linear: $\ddot{O}=C=\ddot{O}$

2. **Polarity of Molecules**

A molecule with a net dipole moment is called polar, as previously mentioned, because it has positive and negative poles. The polarity of a molecule depends on the polarity of the constituent bonds and on the shape of the molecule. A molecule with nonpolar bonds is always nonpolar; a molecule with polar bonds may be polar or nonpolar depending on the orientation of the bond dipoles.

A molecule of two atoms bound by a polar bond must have a net dipole moment and therefore be polar. The two equal and opposite partial charges are localized at the ends of the molecule on the two atoms. A molecule consisting of more than two atoms bound with polar bonds may be either polar or nonpolar, since the overall dipole moment of a molecule is the vector sum of the individual bond dipole moments. If the molecule has a particular shape such that the bond dipole moments cancel each other, i.e., if the vector sum is zero, then the result is a nonpolar molecule. For instance, CCl_4 has four polar C-Cl bonds. According to the VSEPR theory, the shape of CCl_4 is tetrahedral. The four bond dipoles point to the vertices of the tetrahedron and cancel each other, resulting in a nonpolar molecule.

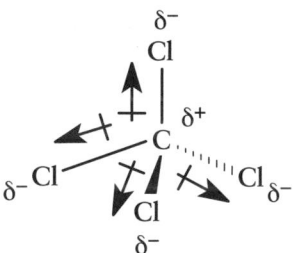

Figure 3.5. No Net Dipole Moment

However, if the orientation of the bond dipoles are such that they do not cancel out, the molecules will have a net dipole moment and therefore be polar. For instance, H_2O has two polar O−H bonds. According to the VSEPR model, its shape is angular. The two dipoles add together to give a net dipole moment to the molecule, making the H_2O molecule polar.

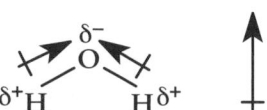

Figure 3.6. Net Dipole Moment

E. ATOMIC AND MOLECULAR ORBITALS

A description of the quantum numbers has already been given in chapter 1. The azimuthal quantum number ℓ describes the orbitals of each n shell. The shapes of these orbitals represent the probability of finding an electron at any given instant. When $\ell = 0$, the orbital is an s orbital. s orbitals are spherically symmetric. The 1s orbital ($n = 1$, $\ell = 0$) is plotted below.

Flashback

Quantum Numbers (chapter 1) revisited:

- For any value of n, there are n values of ℓ ($0 \to n - 1$).

- $\ell = 0 \to s$
  $\ell = 1 \to p$
  $\ell = 2 \to d$

- For any value of ℓ, there are $2\ell + 1$ values of $m\ell$ (number of orbitals); values themselves will range from $-\ell$ to ℓ.

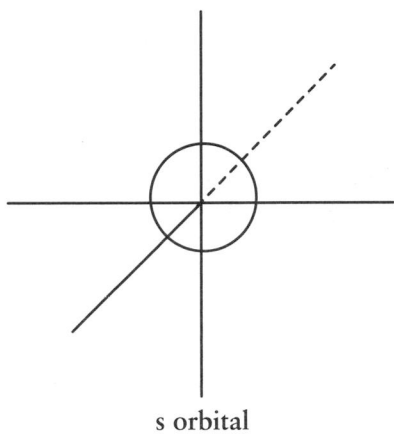

s orbital

Figure 3.7

When $\ell = 1$, there are three possible orbitals (since the magnetic quantum number, m_ℓ may equal -1, 0, or 1). These are called p orbitals and have a dumbbell shape. The three p orbitals, designated p_x, p_y and p_z, are oriented at right angles to each other; the p_x orbital is plotted below.

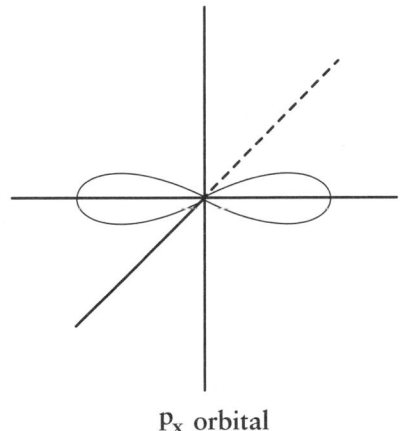

P_x orbital

Figure 3.8

Plus and minus signs, determined from the mathematics of the wave function, are assigned to each lobe of the p orbitals. The shapes of the five d orbitals ($\ell = 2$, $m_\ell = -2, -1, 0, 1, 2$) and the seven f orbitals ($\ell = 3$, $m_\ell = -3, -2, -1, 0, 1, 2, 3$) are more complex and need not be memorized.

When two atoms bond to form a molecule, the atomic orbitals interact to form a **molecular orbital** that describes the probability of finding the bonding electrons. Molecular orbitals are obtained by adding the wave functions of the atomic orbitals. Qualitatively, this is described by the **overlap** of two atomic orbitals. If the signs of the two atomic orbitals are the same, a **bonding orbital** is formed. If the signs are different, an **antibonding orbital** is formed. In addition, two different types of overlap are possible. When orbitals overlap head-to-head, the resulting bond is called a **sigma** (σ) bond. When the orbitals are parallel, a **pi** (π) bond is formed.

Bridge

It is the pi bonds of alkenes, alkynes, aromatic compounds, and carboxylic acid derivates which lend the functionality so important in organic chemistry. Molecular orbitals are discussed further in Organic Chemistry, chapter 3.

THE INTERMOLECULAR FORCES

The attractive forces that exist between molecules are collectively known as **intermolecular forces**. These include **dipole-dipole interactions, hydrogen bonding**, and **dispersion forces**. Dipole-dipole interactions and dispersion forces are often referred to as **van der Waals forces**.

1. **Ion-Dipole Interactions**
   When dipoles are dissolved in solutions where ions are present, ions will arrange themselves with the opposite charged end of the dipole. For example, positive ions will be attracted to and bond with the negative end of the dipole and vice versa.

2. **Dipole-Dipole Interactions**
   Polar molecules tend to orient themselves such that the positive region of one molecule is close to the negative region of another molecule. This arrangement is energetically favorable because an attractive dipole force is formed between the two molecules.

   Dipole-dipole interactions are present in the solid and liquid phases but become negligible in the gas phase because the molecules are generally much farther apart. Polar species tend to have higher boiling points than nonpolar species of comparable molecular weight.

3. **Hydrogen Bonding**

Hydrogen bonding is a specific, unusually strong form of dipole-dipole interaction, which may be either intra- or intermolecular. When hydrogen is bound to a highly electronegative atom such as fluorine, oxygen, or nitrogen, the hydrogen atom carries little of the electron density of the covalent bond. This positively charged hydrogen atom interacts with the partial negative charge located on the electronegative atoms of nearby molecules. Substances which display hydrogen bonding tend to have unusually high boiling points compared with compounds of similar molecular formula that do not hydrogen bond. The difference derives from the energy required to break the hydrogen bonds. Hydrogen bonding is particularly important in the behavior of water, alcohols, amines, and carboxylic acids (see Organic Chemistry section for further discussion).

4. **Dispersion Forces**

The bonding electrons in covalent bonds may appear to be equally shared between two atoms, but at any particular point in time they will be located randomly throughout the orbital. This permits unequal sharing of electrons, causing rapid polarization and counterpolarization of the electron cloud and formation of short-lived dipoles. These dipoles interact with the electron clouds of neighboring molecules, inducing the formation of more dipoles. The attractive interactions of these short-lived dipoles are called dispersion or **London forces.**

Dispersion forces are generally weaker than other intermolecular forces. They do not extend over long distances and are therefore most important when molecules are close together. The strength of these interactions within a given substance depends directly on how easily the electrons in the molecules can move (i.e., be polarized). Large molecules in which the electrons are far from the nucleus are relatively easy to polarize and therefore possess greater dispersion forces. If it were not for dispersion forces, the noble gases would not liquefy at any temperature since no other intermolecular forces exist between the noble gas atoms. The low temperature at which the noble gases liquefy is to some extent indicative of the magnitude of dispersion forces between the atoms.

MCAT Synopsis

These intermolecular forces are the binding forces which keep a substance together in its solid or liquid state (See chapter 8). These same forces determine whether two substances are miscible or immiscible in the solution phase (See chapter 9).

4

COMPOUNDS AND STOICHIOMETRY

A **compound** is a pure substance that is composed of two or more elements in a fixed proportion. Compounds can be broken down chemically to produce their constituent elements or other compounds. All elements, except for some of the noble gases, can react with other elements or compounds to form new compounds. These new compounds can react further to form yet different compounds.

MOLECULES AND MOLES

A **molecule** is a combination of two or more atoms held together by covalent bonds. It is the smallest unit of a compound displaying the properties of that compound. Molecules may contain two atoms of the same element, as in N_2 and O_2, or may be comprised of two or more different atoms, as in CO_2 and $SOCl_2$. Molecules are usually discussed in terms of molecular weights and moles.

Ionic compounds do not form true molecules. In the solid state they can be considered to be a nearly infinite, three dimensional array of the charged particles of which the compound is composed. Since no actual molecule exists, molecular weight becomes meaningless, and the term **formula weight** is used in its place.

A. MOLECULAR WEIGHT

Like atoms, molecules can be characterized by their weight. The molecular weight is the sum of the atomic weights (in amu) of the atoms in the molecule. Similarly, the formula weight of an ionic compound is found by adding the atomic weights according to the empirical formula of the substance.

Example: What is the molecular weight of $SOCl_2$?

Solution: To find the molecular weight of $SOCl_2$, add together the atomic weights of each of the atoms.

$$1S = 1 \times 32 \text{ amu} = 32 \text{ amu}$$
$$1O = 1 \times 16 \text{ amu} = 16 \text{ amu}$$
$$2Cl = 2 \times 35.5 \text{ amu} = \underline{71 \text{ amu}}$$
$$\text{molecular weight} = 119 \text{ amu}$$

B. MOLE

A mole is defined as the amount of a substance that contains the same number of particles that are found in a 12.000 g sample of carbon-12. This quantity, **Avogadro's number,** is equal to 6.022×10^{23}. One mole of a compound has a mass in grams equal to the molecular weight of that compound in amu, and contains 6.022×10^{23} molecules of the compound. For example, 62 g of H_2CO_3 represents 1 mole of carbonic acid and contains 6.022×10^{23} H_2CO_3 molecules. The mass of 1 mole of a compound is called its **molar weight** or **molar mass,** and is usually expressed as g/mol. Therefore, the molar mass of H_2CO_3 is 62 g/mol.

The following formula is used to determine the number of moles that are present:

$$\text{Mol} = \frac{\text{Weight of Sample (g)}}{\text{Molar Weight (g/mol)}}$$

Example: How many moles are in 9.52 g of $MgCl_2$?

Solution: First, find the molar mass of $MgCl_2$.

$$1(24.31 \text{ g/mol}) + 2(35.45 \text{ g/mol}) = 95.21 \text{ g/mol}$$

Now, solve for the number of moles.
$$\frac{9.52}{95.21 \text{ g/mol}} = 0.10 \text{ mol of } MgCl_2$$

C. EQUIVALENT WEIGHT

For some substances, it is useful to define a measure of reactive capacity. This expresses the fact that some molecules are more potent than others in performing certain reactions. An example of this is the ability of different acids to donate protons (H^+ ions) in solution (see chapter 10, Acids and Bases). For instance, 1 mole of HCl can donate 1 mol of hydrogen ions, while 1 mol of H_2SO_4 can donate 2 moles of hydrogen ions. This difference is expressed using the term **equivalent:** 1 mole of HCl contains 1 equivalent of hydrogen ions while 1 mol of H_2SO_4 contains 2 equivalents of hydrogen ions. To determine the number of equivalents a compound contains, a new measure of weight called **gram-equivalent weight (GEW)** was developed.

$$\text{Equivalents} = \frac{\text{Weight of Compound}}{\text{Gram Equivalent Weight}}$$

and

$$\text{Gram Equivalent Weight} = \frac{\text{Molar Mass}}{n}$$

where n is usually either the number of hydrogens used per molecule of acid in a reaction, or the number of hydroxyl groups used per molecule of base in a reaction. This value is strictly dependent on reaction conditions. By using equivalents, it is possible to say that one equivalent of acid will neutralize one equivalent of base, a statement which may not necessarily be true when dealing with moles.

REPRESENTATION OF COMPOUNDS

A. LAW OF CONSTANT COMPOSITION

The **law of constant composition** states that any sample of a given compound will contain the same elements in the identical mass ratio. For instance, every sample of H_2O will contain two atoms of hydrogen for every atom of oxygen, or, in other words, one gram of hydrogen for every eight grams of oxygen.

B. EMPIRICAL AND MOLECULAR FORMULAS

There are two ways to express a formula for a compound. The **empirical formula** gives the simplest whole number ratio of the elements in the compound. The **molecular formula** gives the exact number of atoms of each element in the compound and is usually a multiple of the empirical formula. For example, the empirical formula for benzene is CH, while the molecular formula is C_6H_6. For some compounds, the empirical and molecular formulas are the same, as in the case of H_2O. An ionic compound, such as NaCl or $CaCO_3$, will have only an empirical formula.

C. PERCENT COMPOSITION

The percent composition by mass of an element is the weight percent of the element in a specific compound. To determine the percent composition of an element X in a compound, the following formula is used:

$$\% \text{ Composition} = \frac{\text{Mass of X in Formula}}{\text{Formula Weight of Compound}} \times 100\%$$

The percent composition of an element may be determined using either the empirical or molecular formula. If the percent compositions are known, the empirical formula can be derived. It is possible to determine the molecular formula if both the percent compositions and molecular weight of the compound are known.

Example: What is the percent composition of chromium in $K_2Cr_2O_7$?

Solution: The formula weight of $K_2Cr_2O_7$ is:

$$2(39 \text{ g/mol}) + 2(52 \text{ g/mol}) + 7(16 \text{ g/mol}) = 294 \text{ g/mol}$$

$$\text{Percent composition of Cr} = \frac{2(52 \text{ g/mol})}{294 \text{ g/mol}} = 100$$

$$= 0.354 \times 100$$
$$= 35.4 \text{ percent}$$

Example: What are the empirical and molecular formulas of a compound that contains 40.9 percent carbon, 4.58 percent hydrogen, 54.52 percent oxygen, and has a molecular weight of 264 g/mol?

Method One: First, determine the number of moles of each element in the compound by assuming a 100-gram sample; this converts the percentage of each element present directly into grams of that element. Then convert grams to moles:

$$\text{\# mol of C} = \frac{40.9 \text{ g}}{12 \text{ g/mol}} = 3.41 \text{ mol}$$

$$\text{\# mol of H} = \frac{4.58 \text{ g}}{1 \text{ g/mol}} = 4.58 \text{ mol}$$

$$\text{\# mol of O} = \frac{54.52 \text{ g}}{16 \text{ g/mol}} = 3.41 \text{ mol}$$

Next, find the simplest whole number ratio of the elements by dividing the number of moles by the smallest number obtained in the previous step.

$$\text{C: } \frac{3.41}{3.41} = 1.00 \qquad \text{H: } \frac{4.58}{3.41} = 1.33 \qquad \text{O: } \frac{3.41}{3.41} = 1.00$$

Finally, the empirical formula is obtained by converting the numbers obtained into whole numbers (multiplying them by an integer value).

$$C_1H_{1.33}O_1 \times 3 = C_3H_4O_3$$

$C_3H_4O_3$ is the empirical formula. To determine the molecular formula, divide the molecular weight by the weight represented by the empirical formula. The resultant value is the number of empirical formula units in the molecular formula.

The empirical formula weight of $C_3H_4O_3$ is:

$$3(12 \text{ g/mol}) + 4(1 \text{ g/mol}) + 3(16 \text{ g/mol}) = 88 \text{ g/mol}$$

$$\frac{264 \text{ g/mol}}{88 \text{ g/mol}} = 3$$

$C_3H_4O_3 \times 3 = C_9H_{12}O_9$ is the molecular formula.

Method Two: When the molecular weight is given, it is generally easier to find the molecular formula first. This is accomplished by multiplying the molecular weight by the given percentages to find the grams of each element present in one mole of compound, then dividing by the respective atomic weights to find the mole ratio of the elements:

$$\# \text{ mol of C} = \frac{(0.409)(264) \text{ g}}{12 \text{ g/mol}} = 9 \text{ mol}$$

$$\# \text{ mol of H} = \frac{(0.458)(264) \text{ g}}{1 \text{ g/mol}} = 12 \text{ mol}$$

$$\# \text{ mol of O} = \frac{(0.5452)(264) \text{ g}}{16 \text{ g/mol}} = 9 \text{ mol}$$

Thus the molecular formula, $C_9H_{12}O_9$, is the direct result.

The empirical formula can now be found by reducing the subscript ratio to the simplest integral values.

> **MCAT Synopsis**
>
> The molecular formula is either the same as the empirical formula or a multiple of it. To calculate the molecular formula, you need to know the mole ratio (this will give you the empirical formula) and the molecular weight (molecular wt. ÷ empirical formula wt. will give you the multiplier for the empirical formula → molecular formula conversion).

TYPES OF CHEMICAL REACTIONS

There are many ways in which elements and compounds can react to form other species; memorizing every reaction would be impossible, as well as unnecessary. However, nearly every inorganic reaction can be classified into at least one of four general categories.

> **MCAT Synopsis**
>
> Combination reactions generally have more reactants than products.
>
> $A + B \rightarrow C$

A. COMBINATION REACTIONS

Combination reactions are reactions in which two or more **reactants** form one **product**. The formation of sulfur dioxide by burning sulfur in air is an example of a combination reaction.

$$S\ (s) + O_2\ (g) \rightarrow SO_2\ (g)$$

B. DECOMPOSITION REACTIONS

A **decomposition reaction** is defined as one in which a compound breaks down into two or more substances, usually as a result of heating or electrolysis. An example of a decomposition reaction is the breakdown of mercury (II) oxide (the sign Δ represents the addition of heat).

$$2HgO \ (s) \xrightarrow{\Delta} 2Hg(l) + O_2 \ (g)$$

C. SINGLE DISPLACEMENT REACTIONS

Single displacement reactions occur when an atom (or ion) of one compound is replaced by an atom of another element. For example, zinc metal will displace copper ions in a copper sulfate solution to form zinc sulfate.

$$Zn \ (s) + CuSO_4 \ (aq) \rightarrow Cu \ (s) + ZnSO_4 \ (aq)$$

Single displacement reactions are often further classified as **redox** reactions. (These will be discussed in more detail in chapter 11, Redox Reactions and Electrochemistry.)

D. DOUBLE DISPLACEMENT REACTIONS

In double displacement reactions, also called **metathesis reactions**, elements from two different compounds displace each other to form two new compounds. This type of reaction occurs when one of the products is removed from the solution as a precipitate or gas, or when two of the original species combine to form a weak electrolyte that remains undissociated in solution. For example, when solutions of calcium chloride and silver nitrate are combined, insoluble silver chloride forms in a solution of calcium nitrate.

$$CaCl_2 \ (aq) + 2 \ AgNO_3 \ (aq) \rightarrow Ca(NO_3)_2 \ (aq) + 2 \ AgCl \ (s)$$

NET IONIC EQUATIONS

Because reactions such as displacements often involve ions in solution, they can be written in ionic form. In the example where zinc is reacted with copper sulfate, the **ionic equation** would be:

$$Zn \ (s) + Cu^{2+} \ (aq) + SO_4^{2-} \ (aq) \rightarrow Cu \ (s) + Zn^{2+} \ (aq) + SO_4^{2-} \ (aq)$$

When displacement reactions occur, there are usually **spectator ions** that do not take part in the overall reaction but simply remain in solution throughout. The spectator ion in the equation above is sulfate, which does not undergo any transformation during the reaction. A **net ionic reaction** can be written showing only the species that actually participate in the reaction:

$$Zn \ (s) + Cu^{2+} \ (aq) \rightarrow Cu \ (s) + Zn^{2+} \ (aq)$$

Net ionic equations are important for demonstrating the actual reaction that occurs during a displacement reaction.

NEUTRALIZATION REACTIONS

Neutralization reactions are a specific type of double displacement that occur when an acid reacts with a base to produce a solution of a salt and water. For example, hydrochloric acid and sodium hydroxide will react to form sodium chloride and water.

$$HCl \ (aq) + NaOH \ (aq) \rightarrow NaCl \ (aq) + H_2O \ (l)$$

(This type of reaction will be discussed further in chapter 10, Acids and Bases.)

MCAT Synopsis

Acids and bases combine in neutralization reactions to produce salt and water.

BALANCING EQUATIONS

A. BALANCING EQUATIONS

Chemical equations express how much and which type of reactant must be used to obtain a given quantity of product. From the law of conservation of mass, the mass of the reactants in a reaction must be equal to the mass of the products. More specifically, chemical equations must be balanced so that there are the same number of atoms of each element in the products as there are in the reactants. **Stoichiometric coefficients** are used to indicate the number of moles of a given species involved in the reaction. For example, the reaction for the formation of water is:

$$2 \ H_2 \ (g) + O_2 \ (g) \rightarrow 2 \ H_2O \ (g)$$

The coefficients indicate that two moles of H_2 gas must be reacted with one mole of O_2 gas to produce two moles of water. In general, stoichiometric coefficients are given as whole numbers.

MCAT Favorite

You will rarely need to balance an equation on the MCAT. However, you need to recognize reactions that are or are not balanced. Look at the:

1) charge of each side
2) number of atoms of each element

Example: Balance the following reaction.

$$C_4H_{10} \ (l) + O_2 \ (g) \rightarrow CO_2 \ (g) + H_2O \ (l)$$

Solution: First, balance the carbons in reactants and products.

$$C_4H_{10} + O_2 \rightarrow 4 \ CO_2 + H_2O$$

MCAT Synopsis

When balancing equations, focus on the least represented elements first, and work your way to the most represented element of the reaction (usually oxygen or hydrogen).

Second, balance the hydrogens in reactant and products.

$$C_4H_{10} + O_2 \rightarrow 4\ CO_2 + 5\ H_2O$$

Third, balance the oxygens in the reactants and products.

$$2\ C_4H_{10} + 13\ O_2 \rightarrow 8\ CO_2 + 10\ H_2O$$

Finally, check that all of the elements, and the total charges, are balanced correctly. If there is a difference in total charge between the reactants and products, then the charge will also have to be balanced. (Instructions for balancing charge are found in chapter 11.)

B. APPLICATIONS OF STOICHIOMETRY

Once an equation has been balanced, the ratio of moles of reactant to moles of product is known, and that information can be used to solve many types of stoichiometry problems. It is important to use proper units when solving such problems. If and when you are faced with doing the calculations, the units should cancel out, so that the units obtained in the answer represent those asked for in the problem.

Example: How many grams of calcium chloride are needed to prepare 72 g of silver chloride according to the following equation?

$$CaCl_2\ (aq) + 2AgNO_3\ (aq) \rightarrow Ca(NO_3)_2\ (aq) + 2AgCl\ (s)$$

Solution: Noting first that the equation is balanced, 1 mole of $CaCl_2$ yields 2 moles of AgCl when it is reacted with 2 moles of $AgNO_3$. The molar mass of $CaCl_2$ is 110 g, and the molar mass of AgCl is 144 g.

$$72\ g\ AgCl \times \frac{1\ mol\ AgCl}{144\ g\ AgCl} \times \frac{1\ mol\ CaCl_2}{2\ mol\ AgCl} \times \frac{110\ g\ CaCl_2}{1\ mol\ CaCl_2}$$

Thus, 27.5 g of $CaCl_2$ are needed to produce 72 g of AgCl.

1. Limiting Reactants

When reactants are mixed, they are seldom added in the exact stoichiometric proportions as shown in the balanced equation. Therefore, in most reactions, one reactant will be consumed first. This reactant is known as the **limiting reactant** because it limits the amount of product that can be formed in the reaction. The reactant that remains after all of the limiting reagent is used is called the **excess reactant**.

Pavlov's Dog

When the quantities of two reactants are given, you are dealing with a limiting reactant problem.

Example: If 28 g of Fe react with 24 g of S to produce FeS, what would be the limiting reagent? How many grams of excess reagent would be present in the vessel at the end of the reaction?

The balanced equation is: $Fe + S \xrightarrow{\Delta} FeS$.

Solution: First, determine the number of moles for each reactant.

$$28 \text{ g Fe} \times \frac{1 \text{ mol Fe}}{56 \text{ g}} = 0.5 \text{ mol Fe}$$

$$24 \text{ g S} \times \frac{1 \text{ mol S}}{32 \text{ g}} = 0.75 \text{ mol S}$$

Since 1 mole of Fe is needed to react with 1 mole of S, and there are 0.5 moles Fe for every 0.75 moles S, the limiting reagent is Fe. Thus, 0.5 moles of Fe will react with 0.5 moles of S, leaving an excess of 0.25 moles of S in the vessel. The mass of the excess reagent will be:

$$\text{mass of S} = 0.25 \text{ mol S} \times \frac{32 \text{ g}}{1 \text{ mol S}}$$

$$= 8 \text{ g of S}$$

2. Yields

The **yield** of a reaction, which is the amount of product predicted or obtained when the reaction is carried out, can be determined or predicted from the balanced equation. There are three distinct ways of reporting yields. The **theoretical yield** is the amount of product that can be predicted from a balanced equation, assuming that all of the limiting reagent has been used, that no competing side reactions have occurred, and that all of the product has been collected. The theoretical yield is seldom obtained; therefore, chemists speak of the **actual yield,** which is the amount of product that is isolated from the reaction experimentally.

The term **percent yield** is used to express the relationship between the actual yield and the theoretical yield and is given by the following equation:

$$\text{Percent Yield} = \frac{\text{Actual Yield}}{\text{Theoretical Yield}} \times 100\%$$

Example: What is the percent yield for a reaction in which 27 g of Cu is produced by reacting 32.5 g of Zn in excess $CuSO_4$ solution?

Solution: The balanced equation is as follows:

$$Zn\ (s) + CuSO_4\ (aq) \rightarrow Cu\ (s) + ZnSO_4\ (aq)$$

Calculate the theoretical yield for Cu.

$$32.5\ g\ Zn\ \times\ \frac{1\ mol\ Zn}{65\ g} = 0.5\ mol\ Zn$$

$$0.5\ mol\ Zn\ \times\ \frac{1\ mol\ Cu}{1\ mol\ Zn} = 0.5\ mol\ Cu$$

$$0.5\ mol\ Cu\ \times\ \frac{64\ g}{1\ mol\ Cu} = 32\ g\ Cu\ =\ theoretical\ yield$$

Finally, determine the percent yield.

$$\frac{27\ g}{32\ g}\ \times\ 100\%\ =\ 84\%$$

MCAT Synopsis

Since we are given "excess" copper(II) sulfate, we know that zinc is the limiting reactant.

5

CHEMICAL KINETICS AND EQUILIBRIUM

When studying a chemical reaction, it is important to consider not only the chemical properties of the reactants, but also the **conditions** under which the reaction occurs, the **mechanism** by which it takes place, the rate at which it occurs, and the **equilibrium** (or steady state) toward which it proceeds.

CHEMICAL KINETICS

Chemical kinetics is the study of the rates of reactions, the effect of reaction conditions on these rates, and the mechanisms implied by such observations.

REACTION MECHANISMS

The **mechanism** of a reaction is the actual series of steps through which a chemical reaction occurs. Knowing the accepted mechanism of a reaction often helps to explain the reaction's rate, position of equilibrium, and thermodynamic characteristics (see chapter 6). Consider the reaction below:

$$\text{Overall Reaction: } A_2 + 2\,B \rightarrow 2\,AB$$

This equation seems to imply a mechanism in which two molecules of B collide with one molecule of A_2 to form two molecules of AB. But suppose instead that the reaction actually takes place in two steps.

Step 1:	$A_2 + B \rightarrow A_2B$	(Slow)
Step 2:	$A_2B + B \rightarrow 2\,AB$	(Fast)

Note that these two steps add up to the overall (net) reaction. A_2B, which does not appear in the overall reaction because it is neither a reactant nor a product, is called an **intermediate.** Reaction intermediates are often difficult to detect, but a proposed mechanism can be supported through kinetic experiments.

 Go Online

For an in-depth review of Chemical Kinetics, visit the online workshop.

The slowest step in a proposed mechanism is called the **rate-determining step,** because the overall reaction cannot proceed faster than that step.

REACTION RATES

A. DEFINITION OF RATE

Consider a reaction 2A + B → C, in which 1 mole of C is produced from every 2 moles of A and 1 mole of B. The rate of this reaction may be described in terms of either the disappearance of reactants over time, or the appearance of products over time.

$$rate = \frac{\text{decrease in concentration of reactions}}{\text{time}} = \frac{\text{increase in concentration of products}}{\text{time}}$$

Because the concentration of a reactant decreases during the reaction, a minus sign is placed before a rate that is expressed in terms of reactants. For the reaction above, the rate of reaction with respect to A is $-\Delta[A]/\Delta t$, with respect to B is $-\Delta[B]/\Delta t$, and with respect to C is $\Delta[C]/\Delta t$. In this particular reaction, the three rates are not equal. According to the stoichiometry of the reaction, A is used up twice as fast as B ($-\frac{1}{2}\Delta[A]/\Delta t = -\Delta[B]/\Delta t$), and A is consumed twice as fast as C is produced ($-\frac{1}{2}\Delta[A]/\Delta t = \Delta[C]/\Delta t$). To show a standard rate of reaction in which the rates with respect to all substances are equal, the rate for each substance should be divided by its stoichiometric coefficient.

$$rate = -\frac{1}{2}\frac{\Delta[A]}{\Delta t} = -\frac{\Delta[B]}{\Delta t} = \frac{\Delta[C]}{\Delta t}$$

In general, for the reaction

$$a A + b B \rightarrow c C + d D,$$

$$rate = -\frac{1}{a}\frac{\Delta[A]}{\Delta t} = -\frac{1}{b}\frac{\Delta[B]}{\Delta t} = \frac{1}{c}\frac{\Delta[C]}{\Delta t} = \frac{1}{d}\frac{\Delta[D]}{\Delta t}$$

Rate is expressed in the units of moles per liter per second (mol/L × sec) or molarity per second (molarity/sec).

B. RATE LAW

For nearly all forward, irreversible reactions, the rate is proportional to the product of the concentrations of the reactants, each raised to some power. For the general reaction

$$a A + b B \rightarrow c C + d D$$

the rate is proportional to $[A]^x [B]^y$, that is:

$$rate = k [A]^x [B]^y$$

This expression is the **rate law** for the general reaction above, where k is the **rate constant**. Multiplying the units of k by the concentration factors raised to the appropriate powers gives the rate in units of concentration/time. The exponents x and y are called the **orders of reaction**; x is the order with respect to A and y is the order with respect to B. These exponents may be integers, fractions, or zero, and must be determined experimentally.

It is important to note that the exponents of the rate law are *not* necessarily equal to the stoichiometric coefficients in the overall reaction equation. (The exponents *are* equal to the stoichiometric coefficients of the rate-determining step. If one of the reactants or products in this step is an intermediate not included in the overall reaction, then calculating the rate law in terms of the original reactants is more complex.)

The **overall order of a reaction** (or the **reaction order**) is defined as the sum of the exponents, here equal to x + y.

MCAT Synopsis

Note that the exponents in the rate law are not equal to the stoichiometric coefficients unless the reaction actually occurs via a single step mechanism. Also note that product concentrations never appear in a rate law. Do not confuse a rate law with an equilibrium expression.

MCAT Favorite

Do not assume that the stoichiometric coefficients are the same as the order of each reactant, as they usually are not.

1. **Experimental Determination of Rate Law**

    The values of k, x, and y in the rate law equation (rate $= k [A]^x [B]^y$) must be determined experimentally for a given reaction at a given temperature. The rate is usually measured as a function of the **initial concentrations** of the reactants, A and B.

    Example: Given the data below, find the rate law for the following reaction at 300K.

    $$A + B \rightarrow C + D$$

Trial	$[A]_{initial}(M)$	$[B]_{initial}(M)$	$r_{initial}(M/sec)$
1	1.00	1.00	2.0
2	1.00	2.00	8.1
3	2.00	2.00	15.9

    Solution: First, look for two trials in which the concentrations of all but one of the substances are held constant.

    a)   In Trials 1 and 2, the concentration of A is kept constant while the concentration of B is doubled. The rate increases by a factor of 8.1/2.0, approximately 4. Write down the rate expression of the two trials.

Trial 1: $r_1 = k[A]^x [B]^y = k(1.00)^x (1.00)^y$

Trial 2: $r_2 = k[A]^x [B]^y = k(1.00)^x (2.00)^y$

Divide the second equation by the first.

$$\frac{r_2}{r_1} = \frac{8.1}{2.0} = \frac{k (1.00)^x (2.00)^y}{k (1.00)^x (1.00)^y} = (2.00)^y$$

$$4 = (2.00)^y$$

$$y = 2$$

b) In Trials 2 and 3, the concentration of B is kept constant while the concentration of A is doubled; the rate is increased by a factor of 15.9/8.1, approximately 2. The rate expressions of the two trials are:

Trial 2: $r_2 = k(1.00)^x (2.00)^y$

Trial 3: $r_3 = k(2.00)^x (2.00)^y$

Divide the second equation by the first.

$$\frac{r_3}{r_2} = \frac{15.9}{8.1} = \frac{k (2.00)^x (2.00)^y}{k (1.00)^x (2.00)^y} = (2.00)^x$$

$$2 = (2.00)^x$$

$$x = 1$$

So $r = k[A] [B]^2$

The order of the reaction with respect to A is 1 and with respect to B is 2; the overall reaction order is $1 + 2 = 3$.

To calculate k, substitute the values from any one of the above trials into the rate law, e.g.:

$$2.0 \text{ M/sec} = k \times 1.00 \text{ M} \times (1.00 \text{ M})^2$$
$$k = 2.0 \text{ M}^{-2} \text{ sec}^{-1}$$

Therefore, the rate law is $r = 2.0 \text{ M}^{-2} \text{ sec}^{-1} [A][B]^2$.

C. REACTION ORDERS

Chemical reactions are often classified on the basis of kinetics as zero-order, first-order, second-order, mixed-order, or higher-order reactions. The general reaction $a A + b B \rightarrow c C + d D$ will be used in the discussion below.

1. **Zero-Order Reactions**

   A zero-order reaction has a constant rate, which is independent of the reactants' concentrations. Thus the rate law is: rate = k, where k has units of $Msec^{-1}$. An increase in temperature or a decrease in temperature is the only factor that can change the rate of a zero-order reaction.

2. **First-Order Reactions**

   A first-order reaction (order = 1) has a rate proportional to the concentration of one reactant.

   $$\text{rate} = k[A] \text{ or rate} = k[B]$$

   First-order rate constants have units of sec^{-1}.

   The classic example of a first-order reaction is the process of radioactive decay. The concentration of radioactive substance A at any time t can be expressed mathematically as

   $$[A_t] = [A_o] e^{-kt}$$

   where $[A_o]$ = initial concentration of A
   $[A_t]$ = concentration of A at time t
   k = rate constant
   t = elapsed time

> **Bridge**
>
> For more on radioactive decay, see chapter 12 in the Physics section.

   The half-life ($t_{1/2}$) of a reaction is the time needed for the concentration of the radioactive substance to decrease to one-half of its original value. Half-lives can be calculated from the rate law as follows:

   $$t_{1/2} = \ln 2/k = 0.693/k$$

   where k is the first order rate constant.

3. **Second-Order Reactions**

   A second-order reaction (order = 2) has a rate proportional to the product of the concentration of two reactants, or to the square of the concentration of a single reactant; for example, rate = $k[A]^2$, rate = $k[B]^2$, or rate = $k[A][B]$. The units of second-order rate constants are $M^{-1} sec^{-1}$.

4. **Higher-Order Reactions**

   A higher-order reaction has an order greater than 2.

5. **Mixed-Order Reactions**

   A mixed-order reaction has a fractional order; e.g., rate = $k[A]^{1/3}$.

D. EFFICIENCY OF REACTIONS

1. **Collision Theory of Chemical Kinetics**
    In order for a reaction to occur, molecules must collide with each other. The **collision theory of chemical kinetics** states that the rate of a reaction is proportional to the number of collisions per second between the reacting molecules.

    Not all collisions, however, result in a chemical reaction. An **effective collision** (one that leads to the formation of products) occurs only if the molecules collide with correct orientation and sufficient force to break the existing bonds and form new ones. The minimum energy of collision necessary for a reaction to take place is called the **activation energy, E_a,** or the **energy barrier.** Only a fraction of colliding particles have enough kinetic energy to exceed the activation energy. This means that only a fraction of all collisions are effective. The rate of a reaction can therefore be expressed as:

    $$rate = fZ$$

    where Z is the total number of collisions occurring per second and f is the fraction of collisions that are effective.

2. **Transition State Theory**
    When molecules collide with sufficient energy, they form a **transition state,** in which the old bonds are weakened and the new bonds are beginning to form. The transition state then dissociates into products, and the new bonds are fully formed. For a reaction $A_2 + B_2 \rightarrow 2AB$, the change along the reaction coordinate (a measure of the extent to which the reaction has progressed from reactants to products; see Figures 5.1 and 5.2) can be represented as follows:

    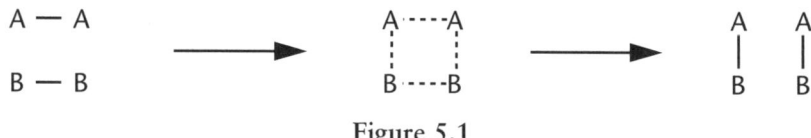

    Figure 5.1

    The **transition state,** also called the **activated complex,** has greater energy than either the reactants or the products and is denoted by the symbol ‡. The activation energy is required to bring the reactants to this energy level. Once an activated complex is formed, it can either dissociate into the products or revert to reactants without any additional energy input. Transition states are distinguished from intermediates in that, existing as they do at energy maxima, transition states do not have a finite lifetime.

A **potential energy diagram** illustrates the relations among the activation energy, the heats of reaction, and the potential energy of the system. The most important factors in such diagrams are the *relative* energies of the products and reactants. The **enthalpy change** of the reaction (**ΔH**) is the difference between the potential energy of the products and the potential energy of the reactants (see chapter 6). A negative enthalpy change indicates an exothermic reaction (where heat is given off) and a positive enthalpy change indicates an endothermic reaction (where heat is absorbed). The activated complex exists at the top of the energy barrier. The difference in potential energies between the activated complex and the reactants is the activation energy of the forward reaction; the difference in potential energies between the activated complex and the products is the activation energy of the reverse reaction.

MCAT Synopsis

$-\Delta H$ = exothermic = heat given off

$+\Delta H$ = endothermic = heat absorbed

For example, consider the formation of HCl from H_2 and Cl_2. The following figure, which gives the energy profile of the reaction

$$H_2 + Cl_2 \rightleftarrows 2\,HCl$$

shows that the reaction is exothermic. The potential energy of the products is less than the potential energy of the reactants; heat is evolved, and the heat of reaction is negative.

MCAT Synopsis

Note that the potential energy of the product can be raised or lowered, thereby changing the value of ΔH, without affecting the value of E_{act} forward, i.e., kinetics and thermodynamics are separate considerations.

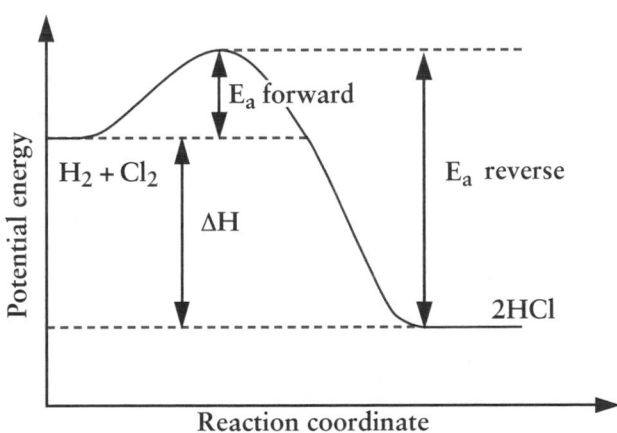

Figure 5.2

The thermodynamic properties of reactions are discussed further in chapter 6.

E. FACTORS AFFECTING REACTION RATE

The rate of a chemical reaction depends upon the individual species undergoing reaction, and upon the reaction environment. The rate of reaction will increase if either of the following occurs: an increase in the number of effective collisions, or a stabilization of the activated complex compared with the reactants.

1. **Reactant Concentrations**

   The greater the concentrations of the reactants (the more particles per unit volume), the greater will be the number of effective collisions per unit time, and therefore the reaction rate will increase for all but zero order reactions. For reactions occurring in the gaseous state, the partial pressures of the reactants can serve as a measure of concentration (see chapter 7).

2. **Temperature**

   For nearly all reactions, the reaction rate will increase as the temperature of the system increases. Since the temperature of a substance is a measure of the particles' average kinetic energy, increasing the temperature increases the average kinetic energy of the molecules. Consequently, the proportion of molecules having energies greater than E_a (thus capable of undergoing reaction) increases with higher temperature.

3. **Medium**

   The rate of a reaction may also be affected by the medium in which it takes place. Certain reactions proceed more rapidly in aqueous solution, whereas other reactions may proceed more rapidly in benzene. The state of the medium (liquid, solid, or gas) can also have a significant effect.

4. **Catalysts**

   Catalysts are substances that increase reaction rate without themselves being consumed; they do this by lowering the activation energy. Catalysts are important in biological systems and in industrial chemistry; enzymes are biological catalysts. Catalysts may increase the frequency of collision between the reactants, change the relative orientation of the reactants making a higher percentage of collisions effective, donate electron density to the reactants, or reduce intramolecular bonding within reactant molecules. Figure 5.3 compares the energy profiles of catalyzed and uncatalyzed reactions.

   The energy barrier for the catalyzed reaction is much lower than the energy barrier for the uncatalyzed reaction. Note that the rates of both the forward and the reverse reactions are increased by catalysis, since E_a of the forward and reverse reactions are lowered by the same amount. Therefore, the presence of a catalyst causes the reaction to proceed more quickly toward equilibrium.

> **Bridge**
>
> For a comprehensive discussion of enzymes, refer to chapter 2 of the Biology section.

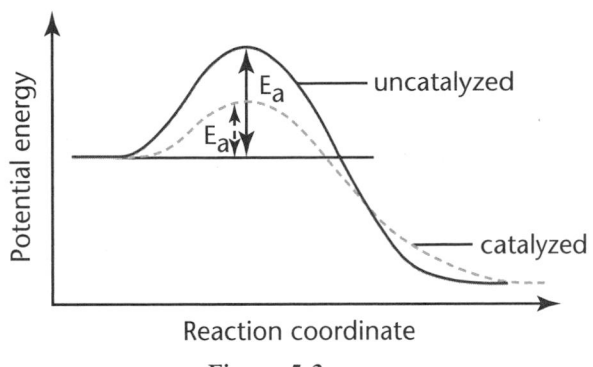

Figure 5.3

EQUILIBRIUM

THE DYNAMIC CONCEPT OF EQUILIBRIUM

So far, reaction rates have been discussed under the assumption that the reactions were **irreversible** (i.e., only proceeded in one direction), and that the reactions proceeded to completion. However, a **reversible** reaction often does not proceed to completion, because (by definition) the products can react to reform the reactants. This is particularly true of reactions occurring in closed systems, where products are not allowed to escape. When there is no **net** change in the concentrations of the products and reactants during a reversible chemical reaction, equilibrium exists. This is not to say that a reaction in equilibrium is static; change continues to occur in both the forward and reverse directions. Equilibrium can be thought of as a balance between the two reaction directions.

Consider the following reaction:

$$A \rightleftarrows B$$

At equilibrium, the concentrations of A and B are constant, yet the reactions A → B and B → A continue to occur at equal rates.

LAW OF MASS ACTION

Consider the following *one-step* reaction:

$$2A \rightleftarrows B + C$$

Since the reaction occurs in one step, the rates of the forward and reverse reaction are given by:

$$rate_f = k_f[A]^2 \text{ and } rate_r = k_r[B][C]$$

When $rate_f = rate_r$, equilibrium is achieved. Since the rates are equal, it can be stated that

$$k_f[A]^2 = k_r[B][C] \text{ or } \frac{k_f}{k_r} = \frac{[B][C]}{[A]^2}$$

Since k_f and k_r are both constants, this equation may be rewritten:

$$K_c = \frac{[B][C]}{[A]^2} \qquad \text{(see below for the general equation)}$$

where K_c is called the **equilibrium constant**, and the subscript c indicates that it is in terms of concentration (when dealing with gases, the equilibrium constant is referred to as K_p, and the subscript p indicates that it is in terms of pressure). For dilute solutions, K_c and K_{eq} are used interchangeably; the symbol K is also often used, although it is not completely correct to do so.

When the forward and reverse reaction rates are equal at equilibrium, the molar concentrations of the reactants and products usually are not equal. This means that the forward and reverse rate constants, k_f and k_r, are also usually unequal. For the *one-step* reaction described above:

$$k_f[A]^2 = k_r[B][C]$$

$$k_f = k_r \frac{[B][C]}{[A]^2}$$

In a reaction of more than one step, the equilibrium constant for the overall reaction is found by multiplying the equilibrium constants for each step of the reaction. When this is done, the equilibrium constant for the overall reaction is equal to the concentrations of products divided by reactants in the overall reaction, each raised to its stoichiometric coefficient.

The forward and reverse rate constants for any step n are designated k_n and k_{-n} respectively. For example, if the reaction

$$a A + b B \rightleftarrows c C + d D$$

occurs in three steps, then

$$K_c = \frac{k_1 k_2 k_3}{k_{-1} k_{-2} k_{-3}} \text{ will equal } \frac{[C]^c[D]^d}{[A]^a[B]^b}$$

This expression is known as the **Law of Mass Action.**

Example: What is the expression for the equilibrium constant for the following reaction?

$$3 H_2 (g) + N_2 (g) \rightleftarrows 2 NH_3 (g)$$

Solution: $K_c = \dfrac{[NH_3]^2}{[H_2]^3[N_2]}$

The **reaction quotient,** Q, is a measure of the degree to which a reaction has gone to completion. Q_c is equal to

$$\dfrac{[C]^c[D]^d}{[A]^a[B]^b}$$

Q_c is a constant only at equilibrium, when it is equal to K_c.

PROPERTIES OF THE EQUILIBRIUM CONSTANT

The equilibrium constant, K_{eq}, has the following characteristics:

- Pure solids and liquids do not appear in the equilibrium constant expression.

- K_{eq} is characteristic of a given system at a given temperature.

- If the value of K_{eq} is very large compared to 1, an equilibrium mixture of reactants and products will contain very little of the reactants compared to the products.

- If the value of K_{eq} is very small compared to 1 (i.e., less than 0.1), an equilibrium mixture of reactants and products will contain very little of the products compared to the reactants.

- If the value of K_{eq} is close to 1, an equilibrium mixture of products and reactants will contain approximately equal amounts of reactants and products.

LE CHÂTELIER'S PRINCIPLE

The French chemist Henry Louis Le Châtelier stated that a system to which a stress is applied tends to change so as to relieve the applied stress. This rule, known as **Le Châtelier's principle,** is used to determine the direction in which a reaction at equilibrium will proceed when subjected to a stress, such as a change in concentration, pressure, temperature, or volume.

A. CHANGES IN CONCENTRATION

Increasing the concentration of a species will tend to shift the equilibrium away from the species that is added to reestablish its equilibrium concentration, and vice versa. For example, in the reaction:

$$A + B \rightleftarrows C + D$$

if the concentration of A and/or B is increased, the equilibrium will shift toward (or favor production of) C and D. Conversely, if the concentration of C and/or D is increased, the equilibrium will shift away from the production of C and D, favoring production of A and B. Similarly, decreasing the concentration of a species will tend to shift the equilibrium toward the production of that species. For example, if A and/or B is removed from the above reaction, the equilibrium will shift so as to favor increasing concentration of A and B.

This effect is often used in industry to increase the yield of a useful product or drive a reaction to completion. If D were constantly removed from the above reaction, the net reaction would produce more D and concurrently more C. Likewise, using an excess of the least expensive reactant would help to drive the reaction forward.

B. CHANGE IN PRESSURE OR VOLUME

In a system at constant temperature, a change in pressure causes a change in volume, and vice versa. Since liquids and solids are practically incompressible, a change in the pressure or volume of systems involving only these phases has little or no effect on their equilibrium. Reactions involving gases, however, may be greatly affected by changes in pressure or volume, since gases are highly compressible.

Pressure and volume are inversely related. An increase in the pressure of a system will shift the equilibrium so as to decrease the number of moles of gas present. This reduces the volume of the system and relieves the stress of the increased pressure. Consider the following reaction:

$$N_2\ (g) + 3\ H_2\ (g) \rightleftarrows 2\ NH_3\ (g)$$

The left side of the reaction has 4 moles of gaseous molecules, whereas the right side has only 2 moles. When the pressure of this system is increased, the equilibrium will shift so that the side of the reaction producing fewer moles is favored. Since there are fewer moles on the right, the equilibrium will shift toward the right. Conversely, if the volume of the same system is increased, its pressure immediately decreases, which, according to Le Châtelier's principle, leads to a shift in the equilibrium to the left.

C. CHANGE IN TEMPERATURE

Changes in temperature also affect equilibrium. To predict this effect, heat may be considered as a product in an exothermic reaction and as a reactant in an endothermic reaction. Consider the following exothermic reaction:

$$A \rightleftarrows B + heat$$

If this system were placed in an ice bath, its temperature would decrease, driving the reaction to the right to replace the heat lost. Conversely, if the system were placed in a boiling-water bath, the reaction equilibrium would shift to the left because of the increased "concentration" of heat.

Not only does a temperature change alter the position of the equilibrium, it also alters the numerical value of the equilibrium constant. In contrast, changes in the concentration of a species in the reaction, in the pressure, or in the volume, will alter the position of the equilibrium without changing the numerical value of the equilibrium constant.

MCAT Synopsis

$$A + B \rightleftarrows C + heat$$

will shift to Ⓡ   will shift to Ⓛ

• If more A or B added	• If more C added
• If C taken away	• If A or B taken away
• If pressure applied or volume reduced (assuming A, B, and C gases)	• If pressure reduced or volume increased (assuming A, B, and C gases)
• If temperature reduced	• If temperature increased

6

THERMOCHEMISTRY

All chemical reactions are accompanied by energy changes. Thermal, chemical, potential, and kinetic energies are all interconvertible, as they must obey the **Law of Conservation of Energy.** Energy changes determine whether reactions can occur and how easily they will do so, thus an understanding of **thermodynamics** is essential to an understanding of chemistry. In chemistry, thermodynamics help determine whether a chemical reaction is **spontaneous,** i.e., if under a given set of conditions it can occur, by itself, without outside assistance. A spontaneous reaction may or may not proceed to completion, depending upon the rate of the reaction, which is determined by chemical kinetics (see chapter 5).

Bridge

Thermodynamics is discussed in detail in chapter 4 of the Physics section.

The application of thermodynamics to chemical reactions is called **thermochemistry.** Several thermodynamic definitions are very useful in thermochemistry. A **system** is the particular part of the universe being studied; everything outside the system is considered the **surroundings** or **environment.** A system may be:

- **isolated**—when it cannot exchange energy or matter with the surroundings, as with an insulated bomb reactor;
- **closed**—when it can exchange energy but not matter with the surroundings, as with a steam radiator;
- **open**—when it can exchange both matter and energy with the surroundings, as with a pot of boiling water.

A system undergoes a **process** when one or more of its properties changes. A process is associated with a change of state. An **isothermal** process occurs when the temperature of the system remains constant; an **adiabatic** process occurs when no heat exchange occurs; and an **isobaric** process occurs when the pressure of the system remains constant. Isothermal and isobaric processes are common, since it is usually easy to control temperature and pressure.

HEAT

A. DEFINITION

Heat is a form of energy that can easily transfer to or from a system, the result of a temperature difference between the system and its surroundings; this transfer will occur spontaneously from a warmer system to a cooler system. According to convention, heat absorbed by a system (from its surroundings) is considered positive, while heat lost by a system (to its surroundings) is considered negative.

Heat change is the most common energy change in chemical processes. Reactions that absorb heat energy are said to be **endothermic**, while those that release heat energy are said to be **exothermic**. Heat is commonly measured in **calories (cal)**, or **Joules (J)**, and more commonly in kcal or kJ (1 cal = 4.184 J).

B. CALORIMETRY

Calorimetry measures heat changes. The terms **constant-volume calorimetry** and **constant-pressure calorimetry** are used to indicate the conditions under which the heat changes are measured. The heat (**q**) absorbed or released in a given process is calculated from the equation:

$$q = mc\Delta T$$

where m is the mass, c is the **specific heat** see Physics, chapter 4, Thermodynamics), and ΔT is the change in temperature.

Constant-Volume Calorimetry

In constant-volume calorimetry, the volume of the container holding the reacting mixture does not change during the course of the reaction. The heat of reaction is measured using a device called a bomb calorimeter. This apparatus consists of a steel bomb into which the reactants are placed. The bomb is immersed in an insulated container containing a known amount of water. The reactants are electrically ignited and heat is absorbed or evolved as the reaction proceeds. The heat of the reaction, q_{rxn}, can be determined as follows. Since no heat enters or leaves the system, the net heat change for the system is zero; therefore, the heat change for the reaction is compensated for by the heat change for the water and the bomb, which is easy to measure.

$$q_{system} = q_{rxn} + q_{water} + q_{steel} = 0$$

Thus:
$$q_{rxn} = -(q_{water} + q_{steel})$$
$$= -(m_{water}\, c_{water}\, \Delta T + m_{steel}\, c_{steel}\, \Delta T)$$

Note that the overall system, as defined, is adiabatic, since no net heat gain or loss occurs. However, the heat exchange between the various components makes it possible to determine the heat of reaction.

STATES AND STATE FUNCTIONS

The state of a system is described by the macroscopic properties of the system. Examples of macroscopic properties include temperature (T), pressure (P), and volume (V). When the state of a system changes, the values of the properties also change. Properties whose magnitude depends only on the initial and final states of the system, and not on the path of the change (how the change was accomplished), are known as **state functions**. Pressure, temperature, and volume are important state functions. Other examples are **enthalpy (H)**, **entropy (S)**, **free energy (G)** (all discussed below), and **internal energy (E or U)**. Although independent of path, state functions are not necessarily independent of one another.

A set of **standard conditions** (25°C and 1 atm) is normally used for measuring the enthalpy, entropy, and free energy of a reaction. A substance in its most stable form under standard conditions is said to be in its **standard state**. Examples of substances in their standard states include hydrogen as H_2 (*g*), water as H_2O (*l*), and salt as NaCl (*s*). The changes in enthalpy, entropy, and free energy that occur when a reaction takes place under standard conditions are called the **standard enthalpy**, **standard entropy**, and **standard free energy** changes respectively, and are symbolized by $\Delta H°$, $\Delta S°$, and $\Delta G°$.

> **MCAT Synopsis**
>
> Standard conditions in thermodynamics must not be confused with standard temperature and pressure (STP) in gas law calculations. (See chapter 7.)

A. ENTHALPY

Most reactions in the lab occur under constant pressure (at 1 atm, in open containers). To express heat changes at constant pressure, chemists use the term **enthalpy (H)**. The change in enthalpy (ΔH) of a process is equal to the heat absorbed or evolved by the system at constant pressure. The enthalpy of a process depends only on the enthalpies of the initial and final states, *not* on the path. Thus to find the enthalpy change of a reaction, ΔH_{rxn}, one must subtract the enthalpy of the reactants from the enthalpy of the products:

$$\Delta H_{rxn} = H_{products} - H_{reactants}$$

A positive ΔH corresponds to an endothermic process, and a negative ΔH corresponds to an exothermic process.

Unfortunately, it is not possible to measure H directly; only ΔH can be measured, and even then, only for certain fast and spontaneous processes. Thus several standard methods have been developed to calculate ΔH for any process.

1. **Standard Heat of Formation**
   The enthalpy of formation of a compound, $\Delta H°_f$, is the enthalpy change that would occur if one mole of a compound were formed directly from its elements in their standard states. Note that $\Delta H°_f$ of

an element in its standard state is zero. The $\Delta H°_f$ of most known substances is tabulated.

2. **Standard Heat of Reaction**

The standard heat of a reaction, $\Delta H°_{rxn}$, is the hypothetical enthalpy change that would occur if the reaction were carried out under standard conditions; i.e., when reactants in their standard states are converted to products in their standard states at 298K. It can be expressed as:

$$\Delta H°_{rxn} = \text{(sum of } \Delta H°_f \text{ of products)} - \text{(sum of } \Delta H°_f \text{ of reactants)}$$

3. **Hess's Law**

Hess's law states that enthalpies of reactions are additive. When thermochemical equations (chemical equations for which energy changes are known) are added to give the net equation for a reaction, the corresponding heats of reaction are also added to give the net heat of reaction. Because enthalpy is a state function, the enthalpy of a reaction does not depend on the path taken but depends only on the initial and final states. For example, consider the reaction:

$$Br_2 \ (l) \rightarrow Br_2 \ (g) \quad \Delta H = (31 \text{ kJ/mol})(1 \text{ mol}) = 31 \text{ kJ}$$

The enthalpy change of the above reaction, called the **heat of vaporization, $\Delta H°_{vap}$**, will always be 31 kJ/mol provided that the same initial and final states, $Br_2 \ (l)$ and $Br_2 \ (g)$ respectively, exist at standard conditions. $Br_2 \ (l)$ could instead be decomposed to Br atoms and then recombined to form $Br_2 \ (g)$, but since the net reaction is the same, the change in enthalpy will always be the same.

$$
\begin{aligned}
Br_2 \ (l) &\rightarrow 2 \ Br \ (g) & \Delta H_1 \\
2 \ Br \ (g) &\rightarrow Br_2 \ (g) & \Delta H_2 \\
\hline
Br_2 \ (l) &\rightarrow Br_2 \ (g) & \Delta H = \Delta H_1 + \Delta H_2 = 31 \text{ kJ}
\end{aligned}
$$

Example: Given the following thermochemical equations:

a) $C_3H_8 \ (g) + 5 \ O_2 \ (g) \rightarrow 3 \ CO_2 \ (g) + 4 \ H_2O \ (l) \quad \Delta H_a = -2220.1 \text{ kJ}$

b) $C \ (graphite) + O_2 \ (g) \rightarrow CO_2 \ (g) \quad\quad\quad\quad\quad\quad \Delta H_b = -393.5 \text{ kJ}$

c) $H_2 \ (g) + 1/2 \ O_2 \ (g) \rightarrow H_2O \ (l) \quad\quad\quad\quad\quad\quad \Delta H_c = -285.8 \text{ kJ}$

Calculate ΔH for the reaction:

d) $3 \ C \ (graphite) + 4 \ H_2 \ (g) \rightarrow C_3H_8 \ (g)$

Solution: Equations a, b, and c must be combined to obtain equation d. Since equation d contains only C, H_2, and C_3H_8, we must eliminate O_2, CO_2, and H_2O from the first three equations. Equation a is reversed to get C_3H_8 on the product side (this gives equation e).

Next, equation b is multiplied by 3 (this gives equation f) and c by 4 (this gives equation g). The following addition is done to obtain the required equation d: 3b + 4c + e.

e) $3 CO_2 (g) + 4 H_2O (l) \rightarrow C_3H_8 (g) + 5 O_2 (g)$ $\Delta H_e = 2220.1$ kJ

f) $3 \times [C (graphite) + O_2 (g) \rightarrow CO_2 (g)]$ $\Delta H_f = 3 \times -393.5$ kJ

g) $4 \times [H_2 (g) + \frac{1}{2} O_2 (g) \rightarrow H_2O (l)]$ $\Delta H_g = 4 \times -285.8$ kJ

$3 C (graphite) + 4 H_2 (g) \rightarrow C_3H_8 (g)$ $\Delta H_d = -103.6$ kJ

where $\Delta H_d = \Delta H_e + \Delta H_f + \Delta H_g$.

It is important to note that the reverse of any reaction has an enthalpy of the same magnitude as that of the forward reaction, but its sign is opposite.

4. **Bond Dissociation Energy**

Heats of reaction are related to changes in energy associated with the break-down and formation of chemical bonds. **Bond energy,** or **bond dissociation energy,** is an average of the energy required to break a particular type of bond in one mole of gaseous molecules. It is tabulated as the positive value of the energy absorbed as the bonds are broken. For example:

$$H_2 (g) \rightarrow 2H (g) \qquad \Delta H = 436 \text{ kJ}$$

A molecule of H_2 gas is cleaved to produce two gaseous, unassociated hydrogen atoms. For each mole of H_2 gas cleaved, roughly 436 kJ of energy is absorbed by the system. The reaction is therefore endothermic. For bonds found in other than diatomic molecules, many compounds have been measured and the energy requirements averaged. For example, the C-H bond dissociation energy one would find in a table (415 kJ/mol) was compiled from measurements on thousands of different organic compounds.

Bond energies can be used to estimate enthalpies of reactions. The enthalpy change of a reaction is given by:

$$\Delta H_{rxn} = (\Delta H \text{ of bonds broken}) - (\Delta H \text{ of bonds formed})$$
$$= \text{total energy input} - \text{total energy released}$$

Example: Calculate the enthalpy change for the following reaction:

$$C\ (s) + 2\ H_2\ (g) \rightarrow CH_4\ (g) \quad \Delta H = ?$$

Bond dissociation energies of H–H and C–H bonds are 436 kJ/mol and 415 kJ/mol, respectively.

$$\Delta H_f \text{ of } C\ (g) = 715 \text{ kJ/mol}$$

Solution: CH_4 is formed from free elements in their standard states (C in solid and H_2 in gaseous state).

Thus here, $\Delta H_{rxn} = \Delta H_f$

The reaction can be written in three steps:

a) $C\ (s) \rightarrow C\ (g)$ $\quad\quad\quad\quad\quad \Delta H_1$
b) $2\ [H_2\ (g) \rightarrow 2\ H\ (g)]$ $\quad\quad\quad 2\Delta H_2$
c) $C\ (g) + 4\ H\ (g) \rightarrow CH_4\ (g)$ $\quad \Delta H_3$

and $\Delta H_f = [\Delta H_1 + 2\Delta H_2] + [\Delta H_3]$

$$\Delta H_1 = \Delta H_f\ C\ (g) = 715 \text{ kJ/mol,}$$

ΔH_2 is the energy required to break the H–H bond of one mole of H_2. So:

$$\Delta H_2 = \text{bond energy of } H_2$$
$$= 436 \text{ kJ/mol}$$

ΔH_3 is the energy released when 4 C–H bonds are formed. So:

$$\Delta H_3 = -(4 \times \text{bond energy of C–H})$$
$$= -(4 \times 415 \text{ kJ/mol})$$
$$= -1{,}660 \text{ kJ/mol}$$

(Note: Since energy is released when bonds are formed, ΔH_3 is negative.)

Therefore:

$$\Delta H_{rxn} = \Delta H_f = [715 + 2(436)] - (1660) \text{ kJ/mol}$$
$$= -73 \text{ kJ/mol}$$

5. **Heats of Combustion**

One more type of standard enthalpy change which is often used is the standard heat of combustion, $\Delta H°_{comb}$. As stated earlier, a requirement for relatively easy measurement of ΔH is that the reaction be fast and spontaneous; combustion generally fits this description. The reactions used in the C_3H_8 (g) example above were combustion reactions, and the corresponding values ΔH_a, ΔH_b, and ΔH_c were thus heats of combustion.

B. ENTROPY

Entropy (S) is a measure of the disorder, or randomness, of a system. The units of entropy are energy/temperature, commonly J/K or cal/K. The greater the order in a system, the lower the entropy; the greater the disorder or randomness, the higher the entropy. At any given temperature, a solid will have lower entropy than a gas, because individual molecules in the gaseous state are moving randomly, while individual molecules in a solid are constrained in place. Entropy is a state function, so a change in entropy depends only on the initial and final states:

$$\Delta S = S_{final} - S_{initial}$$

A change in entropy is also given by:

$$\Delta S = \frac{q_{rev}}{T}$$

where q_{rev} is the heat added to the system undergoing a reversible process (a process that proceeds with infinitesimal changes in the system's conditions) and T is the absolute temperature.

A standard entropy change for a reaction, $\Delta S°$, is calculated using the standard entropies of reactants and products:

$$\Delta S°_{rxn} = (\text{sum of } S°_{products}) - (\text{sum of } S°_{reactants})$$

The second law of thermodynamics states that all spontaneous processes proceed such that the entropy of the system plus its surroundings (i.e., the entropy of the universe) increases:

$$\Delta S_{universe} = \Delta S_{system} + \Delta S_{surroundings} > 0$$

A system reaches its maximum entropy at **equilibrium**, a state in which no observable change takes place as time goes on. For a reversible process, $\Delta S_{universe}$ is zero:

$$\Delta S_{universe} = \Delta S_{system} + \Delta S_{surroundings} = 0$$

A system will spontaneously tend toward an equilibrium state if left alone.

> **MCAT Synopsis**
>
> Entropy can be thought of as synonymous with chaos and disorder.

> **MCAT Synopsis**
>
> Entropy changes accompanying phase changes (see chapter 8) can be easily estimated, at least qualitatively. For example, freezing is accompanied by a decrease in entropy as the relatively disordered liquid becomes a well-ordered solid. Meanwhile, boiling is accompanied by a large increase in entropy as the liquid becomes a much more highly disordered gas. For any substance, sublimation will be the phase transition with the greatest entropy change.

C. GIBBS FREE ENERGY

1. Spontaneity of Reaction

The thermodynamic state function, **G** (known as the **Gibbs Free Energy**), combines the two factors which affect the spontaneity of a reaction—changes in enthalpy, ΔH, and changes in entropy, ΔS. The change in the free energy of a system, ΔG, represents the maximum amount of energy released by a process, occurring at constant temperature and pressure, that is available to perform useful work. ΔG is defined by the equation:

$$\Delta G = \Delta H - T\Delta S$$

where T is the absolute temperature and $T\Delta S$ represents the total amount of heat absorbed by a system when its entropy increases reversibly.

In the equilibrium state, free energy is at a minimum. A process can occur spontaneously if the Gibbs function decreases, i.e., $\Delta G < 0$.

a) If ΔG is negative, the reaction is spontaneous.
b) If ΔG is positive, the reaction is not spontaneous.
c) If ΔG is zero, the system is in a state of equilibrium;
    thus, $\Delta G = 0$ and $\Delta H = T\Delta S$.

Because the temperature is always positive, i.e., in Kelvins, the effects of the signs of ΔH and ΔS and the effect of temperature on spontaneity can be summarized as follows:

ΔH	ΔS	Outcome
−	+	Spontaneous at all temperatures
+	−	Nonspontaneous at all temperatures
+	+	Spontaneous only at high temperatures
−	−	Spontaneous only at low temperatures

It is very important to note that the **rate** of a reaction depends on the **activation energy,** not the ΔG.

2. Standard Free Energy

Standard free energy, $\Delta G°$, is defined as the ΔG of a process occurring at 25°C and 1 atm pressure, and for which the concentrations of any solutions involved are 1 M. The **standard free energy of formation** of a compound, $\Delta G°_f$, is the free-energy change that occurs when 1 mol of a compound in its standard state is formed from its elements in their standard states under standard conditions. The

form (and, therefore, its standard state) is zero. The standard free energy of a reaction, $\Delta G°_{rxn}$, is the free energy change that occurs when that reaction is carried out under standard state conditions; i.e., when the reactants in their standard states are converted to the products in their standard states, at standard conditions of T and P. For example: under standard conditions conversion of C (*diamond*) to C (*graphite*) is spontaneous. However, its rate is so slow that the rxn is never observed.

$\Delta G°_{rxn}$ 5 (sum of $\Delta G°_f$ of products) 2 (sum of $\Delta G°_f$ of reactants).

3. Reaction Quotient

$\Delta G°_{rxn}$ can also be derived from the equilibrium constant for the equation:

$$\Delta G° \; 5 \; 2RT \ln K_{eq}$$

where K_{eq} is the equilibrium constant, R is the gas constant, and T is the temperature in K.

Once a reaction commences, however, the standard state conditions no longer hold. K_{eq} must be replaced by another parameter, the **reaction quotient (Q).** For the reaction, a A 1 b B $\rightleftarrows$ c C 1 d D,

$$Q = \frac{\left[C\right]^c \left[D\right]^d}{\left[A\right]^c \left[B\right]^b}$$

Likewise, ΔG must be used in place of $\Delta G°$. The relationship between the two is as follows:

$$\Delta G \; 5 \; \Delta G° \; 1 \; RT \ln Q$$

where R is the gas constant and T is the temperature in K.

4. Examples
    a. Vaporization of water at one atmosphere pressure

$$H_2O \; (l) \; 1 \; heat \rightarrow H_2O \; (g)$$

When water boils, hydrogen bonds (H-bonds) are broken. Energy is absorbed (the reaction is endothermic), and thus ΔH is positive. Entropy increases as the closely packed molecules of the liquid become the more randomly moving molecules of a gas; thus, $T\Delta S$ is also positive. Since ΔH and $T\Delta S$ are each positive, the reaction will proceed spontaneously only if $T\Delta S > \Delta H$. This is true only at temperatures above 100°C. Below 100°C, ΔG is positive and the water remains a liquid. At 100°C, ΔH = TΔS and ΔG = 0: an equilibrium is established between water and water vapor. The opposite is true when water vapor condenses: H-bonds are formed, and energy is released; the reaction is exothermic (ΔH is negative) and entropy decreases, as a liquid is forming from a gas (TΔS is negative). Condensation will be spontaneous only if ΔH < TΔS. This is the case at temperatures below 100°C; above 100°C, TΔS is more negative than H, ΔG is positive, and condensation is not spontaneous. Again, at 100°C, an equilibrium is established.

b. The combustion of C_6H_6 (benzene)

$$2 \, C_6H_6 \, (l) + 15 \, O_2 \, (g) \rightarrow 12 \, CO_2 \, (g) + 6 \, H_2O \, (g) + heat$$

In this case, heat is released (ΔH is negative) as the benzene burns and the entropy is increased (TΔS is positive), because two gases (18 moles total) have greater entropy than a gas and a liquid (15 moles gas and 2 liquid). ΔG is negative and the reaction is spontaneous.

7

THE GAS PHASE

Matter can exist in three different physical forms, called **phases** or **states: gas, liquid,** and **solid.** Liquids and solids will be discussed in chapter 8.

The gaseous phase, the subject of this chapter, is the simplest to understand, since all gases display similar behavior and follow similar laws regardless of their identity. The atoms or molecules in a gaseous sample move rapidly and are far apart from each other. In addition, only very weak intermolecular forces exist between gas particles; this results in certain characteristic physical properties, such as the ability to expand to fill any volume and to take on the shape of a container. Further, gases are easily, though not infinitely, compressible.

The state of a gaseous sample is generally defined by four variables: pressure (P), volume (V), temperature (T), and number of moles (n). Gas pressures are usually expressed in units of atmospheres (atm) or millimeters of mercury (mm Hg or torr), which are related as follows:

$$1 \text{ atm} = 760 \text{ mm Hg} = 760 \text{ torr}$$

Volume is generally expressed in liters (L) or milliliters (mL). The temperature of a gas is usually given in Kelvin (K, **not** °K). Gases are often discussed in terms of **standard temperature and pressure (STP),** which refers to conditions of 273.15K (0°C) and 1 atm.

Note: It is important not to confuse **STP** with **standard conditions**—the two standards involve different temperatures and are used for different purposes. STP (0°C or 273K) is generally used for gas law calculations; standard conditions (25°C or 298K) is used when measuring standard enthalpy, entropy, Gibbs's free energy, and voltage.

> **MCAT Favorite**
>
> STP is different from standard state. Temperature at STP is 0°C, i.e. 273.15K. Temperature at standard state is 25°C.

IDEAL GASES

When examining the behavior of gases under varying conditions of temperature and pressure, scientists speak of ideal gases. An ideal gas represents a hypothetical gas whose molecules have no intermolecular forces and occupy no volume. Although gases actually deviate from this idealized behavior, at relatively low pressures (atmospheric pressure) and high temperatures many gases behave in a nearly ideal fashion. Therefore, the assumptions used for ideal gases can be applied to real gases with reasonable accuracy.

A. BOYLE'S LAW

> **MCAT Favorite**
>
> Boyle's Law states that pressure and volume are inversely related, i.e., when one increases, the other decreases.

Experimental studies performed by Robert Boyle in 1660 led to the formulation of Boyle's Law. His work showed that for a given gaseous sample held at constant temperature (isothermal conditions), the volume of the gas is inversely proportional to its pressure:

$$PV = k \text{ or } P_1V_1 = P_2V_2$$

where k is a proportionality constant and the subscripts 1 and 2 represent two different sets of conditions. A plot of pressure versus volume for a gas is shown in Figure 7.1.

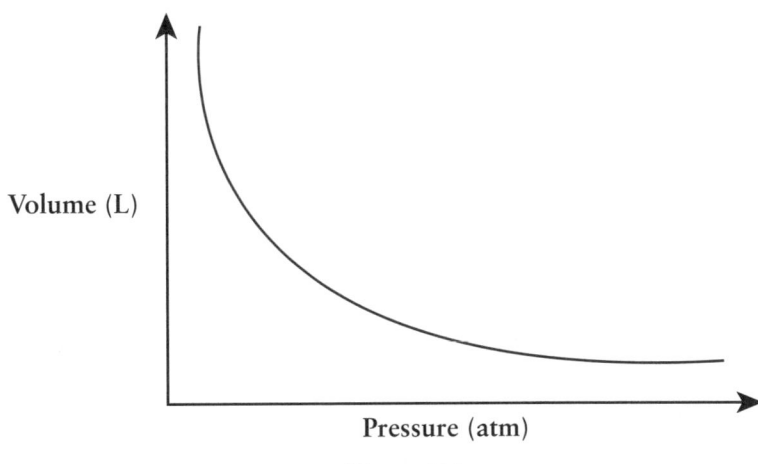

Volume (L)

Pressure (atm)

Figure 7.1

Example: Under isothermal conditions, what would be the volume of a 1 L sample of helium if its pressure is changed from 12 atm to 4 atm?

Solution: $P_1 = 12$ atm $\qquad P_2 = 4$ atm

$\qquad\qquad\qquad V_1 = 1$ L $\qquad\quad V_2 = X$

$\qquad\qquad\qquad P_1V_1 = P_2V_2$

$\qquad 12$ atm $(1$ L$) = 4$ atm (X)

$$\frac{12}{4}L = X$$

$$X = 3 \text{ L}$$

B. LAW OF CHARLES AND GAY-LUSSAC

The Law of Charles and Gay-Lussac, or simply Charles' Law, was developed during the early 19th century. The law states that at constant pressure, the volume of a gas is directly proportional to its absolute temperature. The absolute temperature is the temperature expressed in Kelvin, which can be calculated from the expression $T_K = T_{°C} + 273.15$.

$$\frac{V}{T} = k \text{ or } \frac{V_1}{T_1} = \frac{V_2}{T_2}$$

where k is a constant and the subscripts 1 and 2 represent two different sets of conditions. A plot of temperature versus volume is shown in Figure 7.2.

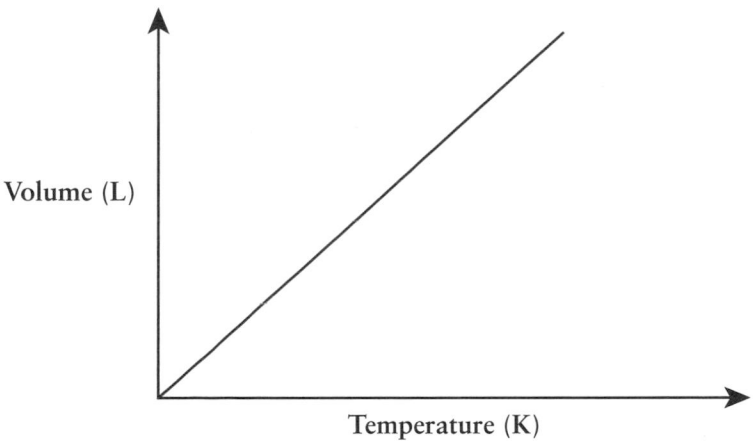

Volume (L)

Temperature (K)

Figure 7.2

Example: If the absolute temperature of 2 L of gas at constant pressure is changed from 283.15K to 566.30K, what would be the final volume?

Solution:

$$T_1 = 283.15K \qquad V_1 = 2\,L$$

$$T_2 = 566.30K \qquad V_2 = X$$

$$\frac{V_1}{T_1} = \frac{V_2}{T_2}$$

$$\frac{2\,L}{283.15K} = \frac{X}{566.30K}$$

$$X = \frac{2\,L\,(566.30K)}{283.15K}$$

$$X = 4\,L$$

C. AVOGADRO'S PRINCIPLE

In 1811, Amedeo Avogadro proposed that for all gases at a constant temperature and pressure, the volume of the gas will be directly proportional to the number of moles of gas present; therefore, all gases have the same number of moles in the same volume.

$$\frac{n}{V} = k \ or \ \frac{n_1}{V_1} = \frac{n_2}{V_2}$$

The subscripts 1 and 2 once again apply to two different sets of conditions with the same temperature and pressure.

D. IDEAL GAS LAW

The ideal gas law combines the relationships outlined in Boyle's Law, Charles' Law, and Avogadro's Principle to yield an expression which can be used to predict the behavior of a gas. The ideal gas law shows the relationship among four variables that define a sample of gas—pressure (P), volume (V), temperature (T), and number of moles (n)—and is represented by the equation

$$PV = nRT$$

The constant R is known as the **gas constant**. Under STP conditions (273.15K and 1 atmosphere), 1 mole of gas was shown to have a volume of 22.4 L. Substituting these values into the ideal gas equation gave $R = 8.21 \times 10^{-2}$ L • atm/(mol • K).

The gas constant may be expressed in many other units: another common value is 8.314 J/(K • mol), which is derived when SI units of Pascals (for pressure) and cubic meters (for volume) are substituted into the ideal gas law. **When carrying out calculations based on the ideal gas law,**

it is important to choose a value of R that matches the units of the variables.

Example: What volume would 12 g of helium occupy at 20°C and a pressure of 380 mm Hg?

Solution: The ideal gas law can be used, but first, all of the variables must be converted to yield units that will correspond to the expression of the gas constant as 0.0821 L • atm/(mol • K).

$$P = 380 \text{ mm Hg} \times \frac{1 \text{atm}}{760 \text{ mm Hg}} = 0.5 \text{ atm}$$

$$T = 20°C + 273.15 = 293.15K$$

$$n = 12g \text{ He} \times \frac{1 \text{ mol He}}{4.0 \text{ g}} = 3 \text{ mol He}$$

Substituting into the ideal gas equation:

$$PV = nRT$$

$$(0.5 \text{ atm})(V) = (3 \text{ mol})(0.0821 \text{ L} \bullet \text{atm/(mol} \bullet \text{K})(293.15K)$$

$$V = 144.4 \text{ L}$$

In addition to standard calculations to determine the pressure, volume, or temperature of a gas, the ideal gas law may be used to determine the density and molar mass of the gas.

1. Density
   Density is defined as the mass per unit volume of a substance and, for gases, is usually expressed in units of g/L. By rearrangement, the ideal gas equation can be used to calculate the density of a gas.

$$PV = nRT$$

where $n = \dfrac{m}{MM} \quad \dfrac{(\text{mass in g})}{(\text{molar mass})}$

therefore $PV = \dfrac{m}{MM} RT$

and $d = \dfrac{m}{V} = \dfrac{P(MM)}{RT}$

Another way to find the density of a gas is to start with the volume of a mole of gas at STP, 22.4 L, calculate the effect of pressure and temperature on the volume, and finally calculate the density by dividing the mass by the new volume. The following equation, derived from Boyle's and Charles's Laws, is used to relate changes in the temperature, volume and pressure of a gas:

$$\frac{P_1 V_1}{T_1} = \frac{P_2 V_2}{T_2}$$

where the subscripts 1 and 2 refer to the two states of the gas (at STP and under the actual conditions). To calculate a change in volume, the equation is rearranged as follows.

$$V_2 = V_1 \left(\frac{P_1}{P_2}\right)\left(\frac{T_2}{T_1}\right)$$

V_2 is then used to find the density of the gas under nonstandard conditions.

$$d = \frac{m}{V_2}$$

If you *visualize* how the changes in pressure and temperature affect the volume of the gas, you can check to be sure you have not accidentally confused the pressure or temperature value that belongs in the numerator with the one that belongs in the denominator.

Example: What is the density of HCl gas at 2 atm and 45°C?

Solution: At STP, a mole of gas occupies 22.4 liters. Since the increase in pressure to 2 atm decreases volume, 22.4 L must be multiplied by $\left(\frac{1\ atm}{2\ atm}\right)$. And since the increase in temperature increases volume, the temperature factor will be $\left(\frac{318K}{273K}\right)$.

$$V_2 = \left(\frac{22.4\ L}{mol}\right)\left(\frac{1\ atm}{2\ atm}\right)\left(\frac{318K}{273K}\right) = 13.0\ L/mol$$

$$d = \left(\frac{36\ g/mol}{13.0\ L/mol}\right) = 2.77\ g/L$$

2. Molar Mass

Sometimes the identity of a gas is unknown, and the molar mass (see chapter 4) must be determined in order to identify it. Using the equation for density derived from the ideal gas law, the molar mass of a gas can be determined experimentally as follows. The pressure and temperature of a gas contained in a bulb of a given volume are measured, and the weight of the bulb plus sample is found. Then, the bulb is evacuated, and the empty bulb is weighed. The weight of the bulb plus sample minus the weight of the bulb yields the weight of the sample. Finally, the density of the sample is determined by dividing the weight of the sample by the volume of the bulb. The density at STP is calculated. The molecular weight is then found by multiplying the number of grams per liter by 22.4 liters per mole.

Example: What is the molar mass of a 2 L sample of gas that weighs 8 g at a temperature of 15°C and a pressure of 1.5 atm?

$$d = \frac{8\ g}{2\ L} \text{ at } 15°C \text{ and } 1.5 \text{ atm}$$

$$V_{STP} = (2\ L)\left(\frac{273\ K}{288\ K}\right)\left(\frac{1.5\ atm}{1\ atm}\right) = 2.84\ L$$

$$\frac{8\ g}{2.84\ L} = 2.82\ g/L \text{ at STP}$$

$$\left(\frac{2.82\ g}{L}\right)\left(\frac{22.4\ L}{mol}\right) = 63.2\ g/mol$$

DALTON'S LAW OF PARTIAL PRESSURES

When two or more gases are found in one vessel without chemical interaction, each gas will behave independently of the other(s). Therefore, the pressure exerted by each gas in the mixture will be equal to the pressure that gas would exert if it were the only one in the container. The pressure exerted by each individual gas is called the **partial pressure** of that gas. In 1801, John Dalton derived an expression, now known as **Dalton's Law of Partial Pressures,** which states that the total pressure of a gaseous mixture is equal to the sum of the partial pressures of the individual components. The equation is:

$$P_T = P_A + P_B + P_C + \cdots$$

The partial pressure of a gas is related to its mole fraction and can be determined using the following equations:

$$P_A = P_T X_A$$

where $$X_A = \frac{n_A}{n_T} \frac{\text{(moles of A)}}{\text{(total moles)}}$$

Example: A vessel contains 0.75 mol of nitrogen, 0.20 mol of hydrogen, and 0.05 mol of fluorine at a total pressure of 2.5 atm. What is the partial pressure of each gas?

First calculate the mole fraction of each gas.

> **MCAT Synopsis**
>
> At high temperature and low pressure, deviations from ideality are usually small; good approximations can still be made from the ideal gas law.

$$X_{N_2} = \frac{0.75 \text{ mol}}{1.0 \text{ mol}} = 0.75 \quad X_{H_2} = \frac{0.20 \text{ mol}}{1.0 \text{ mol}} = 0.20 \quad X_{F_2} = \frac{0.05 \text{ mol}}{1.0 \text{ mol}} = 0.05$$

Then calculate the partial pressure.

$$P_A = X_A P_T$$

$$P_{N_2} = (2.5 \text{ atm})(0.75) \qquad P_{H_2} = (2.5 \text{ atm})(0.20) \qquad P_{F_2} = (2.5 \text{ atm})(0.05)$$

$$= 1.875 \text{ atm} \qquad\qquad = 0.5 \text{ atm} \qquad\qquad = 0.125 \text{ atm}$$

REAL GASES

In general, the ideal gas law is a good approximation of the behavior of real gases, but all real gases deviate from ideal gas behavior to some extent, particularly when the gas atoms or molecules are forced into close proximity under high pressure and at low temperature, so that molecular volume and intermolecular attractions become significant.

A. DEVIATIONS DUE TO PRESSURE

As the pressure of a gas increases, the particles are pushed closer and closer together. As the condensation pressure for a given temperature is approached, intermolecular attraction forces become more and more significant until the gas condenses into the liquid state (see Gas-Liquid Equilibrium in chapter 8).

At moderately high pressure (a few hundred atmospheres) a gas's volume is less than would be predicted by the ideal gas law, due to intermolecular attraction. At extremely high pressure the size of the particles becomes relatively large compared to the distance between them, and this causes the gas to take up a larger volume than would be predicted by the ideal gas law.

B. DEVIATIONS DUE TO TEMPERATURE

As the temperature of a gas is decreased, the average velocity of the gas molecules decreases, and the attractive intermolecular forces become increasingly significant. As the condensation temperature is approached for a given pressure, intermolecular attractions eventually cause the gas to condense to a liquid state (see Gas-Liquid Equilibrium in chapter 8).

As the temperature of a gas is reduced toward its condensation point (which is the same as its boiling point), intermolecular attraction causes the gas to have a smaller volume than would be predicted by the ideal gas law. The closer the temperature of a gas is to its boiling point, the less ideal is its behavior.

C. VAN DER WAALS EQUATION OF STATE

Several real gas equations, or gas laws, exist which attempt to correct for the deviations from ideality which occur when a gas does not closely follow the ideal gas law. The van der Waals equation is a case in point.

$$\left(P + \frac{n^2 a}{V^2}\right)(V - nb) = nRT$$

In this equation, *a* and *b* are physical constants, experimentally determined for each gas. The *a* term corrects for the attractive forces between molecules, and as such will be small in value for a gas such as helium, larger for more polarizable gases such as Xe or N_2, and larger yet for polar molecules such as HCl or NH_3. The *b* term corrects for the volume of the molecules themselves. Larger values of *b* are thus found for larger molecules. Numerical values for *a* are generally much larger than those for *b*.

Example: Find the correction in pressure necessary for the deviation from ideality for 1.00 moles of ammonia in a 1.00 liter flask at 0°C. (For NH_3, a = 4.2, b = 0.037)

Solution: According to the ideal gas law,

P = nRT/V = (1.00)(.0821)(273)/(1.00) = 22.4 atm, while according to the van der Waals equation,

$$P = \frac{nRT}{(V - nb)} - \frac{n^2 a}{V^2} = \frac{(1.00)(0.821)(273)}{(1.00 - 0.037)} - \frac{1.00^2 (4.2)}{1.00^2}$$

= 23.3 – 4.2 = 19.1 atm.

The pressure is thus 3.3 atm less than would be predicted from the ideal gas law, or an error of 15 percent.

KINETIC MOLECULAR THEORY OF GASES

As indicated by the gas laws, all gases show similar physical characteristics and behavior. A theoretical model to explain the behavior of gases was developed during the second half of the 19th century. The combined efforts of Boltzmann, Maxwell, and others led to a simple explanation of gaseous molecular behavior based on the motion of individual molecules. This model is called the **Kinetic Molecular Theory of Gases.** Like the gas laws, this theory was developed in reference to ideal gases, although it can be applied with reasonable accuracy to real gases as well.

A. ASSUMPTIONS OF THE KINETIC MOLECULAR THEORY

1. Gases are made up of particles whose volumes are negligible compared to the container volume.
2. Gas atoms or molecules exhibit no intermolecular attractions or repulsions.
3. Gas particles are in continuous, random motion, undergoing collisions with other particles and the container walls.
4. Collisions between any two gas particles are elastic, meaning that there is no overall gain or loss of energy.
5. The average kinetic energy of gas particles is proportional to the absolute temperature of the gas, and is the same for all gases at a given temperature.

B. APPLICATIONS OF THE KINETIC MOLECULAR THEORY OF GASES

1. **Average Molecular Speeds**

   According to the kinetic molecular theory of gases, the average kinetic energy of a gas particle is proportional to the absolute temperature of the gas:

   $$KE = \frac{1}{2} mv^2 = \frac{3}{2} kT$$

   where k is the Boltzmann constant. This equation also shows that the speed of a gas molecule is related to its absolute temperature. However, because of the large number of rapidly and randomly moving gas particles, the speed of an individual gas molecule is nearly impossible to define. Therefore, the speeds of gases are defined in terms of their average molecular speed ($\bar{c}$), which represents the mathematical average of all the speeds of the gas particles in the sample. This is given by the following equation:

   $$\bar{c} = \left(\frac{3RT}{MM}\right)^{\frac{1}{2}} \text{ where R = gas constant}$$

   MM = molecular mass

   A **Maxwell-Boltzmann distribution curve** shows the distribution of speeds of gas particles at a given temperature. Figure 7.3 shows a distribution curve of molecular speeds at two temperatures, T_1 and T_2, where $T_2 > T_1$. Notice that the bell-shaped curve flattens and shifts to the right as the temperature increases, indicating that at higher temperatures more molecules are moving at high speeds.

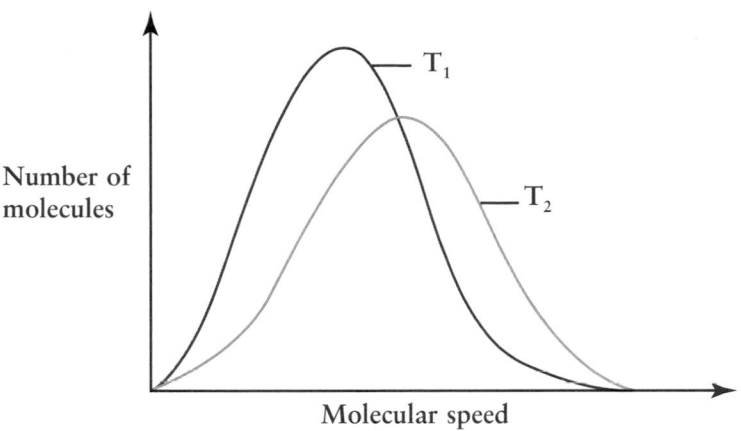

Figure 7.3

Example: What is the average speed of sulfur dioxide molecules at 37°C?

Solution: The gas constant R = 8.314 J/(K • mol) should be used and MM must be expressed in kg/mol.

$$\bar{c} = \left(\frac{3RT}{MM}\right)^{\frac{1}{2}}$$

$$\bar{c} = \left[\frac{3(8.314 \text{ J/K mol})(310.15 \text{ K})}{0/.064 \text{ kg/mol}}\right]^{\frac{1}{2}}$$

$$\bar{c} = \sqrt{120871.3 \text{ J/kg}}$$

Use the conversion factor 1 J = 1 kg • m²/s²:

$$\bar{c} = \sqrt{120871.3 \text{ kg} \bullet \text{m}^2/\text{s}^2 \bullet \text{kg}}$$

$$\bar{c} = 347.7 \text{ m/s}$$

2. Graham's Law of Diffusion and Effusion

   a. Diffusion

   Diffusion occurs when gas molecules diffuse through a mixture. Diffusion accounts for the fact that an open bottle of perfume can quickly be smelled across a room. The kinetic molecular theory of gases predicted that heavier gas molecules diffuse more slowly than lighter ones because of their differing average speeds. In 1832, Thomas Graham showed mathematically that under isothermal and isobaric conditions, the rates at which two gases diffuse are inversely proportional to the square root of their molar masses. Thus:

$$\frac{r_1}{r_2} = \left(\frac{MM_2}{MM_1}\right)^{\frac{1}{2}} = \sqrt{\frac{MM_2}{MM_1}}$$

where r_1 and MM_1 represent the diffusion rate and molar mass of gas 1, and r_2 and MM_2 represent the diffusion rate and molar mass of gas 2.

b. Effusion

Effusion is the flow of gas particles under pressure from one compartment to another through a small opening. Graham used the kinetic molecular theory of gases to show that for two gases at the same temperature, the rates of effusion are proportional to the average speeds. He then expressed the rates of effusion in terms of molar mass and found that the relationship is the same as that for diffusion:

$$\frac{r_1}{r_2} = \left(\frac{MM_2}{MM_1}\right)^{\frac{1}{2}}$$

8

PHASES AND PHASE CHANGES

When the attractive forces between molecules (i.e., van der Waals forces) overcome the kinetic energy that keeps them apart, the molecules move closer together such that they can no longer move about freely, entering the **liquid** or **solid** phase. Because of their smaller volume relative to gases, liquids and solids are often referred to as the **condensed phases.**

LIQUIDS

In a liquid, atoms or molecules are held close together with little space between them. As a result, liquids have definite volumes and cannot easily be expanded or compressed. However, the molecules can still move around and are in a state of relative disorder. Consequently, the liquid can change shape to fit its container, and its molecules are able to **diffuse** and **evaporate.**

One of the most important properties of liquids is their ability to mix, both with each other and with other phases, to form **solutions** (see chapter 9). The degree to which two liquids can mix is called their **miscibility.** Oil and water are almost completely **immiscible;** that is, their molecules tend to repel each other due to their polarity difference. Oil and water normally form separate layers when mixed, with oil on top because it is less dense. Under extreme conditions, such as violent shaking, two immiscible liquids can form a fairly homogeneous mixture called an **emulsion.** Although they look like solutions, emulsions are actually mixtures of discrete particles too small to be seen distinctly.

SOLIDS

In a solid, the attractive forces between atoms, ions, or molecules are strong enough to hold them rigidly together; thus the particles' only motion is vibration about fixed positions, and the kinetic energy of solids is predominantly vibrational energy. As a result, solids have definite shapes and volumes.

A solid may be **crystalline** or **amorphous.** A crystalline solid, such as NaCl, possesses an ordered structure; its atoms exist in a specific three-dimensional geometric arrangement with repeating patterns of atoms, ions, or molecules. An amorphous solid, such as glass, has no ordered three-dimensional arrangement, although the molecules are also fixed in place.

Most solids are crystalline in structure. The two most common forms of crystals are **metallic** and **ionic** crystals.

Ionic solids are aggregates of positively and negatively charged ions; there are no discrete molecules. The physical properties of ionic solids include high melting points, high boiling points, and poor electrical conductivity in the solid phase. These properties are due to the compounds' strong electrostatic interactions, which also cause the ions to be relatively immobile. Ionic structures are given by empirical formulas that describe the ratio of atoms in the lowest possible whole numbers. For example, the empirical formula $BaCl_2$ gives the ratio of barium to chloride within the crystal.

Metallic solids consist of metal atoms packed together as closely as possible. Metallic solids have high melting and boiling points as a result of their strong covalent attractions. Pure metallic structures (consisting of a single element) are usually described as layers of spheres of roughly similar radii.

The repeating units of crystals (both ionic and metallic) are represented by **unit cells.** There are many types of unit cells. We will now consider only the three cubic unit cells: **simple cubic, body-centered cubic,** and **face-centered cubic.**

Atoms are represented as points, but are actually adjoining spheres. Each unit cell is surrounded by similar units. In the ionic unit cell, the spaces between points (anions) are filled with other ions (cations).

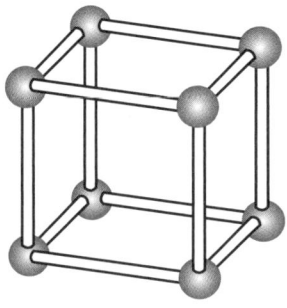
simple cubic

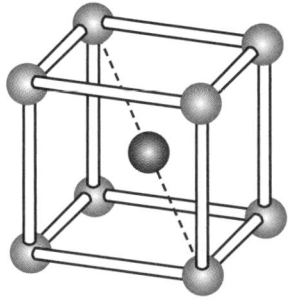
body-centered
cubic

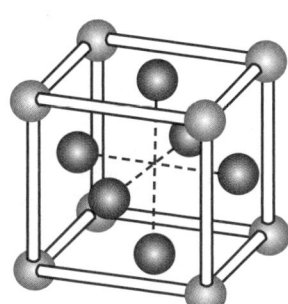
face-centered
cubic

Figure 8.1

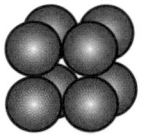
simple cubic

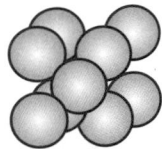
body-centered
cubic

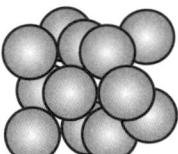
face-centered
cubic

Figure 8.2

PHASE EQUILIBRIA

In an isolated system, phase changes (solid to liquid to gas) are reversible, and an equilibrium exists between phases. For example, at 1 atm and 0°C in an isolated system, an ice cube floating in water is in equilibrium. Some of the ice may absorb heat and melt, but an equal amount of water will release heat and freeze. Thus, the relative amounts of ice and water remain constant.

A. GAS-LIQUID EQUILIBRIUM

The temperature of a liquid is related to the average kinetic energy of the liquid molecules; however, the kinetic energy of the molecules will vary. A few molecules near the surface of the liquid may have enough energy to leave the liquid phase and escape into the gaseous phase. This process is known as **evaporation** (or **vaporization**). Each time the liquid loses a high-energy particle, the temperature of the remaining liquid decreases; thus, evaporation is a cooling process. Given enough kinetic energy, the liquid will completely evaporate.

If a cover is placed on a beaker of liquid, the escaping molecules are trapped above the solution. These molecules exert a countering pressure, which forces some of the gas back into the liquid phase; this process is called **condensation.** Atmospheric pressure acts on a liquid in a similar fashion as a solid lid. As evaporation and condensation proceed, an equilibrium is reached in which the rates of the two processes become equal. Once this equilibrium is reached, the pressure that the gas exerts over the liquid is called the **vapor pressure** of the liquid. Vapor pressure increases as temperature increases, since more molecules have sufficient kinetic energy to escape into the gas phase. The temperature at which the vapor pressure of the liquid equals the external pressure is called the **boiling point.**

B. LIQUID-SOLID EQUILIBRIUM

The liquid and solid phases can also coexist in equilibrium (e.g., the ice-water mixture discussed above). Even though the atoms or molecules of a solid are confined to definite locations, each atom or molecule can undergo motions about some equilibrium position. These motions (vibrations) increase when heat is applied. If atoms or molecules in the solid phase absorb enough energy in this fashion, the solid's three-dimensional structure breaks down and the liquid phase begins. The transition from solid to liquid is called **fusion** or **melting.** The reverse process, from liquid to solid, is called **solidification, crystallization,** or **freezing.** The temperature at which these processes occur is called the **melting point** or **freezing point,** depending on the direction of the transition. Whereas pure crystals have distinct, very sharp melting points, amorphous solids, such as glass, tend to melt over a larger range of temperatures, due to their less-ordered molecular distribution.

C. GAS-SOLID EQUILIBRIUM

A third type of phase equilibrium is that between a gas and a solid. When a solid goes directly into the gas phase, the process is called **sublimation.** Dry ice (solid CO_2) sublimes; the absence of the liquid phase makes it a convenient refrigerant. The reverse transition, from the gaseous to the solid phase, is called **deposition.**

D. THE GIBBS FUNCTION

The thermodynamic criterion for each of the above equilibria is that the change in Gibbs free energy must equal zero; $\Delta G = 0$. For an equilibrium between a gas and a solid:

$$\Delta G = G\ (g) - G\ (s),$$

$$\text{so } G\ (g) = G\ (s) \text{ at equilibrium.}$$

The same is true of the Gibbs functions for the other two equilibria.

E. HEATING CURVES

When a compound is heated, the temperature rises until the melting or boiling points are reached. Then the temperature remains constant as the compound is converted to the next phase, i.e., liquid or gas, respectively. Once the entire sample is converted, then the temperature begins to rise again (Figure 8.3).

PHASE DIAGRAMS

A. SINGLE COMPONENT

A standard **phase diagram** depicts the phases and phase equilibria of a substance at defined temperatures and pressures. In general, the gas phase is found at high temperature and low pressure; the solid phase at low temperature and high pressure; and the liquid phase is found at high temperature and high pressure. A typical phase diagram is shown in Figure 8.4.

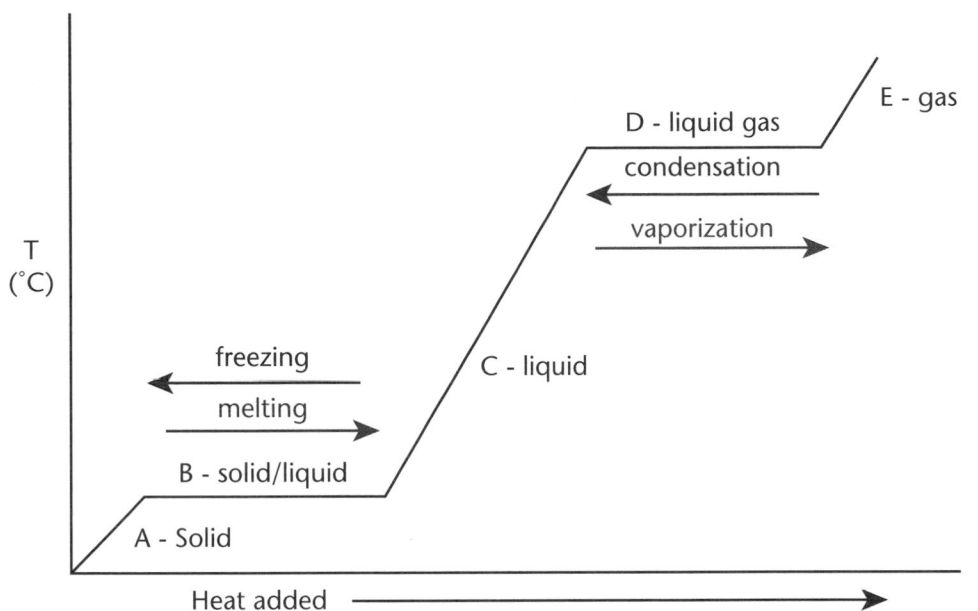

Figure 8.3: Heating Curves

The three phases are demarcated by lines indicating the temperatures and pressures at which two phases are in equilibrium. Line A represents freezing/melting, line B evaporation/condensation, and line C sublimation/deposition. The intersection of the three lines is called the **triple point**. At this temperature and pressure, unique for a given substance, all three phases are in equilibrium. The point at B is known as the **critical point**, the temperature and pressure above which no distinction between liquid and gas is possible.

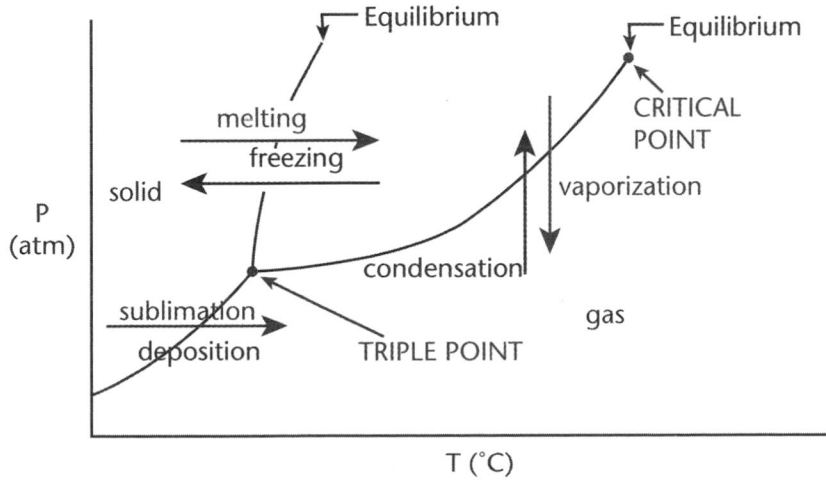

Figure 8.4: Gas-Liquid Equilibrium

B. MULTIPLE COMPONENTS

The phase diagram for a mixture of two or more components (Figure 8.5) is complicated by the requirement that the composition of the mixture, as well as the temperature and pressure, must be specified. Consider a solution of two liquids, A and B. The vapor above the solution is a mixture of the vapors of A and B. The pressures exerted by vapor A and vapor B on the solution are the vapor pressures that each exerts above its individual liquid phase. **Raoult's Law** (described below) enables one to determine the relationship between the vapor pressure of vapor A and the concentration of liquid A in the solution.

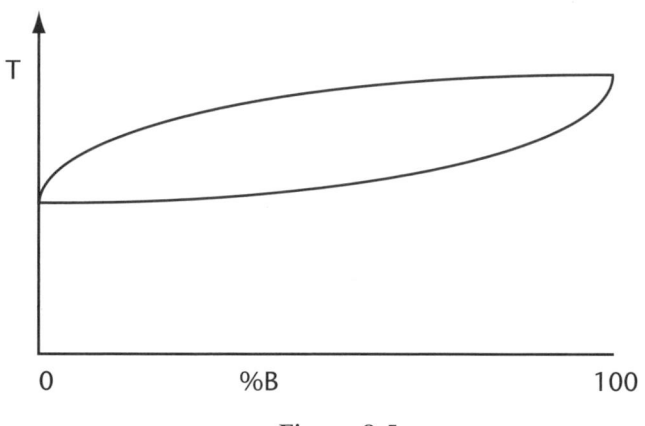

Figure 8.5

Curves such as this show the different compositions of the liquid phase and the vapor phase above a solution; the upper curve is that of the vapor while the lower curve is that of the liquid. It is this difference in composition which forms the basis of distillation, an important separation technique in organic chemistry.

COLLIGATIVE PROPERTIES

Colligative properties are physical properties derived solely from the number of particles present, not the nature of those particles. These properties are usually associated with dilute solutions (see chapter 9).

A. FREEZING-POINT DEPRESSION

Pure water (H_2O) freezes at 0°C; however, for every mole of solute particles dissolved in 1 L of water, the freezing point is lowered by 1.86°C. This is because the solute particles interfere with the process of crystal formation that occurs during freezing; the solute particles lower the temperature at which the molecules can align themselves into a crystalline structure.

The formula for calculating this **freezing-point depression** is:

$$\Delta T_f = K_f m$$

where ΔT_f is the freezing-point depression, K_f is a proportionality constant characteristic of a particular solvent, and m is the molality of the solution (mol solute/kg solvent; see chapter 9). The K_f for water—which you do not need to memorize for the MCAT—is $1.86°Cm^{-1}$. Each solvent has its own characteristic K_f.

B. BOILING-POINT ELEVATION

A liquid boils when its vapor pressure equals the atmospheric pressure. If the vapor pressure of a solution is lower than that of the pure solvent, more energy (and consequently a higher temperature) will be required before its vapor pressure equals atmospheric pressure. The extent to which the boiling point of a solution is raised relative to that of the pure solvent is given by the following formula:

$$\Delta T_b = K_b m$$

where ΔT_b is the boiling-point elevation, K_b is a proportionality constant characteristic of a particular solvent, and m is the molality of the solution. The K_b for water is $0.51°Cm^{-1}$.

C. OSMOTIC PRESSURE

Consider a container separated into two compartments by a semiper-meable membrane (which, by definition, selectively permits the pas-sage of certain molecules). One compartment contains pure water, while the other contains water with dissolved solute. The membrane allows water but not solute to pass through. Because substances tend to flow, or **diffuse**, from higher to lower concentrations (which increas-es entropy), water will diffuse from the compartment containing pure water to the compartment containing the water-solute mixture. This net flow will cause the water level in the compartment containing the solution to rise above the level in the compartment containing pure water.

Because the solute cannot pass through the membrane, the concentra-tions of solute in the two compartments can never be equal. However, the pressure exerted by the water level in the solute-containing compartment will eventually oppose the influx of water; thus, the water level will rise only to the point at which it exerts a sufficient pressure to counterbalance

> **Bridge**
>
> Osmosis is discussed in detail in chapter 1 of the Biology section.

> **MCAT Synopsis**
>
> Remember to always use Kelvin temperature if T is in an equation!.

the tendency of water to flow across the membrane. This pressure is defined as the **osmotic pressure (Π)** of the solution, and is given by the formula:

$$\Pi = \textbf{MRT}$$

where M is the molarity of the solution (see chapter 9), R is the ideal gas constant, and T is the temperature on the Kelvin scale. This equation clearly shows that molarity and osmotic pressure are directly proportional, i.e., as the concentration of the solution increases, the osmotic pressure also increases. Thus, the osmotic pressure depends only on the amount of solute, not its identity.

D. VAPOR-PRESSURE LOWERING (RAOULT'S LAW)

When solute B is added to pure solvent A, the vapor pressure of A above the solvent decreases (see Figure 8.4). If the vapor pressure of A above pure solvent A is designated by $P°_A$ and the vapor pressure of A above the solution containing B is P_A, the vapor pressure decreases as follows:

$$\Delta P = P°_A - P_A$$

In the late 1800s, the French chemist François Marie Raoult determined that this vapor pressure decrease is also equivalent to:

$$\Delta P = X_B P°_A$$

where X_B is the mole fraction of the solute B in solvent A. Since $X_B = 1 - X_A$ and $\Delta P = P°_A - P_A$, substitution into the above equation leads to the common form of Raoult's Law:

$$P_A = X_A P°_A$$

Similarly, the expression for the vapor pressure of the solute in solution (assuming it is volatile) is given by:

$$P_B = X_B P°_B$$

Raoult's Law holds only when the attraction between molecules of the different components of the mixture is equal to the attraction between the molecules of any one component in its pure state. When this condition does not hold, the relationship between mole fraction and vapor pressure will deviate from Raoult's Law. Solutions that obey Raoult's Law are called **ideal solutions.**

9

SOLUTIONS

Solutions are **homogeneous** (everywhere the same) mixtures of substances that combine to form a single phase, generally the liquid phase. Many important chemical reactions, both in the laboratory and in nature, take place in solution (including almost all reactions in living organisms).

NATURE OF SOLUTIONS

A solution consists of a **solute** (e.g., NaCl, NH_3, or $C_{12}H_{22}O_{11}$) dispersed (dissolved) in a **solvent** (e.g., H_2O or benzene). The solvent is the component of the solution whose phase remains the same after mixing. If the two substances are already in the same phase, the solvent is the component present in greater quantity. Solute molecules move about freely in the solvent and can interact with other molecules or ions; consequently, chemical reactions occur easily in solution.

A. SOLVATION

The interaction between solute and solvent molecules is known as **solvation** or **dissolution;** when water is the solvent, it is called **hydration** and the resulting solution is known as an **aqueous solution.** Solvation is possible when the attractive forces between solute and solvent are stronger than those between the solute particles. For example, when NaCl dissolves in water, its component ions dissociate from one another and become surrounded by water molecules. Because water is polar, ion-dipole interactions can occur between the Na^+ and Cl^- ions and the water molecules. For nonionic solutes, solvation involves van der Waals forces between the solute and solvent molecules. The general rule is that like dissolves like; ionic and polar solutes are soluble in polar solvents, and nonpolar solutes are soluble in nonpolar solvents.

Go Online

For more on the properties of solutions, visit the online workshop.

B. SOLUBILITY

The **solubility** of a substance is the maximum amount of that substance that can be dissolved in a particular solvent at a particular temperature. When this maximum amount of solute has been added, the solution is in equilibrium and is said to be **saturated**; if more solute is added, it will not dissolve. For example, at 18°C, a maximum of 83 g of glucose ($C_6H_{12}O_6$) will dissolve in 100 mL of H_2O. Thus the solubility of glucose is 83 g/100 mL. If more glucose is added, it will remain in solid form, precipitating to the bottom of the container. A solution in which the proportion of solute to solvent is small is said to be **dilute**, and one in which the proportion is large is said to be **concentrated**.

C. AQUEOUS SOLUTIONS

The most common class of solutions are the aqueous solutions, in which the solvent is water. The aqueous state is denoted by the symbol (*aq*). In discussing the chemistry of aqueous solutions, it is useful to know how soluble various salts are in water; this information is given by the solubility rules below.

1. All salts of alkali metals are water soluble.
2. All salts of the ammonium ion (NH_4^+) are water soluble.
3. All chlorides, bromides, and iodides are water soluble, with the exceptions of Ag^+, Pb^{2+}, and Hg_2^{2+}.
4. All salts of the sulfate ion (SO_4^{2-}) are water soluble, with the exceptions of Ca^{2+}, Sr^{2+}, Ba^{2+}, and Pb^{2+}.
5. All metal oxides are insoluble, with the exception of the alkali metals and CaO, SrO , and BaO, all of which hydrolyze to form solutions of the corresponding metal hydroxides.
6. All hydroxides are insoluble, with the exception of the alkali metals and Ca^{2+}, Sr^{2+}, and Ba^{2+}.
7. All carbonates (CO_3^{2-}), phosphates (PO_4^{3-}), sulfides (S^{2-}), and sulfites (SO_3^{2-}) are insoluble, with the exception of the alkali metals and ammonium.

IONS

Ionic solutions are of particular interest to chemists because certain important types of chemical interactions—acid-base reactions and oxidation-reduction reactions, for instance—take place in ionic solutions. Ions and their properties in solution will be introduced here; the chemical reactions mentioned are discussed in detail in chapter 10, Acids and Bases, and chapter 11, Redox Reactions and Electrochemistry.

A. CATIONS AND ANIONS

Ionic compounds are made up of **cations** and **anions,** where a cation is a positive ion and an anion is a negative ion. The nomenclature of ionic compounds is based on the names of the component ions.

1. For elements (usually metals) that can form more than one positive ion, the charge is indicated by a Roman numeral in parentheses following the name of the element.

Fe^{2+} Iron (II) Cu^+ Copper (I)
Fe^{3+} Iron (III) Cu^{2+} Copper (II)

2. An older but still commonly used method is to add the endings **-ous** or **-ic** to the root of the Latin name of the element, to represent the ions with lesser or greater charge respectively.

Fe^{2+} Ferrous Cu^+ Cuprous
Fe^{3+} Ferric Cu^{2+} Cupric

3. Monatomic anions are named by dropping the ending of the name of the element and adding **-ide.**

H^- Hydride S^{2-} Sulfide
F^- Fluoride N^{3-} Nitride
O^{2-} Oxide P^{3-} Phosphide

4. Many polyatomic anions contain oxygen and are therefore called **oxyanions.** When an element forms two oxyanions, the name of the one with less oxygen ends in **-ite** and the one with more oxygen ends in **-ate.**

NO_2^- Nitrite SO_3^{2-} Sulfite
NO_3^- Nitrate SO_4^{2-} Sulfate

5. When the series of oxyanions contains four oxyanions, prefixes are also used. **Hypo-** and **per-** are used to indicate less oxygen and more oxygen, respectively.

ClO^- Hypochlorite
ClO_2^- Chlorite
ClO_3^- Chlorate
ClO_4^- Perchlorate

6. Polyatomic anions often gain one or more H^+ ions to form anions of lower charge. The resulting ions are named by adding the word

hydrogen or dihydrogen to the front of the anion's name. An older method uses the prefix **bi-** to indicate the addition of a single hydrogen ion.

HCO_3^- Hydrogen carbonate or bicarbonate

HSO_4^- Hydrogen sulfate or bisulfate

$H_2PO_4^-$ Dihydrogen phosphate

B. ION CHARGES

Metals, which are found in the left part of the periodic table, generally form positive ions, whereas nonmetals, which are found in the right part of the periodic table, generally form negative ions. Note, however, the existence of anions that contain metallic elements, e.g., MnO_4^- (permanganate) and CrO_4^{2-} (chromate). All elements in a given group tend to form monatomic ions with the same charge. Thus ions of alkali metals (Group I) usually form cations with a single positive charge, the alkaline earth metals (Group II) form cations with a double positive charge, and the halides (Group VII) form anions with a single negative charge. Though other main group elements follow this trend, the intermediate electronegativity of such elements (making them less likely to form ionic compounds) and the transition from metallic to nonmetallic character complicates the picture.

> **MCAT Synopsis**
>
> Oxyanions of transition metals like the MnO_4^- and CrO_4^{2-} ions shown here have an inordinately high oxidation number on the metal. As such, they tend to gain electrons in order to reduce this oxidation number, and thus make good oxidizing agents. (See chapter 11.)

C. ELECTROLYTES

The electrical conductivity of aqueous solutions is governed by the presence and concentration of ions in solution. Therefore, pure water does not conduct an electrical current well since the concentrations of hydrogen and hydroxide ions are very small. Solutes whose solutions are conductive are called **electrolytes**. A solute is considered a **strong electrolyte** if it dissociates completely into its constituent ions. Examples of strong electrolytes include ionic compounds, such as NaCl and KI, and molecular compounds with highly polar covalent bonds that dissociate into ions when dissolved, such as HCl in water. A **weak electrolyte**, on the other hand, ionizes or hydrolyzes incompletely in aqueous solution and only some of the solute is present in ionic form. Examples include acetic acid and other weak acids, ammonia and other weak bases, and $HgCl_2$. Many compounds do not ionize at all in aqueous solution, retaining their molecular structure in solution, which usually limits their solubility. These compounds are called nonelectrolytes and include many nonpolar gases and organic compounds, such as oxygen and sugar.

> **MCAT Synopsis**
>
> Since electrolytes ionize in solution, they will produce a larger effect on colligative properties (see chapter 8) than one would expect from the given concentration.

CONCENTRATION

A. UNITS OF CONCENTRATION

Concentration denotes the amount of solute dissolved in a solvent. The concentration of a solution is most commonly expressed as **percent composition by mass, mole fraction, molarity, molality,** or **normality.**

1. **Percent Composition by Mass**

    The percent composition by mass (percent) of a solution is the mass of the solute divided by the mass of the solution (solute plus solvent), multiplied by 100.

    Example: What is the percent composition by mass of a salt wate solution if 100 g of the solution contains 20 g of NaCl?

    Solution:

    $$\frac{20 \text{ g NaCl}}{100 \text{ g}} \times 100 = 20\% \text{ NaCl solution}$$

2. **Mole Fraction**

    The mole fraction (**X**) of a compound is equal to the number of moles of the compound divided by the total number of moles of all species within the system. The sum of the mole fractions in a system will always equal 1.

    Example: If 92 g of glycerol is mixed with 90 g of water, what will be the mole fractions of the two components? (MW of $H_2O = 18$; MW of $C_3H_8O_3 = 92$.)

    Solution:

    $$90 \text{ g water} = 90 \text{ g} \times \frac{1 \text{ mol}}{18 \text{ g}} = 5 \text{ mol}$$

    $$92 \text{ g glycerol} = 92 \text{ g} \times \frac{1 \text{ mol}}{92 \text{ g}} = 1 \text{ mol}$$

    $$\text{Total mol} = 5 + 1 = 6 \text{ mol}$$

    $$X_{water} = \frac{5 \text{ mol}}{6 \text{ mol}} = .833$$

    $$X_{glycerol} = \frac{1 \text{ mol}}{6 \text{ mol}} = .167$$

    $$X_{water} + X_{glycerol} = .833 + .167 = 1.000$$

3. Molarity

The molarity (**M**) of a solution is the number of moles of solute per liter of **solution.** Solution concentrations are usually expressed in terms of molarity. Molarity depends on the volume of the solution, not on the volume of solvent used to prepare the solution.

Example: If enough water is added to 11 g of $CaCl_2$ to make 100 mL of solution, what is the molarity of the solution?

Solution:

$$\frac{11 \text{ g } CaCl_2}{110 \text{ g } CaCl_2/\text{mol } CaCl_2} = 0.10 \text{ mol } CaCl_2$$

$$100 \text{ mL} \times \frac{1L}{1,000 \text{ mL}} = 0.10 \text{ L}$$

$$\text{molarity} = \frac{0.10 \text{ mol}}{0.10 \text{ L}} = 1.0 \text{ M}$$

4. Molality

The molality (**m**) of a solution is the number of moles of solute per kilogram of **solvent.** For dilute aqueous solutions at 25°C the molality is approximately equal to the molarity, because the density of water at this temperature is 1 kilogram per liter. But note that this is an approximation and true only for **dilute aqueous** solutions.

Example: If 10 g of NaOH are dissolved in 500 g of water, what is the molality of the solution?

Solution:

$$\frac{10 \text{ g NaOH}}{40 \text{ g NaOH/mol NaOH}} = 0.25 \text{ mol NaOH}$$

$$500 \text{ g} \times \frac{1kg}{1,000 \text{ g}} = 0.50 \text{ kg}$$

$$\text{molality} = \frac{0.25 \text{ mol}}{0.50 \text{ kg}} = 0.50 \text{ mol/kg} = 0.50 \text{ m}$$

5. Normality

The normality (**N**) of a solution is equal to the number of gram equivalent weights of solute per liter of solution. A gram equivalent weight, or equivalent, is a measure of the reactive capacity of a molecule (see Chapter 4, Compounds and Stoichiometry).

To calculate the normality of a solution, we must know for what purpose the solution is being used, because it is the concentration of the reactive species with which we are concerned. Normality is unique among concentration units in that it is reaction dependent. For example, a 1 molar solution of sulfuric acid would be 2 normal for acid-base reactions (because each mole of sulfuric acid provides 2 moles of H^+ ions) but is only 1 normal for a sulfate precipitation reaction (because each mole of sulfuric acid only provides 1 mole of sulfate ions).

B. DILUTION

A solution is **diluted** when solvent is added to a solution of high concentration to produce a solution of lower concentration. The concentration of a solution after dilution can be conveniently determined using the equation below:

$$M_i V_i = M_f V_f$$

where M is molarity, V is volume, and the subscripts i and f refer to initial and final values, respectively.

> **MCAT Favorite**
>
> This equation is worthy of memorization. Note that it works for any units of concentration, not just molarity.

Example: How many mL of a 5.5 M NaOH solution must be used to prepare 300 mL of a 1.2 M NaOH solution?

Solution:

$$5.5\text{ M} \times V_i = 1.2\text{ M} \times 0.3\text{ L}$$

$$V_i = \frac{1.2\text{ M} \times 0.3\text{ L}}{5.5\text{ M}}$$

$$V_i = 0.065\text{ L} = 65\text{ mL}$$

SOLUTION EQUILIBRIA

The process of solvation, like other reversible chemical and physical changes, tends toward an equilibrium. Immediately after solute has been introduced into a solvent, most of the change taking place is dissociation, because no dissolved solute is initially present. However, according to Le Châtelier's principle, as solute dissociates, the reverse reaction (precipitation of the solute) also begins to occur. Eventually an equilibrium is reached, with the rate of solute dissociation equal to the rate of precipitation, and the net concentration of the dissociated solute remains unchanged regardless of the amount of solute added.

An ionic solid introduced into a polar solvent dissociates into its component ions. The dissociation of such a solute in solution may be represented by

$$A_m B_n\ (s) \rightleftharpoons mA^{n+}\ (aq) + nB^{m-}\ (aq)$$

A. THE SOLUBILITY PRODUCT CONSTANT

A slightly soluble ionic solid exists in equilibrium with its saturated solution. In the case of AgCl, for example, the solution equilibrium is as follows:

$$AgCl\ (s) \rightleftharpoons Ag^+\ (aq) + Cl^-\ (aq)$$

The **ion product, I.P.,** of a compound in solution is defined as follows:

$$I.P. = [A^{n+}]^m[B^{m-}]^n$$

The same expression for a saturated solution at equilibrium defines the **solubility product constant, K_{sp}.**

$$K_{sp} = [A^{n+}]^m[B^{m-}]^n \text{ in a saturated solution}$$

However, I.P. is defined with respect to initial concentrations and does not necessarily represent either an equilibrium or a saturated solution, while K_{sp} does; at any point other than at equilibrium, the ion product is often referred to as Q_{sp}.

Each salt has its own distinct K_{sp} at a given temperature. If at a given temperature a salt's I.P. is equal to its K_{sp}, the solution is saturated, and the rate at which the salt dissolves equals the rate at which it precipitates out of solution. If a salt's I.P. exceeds its K_{sp}, the solution is supersaturated (holding more salt than it should be able to at a given temperature) and unstable. If the supersaturated solution is disturbed by adding more salt, other solid particles, or jarring the solution by a sudden decrease in temperature, the solid salt will precipitate until I.P. equals the K_{sp}. If I.P. is less than K_{sp}, the solution is unsaturated and no precipitate will form.

> **MCAT Synopsis**
>
> If the solution is supersaturated, $Q_{sp} > K_{sp}$, precipitation will occur.
>
> If the solution is undersaturated $Q_{sp} < K_{sp}$, the solute will continue to dissolve.
>
> If the solution is saturated, $Q_{sp} = K_{sp}$, then the solution is at equilibrium.

Example: The solubility of $Fe(OH)_3$ in an aqueous solution was determined to be 4.5×10^{-10} mol/L. What is the value of the K_{sp} for $Fe(OH)_3$?

Solution: The molar solubility (the solubility of the compound in mol/L) is given as 4.5×10^{-10} M. The equilibrium concentration of each ion can be determined from the molar solubility and the balanced dissociation reaction of $Fe(OH)_3$. The dissociation reaction is:

$$Fe(OH)_3\ (s) \rightleftharpoons Fe^{3+}\ (aq) + 3OH^-\ (aq)$$

Thus, for every mol of $Fe(OH)_3$ that dissociates, one mol of Fe^{3+} and three mol of OH^- are produced. Since the solubility is 4.5×10^{-10} M, the K_{sp} can be determined as follows:

$$K_{sp} = [Fe^{3+}][OH^-]^3$$

$[OH^-] = 3[Fe^{3+}]; \qquad [Fe^{3+}] = 4.5 \times 10^{-10}$ M

$$K_{sp} = [Fe^{3+}](3[Fe^{3+}])^3 = 27[Fe^{3+}]^4$$

$$K_{sp} = (4.5 \times 10^{-10})[3(4.5 \times 10^{-10})]^3 = 27(4.5 \times 10^{-10})^4$$

$$K_{sp} = 1.1 \times 10^{-36}$$

> **MCAT Synopsis**
>
> Every slightly soluble salt of general formula MX_3 will have $K_{sp} = 27x^4$, where x is the molar solubility.

Example: What are the concentrations of each of the ions in a saturated solution of $PbBr_2$, given that the K_{sp} of $PbBr_2$ is 2.1×10^{-6}? If 5 g of $PbBr_2$ are dissolved in water to make 1 L of solution at 25°C, would the solution be saturated, unsaturated, or supersaturated?

Solution: The first step is to write out the dissociation reaction:

$$PbBr_2\ (s) \rightleftharpoons Pb^{2+}\ (aq) + 2Br^-\ (aq)$$

$$K_{sp} = [Pb^{2+}][Br^-]^2$$

Let x equal the concentration of Pb^{2+}. Then $2x$ equals the concentration of Br^- in the saturated solution at equilibrium (as $[Br^-]$ is 2 times $[Pb^{2+}]$).

$$(x)(2x)^2 = 4x^3$$

$$2.1 \times 10^{-6} = 4x^3$$

Solving for x, the concentration of Pb^{2+} in a saturated solution is 8.07×10^{-3} M and the concentration of Br^- ($2x$) is 1.61×10^{-2} M.

Next, we convert 5 g of $PbBr_2$ into moles:

$$5\ g \times \frac{1\ mol\ PbBr_2}{367\ g} = 1.36 \times 10^{-2}\ mol$$

> **MCAT Synopsis**
>
> Every slightly soluble salt of general formula MX_2 will have $K_{sp} = 4x^3$, where x is the molar solubility.

1.36×10^{-2} mol of $PbBr_2$ is dissolved in 1 L of solution, so the concentration of the solution 1.36×10^{-2} M. Since this is higher than the concentration of a saturated solution, this solution would be supersaturated.

B. FACTORS AFFECTING SOLUBILITY

The solubility of a substance varies depending on the temperature of the solution, the solvent, and, in the case of a gas-phase solute, the pressure. Solubility is also affected by the addition of other substances to the solution. The solubility of a salt is considerably reduced when it is dissolved in a solution that already contains one of its ions, rather than in a pure solvent. For example, if a salt such as CaF_2 is dissolved in a solution already containing Ca^{2+} ions, the dissociation equilibrium will shift toward the production of the solid salt. This reduction in solubility, called the **common ion effect**, is another example of Le Châtelier's principle.

Example: The K_{sp} of AgI in aqueous solution is 1×10^{-16} mol/L. If a 1×10^{-5} M solution of $AgNO_3$ is saturated with AgI, what will be the final concentration of the iodide ion?

Solution: The concentration of Ag^+ in the original $AgNO_3$ solution will be 1×10^{-5} mol/L. After AgI is added to saturation, the iodide concentration can be found by the formula:

$$1 \times 10^{-16} = [Ag^+][I^-]$$

$$= (1 \times 10^{-5})[I^-]$$

$$[I^-] = 1 \times 10^{-11} \text{ mol/L}$$

If the AgI had been dissolved in pure water, the concentration of both Ag^+ and I^- would have been 1×10^{-8} mol/L. The presence of the common ion, silver, at a concentration one thousand times higher than what it would normally be in a silver iodide solution, has reduced the iodide concentration to one thousandth of what it would have been otherwise. An additional 1×10^{-11} mol/L of silver will, of course, dissolve in solution along with the iodide ion, but this will not significantly affect the final silver concentration, which is much higher.

MCAT Synopsis

Every slightly soluble salt of general formula MX will have $K_{sp} = x^2$, where x is the molar solubility.

10

ACIDS AND BASES

Many important reactions in chemical and biological systems involve two classes of compounds called **acids** and **bases.** Acids and bases cause color changes in certain compounds called **indicators**, which may be in solution or on paper. A particular common indicator is litmus paper, which turns red in acidic solution and blue in basic solution. A more extensive discussion of the chemical properties of acids and bases is outlined below.

DEFINITIONS

A. ARRHENIUS DEFINITION

The first definitions of acids and bases were formulated by Svante Arrhenius toward the end of the 19th century. Arrhenius defined an acid as a species that produces H^+ (a proton) in an aqueous solution, and a base as a species that produces OH^- (a hydroxide ion) in an aqueous solution. These definitions, though useful, fail to describe acidic and basic behavior in nonaqueous media.

B. BRØNSTED-LOWRY DEFINITION

A more general definition of acids and bases was proposed independently by Johannes Brønsted and Thomas Lowry in 1923. A Brønsted-Lowry acid is a species that donates protons, while a Brønsted-Lowry base is a species that accepts protons. For example, NH_3 and Cl^- are both Brønsted-Lowry bases because they accept protons. However, they cannot be called Arrhenius bases since in aqueous solution they do not dissociate to form OH^-. The advantage of the Brønsted-Lowry concept of acids and bases is that it is not limited to aqueous solutions.

Brønsted-Lowry acids and bases always occur in pairs, called **conjugate acid-base pairs.** The two members of a conjugate pair are related by the transfer of a proton. For example, H_3O^+ is the conjugate acid of the base H_2O, and NO_2^- is the conjugate base of HNO_2.

$$H_3O^+ \ (aq) \ \rightleftarrows \ H_2O \ (aq) + H^+ \ (aq)$$

$$HNO_2 \ (aq) \ \rightleftarrows \ NO_2^- \ (aq) + H^+ \ (aq)$$

C. LEWIS DEFINITION

At approximately the same time as Brønsted and Lowry, Gilbert Lewis also proposed definitions of acids and bases. Lewis defined an acid as an electron-pair acceptor, and a base as an electron-pair donor. Lewis's are the most inclusive definitions. Just as every Arrhenius acid is a Brønsted-Lowry acid, every Brønsted-Lowry acid is also a Lewis acid (and likewise for bases). However, the Lewis definition encompasses some species not included within the Brønsted-Lowry definition. For example, BCl_3 and $AlCl_3$ can each accept an electron pair and are therefore Lewis acids, despite their inability to donate protons.

NOMENCLATURE OF ARRHENIUS ACIDS

The name of an acid is related to the name of the parent anion (the anion that combines with H^+ to form the acid). Acids formed from anions whose names end in -ide have the prefix **hydro-** and the ending -ic.

F^-	Fluoride	HF	Hydrofluoric acid
Br^-	Bromide	HBr	Hydrobromic acid

Acids formed from oxyanions are called **oxyacids**. If the anion ends in -ite (less oxygen), then the acid will end with **-ous acid.** If the anion ends in -ate (more oxygen), then the acid will end with **-ic acid.** Prefixes in the names of the anions are retained. Some examples:

ClO^-	Hypochlorite	HClO	Hypochlorous acid
ClO_2^-	Chlorite	$HClO_2$	Chlorous acid
ClO_3^-	Chlorate	$HClO_3$	Chloric acid
ClO_4^-	Perchlorate	$HClO_4$	Perchloric acid
NO_2^-	Nitrite	HNO_2	Nitrous acid
NO_3^-	Nitrate	HNO_3	Nitric acid

MCAT Synopsis

Some exceptions to the rules exist. For instance, MnO_{4-} is called permanganate even though there are no "manganate" or "manganite" ions.

PROPERTIES OF ACIDS AND BASES

A. HYDROGEN ION EQUILIBRIA (pH AND pOH)

Hydrogen ion concentration, $[H^+]$, is generally measured as **pH**, where:

$$pH = -\log[H^+] = \log(1/[H^+])$$

Likewise, hydroxide ion concentration, $[OH^-]$, is measured as **pOH** where:

$$pOH = -\log[OH^-] = \log(1/[OH^-])$$

In any aqueous solution, the H_2O solvent dissociates slightly:

$$H_2O(l) \rightleftarrows H^+(aq) + OH^-(aq)$$

This dissociation is an equilibrium reaction and is therefore described by a constant, K_w, **the water dissociation constant.**

$$K_w = [H^+][OH^-] = 10^{-14}$$

Rewriting this equation in logarithmic form gives:

$$pH + pOH = 14$$

In pure H_2O, $[H^+]$ is equal to $[OH^-]$, since for every mole of H_2O that dissociates, one mole of H^+ and one mole of OH^- are formed. A solution with equal concentrations of H^+ and OH^- is neutral, and has a pH of $7(-\log 10^{-7} = 7)$. A pH below 7 indicates a relative excess of H^+ ions, and therefore an acidic solution; a pH above 7 indicates a relative excess of OH^- ions, and therefore a basic solution.

Math Note: Estimating p-scale values

A useful skill for various problems involving acids and bases, as well as their corresponding buffer solutions, is the ability to quickly convert pH, pOH, pK_a, and pK_b into nonlogarithmic form and vice versa.

When the original value is a power of ten, the operation is relatively simple; changing the sign on the exponent gives the corresponding p-scale value directly. For example:

$$\text{If } [H+] = 0.001, \text{ or } 10^{-3}, \text{ then } pH = 3.$$

$$\text{If } K_b = 1.0 \times 10^{-7}, \text{ then } pK_b = 7.$$

> **MCAT Synopsis**
>
> Recall that a fundamental property of logarithms is that the log of a product is equal to the sum of the logs, i.e., $\log(xy) = \log x + \log y$.

> **MCAT Synopsis**
>
> Other important properties of logarithms include:
>
> $\log x^n = n\log x$, and $\log 10^x = x$. From these two properties one can derive the particularly useful relationship: $-\log 10^{-x} = x$.

MCAT PREMIER PROGRAM

More difficulty arises (in the absence of a calculator) when the original value is not an exact power of 10; exact calculation would be excessively onerous, but a simple method of approximation exists. If the nonlogarithmic value is written in proper scientific notation, it will look like: $n \times 10^{-m}$, where n is a number between 1 and 10. The log of this product can be written as: $\log(n \times 10^{-m}) = -m + \log n$, and the negative log is thus $m - \log n$. Now, since n is a number between 1 and 10, its logarithm will be a fraction between 0 and 1, thus $m - \log n$ will be between $m - 1$ and m. Further, the larger n is, the larger the fraction $\log n$ will be, and therefore the closer to $m - 1$ our answer will be.

Example: If $Ka = 1.8 \times 10^{-5}$, then $pKa = 5 - \log 1.8$. Since 1.8 is small, its log will be small, and the answer will be closer to 5 than to 4. (The actual answer is 4.74.)

B. STRONG ACIDS AND BASES

Strong acids and bases are those that completely dissociate into their component ions in aqueous solution. For example, when NaOH is added to water, it dissociates completely:

$$NaOH\ (s) + excess\ H_2O\ (l) \rightarrow Na^+\ (aq) + OH^-\ (aq)$$

Hence, in a 1 M solution of NaOH, complete dissociation gives 1 mole of OH^- ions per liter of solution.

$$pH = 14 - (-\log[OH^-]) = 14 + \log[1] = 14$$

Virtually no undissociated NaOH remains. Note that the $[OH^-]$ contributed by the dissociation of H_2O is considered to be negligible in this case. The contribution of OH^- and H^+ ions from the dissociation of H_2O can be neglected only if the concentration of the acid or base is greater than 10^{-7} M. For example, the pH of a 1×10^{-8} M HCl solution (HCl is a strong acid) might appear to be 8, since $[-\log (1 \times 10^{-8})] = 8$. However, a pH of 8 is in the basic pH range, and an HCl solution is not basic. The discrepancy arises from the fact that at low HCl concentrations, H^+ from the dissociation of water does contribute significantly to the total $[H^+]$. The $[H^+]$ from the dissociation of water is less than 1×10^{-7} M due to the common ion effect. The total concentration of H^+ can be calculated from

$K_w = (x + 1 \times 10^{-8})(x) = 1.0 \times 10^{-14}$, where $x = [H^+] = [OH^-]$ (both from the dissociation of water molecules).

390

Solving for x gives $x = 9.5 \times 10^{-8}$ M,

so $[H^+]_{total} = (9.5 \times 10^{-8} + 1 \times 10^{-8})$ M $= 1.05 \times 10^{-7}$ M

and pH $= -\log(1.05 \times 10^{-7}) = 6.98$, slightly less than 7, as should be expected for a very dilute, yet acidic solution.

Strong acids commonly encountered in the laboratory include $HClO_4$ (perchloric acid), HNO_3 (nitric acid), H_2SO_4 (sulfuric acid), and HCl (hydrochloric acid). Commonly encountered strong bases include NaOH (sodium hydroxide), KOH (potassium hydroxide), and other soluble hydroxides of Group IA and IIA metals. Calculation of the pH and pOH of strong acids and bases assumes complete dissociation of the acid or base in solution: $[H^+]$ = normality of strong acid and $[OH^-]$ = normality of strong base.

C. WEAK ACIDS AND BASES

Weak acids and bases are those that only partially dissociate in aqueous solution. A weak monoprotic acid, HA, in aqueous solution will achieve the following equilibrium after dissociation (H_3O^+ is equivalent to H^+ in aqueous solution.):

$$HA\ (aq) + H_2O\ (l) \rightleftharpoons H_3O^+\ (aq) + A^-\ (aq)$$

The **acid dissociation constant, K_a,** is a measure of the degree to which an acid dissociates.

$$K_a = \frac{[H_3O^+][A^-]}{[HA]}$$

The weaker the acid, the smaller the K_a. Note that K_a does not contain an expression for the pure liquid, water.

A weak monovalent base, BOH, undergoes dissociation to give B^+ and OH^-. The **base dissociation constant, K_b,** is a measure of the degree to which a base dissociates. The weaker the base, the smaller its K_b. For a monovalent base, K_b is defined as follows:

$$K_b = \frac{[B^+][OH^-]}{[BOH]}$$

A **conjugate acid** is defined as the acid formed when a base gains a proton. Similarly, a **conjugate base** is formed when an acid loses a proton. For example, in the HCO_3^-/CO_3^{2-} conjugate acid/base pair, CO_3^{2-} is the conjugate base and HCO_3^- is the conjugate acid:

$$HCO_3^- \ (aq) \rightleftarrows H^+ \ (aq) + CO_3^{2-} \ (aq)$$

To find the K_a of the conjugate acid HCO_3^-, the reaction with water must be considered.

$$HCO_3^- \ (aq) + H_2O \ (l) \rightleftarrows H_3O^+ \ (aq) + CO_3^{2-} \ (aq)$$

Likewise, for the K_b of CO_3^{2-}:

$$CO_3^{2-} \ (aq) + H_2O \ (l) \rightleftarrows HCO_3^- \ (aq) + OH^- \ (aq)$$

In a conjugate acid/base pair formed from a weak acid, the conjugate base is generally stronger than the conjugate acid. Thus, for HCO_3^- and CO_3^{2-}, the reaction of CO_3^{2-} (the conjugate base) in water to produce HCO_3^- (the conjugate acid) and OH^- occurs to a great extent (i.e., is more favorable) than the reverse reaction.

The equilibrium constants for these reactions are as follows:

$$K_a = \frac{\left[H^+ \right]\left[CO_3^{2-} \right]}{\left[HCO_3^- \right]} \text{ and } K_b = \frac{\left[HCO_3^- \right]\left[OH^- \right]}{\left[CO_3^{2-} \right]}$$

Adding the two reactions shows that the net reaction is simply the dissociation of water:

$$H_2O \ (l) \rightleftarrows H^+ \ (aq) + OH^- \ (aq)$$

The equilibrium constant for this net reaction is $K_w = [H^+][OH^-]$, which is the product of K_a and K_b. Thus, if the dissociation constant either for an acid or for its conjugate base is known, then the dissociation constant for the other can be determined, using the equation:

$$K_a \times K_b = K_w = 1 \times 10^{-14}$$

Thus K_a and K_b are inversely related. In other words, if K_a is large (the acid is strong), then K_b will be small (the conjugate base will be weak), and vice versa.

D. APPLICATIONS OF K_a AND K_b

To calculate the concentration of H^+ in a 2.0 M aqueous solution of acetic acid, CH_3COOH ($K_a = 1.8 \times 10^{-5}$), first write the equilibrium reaction:

$$CH_3COOH \ (aq) \ \rightleftarrows \ H^+ \ (aq) + CH_3COO^- \ (aq)$$

Next, write the expression for the acid dissociation constant:

$$K_a = \frac{\left[H^+\right]\left[CH_3COO^-\right]}{\left[CH_3COOH\right]} = 1.8 \times 10^{-5}$$

Since acetic acid is a weak acid, the concentration of CH_3COOH at equilibrium is equal to its initial concentration, 2.0 M, less the amount dissociated, x. Likewise $[H^+] = [CH_3COO^-] = x$, since each molecule of CH_3COOH dissociates into one H^+ ion and one CH_3COO^- ion. Thus, the equation can be rewritten as follows:

$$K_a = \frac{\left[x\right]\left[x\right]}{\left[2.0 - x\right]} = 1.8 \times 10^{-5}$$

We can approximate that $2.0 - x \approx 2.0$ since acetic acid is a weak acid, and only slightly dissociates in water. This simplifies the calculation of x:

$$K_a = \frac{\left[x\right]\left[x\right]}{\left[2.0\right]} = 1.8 \times 10^{-5}$$
$$x = 6.0 \times 10^{-3} M$$

The fact that [x] is so much less than the initial concentration of acetic acid (2.0 M) validates the approximation; otherwise, it would have been necessary to solve for x using the quadratic formula. (A rule of thumb is that the approximation is valid as long as x is less than 5 percent of the initial concentration.)

SALT FORMATION

Acids and bases may react with each other, forming a salt and (often, but not always) water, in what is termed a **neutralization reaction** (see chapter 4). For example,

$$HA + BOH \rightarrow BA + H_2O$$

The salt may precipitate out or remain ionized in solution, depending on its solubility and the amount produced. Neutralization reactions generally go to completion. The reverse reaction, in which the salt ions react with water to give back the acid or base, is known as **hydrolysis.**

Four combinations of strong and weak acids and bases are possible:

1. strong acid + strong base: e.g., $HCl + NaOH \rightarrow NaCl + H_2O$
2. strong acid + weak base: e.g., $HCl + NH_3 \rightarrow NH_4Cl$
3. weak acid + strong base: e.g., $HClO + NaOH \rightarrow NaClO + H_2O$
4. weak acid + weak base: e.g., $HClO + NH_3 \rightleftarrows NH_4ClO$

The products of a reaction between equal concentrations of a strong acid and a strong base are a salt and water. The acid and base neutralize each other, so the resulting solution is neutral (pH = 7), and the ions formed in the reaction do not react with water. The product of a reaction between a strong acid and a weak base is also a salt but usually no water is formed since weak bases are usually not hydroxides; however, in this case, the cation of the salt will react with the water solvent, reforming the weak base. This reaction constitutes hydrolysis. For example:

$$HCl\ (aq) + NH_3\ (aq) \rightleftarrows NH_4^+\ (aq) + Cl^-\ (aq) \quad \text{Reaction I}$$

$$NH_4^+\ (aq) + H_2O\ (aq) \rightleftarrows NH_3\ (aq) + H_3O^+\ (aq) \quad \text{Reaction II}$$

NH_4^+ is the conjugate acid of a weak base (NH_3), and is therefore stronger than the conjugate base (Cl^-) of the strong acid HCl. NH_4^+ will thus react with OH^-, reducing the concentration of OH^-. There will thus be an excess of H^+, which will lower the pH of the solution.

On the other hand, when a weak acid reacts with a strong base the solution is basic, due to the hydrolysis of the salt to reform the acid, with the concurrent formation of hydroxide ion from the hydrolyzed water molecules. The pH of a solution containing a weak acid and a weak base depends on the relative strengths of the reactants. For example, the acid HClO has a $K_a = 3.2 \times 10^{-8}$, and the base NH_3 has a $K_b = 1.8 \times 10^{-5}$. Thus an aqueous solution of HClO and NH_3 is basic since K_a for HClO is less than K_b for NH_3.

POLYVALENCE AND NORMALITY

The relative acidity or basicity of an aqueous solution is determined by the relative concentrations of **acid** and **base equivalents.** An acid equivalent is equal to one mole of H^+ (or H_3O^+) ions; a base equivalent is equal to one mole of OH^- ions. Some acids and bases are polyvalent, that is, each mole of the acid or base liberates more than one acid or base equivalent. For example, the diprotic acid H_2SO_4 undergoes the following dissociation in water:

$$H_2SO_4\ (aq) \rightarrow H^+\ (aq) + HSO_4^-\ (aq)$$

$$HSO_4^-\ (aq) \rightleftarrows H^+\ (aq) + SO_4^{2-}\ (aq)$$

One mole of H_2SO_4 can thus produce 2 acid equivalents (2 moles of H^+). The acidity or basicity of a solution depends upon the concentration of acidic or basic equivalents that can be liberated. The quantity of acidic or basic capacity is directly indicated by the solution's normality (see chapter 9, Solutions). Since each mole of H_3PO_4 can liberate 3 moles (equivalents) of H^+, a 2 M H_3PO_4 solution would be 6 N (6 normal).

Flashback

Remember gram equivalent weight from chapter 4?

Another useful measurement is equivalent weight. For example, the gram molecular weight of H_2SO_4 is 98 g/mol. Since each mole liberates 2 acid equivalents, the gram equivalent weight of H_2SO_4 would be $\frac{98}{2} = 49g$; that is, the dissociation of 49 g of H_2SO_4 would release one acid equivalent. Common polyvalent acids include H_2SO_4, H_3PO_4, and H_2CO_3.

AMPHOTERIC SPECIES

An **amphoteric**, or **amphiprotic**, species is one that can act either as an acid or a base, depending on its chemical environment. In the Brønsted—Lowry sense, an amphoteric species can either gain or lose a proton. Water is the most common example. When water reacts with a base, it behaves as an acid:

$$H_2O + B^- \rightleftarrows HB + OH^-$$

When water reacts with an acid, it behaves as a base:

$$HA + H_2O \rightleftarrows H_3O^+ + A^-$$

The partially dissociated conjugate base of a polyprotic acid is usually amphoteric (e.g., HSO_4^- can either gain an H^+ to form H_2SO_4, or lose an H^+ to form SO_4^{2-}). The hydroxides of certain metals, e.g., Al, Zn, Pb, and Cr, are also amphoteric. Furthermore, species that can act as either oxidizing or reducing agents (see chapter 11, Redox Reactions and Electrochemistry) are considered to be amphoteric as well, since by accepting or donating electron pairs they act as Lewis acids or bases, respectively.

TITRATION AND BUFFERS

Titration is a procedure used to determine the molarity of an acid or base. This is accomplished by reacting a known volume of a solution of unknown concentration with a known volume of a solution of known concentration. When the number of acid equivalents equals the number of base equivalents added, or vice versa, the **equivalence point** is reached. It is important to emphasize that, while a strong acid/strong base titration will have an equivalence point at pH 7, the equivalence point **need not** always occur at pH 7. Also, when titrating polyprotic acids or bases, there are several equivalence points, as each different acidic or basic species is titrated separately (see Polyprotic Acids and Bases later in this chapter).

The equivalence point in a titration is estimated in two common ways: either by using a graphical method, plotting the pH of the solution as a function of added titrant by using a **pH meter** (e.g. Figure 10.1 below), or by watching for a color change of an added **indicator**. Indicators are weak organic acids or bases that have different colors in their undissociated and dissociated states. Indicators are used in low concentrations and therefore do not significantly alter the equivalence point. The point at which the indicator actually changes color is not the equivalence point but is called the end point. If the titration is performed well, the volume difference (and therefore the error) between the end point and the equivalence point is usually small and may be corrected for, or ignored.

A. STRONG ACID AND STRONG BASE

Consider the titration of 10 mL of a 0.1 N solution of HCl with a 0.1 N solution of NaOH. Plotting the pH of the reaction solution versus the quantity of NaOH added gives the following curve:

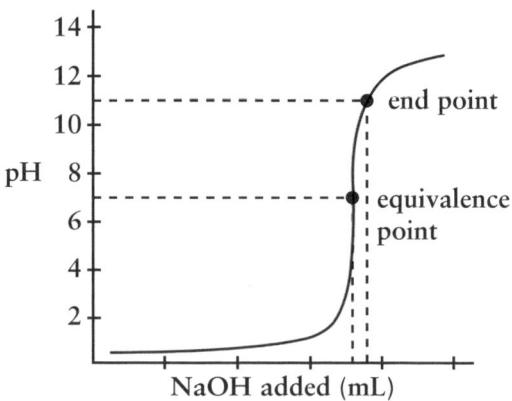

Figure 10.1. Titration of HCl with NaOH

Because HCl is a strong acid and NaOH is a strong base, the equivalence point of the titration will be at pH 7 and the solution will be neutral. Note that the endpoint shown is close to, but not exactly equal to, the equivalence point; selection of a better indicator, say one that changes colors at pH 8, would have given a better approximation.

In the early part of the curve (when little base has been added), the acidic species predominates, and so the addition of small amounts of base will not appreciably change either the [OH⁻] or the pH. Similarly, in the last part of the titration curve (when an excess of base has been added), the addition of small amounts of base will not change the [OH⁻] significantly, and the pH remains relatively constant. The addition of base most alters the concentrations of H^+ and OH^- near the equivalence point, and thus the pH changes most drastically in that region.

B. WEAK ACID AND STRONG BASE

Titration of a weak acid, HA, with a strong base produces the following titration curve:

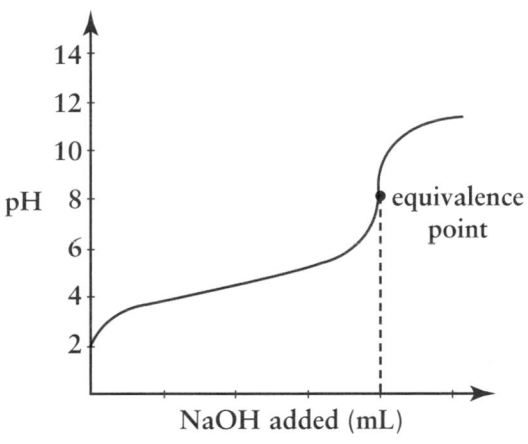

Figure 10.2. Titration of a Weak Acid, HA, with NaOH

Comparing Figure 10.2 with Figure 10.1 shows that the initial pH of the weak acid solution is greater than the initial pH of the strong acid solution. The pH changes most significantly early on in the titration, and the equivalence point is in the basic range.

C. BUFFERS

A **buffer solution** consists of a mixture of a weak acid and its salt (which consists of its conjugate base and a cation), or a mixture of a weak base and its salt (which consists of its conjugate acid and an anion). Two examples of buffers are: a solution of acetic acid (CH_3COOH) and its salt, sodium acetate ($CH_3COO^-Na^+$); and a solution of ammonia (NH_3) and its salt, ammonium chloride ($NH_4^+Cl^-$). Buffer solutions have the useful property of resisting changes in pH when small amounts of acid or base are added.

Consider a buffer solution of acetic acid and sodium acetate:

$$CH_3COOH \rightleftarrows H^+ + CH_3COO^-$$

When a small amount of NaOH is added to the buffer, the OH^- ions from the NaOH react with the H^+ ions present in the solution; subsequently, more acetic acid dissociates (equilibrium shifts to the right), restoring the $[H^+]$. Thus, an increase in $[OH^-]$ does not appreciably change pH. Likewise, when a small amount of HCl is added to the buffer, H^+ ions from the HCl react with the acetate ions to form acetic acid. Thus $[H^+]$ is kept relatively constant and the pH of the solution is relatively unchanged.

The **Henderson-Hasselbalch equation** is used to estimate the pH of a solution in the buffer region where the concentrations of the species and its conjugate are present in approximately equal concentrations. For a weak acid buffer solution:

$$pH = pK_a + \log \frac{[\text{conjugate base}]}{[\text{weak acid}]}$$

Note that when [conjugate base] = [weak acid] (in a titration, halfway to the equivalent point) the pH = pK_a because the log 1 = 0. Likewise, for a weak base buffer solution:

$$pOH = pK_b + \log \frac{[\text{conjugate acid}]}{[\text{weak base}]}$$

and pOH = pK_b when [conjugate acid] = [weak base].

MCAT Synopsis

The Henderson-Hasselbalch equation is also useful in the creation of buffer solutions other than those formed during the course of a titration. By careful selection of the weak acid (or base) and its salt, a buffer at almost any pH can be produced.

D. POLYPROTIC ACIDS AND BASES

The titration curve for a polyprotic acid or base looks different from that for a monoprotic acid or base. Figure 10.3 shows the titration of Na_2CO_3 with HCl in which the polyprotic acid H_2CO_3 is the ultimate product.

In region I, little acid has been added and the predominant species is CO_3^{2-}. In region II, more acid has been added and the predominant species are CO_3^{2-} and HCO_3^-, in relatively equal concentrations. The flat part of the curve is the first buffer region, corresponding to the pK_a of HCO_3^- ($K_a = 5.6 \times 10^{-11}$ implies $pK_a = 10.25$).

Region III contains the equivalence point, at which all of the CO_3^{2-} is titrated to HCO_3^-. As the curve illustrates, a rapid change in pH occurs at the equivalence point; in the latter part of region III, the predominant species is HCO_3^-.

In region IV, the acid has neutralized approximately half of the HCO_3^-, and now H_2CO_3 and HCO_3^- are in roughly equal concentrations. This flat region is the second buffer region of the titration curve, corresponding to the pK_a of H_2CO_3 ($K_a = 4.3 \times 10^{-7}$ implies $pK_a = 6.37$). In region V, the equivalence point for the entire titration is reached, as all of the HCO_3^- is converted to H_2CO_3. Again, a rapid change in pH is observed near the equivalence point as acid is added.

Clinical Correlate

Blood pH is maintained in a relatively small range (slightly above 7) by a bicarbonate buffer system. This homeostasis (see Biology chapter 10) can be upset, leading to a condition known as acidosis.

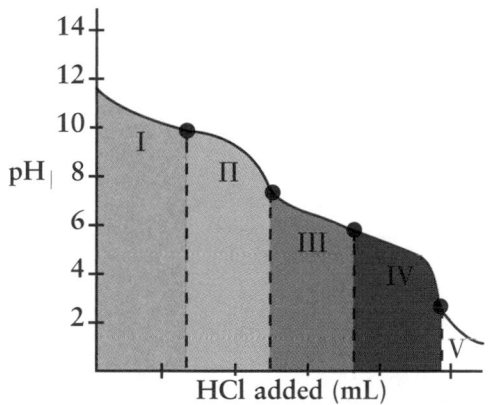

Figure 10.3. Titration of Na_2CO_3 with HCl

11

REDOX REACTIONS AND ELECTROCHEMISTRY

Electrochemistry is the study of the relationships between chemical reactions and electrical energy. **Electrochemical reactions** include spontaneous reactions that produce electrical energy, and nonspontaneous reactions that use electrical energy to produce a chemical change. Both types of reactions always involve a transfer of electrons with conservation of charge and mass.

OXIDATION-REDUCTION REACTIONS

A. OXIDATION AND REDUCTION

The law of conservation of charge states that an electrical charge can be neither created nor destroyed. Thus, an isolated loss or gain of electrons cannot occur; **oxidation** (loss of electrons) and **reduction** (gain of electrons) must occur simultaneously, resulting in an electron transfer called a **redox reaction**. An **oxidizing agent** causes another atom in a redox reaction to undergo oxidation, and is itself reduced. A **reducing agent** causes the other atom to be reduced, and is itself oxidized.

B. ASSIGNING OXIDATION NUMBERS

It is important, of course, to know which atom is oxidized and which is reduced. **Oxidation numbers** are assigned to atoms in order to keep track of the redistribution of electrons during a chemical reaction. From the oxidation numbers of the reactants and products, it is possible to determine how many electrons are gained or lost by each atom. The oxidation number of an atom in a compound is assigned according to the following rules:

1. **The oxidation number of free elements is zero.** For example, the atoms in N_2, P_4, S_8, and He all have oxidation numbers of zero.

2. **The oxidation number for a monatomic ion is equal to the charge of the ion.** For example, the oxidation numbers for Na^+, Cu^{2+}, Fe^{3+}, Cl^-, and N^{3-} are +1, +2, +3, −1, and −3, respectively.

> **KAPLAN) EXCLUSIVE**
>
> OIL RIG stands for "Oxidation Is Loss, Reduction Is Gain," of electrons that is.
>
> Alternatively, reduction is just what it sounds like: reduction of charge.

3. **The oxidation number of each Group IA element in a compound is +1. The oxidation number of each Group IIA element in a compound is +2.**

4. **The oxidation number of each Group VIIA element in a compound is –1, except when combined with an element of higher electronegativity.** For example, in HCl, the oxidation number of Cl is –1; in HOCl, however, the oxidation number of Cl is +1.

5. **The oxidation number of hydrogen is –1 in compounds with less electronegative elements than hydrogen (Groups IA and IIA.)** Examples include NaH and CaH_2. The more common oxidation number of hydrogen is +1.

6. **In most compounds, the oxidation number of oxygen is –2.** This is not the case, however, in molecules such as OF_2. Here, because F is more electronegative than O, the oxidation number of oxygen is +2. Also, in peroxides such as BaO_2, the oxidation number of O is –1 instead of –2 because of the structure of the peroxide ion, $[O–O]^{2-}$. (Note that Ba, a group IIA element, can not be a +4 cation.)

7. **The sum of the oxidation numbers of all the atoms present in a neutral compound is zero. The sum of the oxidation numbers of the atoms present in a polyatomic ion is equal to the charge of the ion.** Thus, for SO_4^{2-}, the sum of the oxidation numbers must be –2.

Example: Assign oxidation numbers to the atoms in the following reaction in order to determine the oxidized and reduced species and the oxidizing and reducing agents.

$$SnCl_2 + PbCl_4 \rightarrow SnCl_4 + PbCl_2$$

Solution: All these species are neutral, so the oxidation numbers of each compound must add up to zero. In $SnCl_2$, since there are two chlorines present, and chlorine has an oxidation number of –1, Sn must have an oxidation number of +2. Similarly, the oxidation number of Sn in $SnCl_4$ is +4; the oxidation number of Pb is +4 in $PbCl_4$ and +2 in $PbCl_2$. Notice that the oxidation number of Sn goes from +2 to +4; it loses electrons and thus is oxidized, making it the reducing agent. Since the oxidation number of Pb has decreased from +4 to +2, it has gained electrons and been reduced. Pb is the oxidizing agent. The sum of the charges on both sides of the reaction is equal to zero, so charge has been conserved.

C. BALANCING REDOX REACTIONS

By assigning oxidation numbers to the reactants and products, one can determine how many moles of each species are required for conservation of charge and mass, which is necessary to balance the equation. To balance a redox reaction, both the net charge and the number of atoms must be equal on both sides of the equation. The most common method for balancing redox equations is the **half-reaction method**, also known as the **ion-electron method**, in which the equation is separated into two half-reactions—the oxidation part and the reduction part. Each half-reaction is balanced separately, and they are then added to give a balanced overall reaction. Consider a redox reaction between $KMnO_4$ and HI in an acidic solution.

$$MnO_4^- + I^- \rightarrow I_2 + Mn^{2+}$$

Step 1: Separate the two half-reactions.

$$I^- \rightarrow I_2$$
$$MnO_4^- \rightarrow Mn^{2+}$$

Step 2: Balance the atoms of each half-reaction. First, balance all atoms except H and O. Next, in an acidic solution, add H_2O to balance the O atoms and then add H^+ to balance the H atoms. (In a basic solution, use OH^- and H_2O to balance the O's and H's.)

To balance the iodine atoms, place a coefficient of 2 before the I^- ion.

$$2 I^- \rightarrow I_2$$

For the permanganate half-reaction, Mn is already balanced. Next, balance the oxygens by adding $4H_2O$ to the right side.

$$MnO_4^- \rightarrow Mn^{2+} + 4H_2O$$

Finally, add H+ to the left side to balance the 4 H_2Os. These two half-reactions are now balanced.

$$MnO_4^- + 8 H^+ \rightarrow Mn^{2+} + 4H_2O$$

Step 3: Balance the charges of each half-reaction. The reduction half-reaction must consume the same number of electrons as are supplied by the oxidation half. For the oxidation reaction, add 2 electrons to the right side of the reaction:

$$2 I^- \rightarrow I_2 + 2e^-$$

For the reduction reaction, a charge of +2 must exist on both sides. Add 5 electrons to the left side of the reaction to accomplish this:

$$5 \text{ e}^- + 8 \text{ H}^+ + MnO_4^- \rightarrow Mn^{2+} + 4 \text{ H}_2O$$

Next, both half-reactions must have the same number of electrons so that they will cancel. Multiply the oxidation half by 5 and the reduction half by 2.

$$5(2I^- \rightarrow I_2 + 2e^-)$$
$$2(5e^- + 8H^+ + MnO_4^- \rightarrow Mn^{2+} + 4 \text{ H}_2O)$$

Step 4:   Add the half-reactions:

$$10 \text{ I}^- \rightarrow 5 \text{ I}_2 + 10 \text{ e}^-$$
$$16 \text{ H}^+ + 2 \text{ MnO}_4^- + 10 \text{ e}^- \rightarrow 2 \text{ Mn}^{2+} + 8 \text{ H}_2O$$

The final equation is:

$$10 \text{ I}^- + 10 \text{ e}^- + 16 \text{ H}^+ + 2 \text{ MnO}_4^- \rightarrow 5 \text{ I}_2 + 2 \text{ Mn}^{2+} + 10 \text{ e}^- + 8 \text{ H}_2O$$

To get the overall equation, cancel out the electrons and any H_2Os, H^+s, or OH^-s that appear on both sides of the equation.

$$10 \text{ I}^- + 16 \text{ H}^+ + 2 \text{ MnO}_4^- \rightarrow 5 \text{ I}_2 + 2 \text{ Mn}^{2+} + 8 \text{ H}_2O$$

Step 5:   Finally, confirm that mass and charge are balanced. There is a +4 net charge on each side of the reaction equation, and the atoms are stoichiometrically balanced.

ELECTROCHEMICAL CELLS

Electrochemical cells are contained systems in which a redox reaction occurs. There are two types of electrochemical cells, **galvanic cells** (also known as **voltaic cells**), and **electrolytic cells**. Spontaneous reactions occur in galvanic cells, and nonspontaneous reactions in electrolytic cells. Both types contain **electrodes** at which oxidation and reduction occur. For all electrochemical cells, the electrode at which oxidation occurs is called the **anode**, and the electrode where reduction occurs is called the **cathode.**

A. GALVANIC CELLS

A redox reaction occurring in a **galvanic cell** has a negative ΔG and is therefore a **spontaneous reaction**. Galvanic cell reactions supply energy and are used to do work. This energy can be harnessed by placing the oxidation and reduction half-reactions in separate containers called **half-cells**. The half-cells are then connected by an apparatus that allows for the flow of electrons.

A common example of a galvanic cell is the Daniell cell in Figure 11.1.

In the Daniell cell, a zinc bar is placed in an aqueous $ZnSO_4$ solution, and a copper bar is placed in an aqueous $CuSO_4$ solution. The anode of this cell is the zinc bar where Zn (s) is oxidized to Zn^{2+} (aq). The cathode is the copper bar, and it is the site of the reduction of Cu^{2+} (aq) to Cu (s). The half-cell reactions are written as follows:

$$Zn\ (s) \rightarrow Zn^{2+}\ (aq) + 2e^- \rightarrow (anode)$$
$$Cu^{2+}\ (aq) + 2e \rightarrow Cu\ (s) \rightarrow (cathode)$$

If the two-half cells were not separated, the Cu^{2+} ions would react directly with the zinc bar and no useful electrical work would be obtained. To complete the circuit, the two solutions must be connected. Without connection, the electrons from the zinc oxidation half reaction would not be able to get to the copper ions, thus a wire (or other conductor) is necessary. If only a wire were provided for this electron flow, the reaction would soon cease anyway because an excess negative charge would build up in the solution surrounding the cathode and an excess positive charge would build up in the solution surrounding the anode. This charge gradient is dissipated by the presence of a **salt bridge**, which permits the exchange of cations and anions. The salt bridge contains an inert electrolyte, usually KCl or NH_4NO_3, whose ions will not react with the electrodes or with the ions in solution. At the same

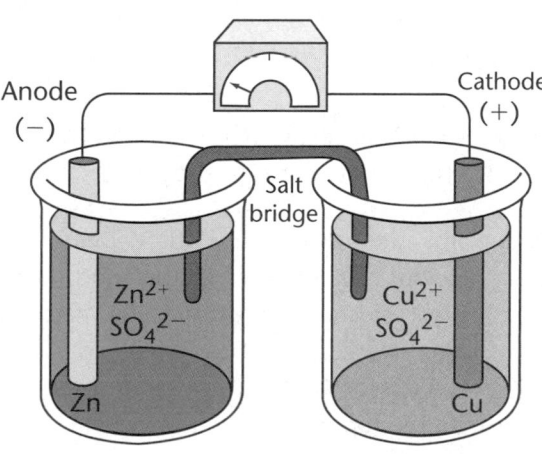

Figure 11.1: Daniell Cell

time the anions from the salt bridge (e.g., Cl^-) diffuse from the salt bridge of the Daniell cell into the $ZnSO_4$ solution to balance out the charge of the newly created Zn^{2+} ions, the cations of the salt bridge (e.g., K^+) flow into the $CuSO_4$ solution to balance out the charge of the SO_4^{2-} ions left in solution when the Cu^{2+} ions deposit as copper metal.

During the course of the reaction, electrons flow from the zinc bar (anode) through the wire and the voltmeter, toward the copper bar (cathode). The anions (Cl^-) flow externally (via the salt bridge) into the $ZnSO_4$, and the cations (K^+) flow into the $CuSO_4$. This flow depletes the salt bridge and, along with the finite quantity of Cu^{2+} in the solution, accounts for the relatively short lifetime of the cell.

A **cell diagram** is a shorthand notation representing the reactions in an electrochemical cell. A cell diagram for the Daniell cell is as follows:

$$Zn\ (s)\ \big|\ Zn^{2+}(x\text{M } SO_4^{2-})\ \big\|\ Cu^{2+}(y\text{M } SO_4^{2-})\ \big|\ Cu\ (s)$$

The following rules are used in constructing a cell diagram:

1. The reactants and products are always listed from left to right in the form:

$$\text{anode}\ \big|\ \text{anode solution}\ \big\|\ \text{cathode solution}\ \big|\ \text{cathode}$$

2. A single vertical line indicates a phase boundary.
3. A double vertical line indicates the presence of a salt bridge or some other type of barrier.

B. ELECTROLYTIC CELLS

A redox reaction occurring in an **electrolytic cell** has a positive ΔG and is therefore **nonspontaneous**. In **electrolysis**, electrical energy is required to induce reaction. The oxidation and reduction half-reactions are usually placed in one container.

An example of an electrolytic cell, in which molten NaCl is electrolyzed to form $Cl_2\ (g)$ and Na (l), is shown in Figure 11.2.

In this cell, Na^+ ions migrate towards the cathode, where they are reduced to Na (l). Similarly, Cl^- ions migrate towards the anode, where they are oxidized to $Cl_2\ (g)$. This cell is used in industry as the major means of sodium and chlorine production. Note that sodium is a liquid at the temperature of molten NaCl; it is also less dense than the molten salt, and thus is easily removed as it floats to the top of the reaction vessel.

> **Note**
>
> $(1.6 \times 10^{-19})(6.022 \times 10^{23})$
> $= 96,487$ C/mol e^-
>
> This number is called **Faraday's constant**, and one **Faraday (F)** is equivalent to the amount of charge contained in one mole of electrons (1 F = 96,487 coulombs, or J/V).

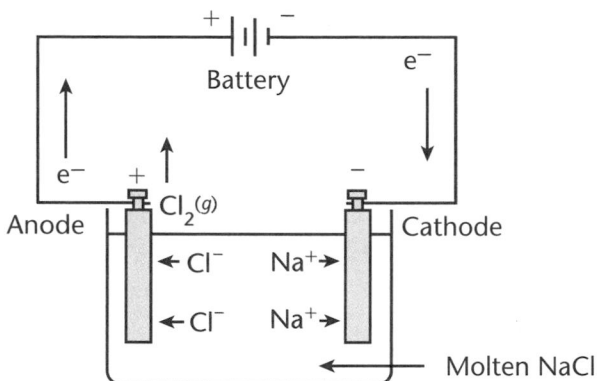

Figure 11.2: Example of an Electrolytic Cell

C. ELECTRODE CHARGE DESIGNATIONS

The anode of an **electrolytic cell** is considered **positive**, since it is attached to the positive pole of the battery and so attracts anions from the solution. The anode of a **galvanic cell**, on the other hand, is considered **negative** because the **spontaneous** oxidation reaction that takes place at the galvanic cell's anode is the original source of that cell's negative charge, i.e., is the source of electrons. In spite of this difference in designating charge, oxidation takes place at the anode in both types of cells, and electrons always flow through the wire from the anode to the cathode.

In a galvanic cell, charge is spontaneously created as electrons are released by the oxidizing species at the anode; since this is the source of electrons, the anode of a galvanic cell is considered the negative electrode.

In an electrolytic cell, electrons are forced through the cathode where they encounter the species that is to be reduced. Here it is the cathode that is providing electrons, and thus the cathode of an electrolytic cell is considered the negative electrode. Alternatively, one can think of the cathode as the electrode attached to the negative pole of the battery (or other power source) used for the electrolysis.

In either case, a simple mnemonic is that the CAThode attracts the CATions. In the Daniell Cell, for example, the electrons created at the anode as the zinc oxidizes travel through the wire to the copper half cell where they attract copper (II) cations to the cathode.

One common topic in which this distinction arises is electrophoresis, a technique often used to separate amino acids based on their isoelectronic points, or pIs (see Organic Chemistry chapter 12). The positively charged amino acids, i.e., those that are protonated at the pH of the solution, will

> **MCAT Synopsis**
>
> In an electrolytic cell, the anode is positive and the cathode is negative. In a galvanic cell, the anode is negative and the cathode is positive. However, in both types of cells, reduction occurs at the cathode and oxidation occurs at the anode.

migrate toward the cathode; negatively charged amino acids, i.e., those that are deprotonated at the solution pH, migrate instead toward the anode.

REDUCTION POTENTIALS AND THE ELECTROMOTIVE FORCE

A. REDUCTION POTENTIALS

Sometimes when electrolysis is carried out in an aqueous solution, water rather than the solute is oxidized or reduced. For example, if an aqueous solution of NaCl is electrolyzed, water may be reduced at the cathode to produce H_2 (g) and OH^- ions, instead of Na^+ being reduced to Na (s), as occurs in the absence of water. The species in a reaction that will be oxidized or reduced can be determined from the **reduction potential** of each species, defined as the tendency of a species to acquire electrons and be reduced. Each species has its own intrinsic reduction potential; the more positive the potential, the greater the species' tendency to be reduced.

A reduction potential is measured in volts (V) and is defined relative to the **standard hydrogen electrode (SHE)**, which is arbitrarily given a potential of 0.00 volts. **Standard reduction potential, ($E°$),** is measured under **standard conditions**: 25°C, a 1 M concentration for each ion participating in the reaction, a partial pressure of 1 atm for each gas that is part of the reaction, and metals in their pure state. The relative reactivities of different half-cells can be compared to predict the direction of electron flow. A higher or more positive $E°$ means a greater tendency for reduction to occur, while a lower $E°$ means a greater tendency for oxidation to occur.

Example: Given the following half-reactions and $E°$ values, determine which species would be oxidized and which would be reduced.

$Ag^+ + e \rightarrow Ag$ (s) $E° = +0.80$ V

$Tl^+ + e- \rightarrow Tl$ (s) $E° = -0.34$ V

Solution: Ag^+ would be reduced to Ag (s) and Tl (s) would be oxidized to Tl^+, since Ag^+ has the higher $E°$. Therefore, the reaction equation would be:

$Ag^+ + Tl$ (s) $\rightarrow Tl^+ + Ag$ (s)

which is the sum of the two spontaneous half-reactions.

It should be noted that reduction and oxidation are opposite processes. Therefore, in order to obtain the oxidation potential of a given half-reaction, the reduction half reaction and the sign of the reduction potential are both reversed. For instance, from the example above, the oxidation half reaction and oxidation potential of Tl (s) are:

$$Tl\ (s) \rightarrow Tl^+ + e^- \qquad E° = +0.34\ V$$

B. THE ELECTROMOTIVE FORCE

Standard reduction potentials are also used to calculate the **standard electromotive force (EMF or $E°_{cell}$)** of a reaction, the difference in potential between two half-cells. The EMF of a reaction is determined by adding the standard reduction potential of the reduced species and the standard oxidation potential of the oxidized species. When adding standard potentials, *do not* multiply by the number of moles oxidized or reduced.

$$EMF = E°_{red} + E°_{ox} \qquad \text{(Equation 1)}$$

The standard EMF of a galvanic cell is positive, while the standard EMF of an electrolytic cell is negative.

Example: Given that the standard reduction potentials for Sm^{3+} and $[RhCl_6]^{3-}$ are −2.41 V and +0.44 V respectively, calculate the EMF of the following reaction:

$$Sm^{3+} + Rh + 6\ Cl^- \rightarrow [RhCl_6]^{3-} + Sm$$

Solution: First, determine the oxidation and reduction half-reactions. As written, the Rh is oxidized and the Sm^{3+} is reduced. Thus the Sm^{3+} reduction potential is used as is, while the reverse reaction for Rh, $[RhCl_6]^{3-} \rightarrow Rh + 6\ Cl^-$, applies and the oxidation potential of $[RhCl_6]^{3-}$ must be used. Then, using Equation 1, the EMF can be calculated to be (−2.41 V) + (−0.44 V) = −2.85 V. The cell is thus electrolytic as written. From this result, it is evident that the reaction would proceed spontaneously to the left, in which case the Sm would be oxidized while $[RhCl_6]^{3-}$ would be reduced.

THERMODYNAMICS OF REDOX REACTIONS

A. EMF AND GIBBS FREE ENERGY

The thermodynamic criterion for determining the spontaneity of a reaction is ΔG, Gibbs free energy, the maximum amount of useful work produced by a chemical reaction. In an electrochemical cell, the work done

> Flashback
>
> Recall that if ΔG is positive, the reaction is not spontaneous; if ΔG is negative, the reaction is spontaneous.

is dependent on the number of coulombs and the energy available. Thus, ΔG and EMF are related as follows:

$$\Delta G = -nFE_{cell} \qquad \text{(Equation 2)}$$

where n is the number of moles of electrons exchanged, F is Faraday's constant, and E_{cell} is the EMF of the cell. **Keep in mind that if Faraday's constant is expressed in coulombs (J/V), then ΔG must be expressed in J, not kJ.**

If the reaction takes place under standard conditions (25°C, 1 atm pressure, and all solutions at 1M concentration), then the ΔG is the standard Gibbs free energy and E_{cell} is the standard cell potential. The above equation then becomes:

$$\Delta G° = -nFE°_{cell} \qquad \text{(Equation 3)}$$

B. THE EFFECT OF CONCENTRATION ON EMF

Thus far, only the calculations for the EMF of cells in unit concentrations (all the ionic species present have a molarity of 1 and all gases are at a pressure of 1 atm) have been discussed. However, concentration does have an effect on the EMF of a cell: EMF varies with the changing concentrations of the species involved. It can also be determined by the use of the **Nernst equation:**

$$E_{cell} = E°_{cell} - (RT/nF)(\ln Q)$$

Q is the reaction quotient for a given reaction. For example, in the following reaction:

$$a\,A + b\,B \rightarrow c\,C + d\,D$$

the reaction quotient would be:

$$Q = \frac{[C]^c[D]^d}{[A]^a[B]^b}$$

The EMF of a cell can be measured by a **voltmeter**. A **potentiometer is** a kind of voltmeter that draws no current, and gives a more accurate reading of the difference in potential between two electrodes.

C. EMF AND THE EQUILIBRIUM CONSTANT (K_{eq})

For reactions in solution, $\Delta G°$ can be determined in another manner, as follows:

$$\Delta G° = -RT \ln K_{eq} \qquad \text{(Equation 4)}$$

where R is the gas constant 8.314 J/(K•mol), T is the temperature in K, and K_{eq} is the equilibrium constant for the reaction.

If Equations 3 and 4 are combined, then:

$$\Delta G° = -nFE°_{cell} = -RT \ln K_{eq}$$

or simply:

$$nFE°_{cell} = RT \ln K_{eq} \qquad \text{(Equation 5)}$$

If the values for n, T, and K_{eq} are known, then the $E°_{cell}$ for the redox reaction can be readily calculated.

> **MCAT Synopsis**
>
> If $E°_{cell}$ is positive, then ln K is positive. This means that K must be greater than one, and that the equilibrium must lie toward the right, i.e., products are favored.

General Chemistry
Practice Set

Use this practice set to evaluate your mastery of the general chemistry section of the test.

Read the explanations to all the practice problems, and revisit the chapters that relate to weak areas.

Good luck.

General Chemistry Practice Set

Passage 1 (Questions 1–4)

One of the first attempts at quantitative analysis of organic materials was made by Lavoisier in the late 1700s while he was investigating combustion. After carefully measuring the weight of a sample of charcoal and allowing it to combust in the presence of a known volume of oxygen, he was able to determine the percent composition of the charcoal by measuring the amounts of CO_2 and H_2O produced. He then tested a number of other organic materials in the same fashion.

A generalized design for a combustion apparatus that might be used today is illustrated in the figure below. A sample of an unknown compound is placed in a furnace. Oxygen flows past the sample and through the apparatus. The combustion products, H_2O and CO_2, flow out of the furnace along with the excess oxygen, and are absorbed by magnesium perchlorate and sodium hydroxide, respectively. The figure below shows these absorbing compounds in sections of tube that are arranged in series with the furnace chamber.

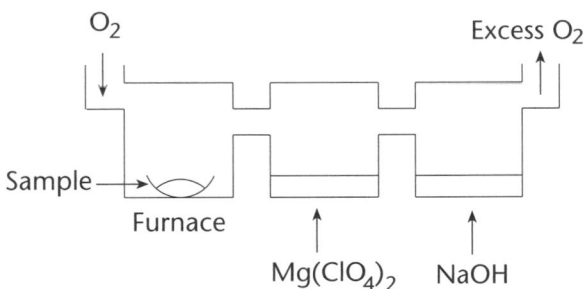

Table 1 gives the results of combusting 3.0 g of an unknown organic compound in an apparatus similar to the one shown above.

Table 1

Absorbing species	Initial weight	Final weight
$Mg(ClO_4)_2$	25.7 g	27.5 g
NaOH	22.0 g	26.4 g

1. How many moles of CO_2 are produced by combustion of the unknown compound?

   A. 0.10
   B. 0.17
   C. 0.20
   D. 2.00

2. In the perchlorate ion, shown below, where is the negative charge predominantly located?

$$\left[\begin{array}{c} :\!\overset{\displaystyle ..}{O}\!: \\ | \\ \overset{..}{\underset{..}{O}}\!=\!Cl\!=\!\overset{..}{\underset{..}{O}} \\ \| \\ :\!\overset{..}{O}\!: \end{array} \right]^{-}$$

   A. On the chlorine atom
   B. On the oxygen atom shown at the top of the diagram
   C. Distributed evenly among the four oxygen atoms
   D. Distributed evenly among all five atoms

3. The equation for the absorption of CO_2 by NaOH in the furnace chamber is:

$$NaOH + CO_2 \rightarrow NaHCO_3$$

   Which of the following formulas could be used to find the percentage of NaOH converted to $NaHCO_3$?

   A. $\dfrac{(\text{grams } CO_2 \text{ absorbed})(100)}{(\text{molar mass } CO_2)(\text{initial moles NaOH})}$

   B. $\dfrac{(\text{grams } CO_2 \text{ absorbed})(100)}{(\text{molar mass } CO_2)(\text{initial grams NaOH})}$

   C. $\dfrac{(\text{grams } CO_2 \text{ absorbed})(100)}{(\text{molar mass } NAHCO_3)(\text{initial grams NaOH})}$

   D. $\dfrac{(\text{grams } CO_2 \text{ absorbed})(100)}{(\text{molar mass } NAHCO_3)(\text{initial moles NaOH})}$

4. When the procedure described in the passage is used to analyze an unknown hydrocarbon, which of the following can always be determined?

   A. The empirical formula only
   B. The molecular formula only
   C. Both the empirical and molecular formulas
   D. Neither the empirical nor the molecular formula

Questions 5 through 7 are NOT based on a descriptive passage.

5. Despite the fact that they are both triatomic, BeF_2 is linear and SO_2 is bent. Which of the following explains the difference between the geometries of these molecules?

   A. Be has lone electron pairs while S does not.
   B. S has lone electron pairs while Be does not.
   C. Be is sp hybridized while S is sp^3 hybridized.
   D. S is sp hybridized while Be is sp^3 hybridized.

6. How will the reaction rate at equilibrium be affected if a catalyst is added to the system?

   A. Both the forward and reverse rates increase until the catalyst is consumed.
   B. Both the forward and reverse rates increase although no net change in product or reactant concentration is observed.
   C. Neither the forward nor reverse rate changes since catalysts do not affect the equilibrium of a reaction.
   D. Neither the forward nor reverse rate changes because the product and reactant concentrations change inversely with the rate constants.

7. Three balloons are filled with three different gases so that they are equal in volume at 80°C. The temperature is then decreased to 0°C, and the volume and mass of the contents of each balloon are recorded. Which of the following statements correctly describes the results?

   A. The contents will be equal in both mass and volume.
   B. The contents will be equal in mass but will differ in volume.
   C. The contents will differ in mass but will be equal in volume.
   D. The contents will differ in both mass and volume.

Passage II (Questions 8–14)

Acid/base indicators are used to detect the equivalence points in titration procedures. Indicators, which are weak organic acids or bases, change color in the vicinity of their equivalence points. A weak organic acid indicator will dissociate according to the following reaction:

$$HInd \rightleftarrows H^+ + Ind^-$$

Reaction 1

The undissociated and dissociated forms are referred to, respectively, as the "acidic" and "basic" forms of the indicator. Since these forms have different colors, the color change allows a chemist to localize the equivalence point. The dissociation constant of the acidic form can be expressed by the following equation:

$$K_a = \frac{[H^+][Ind^-]}{[H\,Ind]}$$

Equation 1

and the relationship between the concentrations of the dissociated and undissociated forms is therefore:

$$\frac{[Ind^-]}{[HInd]} = \frac{K_a}{[H^+]}$$

Equation 2

For a given indicator, the ratio $[Ind^-]/[HInd]$ depends only on the pH, since K_a is a constant. Since the equivalence point is characterized by a very sharp pH change, the color of the indicator solution changes rapidly when the pH reaches the equivalence point.

Table 1 lists some widely used indicators and the pH ranges at which each one undergoes transformation from its acidic to its basic form and vice versa.

Table 1

Indicator	Effective pH range	Color change (acid $\rightleftarrows$ base)
Methyl orange	3.2–4.4	Red $\rightleftarrows$ Yellow
Bromocresol green	4.0–5.6	Yellow $\rightleftarrows$ Blue
Bromothynol blue	6.0–7.6	Yellow $\rightleftarrows$ Blue
Phenolphthalein	8.2–10.0	Colorless $\rightleftarrows$ Pink
Thymolphthelein	9.3–10.5	Colorless $\rightleftarrows$ Blue

8. Based on the passage, which of the following are true?

   I. $K_a(HInd) < K_a(HCl)$
  II. $pK_a(HInd) > pK_a(HCl)$
 III. $pK_a(HInd) < pK_a(HCl)$
 IV. $pK_b(Ind-) < pK_b(Cl^-)$

  A. I and II only
  B. I and III only
  C. II and IV only
  D. I, II, and IV only

9. A dilute solution of Ind^-Na^+ is likely to be:

  A. acidic.
  B. basic.
  C. neutral.
  D. Cannot be detemined.

10. Given that the $K_a(HInd) = 10^{-8}$, the equivalence point on the titration below corresponds to what sort of change in the $[Ind^-]/[HInd]$ ratio?

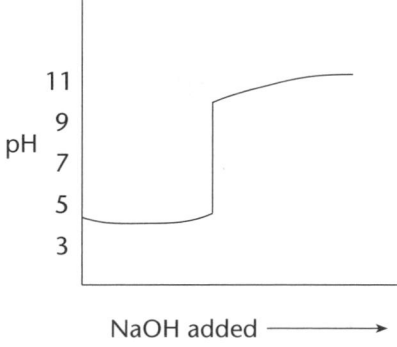

  A. A 1,000-fold increase
  B. A 1,000-fold decrease
  C. A 100,000-fold increase
  D. A 100,000-fold decrease

11. Phenolphthalein is a poor indicator for the titration of an ammonia solution with HCl described by the graph below. This is because its effective pH range coincides with:

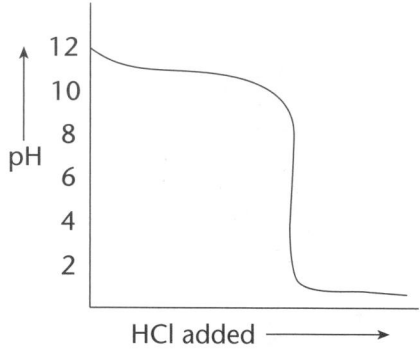

HCl added ⟶

A. the region in which $[Cl^-]/[HCl]$ is low.
B. the region in which $[NH_3]/[NH_4^+]$ is high.
C. the region in which $[NH_3]/[NH_4^+]$ is low.
D. the region in which $[NH_3][NH_4^+]$ is close to 1.

12. Hydrogen sulfide has a pK_{a1} of 7 and a pK_{a2} of 13. What will be the concentration of S^{2-} in a 1 M solution of H_2S when the pH of the solution is 7?

A. 0
B. 1×10^{-13}
C. 5×10^{-7}
D. 1×10^{-6}

13. For the titration of sodium acetate with HCl, which of the following equations holds true as the reaction proceeds toward the equivalence point?

A. $pOH = -log[CH_3COOH]$
B. $pOH = -log[CH_3COO^-]$
C. $pOH = pK_a(CH_3COOH) + log([CH_3COO^-]/[CH_3COOH])$
D. $pOH = pK_b(CH_3COO^-) + log([CH_3COOH]/[CH_3COO^-])$

14. The second dissociation constant of H_2SO_4 is 1.2×10^{-2} mol/L. What are the most likely concentrations of H_2SO_4, HSO_4^-, and SO_4^{2-} in a 0.1 M solution of H_2SO_4?

A. 0.00 M H_2SO_4, 0.09 M HSO_4^-, 0.01 M SO_4^{2-}
B. 0.00 M H_2SO_4, 0.02 M HSO_4^-, 0.08 M SO_4^{2-}
C. 0.01 M H_2SO_4, 0.06 M HSO_4^-, 0.03 M SO_4^{2-}
D. 0.033 M H_2SO_4, 0.033 M HSO_4^-, 0.033 M SO_4^{2-}

Passage III (Questions 15–19)

By the late 1860s, researchers had noticed patterns in the properties of some of the known chemical elements. In 1869, Dmitri Mendeleev arranged the known elements into a table with several columns in order of increasing atomic weight and found that similarities in elements' properties correlated with their positions in the table. He used this table to predict the properties of elements that had yet to be discovered; many of his predictions have proved quite accurate. It was found that an element's place in the periodic table correlates with the electronic structure of its valence shell. In a modern periodic table, each element shares some chemical properties with other elements in the same column.

- The alkali metals in Column 1 are able to decompose water, and may also react with oxygen in the air; they are therefore usually stored under mineral oil.
- The alkaline earth metals of Column 2 are less reactive, but do form oxides or nitrides when exposed to air.
- The transition elements in Columns 3−12 are related in electronic structure but nonetheless show considerable variation between columns. Silver and gold are the least reactive of the transition metals in their respective periods.
- The rare earth elements, listed below the table, form two sets, each with similar properties: the lanthanide elements are found in nature, but the actinides, to the right of uranium, are synthetic.
- The elements in Columns 13−16 include several of the most common on the earth's surface. Half

these elements are nonmetals; metallic characteristics increase toward the bottom left of this part of the table. Some, such as phosphorus and sulfur, occur in multiple forms, known as allotropes, that have different physical and chemical properties.

- The halogens in Column 17 are reactive nonmetals; fluorine and chlorine are gaseous, bromine is liquid, and iodine is solid under standard conditions.
- The noble gases in Column 18 do not normally ionize and are so unreactive that nineteenth-century scientists were unaware that they even existed.

15. How many valence electrons are present in the elements in Column 13?

A. 1
B. 3
C. 13
D. The number depends on the particular element.

16. The passage suggests that the least reactive transition metal in Period 4 should be:

A. K.
B. Mn.
C. Cu.
D. Zn.

17. Based on information in the passage, which of the following is most likely true of selenium (Se, 34)?

A. It is a common element that occurs as an oxide in most igneous rocks.
B. Under standard conditions, it is a dense liquid.
C. It is a metal that burns spontaneously in air.
D. It occurs in several allotropic forms.

18. Which of the following elements has the highest second ionization energy?

A. Cl
B. Ar
C. K
D. Ca

19. What is the chief difference between the ordering of elements in Mendeleev's periodic table and the modern periodic table?

A. Mendeleev did not make space in his periodic table for undiscovered elements.
B. Mendeleev left out the noble gases.
C. Recalculations of atomic weight using modern equipment have been used to reorder Mendeleev's table.
D. The modern table is ordered by increasing atomic number which does not follow exactly with increasing atomic weight.

Questions 20 and 21 are NOT based on a descriptive passage.

20. The pH of a solution of $CH_3COO^-Na^+$ was found to rise as the solution was gently heated. Which of the following best explains this observation?

A. The evaporation of acetic acid increases with temperature.
B. Sodium acetate is more soluble at lower temperatures.
C. The hydrolysis of sodium acetate is an exothermic process.
D. The hydrolysis of sodium acetate is a nonspontaneous process.

21. Hg_2Cl_2 is usually stored in amber colored bottles, because, when it is exposed to light, it slowly decomposes by the following reaction:

$$Hg_2Cl_2 \xrightarrow{h\nu} HgCl_2 + Hg\ (l)$$

This reaction is:

I. a single displacement reaction.
II. a double displacement reaction.
III. a disproportionation reaction.
IV. endothermic.

A. I only
B. II only
C. I and IV only
D. III and IV only

Passage IV (Questions 22–26)

The extent to which a liquid vaporizes—that is, the position of the equilibrium between the liquid and its vapor—depends on the strength of its intermolecular forces. The behavior of a mixture of liquids in equilibrium with their vapors can be described by two laws, named after the scientists who first proposed them. Dalton's law states that the total pressure of a mixture of gases is given by the sum of the partial pressures of the component gases, or:

$$P = P_A + P_B + P_C + \ldots$$

Equation 1

where P is the total pressure and P_x is the partial pressure of component X. The partial pressure of one component in a mixture of gases is defined as the pressure that would be exerted by the same amount of gas if it were the only one present in the same volume. Raoult's law predicts that where the gases are in equilibrium with their liquid forms, the partial pressure of each one will be equal to its mole fraction in solution multiplied by the vapor pressure of the pure liquid, or:

$$P = (X_A \times P_A^{\circ}) + P_B$$

Equation 2

where X_A is the mole fraction of component A and P_A° is the vapor pressure of pure A. The following experiment was designed to test the accuracy of these laws for acetone, n-pentane, and chloroform, using the apparatus shown in Figure 1.

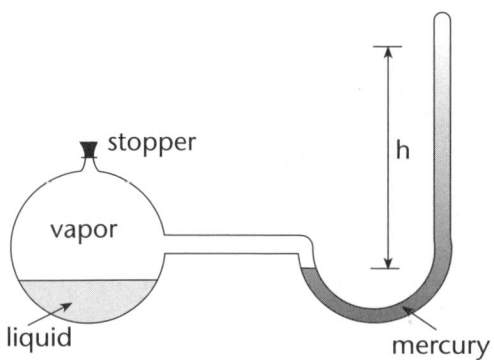

Figure 1

The experiment was designed to measure the vapor pressures of the three pure liquids and of a series of chloroform/acetone and n-pentane/acetone mixtures. For each measurement, all air was removed so that the flask contained only the liquid sample and vapor produced by the sample. Once the mercury stabilized, indicating that the system had come to equilibrium, the difference in the heights of the two columns, h, was read from the apparatus, giving the vapor pressure in mm Hg. The results are shown in Figure 2.

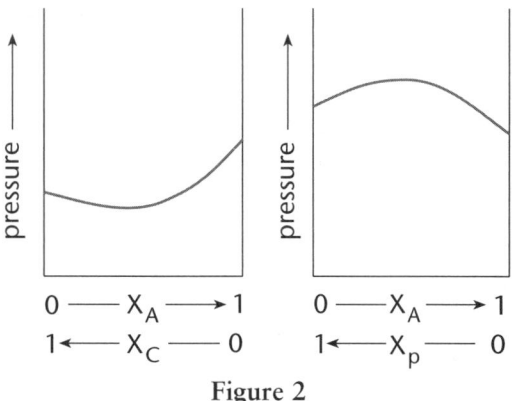

Figure 2

X_A = mole fraction of acetone
X_C = mole fraction of chloroform
X_P = mole fraction of n-pentane

22. Acetone has a lower vapor pressure than pure n-pentane at the same temperature because:

 A. the carbon-oxygen bond is weaker than the carbon-hydrogen bond.
 B. acetone has a lower molecular weight and therefore is more easily vaporized.
 C. n-pentane is more strongly hydrogen-bonded.
 D. acetone is polar and therefore has stronger intermolecular attractions.

23. Which of the following diagrams shows the variation of vapor pressure with composition that would be predicted by Dalton's and Raoult's laws for a mixture of chloroform and acetone?

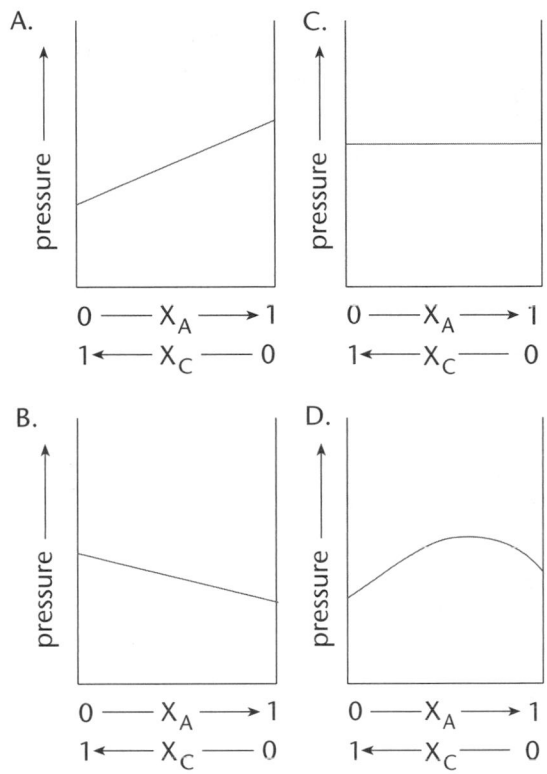

24. Which of the following is the best explanation of the divergence of the experimental data from the results predicted by Dalton's and Raoult's laws?

A. There are differences in the amount of attraction between molecules in the liquid.
B. There are differences in the amount of attraction between molecules in the vapor.
C. The compound with a higher molecular weight has a lower mole fraction near the surface.
D. Mixing the two liquids causes a change in temperature.

25. To get an accurate value for the mixture's vapor pressure using the apparatus in Figure 1, which of the following must be true?

A. The vapors must obey the ideal gas law.
B. The mercury must exert no measurable vapor pressure.
C. The width of the tube must be the same each time the experiment is performed.
D. Other gases must be excluded from the flask.

26. When n-pentane (density 0.63 g/mL) and water are mixed, they separate into two phases, each consisting of one compound with a very small amount of the other compound dissolved in it. Which of the following would be the most likely result if various mole fractions of these two compounds were mixed and the resulting vapor pressures graphed?

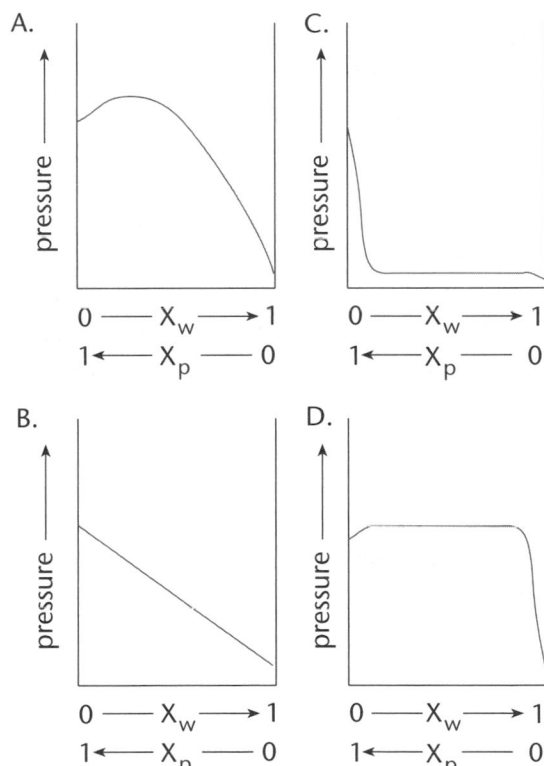

Chlorosis is a plant disease in which the leaves contain insufficient chlorophyll. It is caused by a plant's inability to absorb adequate quantities of certain micronutrients, particularly iron, and develops most frequently in plants such as rhododendrons that require high levels of soluble iron in the soil. Unfortunately, adding iron to the soil usually does not cure chlorosis; iron is usually present in sufficient quantities, but in forms that make it unavailable to plants. Instead, conditions must be created that will allow iron to be converted into an available form.

Because many of the reactions of iron in soil include protons or hydroxide ions as reactants or products, the reduction potentials of these reactions vary with pH. Moreover, since many half-reactions occur simultaneously in soil, the spontaneity of a particular half-reaction depends on the net reduction potential of the soil solution rather than on the potential of another single half-reaction. In a soil whose pH and reduction potential are sufficiently high, Fe^{2+} iron is oxidized to form ferric oxides and hydroxides, which are unavailable to plants. In its reduced, ferrous form, iron remains dissociated in the pH ranges commonly found in soil and is thus available to plants. Well-aerated soils have high reduction potentials, and thus may have little available iron. Increased soil wetness decreases both pH and soil reduction potential, making iron more available; ground water is more reducing than rain water because its oxygen content is lower. Iron availability is also affected by movement within the water table, which may remove reduced iron from a particular area. On higher ground, a temporary water table may form after rain under certain conditions; iron may then migrate, and accumulate and oxidize in other areas as the soil dries.

Table 1 shows the pH values above which each of three half-reactions proceeds to the right for the given net soil reduction potentials.

Table 1

Soil reduction potential (V)	pH range in which the reaction product predominates*		
	$Fe^{2+}\rightarrow$ $Fe(OH)_3$	$Fe^{2+}\rightarrow$ $Fe(OH)_2$	$Fe(OH)_2\rightarrow$ $Fe(OH)_3$
+0.3	>4.5	---	---
+0.2	>5.1	---	---
+0.1	>5.6	---	---
0.0	>6.2	---	---
−0.1	>6.7	---	---
−0.2	---	>7.0	>8.0
−0.3	---	>7.0	>9.7

*Values are for an Fe^{2+} concentration of 0.005 M, with O_2 at its atmospheric partial pressure of 0.21 atm.

27. Which of the following chemicals is most likely to cure chlorosis in rhododendrons growing in well-drained soil?

  A. $CaCO_3$
  B. Fe_2O_3
  C. $Fe(OH)_2$
  D. $(NH_4)_2SO_4$

28. Under which of the following conditions are vulnerable plants most likely to be harmed by exposure to *too much* soluble iron?

  A. On a hilltop in a rainforest
  B. On a flat lowland during a wet period
  C. On a flat lowland during a drought
  D. On a well-drained highland just after a rain

29. For the reaction

$$Fe(OH)_2 \rightleftarrows Fe^{2+} + 2\ OH^-$$

the table lists the same pH range for two different soil reduction potentials. This indicates that:

  A. the soil pH does not affect the reaction.
  B. the soil reduction potential does not affect the reaction.
  C. neither soil pH nor soil reduction potential affects the reaction.
  D. both soil pH and soil reduction potential affect the reaction, but the changes are not correlated.

30. Based on the passage, what effect does water from subterranean sources have on the oxidation state of iron in soil?

   A. It decreases the reduction potential of the soil solution, so iron is reduced.
   B. It decreases the reduction potential of the soil solution, so iron is oxidized.
   C. It increases the reduction potential of the soil solution, so iron is reduced.
   D. It increases the reduction potential of the soil solution, so iron is oxidized.

31. Which of the following equations could be used to calculate the values in Table 1?

   A. $E = A/[(1/n_2)^2 - (1/n_1)^2]$
   B. $E° = -\Delta G°/nF$
   C. $E = E° - (2.3RT/nF)(\log Q)$
   D. $E_h = h^2/4\pi m_c a_o^2$

Questions 32 through 34 are NOT based on a descriptive passage.

32. The following is the rate expression for a certain reaction:

$$rate = k[A][B]$$

   What is the rate expression for this reaction if a catalyst is added?

   A. $rate = k[A][B][catalyst]$
   B. $rate = k[A][B]/[catalyst]$
   C. $rate = k_c[A][B]$ where $k_c > k$
   D. $rate = k_c[A][B]$ where $k_c < k$

33. Which of the following describes the energy change that takes place when a bond is formed between two atoms?

   A. ΔH is positive, because energy is absorbed.
   B. ΔH is positive, because energy is released.
   C. ΔH is negative, because energy is absorbed.
   D. ΔH is negative, because energy is released.

34. Which of the following is NOT true of an element that is very highly electronegative?

   A. Its electron affinity is likely to be near zero.
   B. It is likely to have a high ionization energy.
   C. It is likely to have a small atomic radius.
   D. It is likely to be located in the upper right hand corner of the periodic table.

General Chemistry Practice Set:
Answers and Explanations

ANSWER KEY

1. A	10. C	19. D	27. D
2. C	11. D	20. A	28. B
3. A	12. C	21. D	29. B
4. A	13. D	22. D	30. A
5. B	14. A	23. A	31. C
6. B	15. B	24. A	32. C
7. C	16. C	25. D	33. D
8. D	17. D	26. D	34. A
9. B	18. C		

EXPLANATIONS

Passage I (Questions 1–4)

1. A The passage states that CO_2 produced by the combustion process is absorbed by the NaOH. You may remember that carbon dioxide and sodium hydroxide combine to form sodium bicarbonate, but you don't need to know that to answer the question. What is important is that, as the table shows, the weight of the NaOH sample increases by 4.4 grams during the course of the experiment; this means that 4.4 grams of carbon dioxide have been absorbed. You can determine easily, using the periodic table, that a mole of carbon dioxide weighs 44 grams: 12 grams for a mole of carbon plus 32 grams for the two moles of oxygen contained in a single mole of CO_2. So 4.4 grams of CO_2 is 0.1 moles, and choice (A) is correct.

2. C To answer this, you first have to figure out the relative electronegativities of oxygen and chlorine. You can remember that oxygen is more electronegative than chlorine by the fact that oxygen is one of three elements (oxygen, nitrogen, and fluorine) that are electronegative enough to induce hydrogen bonding. Therefore the negative charge couldn't be predominantly on the chlorine, nor could it be distributed evenly among all five atoms,

so choices (A) and (D) must be wrong. Choice (B) is wrong because the diagram shows only one of four resonance forms of perchlorate. Since all the oxygens are equivalent, it would be impossible for one of them to have a bonding structure different from that of the others. The actual perchlorate ion is a hybrid of four resonance structures, each with the negative charge on a different oxygen. Therefore, choice (C) is correct.

3. A To find the percentage of NaOH that is converted into $NaHCO_3$, it is necessary to divide the amount of NaOH converted into $NaHCO_3$ by the initial amount of NaOH. You have the initial amount of NaOH in grams, but you aren't given the amount of NaOH converted to $NaHCO_3$. However, you can calculate this from the amount of CO_2 absorbed since the number of moles of carbon dioxide absorbed is the same as the number of moles of NaOH converted. You can see this from the 1:1 stoichiometry in the reaction. However, this ratio is a molar ratio, and from the table, you can only get the grams of CO_2 absorbed. However, from the fact that this number is in the numerator of all the answer choices, you know that it is the place to start. The other factor that is in all the answer choices is a 100 in each numerator. (That's there to convert the calculation to a percentage.) Now, consider the denominator of each answer choice. The ratio you're using to find the number of moles of NaOH converted is a molar ratio, so you need to change the grams of CO_2 into moles of CO_2. Divide by the molar mass of CO_2. Grams of CO_2 divided by grams per mole of CO_2 gives moles of CO_2, and by the stoichiometric ratio, that is equal to moles of NaOH converted in this experiment. So you can eliminate choices (C) and (D) which don't have the molar mass of CO_2 in the denominator. That leaves choices (A) and (B). Divide the amount of NaOH converted by the initial amount of NaOH, and the amount of NaOH converted is in moles, so the answer must be choice (A). You can't get a valid percentage if the numbers you use have different units, so choice (A), which divides moles by moles, is the right answer.

4. A Only the empirical formula can always be found using the procedure described in the passage. The empirical formula is the simplest whole-number ratio of elements in the compound. The procedure described in the passage makes it possible to calculate the number of moles of carbon in the sample from the amount of carbon dioxide absorbed by the NaOH, and to calculate the number of moles of hydrogen in the sample from the amount of water absorbed by the magnesium perchlorate. The procedure does not include any means of determining the amounts of any other elements that may be present in the sample, but if the sample is a hydrocarbon, then it contains only hydrogen and carbon. Knowing the ratio of these two elements allows us to determine the empirical formula. Whether we will also be able to determine the molecular formula depends on the ratio of carbon to hydrogen that we find. For example, if the molar ratio of carbon to hydrogen is 5:12, the compound can only be pentane, but if the ratio of moles of carbon to moles of hydrogen is 1:2, the compound could be anything that contains ethene, with 2 carbons and 4 hydrogens, or propene, with 3 carbons and 6 hydrogens, or cyclohexane, with 6 carbons and 12 hydrogens, and so on.

Discrete Questions

5. B Answering this question requires you to think a little bit about the things that determine a molecule's shape. The orientation of atoms in a molecule will be influenced by the electron repulsions between the atoms as well as by the bonding. The valence shell electron pair repulsion, or VSEPR theory, has been developed to explain the shapes molecules take. The important thing here is that the constituent atoms bonded to the central atom will arrange themselves so as to be as far away from each other as possible. However, constituent atoms will space themselves away from lone-pair valence electrons on the central atom as well.

Beryllium only has two valence electrons, both of which are involved in bonding to the two fluorine atoms, so it doesn't have any lone pairs and adopts a linear shape, putting the two fluorines on opposite sides of the central beryllium. However, sulfur has six valence electrons, only four of which are involved in bonding to the two oxygen atoms, leaving one lone pair of electrons for the oxygens to contend with. As a result, the 2 oxygens and the 1 pair of electrons space themselves approximately 120° from each other in a plane around the sulfur, giving the molecule a bent shape.

Choices (C) and (D) are wrong because the Be orbitals don't hybridize to form the bonds with the fluorines. The Be's s-subshell binds directly to fluorine p-shells. Additionally, the hybridization of the sulfur is actually sp^2.

6. B To answer this question, you need to know a little bit about catalysts and equilibrium. You have to remember that at equilibrium, the forward and reverse reactions of system are happening at the same rate. So at equilibrium, the reaction does not seem to be proceeding in any direction because the concentrations of products and reactants are balanced. If this balance is upset, the system will adjust itself to reach equilibrium again. Catalysts lower the activation energy of a reaction, making it easier for the reaction to proceed. Catalysts thus increase the rate of a reaction without affecting the equilibrium of a system or altering the rate constants. Both the forward and reverse reactions are faster, but there is still no change in the concentrations of the products or reactants, just like in the uncatalyzed system. Also, by definition, catalysts are not consumed in a reaction.

7. C The contents of the balloons will differ in mass but will be equal in volume. Equal volumes of different gases, at the same temperature and pressure, contain an equal number of moles, but not an equal mass. Since these are three different gases, they will almost certainly have different molecular weights, and therefore different molar masses. However, each balloon will contain the same number of moles of gas molecules. Since the balloons contain different masses of gas, choices (A) and (B) can be eliminated. To choose between the remaining two possibilities, decide how the change in temperature will affect the gas volumes. Since the volume and the temperature of a gas are directly proportional at constant pressure, and since the initial volume was the same, the final volume must also be the same for all three gases. Therefore, choice (D) is wrong and choice (C) is correct.

Passage II (Questions 8–14)

8. D These statements all compare various constants for a general indicator with the same constants for HCl. K_a, K_b, pK_a, and pK_b are all different ways of describing the strength of acids and bases, so the first step to answering this question is to think about the relative strengths of HInd and HCl. Since HInd tends to give up a proton, it's an acid, so, as the passage tells you, HInd must be a weak acid. You should know that HCl is a common strong acid, so it is safe to assume that HCl is a stronger acid than HInd. Now all you have to do is relate this fact to the constants in the statements. Statement I compares the K_a values of HInd and HCl. The K_a is the dissociation constant for an acid, and the passage gives you the expression for it. The stronger an acid, the more dissociated it will be, and you can see from the equation that a more dissociated acid will have a higher K_a. Since HInd is the weaker acid, its K_a will be lower than HCl's, so Statement I is true. Statement II compares the pK_a values. Remember that the pK_a is the negative log of the K_a, so the strong acids, with high K_a's, will have low pK_a's. This is easy to remember because pK_a is like pH. The more acidic a solution is, the lower the pH is, so a strong acid has a low pK_a. Since HInd is the weaker acid, it'll have the higher pK_a, so Statement II is true as well. Statement III is the opposite of Statement II, so it must be false. The last statement compares the pK_b's of the indicator anion and the chloride anion, which are the conjugate bases of the two acids. Remember, the stronger the acid, the weaker the conjugate base. This means that the chloride ion must be a weak

base and the Ind⁻ anion is a stronger base, since HInd is a weak acid. So how will their pK_b values compare? pK_b indicates base strength just like pK_a indicates acid strength: and the lower the pK_b, the stronger the base. Since the indicator anion is the stronger base, it will have the lower pK_b, and Statement IV is true. So Statements I, II, and IV are true, and the correct choice is D.

9. B When the sodium salt of an indicator anion is dissolved in pure water, the indicator anion, which is a relatively strong base, will split water molecules in order to combine with hydrogen ions, thereby releasing hydroxide that will make the solution basic. The sodium cation will not bind to the released hydroxide. Sodium hydroxide is a strong base that dissociates completely in water, so the sodium ion remains dissociated in solution. Since there will be more free hydroxide ions than free hydrogen ions, the resulting solution will be basic, and so choice (B) is correct.

10. C The ratio of Ind⁻ anions to undissociated HInd molecules will increase 100,000-fold, or by a factor of 10^5. At the equivalence point, the graph shows that the pH suddenly increases from 5 to 10. This means the hydrogen ion concentration has decreased from 10^{-5} to 10^{-10}. This decrease in the hydrogen ion concentration will cause HInd molecules to dissociate, so the concentration of indicator anions will increase and the concentration of undissociated indicator molecules will decrease. To see the magnitude of this change, consider Equation 2. According to this equation, the ratio of Ind⁻ over HInd is equal to the K_a divided by the hydrogen ion concentration. So this ratio, just before the equivalence point is reached, is $10^{-8}/10^{-5}$, and a moment later the ratio is $10^{-8}/10^{-10}$. The before and after ratios, when worked out, come to 10^{-3} before and 10^2 afterward. This is an increase of 10^5, which comes to 100,000, so the ratio of Ind⁻ to HInd has increased by a factor of 100,000, and choice (C) is correct.

11. D The graph for this question shows the titration of an ammonia solution with HCl. Since you aren't given the base constant for ammonia, the question has to be answered on the basis of the information you can extract from the graph. In order for an indicator to be effective in determining the equivalence point, it must change color in a range that includes that point. The pH range given for phenolphthalein in Table 1 is 8.2 to 10. In this graph, the curve is relatively flat over this pH range. The equivalence point, which the indicator would be used to identify, is shown by the sharp vertical drop on the graph, which begins at a lower pH. Because the pH of the equivalence point doesn't fall into the transition pH range of phenolphthalein, it would be the wrong indicator for this titration. All the answer choices are stated in terms of concentration ratios, so you have to relate this information to the concentrations of the various species. Since the part of the graph ranging from pH 10 to 8.2 is relatively flat, very little change in pH is taking place for any given amount of HCl that is added in this region, which indicates that the ammonia solution is functioning as a buffer here. A solution can buffer added strong acid in the range in which the a weak base is being converted to its conjugate acid. So, as HCl is added, the hydrogen ions are combining with ammonia to form the ammonium ion. In the pH range in which this process is occurring, both the conjugate acid and the base will be present in the solution. So choice (D) is correct; the conjugate acid and base concentrations will be about equal in this range. Choice (B), with a higher concentration of the base, describes the far left side of the graph, where very little HCl has been added and the pH is still above 10; choice (C) describes the part of the graph near and to the right of the equivalence point, where the concentration of the conjugate acid is high. Finally, choice (A) would imply that HCl was a weak acid, since a low Cl⁻ to HCl ratio would indicate that HCl was not very highly dissociated. Since HCl is actually a strong acid that dissociates completely, the ratio of dissociated chloride to undissociated HCl is always high, so choice (A) is wrong.

12. C The hydrogen sulfide solution described in this question has a first pK_a of 7 and a second pK_a of 13. The pK_a, remember, is the negative log of the K_a. So this acid has a first K_a of 10^{-7}, and a second K_a of 10^{-13}. What this means is that at pH 7, the concentration of H_2S is equal to the concentration of its monoprotic conjugate base, the HS^- ion; and at pH 13, the concentration of the HS^- ion is equal to the concentration of its conjugate base, the sulfide ion. Since the solution was one molar for H_2S before any dissociation, at pH 7 the concentrations of H_2S and of HS^- must each be 0.5 moles per liter. This might lead you to believe that the concentration of the sulfide anion is zero at pH 7. It's true that the concentration of sulfide is very close to zero, but, since the second K_a is a constant that is always equal to 1×10^{-13}, an extremely small amount of the HS^- must dissociate into sulfide ions and protons. The concentrations of H_2S, HS^-, and sulfide will all equilibrate in such a way that both the first and second equilibrium constants are maintained, given the pH, which is being maintained at 7. So the concentration of sulfide is non-zero and (A) is wrong.

Now, find an expression for the concentration of sulfide and solve it. Start from the acid dissociation constants for each step in this diprotic dissociation. From Equation 1, you know that the first K_a is equal to the H^+ ion concentration, times the HS^- concentration divided by the H_2S concentration and that the second K_a is equal to the H^+ concentration times the S^{2-} concentration divided by the HS^- concentration. Since these two are simultaneous equations, you can solve the K_{a2} equation for the concentration of HS^- and substitute that value into the expression for K_{a1}. That gives us K_{a1} equal to the concentration of H^+ squared x the concentration of S^{2-} divided by the quantity K_{a2} times the concentration of H_2S. If you solve this equation for the concentration of S^{2-}, you get that is equal to K_{a1} times K_{a2} times the concentration of H_2S divided by the concentration of H^+ squared. Plug in the values you know. K_{a1} is 10^{-7}, K_{a2} is 10^{-13}, the concentration of H^+ is 10^{-7} since the pH is seven, and the concentration of H_2S is 0.5. Actually, it is slightly lower than 0.5, but that "lower" will be very small, and so can be ignored in this calculation. 0.5×10^{-6}, which is the same as 5×10^{-7}, choice (C).

13. D The pOH of a solution is the negative log of the hydroxide concentration in solution. You can see that OH⁻ is generated in this solution through the formula $CH_3COO^- + H_2O$ yields CH_3COOH and OH⁻. Since the concentration of water remains essentially constant, don't consider it, and the K_b is given by the concentration of acetic acid x the concentration of hydroxide/the concentration of acetate. To get the pOH from this equation, solve for the concentration of hydroxide, and then take the negative log of that value to get the pOH. Rearrange the equation to get the concentration of hydroxide equal to the K_b of acetate x the concentration of acetate divided by the concentration of acetic acid. By taking the negative log of both sides, we get pOH equal to the pK_b of acetate plus the log of the ratio of the concentration acetic acid to the concentration of acetate. Subtracting a log is equivalent to adding the inverse of the log, so combine the concentrations of acetate and acetic acid into a fraction with acetate in the denominator, and take the log of the total fraction This corresponds to correct choice (D).

14. A Sulfuric acid is a strong acid, so when it's dissolved in water, one of its hydrogen ions dissociates essentially completely. Of course, no dissociation is ever absolutely complete, but the amount of totally undissociated sulfuric acid will be extremely small. Choice (C) shows 1/10 of the sulfuric acid remaining totally undissociated, and choice (D) shows 1/3 remaining undissociated, so both these choices are safe to eliminate. The concentration of undissociated sulfuric acid is close enough to zero to assume that there is no undissociated acid as in A and B. Now you only need to decide what happens to the hydrogen sulfate ion. In choice (B) the sulfate ion concentration in the solution is higher than that of the hydrogen sulfate, while in choice (A), the opposite is true. The conjugate base of an amphoteric acid is always a far weaker acid than the original acid, and loses its proton much less readily. In this case, after the first proton has been lost, the solution has a concentration of hydrogen ions of 0.1 molar, making this an extremely acidic solution. In such a strong acid, it isn't likely that a weak acid will dissociate too much. If the solution were basic, or if the protons

were being neutralized as they dissociated, as with a titration, the hydrogen sulfate would dissociate to replace the protons being taken out of solution, but that isn't what's happening here. Mathematically, you know that the second dissociation constant, 1.2×10^{-2}, is equal to the hydrogen ion concentration × the sulfate ion concentration divided by the hydrogen sulfate concentration. Estimating that the hydrogen ion concentration is close to 0.1 from the first acid dissociation, you see that the ratio of sulfate to hydrogen sulfate is 0.12, or less than 1. That tells you that the hydrogen sulfate concentration must be greater than the sulfate concentration, and only choice (A) of the remaining choices can be correct.

Passage III (Questions 15-19)

15. B The elements in column 13 have 3 valence electrons. All of the elements in one column, or group, of the periodic table will have the same number of valence electrons, so choice (D) is incorrect. The valence shell is the outer energy shell of an atom, the one with the highest principle quantum number. For elements in columns 13 through 18, the valence shells are the s and p subshells. The outermost d subshell isn't part of the valence shell of the elements outside the transition series, since it is always filled after the s subshell of the next higher energy level has already been filled. Any element in column 13 will have 2 valence electrons in an s orbital and one in a p orbital; if you didn't know this offhand, you could figure it out from the periodic table. The total number of valence electrons for each element in column 13 is therefore 3, so choices (A) and (C) are incorrect, and choice (B) is correct.

16. C To find the correct answer here, you have to use the information given in the passage about elements in the same column having similar properties. Reasoning from your general knowledge of the periodic table alone isn't adequate. The passage tells you that gold and silver are the least reactive metals in their periods. By analogy, it seems reasonable that the element directly above them, copper, should be the least reactive metal in its period also. The other choices aren't as plausible. Choice (A), potassium, is an alkali metal, not a transition element, and anyway, the elements in this first group are described as very reactive. The other three choices are all transition metals, but not from the same group as silver and gold. You might have chosen choice (D), zinc, on the ground that elements further to the right in the periodic table tend to be more electronegative, which in the case of a metal would make it less reactive. However, the increase in electronegativity toward the right side of the periodic table is a general tendency, not an absolute rule. Copper is actually slightly more electronegative than zinc, even though zinc is further to the right in the table.

17. D Here again, the key to finding the correct answer is the statement that elements that belong to the same group tend to show similarities. Selenium is a member of the group that also contains oxygen and sulfur, so it should be similar in some way to these elements. Since the passage says that sulfur occurs in several allotropic forms, this might well be true of selenium also, so choice (D) is the correct answer.

Choice (A) might sound plausible, especially if you happen to know that selenium is a nutrient found in soil. But the passage doesn't say anything about selenium oxides being found in rock, and you wouldn't be expected to know something like that even if it were true, since this would be detailed information about geology, not chemistry. In passage-related questions such as this, stick to the information in the passage. Choice (B) is wrong because there is nothing in the passage to suggest that selenium should be a liquid. The only reason you might have for selecting Choice (B) is that bromine, which occurs to the right of selenium in the periodic table, is liquid under standard conditions; but the passage says that elements are similar to other elements in their *group*, not their *period*. Choice (C) also might seem tempting, since the borderline between metals and nonmetals cuts diagonally across the right side of the periodic table, and selenium is close to this line. But this choice can be discounted because the passage gives no evidence that

elements in this portion of the table are highly reactive with air; high reactivity with water and/or with air is mentioned only as a characteristic of the alkali metals and the alkaline earth metals in Columns 1 and 2.

18. C A second ionization energy is the energy needed to remove a second electron from an element, after one electron has already been removed. If you look up the four choices in the periodic table, the order in which they are listed should stand out: they are the elements with atomic numbers 17, 18, 19, and 20. In their elemental states, the numbers of valence electrons that these elements possess are, respectively, 7, 8, 1, and 2. With 1 electron removed, chlorine and argon will have 6 and 7 valence electrons respectively. Removing one electron from potassium will strip it of its one valence electron, leaving it with a complete octet in its next-lowest energy level. Calcium will be left with one valence electron. Since potassium's loss of one electron will leave it with a complete octet, and since a complete octet is the most stable electron configuration, removing a second electron from potassium will require more energy than will removing a second electron from any of the other three elements. So potassium, choice (C), has the highest second ionization energy, and is therefore the correct choice. You rarely need to worry about the second ionization energy of Cl, Ar, or K, because the first electron is so hard to remove from Cl and Ar, and the second electron is so hard to remove from K, but the question presupposes that you can remove these electrons. Basically, it is asking you to identify a trend based on the periodic table, not on your experience or on practicality.

19. D You are told in the passage that Mendeleev ordered the elements on his periodic table according to atomic weight. You are also told that he used his table to predict, with surprising accuracy, the properties of elements that hadn't been discovered yet. That discounts choice (A) since it implies that Mendeleev knew that he *didn't* know the identities of all the elements. However, the modern periodic table, as you probably know, is ordered by atomic number. There are three places in the periodic table where this order does not match up exactly to increasing atomic weight.

Potassium, which is lighter than argon, has one more proton and thus a greater atomic number. This is true for nickel and cobalt and for iodine and tellurium. So, even though Mendeleev actually did put iodine in the correct column because of its reactive similarity to other halogens, there were exceptions to his ordering scheme. The definition of element ordering changed so that these elements no longer represented exceptions, so choice (D) is correct. You may have gotten confused by choice (B), the noble gases, because the passage told you that 19th century scientists were unaware of their existence. However, when they were discovered, they fell pretty well in line with Mendeleev's ordering scheme, except for argon, which we've already discussed. Choice (C) says that Mendeleev's order was wrong because he had the wrong atomic weights. Nothing in the passage leads you to believe this, and your outside knowledge of the periodic table actually discounts it, since you know that the table is now ordered by atomic number.

Discrete Questions

20. A Although this question appears to be simply about pH, finding the solution actually requires you to apply Le Châtelier's principle, which states that a system at equilibrium responds to an applied stress by attempting to relieve that stress. When sodium acetate is dissolved in water, some of the acetate combines with protons from water molecules to form acetic acid, splitting the water molecules and releasing hydroxide ions. The sodium ion, meanwhile, remains dissociated in solution. Since hydroxide ions are liberated from water molecules, the solution becomes basic. When the solution is gently heated, as described in the question, both water and acetic acid will evaporate. The evaporation of the water shifts the equilibrium of the equation for the dissociation of water to the left, as some hydroxide ions combine with protons to form more water molecules, but this one-to-one combination of protons with hydroxide ions has no effect on the pH. However, the evaporation of acetic acid causes more acetate ions to combine with protons from water molecules to replace the missing acetic acid. As the acetic acid continues to evaporate, hydroxide ions will accumulate in the solution. Thus the net concentration of hydroxide ions will increase as the solution is heated, and the pH will rise. Eventually, the increase in hydroxide concentration will shift the equation for the hydrolysis of acetate to the left, preventing further hydrolysis and establishing a new equilibrium at the higher temperature. However, the pH will be much higher than it had been before the heating of the solution began. So choice (A) is correct. Choice (B) is wrong because, even if heating did make the sodium acetate less soluble, and so caused some of it to precipitate out of solution, that would shift the equilibrium away from the formation of hydroxide, so this should decrease the pH of the solution. Furthermore, solids become more soluble, if anything, as temperature is increased; only gases are more soluble at lower temperatures. If the process of hydrolysis were exothermic, as stated in choice (C), then a higher temperature would cause the equilibrium to shift toward a decrease in hydrolysis, and this would also decrease the pH. So whether the process is exothermic or not, this couldn't explain an increase in pH with temperature. As for choice (D), in order for hydrolysis of the acetate ion to be nonspontaneous under standard conditions, acetate would have to be a very weak base and acetic acid would have to be a strong acid. Since acetic acid is a weak acid, choice (D) is wrong.

21. D A single displacement reaction, Option I, is one in which one element in a compound is replaced by another element. This reaction doesn't qualify because, although the mercury ions undergo a change of valence, one of them remains part of the molecule. Therefore, Option I is incorrect. Nor is the reaction a double displacement, since in double displacement reactions elements from two different compounds replace each other to form 2 new compounds, so Option II is also untrue. A disproportionation reaction, Option III, is a redox reaction in which the valence of one element changes in two directions; that is, one atom of the element is oxidized while another is reduced. Here, the two mercury atoms start out in a +1 oxidation state, and finish with one oxidized to +2 and the other reduced to 0. Thus, Option III is correct. And Option IV is also true: The reaction takes place progressively in the presence of light, indicating that light energy must be absorbed continuously for the reaction to occur. Since energy must be added for a reaction to occur, the reaction must be endothermic. We know the light can't be acting simply as a catalyst for an exothermic reaction, because if that were the case then the energy produced by the reaction would cause the rate to increase, and light would be needed only initially. So Option IV is true; this reaction must be endothermic. Since Options III and IV are true, the correct choice is D.

Passage IV (Questions 22–26)

22. D The vapor pressure of a liquid is determined by the strength of the forces between the molecules in the liquid phase. The stronger the forces are, the harder it is to separate the molecules and vaporize the liquid, and the lower the vapor pressure. The relative strengths of bonds within the molecules, discussed in choice (A), does not affect the vapor pressure, so choice (A) is wrong. It's true that acetone has a lower molecular weight than pentane, as in choice (B), and compounds with lower molecular weights do tend to have higher vapor pressures, because a smaller compound tend to have weaker dispersion forces between molecules, which is an intermolecular force. However, acetone has a lower vapor pressure than *n*-pentane, which means that it doesn't vaporize more easily, so choice (B) must be wrong. Choice (B) would be true if dispersion forces were the only kind, or even the strongest kind, of intermolecular forces. Since they are not, one of these other forces must be at work here. Choice (C) suggests that the vapor pressure difference is due to greater hydrogen bonding in *n*-pentane. Hydrogen bonding only occurs when hydrogens are bonded to a highly electronegative atom like fluorine, nitrogen, or oxygen, creating a very strong partial positive charge. Since pentane contains only carbon and hydrogen atoms, and carbon isn't electronegative enough to induce hydrogen bonding, choice (C) must be wrong. This

leaves choice (D) as the only possible answer. Choice (D) is true because acetone is indeed a polar molecule, while *n*-pentane is not. The interactions between the acetone molecules in the liquid phase are dipole-dipole interactions, and these are much stronger than the dispersion forces that hold *n*-pentane molecules in the liquid phase.

23. A Raoult's law predicts that the vapor pressure of the each component of the mixture will vary linearly with its mole fraction. This means that the vapor pressure for any component A will be zero when the mole fraction of A is 0, and will increase linearly to the normal vapor pressure of A when its mole fraction is 1. Dalton's law predicts that the vapor pressure of a mixture will be the sum of the vapor pressures of the components. Since the vapor pressure of each component of the mixture varies linearly, and the total vapor pressure is found by adding the partial pressures of the two components, it follows that the total vapor pressure must vary linearly between the vapor pressure of pure chloroform and that of pure acetone. You can prove this by substituting the expression for the vapor pressure of these two components in various ratios, as given by Raoult's law, into Dalton's law. This is the situation shown by Diagram A. Diagram B shows pure chloroform having a higher vapor pressure than pure acetone, which conflicts with Figure 2. Diagram C shows the two liquids having identical vapor pressures, which is wrong, and Diagram D shows a nonlinear relationship, which is also wrong.

24. A The vapor pressure of a liquid is dependent on the intermolecular attractions between its molecules. The stronger these attractions, the less likely is it that a molecule will escape from the liquid into the gas phase. When two different liquids are mixed, the attraction between the different kinds of molecules could be either stronger or weaker than the attraction between the molecules of the pure compound. If the intermolecular attractions are stronger in the mixture, then the molecules won't escape as often, and the vapor pressure of the mixture will be lower, like in the mixture of chloroform and acetone. If the intermolecular attractions are weaker in the mixture, then more molecules will vaporize and the vapor pressure will be higher. So choice (A) is correct. Intermolecular attractions are of little importance in the gas phase because the distance between molecules is too great. Intermolecular forces are only effective over small distances. Therefore the effect of intermolecular attraction on vapor pressure occurs almost exclusively in the liquid phase, eliminating choice (B). Choice (C) is wrong because, assuming the two liquids are completely miscible, the liquids are completely mixed. You could have also figured this out by looking at the experimental results shown in Figure 2. In the graph on the left, if the heavier chloroform sank to the bottom, a higher mole fraction of acetone, which has a higher vapor pressure, should cause the graph to diverge upward, not downward. In the graph on the right, it is the heavier pentane that would sink if this happened, causing the graph to diverge downward, since acetone's vapor pressure is lower. Choice (D) is wrong because the whole point of the experiment is to learn the effect of mixing two substances on their vapor pressure. There is no chemical reaction, so heat can't be produced. The only way physical mixing could bring about a change in temperature would be if there was a change in hydrogen bonding so that energy was absorbed or released, but the compounds in these mixtures don't form hydrogen bonds. Additionally, as far as you know, the flask is not insulated, so any small change in temperature would be quickly offset by the temperature of the surroundings.

25. D   Other gases must be excluded from the flask for the experimental results to be accurate. Since the vapor pressure is measured by the difference between the heights of the mercury in the two columns on either side of the curved part of the tube, the entire difference in height is attributed to the vapor pressure of the liquid sample. If the vapor pressure were measured as the difference between the height of the mercury before and after the liquid was added to the flask, then it would be possible to get accurate results without excluding other gases, because the vapor pressure from other gases would be subtracted out as the "before" reading. This isn't done, so it is necessary to use an experimental technique that excludes all

other gases from the flask, and that's choice (D). The reason choice (A) is wrong is that the purpose of this experiment is simply to measure the vapor pressure under the given conditions, not to explain why you get the results you do. This measurement will be accurate regardless of the adhesion to the ideal gas law. In fact, since the vapor is in equilibrium with its liquid phase, it will deviate somewhat from the behavior of an ideal gas. Choice (B) is incorrect because, in the apparatus shown, mercury can vaporize above both sides of the U-shaped tube, so any vapor pressure due to mercury on one side of the tube will be counterbalanced by an equal mercury vapor pressure on the other side of the tube. Therefore, any vapor pressure due to mercury won't affect the experimental results. In practice, the vapor pressure of mercury is very low, so it won't pose much of a problem. Finally, choice (C) is wrong because the height of mercury produced in a tube by gas pressure is independent of the width of the tube. A familiar example of this effect is that a barometer always shows the same height of mercury for a given air pressure, regardless of the width of the barometer tube.

26. D   The density of pentane, given in the question, is a major clue. The question tells you that pentane and water, when mixed, separate into two separate phases, each of which is almost, but not quite, pure. Basically, it's like mixing oil and water. One floats on top of the other. You should remember that water has a density of one gram per milliliter; since pentane is less dense than water, the pentane will float above the phase containing mostly water. In a mixture of pentane and water, the pentane will cover the entire surface unless its mole fraction is so small that there isn't enough of it to cover the surface. So, for most of the readings, the nearly pure pentane will be present at the liquid-gas interface, and the vapor pressure measured will only be dependent on this phase. The reading for the sample containing 100 percent water will, of course, be equal to the vapor pressure of water. If a reading is taken for a mixture containing so little pentane that it doesn't cover the surface, this will produce a reading somewhere between that of pentane and water. So the graph will appear as a straight line at or close to the level of the vapor pressure of pentane, except for the very low mole fractions of pentane. At this point, the line will drop down to the vapor pressure of water. This is shown in choice (D). The vapor pressure shown across most of the graph is actually slightly higher than the vapor pressure of pure pentane, indicating that the small amount of water in this phase increases the vapor pressure of the pentane. Choices (A) and (B) don't take into account the fact that the pentane usually covers the water, so the mixture will seem like a pure compound with one vapor pressure. Choice (C) shows what the graph would look like if the phase containing mostly water floated on top of the phase containing mostly pentane, but that conflicts with the known densities of these compounds.

Passage V (Questions 27–31)

27. D According to the passage, iron deficiency is caused not by a lack of iron in the soil but by lack of iron availability. Iron in the form of dissolved ferrous ion is available to plants, but both ferrous and ferric hydroxides are solids, so iron is not available in these forms. Adding more of these solids to the soil won't help. If the soil could convert these solids to a usable form, it could use the oxides that are presumably already in the soil, so we can eliminate (B) and (C). Choice (A), calcium carbonate, consists of a strong base and a weak acid. Adding calcium carbonate would make the soil more alkaline, that is, raise the pH. The table shows that for soil with any given reduction potential, iron will occur in the form of either ferric or ferrous hydroxide above a certain pH, while the free ferrous ion will predominate at lower pH values. Therefore, the alkaline soil created by adding calcium carbonate would make iron less available, so choice (A) is wrong. Choice (D), ammonium sulfate, combines the conjugate base of a strong acid, sulfate, with the ammonium ion, which is the conjugate acid of a weak base. The ammonium ion would combine with hydroxide ions in the soil to form ammonia and water, making the soil less alkaline. The

increased acidity would encourage the increase of the concentration of free iron II ions. Of the choices given, this would be the most effective way to cure the rhododendrons' chlorosis by getting the plant more iron II.

28. B Finding the correct answer to this question requires some reasoning ability. Basically, this question just asks which conditions have the greatest concentration of free Fe^{2+} ions. Remember, the passage states that iron is reduced to the more available ferrous form in wet soil, so choice (C) is probably wrong since it will have very little Fe^{2+}. So, which of the other three situations would tend to make the concentration of iron II excessive enough to cause harm to plants? According to the passage, water from subterranean sources is more reducing than rainwater, but the passage also states that soluble iron can migrate away from an area if the iron is below the water table. This could happen in any of these three situations, but it would be more likely in the cases of the hilltop and the well-drained highland, since the water has someplace else to go, downhill or wherever the drainage takes it. Although the passage states that a temporary water table can form on high ground after rain, it still isn't likely that too much soluble iron would accumulate in the soil described in choice (D), since this ground is described as being well-drained. In the flat lowland, water that is low in oxygen content, and therefore more reducing, may accumulate, increasing the concentration of available iron. The combination of wet soil and poor drainage provides an environment in which the concentration of available iron may rise high enough to be harmful to plants not adapted to this environment, so choice (B) is correct.

29. B   There is no exchange of electrons, so the oxidation number of the ferrous ion doesn't change, and no redox reaction takes place. That means the transition between the ferrous ion and ferrous hydroxide is simply a precipitation or solvation event, so the equilibrium is determined simply by the K_{sp}. As a result, the soil reduction potential doesn't affect the reaction's equilibrium. When the concentration of the ferrous ion is given, as it is in Table 1, the hydroxide ion concentration at which precipitation occurs can be calculated from the equilibrium constant, without considering the reduction potential. However, since the hydroxide ion is a part of this precipitation, the pH of the soil will affect the precipitation or solvation of the ferrous hydroxide. The lower the pH, the greater the amount of dissociated ferrous hydroxide. So, since the soil's pH has an effect and the soil's reduction potential does not, the correct choice is (B).

30. A   The passage doesn't give you the iron half-reactions that occur in soil or the reduction potentials for these reactions. Instead, you're told that when iron is oxidized, the other half-reaction is not a single reaction, but a composite of all the half reactions going on in the soil solution. The second paragraph tells you that increased soil wetness decreases the soil reduction potential, so you can eliminate choices (C) and (D). Increased soil wetness increases the amount of available iron. Since the ferrous ion is the form of iron available to plants, you want the iron to be in the +2 oxidation, so the water from subterranean sources must help reduce the iron from +3 to +2. Since iron is being reduced, choice (A) must be correct. This should make sense overall because in order for iron to be reduced as part of a single reaction in a test tube, the reduction potential of the iron would have to be higher than the reduction potential of the element being oxidized. The lower the reduction potential of a species, the more likely it is to become oxidized and thus the more likely it is to act as a reducing agent. So since ground water increases the availability of reduced iron, it decreases the reduction potential of the soil.

31. C   To find the answer to this question, you have to understand how reduction potentials are calculated under nonstandard conditions. The column below each half-reaction in Table 1 shows the pH values above which the product of the half-reaction is present in greater concentration than the reactant. Choice (A) doesn't have factors for iron concentration or changing pH, so it is wrong. In fact, this equation is the equation for the energy difference between electron states in a hydrogen atom. Choice (B) relates the standard reduction potential of a reaction to the Gibbs free energy. The passage and the table describe nonstandard conditions and we haven't got any free-energy information, so choice (B) is probably wrong. Choice (C) starts with the reduction potential of a half-reaction under standard conditions, $E°$, which can be looked up in a table, and then calculates the actual reduction potential based on how far the actual conditions diverge from standard conditions. Q is the reaction quotient, which relates the concentrations of reactants and products present, whether the conditions are standard or not. Since Q will factor in the concentrations of hydrogen ions as part of the reactants and products of the reaction, it will account for changing pH and this expression could be used to find the pH values in Table 1, assuming that the concentration of iron and the pH of the soil is known. So, choice (C), which is really just the Nernst equation, is correct. Choice (D) is an equation used in atomic physics that you don't need to know about; it's the definition of an energy unit called a hartree. The appearance of Planck's constant, h, the mass of an electron m_e, and p are pretty dead giveaways that this expression will not be useful for our purposes.

Discrete Questions

32. C   To answer this question, you need to remember what a catalyst does to a reaction and its rate. A catalyst is a substance that increases the rate of a reaction without being consumed itself. So by adding a catalyst, you are speeding up the reaction. So you can eliminate choice (D), since it is slower than the original rate. If the new rate constant is less than the original one, then the new rate will be slower. Notice that you cannot eliminate choice (B) by this line of reasoning because the concentration of the catalyst could be less than one, which would increase the rate. However, choices (A) and (B) can both be eliminated because they figure in the concentration of the catalyst directly. It is true that the degree of catalysis can vary with the concentration of the catalyst, but you don't know whether this is a direct or indirect relationship. Further, since the concentration of the catalyst doesn't change because the catalyst is not consumed by the reaction, the factor is constant through the reaction. So, however the catalyst affects the rate, it is best to factor it into the rate constant. That's why in choices (C) and (D), the rate constant is k_c instead of the original k. However, k_c will always be greater than k because the rate increases. Therefore, (C) is the best answer.

33. **D** When a bond is formed, energy is released, and therefore ΔH (the change in enthalpy) is negative. This is easily understood by considering the bonding theory of molecular orbitals. When two atoms form a bond, two atomic orbitals, one from each atom, form two molecular orbitals, both of which encompass both atoms. One of the new orbitals is a bonding orbital and the other is an antibonding orbital. Compared to the atomic orbitals from which the new molecular orbitals were formed, the bonding orbital has a lower energy level, while the antibonding orbital has a higher energy level. The two electrons normally go into the lower-energy, bonding orbital. This forms the new bond and releases energy. The amount of energy released is the difference between the energy levels of the two atomic orbitals, added together, and the energy level of the new molecular orbital. The higher-energy, antibonding molecular orbital is normally empty. However, if one or both of the electrons absorbs energy from an outside source, such as light or applied heat, the electron may then have enough energy to enter the antibonding orbital. When an electron enters an antibonding orbital, energy is absorbed. However, the antibonding orbital doesn't form a bond; instead, the two atoms will separate. So if a bond is formed, the electrons must have entered the bonding orbital. Since the reactants go to a lower energy state, energy is released, so choice (D) is correct.

34. **A** If an element is very highly electronegative, its electron affinity won't be near zero. Electron affinity is a measure of the ease with which an atom can accept an electron in terms of the amount of energy released when a neutral atom accepts an additional electron. An atom that is highly electronegative can, of course, accept an electron very easily, so it will release a larger amount of energy. There are two ways of measuring electron affinity. According to one convention, increasing electron affinity is indicated by increasingly high positive numbers; according to the other convention, an increase in electron affinity is indicated by more negative numbers. The reason for the second convention is that increased electron affinity means more energy is released, and energy leaving a system means that the ΔH is negative. What both these conventions have in common is that the electron affinity is closer to zero for those elements that accept an electron less readily. A highly electronegative element, therefore, will have an electron affinity that is not close to zero, so choice (A) is our answer. Choice (B) is a true statement. The ionization energy is the amount of energy that must be added to the atom to remove an electron. The more electronegative the atom, the more it wants to keep electrons, and so more energy is needed to remove an electron. Choice (C) is also true. In highly electronegative elements, the valence electrons are strongly attracted to the nucleus, so the atomic radii are small. In addition, the most electronegative elements are in the higher periods, so they have fewer electron shells, which helps make their radii small. Choice (D) is also true. The most electronegative elements are found in the upper right corner of the periodic table. Fluorine is the most electronegative element and elements tend to become more electronegative the closer they get to fluorine, which is located in the upper right of the periodic table.

ORGANIC CHEMISTRY

PERIODIC TABLE OF THE ELEMENTS

Period

1 IA 1A																	18 vIIIA 8A
1 1 H 1.008	2 IIA 2A											13 IIIA 3A	14 IVA 4A	15 VA 5A	16 VIA 6A	17 VIIA 7A	**1** 2 He 4.003
2 3 Li 6.941	4 Be 9.012											5 B 10.81	6 C 12.01	7 N 14.01	8 O 16.00	9 F 19.00	10 Ne 20.18
3 11 Na 22.99	12 Mg 24.31	3 IIIB 3B	4 IVB 4B	5 VB 5B	6 VIB 6B	7 VIIB 7B	8 ------- VIII -- ------- 8 -------	9	10 -----	11 IB 1B	12 IIB 2B	13 Al 26.98	14 Si 28.09	15 P 30.97	16 S 32.07	17 Cl 35.45	18 Ar 39.95
4 19 K 39.10	20 Ca 40.08	21 Sc 44.96	22 Ti 47.88	23 V 50.94	24 Cr 52.00	25 Mn 54.94	26 Fe 55.85	27 Co 58.47	28 Ni 58.69	29 Cu 63.55	30 Zn 65.39	31 Ga 69.72	32 Ge 72.59	33 As 74.92	34 Se 78.96	35 Br 79.90	36 Kr 83.80
5 37 Rb 85.47	38 Sr 87.62	39 Y 88.91	40 Zr 91.22	41 Nb 92.91	42 Mo 95.94	43 Tc (98)	44 Ru 101.1	45 Rh 102.9	46 Pd 106.4	47 Ag 107.9	48 Cd 112.4	49 In 114.8	50 Sn 118.7	51 Sb 121.8	52 Te 127.6	53 I 126.9	54 Xe 131.3
6 55 Cs 132.9	56 Ba 137.3	57 La* 138.9	72 Hf 178.5	73 Ta 180.9	74 W 183.9	75 Re 186.2	76 Os 190.2	77 Ir 190.2	78 Pt 195.1	79 Au 197.0	80 Hg 200.5	81 Tl 204.4	82 Pb 207.2	83 Bi 209.0	84 Po (210)	85 At (210)	86 Rn (222)
7 87 Fr (223)	88 Ra (226)	89 Ac~ (227)	104 Rf (257)	105 Db (260)	106 Sg (263)	107 Bh (262)	108 Hs (265)	109 Mt (266)	110 --- ()	111 --- ()	112 --- ()	114 --- ()		116 --- ()		118 --- ()

Lanthanide Series*

58 Ce 140.1	59 Pr 140.9	60 Nd 144.2	61 Pm (147)	62 Sm 150.4	63 Eu 152.0	64 Gd 157.3	65 Tb 158.9	66 Dy 162.5	67 Ho 164.9	68 Er 167.3	69 Tm 168.9	70 Yb 173.0	71 Lu 175.0

Actinide Series~

90 Th 232.0	91 Pa (231)	92 U (238)	93 Np (237)	94 Pu (242)	95 Am (243)	96 Cm (247)	97 Bk (247)	98 Cf (249)	99 Es (254)	100 Fm (253)	101 Md (256)	102 No (254)	103 Lr (257)

NOMENCLATURE

Nomenclature, the set of accepted conventions for naming compounds, is crucial to a discussion of organic chemistry. The rules of nomenclature presented in this chapter are for general cases only. More specific examples will be discussed in the chapters dealing with particular types of compounds.

You may see specific nomenclature questions on the MCAT, such as "Name the following compound," or "Which structure represents the following named compound?" But more importantly, nomenclature represents the basic language of organic chemistry. If you don't know it, you may feel like you're taking a test in a foreign language—which, in a way, you would be!

ALKANES

Alkanes are the simplest organic molecules, consisting only of carbon and hydrogen atoms held together by single bonds.

A. STRAIGHT-CHAIN ALKANES

The names of the four simplest alkanes are:

CH_4	CH_3CH_3	$CH_3CH_2CH_3$	$CH_3CH_2CH_2CH_3$
methane	ethane	propane	butane

The names of the longer-chain alkanes consist of prefixes derived from the Greek root for the number of carbon atoms, with the ending **-ane**.

C_5H_{12} = **pent**ane
C_6H_{14} = **hex**ane
C_7H_{16} = **hept**ane
C_8H_{18} = **oct**ane

C_9H_{20} = **non**ane
$C_{10}H_{22}$ = **dec**ane
$C_{11}H_{24}$ = **undec**ane
$C_{12}H_{26}$ = **dodec**ane

These prefixes are applicable to more complex organic molecules and should be memorized.

> **MCAT Synopsis**
>
> All straight-chain alkanes have the general formula C_nH_{2n+2} (n is an integer).

B. BRANCHED-CHAIN ALKANES

The International Union of Pure and Applied Chemistry (IUPAC) has proposed a set of simple rules for naming complex molecules. This basic system can be used to name all classes of organic compounds. Throughout these notes, the IUPAC names will be listed as the primary name, and common names will appear in parentheses.

1. **Find the longest chain in the compound.**

   The longest continuous carbon chain within the compound is taken as the backbone. If there are two or more chains of equal length, the most highly substituted chain takes precedence. The longest chain may not be obvious from the structural formula as it is drawn. For example, the backbone shown below is an octane (it contains eight carbon atoms).

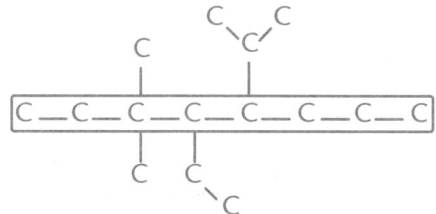

Figure 1.1

2. **Number the chain.**

   Number the chain from one end in such a way that the lowest set of numbers is obtained for the substituents.

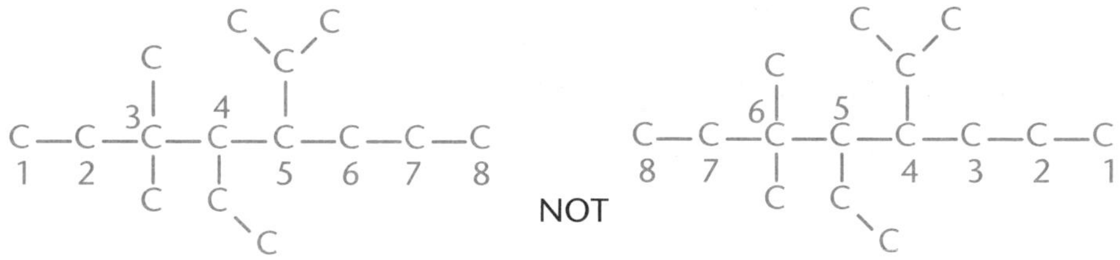

NOT

Figure 1.2

3. **Name the substituents.**

   Substituents are named according to their appropriate prefix with the ending **-yl**. More complex substituents are named as derivatives of the longest chain in the group.

$$CH_3- \qquad CH_3CH_2- \qquad CH_3CH_2CH_2-$$
$$\text{methyl} \qquad \text{ethyl} \qquad \textit{n}\text{-propyl}$$

   The prefix *n*- in the above example indicates an unbranched ("normal") compound. There are special names for some common branched alkanes, and these are usually used in the naming of substituents.

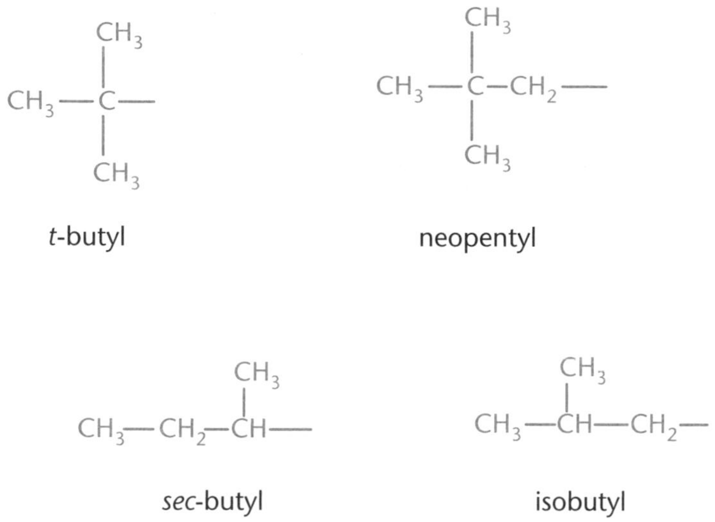

t-butyl
neopentyl
isopropyl
sec-butyl
isobutyl

Figure 1.3

> **MCAT Synopsis**
>
> You should memorize these common structures.

If there are two or more equivalent groups, the prefixes **di-**, **tri-**, **tetra-**, etc., are used.

4. **Assign a number to each substituent.**
   Each substituent is assigned a number to identify its point of attachment to the principal chain. If the prefixes **di-**, **tri-**, **tetra-**, etc., are used, a number is still necessary for each individual group.

5. **Complete the name.**
   List the substituents in alphabetical order with their corresponding numbers. Prefixes such as *di-*, *tri-*, etc., as well as the hyphenated prefixes (*tert-* [or *t-*], *sec-*, *n-*) are ignored in alphabetizing. In contrast, **cyclo-**, **iso-**, and **neo-** are considered part of the group name, and are alphabetized. Commas should be placed between numbers, and dashes should be placed between numbers and words. For example:

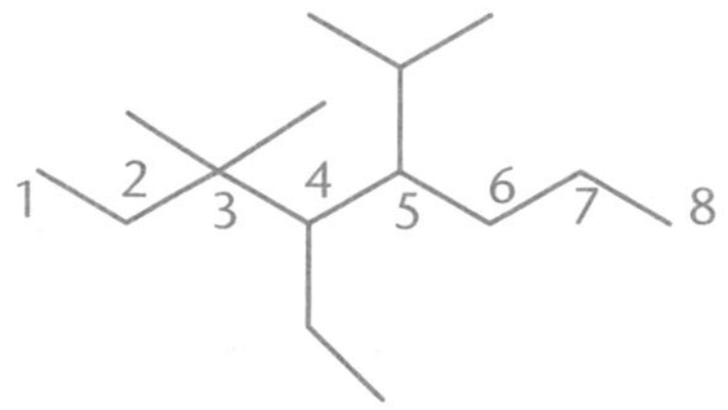

1
2
3
4
5
6
7
8

4-ethyl-5-isopropyl-3,3-dimethyl octane

Figure 1.4

You may also need to indicate the isomer you are describing, e.g., *cis* or *trans, R* or *S*, etc. Isomers will be discussed in detail in chapter 2.

C. CYCLOALKANES

Alkanes can form rings. These are named according to the number of carbon atoms in the ring with the prefix **cyclo-**.

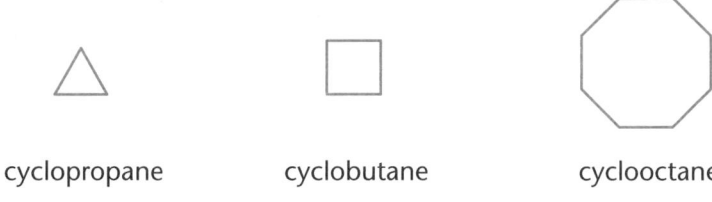

cyclopropane   cyclobutane   cyclooctane

Figure 1.5

Substituted cycloalkanes are named as derivatives of the parent cyclo-alkane. The substituents are named, and the carbon atoms are numbered around the ring *starting from the point of greatest substitution.* Again, the goal is to provide the lowest series of numbers as in Rule 2 on page 432.

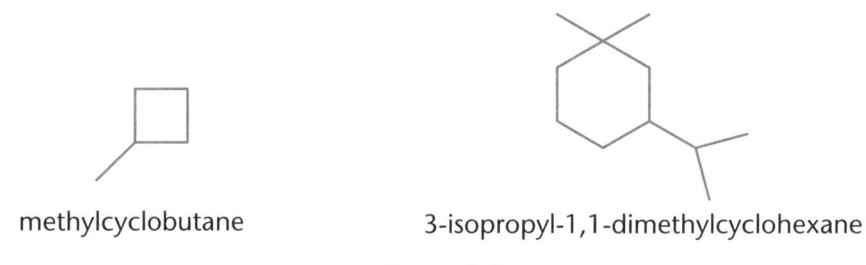

methylcyclobutane   3-isopropyl-1,1-dimethylcyclohexane

Figure 1.6

MORE COMPLICATED MOLECULES

Organic molecules that are more complicated than simple alkanes can also be named using this 5-step process, with a few additional considerations.

MULTIPLE BONDS

A. ALKENES

Alkenes (or **olefins**) are compounds containing carbon-carbon double bonds. The nomenclature rules are essentially the same as for alkanes, except that the ending **-ene** is used rather than **-ane**. (Exceptions: The common names *ethylene* and *propylene* which are used preferentially over the IUPAC names *ethene* and *propene*).

When identifying the carbon backbone, select the longest chain that contains the double bond (or the greatest number of double bonds, if more than one is present).

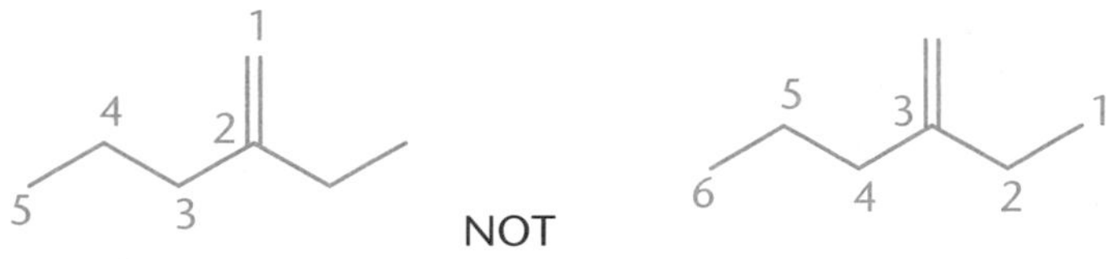

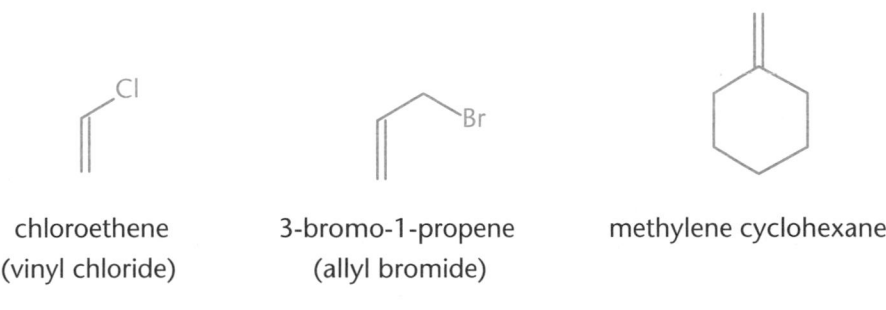

NOT

Figure 1.7

Number the backbone so that the double bond receives the lowest number possible. Remember that multiple double bonds must be named using the prefixes *di-, tri-,* etc. and that each must receive a number. Also, you may need to name the configurational isomer (*cis/trans, Z/E*). This topic will be discussed further in chapter 2.

Substituents are named as they are for alkanes, and their positions are specified by the number of the backbone carbon atom to which they are attached.

Frequently, an alkene group must be named as a substituent. In these cases, the systematic names may be used, but common names are more popular. **Vinyl-** derivatives are monosubstituted ethylenes (**ethenyl-**), and **allyl-**derivatives are propylenes substituted at the C–3 position (**2-propenyl-**). **Methylene-** refers to the –CH$_2$ group.

| chloroethene | 3-bromo-1-propene | methylene cyclohexane |
| (vinyl chloride) | (allyl bromide) | |

Figure 1.8

B. CYCLOALKENES

Cycloalkenes are named like cycloalkanes but with the suffix **-ene** rather than **-ane**. If there is only one double bond and no other substituents, a number is not necessary.

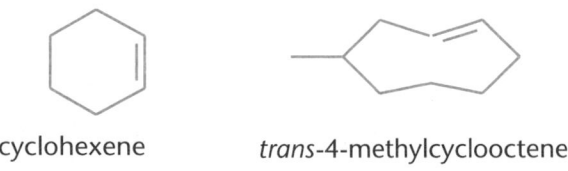

cyclohexene   *trans*-4-methylcyclooctene

Figure 1.9

MCAT Synopsis

Straight chain alkynes have the general formula C_nH_{2n-2} (n is an integer).

C. ALKYNES

Alkynes are compounds that possess carbon-carbon triple bonds. The suffix **-yne** replaces *-ane* in the parent alkane. The position of the triple bond is indicated by a number when necessary. The common name for ethyne is **acetylene**, and this name is used almost exclusively.

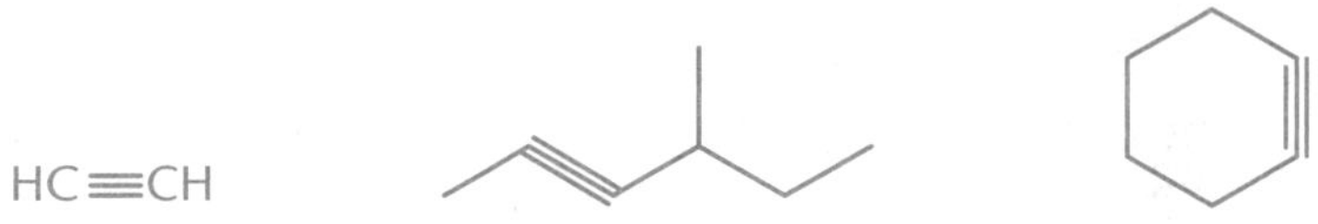

ethyne (acetylene) | 4-methyl-2-hexyne | cyclohexyne

Figure 1.10

SUBSTITUTED ALKANES

A. HALOALKANES

Compounds that contain a halogen substituent are named as **haloalkanes**. The appendages are numbered and alphabetized as alkyl groups are treated. Notice that the presence of the halide does not dramatically affect the numbering of the chain—you should still proceed so that substituents receive the lowest possible numbers. For example:

2-chloro-3-iodopentane | 1-chloro-2-methylcyclohexane

Figure 1.11

Alternatively, the haloalkane may be named as an **alkyl halide**. In this system, chloroethane is called **ethyl chloride**. Other examples are:

2-bromo-2-methylpropane (*t*-butyl bromide) | 2-iodopropane (isopropyl iodide)

Figure 1.12

B. ALCOHOLS

In the IUPAC system, **alcohols** are named by replacing the **-e** of the corresponding alkane with **-ol**. The chain is numbered in such a way that the carbon attached to the hydroxyl group (–OH) receives the lowest number possible.

MCAT Synopsis

–OH has priority over a multiple bond when numbering the chain.

In compounds that possess a multiple bond and a hydroxyl group, numerical priority is given to the carbon attached to the –OH.

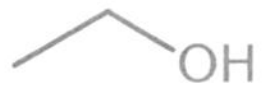

ethanol

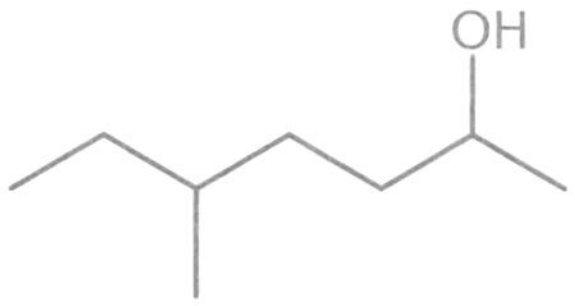

5-methyl-2-heptanol

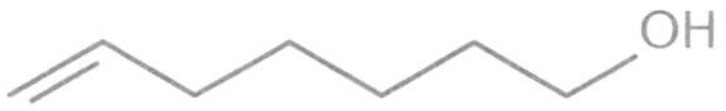

hept-6-en-1-ol

Figure 1.13

A common system of nomenclature exists for alcohols in which the name of the alkyl group is combined with the word *alcohol*. These common names are used for simple alcohols. For example, methanol may be named "methyl alcohol," while 2-propanol may also be named "isopropyl alcohol."

Molecules with two hydroxyl groups are called **diols** (or **glycols**) and are named with the suffix **-diol**. Two numbers are necessary to locate the two functional groups. Diols with hydroxyl groups on adjacent carbons are referred to as **vicinal**, and diols with hydroxyl groups on the same carbon are **geminal**. Geminal diols (also called **hydrates**) are not commonly observed because they spontaneously lose water (**dehydrate**) to produce carbonyl compounds (containing C=O; see chapter 8).

C. ETHERS

In the IUPAC system, **ethers** are named as derivatives of alkanes, and the larger alkyl group is chosen as the backbone. The ether functionality is specified as an **alkoxy**- prefix, indicating the presence of an ether (*-oxy-*), and the corresponding smaller alkyl group (*alk-*). The chain is numbered to give the ether the lowest position. Common names for ethers are frequently used. They are derived by naming the two alkyl groups in alphabetical order and adding the word *ether*. The generic term *ether* refers to diethyl ether, a commonly used solvent.

For **cyclic ethers**, numbering of the ring begins at the oxygen and proceeds to provide the lowest numbers for the substituents. Three-membered rings are termed **oxiranes** by IUPAC, although they are commonly called **epoxides**.

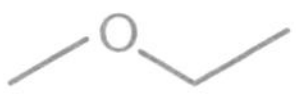

methoxyethane
(ethyl methyl ether)

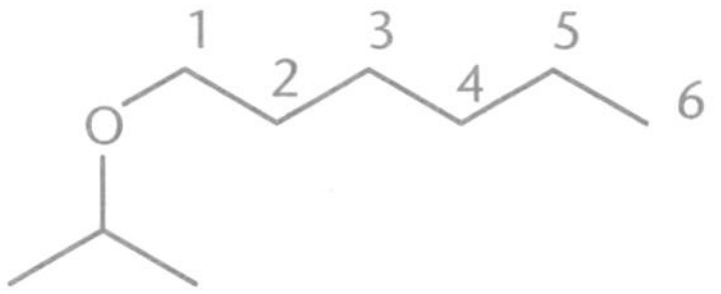

1-isopropoxyhexane
(n-hexyl isopropyl ether)

> **MCAT Synopsis**
>
> Cyclic ethers with three members are *epoxides*.

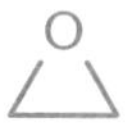

oxirane
(ethylene oxide)

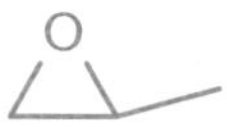

2-methyloxirane
(propylene oxide)

Figure 1.14

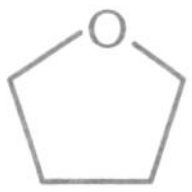

tetrahydrofuran
(THF)

Figure 1.15

> **MCAT Synopsis**
>
> An aldehyde is a terminal functional group: it defines the C-1 of the backbone.

D. ALDEHYDES AND KETONES

Aldehydes are named according to the longest chain containing the aldehyde functional group. The suffix **-al** replaces the **-e** of the corresponding alkane. The carbonyl carbon receives the lowest number, although numbers are not always necessary since by definition an aldehyde is terminal and receives the number 1.

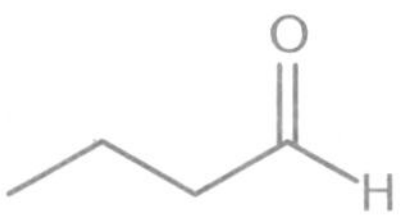

n-butanal

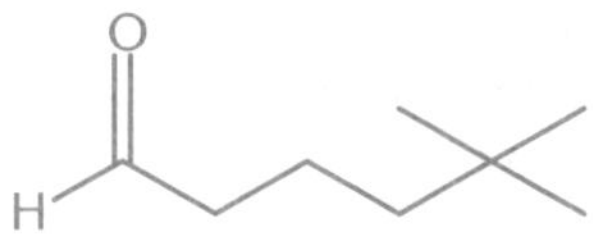

5,5-dimethylhexanal

Figure 1.16

The common names *formaldehyde*, *acetaldehyde*, and *propionaldehyde* are used almost exclusively instead of the IUPAC names *methanal*, *ethanal*, and *propanal*, respectively.

MCAT Synopsis

The carbonyl in a ketone should receive the lowest number possible unless there is a higher priority group.

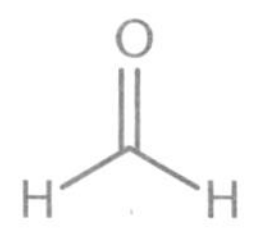

methanal
(formaldehyde)

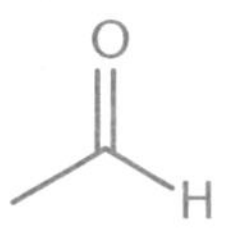

ethanal
(acetaldehyde)

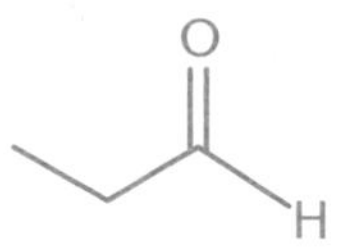

propanal
(propionaldehyde)

Figure 1.17

Ketones are named analogously, with **-one** as a suffix. The carbonyl group has to be assigned the lowest possible number. In complex molecules, the carbonyl group can be named as a prefix with the term **oxo-**. Alternatively, the individual alkyl groups may be listed in alphabetical order, followed by the word **ketone**.

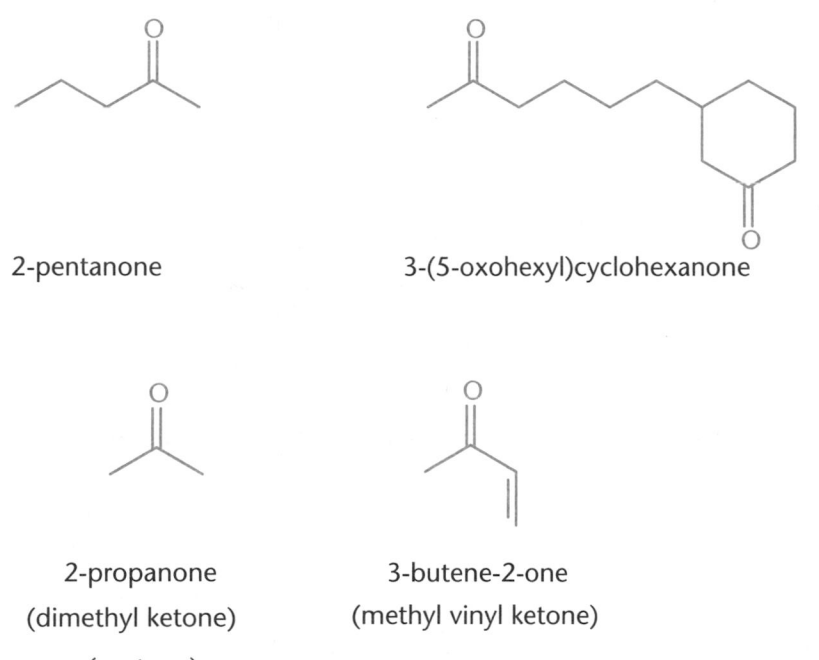

2-pentanone

3-(5-oxohexyl)cyclohexanone

2-propanone
(dimethyl ketone)
(acetone)

3-butene-2-one
(methyl vinyl ketone)

Figure 1.18

A commonly used alternative to the numerical designation of substituents is to term the carbon atom adjacent to the carbonyl carbon as α and the carbon atoms successively along the chain as β, γ, δ, etc. This system is encountered with dicarbonyl compounds and halocarbonyl compounds.

E. CARBOXYLIC ACIDS

Carboxylic acids are named with the ending **-oic** and the word **acid** replacing the **-e** ending of the corresponding alkane. Carboxylic acids are terminal functional groups and, like aldehydes, are numbered one (1). The common names formic acid (methanoic acid), acetic acid (ethanoic acid), and propionic acid (propanoic acid) are used almost exclusively.

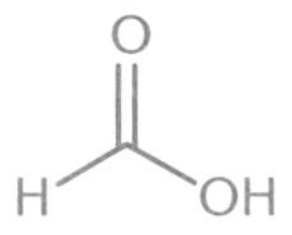

methanoic acid (formic acid)

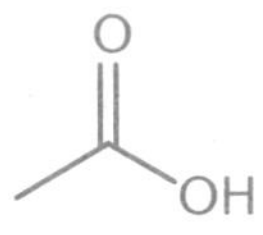

ethanoic acid (acetic acid)

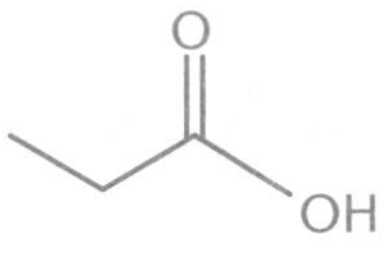

propanoic acid (propionic acid)

Figure 1.19

F. AMINES

The longest chain attached to the nitrogen atom is taken as the backbone. For simple compounds, name the alkane and replace the final "e" with "amine."

MCAT Synopsis

When additional alkyl groups are attached to the nitrogen, use the prefix N–.

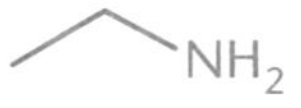

ethanamine

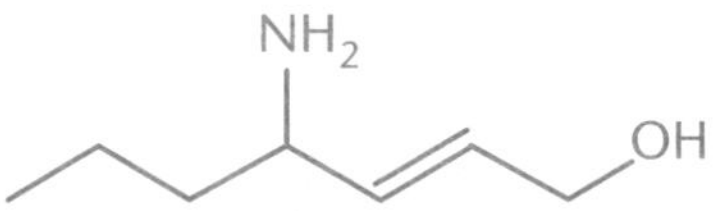

4-aminohept-2-en-1-ol

Figure 1.20

To specify the location of an additional alkyl group that is attached to the nitrogen, the prefix ***N***- is used:

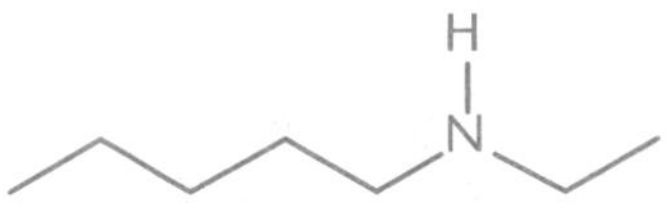

N-ethylpentanamine
(ethylpentylamine)

Figure 1.21

SUMMARY OF FUNCTIONAL GROUPS

Table 1.1 lists the major functional groups you need to known for the MCAT.

Table 1.1

Functional Group	Structure	IUPAC Prefix	IUPAC Suffix
Carboxylic acid	R–C(=O)–OH	carboxy-	-oic acid
Ester	R–C(=O)–OR	alkoxycarbonyl-	-oate
Acyl halide	R–C(=O)–X	halocarbonyl-	-oyl halide
Amide	R–C(=O)–NH$_2$	amido-	-amide
Nitrile/Cyanide	RC≡N	cyano-	-nitrile
Aldehyde	R–C(=O)–H	oxo-	-al
Ketone	R–C(=O)–R	oxo-	-one
Alcohol	ROH	hydroxy-	-ol
Thiol	RSH	sulfhydryl-	-thiol
Amine	RNH$_2$	amino-	-amine
Imine	R$_2$C=NR'	imino-	-imine
Ether	ROR	alkoxy-	-ether
Sulfide	R$_2$S	alkylthio-	
Halide	-I, -Br, -Cl, -F	halo-	
Nitro	RNO$_2$	nitro-	
Azide	RN$_3$	azido-	
Diazo	RN$_2$+	diazo-	

1SOMERS

Isomers are chemical compounds that have the same molecular formula but differ in structure—that is, in their atomic connectivity, rotational orientation, or the 3-dimensional position of their atoms. Isomers may be extremely similar, sharing most or all of their physical and chemical properties, or they may be very different.

```
                              Stereoisomers
Most                         ┌──────┴──────┐         Most
Different                    │             │        \Similar
     ◄──────────┼────────────┼─────────────┼──────────►
     Structural          Diastereomers  Enantiomers  Conformation
                         (including
                         geometric isomers)
```

Structural isomers are the most unlike each other, while conformational isomers are the most similar.

STRUCTURAL ISOMERISM

Structural isomers are compounds that share only their molecular formula. Because their atomic connections may be completely different, they often have very different chemical and physical properties (such as melting point, boiling point, solubility, etc.). For example, five different structures exist for compounds with the formula C6H14.

MCAT Synopsis

Structural isomers share only their molecular formula; their atomic connectivity is different. Therefore, they may have very different chemical and physical properties.

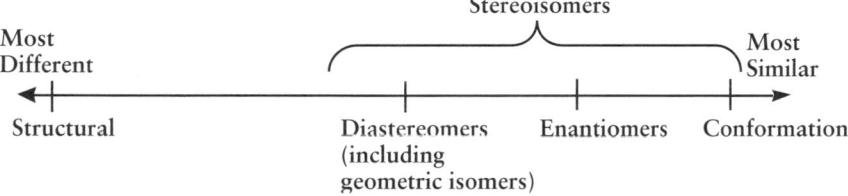

n-hexene   2-methylpentane

3-methylpentane   2,3-methylpentane   2,2-methylpentane

Figure 2.1

All have the same formula, but they differ in their carbon framework and in the number and type of atoms bonded to each other.

STEREOISOMERISM

Stereoisomers are compounds that differ from each other only in the way that their atoms are oriented in space. Geometric isomers; enantiomers, diastereomers, and *meso* compounds; and conformational isomers all fall under this heading.

ISOMERS

STRUCTURAL ISOMERS (constitutional isomers)   STEREOISOMERS

CONFIGURATIONAL ISOMERS   CONFORMATIONAL ISOMERS

DIASTEREOMERS   ENANTIOMERS

GEOMETRIC ISOMERS

Figure 2.2

A. GEOMETRIC ISOMERS

Geometric isomers are compounds that differ in the position of substituents attached to a double bond. If two substituents are on the same side, the double bond is called **cis**. If they are on opposite sides, it is a **trans** double bond.

For compounds with polysubstituted double bonds, the situation can be confusing, and an alternative method of naming is employed. The highest priority substituent attached to each double bonded carbon has to be determined: The higher the atomic number, the higher the priority, and if the atomic numbers are equal, priority is determined by the substituents of these atoms. The alkene is called (*Z*) (from German *zusammen*, meaning "together") if the two highest priority substituents on each carbon lie on the same side of the double bond, and (*E*) (from German *entgegen*, meaning opposite) if they are on opposite sides.

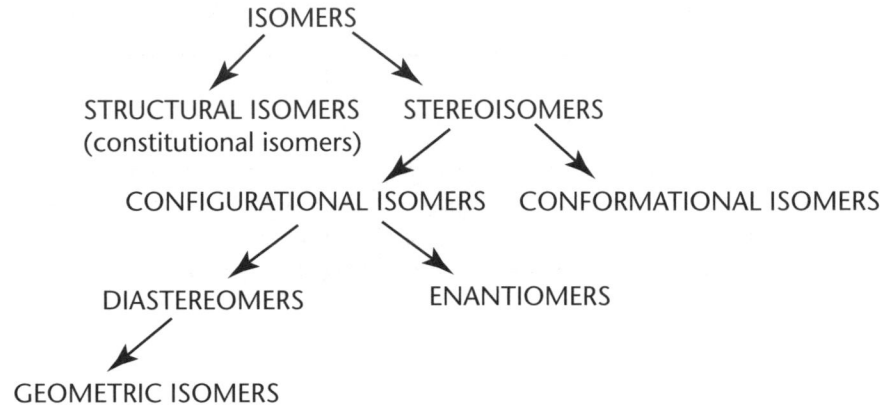

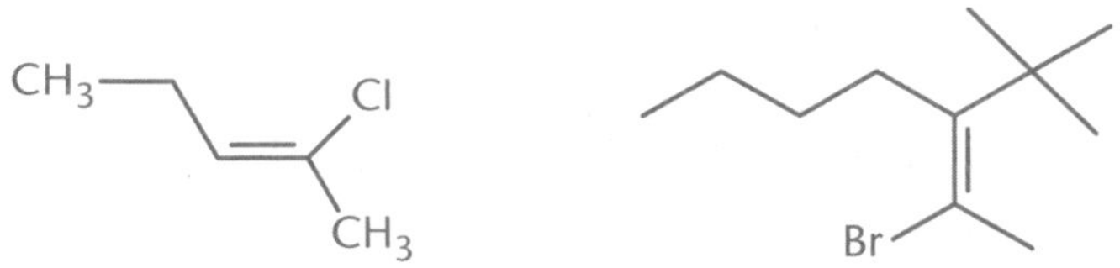

(*Z*)-2-chloro-2-pentene   (*E*)-2-bromo-3-*t*-butyl-2-heptene

Figure 2.3

B. CHIRALITY

An object that is not superimposable upon its mirror image is called **chiral**. Familiar chiral objects are your right and left hands. Although essentially identical, they differ in their ability to fit into a right-handed glove. They are mirror images of each other, yet cannot be superimposed. **Achiral** objects are mirror images that can be superimposed; for example, the letter A is identical to its mirror image and therefore achiral.

MCAT Synopsis

Chirality = handedness. Nonsuperimposable mirror images exist—like your right and left hands.

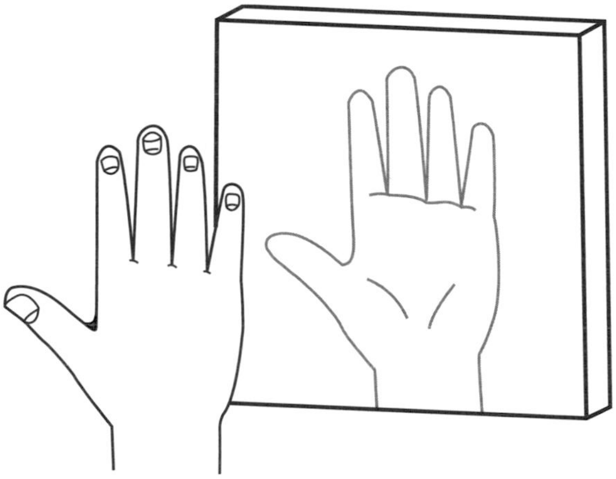

Figure 2.4

In organic chemistry, chirality is most frequently encountered when carbon atoms have four different substituents. Such a carbon atom is called *asymmetric* because it lacks a plane or point of symmetry. For example, the C-1 carbon atom in 1-bromo-1-chloroethane has four different substituents. The molecule is chiral because it is not superimposable on its mirror image. Chiral objects that are non-superimposable mirror images are called **enantiomers** and are a specific type of stereoisomer.

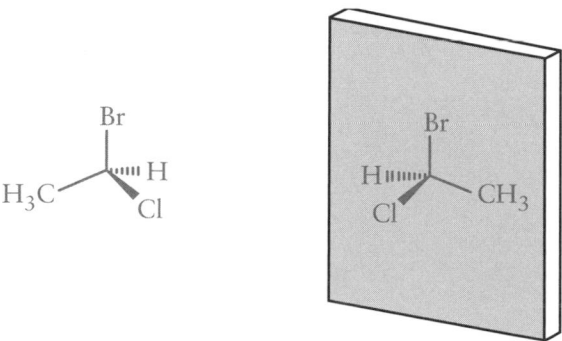

MCAT Synopsis

A carbon must have four different substituents to be a chiral center.

Figure 2.5

MCAT Synopsis

Rotating a molecule in space does not change its chirality.

A carbon atom with only three different substituents, such as 1,1-dibromoethane, has a plane of symmetry and is therefore achiral. A simple 180° rotation along the *y*-axis allows the compound to be superimposed upon its mirror image.

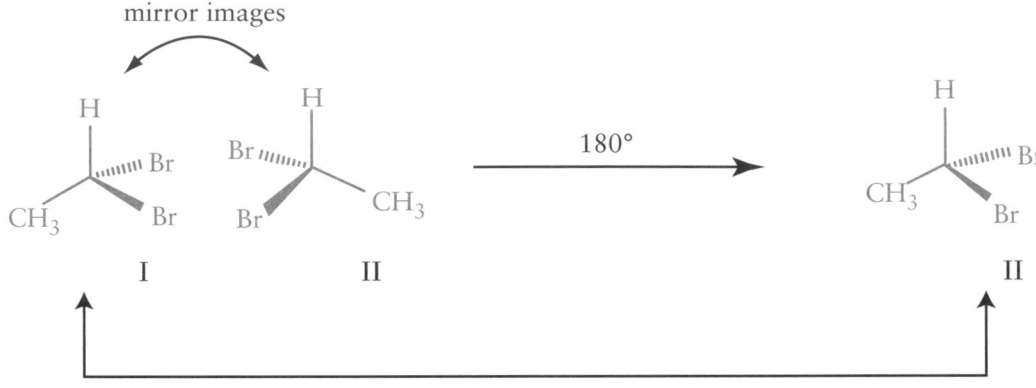

Superimposable

Figure 2.6

1. **Relative and Absolute Configuration**

The **configuration** is the spatial arrangement of the atoms or groups of a stereoisomer. The **relative configuration** of a chiral molecule is its configuration in relation to another chiral molecule. The **absolute configuration** of a chiral molecule describes the spatial arrangement of these atoms or groups. There is a set sequence to determine the absolute configuration of a molecule at a single chiral center:

Step 1:

Assign priority to the four substituents, looking only at the first atom that is directly attached to the chiral center. Higher atomic number takes precedence over lower atomic number. If the atomic numbers are equal, then priority is determined by the substituents attached to these atoms. For example:

> ### MCAT Synopsis
> When assigning priority, look only at the first atom attached to the chiral carbon, not at the group as a whole! The higher the atomic number, the higher the priority—this same system is used when determining Z and E.

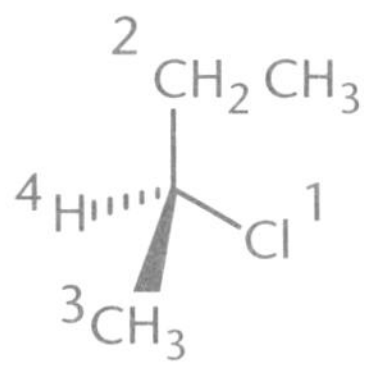

$$\overset{2}{CH_2}CH_3$$
$$\overset{4}{H}\text{''''}\overset{}{\underset{\underset{3}{CH_3}}{}}Cl\ ^1$$

Figure 2.7

Step 2:

Orient the molecule in space so that the line of sight proceeds down the bond from the asymmetric carbon atom (the chiral center) to the substituent with lowest priority. The three substituents with highest priority should radiate from the asymmetric atom like the spokes of a wheel.

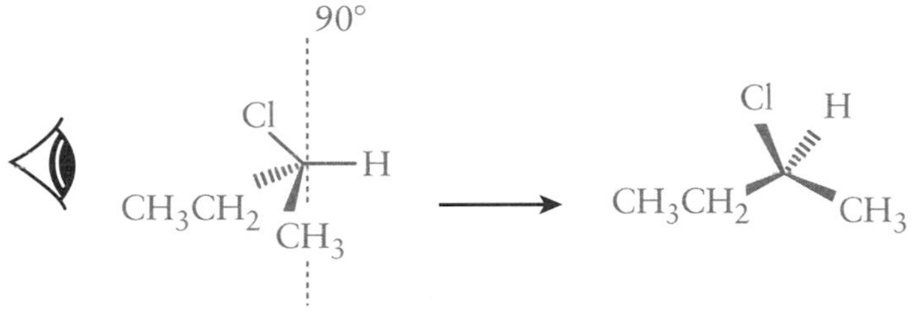

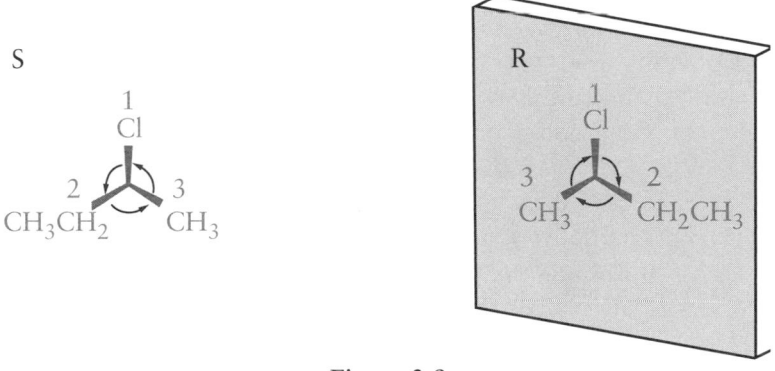

Figure 2.8

Step 3:

Proceeding from highest priority (#1) on down, determine the order of substituents around the wheel as either clockwise or counterclockwise. If the order is clockwise, the asymmetric atom is called ***R*** (from Latin *rectus,* meaning "right"). If it is counterclockwise, it is called ***S*** (from Latin *sinister,* meaning "left").

Figure 2.9

Step 4:

Provide a full name for the compound. The terms *R* and *S* are put in parentheses and separated from the rest of the name by a dash. If there is more than one asymmetric carbon, location is specified by a number preceding the *R* or *S* within the parentheses, without a dash.

2. **Fischer Projections**

A three-dimensional molecule can be conveniently represented in two dimensions in a **Fischer projection**. In this system, horizontal lines indicate bonds that project out from the plane of the page, while vertical lines indicate bonds behind the plane of the page. The

> **MCAT Synopsis**
>
> *R* and *S* are conventions of notation. They do not predict the direction of light rotation.

> **MCAT Synopsis**
>
> To determine the absolute configuration at a single chiral center:
>
> 1. Assign priority by atomic number.
> 2. Orient the molecule with the lowest priority substituent in the back.
> 3. Move around the molecule from highest to lowest priority (1 → 2 → 3).
> 4. Clockwise = *R*
>   Counterclockwise = *S*.

point of intersection of the lines represents a carbon atom. They can be interconverted by interchanging any two pairs of substituents, or by rotating the projection in the plane of the page by 180°. If only one pair of substituents is interchanged, or if the molecule is rotated by 90°, the mirror image of the original compound is obtained.

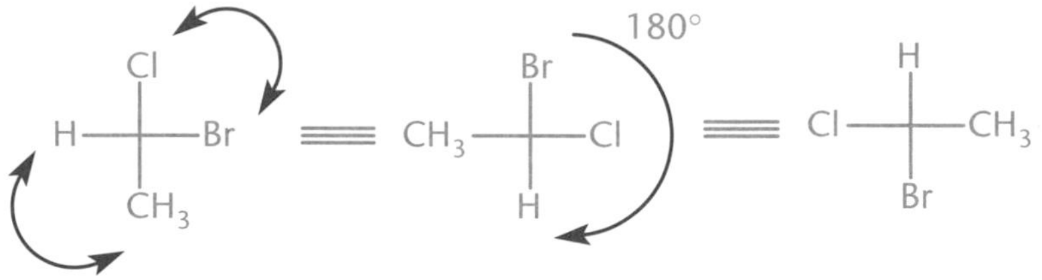

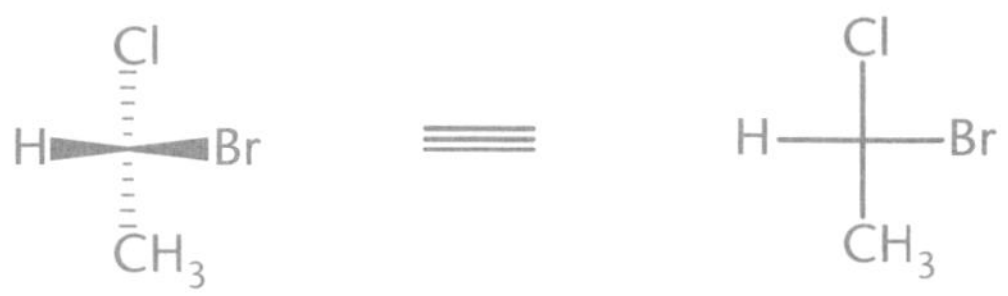

Figure 2.10

> **MCAT Synopsis**
>
> Differences in chirality (handedness) can produce isomers such as *enantiomers* (nonsuperimposable mirror images) as well as *diastereomers* (isomers that differ in their chirality but are not mirror images). *Meso compounds* contain chiral centers but are not optically active due to an internal mirror plane of symmetry.

This provides another way to determine the chirality at a chiral center. If the lowest priority substituent is on the vertical axis, it is already pointing away from you. Simply picture moving from #1 → #2 → #3, and you'll be able to name the center.

However, if the lowest priority substituent is on the horizontal axis, it is pointing towards you, and so the situation is trickier. Here are some ways to handle this situation:

1) Go ahead and imagine rotating from #1 → #2 → #3. Obtain a designation (*R* or *S*). The *true* designation will be the opposite of what you have just obtained.
2) Alternatively, make a single switch—move the low priority substituent so that it is on the vertical axis. Obtain the designation (*R* or *S*). Again, the *true* designation will be the opposite of what you have just obtained.
3) Another approach is to make two switches or interconversions—that is, move the low-priority atom to the vertical axis and "trade" some other pair of atoms at the same time. This new molecule has the same configuration as the molecule you started with. So you can go ahead and determine the correct designation right away.

3. Optical Activity

Enantiomers have identical chemical and physical properties with one exception: **optical activity**. A compound is optically active if it has the ability to rotate plane-polarized light. Ordinary light is unpolarized. It consists of waves vibrating in all possible planes perpendicular to its direction of motion. A polarizer allows light waves oscillating only in a particular direction to pass, producing plane-polarized light.

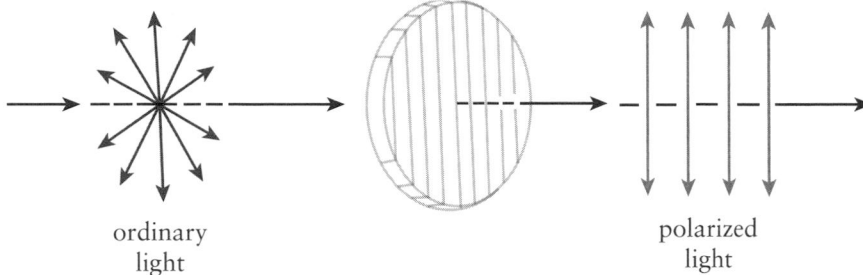

ordinary
light

polarized
light

Figure 2.11

If plane-polarized light is passed through an optically active compound, the orientation of the plane is rotated by an angle α. The enantiomer of this compound will rotate light by the same amount, but in the opposite direction. A compound that rotates the plane of polarized light to the right, or clockwise (from the point of view of an observer seeing the light approach), is **dextrorotatory** and is indicated by (+). A compound that rotates light toward the left, or counterclockwise, is **levorotatory** and is labeled (–). The direction of rotation cannot be determined from the structure of a molecule and must be determined experimentally.

The amount of rotation depends on the number of molecules that a light wave encounters. This depends on two factors: the concentration of the optically active compound and the length of the tube through which the light passes. Chemists have set standard conditions of 1 g/mL for concentration and 1 dm for length in order to compare the optical activities of different compounds. Rotations measured at different concentrations and tube lengths can be converted to a standardized **specific rotation** (α) using the following equation:

$$\text{specific rotation } ([\alpha]) = \frac{\text{observed rotation } (\alpha)}{\text{concentration (g/mL)} \times \text{length (dm)}}$$

A **racemic mixture**, or **racemic modification**, is a mixture of equal concentrations of both the (+) and (–) enantiomers. The rotations cancel each other and no optical activity is observed.

C. OTHER CHIRAL COMPOUNDS
1. Diastereomers
For any molecule with n chiral centers, there are 2^n possible stereoisomers. Thus, if a compound has two chiral carbon atoms, it has four possible stereoisomers (see Figure 2.12).

MCAT Favorite

The direction of rotation can only be determined experimentally. *S* or *R* says nothing about the direction of rotation.

MCAT Synopsis

A racemic mixture displays no optical activity.

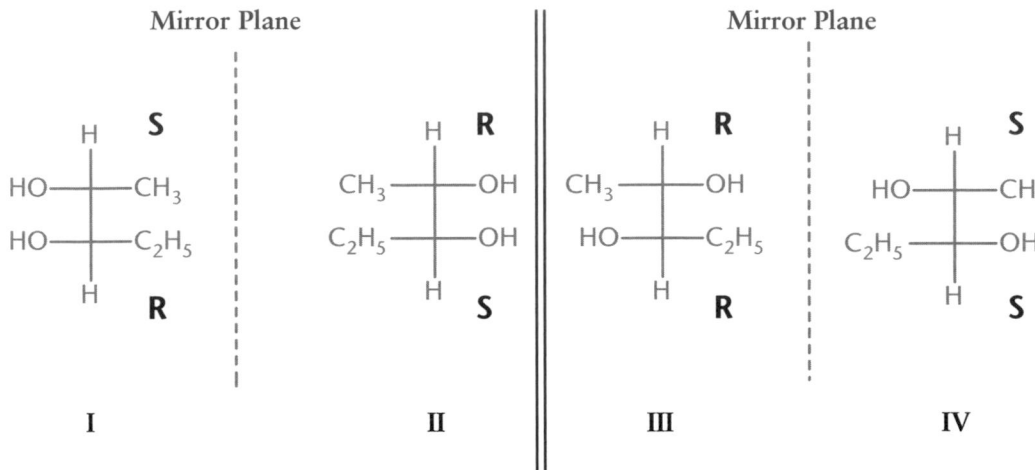

Figure 2.12

I and II are mirror images of each other and are therefore enantiomers. Similarly, III and IV are enantiomers. However, I and III are not. They are stereoisomers that are not mirror images, and so they are called **diastereomers**. Notice that other combinations of nonmirror image stereoisomers are also diastereomeric. Hence I and IV, II and III, I and III, and II and IV are all pairs of diastereomers.

2. **Meso Compounds**

    The criterion for optical activity of a molecule containing a single chiral center is that it has no plane of symmetry. The same criterion applies to a molecule with two or more chiral centers. If a plane of symmetry exists, the molecule is not optically active, even though it possesses chiral centers. Such a molecule is called a *meso* compound. For example:

    D- and L-tartaric acid are both optically active, but *meso*-tartaric acid

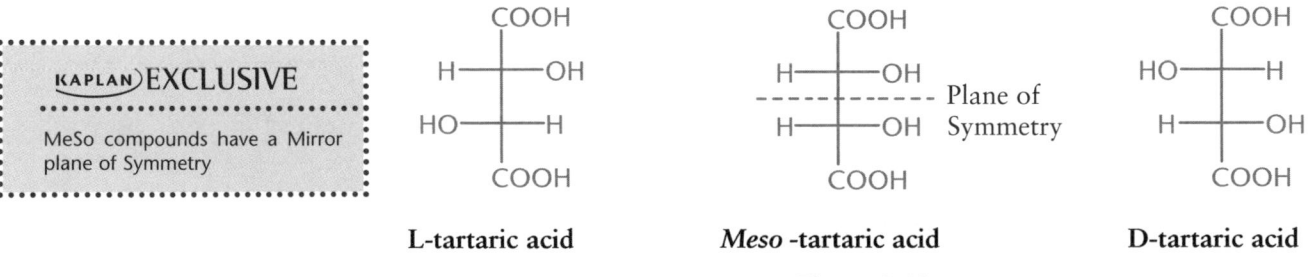

L-tartaric acid   *Meso*-tartaric acid   **D-tartaric acid**

Figure 2.13

has a plane of symmetry and is not optically active. Although *meso*-tartaric acid has two chiral carbon atoms, the lack of optical activity is a function of the molecule as a whole.

D. CONFORMATIONAL ISOMERISM

Conformational isomers are compounds that differ only by rotation about one or more single bonds. Essentially, these isomers represent the same compound in a slightly different position—analogous to a person who may be either standing up or sitting down. These different conformations can be seen when the molecule is depicted in a **Newman projection,** in which the line of sight extends along a carbon-carbon bond axis. The conformations are encountered as the molecule is rotated about this axis. The classic example for demonstrating conformational isomerism in a straight chain is *n*-butane. In a Newman projection, the line of sight extends through the C-2—C-3 bond axis.

MCAT Synopsis

Think of conformational isomers as being different positions (conformations) of a compound—like a person who may be standing up or sitting down. Thus, they are often easily interconverted.

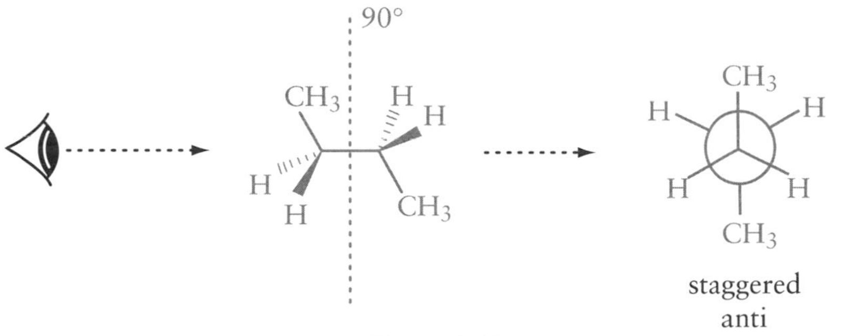

Figure 2.14

1. Straight-Chain Conformations

The most stable conformation is when the two methyl groups (C-1 and C-4) are oriented 180° from each other. There is no overlap of atoms along the line of sight (besides C-2 and C-3), so the molecule is said to be in a **staggered** conformation. Specifically, it is called the ***anti*** conformation, because the two methyl groups are antiperiplanar to each other. This particular orientation is very stable and thus represents an energy minimum because all atoms are far apart, minimizing repulsive steric interactions.

The other type of staggered conformation, called ***gauche,*** occurs when the two methyl groups are 60° apart. In order to convert from the *anti* to the *gauche* conformation, the molecule must pass through an **eclipsed** conformation, in which the two methyl groups are 120° apart and overlap with the H atoms on the adjacent carbon. When the two methyl groups overlap with each other, the molecule is said to be **totally eclipsed** and is in its highest energy state.

KAPLAN EXCLUSIVE

It's "gauche" (or inappropriate) for one methyl group to stand too close to another group!

MCAT Synopsis

Notice that the anti isomer has the lowest energy, while the totally eclipsed isomer has the highest energy.

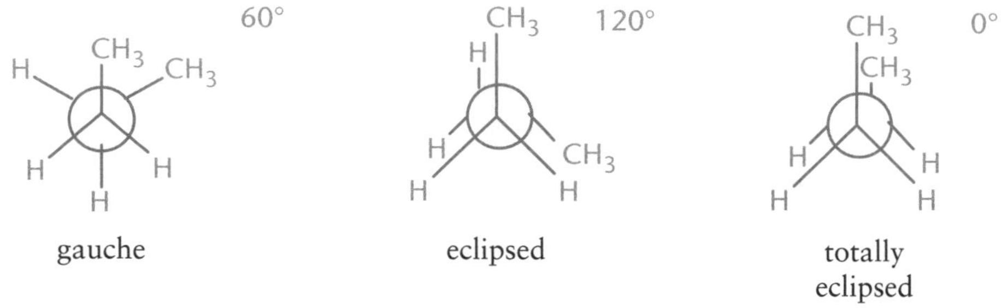

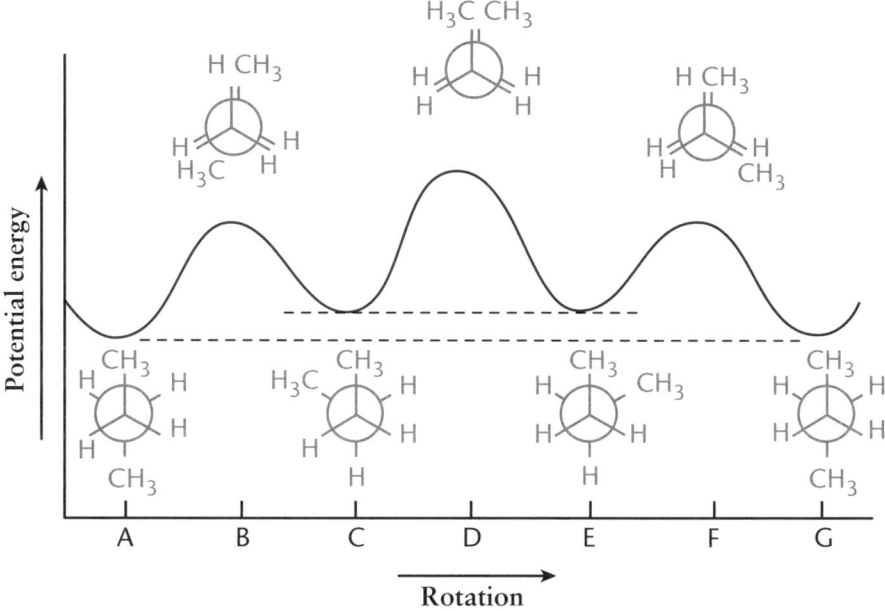

Figure 2.15

A plot of potential energy versus the degree of rotation about the C-2—C-3 bond shows the relative minima and maxima the molecule encounters throughout its various conformations.

Figure 2.16

It is important to note that these barriers are rather small (3–4 kcal/mol) and are easily overcome at room temperature. Very low temperatures will slow conformational interconversion. If the molecules do not possess sufficient energy to cross the energy barrier, they may not rotate at all.

2. **Cyclic Conformations**
   a. **Strain Energies**
   In cycloalkanes, ring strain arises from three factors: angle strain, torsional strain, and nonbonded strain. Angle strain results when bond angles deviate from their ideal values; torsional strain results when cyclic molecules must assume conformations that have eclipsed interactions; and nonbonded strain (van der Waals

repulsion) results when atoms or groups compete for the same space. In order to alleviate these three types of strain, cycloalkanes attempt to adopt nonplanar conformations. Cyclobutane puckers into a slight V shape, cyclopentane adopts what is called the **envelope** conformation, and cyclohexane exists mainly in three conformations called the **chair,** the **boat,** and the **twist** or **skew-boat**.

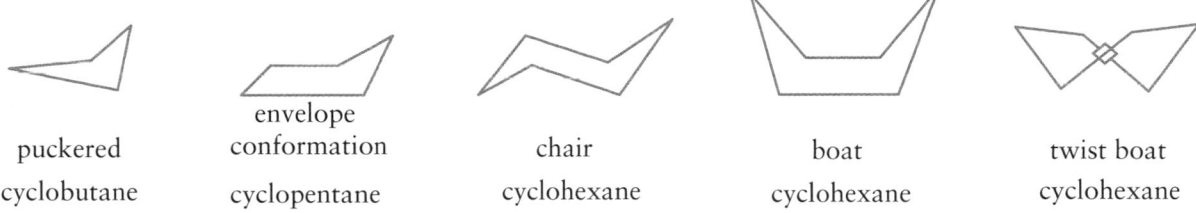

| puckered cyclobutane | envelope conformation cyclopentane | chair cyclohexane | boat cyclohexane | twist boat cyclohexane |

Conformations of cyclic hydrocarbons

Figure 2.17

b. Cyclohexane

i. Unsubstituted

The most stable conformation of cyclohexane is the chair conformation. In this conformation, all three types of strain are eliminated. The hydrogen atoms that are perpendicular to the plane of the ring are called **axial,** and those parallel are called **equatorial**. The axial-equatorial orientations alternate around the ring.

The boat conformation is adopted when the chair "flips" and converts to another chair. In such a process, hydrogen atoms that were equatorial become axial, and vice versa, in the new chair. In the boat conformation, all of the atoms are eclipsed, creating a high-energy state. To avoid this strain, the boat can twist into a slightly more stable form called the twist or skew-boat conformation.

ii. Monosubstituted

The interconversion between the two chairs can be slowed or even prevented if a sterically bulky group is attached to the ring. The equatorial position is favored over the axial position because of steric repulsion with other axial substituents. Hence, a large group such as *t*-butyl can lock the molecule in one conformation.

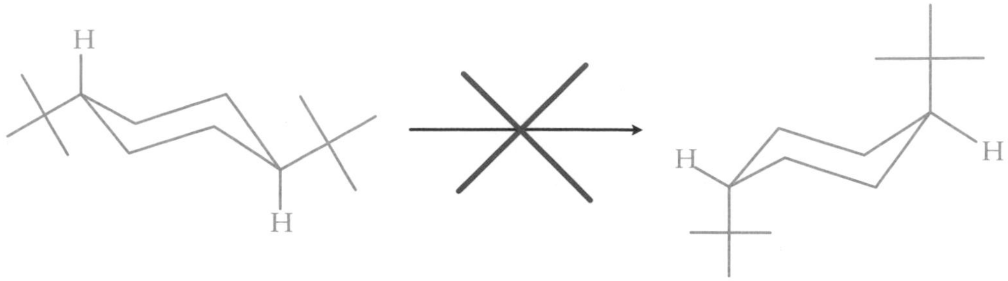

Bulky groups prefer equatorial positions

Figure 2.18

> **MCAT Synopsis**
>
> A bulky substituent can prevent the ring from adopting certain conformations.

iii. **Disubstituted**

Different isomers can exist for disubstituted cycloalkanes. If both substituents are located on the same side of the ring, the molecule is called ***cis***; if the two groups are on opposite sides of the ring, it is called ***trans***.

> **MCAT Synopsis**
>
> *Cis* and *trans* apply to cycloalkanes too!

cis-1,2-dimethylcyclohexane *trans*-1,2-dimethylcyclohexane

Figure 2.19

In *trans*-1,4-dimethylcyclohexane, both of the methyl groups are equatorial in one chair conformation and axial in the other, but in either case they point in opposite directions relative to the plane of the ring.

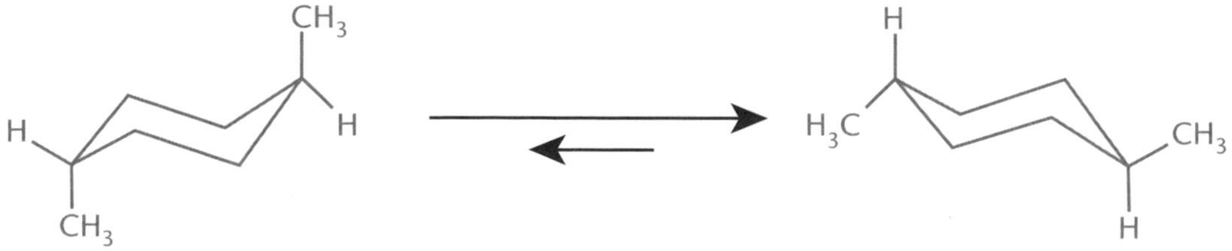

trans-1,4-dimethylcyclohexane

Figure 2.20

3

BONDING

As discussed in General Chemistry, there are two types of chemical bonds: **ionic**, in which an electron is transferred from one atom to another, and **covalent**, in which pairs of electrons are shared between two atoms. In organic chemistry, it is important to understand the details of covalent bonding, as these play a crucial role in determining the properties and reactions of organic compounds.

ATOMIC ORBITALS

The first three quantum numbers, n, l, and m, describe the size, shape, and number of the atomic orbitals that an element possesses. The number n, which can equal 1, 2, 3, . . . , corresponds to the energy levels in an atom and is essentially a measure of size. Within each electron shell, there can be several types of orbitals (s, p, d, f, g, . . . , corresponding to the quantum numbers $l = 0, 1, 2, 3, 4, . . . $). Each type of atomic orbital has a specific shape. An s orbital is spherical and symmetrical, and it is centered around the nucleus. A p orbital is composed of two lobes located symmetrically about the nucleus and contains a **node** (an area in which the probability of finding an electron is zero). A d orbital is composed of four symmetrical lobes and contains two nodes. Both d and f orbitals are complex in shape and are rarely encountered in organic chemistry.

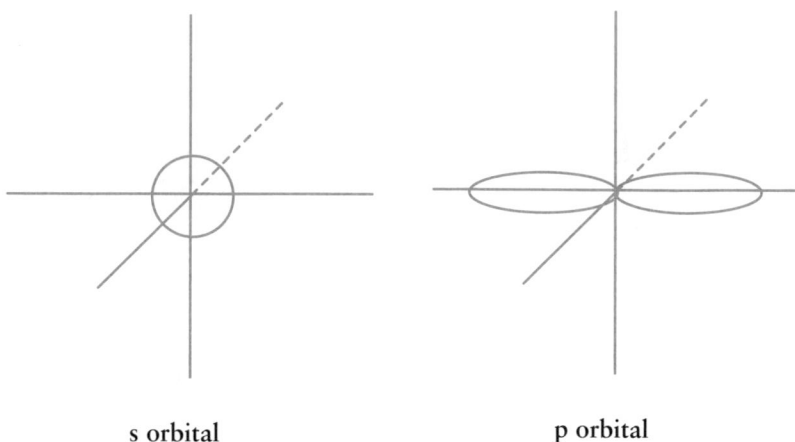

s orbital   p orbital

Figure 3.1

MOLECULAR ORBITALS

A. SINGLE BONDS

Two atomic orbitals can be combined to form what is called a **molecular orbital (MO)**. Molecular orbitals are obtained mathematically by adding the wave functions of the atomic orbitals. If the signs of the wave functions are the same, a lower-energy **bonding orbital** is produced. If the signs are different, a higher-energy **antibonding orbital** is produced. This is represented schematically by the addition of two s orbitals. Two p orbitals or one p and one s orbital can be combined in a similar fashion.

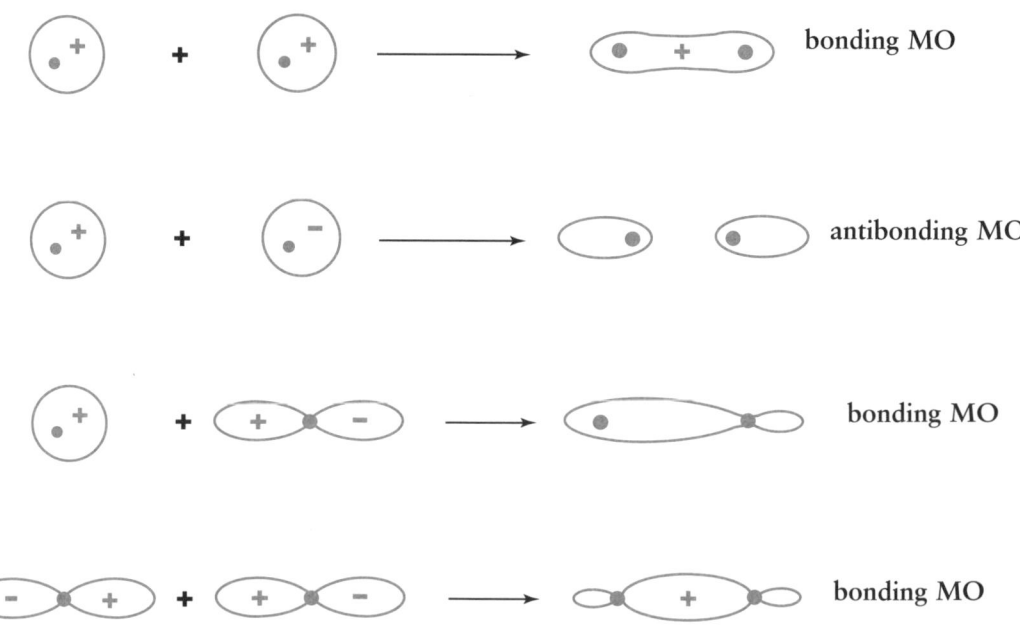

Figure 3.2

When a molecular orbital is formed by head-to-head overlap as in Figure 3.2, the resulting bond is called a **sigma (σ) bond**. All single bonds are sigma bonds, accommodating two electrons. Shorter single bonds are stronger than longer single bonds.

B. DOUBLE AND TRIPLE BONDS

When two p orbitals overlap in a parallel fashion, a bonding MO is formed, called a **pi (π) bond**. When both a sigma and a pi bond exist between two atoms, a **double bond** is formed. When a sigma bond and two pi bonds exist, a **triple bond** is formed. As can be seen in Figure 3.3, the overlap of the p orbitals involved in a p bond hinder rotation about double and triple bonds.

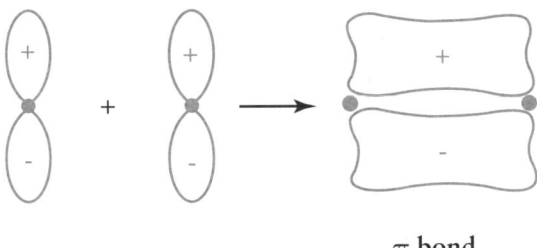

π bond

Figure 3.3

A pi bond cannot exist independently of a sigma bond. Only after the formation of a sigma bond will the p orbitals of adjacent carbons be parallel, because without the bond the three p orbitals are orthogonal to one another.

In general, pi bonds are weaker than sigma bonds; it is possible to break one bond of a double bond, leaving a single bond intact.

HYBRIDIZATION

The carbon atom has the electron configuration $1s^2 2s^2 2p^2$ and therefore needs four electrons to complete its octet. A typical molecule formed by carbon is methane, CH_4. Experimentation shows that the four sigma bonds in methane are equal. This is inconsistent with the unsymmetrical distribution of valence electrons: two electrons in the 2s orbital, one in the p_x orbital, one in the p_y orbital, and none in the p_z orbital.

A. sp³

The theory of **orbital hybridization** was developed to account for this discrepancy. Hybrid orbitals are formed by mixing different types of atomic orbitals. If one s orbital and three p orbitals are mathematically combined, the result is four sp³ hybrid orbitals that have a new shape.

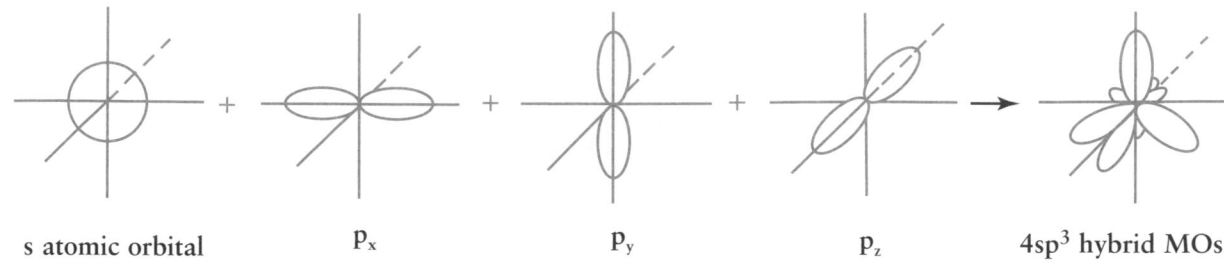

| s atomic orbital | p_x | p_y | p_z | 4sp³ hybrid MOs |

Figure 3.4

These four orbitals will point toward the vertices of a tetrahedron, minimizing repulsion. This explains the preferred tetrahedral geometry adopted by carbon.

The hybridization is accomplished by promoting one of the 2s electrons into the $2p_z$ orbital (see Figure 3.5). This produces four valence orbitals, each with one electron, which can be mathematically mixed to provide the hybrids.

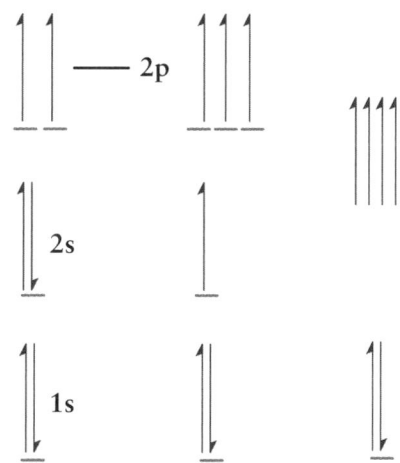

| unhybridized ground state | unhybridized excited state | hybridized ground state |

Figure 3.5

B. sp²

Although carbon is most often found with sp³ hybridization, there are other possibilities. If one s orbital and two p orbitals are mixed, three sp² hybrid orbitals are obtained.

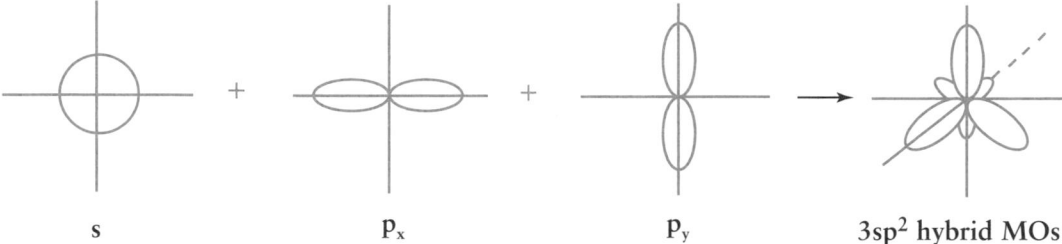

s P_x P_y $3sp^2$ hybrid MOs

Figure 3.6

This occurs, for example, in ethylene. The third p orbital of each carbon atom is left unhybridized and participates in the pi bond. The three sp^2 orbitals are 120° apart, allowing maximum separation. These orbitals participate in the formation of the C–C and C–H single bonds.

C. sp

If two p orbitals are used to form a triple bond, and the remaining p orbital is mixed with an s orbital, two sp hybrid orbitals are obtained. They are oriented 180° apart, explaining the linear structure of molecules like acetylene.

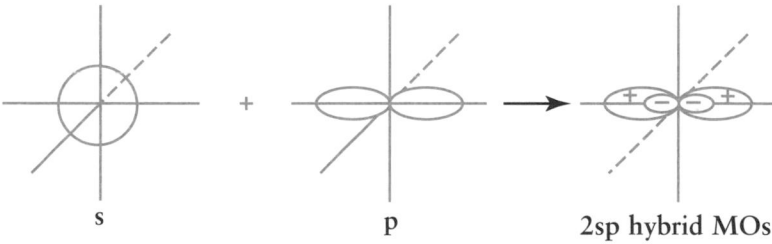

s   p   2sp hybrid MOs

Figure 3.7

BONDING SUMMARY

The following table summarizes the major features of bonding in organic molecules.

Bond Order	Component Bonds	Hybridization	Angles	Examples
single	sigma	sp^3	109.5°	C–C; C–H
double	sigma pi	sp^2	120°	C=C; C=O
triple	sigma pi pi	sp	180°	C≡C; C≡N

4

ALKANES

Alkanes are fully saturated hydrocarbons, compounds consisting only of hydrogen and carbon atoms joined by single bonds. Their general formula is C_nH_{2n+2}, which means they have the maximum possible number of hydrogen atoms attached to each carbon atom.

NOMENCLATURE

Once again, be sure that you are familiar with the common, frequently encountered names. These include:

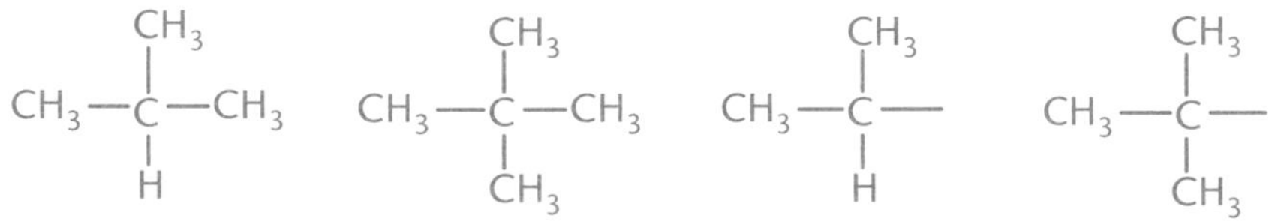

isobutane   neopentane   isopropyl   t-butyl

Figure 4.1

Carbon atoms can be characterized by the number of other carbon atoms to which they are directly bonded. A **primary** carbon atom (written as **1°**) is bonded to only one other carbon atom. A **secondary (2°)** carbon is bonded to two; a **tertiary (3°)** to three, and a **quaternary (4°)** to four other carbon atoms. In addition, hydrogen atoms attached to 1°, 2°, or 3° carbon atoms are referred to as 1°, 2°, or 3°, respectively.

> **MCAT Favorite**
>
> The ability to identify 1°, 2°, and 3° carbons is crucial to determining the products of many chemical reactions and to understanding NMR Spectroscopy.

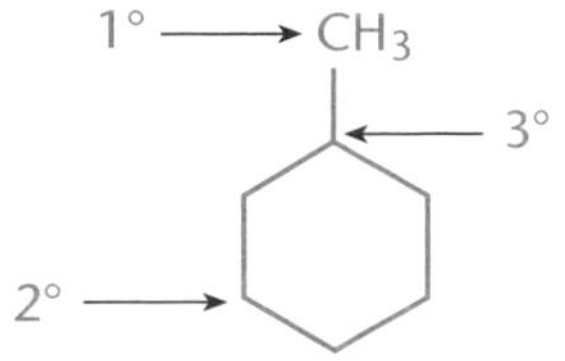

Figure 4.2

PHYSICAL PROPERTIES

The physical properties of alkanes vary in a regular manner. In general, as the molecular weight increases, the melting point, boiling point, and density also increase. At room temperature, the straight-chain compounds C_1 through C_4 are gases, C_5 through C_{16} are liquids, and the longer-chain compounds are waxes and harder solids. Branched molecules have slightly lower boiling and melting points than their straight-chain isomers. Greater branching reduces the surface area of a molecule, decreasing the weak intermolecular attractive forces (van der Waals forces). Hence, the molecules are held together less tightly, effectively lowering the boiling point. In addition, branched molecules are more difficult to pack into a tight, three-dimensional structure. This difficulty is reflected in the lower melting points of branched alkanes.

> **In a Nutshell**
>
> ↑ chain length   ↑ b.p.
>   ↑ m.p.
>   ↑ density
> ↑ branching   ↓ b.p.
>   ↓ m.p.
>   ↓ density

REACTIONS

A. FREE RADICAL HALOGENATION

One frequently encountered reaction of alkanes are **halogenations**, in which one or more hydrogen atoms are replaced by halogen atoms (Cl, Br, or I) via a **free-radical substitution** mechanism. These reactions involve three steps:

1. **Initiation**—Diatomic halogens are homolytically cleaved by either heat or light (hν), resulting in the formation of free radicals. Free radicals are neutral species with unpaired electrons (such as Cl• or R_3C•). They are extremely reactive and readily attack alkanes.

$$\text{Initiation: } X_2 \xrightarrow[\text{or } \Delta]{h\nu} 2X\bullet$$

2. **Propagation**—A propagation step is one in which a radical produces another radical that can continue the reaction. A free radical reacts with an alkane, removing a hydrogen atom to form HX, and creating an alkyl radical. The alkyl radical can then react with X_2 to form an alkyl halide, generating X•.

Propagation: $X\bullet + RH \rightarrow HX + R\bullet$
                                    $R\bullet + X_2 \rightarrow RX + X\bullet$

3. **Termination**—Two free radicals combine with one another to form a stable molecule.

Termination: $2X\bullet \rightarrow X_2$
                                    $X\bullet + R\bullet \rightarrow RX$
                                    $2R\bullet \rightarrow R_2$

A single free radical can initiate many reactions before the reaction chain is terminated.

Larger alkanes have many hydrogens that the free radical can attack. Bromine radicals react fairly slowly, and primarily attack the hydrogens on the carbon atom that can form the most stable free radical, i.e., the most substituted carbon atom.

$$\bullet CR_3 > \bullet CR_2H > \bullet CRH_2 > \bullet CH_3$$
$$3° > 2° > 1° > \text{methyl}$$

Thus, a tertiary radical is the most likely to be formed in a free-radical bromination reaction.

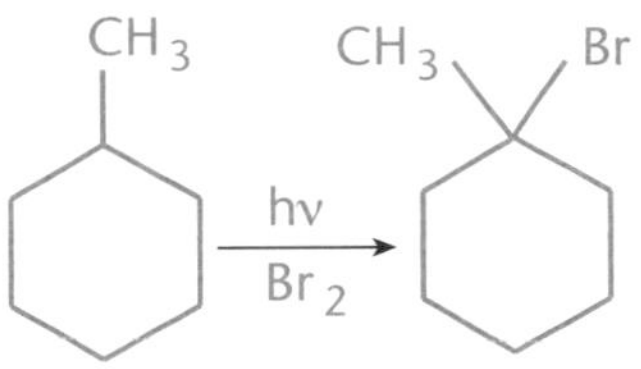

Figure 4.3

Free-radical chlorination is a more rapid process and thus depends not only on the stability of the intermediate, but on the number of hydrogens present. Free-radical chlorination reactions are likely to replace primary hydrogens because of their abundance, despite the relative instability of primary radicals. Unfortunately, free-radical chlorination reactions produce mixtures of products, and are preparatively useful only when just one type of hydrogen is present.

B. COMBUSTION

The reaction of alkanes with molecular oxygen, to form carbon dioxide, water, and heat, is a process of great practical importance. It is an unusual reaction because heat, not a chemical species, is generally the desired product. The reaction mechanism is very complex and is believed to proceed through a radical process. The equation for the complete **combustion** of propane is:

$$C_3H_8 + 5O_2 \rightarrow 3CO_2 + 4H_2O + \text{heat}$$

Combustion is often incomplete, producing significant quantities of carbon monoxide instead of carbon dioxide. This frequently occurs, for example, in the burning of gasoline in an internal combustion engine.

MCAT Synopsis

Free radicals, as well as carbocations, follow the same patterns of stability:

3° > 2° > 1° > methyl

Real World Analogy

Nitrogen in the air is also often oxidized in the internal combustion engine. Various nitrogen oxides are major contributors to air pollution.

C. PYROLYSIS

Pyrolysis occurs when a molecule is broken down by heat. Pyrolysis, also called **cracking**, is most commonly used to reduce the average molecular weight of heavy oils and to increase the production of the more desirable volatile compounds. In the pyrolysis of alkanes, the C–C bonds are cleaved, producing smaller-chain alkyl radicals. These radicals can recombine to form a variety of alkanes:

$$CH_3CH_2CH_3 \xrightarrow{\Delta} CH_3\bullet + \bullet CH_2CH_3$$

$$2\ CH_3\bullet \longrightarrow CH_3CH_3$$

$$2\ \bullet CH_2CH_3 \longrightarrow CH_3CH_2CH_2CH_3$$

Figure 4.4

Alternatively, in a process called **disproportionation**, a radical transfers a hydrogen atom to another radical, producing an alkane and an alkene:

$$CH_3\bullet + \bullet CH_2CH_3 \rightarrow CH_4 + CH_2 = CH_2$$

Figure 4.5

SUBSTITUTION REACTIONS OF ALKYL HALIDES

Alkyl halides and indeed other substituted carbon atoms can take part in reactions known as *nucleophilic substitutions*. **Nucleophiles** ("nucleus lovers") are electron-rich species that are attracted to positively polarized atoms.

A. NUCLEOPHILES

> ### MCAT Synopsis
>
> In protic solvents (solvents capable of hydrogen bonding), larger atoms are better nucleophiles. In aprotic solvents, more basic atoms are better nucleophiles.

1. **Basicity**
   If the nucleophiles have the same attacking atom (for example, oxygen) then nucleophilicity is roughly correlated to basicity. In other words, the stronger the base, the stronger the nucleophile. For example, nucleophilic strength decreases in the order:

$$RO^- > HO^- > RCO_2^- > ROH > H_2O$$

2. **Size and Polarizability**
   If the attacking atoms differ, nucleophilic ability doesn't necessarily correlate to basicity. In a protic solvent, large atoms tend to be better nucleophiles as they can shed their solvent molecules and are more polarizable. Hence, nucleophilic strength decreases in the order:

$$CN^- > I^- > RO^- > HO^- > Br^- > Cl^- > F^- > H_2O$$

In aprotic solvents however, the nucleophiles are "naked"; they are not solvated. In this situation, nucleophilic strength is related to basicity. For example in DMSO, the order of nucleophilic strength is the same as base strength:

$$F^- > Cl^- > Br^- > I^-$$

Note that this is the opposite of what happens in polar solvents.

B. LEAVING GROUPS

The ease with which nucleophilic substitution takes place is also dependent on the leaving group. The best leaving groups are those that are weak bases, as these can accept an electron pair and dissociate to form a stable species. In the case of the halogens, therefore, this is the opposite of base strength:

MCAT Synopsis

Weak bases make good leaving groups.

$$I^- > Br^- > Cl^- > F^-$$

C. S_N1 REACTIONS

S_N1 is the designation for **unimolecular nucleophilic substitution** reaction. It is called unimolecular because the rate of the reaction is dependent upon only one species. Generally, the rate-determining step is the dissociation of this species to form a stable, positively charged ion called a **carbocation** or **carbonium ion.**

1. Mechanism of S_N1 Reactions

S_N1 reactions involve two steps: the dissociation of a molecule into a carbocation and a good leaving group, followed by the combination of the carbocation with a strong nucleophile.

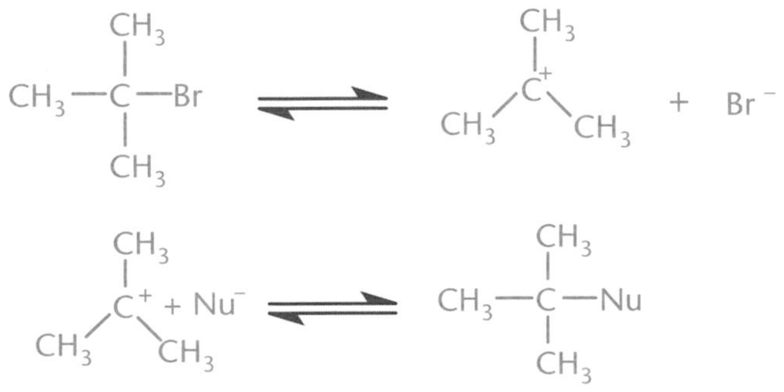

Figure 4.6

In the first step, a carbocation is formed. Carbocations are stabilized by polar solvents that have lone electron pairs to donate (e.g., water, acetone). Carbocations are also stabilized by charge delocalization.

More highly substituted cations are therefore more stable. The order of stability for carbocations is:

tertiary > secondary > primary > methyl

To get the desired product, the original substituent should be a better leaving group than the nucleophile, so that at equilibrium, RNu is the main product. Conditions are usually chosen so that the second step of the reaction is essentially irreversible.

2. Rate of S_N1 Reactions

The rate at which a reaction occurs can never be greater than the rate of its slowest step. Such a step is termed the **rate-limiting** or **rate-determining step** of the reaction, because it limits the speed of the reaction. In an S_N1 reaction, the slowest step is the dissociation of the molecule to form a carbocation, a step that is energetically unfavorable. The formation of a carbocation is therefore the rate-limiting step of an S_N1 reaction. The only reactant in this step is the original molecule, and so the rate of the entire reaction, under a given set of conditions, depends only on the concentration of this original molecule (a so-called *first-order reaction*). The rate is *not* dependent on the concentration or the nature of the nucleophile, because it plays no part in the rate-limiting step.

The rate of an S_N1 reaction can be increased by anything that accelerates the formation of the carbocation. The most important factors are as follows:

a. Structural factors: Highly substituted alkyl halides allow for distribution of the positive charge over a greater number of carbon atoms, and thus form the most stable carbocations.

b. Solvent effects: Highly polar solvents are better at surrounding and isolating ions than are less polar solvents. Polar protic solvents such as water work best since solvation stabilizes the intermediate state.

c. Nature of the leaving group: Weak bases dissociate more easily from the alkyl chain and thus make better leaving groups, increasing the rate of carbocation formation.

Bridge

The kinetics of unimolecular reactions are first order. See General Chemistry chapter 5.

D. S$_N$2 REACTIONS

The formation of a carbocation is not always favorable. Under certain conditions, substitution can proceed by a different mechanism, which does not involve a carbocation. An S$_N$2 (**bimolecular nucleophilic substitution**) reaction involves a nucleophile pushing its way into a compound while simultaneously displacing the leaving group. Its rate-determining, and only, step involves two molecules: the **substrate** and the nucleophile.

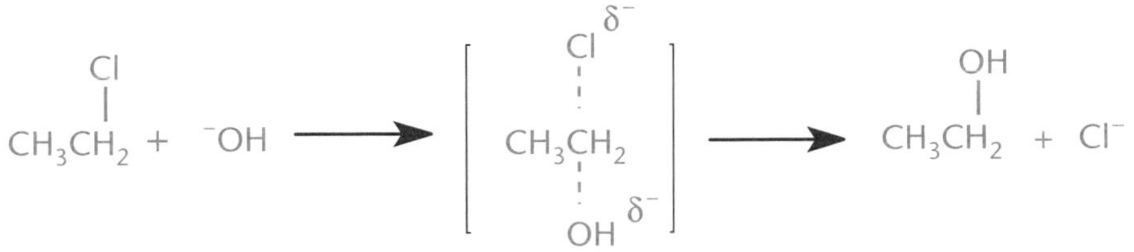

Figure 4.7

1. **Mechanism of S$_N$2 reactions**

In S$_N$2 reactions, the nucleophile actively displaces the leaving group. For this to occur, the nucleophile must be strong, and the reactant cannot be sterically hindered. The nucleophile attacks the reactant from the backside of the leaving group, forming a trigonal bipyramidal **transition state**. As the reaction progresses, the bond to the nucleophile strengthens while the bond to the leaving group weakens. The leaving group is displaced as the bond to the nucleophile becomes complete.

> **MCAT Synopsis**
>
> An intermediate is distinct from a transition state. An intermediate is a well defined species with a finite lifetime. On the other hand, a transition state is a theoretical structure used to define a mechanism.

2. **Rate of S$_N$2 Reactions**

The single step of an S$_N$2 reaction involves *two* reacting species: the substrate (the molecule with a leaving group, usually an alkyl halide), and the nucleophile. The concentrations of both therefore play a role in determining the rate of an S$_N$2 reaction; the two species must "meet" in solution, and raising the concentration of either will make such a meeting more likely. Since the rate of the S$_N$2 reaction depends on the concentration of two reactants, it follows **second-order kinetics**.

> **Bridge**
>
> The kinetics of second order reactions such as S$_N$2 are discussed in General Chemistry chapter 5.

S$_N$1 VERSUS S$_N$2

Certain reaction conditions favor one substitution mechanism over the other. It is also possible for both to occur in the same flask. Sterics, nucleophilic strength, leaving group ability, reaction conditions, and solvent effects are all important in determining which reaction will occur.

STEREOCHEMISTRY OF SUBSTITUTION REACTIONS

A. S$_N$1 STEREOCHEMISTRY

S$_N$1 reactions involve carbocation intermediates, which are approximately planar and therefore achiral.

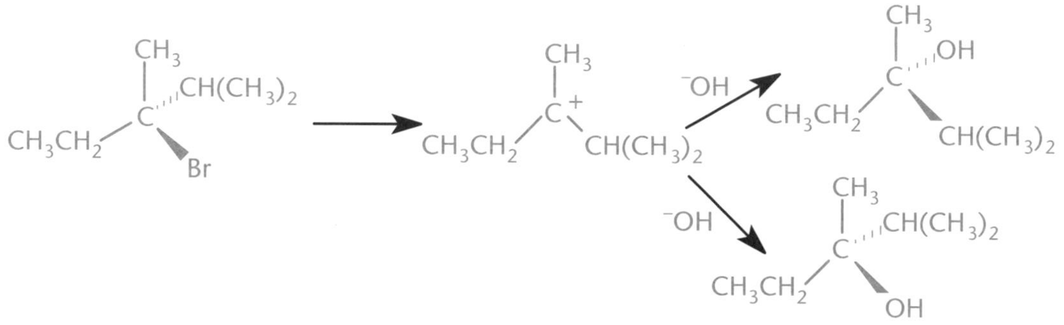

Figure 4.8

Flashback

Refer to chapter 2 for further discussion of optical activity.

If the original compound is optically active because of the reacting chiral center, then a racemic mixture will be produced. S$_N$1 reactions result in a loss of optical activity.

B. S$_N$2 STEREOCHEMISTRY

The single step of an S$_N$2 reaction involves a chiral transition state. Since the nucleophile attacks from one side of the central carbon and the leaving group departs from the opposite side, the reaction "flips" the bonds attached to the carbon.

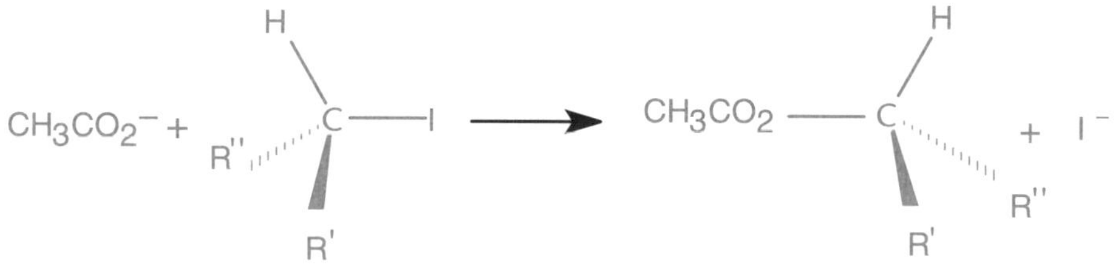

MCAT Synopsis

S$_N$1	S$_N$2
• 2 steps	• 1 step
• Favored in polar protic solvents	• Favored in polar aprotic solvents
• 3° > 2° > 1° > methyl	• 1° > 2° > 3°
• rate = k[RX]	• rate = k[Nu][RX]
• racemic products	• optically active/inverted products
• favored with the use of bulky nucleophiles	

Figure 4.9

If the reactant is chiral, optical activity is usually retained; however, in the case of S$_N$2 reactions, an inversion of configuration occurs.

5

ALKENES AND ALKYNES

ALKENES

Alkenes are hydrocarbons that contain carbon-carbon double bonds. The general formula for a straight-chain alkene with one double bond is C_nH_{2n}. The degree of unsaturation (the number N of double bonds or rings) of a compound of molecular formula C_nH_m can be determined according to the equation:

$$N = \frac{1}{2}(2n + 2 - m)$$

Double bonds are considered functional groups, and alkenes are more reactive than the corresponding alkanes.

NOMENCLATURE

Alkenes, also called **olefins**, may be described by the terms *cis, trans, E,* and *Z*. The common names *ethylene, propylene,* and *isobutylene* are often used over the IUPAC names.

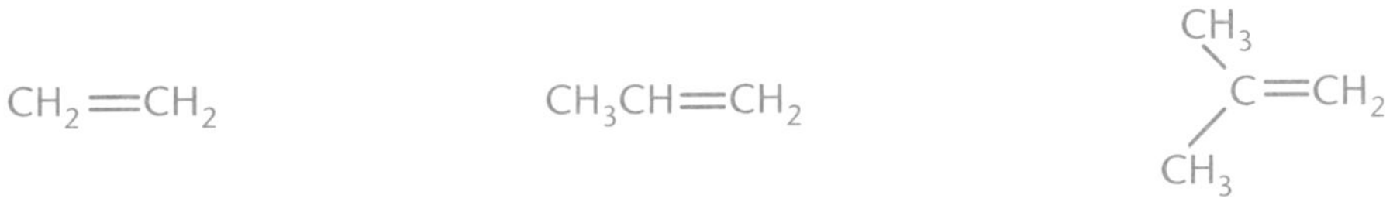

$CH_2\!=\!CH_2$

$CH_3CH\!=\!CH_2$

ethene
(ethylene)

propene
(propylene)

2-methyl-1-propene
(isobutylene)

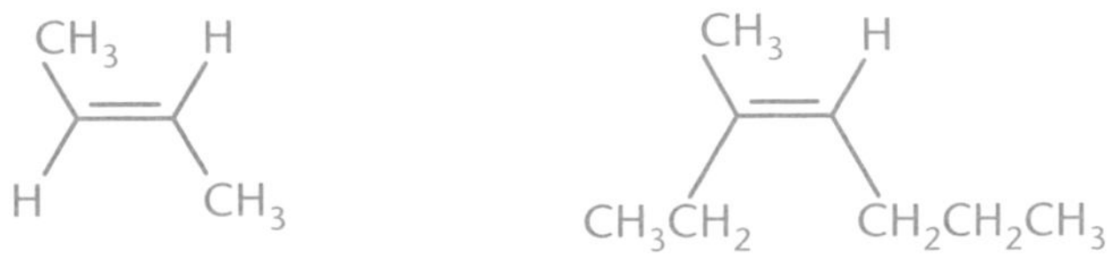

trans-2-butene

(Z)-3-methyl-3-heptene

Figure 5.1

PHYSICAL PROPERTIES

The physical properties of alkenes are similar to those of alkanes. For example, the melting and boiling points increase with increasing molecular weight and are similar in value to those of the corresponding alkanes. Terminal alkenes (or 1-alkenes) usually boil at a lower temperature than internal alkenes, and can be separated by fractional distillation (see chapter 12). *Trans*-alkenes generally have higher melting points than *cis*-alkenes because their higher symmetry allows better packing in the solid state. They also tend to have lower boiling points than *cis*-alkenes because they are less **polar**.

Polarity is a property that results from the asymmetrical distribution of electrons in a particular molecule. In alkenes, this distribution creates dipole moments that are oriented from the electropositive alkyl groups toward the electronegative alkene. In *trans*-2-butene, the two dipole moments are oriented in opposite directions and cancel each other. The compound possesses no net dipole moment and is not polar. On the other hand, *cis*-2-butene has a net dipole moment, resulting from addition of the two smaller dipoles. The compound is polar, and the additional intermolecular forces tend to raise the boiling point.

MCAT Synopsis

Trans-alkenes have higher melting points than *cis*-alkenes due to higher symmetry.

Cis-alkenes have higher boiling points than *trans*-alkenes due to polarity. Internal alkenes have higher boiling points than terminal alkenes.

Flashback

Polarity is discussed in General Chemistry chapter 3.

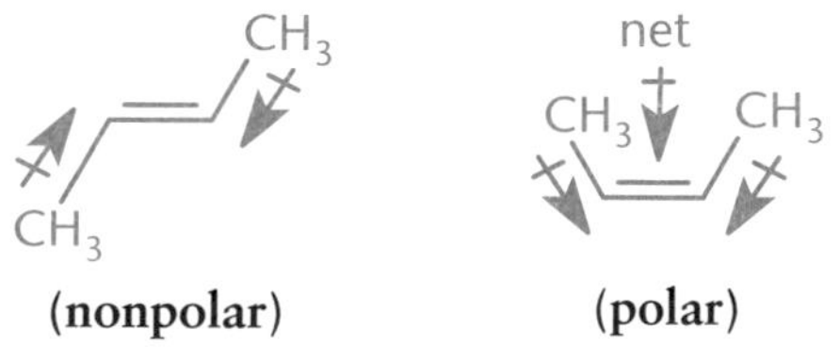

(nonpolar)   **(polar)**

Figure 5.2

SYNTHESIS

Alkenes can be synthesized in a number of different ways. The most common method involves **elimination reactions** of either alcohols or alkyl halides. In these reactions the carbon skeleton loses HX (where X is a halide), or a molecule of water, to form a double bond:

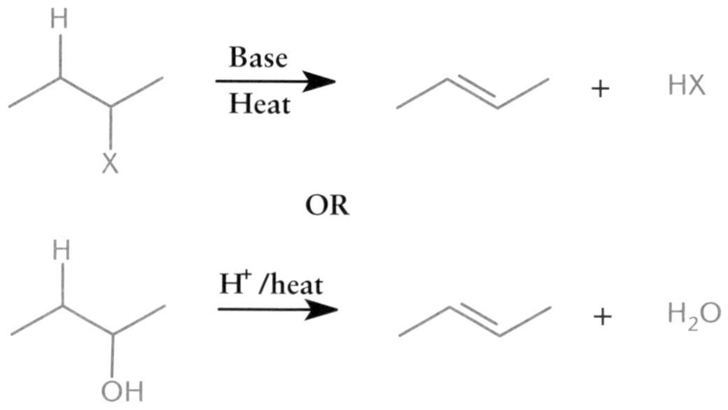

Figure 5.3

Elimination occurs by two distinct mechanisms, unimolecular and bimolecular, which are referred to as **E1** and **E2,** respectively.

A. UNIMOLECULAR ELIMINATION

Unimolecular elimination, which is abbreviated E1, is a two-step process proceeding through a carbocation intermediate. The rate of reaction is dependent on the concentration of only one species, namely the substrate. The elimination of a leaving group and a proton results in the production of a double bond. In the first step, the leaving group departs, producing a carbocation. In the second step, a proton is removed by a base.

E1 is favored by the same factors that favor S_N1: highly polar solvents, highly branched carbon chains, good leaving groups, and weak nucleophiles in low concentration. These mechanisms are therefore competitive, and directing a reaction toward either E1 or S_N1 alone is difficult, although high temperatures tend to favor E1.

B. BIMOLECULAR ELIMINATION

Bimolecular elimination, termed E2, occurs in one step. Its rate is dependent on the concentration of two species, the substrate and the base. A strong base such as the ethoxide ion ($C_2H_5O^-$) removes a proton, while a halide ion *anti* to the proton leaves, resulting in the formation of a double bond.

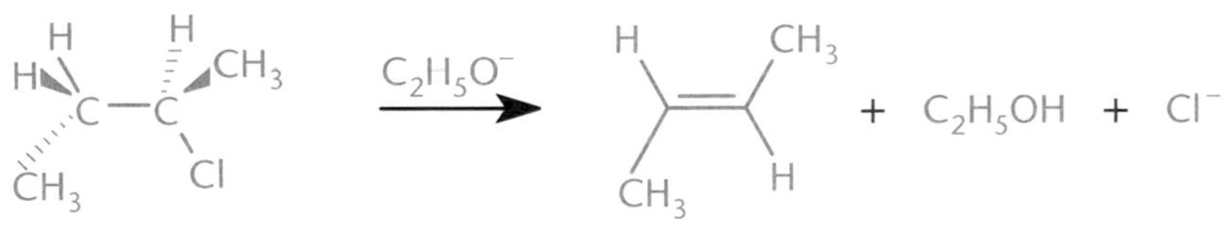

Figure 5.4

Often there are two possible products. In such cases, the more substituted double bond is formed preferentially.

Controlling E2 versus S_N2 is easier than controlling E1 versus S_N1.

1. Steric hindrance does not greatly affect E2 reactions. Therefore, highly substituted carbon chains, which form the most stable alkenes, undergo E2 most easily and S_N2 rarely.

2. A strong base favors E2 over S_N2. S_N2 is favored over E2 by weak Lewis bases (strong nucleophiles).

Other factors, such as the polarity of the solvent and branching of the carbon chain, can be modified in order to reduce the competition between E1 and S_N1 reactions.

REACTIONS

A. REDUCTION

Catalytic hydrogenation is the reductive process of adding molecular hydrogen to a double bond with the aid of a metal catalyst. Typical catalysts are platinum, palladium, and nickel (usually Raney nickel, a special powdered form), but occasionally rhodium, iridium, or ruthenium are used.

MCAT Synopsis

Reactions where one stere-oisomer is favored are termed stereospecific reactions.

The reaction takes place on the surface of the metal. One face of the double bond is coordinated to the metal surface, and thus the two hydrogen atoms are added to the same face of the double bond. This type of addition is called *syn* addition.

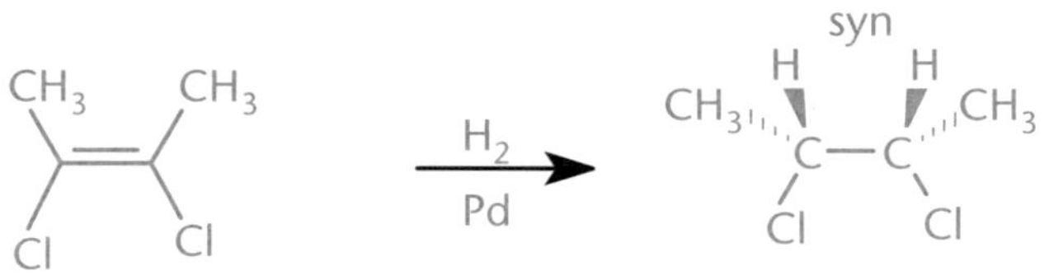

Figure 5.5

B. ELECTROPHILIC ADDITIONS

The π bond is somewhat weaker than the σ bond, and can therefore be broken without breaking the σ bond. As a result, one can *add* compounds to double bonds while leaving the carbon skeleton intact. Though many different **addition reactions** exist, most operate via the same essential mechanism.

MCAT Synopsis

Markovnikov's rule refers to the addition of something (e.g., halide, hydroxyl group) to the most substituted carbon in the double bond.

The electrons of the π bond are particularly exposed and are thus easily attacked by molecules that seek to accept an electron pair (Lewis acids). Because these groups are electron-seeking, they are more often termed **electrophiles** (literally, "lovers of electrons").

1. **Addition of HX**

   The electrons of the double bond act as a Lewis base and react with electrophilic HX molecules. The first step yields a carbocation intermediate after the double bond reacts with a proton. In the second step, the halide ion combines with the carbocation to give an alkyl halide. In cases where the alkene is asymmetrical, the initial protonation proceeds to produce the *most stable carbocation*. The proton will add to the less substituted carbon atom (the carbon atom with the most protons), since alkyl substituents stabilize carbocations. This phenomenon is called **Markovnikov's rule**. An example is:

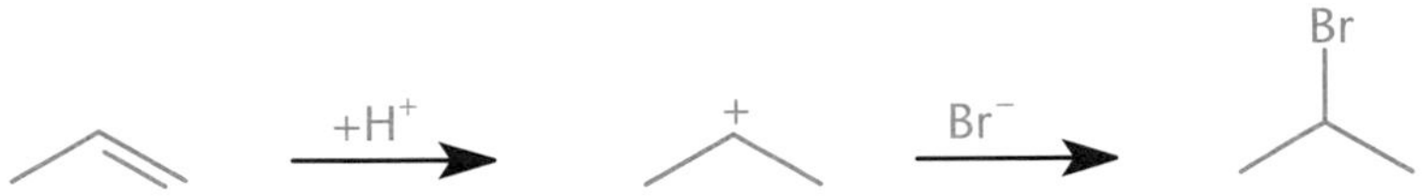

Figure 5.6

2. Addition of X₂

The addition of halogens to a double bond is a rapid process. It is frequently used as a diagnostic tool to test for the presence of double bonds. The double bond acts as a nucleophile and attacks an X_2 molecule, displacing X^-. The intermediate carbocation forms a **cyclic halonium ion,** which is then attacked by X^-, giving the dihalo compound. Note that this addition is *anti,* because the X^- attacks the cyclic halonium ion in a standard S_N2 displacement.

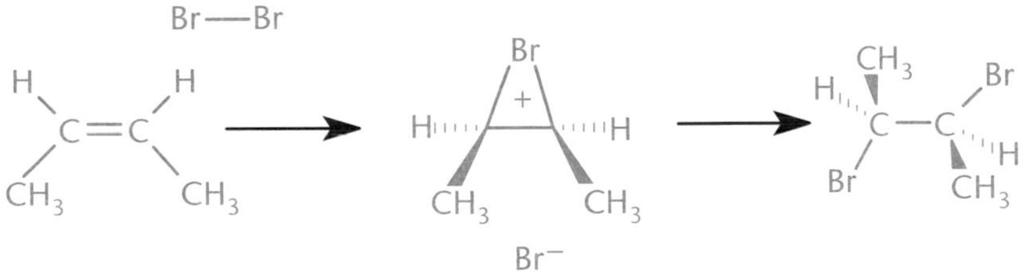

Anti-addition

Figure 5.7

If the reaction is carried out in a nucleophilic solvent, the solvent molecules can compete in the displacement step, producing, for example, a **halo alcohol** (rather than the **dihalo** compound).

3. Addition of H₂O

Water can be added to alkenes under acidic conditions. The double bond is protonated according to Markovnikov's rule, forming the most stable carbocation. This carbocation reacts with water, forming a protonated alcohol, which then loses a proton to yield the alcohol. The reaction is performed at low temperature because the reverse reaction is an acid-catalyzed **dehydration** that is favored by high temperatures.

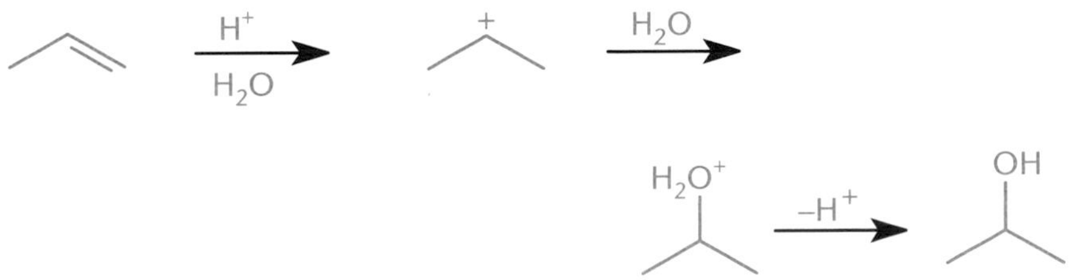

Figure 5.8

Direct addition of water is generally not useful in the laboratory because yields vary greatly with reaction conditions; therefore, this reaction is generally carried out indirectly using mercuric acetate, $Hg(CH_3COO)_2$.

C. FREE RADICAL ADDITIONS

An alternate mechanism exists for the addition of HX to alkenes, which proceeds through **free-radical intermediates**, and occurs when peroxides, oxygen, or other impurities are present. Free-radical additions disobey the Markovnikov rule because X• adds first to the double bond, producing the most stable free radical, whereas H$^+$ adds first in standard electrophilic additions, producing the most stable carbocation. The reaction is useful for HBr, but is not practical for HCl or HI, because the energetics are unfavorable.

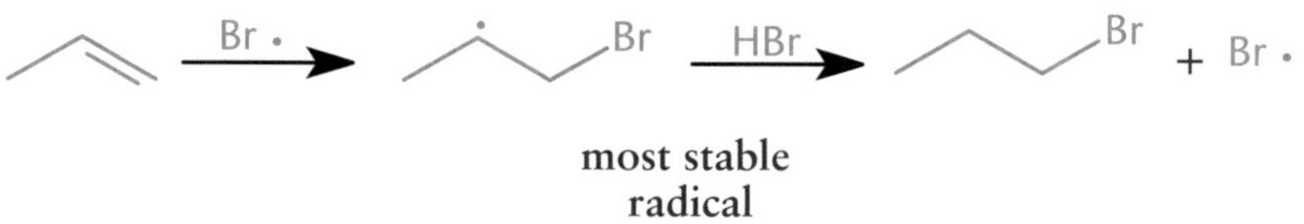

most stable
radical

Figure 5.9

D. HYDROBORATION

Diborane (B_2H_6) adds readily to double bonds. The boron atom is a Lewis acid and attaches to the less sterically hindered carbon atom. The second step is an oxidation-hydrolysis with peroxide and aqueous base, producing the alcohol with overall anti-Markovnikov, *syn* orientation.

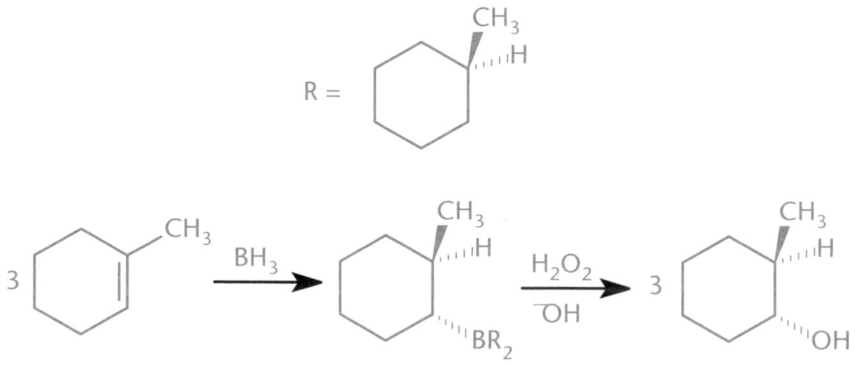

Figure 5.10

E. OXIDATION

1. Potassium Permanganate

Alkenes can be oxidized with KMnO$_4$ to provide different types of products, depending upon the reaction conditions. Cold, dilute, aqueous KMnO$_4$ reacts to produce 1,2 diols (vicinal diols), which are also called glycols, with *syn* orientation:

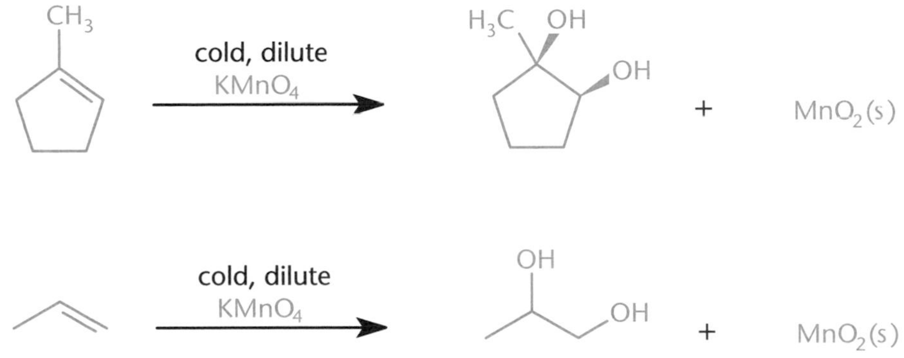

Figure 5.11

If a hot, basic solution of potassium permangenate is added to the alkene and then acidified, nonterminal alkenes are cleaved to form 2 molar equivalents of carboxylic acid, and terminal alkenes are cleaved to form a carboxylic acid and carbon dioxide. If the nonterminal double bonded carbon is disubstituted, however, a ketone will be formed:

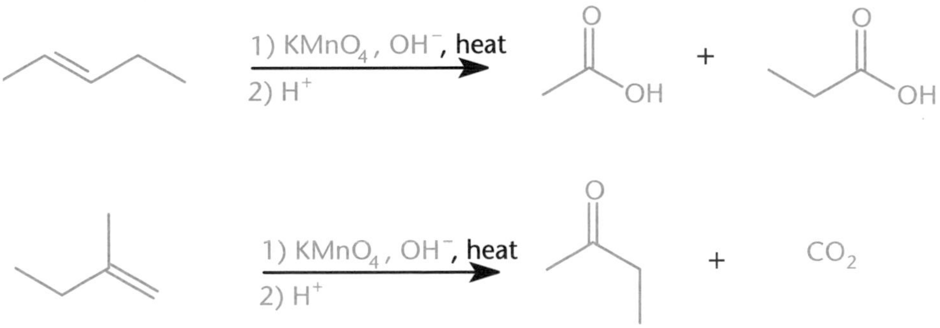

Figure 5.12

2. Ozonolysis

Treatment of alkenes with ozone followed by reduction with zinc and water results in cleavage of the double bond in the following manner:

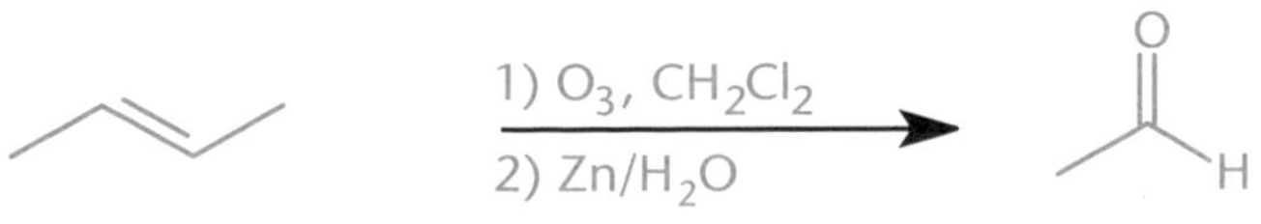

Figure 5.13

If the reaction mixture is reduced with sodium borohydride, NaBH$_4$, the corresponding alcohols are produced:

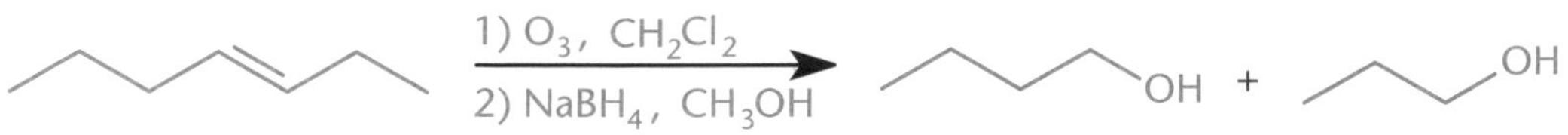

Figure 5.14

3. **Peroxycarboxylic Acids**

    Alkenes can be oxidized with peroxycarboxylic acids. Peroxyacetic acid (CH$_3$CO$_3$H) and *m*-chloroperoxybenzoic acid (mcpba) are commonly used. The products formed are **oxiranes** (also called **epoxides**):

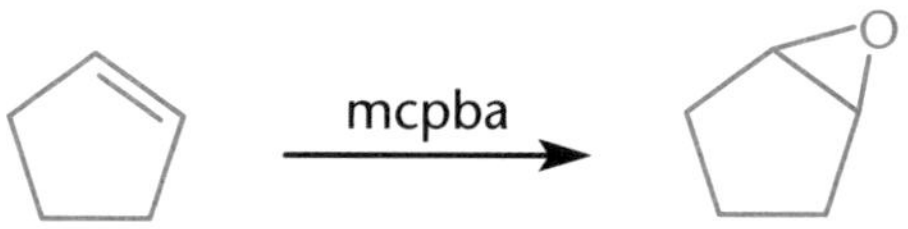

Figure 5.15

F. POLYMERIZATION

Polymerization is the creation of long, high molecular weight chains (**polymers**), composed of repeating subunits (called **monomers**). Polymerization usually occurs through a radical mechanism, although anionic and even cationic polymerizations are commonly observed. A typical example is the formation of polyethylene from ethylene (ethene) that requires high temperatures and pressures:

$$CH_2\!\!=\!\!CH_2 \xrightarrow[\text{high pressure}]{\text{R•, heat}} RCH_2CH_2(CH_2CH_2)_nCH_2CH_2R$$

Figure 5.16

ALKYNES

Alkynes are hydrocarbon compounds that possess one or more carbon-carbon triple bonds.

NOMENCLATURE

The suffix **-yne** is used, and the position of the triple bond is specified when necessary. A common exception to the IUPAC rules is ethyne, which is called *acetylene*. Frequently, compounds are named as derivatives of acetylene.

$$CH_3CH_2CH_2CHC{\equiv}CCH_3 \qquad CH{\equiv}CH \qquad CH_3C{\equiv}CH$$
$$\overset{|}{Cl}$$

4-chloro-2-heptyne　　　　**ethyne**　　　　**propyne**
　　　　　　　　　　　　　　(acetylene)　　　(methylacetylene)

Figure 5.17

PHYSICAL PROPERTIES

The physical properties of the alkynes are similar to the properties of the analogous alkenes and alkanes. In general, the shorter-chain compounds are gases, boiling at somewhat higher temperatures than the corresponding alkenes. Internal alkynes, like alkenes, boil at higher temperatures than terminal alkynes.

Asymmetrical distribution of electron density causes alkynes to have dipole moments which are larger than those of alkenes, but still small in magnitude. Thus, solutions of alkynes can be slightly polar.

Terminal alkynes are fairly acidic, with a pKa of approximately 25. This property is exploited in some of the reactions of alkynes, which will be discussed later.

SYNTHESIS

Triple bonds can be made by the elimination of two molecules of HX from a geminal or vicinal dihalide:

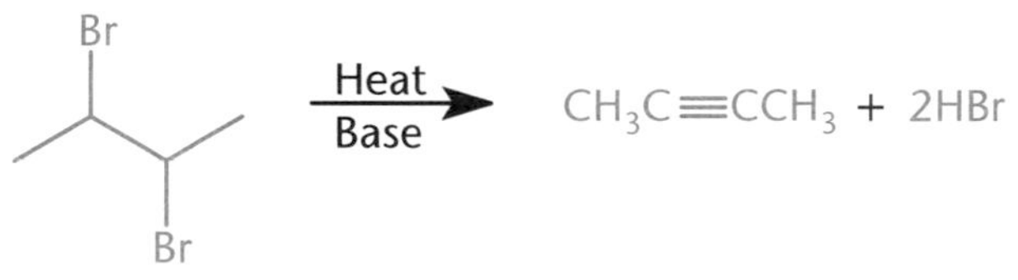

$$\xrightarrow[\text{Base}]{\text{Heat}} \quad CH_3C{\equiv}CCH_3 + 2HBr$$

Figure 5.18

This reaction is not always practical and requires high temperatures and a strong base. A more useful method adds an already existing triple bond into a particular carbon skeleton. A terminal triple bond is converted to a nucleophile by removing the acidic proton with strong base, producing an *acetylide ion*. This ion will perform nucleophilic displacements on alkyl halides at room temperature:

$$CH{\equiv}CH \xrightarrow{n\text{-BuLi}} CH{\equiv}C^- Li^+ \xrightarrow{CH_3Cl} CH{\equiv}CCH_3$$

Figure 5.19

REACTIONS

A. REDUCTION

Alkynes, just like alkenes, can be hydrogenated with a catalyst to produce alkanes. A more useful reaction stops the reduction after addition of just one equivalent of H_2, producing alkenes. This partial hydrogenation can take place in two different ways. The first uses **Lindlar's catalyst**, that is palladium on barium sulfate ($BaSO_4$) with quinoline, a poison that stops the reaction at the alkene stage. Because the reaction occurs on a metal surface, the product alkene is the *cis* isomer. The other method uses sodium in liquid ammonia below –33°C (the boiling point of ammonia), and produces the *trans* isomer of the alkene via a free radical mechanism:

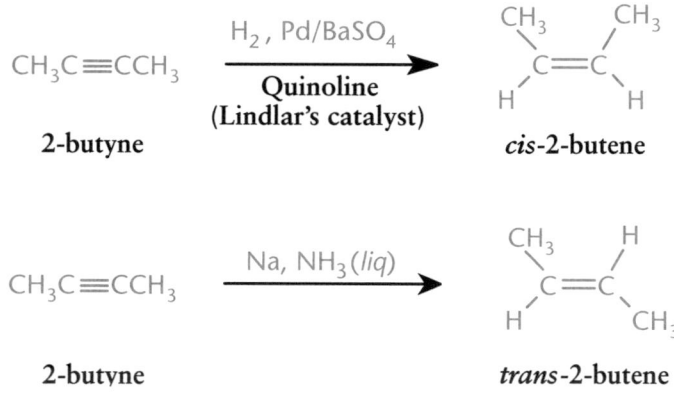

Figure 5.20

B. ADDITION

1. Electrophilic

Electrophilic addition to alkynes occurs in the same manner as it does to alkenes. The reaction occurs according to Markovnikov's rule. The addition can generally be stopped at the intermediate alkene stage, or carried further. The following examples are illustrative:

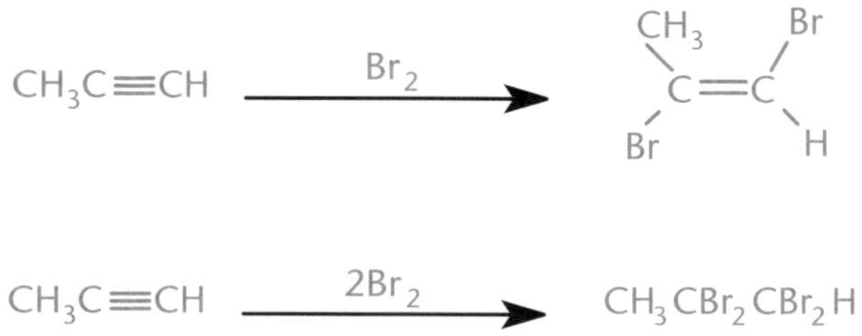

Figure 5.21

2. Free Radical

Radicals add to triple bonds as they do to double bonds—with anti-Markovnikov orientation. The reaction product is usually the *trans* isomer, because the intermediate vinyl radical can isomerize to its more stable form.

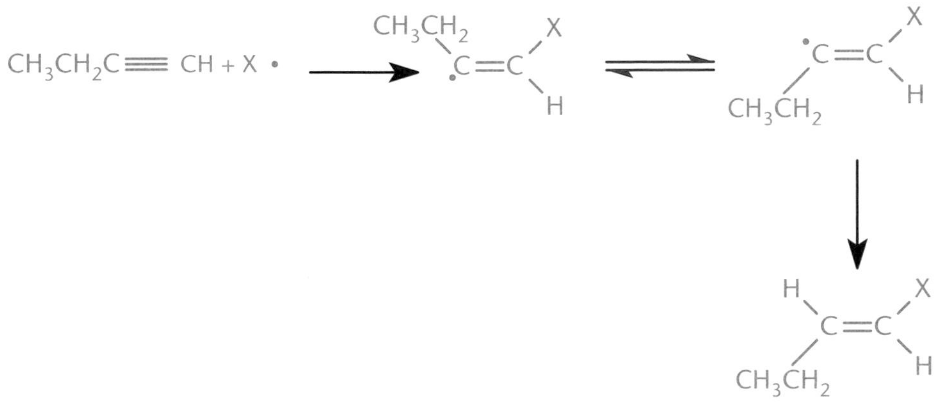

Figure 5.22

C. HYDROBORATION

Addition of boron to triple bonds occurs by the same method as addition of boron to double bonds. Addition is *syn,* and the boron atom adds first. The boron atom can be replaced with a proton from acetic acid, to produce a *cis* alkene:

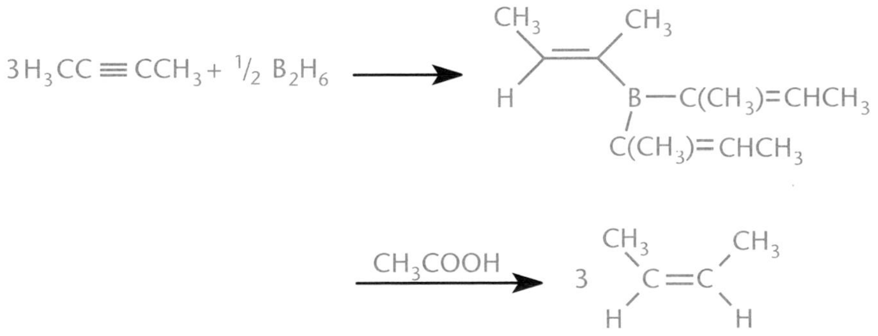

Figure 5.23

With terminal alkynes, a disubstituted borane is used to prevent further boration of the vinylic intermediate to an alkane. The vinylic borane intermediate can be oxidatively cleaved with hydrogen peroxide (H_2O_2), creating an intermediate vinyl alcohol, which rearranges to the more stable carbonyl compound (via **keto-enol tautomerism**).

> **MCAT Synopsis**
>
> Keto-enol tautomerisms will be discussed in chapter 8.

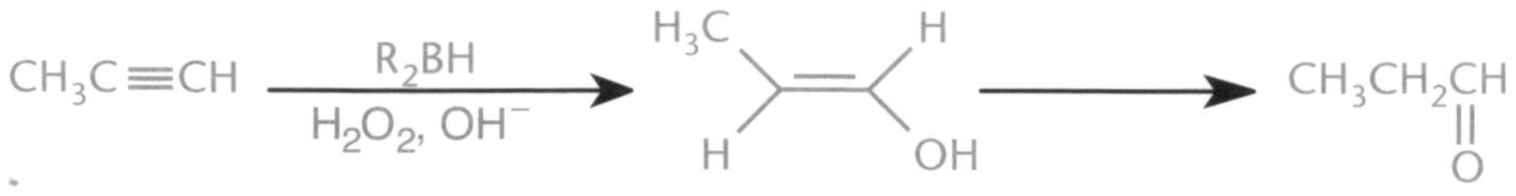

$$CH_3C\equiv CH \xrightarrow[\text{H}_2\text{O}_2,\ \text{OH}^-]{\text{R}_2\text{BH}} \text{(alkene)} \longrightarrow CH_3CH_2CH=O$$

Figure 5.24

D. OXIDATION

Alkynes can be oxidatively cleaved with either basic potassium permanganate (followed by acidification) or ozone.

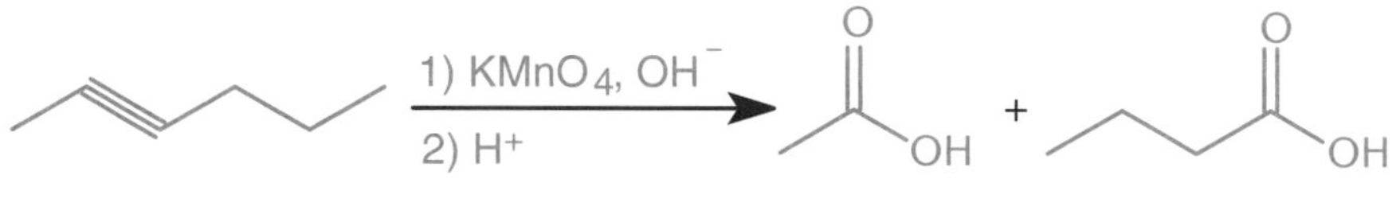

Figure 5.25

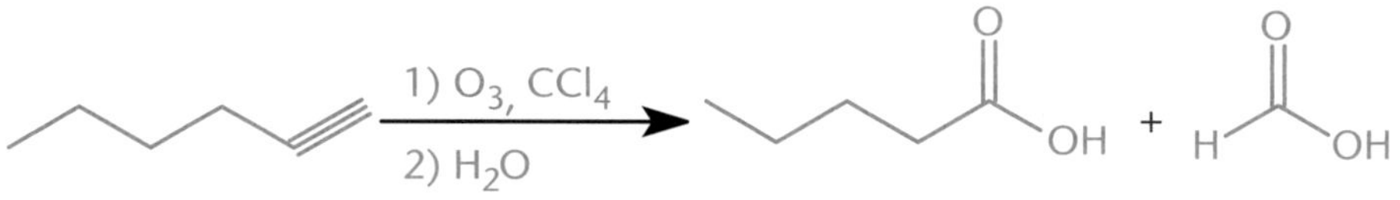

Figure 5.26

6

AROMATIC COMPOUNDS

The terms **aromatic** and **aliphatic,** meaning "fragrant" and "fatty," respectively, were used originally to distinguish types of organic compounds. The terms persist with new definitions. "Aromatic" now describes any unusually stable ring system. These compounds are cyclic, conjugated polyenes that possess $4n + 2$ pi electrons and adopt planar conformations to allow maximum overlap of the conjugated pi orbitals. "Aliphatic" describes all compounds that are not aromatic.

The criterion of $4n + 2$ pi electrons is known as **Hückel's rule**, and is an important indicator of aromaticity. In general, if a cyclic conjugated polyene follows Hückel's rule, then it is an aromatic compound. Neutral compounds, anions, and cations may all be aromatic. Some typical aromatic compounds and ions are:

> **MCAT Synopsis**
>
> n can be any nonnegative integer; thus, $4n + 2$ can be 2, 6, 10, 14, 18, etcetera.

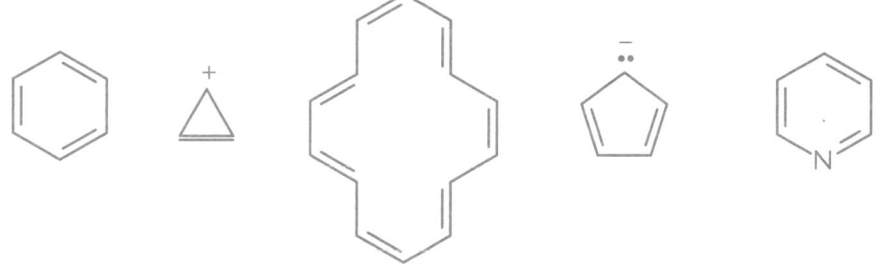

Figure 6.1

A cyclic, conjugated polyene that possesses $4n$ electrons is said to be **antiaromatic** (a cyclic, conjugated polyene that is destabilized). Some typical antiaromatic compounds are:

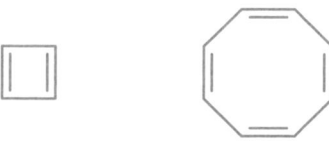

Figure 6.2

NOMENCLATURE

Aromatic compounds are referred to as **aryl** compounds, or **arenes**, and are represented by the symbol **Ar**. Aliphatic compounds are called **alkyl** and are represented by the symbol **R**. Common names exist for many mono- and di-substituted aromatic compounds.

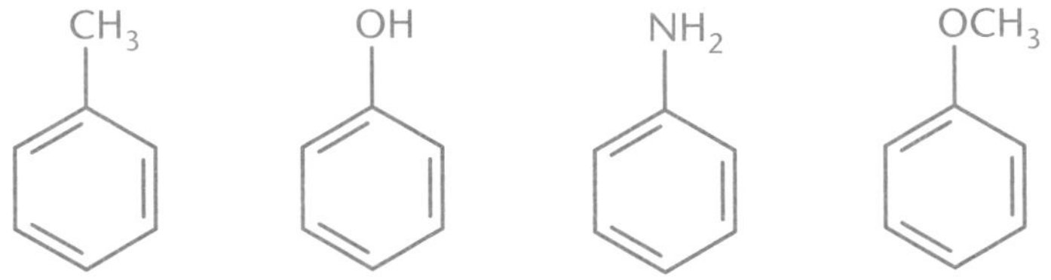

Toluene   Phenol   Aniline   Anisole

Figure 6.3

The benzene group is called a **phenyl** group (**Ph**) when named as a substituent. The term **benzyl** refers to a toluene molecule substituted at the methyl position.

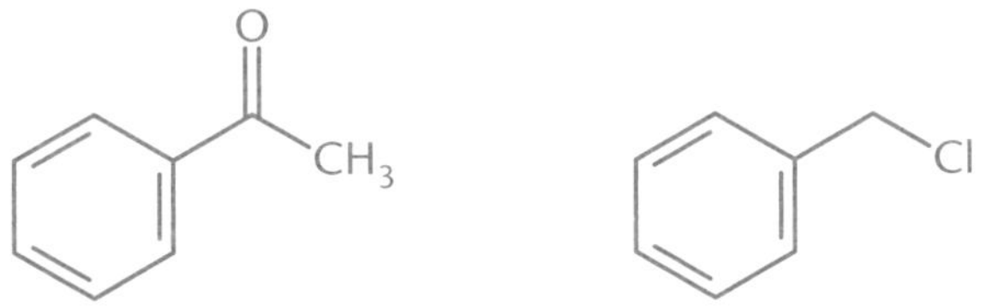

methyl phenyl ketone   benzyl chloride

Figure 6.4

Substituted benzene rings are named as alkyl benzenes, with the substituents numbered to produce the lowest sequence. A 1,2-disubstituted compound is called *ortho-* or *o-*; a 1,3 disubstituted compound is called *meta-* or *m-*; and a 1,4 disubstituted compound is called *para-* or *p-*.

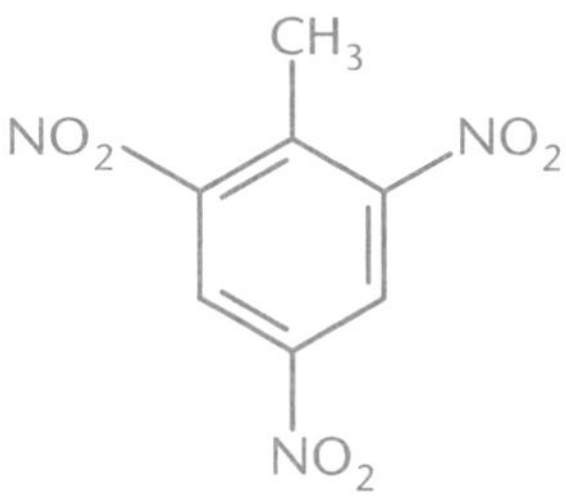

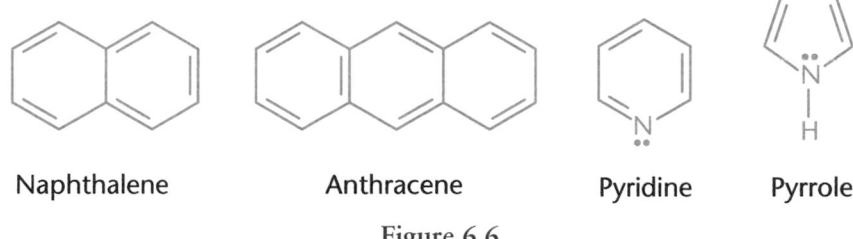

2,4,6-trinitrotoluene (TNT)

o-nitrotoluene

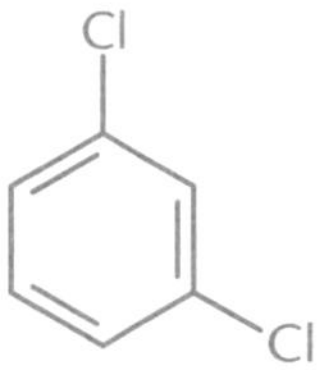

m-dichlorobenzene

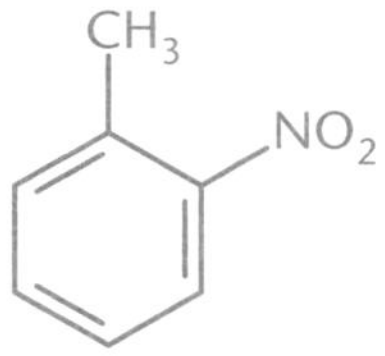

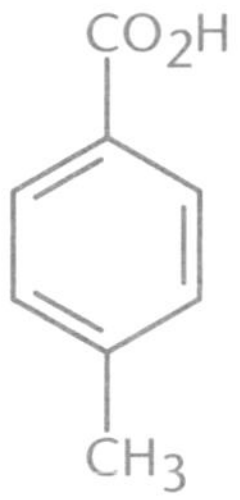

p-methylbenzoic acid

Figure 6.5

There are many polycyclic and heterocyclic aromatic compounds.

Naphthalene

Anthracene

Pyridine

Pyrrole

Figure 6.6

MCAT Synopsis

The nonbonding electron pair in pyridine is in a nitrogen sp^2 orbital. This orbital is perpendicular to the p orbitals around the ring and therefore is not involved in the conjugated pi system. On the other hand, the nonbonding pair in pyrrole is in a nitrogen sp^3 orbital parallel to the ring p orbitals and therefore can participate in the delocalized pi system.

PROPERTIES

The physical properties of aromatic compounds are generally similar to those of other hydrocarbons. By contrast, chemical properties are significantly affected by aromaticity. The characteristic planar shape of benzene permits the ring's six pi orbitals to overlap, delocalizing the electron density. All six carbon atoms are sp^2 hybridized, and each of the six orbitals overlaps equally with its two neighbors. As a result, the delocalized electrons form two "pi electron clouds," one above and one below the plane of the ring. This delocalization stabilizes the molecule, making it fairly unreactive: In particular, benzene does not undergo addition reactions as do alkenes. The same holds true for other aromatic compounds, since the definition of an aromatic compound includes the condition that it have a delocalized pi electron system.

REACTIONS

A. ELECTROPHILIC AROMATIC SUBSTITUTION

The most important reaction of aromatic compounds is electrophilic aromatic substitution. In this reaction an electrophile replaces a proton on an aromatic ring, producing a substituted aromatic compound. The most common examples are halogenation, sulfonation, nitration, and acylation.

1. Halogenation

Aromatic rings react with bromine or chlorine in the presence of a Lewis acid, such as $FeCl_3$, $FeBr_3$, or $AlCl_3$, to produce monosubstituted products in good yield. Reaction of fluorine and iodine with aromatic rings is less useful, as fluorine tends to produce multisubstituted products, and iodine's lack of reactivity requires special conditions for the reaction to proceed.

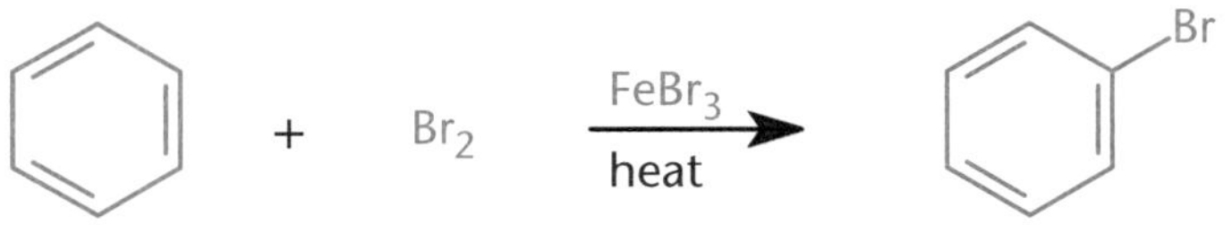

Figure 6.7

2. Sulfonation

Aromatic rings react with fuming sulfuric acid (a mixture of sulfuric acid and sulfur trioxide) to form sulfonic acids.

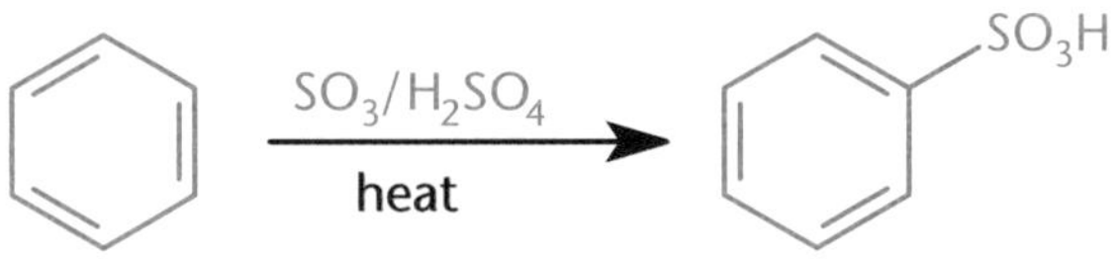

Figure 6.8

3. Nitration

The nitration of aromatic rings is another synthetically useful reaction. A mixture of nitric and sulfuric acids is used to create the nitronium ion, NO_2^+, a strong electrophile. This reacts with aromatic rings to produce nitro compounds.

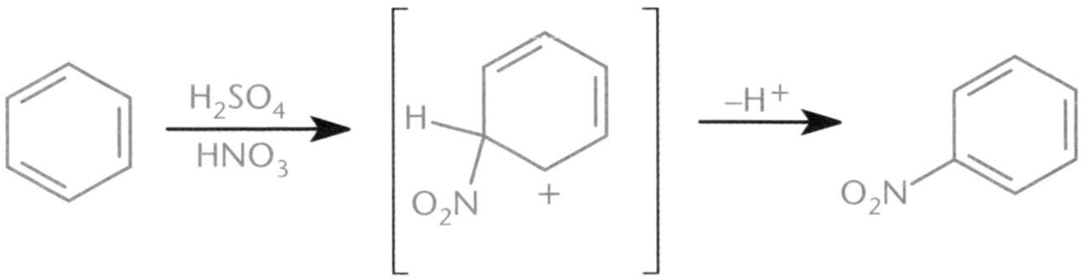

Figure 6.9

4. Acylation (Friedel-Crafts Reactions)

In Friedel-Crafts acylation reaction, a carbocation electrophile, usually an acyl group, is incorporated into the aromatic ring. These reactions are usually catalyzed by Lewis acids such as $AlCl_3$.

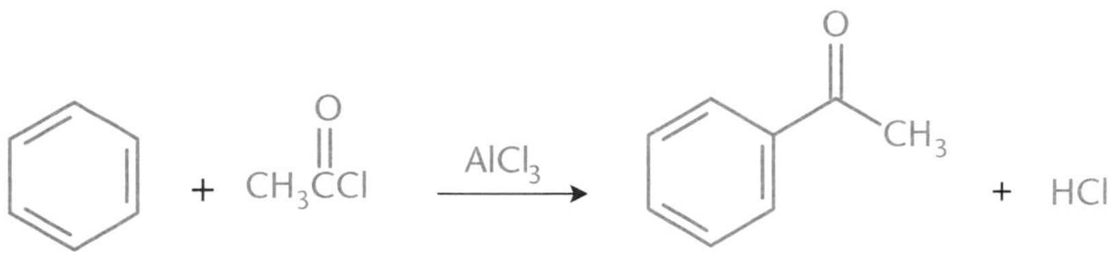

Figure 6.10

5. Substituent Effects

Substituents on an aromatic ring strongly influence the susceptibility of the ring to electrophilic aromatic substitution, and also strongly affect what position on the ring an incoming electrophile is most likely to attack. Substituents can be grouped into three different classes according to whether substitution is enhanced (activating) or inhibited (deactivating), and where the reaction is likely to take place with respect to the group already present. These effects depend on whether the group tends to donate or withdraw electron density, and how it does so; the specifics of these mechanisms will not be discussed here. Arranged in order of decreasing strength of the substituent effect, the three classes are listed below:

a. Activating, *ortho/para*-directing substituents (electron-donating): NH_2, NR_2, OH, NHCOR, OR, OCOR, and R.

b. Deactivating, *ortho/para*-directing substituents (weakly electron-withdrawing): F, Cl, Br, and I.

c. Deactivating, *meta*-directing substituents (electron-withdrawing): NO_2, SO_3H, and carbonyl compounds, including COOH, COOR, COR, and CHO.

> **MCAT Favorite**
>
> Be sure to understand substituent effects:
>
> - activating = ortho/para directing = e⁻ donating
>
> - deactivating = meta directing = e⁻ withdrawing
>
> (Halogens are exceptions: although they are e⁻ withdrawing and deactivators, they are ortho/para directors.)

For example, when toluene undergoes electrophilic aromatic substitution, the methyl group directs substitution to occur at the *ortho* and *para* positions:

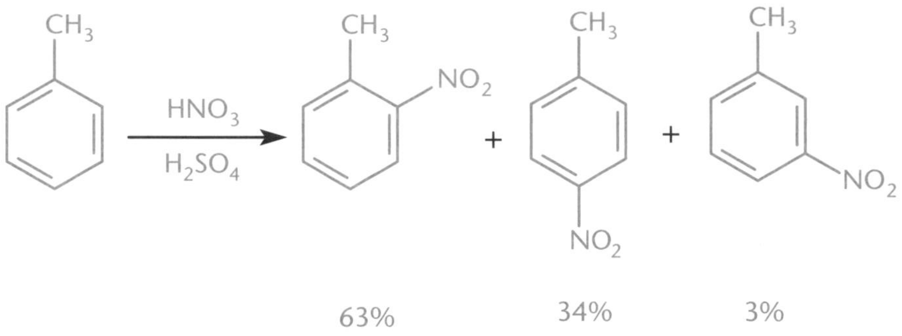

63%   34%   3%

Figure 6.11

B. REDUCTION

1. Catalytic Reduction

Benzene rings can be reduced by catalytic hydrogenation under vigorous conditions (elevated temperature and pressure) to yield cyclohexane. Ruthenium or rhodium on carbon are the most common catalysts; platinum or palladium may also be used.

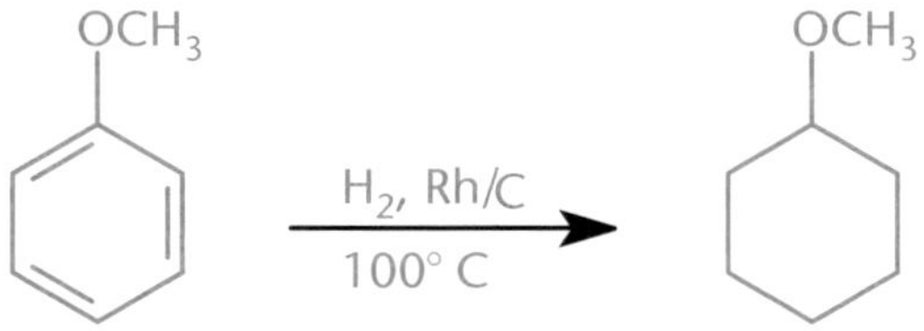

Figure 6.12

7

ALCOHOLS AND ETHERS

ALCOHOLS

Alcohols are compounds with the general formula **ROH**. The functional group **–OH** is called the **hydroxyl** group. An alcohol can be thought of as a substituted water molecule, with an alkyl group R replacing one H atom.

NOMENCLATURE

Alcohols are named in the IUPAC system by replacing the **-e** ending of the root alkane with the ending **-ol**. The carbon atom attached to the hydroxyl group must be included in the longest chain and receives the lowest possible number. Some examples are:

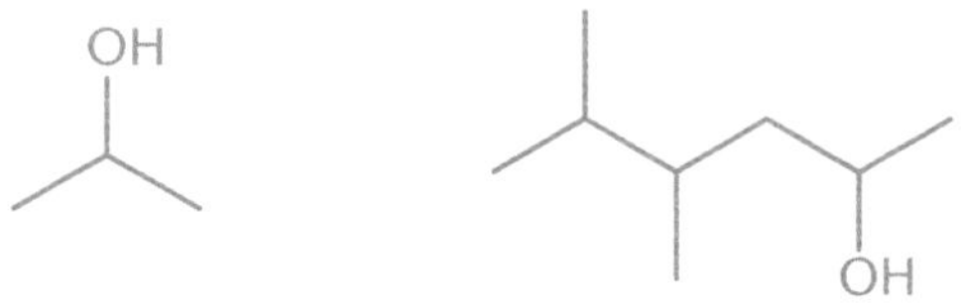

2-propanol   4, 5-dimethyl-2-hexanol

Figure 7.1

Alternatively, the alkyl group can be named as a derivative, followed by the word *alcohol*.

ethyl alcohol   isobutyl alcohol

Figure 7.2

Compounds of the general formula ArOH, with a hydroxyl group attached to an aromatic ring, are called **phenols** (see chapter 6).

> **MCAT Synopsis**
>
> Aromatic alcohols (ArOH) are called phenols. Resonance (through the ring) gives them special properties.

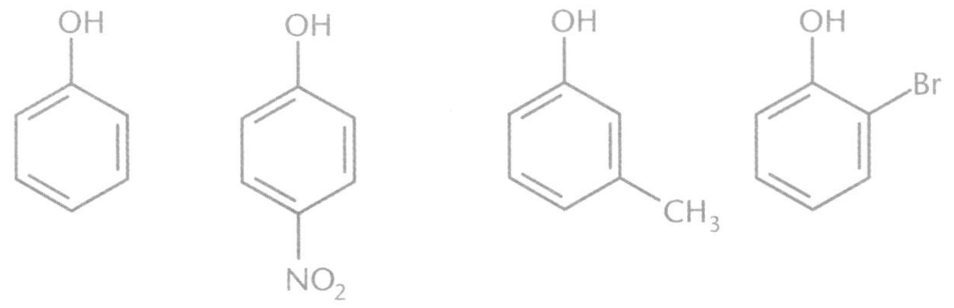

phenol *p*-nitrophenol *m*-cresol (*m*-methylphenol) *o*-bromophenol

Figure 7.3

PHYSICAL PROPERTIES

The boiling points of alcohols are significantly higher than those of the analogous hydrocarbons, due to **hydrogen bonding** (see General Chemistry chapter 3).

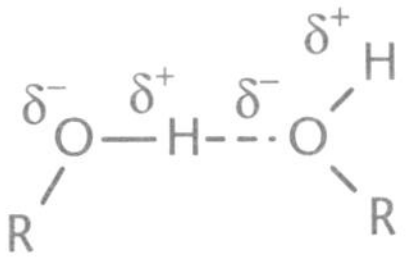

Figure 7.4

Molecules with more than one hydroxyl group show greater degrees of hydrogen bonding, as is evident from the following boiling points.

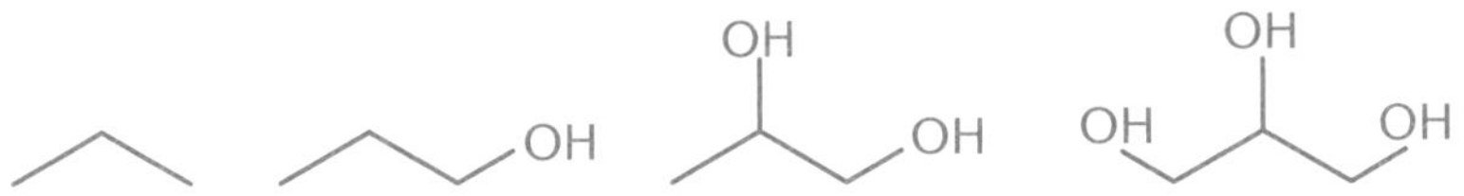

Boiling Point (°C)	–42.1	97.4	189.0	290.0

Figure 7.5

> **KAPLAN EXCLUSIVE**
>
> Hydrogen bonds form on the "phone"—the "FON"!
>
> (Fluorine, Oxygen, Nitrogen)

Hydrogen bonding can also occur when hydrogen atoms are attached to other highly electronegative atoms, such as nitrogen and fluorine. HF has particularly strong hydrogen bonds because the high electronegativity of fluorine causes the HF bond to be highly polarized.

The hydroxyl hydrogen atom is weakly acidic, and alcohols can dissociate into protons and alkoxy ions just as water dissociates into protons and hydroxide ions. pK_a values of several compounds are listed below.

Table 7.1

Dissociation	pK$_a$
$H_2O \rightleftharpoons HO^- + H^+$	15.7
$CH_3OH \rightleftharpoons CH_3O^- + H^+$	15.5
$C_2H_5OH \rightleftharpoons C_2H_5O^- + H^+$	15.9
$i\text{-PrOH} \rightleftharpoons i\text{-PrO}^- + H^+$	17.1
$t\text{-BuOH} \rightleftharpoons t\text{-BuO}^- + H^+$	18.0
$CF_3CH_2OH \rightleftharpoons CF_3CH_2O^- + H^+$	12.4
$PhOH \rightleftharpoons PhO^- + H^+$	≈10.0

Bridge

$pK_a = -\log K_a$

Strong acids have high Ka's and small pKa's. Thus, phenol, which has the smallest pKa, is the most acidic (see Chemistry chapter 10).

The hydroxyl hydrogens of phenols are more acidic than those of alcohols, due to resonance stuctures that distribute the negative charge throughout the ring, thus stabilizing the anion. As a result, these compounds form intermolecular hydrogen bonds and have relatively high melting and boiling points. Phenol is slightly soluble in water (presumably due to hydrogen bonding), as are some of its derivatives. Phenols are much more acidic than aliphatic alcohols and can form salts with inorganic bases such as NaOH.

The presence of other substituents on the ring has significant effects on the acidity, boiling points, and melting points of phenols. As with other aromatic compounds, electron-withdrawing substituents increase acidity, and electron-donating groups decrease acidity.

MCAT Synopsis

Acidity decreases as more alkyl groups are attached because the electron-donating alkyl groups *destabilize* the alkoxide anion. Electron-withdrawing groups stabilize the alkoxy anion, making the alcohol more acidic.

REVIEW

A. KEY REACTION MECHANISMS FOR ALCOHOLS AND ETHERS

As you read about synthesis of (and from) alcohols and ethers, you'll see the same basic reaction mechanisms recurring over and over. Rather than memorizing each reaction individually, try to think of them in broad categories. Focus on how the basic mechanism works and on how this particular reaction exemplifies it. The "Big Three" mechanisms for alcohols and ethers are:

1) S_N1, S_N2: nucleophilic substitution

e.g., $CH_3Br + OH^- \longrightarrow CH_3OH + Br^-$

See chapter 4 for review.

2) Electrophilic addition to a double bond,

e.g. H_2O +

This and other reactions adding H_2O to double bonds are covered in chapter 4.

3) Nucleophilic addition to a carbonyl,

e.g., CH_3MgBr +

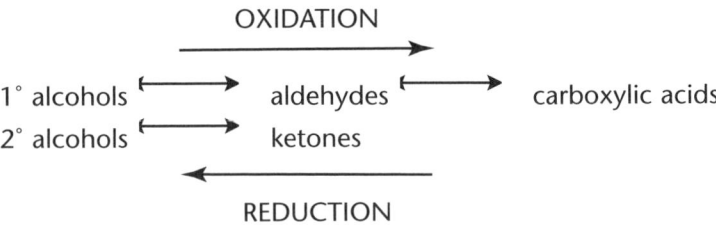

This mechanism is discussed further in chapters 8–10.

Also, when thinking about alcohols, you should keep in mind their place on the oxidation-reduction continuum:

OXIDATION

1° alcohols ⟷ aldehydes ⟷ carboxylic acids
2° alcohols ⟷ ketones

REDUCTION

As you read about the individual reactions in which alcohols participate, try to fit them into this framework (possible for most reactions, though not all).

SYNTHESIS

Alcohols can be prepared from a variety of different types of compounds. Methanol, also called wood alcohol, is obtained from the destructive distillation of wood. It is toxic and can cause blindness if ingested. Ethanol, or grain alcohol, is produced from the fermentation of sugars and can be metabolized by the body; however, in large enough quantities, it too is toxic.

A. ADDITION REACTIONS

Alcohols can be prepared via several reactions which involve addition of water to double bonds (discussed in chapter 5). Alcohols can also be prepared from the addition of organometallic compounds to carbonyl groups (discussed in chapter 10).

B. SUBSTITUTION REACTIONS

Both S_N1 and S_N2 reactions can be used to produce alcohols under the proper conditions (discussed in chapter 4).

C. REDUCTION REACTIONS

Alcohols can be prepared from the reduction of aldehydes, ketones, carboxylic acids, or esters. Lithium aluminum hydride (LiAlH$_4$, or LAH) and sodium borohydride (NaBH$_4$) are the two most frequently used reducing reagents. LAH is more powerful and more difficult to work with, whereas NaBH$_4$ is more selective and easier to handle. For example, LAH will reduce carboxylic acids and esters, while NaBH$_4$ will not.

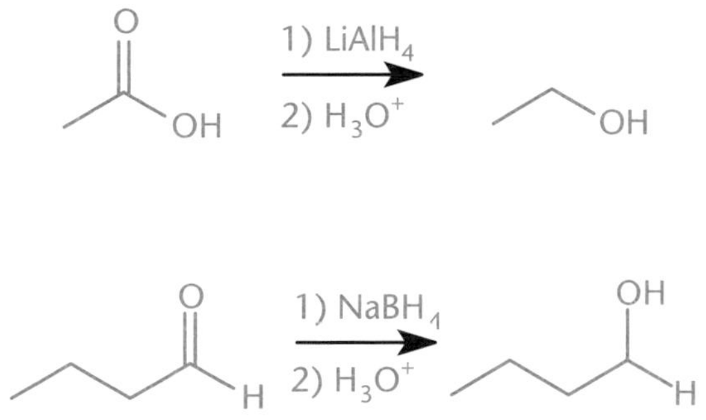

Figure 7.6

D. PHENOL SYNTHESIS

Phenols may be synthesized from arylsulfonic acids with hot NaOH, as described in chapter 6. However, this reaction is useful only for phenol or its alkylated derivatives, as most functional groups are destroyed by the harsh reaction conditions.

A more versatile method of synthesizing phenols is via hydrolysis of diazonium salts.

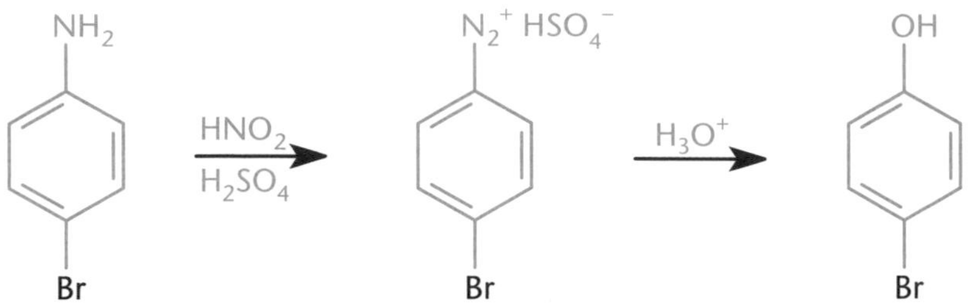

Figure 7.7

REACTIONS

A. ELIMINATION REACTIONS

Alcohols can be **dehydrated** in a strongly acidic solution (usually H_2SO_4) to produce alkenes. The mechanism of this dehydration reaction is E1, and proceeds via the protonated alcohol.

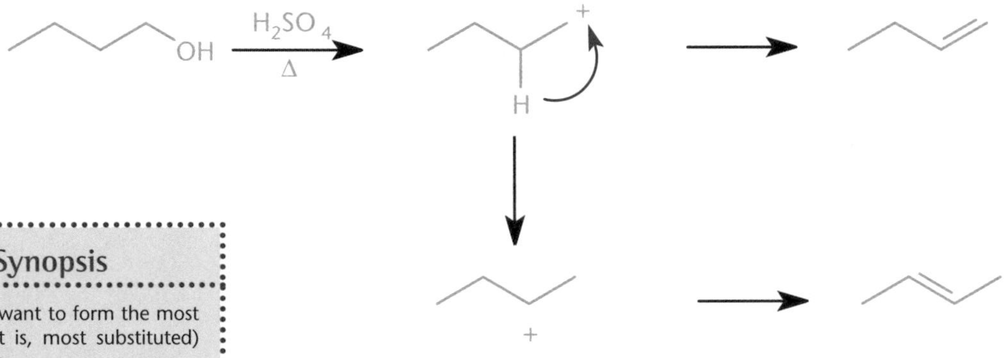

minor

major

Figure 7.8

Notice that two products are obtained, with the more stable alkene being the major product. This occurs via movement of a proton to produce the more stable 2° carbocation. This type of rearrangement is commonly encountered with carbocations.

B. SUBSTITUTION REACTIONS

The displacement of hydroxyl groups in substitution reactions is rare because the hydroxide ion is a poor leaving group. If such a transformation is desired, the hydroxyl group must be made into a good leaving group. Protonating the alcohol makes water the leaving group, which is good for S_N1 reactions; even better, the alcohol can be converted into a tosylate (p-toluenesulfonate) group, which is an excellent leaving group for S_N2 reactions (see Figures 7.9a and 7.9b).

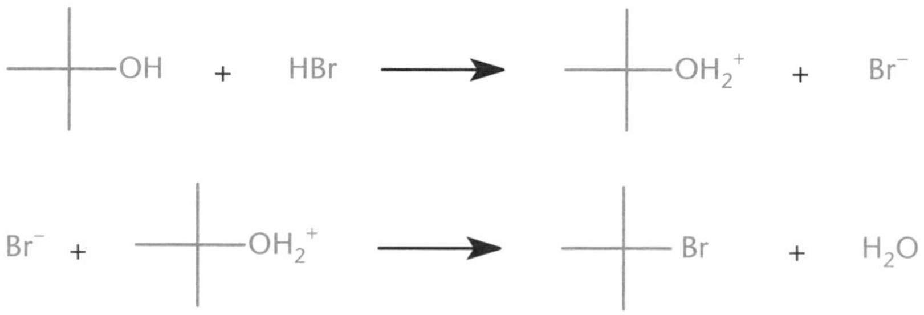

Figure 7.9a

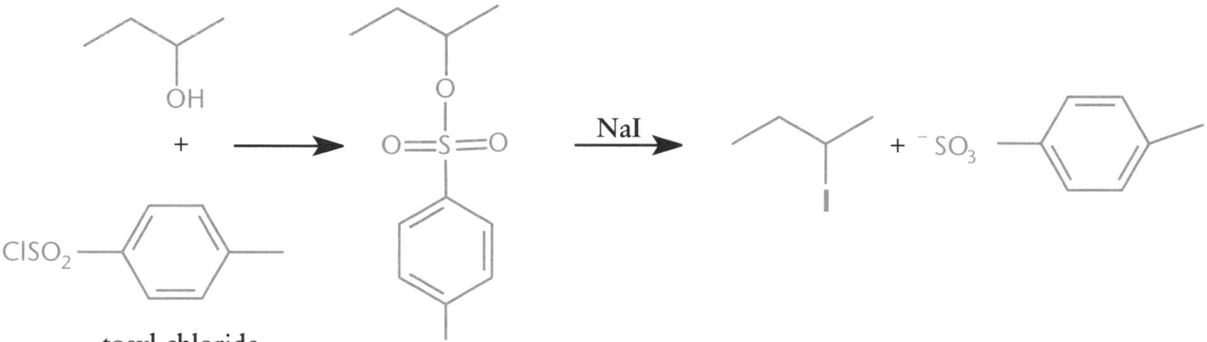

tosyl chloride

Figure 7.9b

A common method of converting alcohols into alkyl halides involves the formation of inorganic esters, which readily undergo S_N2 reactions. Alcohols react with thionyl chloride to produce an intermediate inorganic ester (a chlorosulfite) and HCl. The chloride ion of HCl displaces SO_2 and regenerates Cl⁻, forming the desired alkyl chloride.

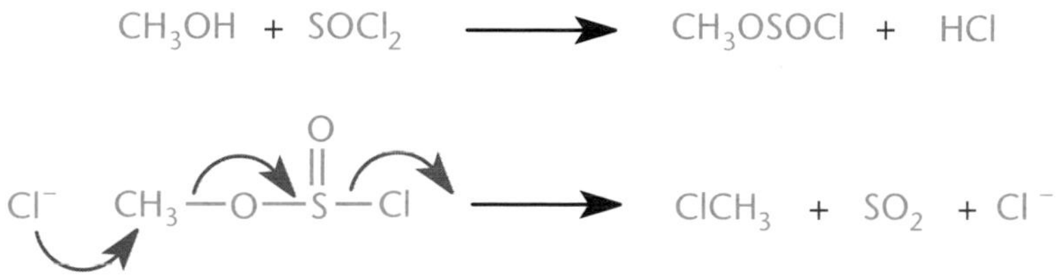

$$CH_3OH + SOCl_2 \longrightarrow CH_3OSOCl + HCl$$

Figure 7.10

An analogous reaction, where the alcohol is treated with PBr_3 instead of thionyl chloride, produces alkyl bromides.

Phenols readily undergo electrophilic aromatic substitution reactions; since it has lone pairs that it can donate to the ring, the –OH group is a strongly activating, *ortho/para*-directing ring substituent (see chapter 6).

MCAT Synopsis

Phenols are good substrates for electrophilic aromatic substitution; the –OH is activating and o, p directing.

C. OXIDATION REACTIONS

The oxidation of alcohols generally involves some form of chromium (VI) as the oxidizing agent, which is reduced to chromium (III) during the reaction. PCC (pyridinium chlorochromate, $C_5H_6NCrO_3Cl$) is commonly used as a mild oxidant. It converts primary alcohols to aldehydes without overoxidation to the acid. (In contrast, $KMnO_4$ is a very strong oxidizing agent that will take the alcohol all the way to the carboxylic acid.) It can also be used to form ketones from 2° alcohols. Tertiary alcohols cannot be oxidized for valence reasons.

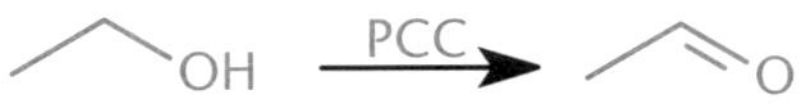

Figure 7.11

Another reagent used to oxidize secondary alcohols is alkali (either sodium or potassium) dichromate salt. This will also oxidize 1° alcohols to carboxylic acids.

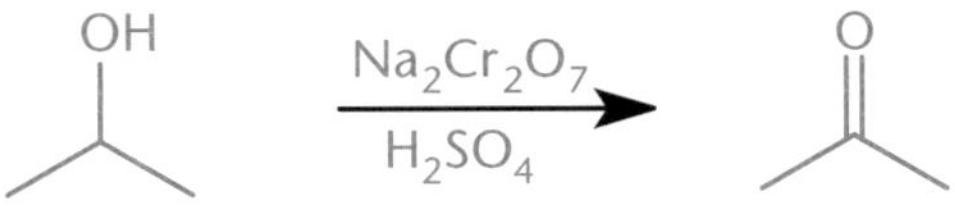

Figure 7.12

A stronger oxidant is chromium trioxide, CrO_3. This is often dissolved with dilute sulfuric acid in acetone; the mixture is called Jones' reagent. It oxidizes primary alcohols to carboxylic acids and secondary alcohols to ketones.

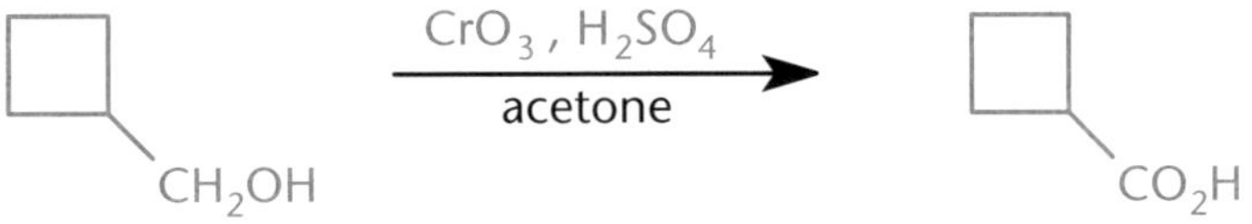

Figure 7.13

Treatment of phenols with oxidizing reagents produces compounds called quinones (2,5-cyclohexadiene-1,4-diones).

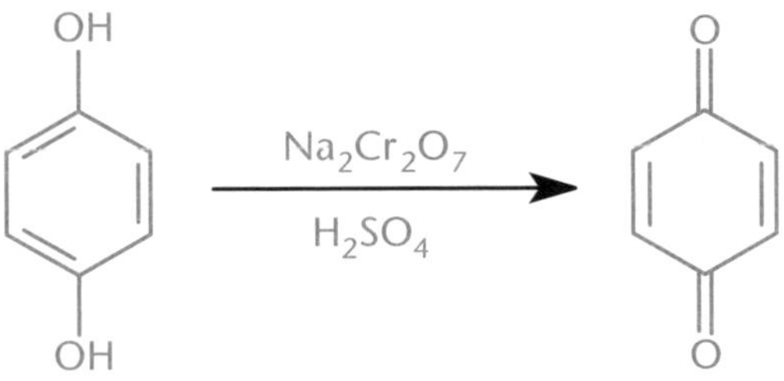

1,4-Benzenediol p-Benzoquinone

Figure 7.14

Pavlov's Dog

When you see a transition metal (such as Cr or Mn) with lots of oxygen (Cr_2O_7, CrO_3, MnO_4), think OXIDATION.

MCAT Synopsis

Alcohols can be formed by and can participate in many of the key reaction mechanisms you've already seen:

1) S_N1, S_N2
   (although –OH must be made into a better leaving group);
2) addition of H_2O to a double bond (including electrophilic addition), and reverse reactions such as E1 (see chapter 5);
3) nucleophilic addition to a carbonyl;

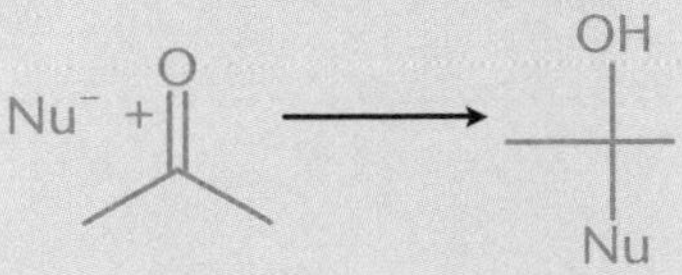

4) oxidation/reduction reactions.

ETHERS

An ether is a compound with two alkyl (or aryl) groups bonded to an oxygen atom. The general formula for an ether is **ROR**. Ethers can be thought of as disubstituted water molecules. The most familiar ether is diethyl ether, once used as a medical anesthetic, and still often used that way in the laboratory.

NOMENCLATURE

Ethers are named according to IUPAC rules as **alkoxyalkanes,** with the smaller chain as the prefix and the larger chain as the suffix. There is a common system of nomenclature in which ethers are named as alkyl alkyl ethers. In this system, methoxyethane would be named ethyl methyl ether. The alkyl substituents are alphabetized.

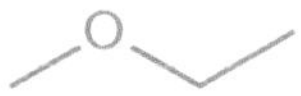

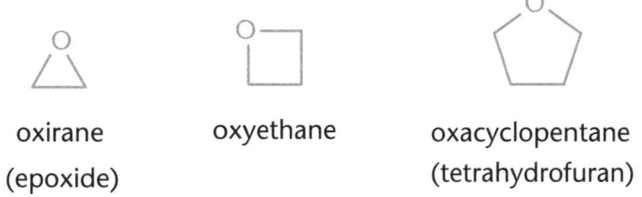

methoxyethane
(ethyl methyl ether)

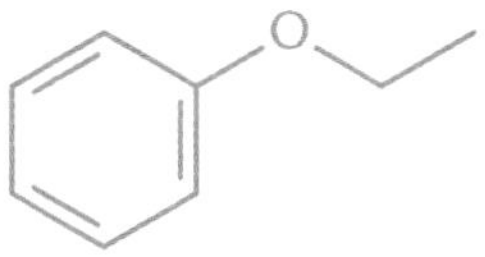

ethoxybenzene
(ethyl phenyl ether)

Figure 7.15

Exceptions to these rules occur for cyclic ethers, for which many common names also exist.

oxirane
(epoxide)

oxyethane

oxacyclopentane
(tetrahydrofuran)

Figure 7.16

MCAT Synopsis

Remember that smaller rings have more angle strain, making them less stable.

PHYSICAL PROPERTIES

Ethers do not undergo hydrogen bonding because they have no hydrogen atoms bonded to the oxygen atoms. Ethers therefore boil at relatively low temperatures compared to alcohols; in fact, they boil at approximately the same temperatures as alkanes of comparable molecular weight.

Ethers are only slightly polar and therefore only slightly soluble in water. They are rather inert to most organic reagents and are frequently used as solvents.

SYNTHESIS

The Williamson ether synthesis produces ethers from the reaction of metal alkoxides with primary alkyl halides or tosylates. The alkoxides behave as nucleophiles, and displace the halide or tosylate via an S_N2 reaction, producing an ether.

MCAT Synopsis

Look! It's S_N2 again! Therefore, you need a strong nucleophile (alkoxides are good) and an unhindered substrate (*not* bulky or highly substituted).

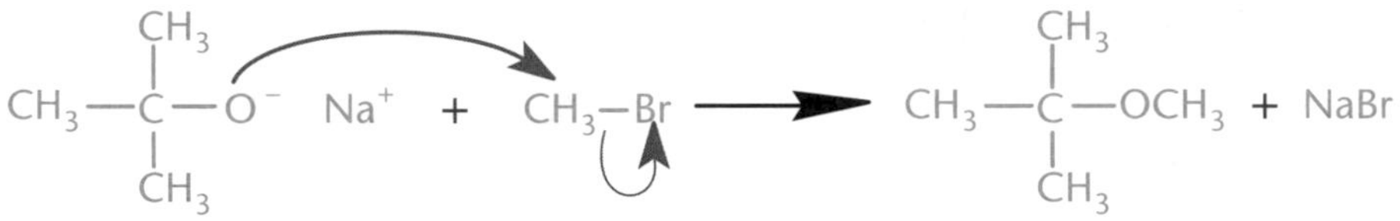

Figure 7.17

It is important to remember that alkoxides will attack only nonhindered halides. Thus, to synthesize a methyl ether, an alkoxide must attack a methyl halide; the reaction cannot be accomplished with methoxide ion attacking a hindered alkyl halide substrate.

The Williamson ether synthesis can also be applied to phenols. Relatively mild reaction conditions are sufficient, due to the phenols' acidity.

MCAT Synopsis

More S_N2! This time, however, it's intramolecular—the nucleophile and leaving group are part of the same molecule.

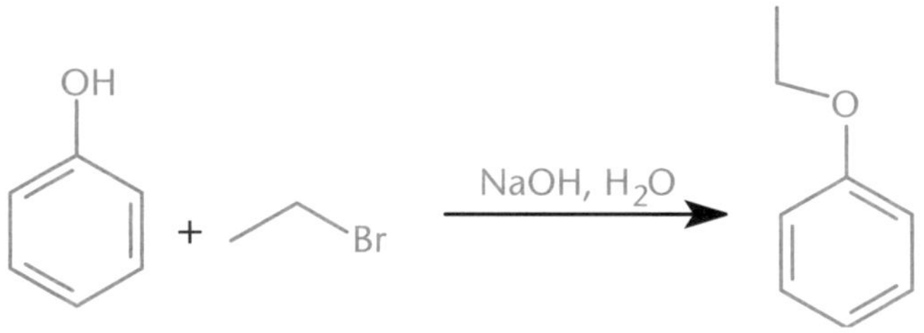

Figure 7.18

Cyclic ethers are prepared in a number of ways. Oxiranes can be synthesized by means of an internal S_N2 displacement.

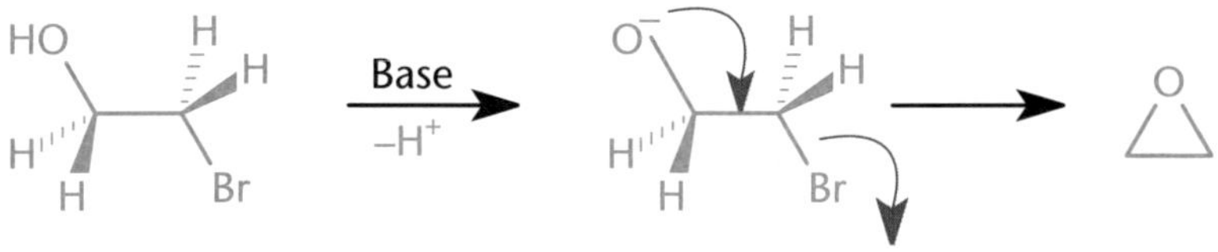

Figure 7.19

Oxidation of an alkene with a **peroxy acid** (general formula RCOOOH) such as mcpba (*m*-chloroperoxybenzoic acid) will also produce an oxirane.

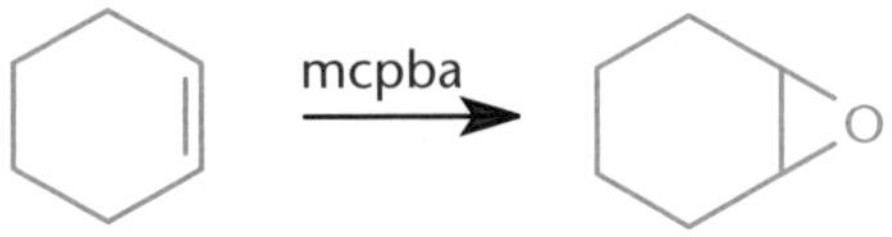

Figure 7.20

REACTIONS

A. PEROXIDE FORMATION

Ethers react with the oxygen in air to form highly explosive compounds called **peroxides** (general formula ROOR).

B. CLEAVAGE

Cleavage of straight-chain ethers will take place only under vigorous conditions: usually at high temperatures in the presence of HBr or HI. Cleavage is initiated by protonation of the ether oxygen. The reaction then proceeds by an S_N1 or S_N2 mechanism, depending on the conditions and the structure of the ether (Figure 7.20). Although not shown below, the alcohol products usually react with a second molecule of hydrogen halide to produce an alkyl halide.

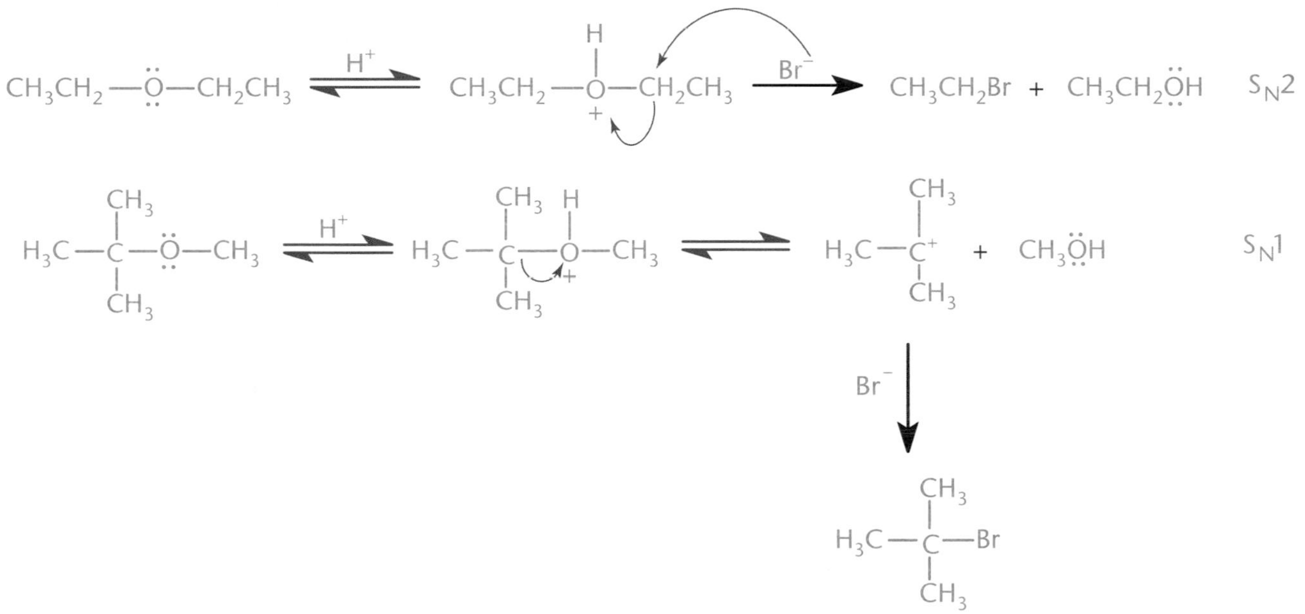

> **MCAT Synopsis**
>
> Remember, strong bases are poor leaving groups. Without protonation, the leaving group would be an alkoxide (strongly basic), and the reaction would be unlikely to proceed.

Figure 7.21

Since epoxides are highly strained cyclic ethers, they are susceptible to S_N2 reactions. Unlike straight-chain ethers, these reactions can be catalyzed by acid or base. In symmetrical epoxides, either carbon can be nucleophilically attacked; but in asymmetrical epoxides, the most substituted carbon is nucleophilically attacked in the presence of acid, and the least substituted carbon is attacked in the presence of base:

> **MCAT Synopsis**
>
> Cleavage of straight chain ethers is acid-catalyzed. Cleavage of cyclic ethers can be acid- or base-catalyzed.

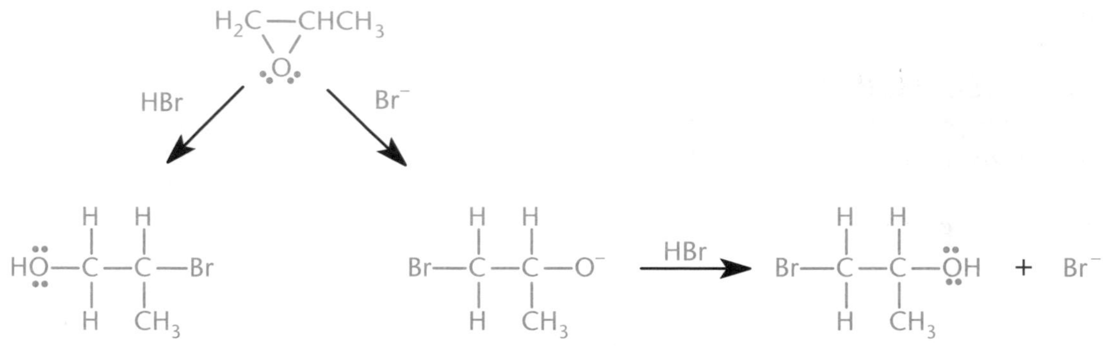

$$H_2C-CHCH_3$$

HBr ... Br⁻

HÖ—C—C—Br

Acid-catalyzed ring opening

Br—C—C—O⁻ →HBr→ Br—C—C—ÖH + Br⁻

Base-catalyzed ring opening

Figure 7.22

> ### MCAT Synopsis
>
> Base-catalyzed cleavage has the most S_N2 character, while acid-catalyzed cleavage seems to have some S_N1 character.

Base-catalyzed cleavage has the most S_N2 character, so it occurs at the least hindered (least substituted) carbon. The basic environment provides the best nucleophile.

In contrast, acid-catalyzed cleavage is thought to have some S_N1 character as well as some S_N2 character. The epoxide O can be protonated, making it a better leaving group. This gives the carbons a bit of positive charge. Since substitution stabilizes this charge (remember, 3° carbons make the best carbocations), the more substituted C becomes a good target for nucleophilic attack.

Don't let epoxides intimidate you; the same basic principles and reaction mechanisms apply, just as we've seen with more simple compounds.

ALDEHYDES AND KETONES

Aldehydes and ketones are compounds that contain the carbonyl group, C=O, a double bond between a carbon atom and an oxygen atom. A ketone has two alkyl or aryl groups bonded to the carbonyl, whereas an aldehyde has one alkyl group and one hydrogen (or, in the case of formaldehyde, two hydrogens) bonded to the carbonyl. The carbonyl group is one of the most important functional groups in organic chemistry. In addition to aldehydes and ketones, it is also found in carboxylic acids, esters, amides, and more complicated compounds.

NOMENCLATURE

In the IUPAC system, aldehydes are named with the suffix -al. The position of the aldehyde group does not need to be specified: it must occupy the terminal (C–1) position. Common names exist for the first five aldehydes: formaldehyde, acetaldehyde, propionaldehyde, butyraldehyde, and valeraldehyde.

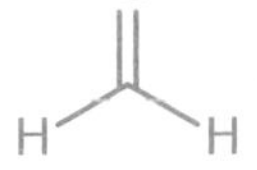

methanal
(formaldehyde)

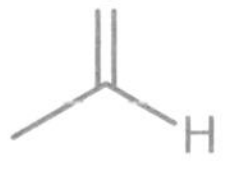

ethanal
(acetaldehyde)

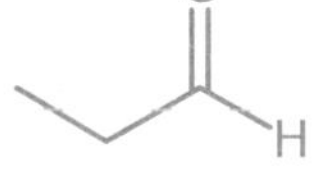

propanal
(propionaldehyde)

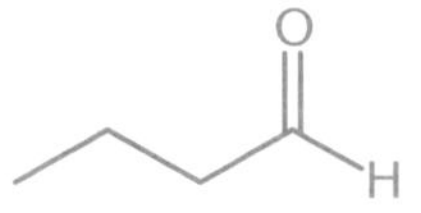

butanal
(butyraldehyde)

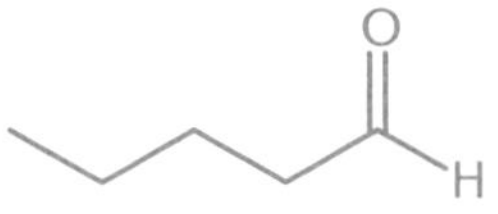

pentanal
(valeraldehyde)

Figure 8.1

In more complicated molecules, the suffix **-carbaldehyde** can be used. In addition, the aldehyde can be named as a functional group with the prefix **formyl-**.

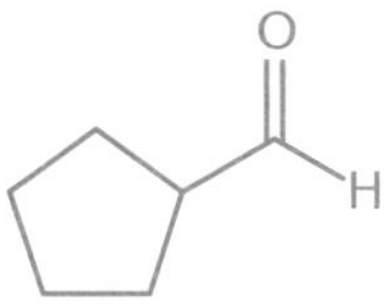

cyclopentanecarbaldehyde

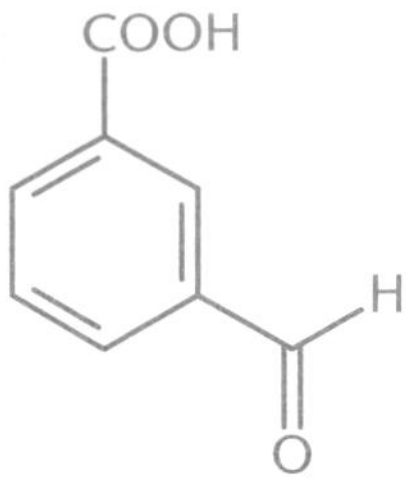

m-formylbenzoic acid

Figure 8.2

Ketones are named with the suffix **-one**. The location of the carbonyl group must be specified with a number, except in cyclic ketones, where it is assumed to occupy the number 1 position. The common system of naming **ketones** lists the two alkyl groups followed by the word *ketone*. When it is necessary to name the carbonyl as a substituent, the prefix **oxo-** is used.

MCAT Synopsis

The carbonyl group has a dipole moment. Oxygen is more electronegative—it is an "electron hog," pulling the electrons away from the carbon.

2-propanone
(dimethyl ketone)
(acetone)

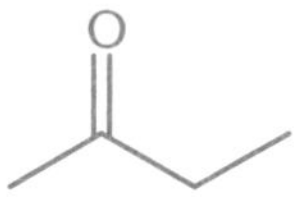

2-butanone
(ethyl methyl ketone)

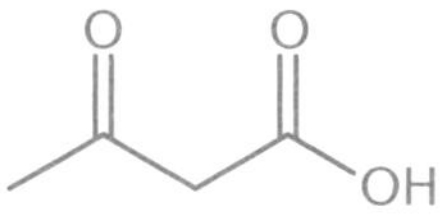

3-oxobutanoic acid

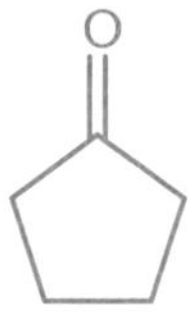

cyclopentanone

Figure 8.3

PHYSICAL PROPERTIES

The physical properties of aldehydes and ketones are governed by the presence of the carbonyl group. The dipole moments that are associated with the polar carbonyl groups align, causing an elevation in boiling point relative to the alkanes. This elevation is less than that in alcohols, as no hydrogen bonding is involved.

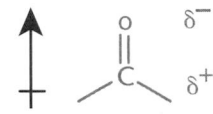

Figure 8.4

> **MCAT Synopsis**
>
> Dipole—dipole interactions elevate the boiling point, but not as strongly as do hydrogen bonds.

SYNTHESIS

There are numerous methods of preparing aldehydes and ketones; three of the most common are described below.

A. OXIDATION OF ALCOHOLS

An aldehyde can be obtained from the oxidation of a primary alcohol; a ketone can be obtained from a secondary alcohol. As mentioned in chapter 7, these reactions are usually performed with PCC, sodium or potassium dichromate, or chromium trioxide (Jones's reagent).

> **MCAT Synopsis**
>
> Primary alcohols can be oxidized to aldehydes. Secondary alcohols can be oxidized to ketones.

Primary Alcohols (1) → Aldehydes (2) → Carboxylic Acids (3)
Secondary Alcohols (1) → Ketone (2)

B. OZONOLYSIS OF ALKENES

Double bonds can be oxidatively cleaved to yield aldehydes and/or ketones, typically with ozone. See chapter 5 for more details.

C. FRIEDEL-CRAFTS ACYLATION

This reaction, discussed in chapter 6, produces ketones of the form R–CO–Ar.

REACTIONS

A. ENOLIZATION AND REACTIONS OF ENOLS

Protons alpha to carbonyl groups are relatively acidic ($pK_a \approx 20$), due to resonance stabilization of the conjugate base. A hydrogen atom that detaches itself from the alpha carbon has a finite probability of reattaching itself to the oxygen instead of the carbon. Therefore, aldehydes and ketones exist in solution as a mixture of two isomers, the familiar **keto** form, and the **enol** form, representing the unsaturated alcohol (**ene** = the double bond, **ol** = the alcohol, so **ene** + **ol** = **enol**). The two isomers, which differ only in the placement of a proton, are called **tautomers**. The equilibrium between the tautomers lies far to the keto side. The process of interconverting from the keto to the enol tautomer is called **enolization**.

> **MCAT Synopsis**
>
> Aldehydes and ketones have the traditional keto form (C=O), as well as the less common enol tautomer (enol = ene + ol). The enol form can act as a nucleophile.

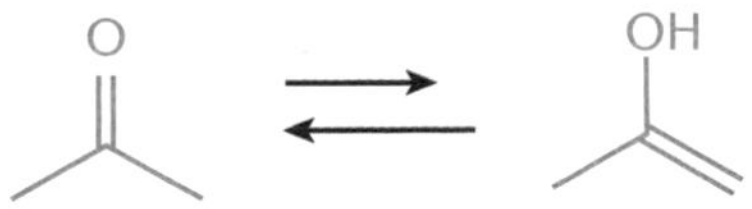

Figure 8.5

Enols are the necessary intermediates in many reactions of aldehydes and ketones. The enolate carbanion, which is nucleophilic, can be created with a strong base such as lithium diisopropyl amide (LDA) or potassium hydride, KH. This nucleophilic carbanion reacts via S_N2 with α,β-unsaturated carbonyl compounds in reactions called **Michael additions**.

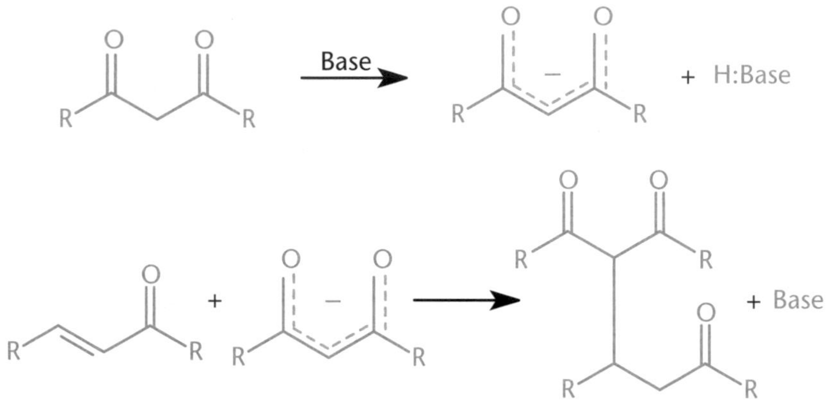

Figure 8.6

B. ADDITION REACTIONS

General Reaction Mechanism: Nucleophilic Addition to a Carbonyl

Many of the reactions of aldehydes and ketones share this general reaction mechanism. Rather than memorizing them all individually, focus on understanding the basic pattern. Then, you can learn how each reaction exemplifies it.

As shown in Figure 8.4 earlier, the C=O bond is polarized, with a partial positive charge on C and a partial negative charge on O. This makes the carbon ripe for nucleophilic attack.

MCAT Synopsis

The carbonyl carbon is a good target for nucleophilic attack.

The nucleophile attacks, forming a bond to the C, which causes the π bond in the C=O to break. This generates a tetrahedral intermediate. If no good leaving group is present, the double bond cannot reform, and so the final product is nearly identical to the intermediate, except that usually the O^- will accept a proton to become a hydroxyl (–OH).

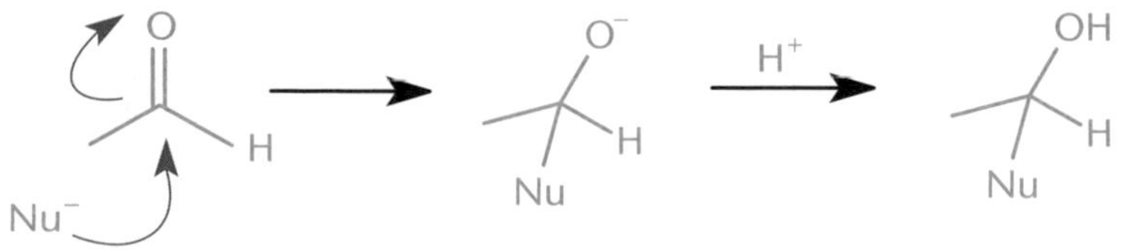

Figure 8.7

Although the figure shows only nucleophilic addition to an aldehyde, this mechanism applies to ketones as well.

1. **Hydration**

   In the presence of water, aldehydes and ketones react to form *gem* diols (1,1-diols). In this case, water acts as the nucleophile attacking at the carbonyl carbon. This hydration reaction proceeds slowly; the rate may be increased by the addition of a small amount of acid or base.

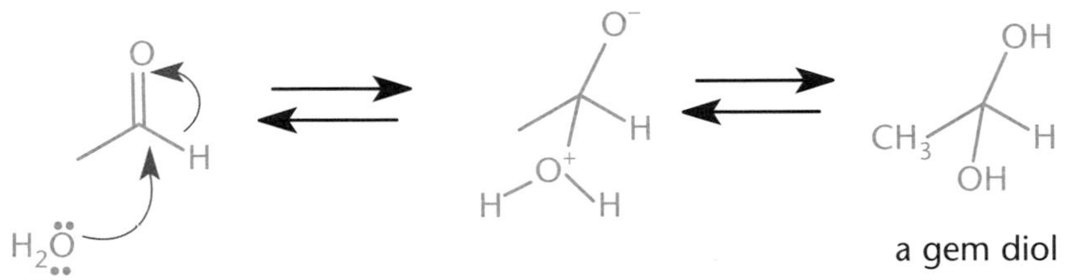

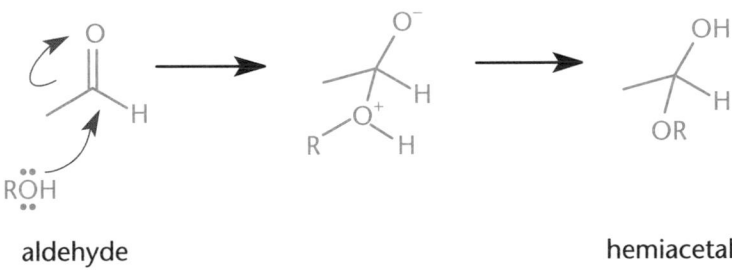

Figure 8.8

a gem diol

2. **Acetal and Ketal Formation**

   A reaction similar to hydration occurs when aldehydes and ketones are treated with alcohols. When one equivalent of alcohol (in this reaction the nucleophile) is added to an aldehyde or ketone, the product is a **hemiacetal** or a **hemiketal**, respectively. When two equivalents of alcohol are added, the product is an **acetal** or a **ketal**, respectively. The reaction mechanism is the same as it is for hydration and is catalyzed by anhydrous acid. Acetals and ketals, comparatively inert, are frequently used as protecting groups for carbonyl functionalities. They can easily be converted back to the carbonyl with aqueous acid.

aldehyde

hemiacetal

Figure 8.9

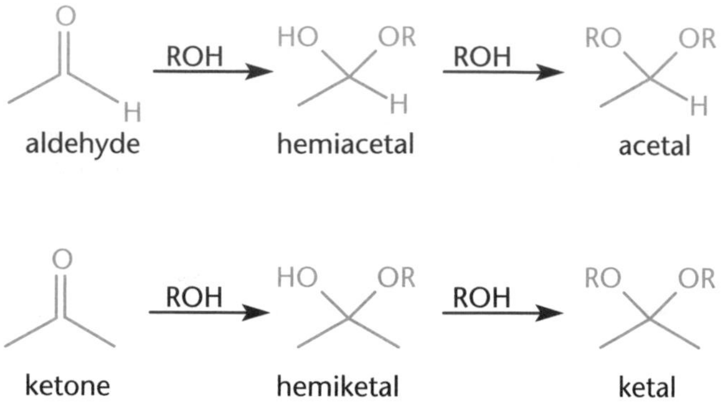

Figure 8.10

3. **Reaction with HCN**

   Aldehydes and ketones react with HCN (hydrogen cyanide) to produce stable compounds called **cyanohydrins**. HCN dissociates and the nucleophilic cyanide anion attacks the carbonyl carbon atom. Protonation of the oxygen produces the cyanohydrin. The cyanohydrin gains its stability from the newly formed C–C bond (in contrast, when a carbonyl reacts with HCl, a weak C–Cl bond is formed, and the resulting chlorohydrin is unstable).

> **MCAT Synopsis**
>
> When CN^- is the nucleophile, cyanohydrins are formed.

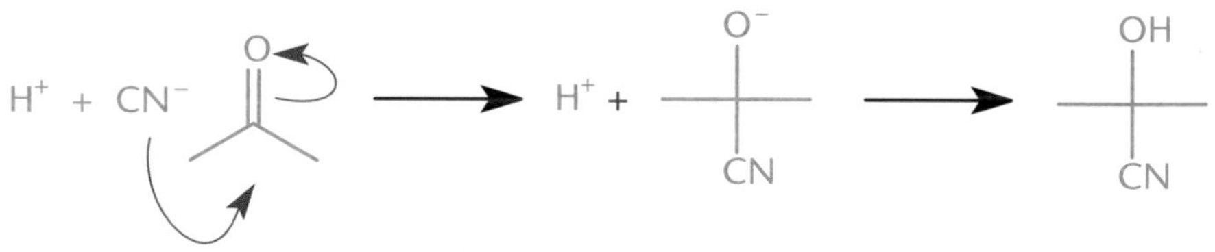

Figure 8.11

4. **Condensations with Ammonia Derivatives**

   Ammonia and some of its derivatives are nucleophiles and can add to carbonyl compounds. In the simplest case, ammonia adds to the carbon atom and water is lost, producing an **imine,** a compound with a nitrogen atom double-bonded to a carbon atom. (A reaction in which water is lost between two molecules is called a **condensation reaction**.)

   In this case, the first part of the reaction follows the mechanism of nucleophilic addition described above. However, after formation of a tetrahedral intermediate, this reaction proceeds further: The C=O double bond reforms and a leaving group is kicked off. This mechanism is called nucleophilic *substitution* on a carbonyl and will be described in greater detail in chapter 9.

   Some common ammonia derivatives that react with aldehydes and ketones are hydroxylamine (H_2NOH), hydrazine (H_2NNH_2), and semicarbazide ($H_2NNHCONH_2$); these form oximes, hydrazones, and semicarbazones, respectively.

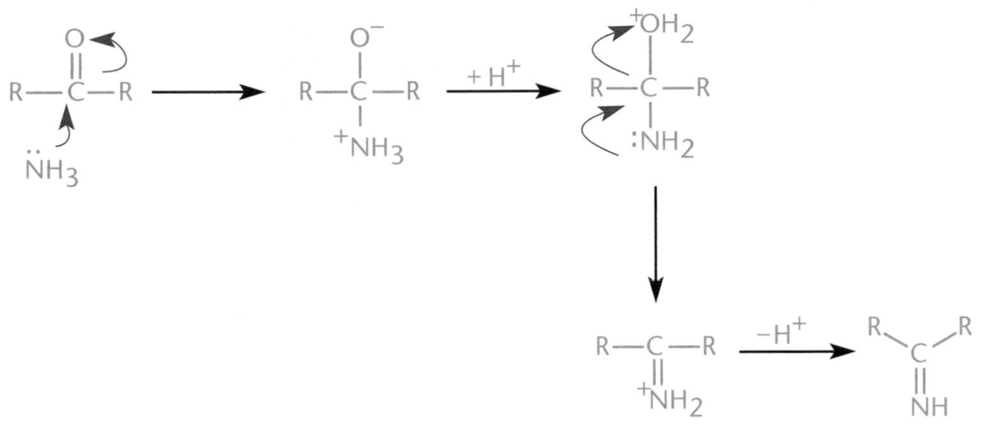

Figure 8.12

Don't worry too much about protons coming and going; there should be plenty in the solution, so you can transiently put them where needed to facilitate this reaction.

Examples of other potential nucleophiles and their respective products are shown below.

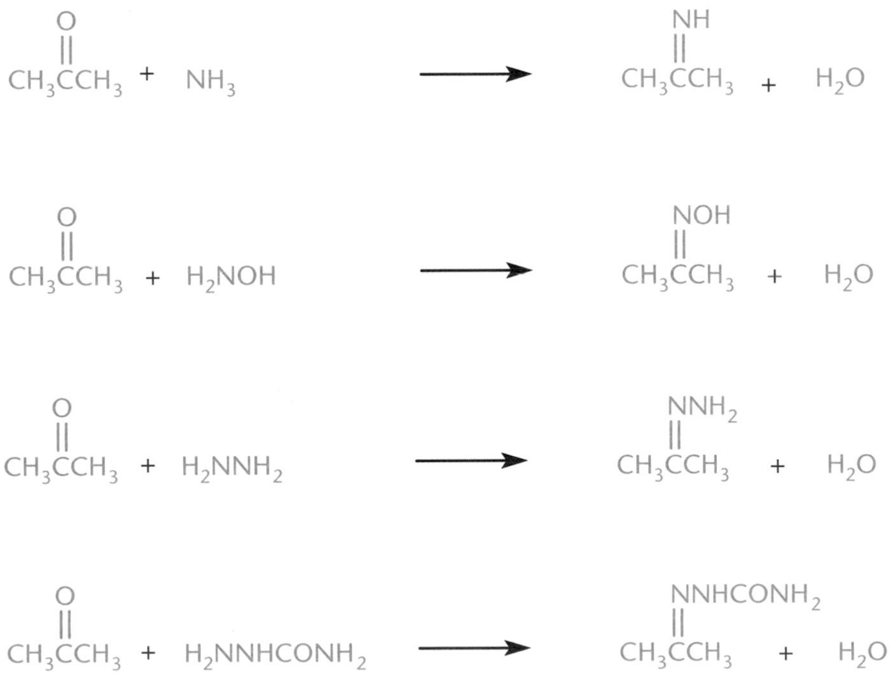

Figure 8.13

C. THE ALDOL CONDENSATION

The aldol condensation is an important reaction that basically follows the mechanism of nucleophilic addition to a carbonyl that was described above. In this case, an aldehyde acts both as nucleophile (enol form) and target (keto form). When acetaldehyde (ethanal) is treated with base, an enolate ion is produced. This enolate ion, being nucleophilic, can react with the carbonyl group of another acetaldehyde molecule. The product is 3-hydroxybutanal, which contains both an alcohol and an aldehyde functionality. This type of compound is called an **aldol**, from **ald**ehyde and alco**hol**. With stronger base and higher temperatures, condensation occurs, producing an α,β-unsaturated aldehyde. This type of condensation reaction has become known as the **aldol condensation**.

3-hydroxybutanal
(an aldol)

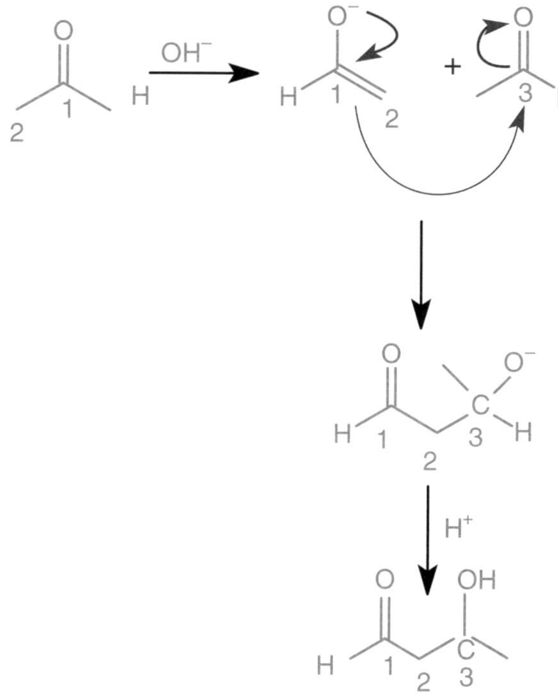

Figure 8.14a

When heated, this molecule can undergo elimination and lose H_2O to form a double bond:

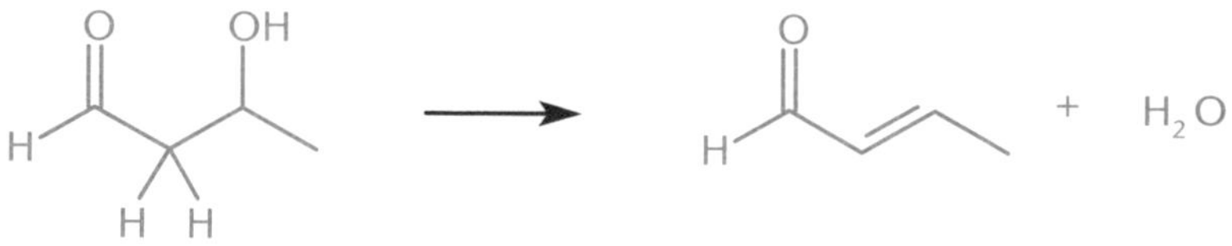

Figure 8.14b

The aldol condensation is most useful when only one type of aldehyde or ketone is present, since mixed condensations usually result in a mixture of products.

D. THE WITTIG REACTION

The **Wittig Reaction** is a method of forming carbon-carbon double bonds by converting aldehydes and ketones into alkenes. The first step involves the formation of a phosphonium salt from the S_N2 reaction of an alkyl halide with the nucleophile triphenylphosphine, $(C_6H_5)_3P$. The phosphonium salt is then deprotonated (losing the proton α to the phosphorus) with a strong base, yielding a neutral compound called an **ylide** (pronounced "ill-id") or **phosphorane**. (The phosphorus atom may be drawn as pentavalent, utilizing the low-lying 3d atomic orbitals.)

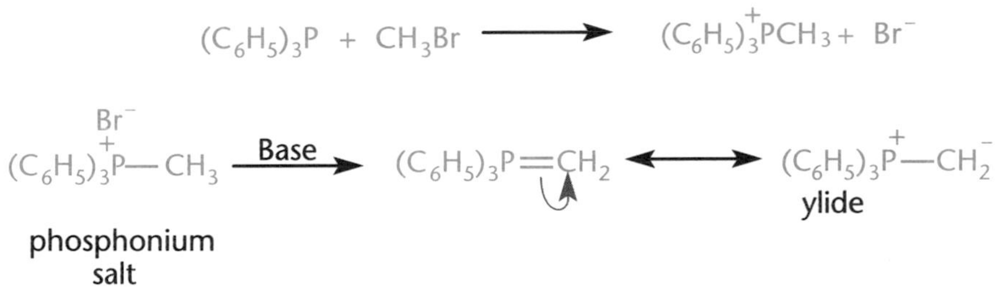

$$(C_6H_5)_3P + CH_3Br \longrightarrow (C_6H_5)_3\overset{+}{P}CH_3 + Br^-$$

Figure 8.15

Notice that an ylide is a type of carbanion and has nucleophilic properties. When combined with an aldehyde or ketone, an ylide attacks the carbonyl carbon, giving an intermediate called a *betaine*, which forms a four-membered ring intermediate called an oxaphosphetane. This decomposes to yield an alkene and triphenylphosphine oxide.

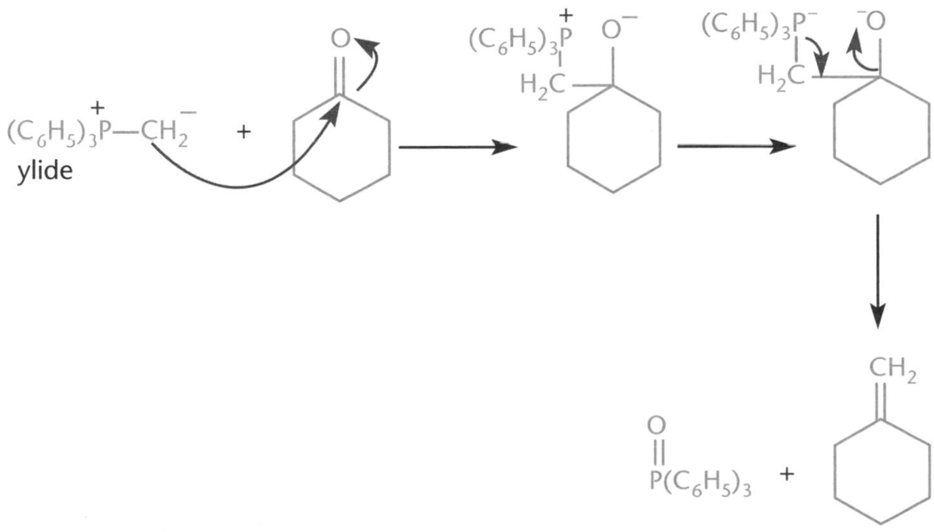

Figure 8.16

The decomposition reaction is driven by the strength of the phosphorus-oxygen bond that is formed.

E. OXIDATION AND REDUCTION

Aldehydes and ketones occupy the middle of the oxidation-reduction continuum. They are more oxidized than alcohols but less oxidized than carboxylic acids.

Aldehydes can be oxidized with a number of different reagents, such as $KMnO_4$, CrO_3, Ag_2O, or H_2O_2. The product of oxidation is a carboxylic acid.

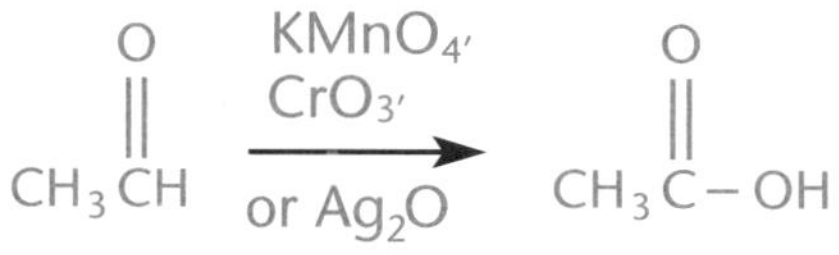

$$CH_3\overset{O}{\underset{\|}{C}}H \xrightarrow[\text{or } Ag_2O]{KMnO_4, \; CrO_3,} CH_3\overset{O}{\underset{\|}{C}}-OH$$

Figure 8.17

A number of different reagents will reduce aldehydes and ketones to alcohols. The most common is lithium aluminum hydride (LAH); sodium borohydride ($NaBH_4$) is often used when milder conditions are needed.

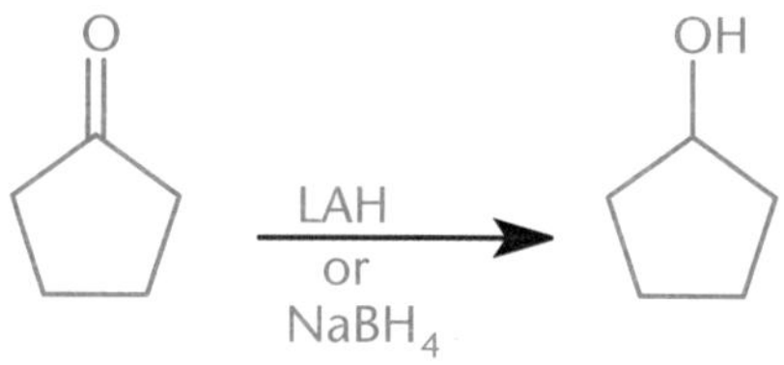

$$\xrightarrow[NaBH_4]{\substack{LAH \\ or}}$$

Figure 8.18

Aldehydes and ketones can be completely reduced to alkanes by two common methods. In the **Wolff-Kishner** Reduction, the carbonyl is first converted to a hydrazone, which releases molecular nitrogen (N_2) when heated and forms an alkane (the protons being abstracted from the solvent). The Wolff-Kishner reaction is performed in basic solution and therefore is useful only when the product is stable under basic conditions.

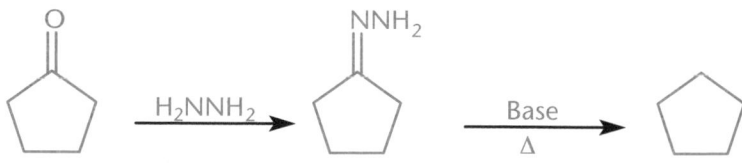

Figure 8.19

> **MCAT Synopsis**
>
> Both aldehydes and ketones can be fully reduced to alkanes:
>
> —Wolff-Kishner (H_2NNH_2);
> —Clemmensen [Hg (Zn), HCl].

An alternative reduction not subject to this restriction is the **Clemmensen Reduction**, in which an aldehyde or ketone is heated with amalgamated zinc in hydrochloric acid.

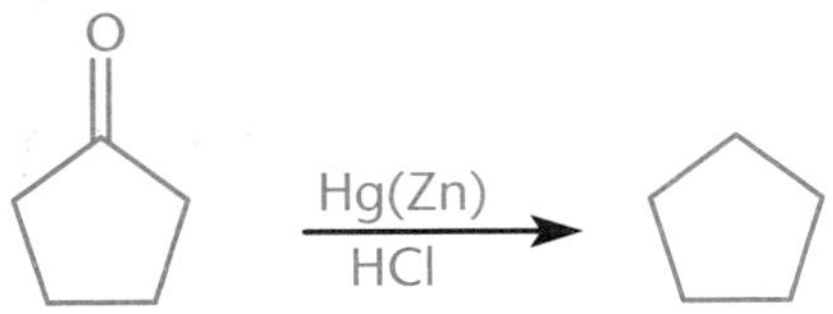

Figure 8.20

9

CARBOXYLIC ACIDS

Carboxylic acids are compounds that contain hydroxyl groups attached to carbonyl groups. This functionality is known as a **carboxyl group**. The hydroxyl hydrogen atoms are acidic, with pK_a values in the general range of 3 to 6. Carboxylic acids occur widely in nature and are synthesized by all living organisms.

NOMENCLATURE

In the IUPAC system of nomenclature, carboxylic acids are named by adding the suffix **-oic acid** to the alkyl root. The chain is numbered so that the carboxyl group receives the lowest possible number. Additional substituents are named in the usual fashion.

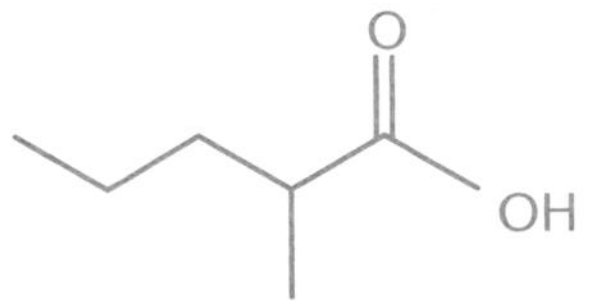

2-methylpentanoic acid 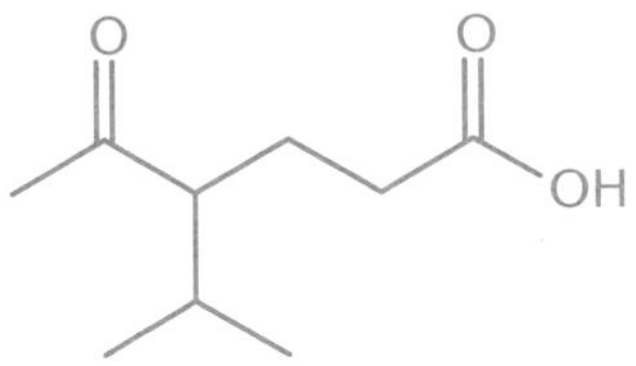   4-isopropyl-5-oxohexanoic acid

Figure 9.1

Carboxylic acids were among the first organic compounds discovered. Their original names continue today in the common system of nomenclature. For example, formic acid (from Latin *formica*, meaning "ant") was found in ants and butyric acid (from Latin *butyrum*, meaning "butter") in rancid butter. The common and IUPAC names of the first three carboxylic acids are listed in Figure 9.2.

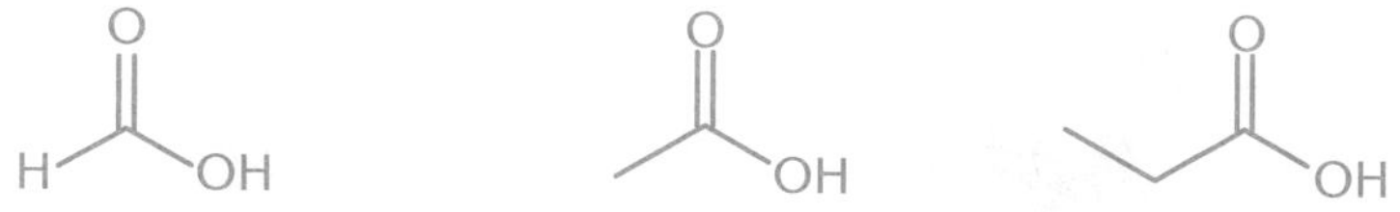

methanoic acid (formic acid)　　ethanoic acid (acetic acid)　　propanoic acid (propionic acid)

Figure 9.2

Cyclic carboxylic acids are usually named as cycloalkane carboxylic acids. The carbon atom to which the carboxyl group is attached is numbered 1. Salts of carboxylic acids are named beginning with the cation, followed by the name of the acid with the ending **-ate** replacing **-ic acid**. Typical examples are:

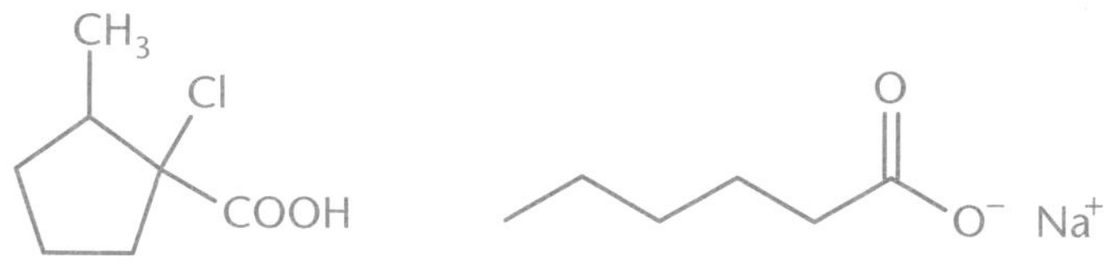

1-chloro-2-methylcyclo-pentane carboxylic acid　　sodium hexanoate

Figure 9.3

Dicarboxylic acids—compounds with two carboxyl groups—are common in biological systems. The first six straight-chain terminal dicarboxylic acids are oxalic, malonic, succinic, glutaric, adipic, and pimelic acids. Their IUPAC names are ethanedioic acid, propanedioic acid, butanedioic acid, pentanedioic acid, hexanedioic acid, and heptanedioic acid.

PHYSICAL PROPERTIES

A. HYDROGEN BONDING

Carboxylic acids are polar and can form hydrogen bonds. As a result, carboxylic acids can form dimers: pairs of molecules connected by hydrogen bonds. The boiling points of carboxylic acids are therefore even higher than those of the corresponding alcohols. The boiling points follow the usual trend of increasing with molecular weight.

B. ACIDITY

The acidity of carboxylic acids is due to the resonance stabilization of the carboxylate anion (the conjugate base). When the hydroxyl proton dissociates from the acid, the negative charge left on the carboxylate group is delocalized between the two oxygen atoms.

MCAT Synopsis

Carboxylic acids are polar and can form hydrogen bonds. Their acidity is due to resonance stabilization and can be enhanced by adding electronegative groups or other potential resonance structures.

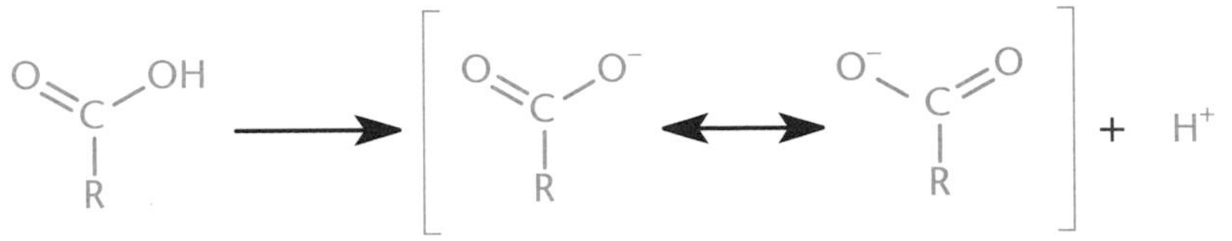

Figure 9.4

Substituents on carbon atoms adjacent to a carboxyl group can influence acidity. Electron-withdrawing groups such as –Cl or –NO_2 further delocalize the negative charge and increase acidity. Electron-donating groups such as –NH_2 or –OCH_3 destabilize the negative charge, making the compound less acidic.

In dicarboxylic acids, one –COOH group (which is electron-withdrawing) influences the other, making the compound more acidic than the analogous monocarboxylic acid. The second carboxyl group is then influenced by the carboxylate anion. Ionization of the second group will create a doubly charged species, in which the two negative charges repel each other. Since this is unfavorable, the second proton is less acidic than that of a monocarboxylic acid.

β-dicarboxylic acids are notable for the high acidity of the α-hydrogens located between the two carboxyl groups (pK$_a$ ~ 10). Loss of this acidic hydrogen atom produces a carbanion that is stabilized by the electron-withdrawing effect of the two carboxyl groups (the same effect seen in β-ketoacids, RC=OCH$_2$ COOH).

> **MCAT Favorite**
>
> Other ways to stabilize the negative charge (and thus increase acidity) are:
> - electron-withdrawing groups (e.g., halides);
> - groups that allow more resonance stabilization (e.g., benzyl or allyl substituents).
>
> The more of such groups that exist, and the closer to the acid they are, the stronger the acid.

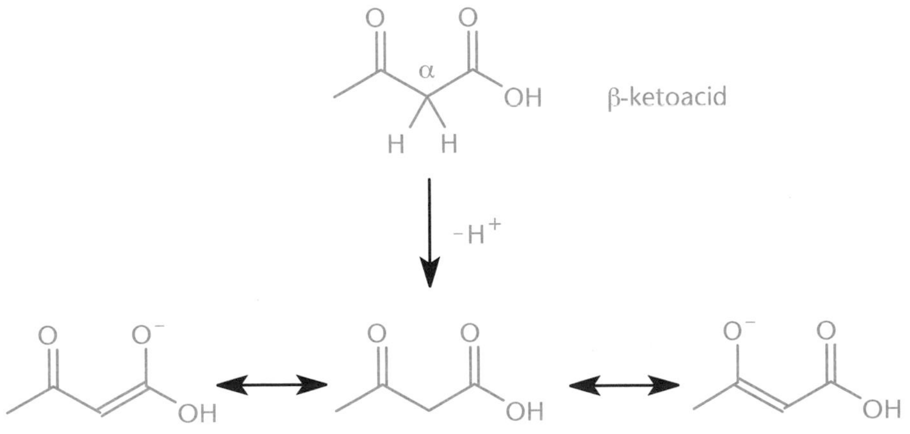

Figure 9.5

Similarly, the β-dicarboxylic acid also has acidic α hydrogens.

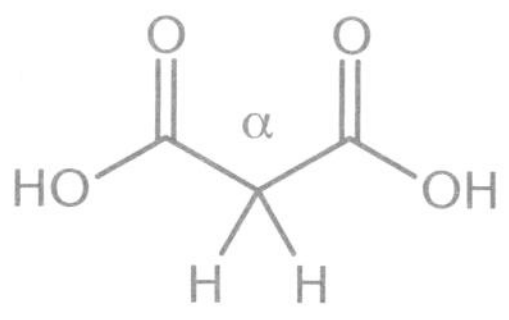

Figure 9.6

SYNTHESIS

KAPLAN EXCLUSIVE

Carboxylic acids are the most oxidized.

A. OXIDATION REACTIONS

Carboxylic acids can be prepared via oxidation of aldehydes, primary alcohols, and certain alkylbenzenes. The oxidant is usually potassium permanganate, $KMnO_4$. Note that secondary and tertiary alcohols cannot be oxidized to carboxylic acids because of valence limitations.

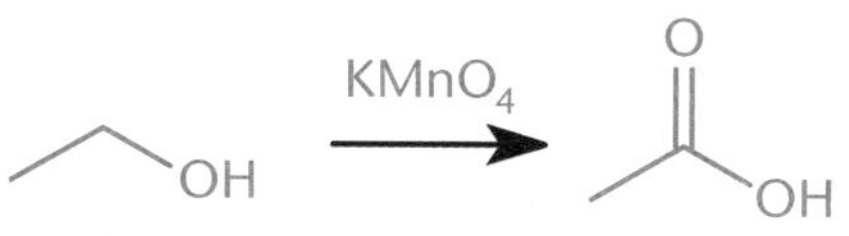

Figure 9.7

B. CARBONATION OF ORGANOMETALLIC REAGENTS

Organometallic reagents, such as Grignard reagents, react with carbon dioxide (CO_2) to form carboxylic acids. This reaction is useful for the conversion of tertiary alkyl halides into carboxylic acids, which cannot be accomplished through other methods. Note that this reaction adds one carbon atom to the chain.

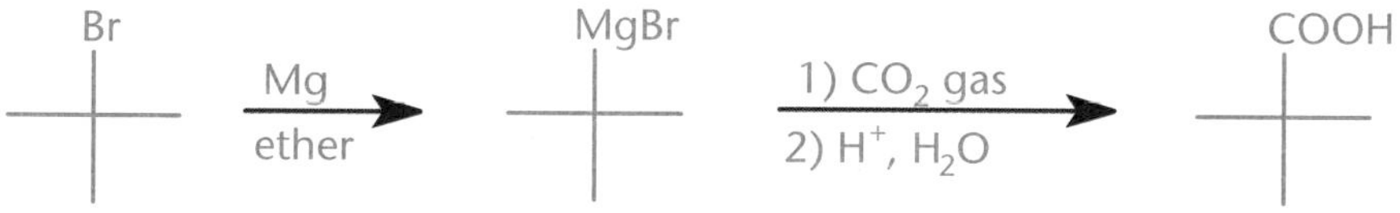

Figure 9.8

C. HYDROLYSIS OF NITRILES

Nitriles, also called cyanides, are compounds containing the functional group –CN. The cyanide anion CN^- is a good nucleophile and will displace primary and secondary halides in typical S_N2 fashion.

Nitriles can be hydrolyzed under either acidic or basic conditions. The products are carboxylic acids and ammonia (or ammonium salts).

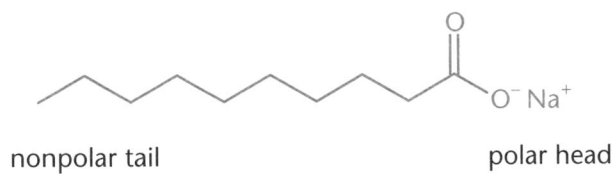

$$CH_3Cl \longrightarrow CH_3CN \longrightarrow CH_3\overset{\displaystyle O}{\overset{\displaystyle \|}{C}}OH + NH_4^+$$

Figure 9.9

This allows for the conversion of alkyl halides into carboxylic acids. As in the carbonation reaction, an additional carbon atom is introduced. For instance, if the desired product is acetic acid, a possible starting material would be methyl iodide.

REACTIONS

A. SOAP FORMATION

When long-chain carboxylic acids react with sodium or potassium hydroxide, they form salts. These salts, called soaps, are able to solubilize nonpolar organic compounds in aqueous solutions because they possess both a nonpolar "tail" and a polar carboxylate "head."

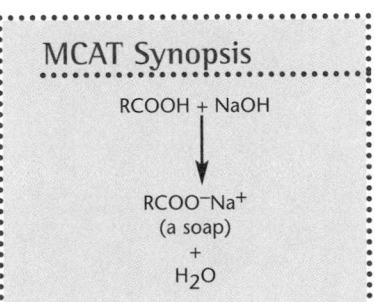

nonpolar tail   polar head

Figure 9.10

When placed in aqueous solution, soap molecules arrange themselves into spherical structures called **micelles**. The polar heads face outward, where they can be solvated by water molecules, and the nonpolar hydrocarbon chains are inside the sphere, protected from the solvent. Nonpolar molecules such as grease can dissolve in the hydrocarbon interior of the spherical micelle, while the micelle as a whole is soluble in water because of its polar shell.

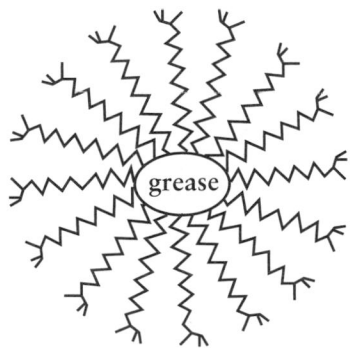

grease

Figure 9.11

B. NUCLEOPHILIC SUBSTITUTION

Many of the reactions that carboxylic acids (and their derivatives) participate in can be described by a single mechanism: nucleophilic substitution. This mechanism is very similar to nucleophilic addition to a carbonyl, shown in the preceding chapter. The key difference: nucleophilic substitution concludes with reformation of the C=O double bond and elimination of a leaving group.

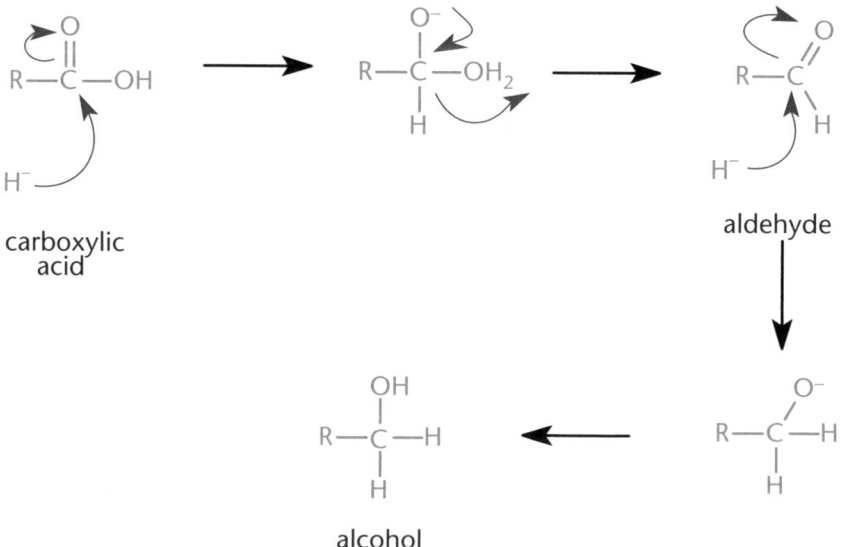

Figure 9.12

1. Reduction

Carboxylic acids occupy the most oxidized side of the oxidation-reduction continuum (see Organic Chemistry chapter 7). Carboxylic acids are reduced with lithium aluminum hydride (LAH) to the corresponding alcohols. Aldehyde intermediates that may be formed in the course of the reaction are also reduced to the alcohol. The reaction occurs by nucleophilic addition of hydride to the carbonyl group.

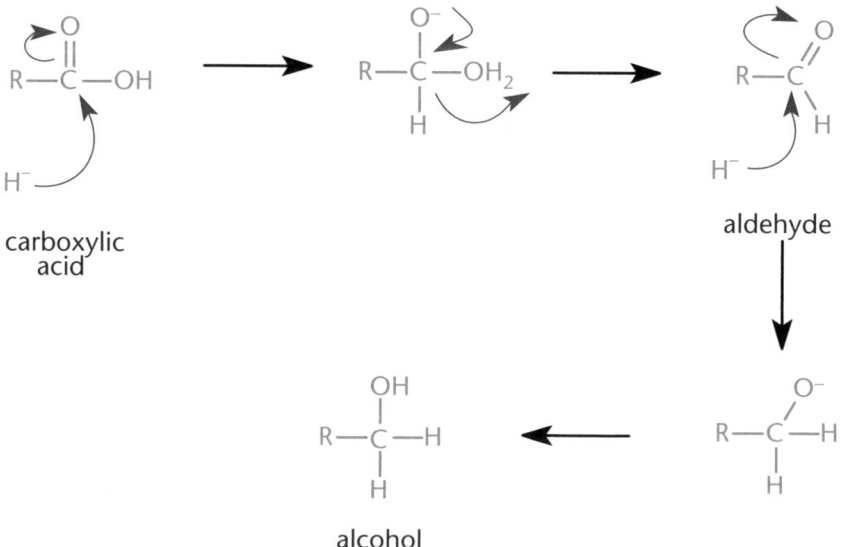

Figure 9.13

2. Ester Formation

Carboxylic acids react with alcohols under acidic conditions to form esters and water. In acidic solution, the O on the C=O can become protonated. This accentuates the polarity of the bond, putting even more positive charge on the C and making it even more susceptible to nucleophilic attack. This condensation reaction occurs most rapidly with primary alcohols.

> **MCAT Synopsis**
>
> Protonating the C=O makes the C even more ripe for nucleophilic attack.

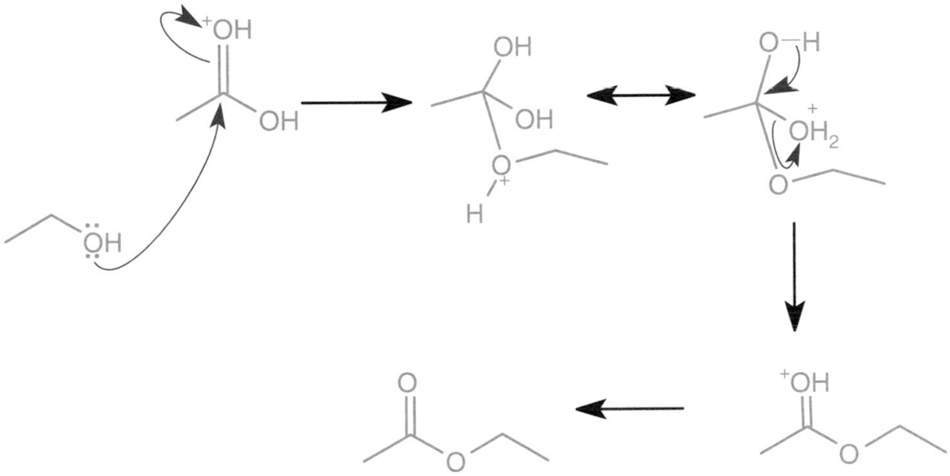

Figure 9.14

3. Acyl Halide Formation

Acyl halides, also called acid halides, are compounds with carbonyl groups bonded to halides. Several different reagents can accomplish this transformation; thionyl chloride, $SOCl_2$, is the most common.

Figure 9.15

> **MCAT Synopsis**
>
> Acid chlorides are among the highest energy (least stable and most reactive) members of the carbonyl family.

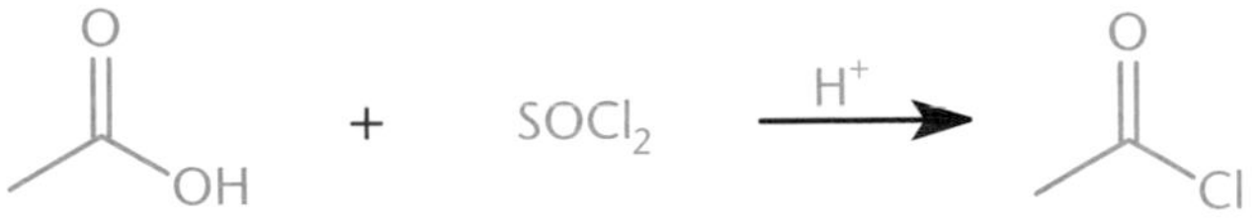

Acid chlorides are very reactive, as the greater electron-withdrawing power of the Cl^- makes the carbonyl carbon more susceptible to nucleophilic attack than the carbonyl carbon of a carboxylic acid. Thus acid chlorides are frequently used as intermediates in the conversion of carboxylic acids to esters and amides.

MCAT Synopsis

Key reactions include:

- soap formation (e.g., when neutralized by NaOH or KOH);
- nucleophilic substitution;
- decarboxylation, in which CO_2 is lost.

C. DECARBOXYLATION

Carboxylic acids can undergo decarboxylation reactions, resulting in the loss of carbon dioxide.

1,3-dicarboxylic acids and other β-keto acids may spontaneously decarboxylate when heated. The carboxyl group is lost and replaced with a hydrogen. The reaction proceeds through a six-membered ring transition state. The enol initially formed tautomerizes to the more stable keto form.

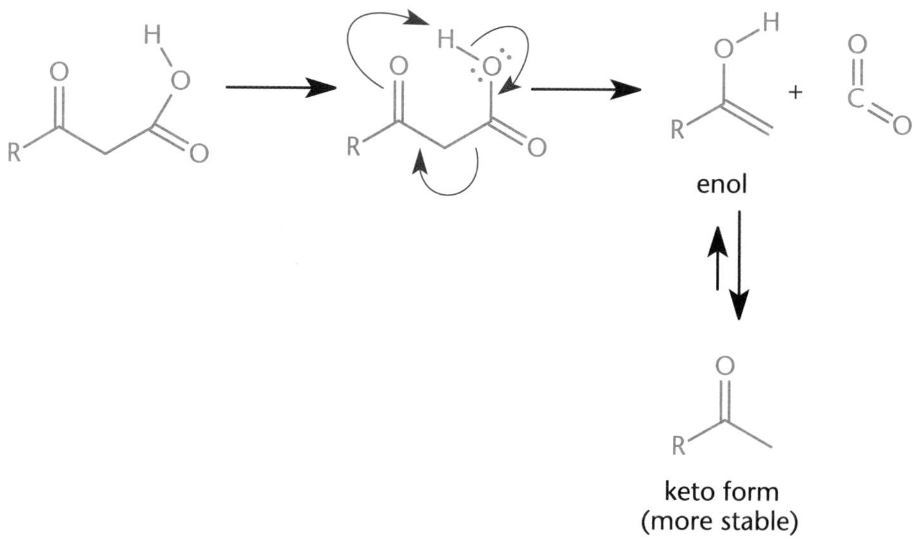

Figure 9.16

Bridge

Decarboxylation is very common in biochemical pathways in the body, such as the Krebs cycle (see Biology chapter 3).

10

CARBOXYLIC ACID DERIVATIVES

Carboxylic acids can be converted into several types of derivatives: **acyl halides, anhydrides, amides**, and **esters**. These are compounds in which the –OH of the carboxyl group has been replaced with **–X, –OCOR, –NH$_2$**, or **–OR**, respectively. They readily undergo nucleophilic substitution reactions, including hydrolysis (H$_2$O as nucleophile) which produces the original carboxylic acid. They also undergo other additions and substitutions, including various interconversions between different acid derivatives. In general, the acyl halides are the most reactive of the carboxylic acid derivatives, followed by the anhydrides, the esters, and the amides.

MCAT Synopsis

Order of reactivity:

acyl halides > anhydrides > esters > amides

ACYL HALIDES

A. NOMENCLATURE

Acyl halides are also called **acid** or **alkanoyl halides**. (The acyl group is RCO–.) They are the most reactive of the carboxylic acid derivatives. They are named in the IUPAC system by changing the *-ic acid* ending of the carboxylic acid to **-yl halide**. Some typical examples are ethanoyl chloride (also called acetyl chloride), benzoyl chloride, and *n*-butanoyl bromide.

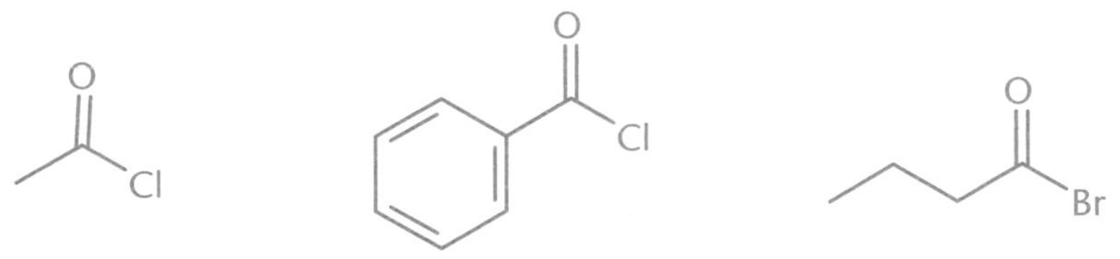

ethanoyl chloride
(acetyl chloride)

benzoyl chloride

n-butanoyl bromide

Figure 10.1

B. SYNTHESIS

The most common acyl halides are the acid chlorides, although acid bromides and iodides are occasionally encountered. They are prepared by reaction of the carboxylic acid with thionyl chloride, $SOCl_2$, producing SO_2 and HCl as side products. Alternatively, PCl_3 or PCl_5 (or PBr_3, to make an acid bromide) will accomplish the same transformation.

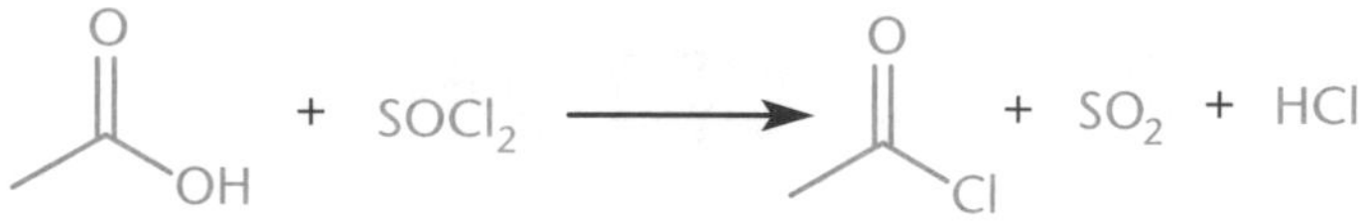

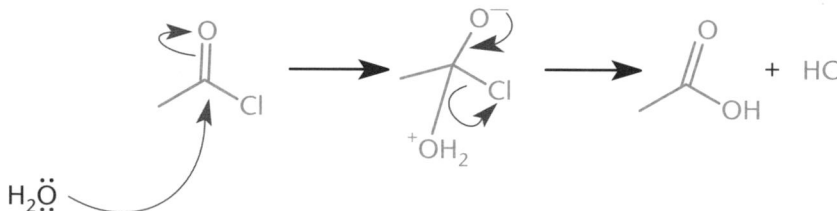

Figure 10.2

C. REACTIONS: NUCLEOPHILIC ACYL SUBSTITUTION

The following reactions of acyl halides proceed via the mechanism of nucleophilic substitution on a carbonyl, shown in detail in chapter 9.

1. **Hydrolysis**

The simplest reaction of acid halides is their reconversion to carboxylic acids. They react very rapidly with water to form the corresponding acid, along with HCl, which is responsible for their irritating odor.

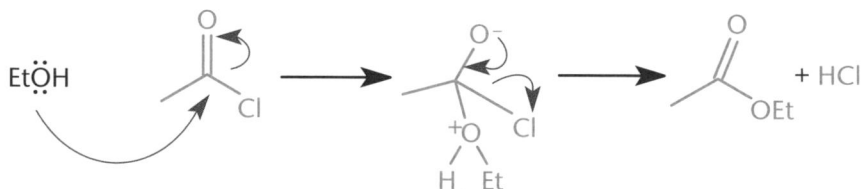

Figure 10.3

> **KAPLAN EXCLUSIVE**
>
> Hydrolysis = hydro + lysis, or cleavage by water.

2. **Conversion into Esters**

Acyl halides can be converted into esters by reaction with alcohols. The same type of nucleophilic attack found in hydrolysis leads to the formation of a tetrahedral intermediate, with the hydroxyl oxygen as the nucleophile. Chloride is displaced and HCl is released as the side-product.

Figure 10.4

3. **Conversion into Amides**

Acyl halides can be converted into amides (compounds of the general formula $RCONR_2$) by an analogous reaction with amines. Nucleophilic amines, such as ammonia, attack the carbonyl group, displacing chloride. The side product is ammonium chloride, formed from excess ammonia and HCl.

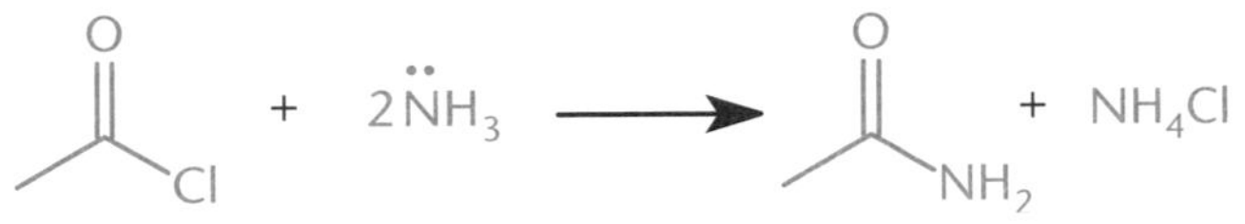

Figure 10.5

D. OTHER REACTIONS

1. Friedel-Crafts Acylation

Aromatic rings can be acylated in a Friedel-Crafts reaction. The mechanism is electrophilic aromatic substitution, and the attacking reagent is an acylium ion, formed by reaction of an acid chloride with $AlCl_3$ or another Lewis acid. The product is an alkyl aryl ketone.

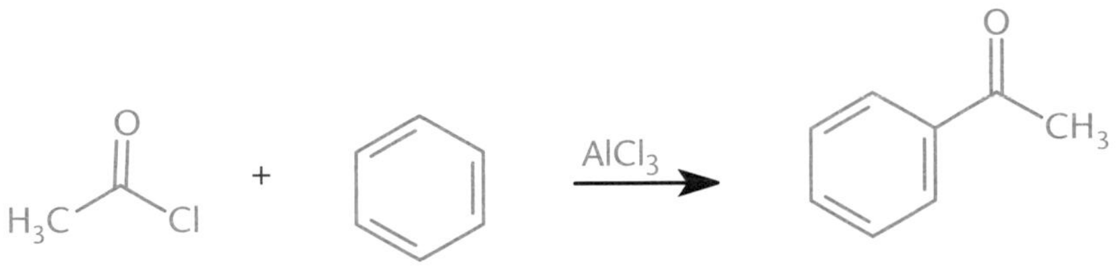

Figure 10.6

> **MCAT Synopsis**
>
> The mechanism for the Friedel-Crafts acylation is electrophilic aromatic substitution.

2. Reduction

Acid halides can be reduced to alcohols, or selectively reduced to the intermediate aldehydes. Catalytic hydrogenation in the presence of a "poison" like quinoline accomplishes the latter transformation. (Compare with Lindlar's catalyst, chapter 5.)

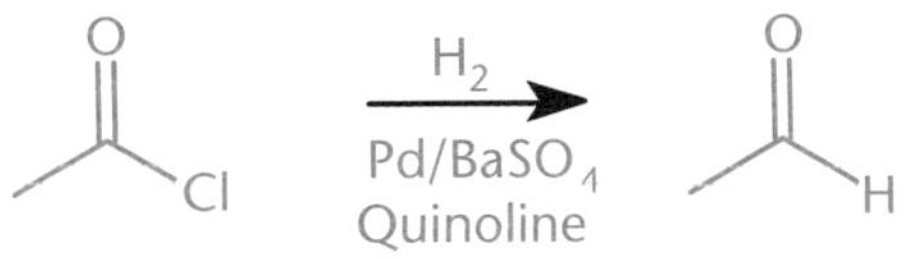

Figure 10.7

> **KAPLAN) EXCLUSIVE**
>
> Anhydride means "without water." Anhydrides are formed by two acid molecules condensing (losing water).

ANHYDRIDES

A. NOMENCLATURE

Anhydrides, also called **acid anhydrides**, are the condensation dimers of carboxylic acids, with the general formula RCOOCOR. They are named by substituting the word **anhydride** for the word *acid* in an alkanoic acid. The most common and important anhydride is acetic anhydride, the dimer of acetic acid. Other common anhydrides, such as succinic, maleic, and phthalic anhydrides, are **cyclic anhydrides** arising from intramolecular condensation or dehydration of diacids (Figure 10.9).

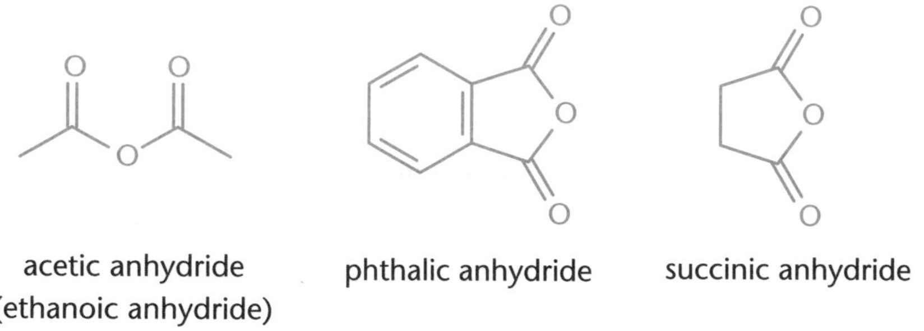

acetic anhydride (ethanoic anhydride) · phthalic anhydride · succinic anhydride

Figure 10.8

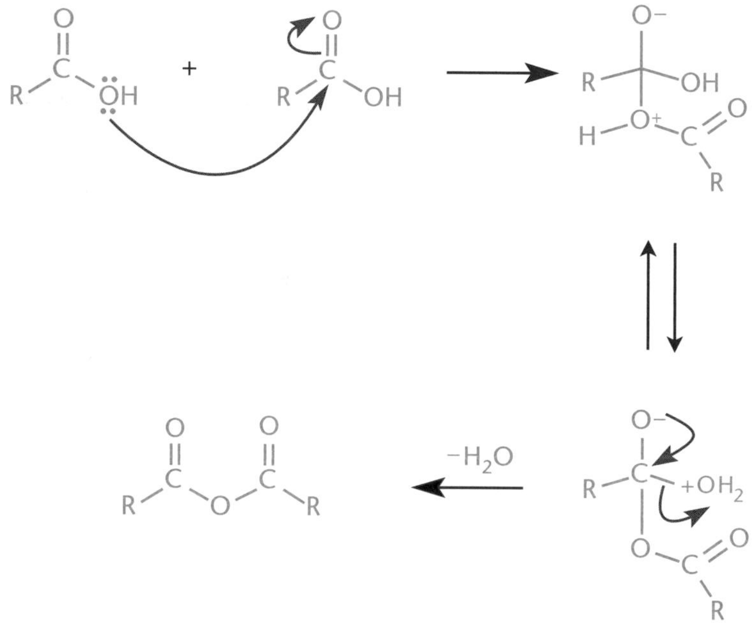

Figure 10.9

Condensation of two carboxylic acid molecules to form an anhydride.

B. SYNTHESIS

Anhydrides can be synthesized by reaction of an acid chloride with a carboxylate salt.

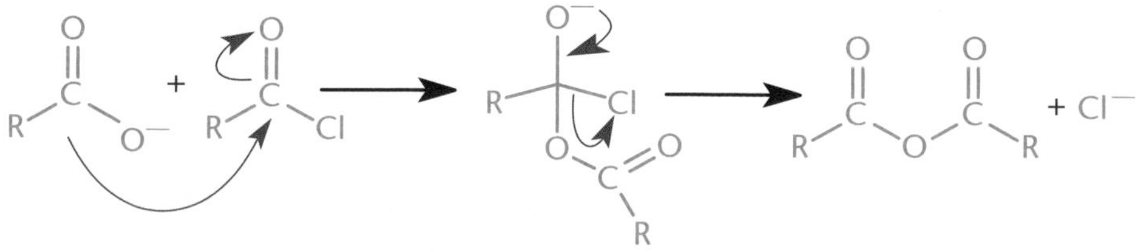

Figure 10.10

Reaction of acid chloride with carboxylate anion to form an anhydride.

Certain cyclic anhydrides can be formed simply by heating carboxylic acids. The reaction is driven by the increased stability of the newly formed ring; hence, only five- and six-membered ring anhydrides are easily made. In this case, the hydroxyl of one –COOH moiety acts as a nucleophile, attacking the carbonyl on the other –COOH moiety.

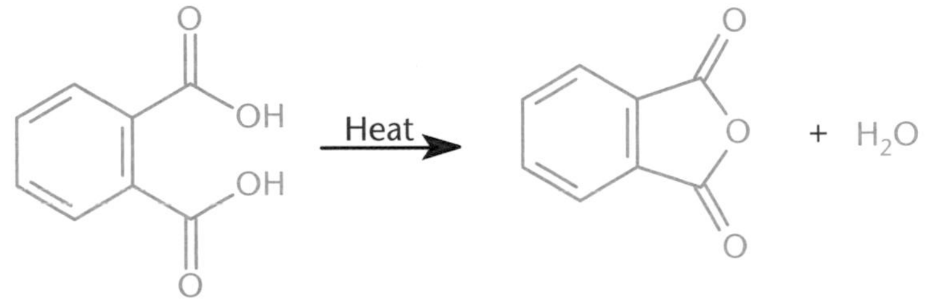

o-phtalic acid   phthalic anhydride

Figure 10.11

C. REACTIONS

Anhydrides react under the same conditions as acid chlorides, but since they are somewhat more stable, they are a bit less reactive. The reactions are slower and produce a carboxylic acid as the side product instead of HCl. Cyclic anhydrides are also subject to these reactions, which cause ring-opening at the anhydride group along with formation of the new functional groups.

1. **Hydrolysis**

   Anhydrides are converted into carboxylic acids when exposed to water.

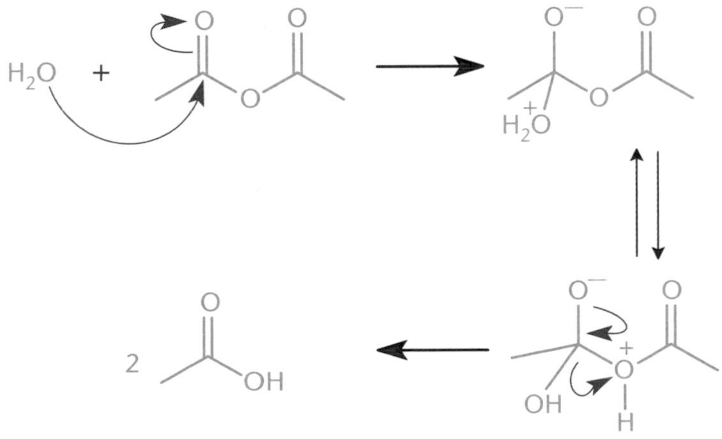

Figure 10.12

Note that in this reaction, the leaving group is actually a carboxylic acid.

2. **Conversion into Amides**
   Anhydrides are cleaved by ammonia, producing amides and ammonium carboxylates.

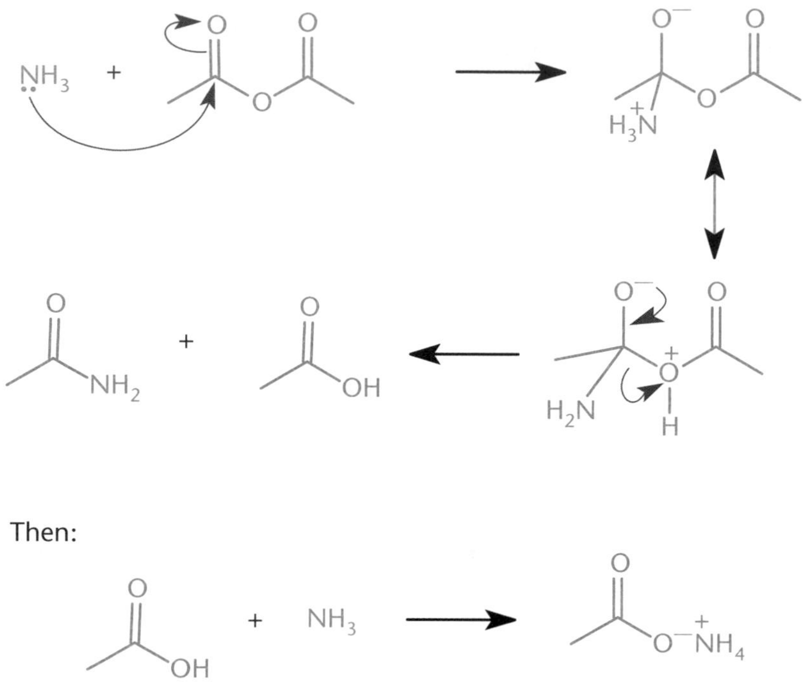

Then:

Figure 10.13

Thus, even though the leaving group is actually a carboxylic acid, the final products are an amide and the ammonium salt of a carboxylate anion.

3. **Conversion into Esters and Carboxylic Acids**
   Anhydrides react with alcohols to form esters and carboxylic acids.

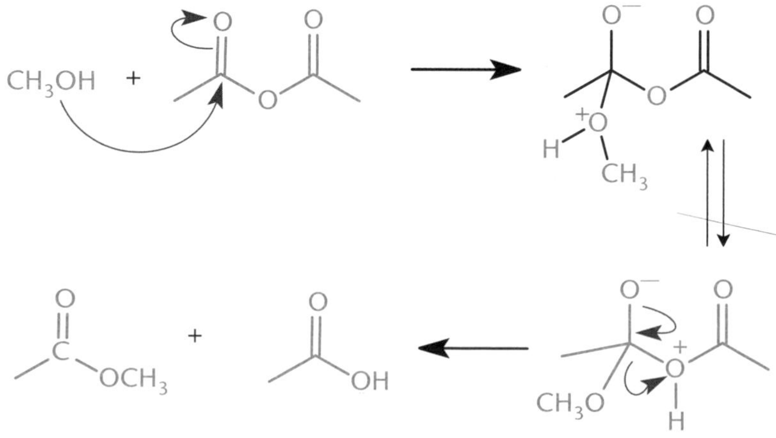

Figure 10.14

4. Acylation

Friedel-Crafts acylation occurs readily with $AlCl_3$ or other Lewis acid catalysts.

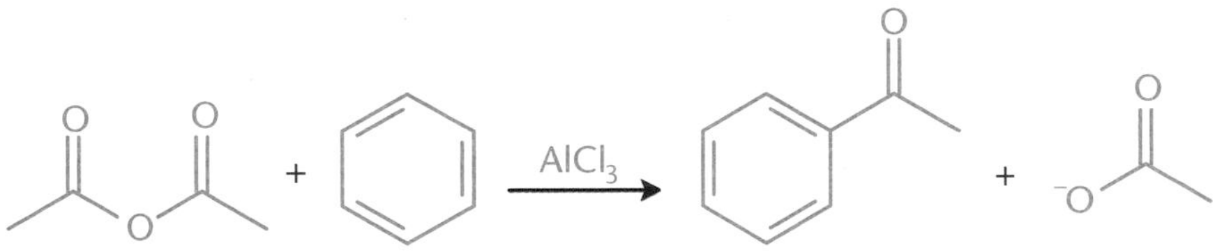

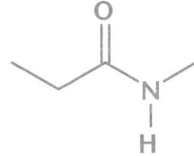

Figure 10.15

> **MCAT Synopsis**
>
> This reaction proceeds via electrophilic aromatic substitution.

AMIDES

A. NOMENCLATURE

Amides are compounds with the general formula $RCONR_2$. They are named by replacing the *-oic* acid ending with **-amide**. Alkyl substituents on the nitrogen atom are listed as prefixes, and their location is specified with the letter *N*. For example:

N-methylpropanamide

Figure 10.16

> **Bridge**
>
> The peptide bond is actually an amide linkage (see chapter 3).

B. SYNTHESIS

Amides are generally synthesized by the reaction of acid chlorides with amines or by the reaction of acid anhydrides with ammonia (see above). Note that loss of hydrogen is required; thus, only primary and secondary amines will undergo this reaction.

C. REACTIONS

1. Hydrolysis

Amides can be hydrolyzed under acidic conditions, via nucleophilic substitution, to produce carboxylic acids or basic conditions to form carboxylates:

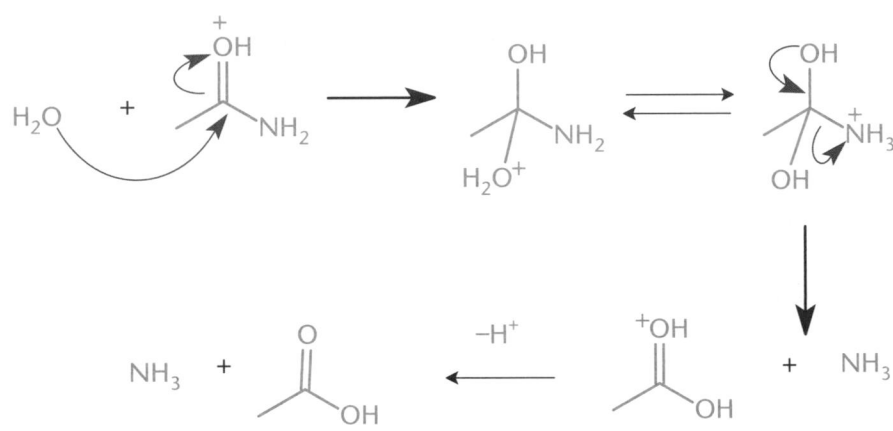

Figure 10.17

2. Hofmann Rearrangement

The **Hofmann rearrangement** converts amides to primary amines with the loss of the carbonyl carbon. The mechanism involves the formation of a **nitrene**, the nitrogen analog of a carbene. The nitrene is attached to the carbonyl group and rearranges to form an **isocyanate**, which, under the reaction condition is hydrolyzed to the amine.

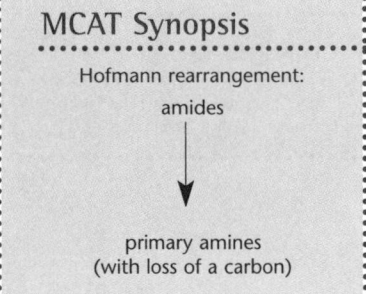

Figure 10.18

3. Reduction

Amides can be reduced with LAH to the corresponding amine. Notice that this differs from the product of the Hofmann rearrangement in that no carbon atom is lost.

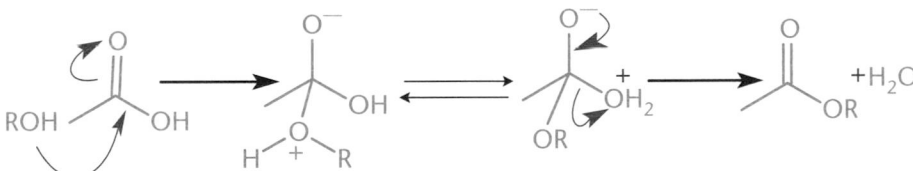

Figure 10.19

ESTERS

A. NOMENCLATURE

Esters are the dehydration products of carboxylic acids and alcohols. They are commonly found in many fruits and perfumes. They are named in the IUPAC system as **alkyl** or **aryl alkanoates.** For example, ethyl acetate, derived from the condensation of acetic acid and ethanol, is called ethyl ethanoate according to IUPAC nomenclature.

B. SYNTHESIS

Mixtures of carboxylic acids and alcohols will condense into esters, liberating water, under acidic conditions. Esters can also be obtained from reaction of acid chlorides or anhydrides with alcohols (see above). Phenolic (aromatic) esters are produced in the same way, although the aromatic acid chlorides are less reactive than aliphatic acid chlorides, so that base must generally be added as a catalyst.

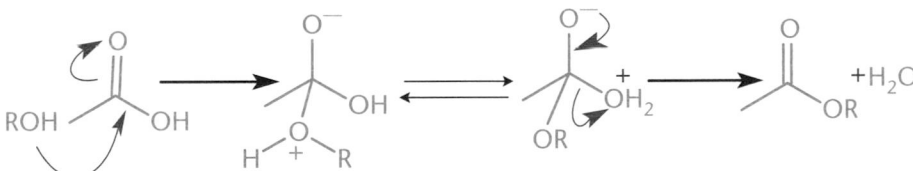

Figure 10.20

C. REACTIONS

1. Hydrolysis

Esters, like the other derivatives of carboxylic acids, can be hydrolyzed, yielding carboxylic acids and alcohols. Hydrolysis can take place under either acidic or basic conditions.

> **MCAT Synopsis**
>
> An acid + an alcohol = an ester

Under acidic conditions:

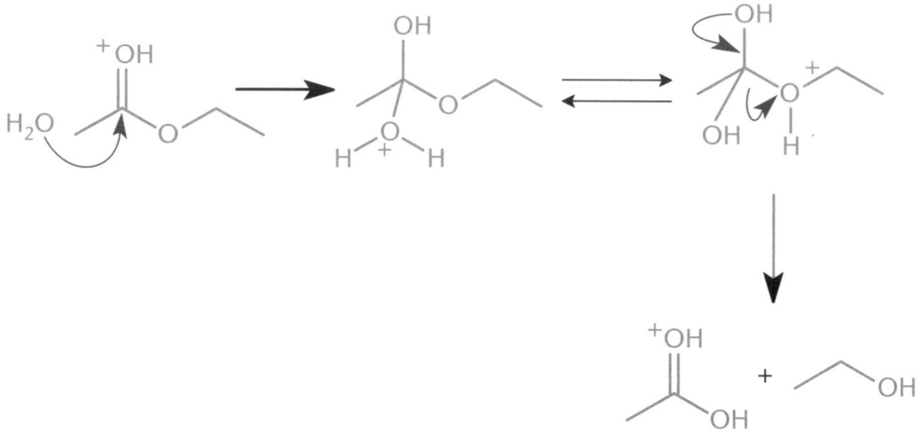

Figure 10.21

The reaction proceeds similarly under basic conditions, except that the oxygen on the C=O is not protonated, and the nucleophile is OH⁻.

Triacylglycerols, also called fats, are esters of long-chain carboxylic acids, often called fatty acids, and glycerol (1,2,3-propanetriol). **Saponification** is the process whereby fats are hydrolyzed under basic conditions to produce soaps. (Note: Acidification of the soap retrieves triacylglycerol.)

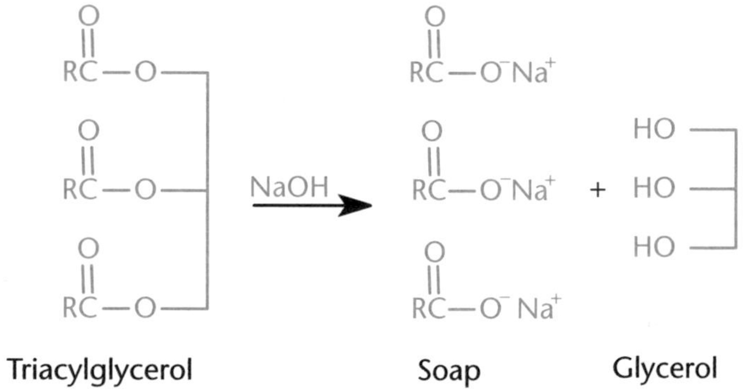

Triacylglycerol   Soap   Glycerol

Figure 10.22

2. **Conversion into Amides**
   Nitrogen bases such as ammonia will attack the electron-deficient carbonyl carbon atom, displacing alkoxide, to yield an amide and an alcohol side-product. Here, ammonia is the nucleophile.

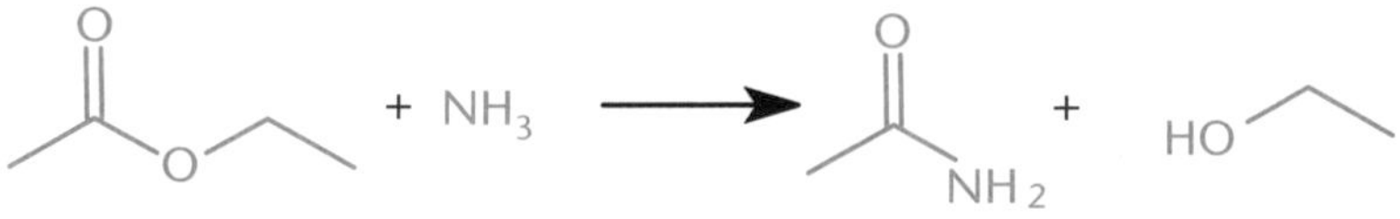

Figure 10.23

3. Transesterification

Alcohols can act as nucleophiles and displace the alkoxy groups on esters. This process, which transforms one ester into another, is called **transesterification**.

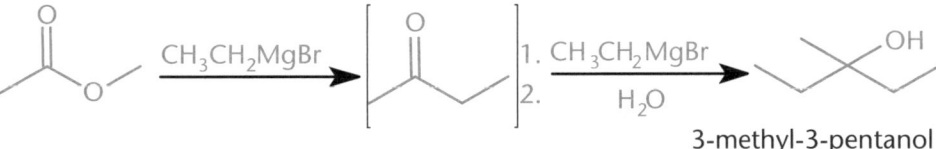

Figure 10.24

4. Grignard Addition

Grignard reagents add to the carbonyl groups of esters to form ketones; however, these ketones are more reactive than the initial esters and are readily attacked by more Grignard reagent. Two equivalents of Grignard reagent can thus be used to produce tertiary alcohols with good yield. (The intermediate ketone can be isolated only if the alkyl groups are sufficiently bulky to prevent further attack.) This reaction proceeds via nucleophilic substitution followed by nucleophilic addition.

MCAT Synopsis

Grignard reagents, RMgX, are essentially equivalent to R⁻ nucleophiles.

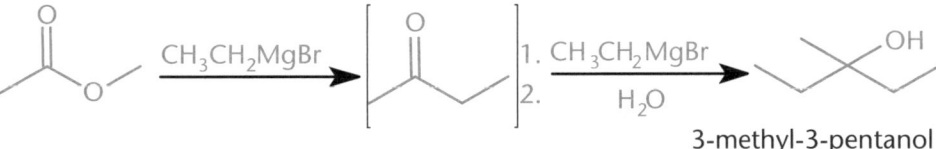

3-methyl-3-pentanol

Figure 10.25

5. Condensation Reactions

An important reaction of esters is the **Claisen condensation**. In the simplest case, two moles of ethyl acetate react under basic conditions to produce a β-keto ester, ethyl 3-oxobutanoate, or acetoacetic ester by its common name. (The Claisen condensation is also called the **acetoacetic ester condensation**.) The reaction proceeds by addition of an enolate anion to the carbonyl group of another ester, followed by displacement of ethoxide ion. This mechanism is analogous to that of the aldol condensation.

MCAT Synopsis

In the Claisen condensation, the enolate ion of one ester acts as a nucleophile, attacking another ester.

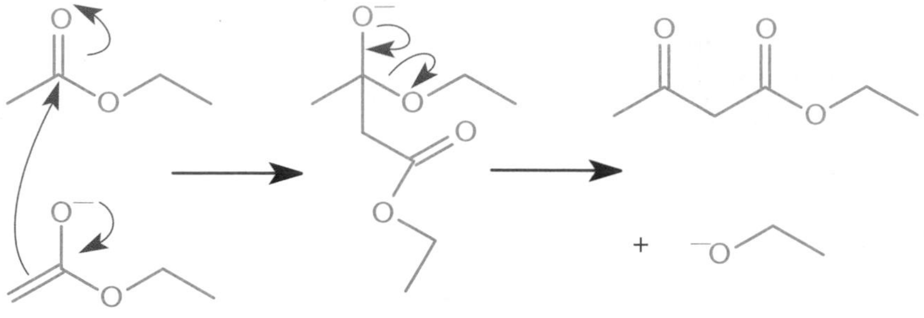

Figure 10.26

6. **Reduction**

   Esters may be reduced to primary alcohols with LAH, but not with $NaBH_4$. This allows for selective reduction in molecules with multiple functional groups.

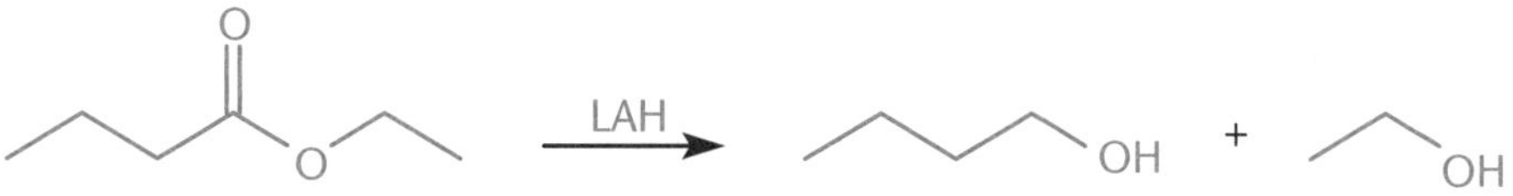

Figure 10.27

MCAT Synopsis

LAH is esentially equivalent to a H^- nucleophile.

D. PHOSPHATE ESTERS

While phosphoric acid derivatives are not carboxylic acid derivatives they form esters similar to those above.

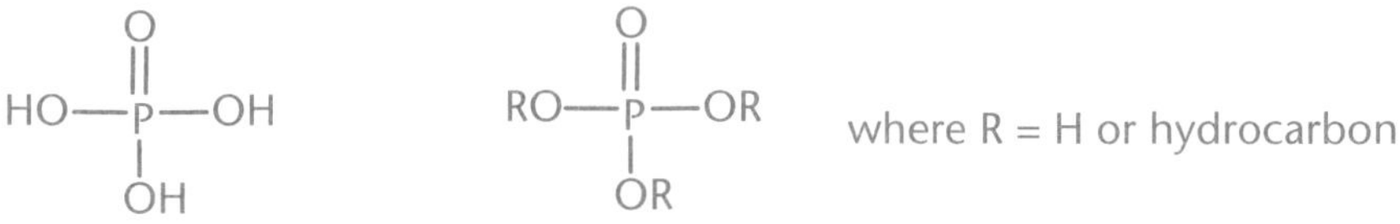

phosphoric acid

phosphoric ester

Figure 10.28

Phosphoric acid and the mono- and diesters are acidic (more so than carboxylic acids) and usually exist as anions. Like all esters, under acidic conditions they can be cleaved into the parent acid (here, H_3PO_4) and alcohols.

Phosphate esters are found in living systems in the form of **phospholipids** (phosphoglycerides), in which glycerol is attached to two carboxylic acids and one phosphoric acid.

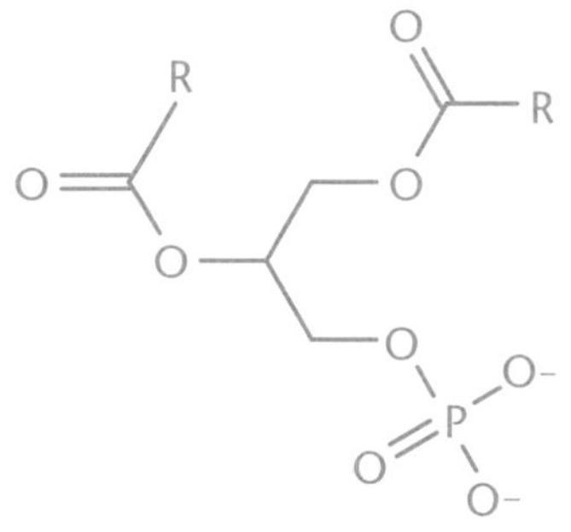

phosphatidic acid
diacylglycerol phosphate
(a phosphoglyceride)

Figure 10.29

Phospholipids are the main component of cell membranes, and phospholipid/carbohydrate polymers form the backbone of nucleic acids, the hereditary material of life. (See chapter 14 and chapter 3 of the Biology section.) The nucleic acid derivative **adenosine triphosphate (ATP)** can give up and regain one or more phosphate groups. ATP facilitates many biological reactions by releasing phosphate groups to other compounds, thereby increasing their reactivities.

> **MCAT Synopsis**
>
> Remember phosphodiester bonds? They hold the backbone of DNA together, connecting nucleotides with covalent linkages.

SUMMARY OF REACTIONS

The most important derivatives of carboxylic acid are acyl halides, anhydrides, esters, and amides. These are listed from most reactive (least stable) to least reactive (most stable).

ACYL HALIDES:

- can be formed by adding $RCOOH + SOCl_2$, PCl_3 or PCl_5, or PBr_3;
- undergo many different nucleophilic substitutions; H_2O yields carboxylic acid, while ROH yields an ester, and NH_3 yields an amide;
- can participate in Friedel-Crafts acylation to form an alkyl aryl ketone;
- can be reduced to alcohols or, selectively, to aldehydes.

ANHYDRIDES:

- can be formed by $RCOOH + RCOOH$ (condensation) or $RCOO^- + RCOCl$ (substitution);
- undergo many nucleophilic substitution reactions, forming products that include carboxylic acids, amides, and esters;
- can participate in Friedel-Crafts acylation.

ESTERS:

- formed by $RCOOH + ROH$ or, better, by acid chlorides or anhydrides + ROH;
- hydrolyze to yield acids + alcohols; adding ammonia yields an amide;
- reaction with Grignard reagent (2 moles) produces a tertiary alcohol;
- In Claisen condensation, analogous to the aldol, the ester acts both as nucleophile and target;
- very important in biological processes, particularly phosphate esters, which can be found in membranes, nucleic acids, and metabolic reactions.

AMIDES:

- can be formed by acid chlorides + amines, or acid anhydrides + ammonia;
- hydrolysis yields carboxylic acids or carboxylate anions;
- can be transformed to primary amines via Hofmann rearrangement or reduction.

11

AMINES AND NITROGEN-CONTAINING COMPOUNDS

NOMENCLATURE

Amines are compounds of the general formula NR_3. They are classified according to the number of alkyl (or aryl) groups to which they are bound. A **primary** (1°) amine is attached to one alkyl group, a **secondary** (2°) amine to two, and a **tertiary** (3°) amine to three. A nitrogen atom attached to four alkyl groups is called a **quaternary ammonium compound**. The nitrogen carries a positive charge; thus, these compounds generally exist as salts.

In the common system, amines are generally named as alkylamines. The groups are designated individually or by using the prefixes di- or tri- if they are the same. In the IUPAC system, amines are named by substituting the suffix -**amine** for the final "e" of the name of the alkane to which the nitrogen is attached. N is used to label substituents attached to the nitrogen in secondary or tertiary amines. The prefix **amino-** is used for naming compounds containg an OH or a CO_2H group. Aromatic amines are named as derivatives of aniline ($C_6H_5NH_2$), the IUPAC name for which is benzenamine.

Formula:	$CH_3CH_2NH_2$	$CH_3CH_2N(CH_3)_2$	$(CH_3)_2NCH_2CH_2CH_2CH_2CH_2CH_3$
IUPAC:	ethanamine	N,N-dimethylethanamine	N,N-dimethylhexanamine
Common:	ethylamine	dimethylethylamine	dimethylhexylamine

Table 11.1

Aromatic amines are named as derivatives of **aniline** ($C_6H_5NH_2$).

There are many other nitrogen-containing organic compounds. **Amides** are the condensation products of carboxylic acids and amines, and have already been discussed in Chapter 10. **Carbamates** are compounds with the general formula RNHC(O)OR'. They are also called **urethanes**, and can form polymers called **polyurethanes**. Carbamates are derived from compounds called **isocyanates**, (general formula RNCO) by the addition of an alcohol.

Enamines are the nitrogen analogs of enols, with an amine group attached to one carbon of a double bond. **Imines** are nitrogen compounds that contain nitrogen-carbon double bonds. **Nitriles**, or **cyanides**, are compounds with a triple bond between a carbon atom and a nitrogen atom. They are named with either the prefix **cyano-** or the suffix **-nitrile**. **Nitro** compounds contain the nitro group, NO_2. **Diazo** compounds contain an N_2 functionality. They tend to lose N_2 to form carbenes. **Azides** are compounds with an N_3 functionality. When azides lose nitrogen (N_2), they form **nitrenes**, the nitrogen analogs of carbenes. Examples of these various compounds are listed below.

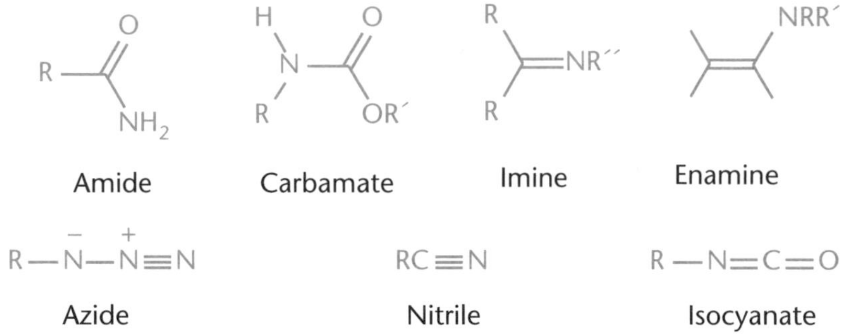

| Amide | Carbamate | Imine | Enamine |

| Azide | | Nitrile | Isocyanate |

Figure 11.1

PROPERTIES

The boiling points of amines are between those of alkanes and alcohols. For example, ammonia boils at $-33°C$, whereas methane boils at $-161°C$ and methanol at $64.5°C$. As molecular weight increases, so do boiling points. Primary and secondary amines can form hydrogen bonds, while tertiary amines cannot; therefore, tertiary amines have lower boiling points. Since nitrogen is not as electronegative as oxygen, the hydrogen bonds of amines are not as strong as those of alcohols.

The nitrogen atom in an amine is approximately sp^3 hybridized. Nitrogen must bond to only three substituents in order to complete its octet; a lone pair occupies the last sp^3 orbital. This lone pair is very important to the chemistry of amines; it is associated with their basic and nucleophilic properties.

Nitrogen atoms bonded to three different substituents are chiral because of the geometry of the orbitals. However, these enantiomers cannot be isolated, because they interconvert rapidly in a process called **nitrogen inversion**: an inversion of the sp^3 orbital occupied by the lone pair. The activation energy for this process is only 6 kcal/mol, and only at very low temperatures is it significantly slowed or stopped.

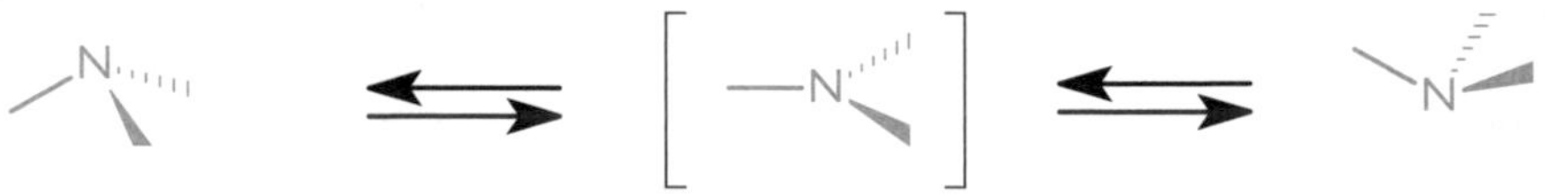

Figure 11.2

Amines are bases and readily accept protons to form ammonium ions. The pK_b values of alkyl amines are around 4, making them slightly more basic than ammonia ($pK_b = 4.76$), but less basic than hydroxide ($pK_b = -1.7$). Aromatic amines such as aniline ($pK_b = 9.42$) are far less basic than aliphatic amines, because the electron-withdrawing effect of the ring reduces the basicity of the amino group. The presence of other substituents on the ring alters the basicity of anilines: electron-donating groups (such as –OH, –CH$_3$, and –NH$_2$) increase basicity, while electron-withdrawing groups (such as NO$_2$) reduce basicity.

Amines also function as very weak acids. The pK_a's of amines are around 35, and a very strong base is required for deprotonation. For example, the proton of diisopropylamine may be removed with butyllithium, forming the sterically hindered base lithium diisopropylamide, LDA.

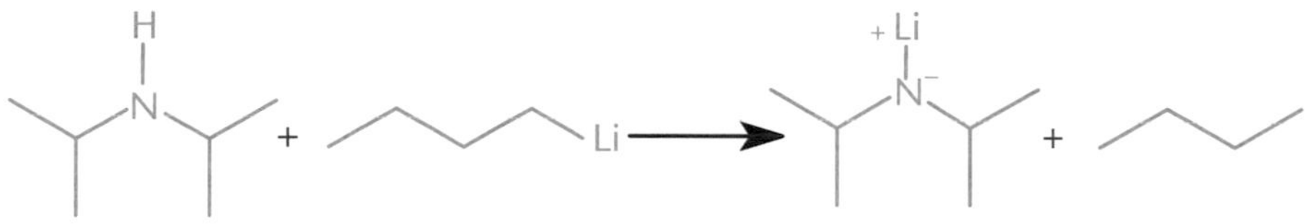

> **Real World Analogy**
>
> An interesting property of several nitrogen containing compounds, such as nitroglycerin and nitrous oxide, is their ability to act as relaxants. Nitroglycerine is given sublingually to relieve coronary artery spasms in people with chest pain, and nitrous oxide (laughing gas) is a common dental anesthetic. Nitroglycerine has the additional property of rapidly decomposing to form gas and is thus fairly explosive.

Figure 11.3

SYNTHESIS

A. ALKYLATION OF AMMONIA

1. Direct

Alkyl halides react with ammonia to produce alkylammonium halide salts. Ammonia functions as a nucleophile and displaces the halide atom. When the salt is treated with base, the alkylamine product is formed.

$$CH_3Br + NH_3 \longrightarrow CH_3\overset{+}{N}H_3Br^- \xrightarrow{NaOH} CH_3NH_2 + NaBr + H_2O$$

Figure 11.4

This reaction often leads to side products, because the alkylamine formed is nucleophilic and can react with the alkyl halide to form more complex products.

2. Gabriel Synthesis

The **Gabriel synthesis** converts a primary alkyl halide to a primary amine. The use of a disguised form of ammonia prevents side-product formation.

o-phthalic acid   phthalimide

good nucleophile

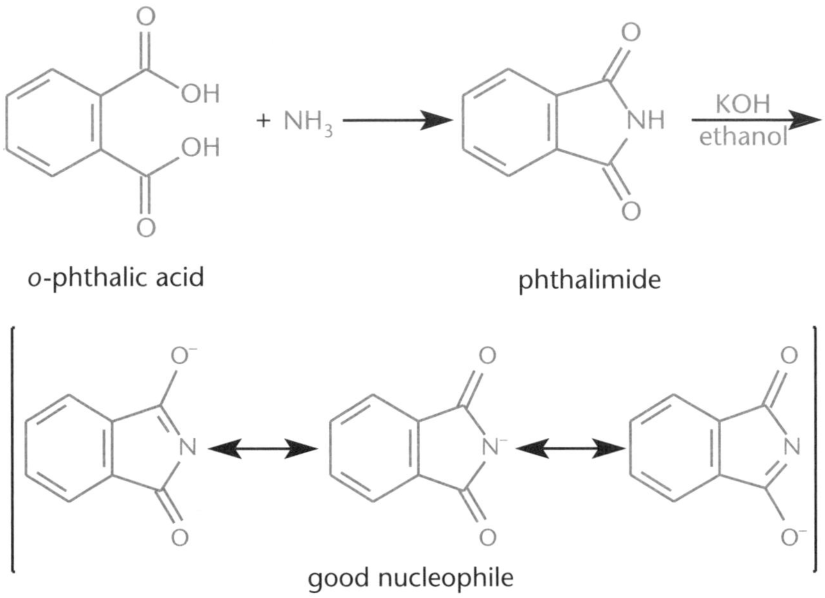

Figure 11.5

Phthalimide, the condensation product of phthalic acid and ammonia, acts as a good nucleophile when deprotonated. It displaces halide ions, forming N-alkylphthalimides, which do not react with other alkyl halides. When the reaction is complete, the N-alkylphthalimide can be hydrolyzed with aqueous base to produce the alkylamine.

Flashback

Addition of ammonia to an alkyl halide and the Gabriel Synthesis are both S_N2 reactions. With its unshared electron pair, ammonia is a very good nucleophile, while the halides are all good leaving groups (see chapter 4).

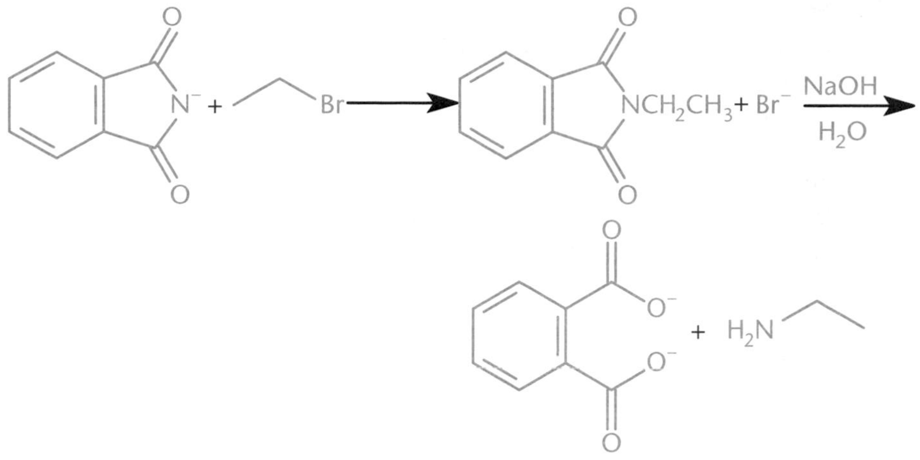

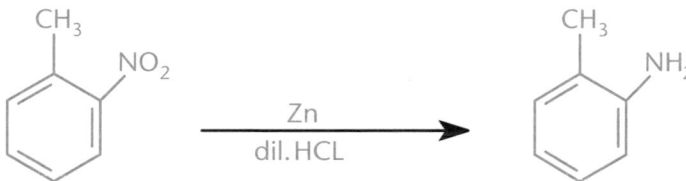

Figure 11.6

B. REDUCTION

Amines can be obtained from other nitrogen-containing functionalities via reduction reactions.

1. From Nitro Compounds:

Nitro compounds are easily reduced to primary amines. The most common reducing agent is iron or zinc and dilute hydrochloric acid, although many other reagents can be used. This reaction is especially useful for aromatic compounds, because nitration of aromatic rings is facile.

Figure 11.7

2. From Nitriles:

Nitriles can be reduced with hydrogen and a catalyst, or with lithium aluminum hydride (LAH), to produce primary amines.

$$CH_3CH_2C\equiv N \xrightarrow{\text{LAH}} CH_3CH_2CH_2NH_2$$

Figure 11.8

> ## MCAT Synopsis
>
> Amines can be formed by:
>
> 1) S_N2 reactions
>   - ammonia reacting with alkyl halides
>   - Gabriel Synthesis
>
> 2) Reduction of:
>   - amides
>   - aniline and its derivatives
>   - nitriles
>   - imines
>
> Amines can be destroyed (converted to alkenes) by exhaustive methylation.

MCAT Synopsis

An imine is a nitrogen double bonded to a carbon and has about the same polarity as a carbonyl functionality.

3. **From Imines**
Amines can be synthesized by **reductive amination**, a process whereby an aldehyde or ketone is reacted with ammonia, a primary amine, or a secondary amine to form a primary, secondary, or tertiary amine, respectively. When the amine reacts with the aldehyde or the ketone, an imine is produced. Consequently, it will undergo hydride reduction in much the same way that a carbonyl does. When the imine is reduced with hydrogen in the presence of a catalyst, an amine is produced.

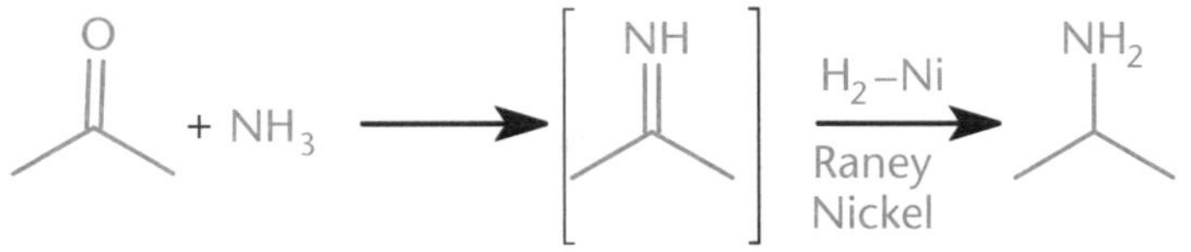

acetone | imine isopropylimine | amine isopropylamine (aminoisopropane)

Figure 11.9

4. **From Amides**
Amides can be reduced with LAH to form amines (see chapter 10).

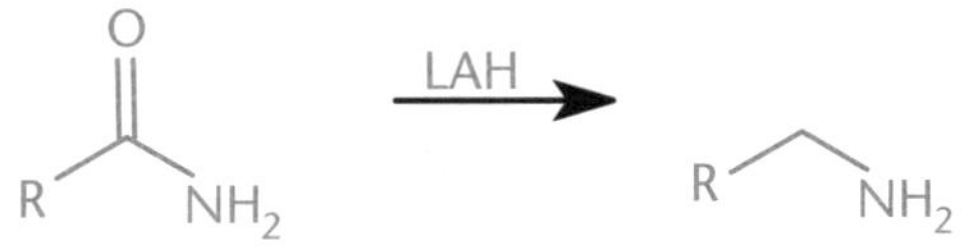

Figure 11.10

REACTIONS

A. EXHAUSTIVE METHYLATION

Exhaustive methylation is also known as **Hofmann elimination**. In this process, an amine is converted to a quaternary ammonium iodide by treatment with excess methyl iodide. Treatment with silver oxide and water converts this to the ammonium hydroxide, which, when heated, undergoes elimination to form an alkene and an amine. The predominant alkene formed is the least substituted, in contrast with normal elimination reactions, where the predominant alkene product is the most substituted.

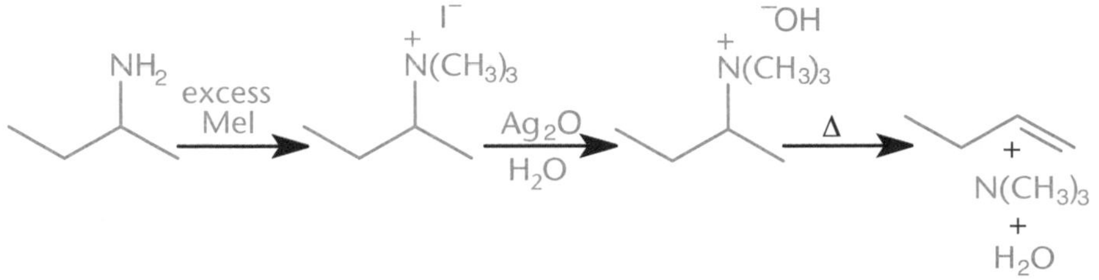

Figure 11.11

12

PURIFICATION AND SEPARATION

Much of organic chemistry is concerned with the isolation and purification of the desired reaction product. A reaction itself may be completed in a matter of minutes, but separating the product from the reaction mixture is often a difficult and rather time-consuming process. Many different techniques have been developed to accomplish this objective: to obtain a pure compound separated from solvents, reagents, and other products.

BASIC TECHNIQUES

A. EXTRACTION

One way of separating a desired product is through **extraction**, the transfer of a dissolved compound (here, the desired product) from one solvent into another in which it is more soluble. Most impurities will be left behind in the first solvent. The two solvents should be immiscible (form two layers that do not mix because of mutual insolubility). The two layers are temporarily mixed together so that solute can pass from one to the other. For example, a solution of isobutyric acid in diethyl ether can be extracted with water. Isobutyric acid is more soluble in water than in ether, and so when the two solvents are placed together, isobutyric acid transfers to the water phase.

> **MCAT Synopsis**
>
> Think of the aqueous and organic layers as being like oil and water in salad dressing: you can shake the mixture to increase their interaction, but ultimately they will separate again.

The water (aqueous) and ether (organic) phases are separated in a specialized piece of glassware called a separatory funnel. Once separated, the isobutyric acid can be isolated from the aqueous phase in pure form. Some isobutyric acid will remain dissolved in the ether phase, so the extraction should be repeated several times with fresh solvent (water). More product can be obtained with successive extractions; i.e., it is more effective to perform three successive extractions of 10 mL each than to perform one extraction of 30 mL. Once the compound has been isolated in its purified form in a solvent, it can then be obtained by evaporation of the solvent.

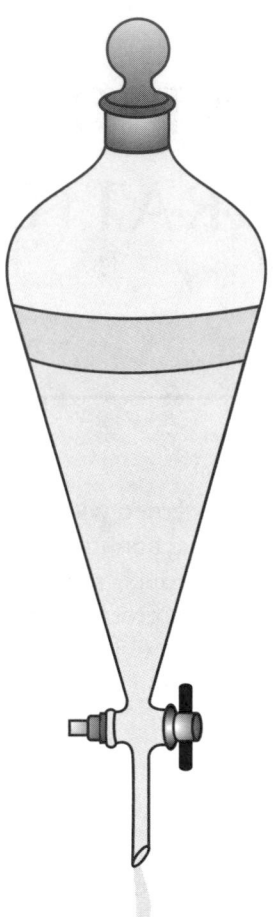

Figure 12.1: Separatory Funnel

An extraction carried out to remove unwanted impurities rather than to isolate a pure product is called a **wash**.

B. FILTRATION

Filtration is used to isolate a solid from a liquid. In this technique, a liquid/solid mixture is poured onto a paper filter that allows only the solvent to pass through. The result of this process is the separation of the solid (often referred to as the residue) from the liquid or **filtrate**. The two basic types of filtration are **gravity filtration** and **vacuum filtration**. In gravity filtration, the solvent's own weight pulls it through the filter. Frequently, however, the pores of the filter become clogged with solid, slowing the rate of filtration. For this reason, in gravity filtration it is generally desirable for the substance of interest to be in solution (dissolved in the solvent), while impurities remain undissolved and can be filtered out. This allows the desired product to flow more easily and rapidly through the apparatus. To ensure that the product remains dissolved, gravity filtration is usually carried out with hot solvent.

In vacuum filtration, the solvent is forced through the filter by a vacuum on the other side. Vacuum filtration is used to isolate relatively large quantities of solid, usually when the solid is the desired product.

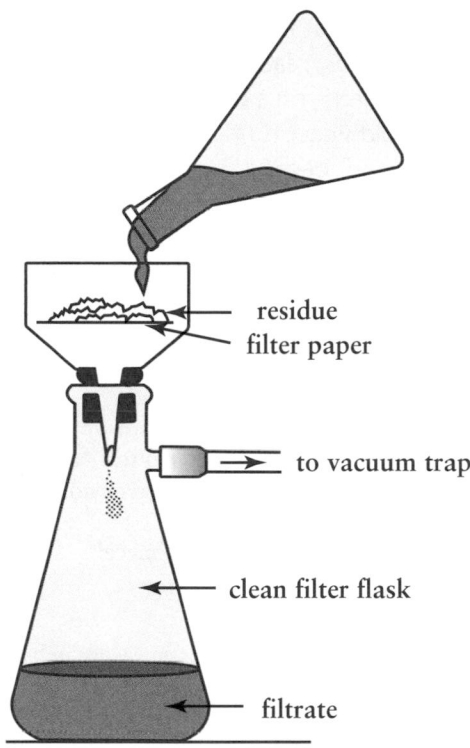

residue
filter paper

to vacuum trap

clean filter flask

filtrate

Figure 12.2: Vacuum Filtration

C. RECRYSTALLIZATION

Recrystallization is a process in which impure crystals are dissolved in a minimum amount of hot solvent. As the solvent is cooled, the crystals reform, leaving the impurities in solution. For recrystallization to be effective, the solvent must be chosen carefully. It must dissolve the solid while it is hot, but not while it is cold. In addition, it must dissolve the impurities at both temperatures, so that they remain in solution. Solvent choice is usually a matter of trial and error, although some generalizations can be made. An estimate of polarity is useful, since polar solvents dissolve polar compounds while nonpolar solvents dissolve nonpolar compounds (see General Chemistry, chapter 9). A solvent with intermediate polarity is generally desirable in recrystallization. In addition, the solvent should have a low enough freezing point that the solution may be sufficiently cooled.

In some instances, a mixed solvent system may be used. Here the crude compound is dissolved in a solvent in which it is highly soluble. Another solvent, in which the compound is less soluble, is then added in drops, just

> **MCAT Synopsis**
>
> Ideally the desired product should have solubility that depends on temperature—it should be more soluble at high temperature, less so at low. In contrast, impurities should be equally soluble at various temperatures.

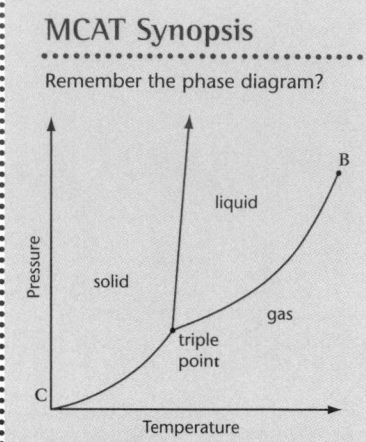
until solid begins to precipitate. The solution is heated a bit more to redissolve the precipitate, and then slowly cooled to induce crystal formation.

D. SUBLIMATION

Sublimation occurs when a heated solid turns directly into a gas, without an intervening liquid stage. It is used as a method of purification because the impurities found in most reaction mixtures will not sublime easily. The vapors are made to condense on a **cold finger**, a piece of glassware packed with dry ice or with cold water running through it. Most sublimations are performed under vacuum, because at higher pressures more compounds will pass through a liquid phase rather than subliming; low pressure also reduces the temperature required for sublimation and thus the danger that the compound will decompose. The optimal conditions depend on the compound to be purified, since each compound has a different phase diagram (see General Chemistry, chapter 8).

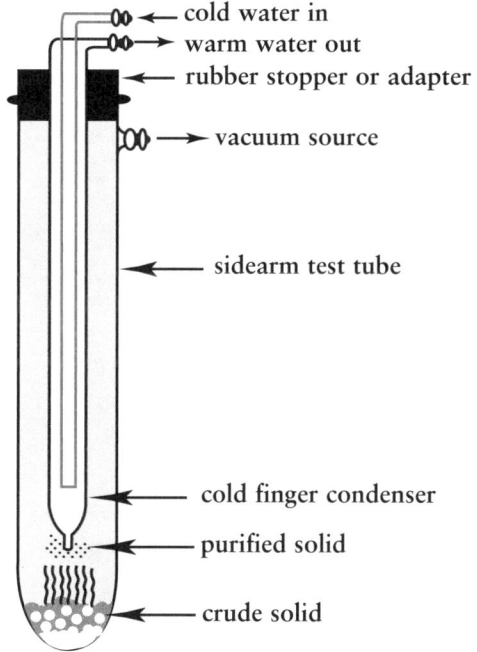

Figure 12.3: Sublimation

E. CENTRIFUGATION

Particles in a solution settle, or **sediment**, at different rates depending upon their mass, their density, and their shape. Sedimentation can be accelerated by **centrifuging** the solution. A centrifuge is an apparatus in which test tubes containing the solution are spun at high speed, which subjects them to centrifugal force. Compounds of greater mass and density settle toward the bottom of the test tubes, while lighter compounds remain near the top. This method of separation is effective for many different types of compounds, and is frequently used in biochemistry to separate cells, organelles, and biological macromolecules.

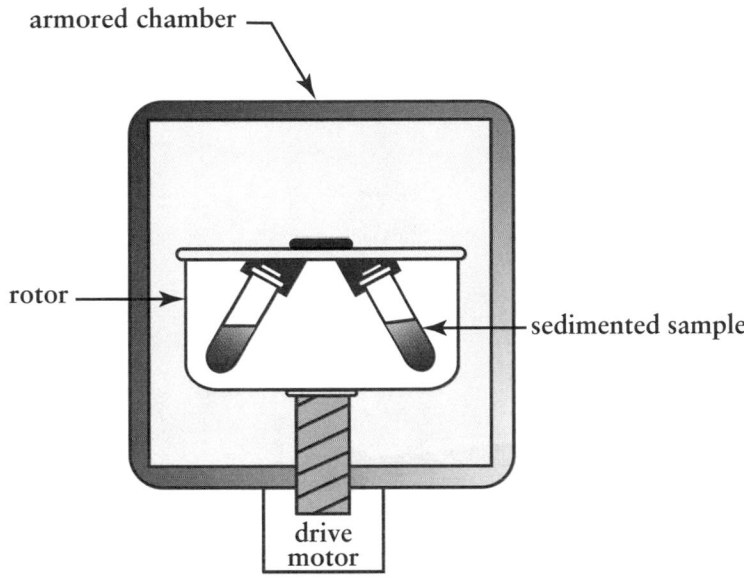

Figure 12.4: Centrifuge

DISTILLATION

Distillation is the separation of one liquid from another through vaporization and condensation. A mixture of two (or more) miscible liquids is slowly heated; the compound with the lowest boiling point is preferentially vaporized, condenses on a water-cooled distillation column, and is separated from the other, higher-boiling compound(s). (Immiscible liquids can be separated in a separatory funnel and thus do not require distillation.)

A. SIMPLE

Simple distillation is used to separate liquids that boil *below* 150°C and at least 25°C apart. The apparatus consists of a distilling flask containing the two liquids, a distillation column consisting of a thermometer and a condenser, and a receiving flask to collect the distillate.

B. VACUUM

Vacuum distillation is used to separate liquids that boil *above* 150°C and at least 25°C apart. The entire system is operated under reduced pressure, lowering the boiling points of the liquids and thus preventing their decomposition due to excessive temperature.

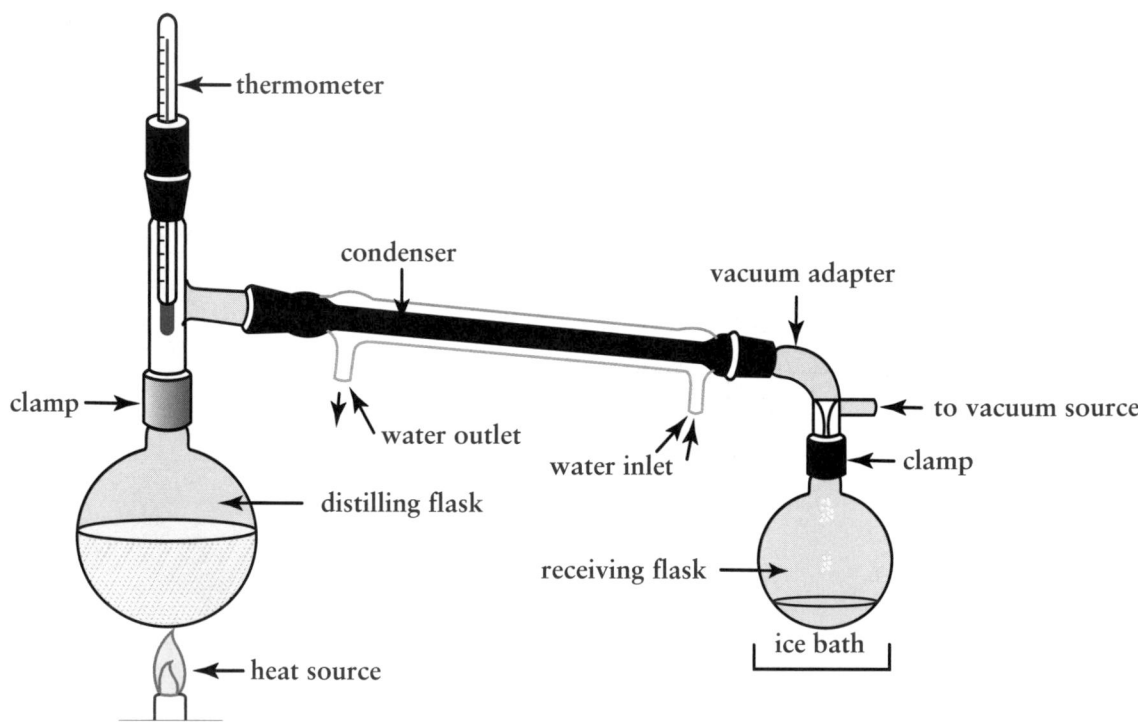

Figure 12.5: Vacuum Distillation

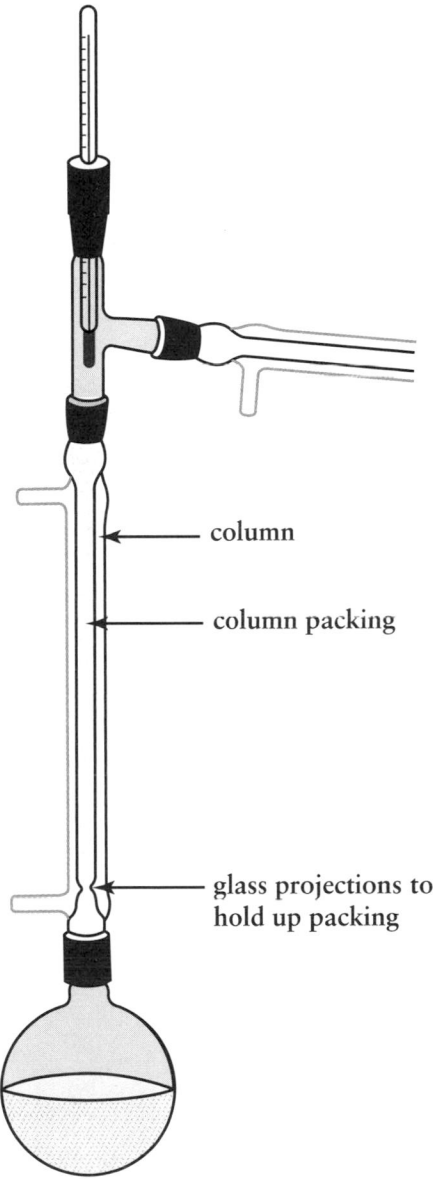

Figure 12.6: Fractional Distillation

C. FRACTIONAL

Fractional distillation is used to separate liquids that boil less than 25°C apart. A fractionating column is used to connect the distilling flask to the distillation column. It is filled with inert objects, such as glass beads, which have a large surface area. The vapors condense on these surfaces, reevaporate, and then condense further up the column. Each time the liquid evaporates, the vapors contain a greater proportion of the lower-boiling component. Eventually, near the top of the fractionating column, the vapor is composed solely of one component, which will condense on the distillation column and collect in the receiving flask.

CHROMATOGRAPHY

A. GENERAL PRINCIPLES

Chromatography is a technique that allows scientists to separate, identify, and isolate individual compounds from a complex mixture based on their differing chemical properties. First, the sample is placed, or loaded, onto a solid medium called the **stationary phase** or **adsorbant**. Then, the **mobile phase**, a liquid (or gas for gas chromatography), is run through the stationary phase, to displace (or **elute**) adhered substances. Different compounds will adhere to the stationary phase with different strengths, and therefore migrate with different speeds. This causes separation of the compounds within the stationary phase, allowing each compound to be isolated.

There are several forms of media used as the stationary phase, which separate compounds based on different chemical properties. How quickly a compound travels through the stationary phase depends on a variety of factors. Commonly, the key is polarity. For instance, thin layer chromatography often uses silica gel, which is highly polar. Thus, polar compounds bind tightly, eluting poorly into the less polar organic solvent. Size or charge may also play a role, as in column chromatography (described in detail below). Newer techniques, such as affinity chromatography, take advantage of unique properties of a substance (such as its strong binding to a specific antibody or to a known receptor or ligand) to bind it tightly to the stationary phase.

Compounds can be distinguished from each other because they travel across the stationary phase (adsorbant) at different rates. In practice, a substance can be identified based on:

- how far it travels in a given amount of time (as in TLC); or
- how rapidly it travels a given distance, e.g., how quickly it elutes off the column (as in GC or column chromatography.)

The four most commonly used types of chromatography are **thin-layer chromatography**, **column chromatography**, **gas chromatography**, and **high-pressure** (or **performance**) **liquid chromatography**.

B. THIN-LAYER CHROMATOGRAPHY

The adsorbant in thin-layer chromatography (TLC) is either a piece of paper or a thin layer of silica gel or alumina on a plastic or glass sheet. The mixture to be separated is placed on the adsorbant; this is called **spotting**, because a small, well defined spot is desirable. The TLC plate is then **developed**: placed upright in a developing chamber (usually a beaker with a lid or a wide-mouthed jar), containing **eluant** (solvent) approximately 1/4 inch deep (this value depends on the size of the plate). It is imperative that

> **MCAT Synopsis**
>
> Key idea: Chromatography separates compounds based on how strongly they adhere to the *solid*, or *stationary*, phase (or, in other words, how easily they come off into the mobile phase).

the initial spots on the plate be above the level of the solvent, or they will simply elute off the plate into the solvent rather than moving neatly up the plate itself. The solvent creeps up the plate by capillary action, moving different compounds at different rates. When the **solvent front** nears the top of the plate, the plate is removed from the chamber and allowed to dry.

Chromatography is often done with silica gel, which is very polar and hydrophilic. The mobile phase, usually an organic solvent of weak to moderate polarity, is then used to "run" the sample through the gel. Nonpolar compounds move very quickly, while polar molecules are stuck tightly to the gel. The more polar the solvent, the faster the sample will migrate. Reverse-phase chromatography is just the opposite. Here the stationary phase is very nonpolar, so polar molecules run very quickly, while non-polar molecules stick more tightly.

The spots of individual compounds (usually white) are not usually visible on the white TLC plate. They are **visualized** by placing the TLC plate under UV light, which will show any compounds that are UV-sensitive (see chapter 13, Spectroscopy); or by allowing iodine, I_2, to stain the spots. Other chemical staining agents include phosphomolybdic acid and vanillin. Note that these compounds destroy the product (usually by oxidation), so that it cannot be recovered for further study.

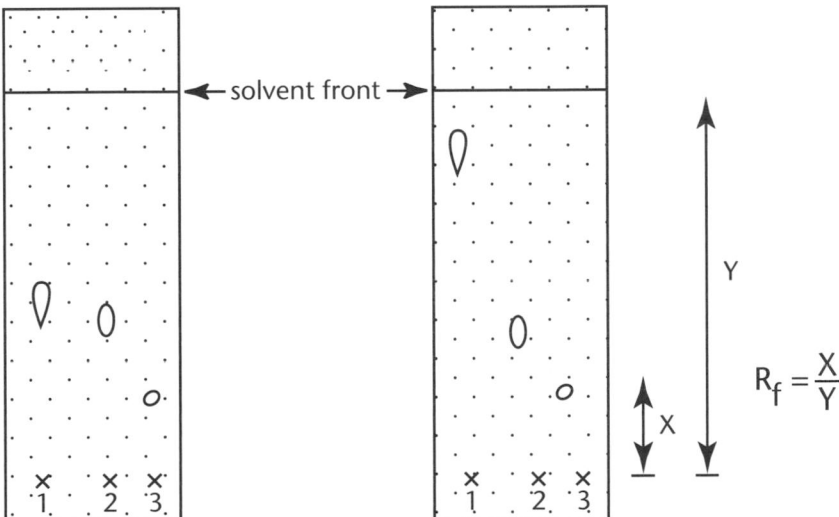

Figure 12.7: Thin Layer Chromatograms

The distance a compound travels, divided by the distance the solvent travels, is called the **R_f value**. This value is relatively constant for a particular compound in a particular solvent, and can therefore be used for identification.

TLC is most frequently used for qualitative identification (i.e., determining the identity of a compound). It can also be used on a larger scale, as a means of purification. **Preparative** or **prep TLC** uses a large TLC plate upon which a sizeable streak of a mixture is placed. As the plate develops, the streak splits into bands of individual compounds, which can be scraped off. Rinsing with a polar solvent will recover the pure compounds from the silica.

C. COLUMN CHROMATOGRAPHY

The principle behind column chromatography is the same as for TLC. Column chromatography, however, uses silica gel or alumina as an adsorbant (not paper), and this adsorbant is in the form of a column (not a layer), allowing much more separation. In TLC the solvent and compounds move up the plate (by capillary action), whereas in column chromatography they move down the column (by gravity). Sometimes the solvent is forced through the column with nitrogen gas; this is called **flash column chromatography**.

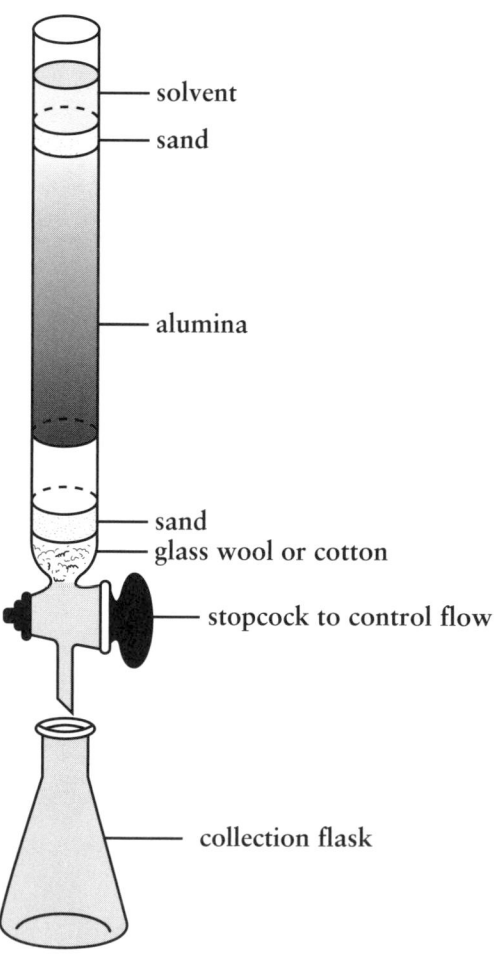

Figure 12.8: Column Chromatography

The solvent drips out the end of the column and fractions are collected in flasks or test tubes. These fractions contain bands corresponding to the different compounds, and when the solvents are evaporated, the compounds can be isolated.

Column chromatography is particularly useful in biochemistry, because it can be used to separate macromolecules such as proteins or nucleic acids. Several techniques exist:

1) In *ion exchange chromatography,* the beads in the column are coated with charged substances, and so they will attract or bind compounds with an opposing charge. For instance, a positively charged column will attract and hold negative substances while letting those with positive charge pass through.

2) In *size-exclusion chromatography,* the column contains beads with many tiny pores. Very small molecules can enter the beads, which slows down their progress, while large molecules move around or between the beads and thus travel through the column faster.

3) In *affinity chromotography,* columns can be "customized" to bind a substance of interest. For example, to purify substance A, a scientist might use a column of beads coated with something that binds A very tightly, such as a receptor for A, A's biological target, or even a specific antibody. A will bind to the column very tightly. It can later be eluted by washing with free receptor (or target or antibody), which will compete with the bead-bound receptor and ultimately free substance A from the column.

D. GAS CHROMATOGRAPHY

Gas chromatography (GC) is another method of qualitative separation. In gas chromatography, also called **vapor-phase chromatography** (VPC), the eluant that passes through the adsorbant is a gas, usually helium or nitrogen. The adsorbant is inside a 30-foot column that is coiled and kept inside an oven to control its temperature. The mixture to be separated is injected into the column and vaporized. The gaseous compounds travel through the column at different rates, because they adhere to the adsorbant to different degrees, and will separate by the time they reach the end of the column. At this point they are registered by a detector, which records the presence of a compound as a peak.

> ### MCAT Synopsis
>
> To identify a compound or distinguish two different compounds, look at their "retention times"— that is, how *long* it took for each to travel through the column.

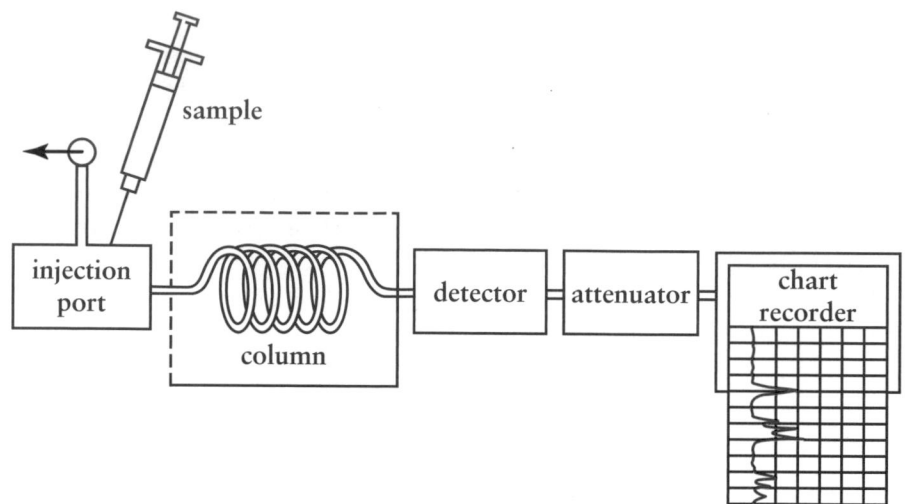

Figure 12.9: Gas Chromatography

GC can be used on a larger scale for quantitative separation, and is then called preparative or prep GC. This is, however, very tedious and difficult to perform.

E. HPLC

HPLC stands for either high-pressure or high-performance liquid chromatography. The eluant is a liquid that travels through a column similar to a GC column, but under pressure. In the past, very high pressures were used; now they are much lower, hence the change from high *pressure* to high *performance*.

In HPLC, a sample is injected into the column and separation occurs as it flows through. The compounds pass through a detector and are collected as the solvent flows out the end of the apparatus. The eluant may vary, as in thin-layer or column chromatography.

ELECTROPHORESIS

When a molecule is placed in an electric field, it will move towards either the cathode or the anode depending on its size and charge. **Electrophoresis** employs this phenomenon to separate macromolecules (usually biological macromolecules) such as proteins or DNA. The migration velocity, v, of a molecule is directly proportional to the electric field strength, E, and to the net charge on the molecule, z, and is inversely proportional to a frictional coefficient, f, which depends on the mass and shape of the migrating molecules.

$$v = \frac{Ez}{f}$$

Therefore, in a constant electric field, highly charged molecules will move most rapidly, as will small molecules.

> **KAPLAN⟩ EXCLUSIVE**
>
> In electrophoresis:
>
> *Anions* are attracted to the *Anode* while
> *Cations* are attracted to the *Cathode*.

> **MCAT Synopsis**
>
> In most forms of electrophoresis, the size of a macromolecule is usually the most important factor—small molecules move faster, while large ones move more slowly and may in fact take hours to leave the well.

A. AGAROSE GEL ELECTROPHORESIS

Agarose gel electrophoresis is used by molecular biologists to separate pieces of **nucleic acid** (usually **deoxyribonucleic acid**, DNA, but sometimes **ribonucleic acid**, RNA, as well; see chapter 15). Agarose is a plant gel, derived from seaweed, that is nontoxic and easy to manipulate (unlike SDS/polyacrylamide). Since every piece of nucleic acid is highly negatively charged, nucleic acids can be separated effectively on the basis of size even without the charge-masking provided by SDS. Agarose gels are stained with a compound called ethidium bromide, which binds to nucleic acids and is visualized by its fluorescence under ultraviolet light. Agarose gel electrophoresis can also be used preparatively, by cutting the desired band out of the gel and eluting out the nucleic acid.

> **KAPLAN) EXCLUSIVE**
>
> SDS–PAGE and agarose gel electrophoresis separate molecules based on *size*.

B. SDS-POLYACRYLAMIDE GEL ELECTROPHORESIS

SDS-polyacrylamide gel electrophoresis separates proteins on the basis of mass, not charge. Polyacrylamide gel is the standard medium for electrophoresis. SDS is sodium dodecyl sulfate, which disrupts noncovalent interactions. It binds to proteins and creates large negative net charges, neutralizing the protein's original net charge. As proteins move through the gel, the only variable affecting their velocity is f, the frictional coefficient, which is dependent on mass. After separation, the gel is stained so that the protein bands can be visualized.

> **MCAT Synopsis**
>
> When pH = pI, a protein stops moving.

C. ISOELECTRIC FOCUSING

A protein may be characterized by its **isoelectric point,** pI, which is the pH at which its net charge (the sum of the charges on all of its component amino acids; see chapter 15) is zero. If a mixture of proteins is placed in an electric field in a gel with a pH gradient, the proteins will move until they reach the point at which the pH is equal to their pI. At this location, the protein will be uncharged and will no longer move in the field. Molecules differing by as little as one charge can be separated in this manner, which is called **isoelectric focusing.**

> **Bridge**
>
> Since amino acids and proteins are organic molecules, the fundamental principles of acid-base chemistry apply to them as well.
>
> - At a low pH, [H+] is relatively high. Thus, at a pH < pI, proteins will tend to be protonated and, as a result, positively charged.
>
> - At a relatively high (basic) pH, [H+] is fairly low and proteins will tend to be de-pronated— thus carrying a negative charge.

SUMMARY OF PURIFICATION METHODS

Method	Use
Extraction	separates dissolved substances based on differential solubility in aqueous versus organic solvents
Filtration	separates solids from liquids
Recrystallization	separates solids based on differential solubility; temperature is important here
Sublimation	separates solids based on their ability to sublime
Centrifugation	separates large things (like cells, organelles and macromolecules) based on mass and density
Distillation	separates liquids based on boiling point, which in turn depends on intermolecular forces
Chromatography	uses a stationary phase and a mobile phase to separate compounds based on how tightly they adhere (generally due to polarity but sometimes size as well)
Electrophoresis	used to separate biological macromolecules (such as proteins or nucleic acids) based on size and sometimes charge

13

SPECTROSCOPY

Once an organic compound is isolated, it must be characterized and identified. If it is a known compound, identification can often be made from elemental analysis or determination of the melting point. With new or more complex compounds, other methods must be used. **Spectroscopy** is the process of measuring the energy differences between the possible states of a molecular system by determining the frequencies of electromagnetic radiation (light) absorbed by the molecules. The possible states are quantized energy levels associated with different types of molecular motion, including molecular rotation, vibration of bonds, and electron movement. Different types of spectroscopy measure these different types of molecular motion, identifying specific functional groups and how they are connected.

Spectroscopy is useful because only a very small quantity of sample is needed. In addition, the sample may be reused after an IR, NMR, or UV spectrum is obtained.

INFRARED

A. BASIC THEORY

Infrared (IR) spectroscopy measures molecular vibrations, which include bond **stretching, bending**, and **rotation**. The useful absorptions of infrared light occur in the 3,000–30,000 nm region, which corresponds to 3,500–300 cm⁻¹ (called **wavenumbers**). When light of these wavelengths/wavenumbers is absorbed, the molecules enter higher (excited) vibrational states.

Bond stretching (which can be of two types: symmetric or asymmetric) involves the largest change in energy and is observed in the region 1,500–4,000 cm⁻¹. Bending vibrations are observed in the region 400–1,500 cm⁻¹. Four different types of vibration that can occur are shown in Figure 13.1.

 Go Online

For more on spectroscopy, visit the online workshop.

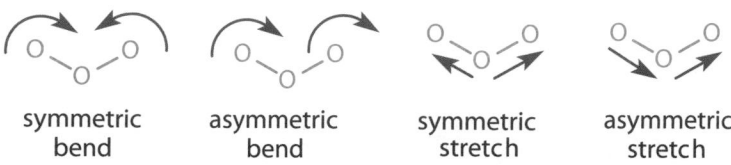

symmetric
bend

asymmetric
bend

symmetric
stretch

asymmetric
stretch

Figure 13.1

In addition to bending and stretching vibrations, more complex vibrations may occur. These can be combinations of bending, stretching, and rotation frequencies or complex frequency patterns caused by the motion of the whole molecule. Absorptions of these types are seen in the region 1,500–400 cm^{-1}. This region of the spectrum is known as the **fingerprint region** and is characteristic of a molecule; it is, therefore, frequently used to identify a substance.

In order for an absorption to be recorded, the motion must result in a change in a bond dipole moment. Molecules comprised of atoms with the same electronegativity, as well as symmetrical molecules, do not experience a changing dipole moment and therefore do not exhibit absorption. For example, O_2 and Br_2 do not absorb, but HCl and CO do.

A typical spectrum is obtained by passing infrared light (of frequencies from approximately 4,000–400 cm^{-1}) through a sample, and recording the absorption pattern. Percent transmittance is plotted versus frequency, where percent transmittance = absorption^{-1} (%T = A^{-1}); absorptions appear as valleys on the spectrum.

B. CHARACTERISTIC ABSORPTIONS

Particular functional groups absorb at localized frequencies. For example, alcohols absorb around 3,300 cm^{-1}, carbonyl groups around 1,700 cm^{-1}, and ethers around 1,100 cm^{-1}. Table 13.1 lists the specific absorptions of key functional groups and their corresponding vibrations.

> **MCAT Synopsis**
>
> Symmetric stretches do not show up in IR spectra since they involve no net change in dipole movement.

> **MCAT Synopsis**
>
> Wave numbers (cm^{-1}) are not the same as frequency.
>
> $v = \dfrac{c}{\lambda}$, while wave number $= \dfrac{1}{\lambda}$

Table 13.1. Common Infrared Absorption Peaks

Functional Group	Frequency (cm^{-1})	Vibration
Alkanes	2,800–3,000	C—H
	1,200	C—C
Alkenes	3,080–3,140	=C—H
	1,645	C=C
Alkynes	2,200	C≡C
	3,300	≡C—H
Aromatic	2,900–3,100	C—H
	1,475–1,625	C—C
Alcohols	3,100–3,500	O—H (broad)
Ethers	1,050–1,150	C—O
Aldehydes	2,700–2,900	(O)C—H
	1,725–1,750	C=O
Ketones	1,700–1,750	C=O
Acids	1,700–1,750	C=O
	2,900–3,300	O—H (broad)
Amines	3,100–3,500	N—H (sharp)

C. APPLICATION

A great deal of information can be obtained from an IR spectrum. Most of the useful functional group information is found between 1,400 and 4,000 cm^{-1}.

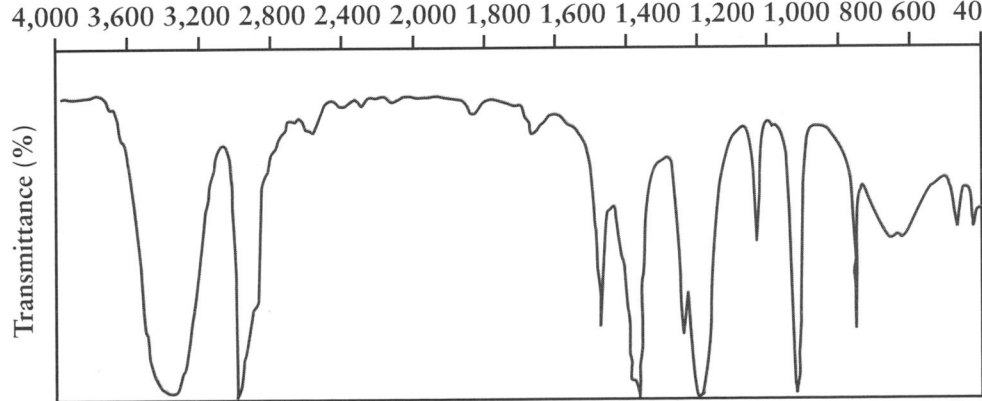

Figure 13.2

Figure 13.2 shows the IR spectrum of an aliphatic alcohol. The large peak at 3,300 cm^{-1} is due to the presence of the hydroxyl group, while the peak at 3,000 cm^{-1} can be attributed to the alkane portion of the molecule.

NUCLEAR MAGNETIC RESONANCE

A. BASIC THEORY

Nuclear Magnetic Resonance (NMR) spectroscopy is one of the most widely used spectroscopic tools in organic chemistry. NMR is based on the fact that certain nuclei have magnetic moments which are normally oriented at random. When such nuclei are placed in a magnetic field, their magnetic moments tend to align either with or against the direction of this applied field. Nuclei whose magnetic moments are aligned with the field are said to be in the α *state* (lower energy), while those whose moments are aligned against the field are said to be in the β *state* (higher energy). If the nuclei are then irradiated with electromagnetic radiation, some will be excited into the β state. The absorption corresponding to this excitation occurs at different frequencies depending on an atom's environment. The nuclear magnetic moments are affected by other nearby atoms that also possess magnetic moments. Hence, a compound may contain many nuclei that resonate at different frequencies, producing a very complex spectrum.

A typical NMR spectrum is a plot of frequency versus absorption of energy during resonance. Frequency *decreases* toward the right. Alternatively, varying magnetic field may be plotted on the *x* axis, *increasing* toward the right. Because different NMR spectrometers operate at different magnetic field strengths, a standardized method of plotting the NMR spectrum has been adopted. An arbitrary variable, called **chemical shift** (represented by the symbol δ), with units of **parts per million (ppm)** of spectrometer frequency, is plotted on the *x* axis.

NMR is most commonly used to study ^{1}H nuclei (protons) and ^{13}C nuclei, although any atom possessing a nuclear spin (any nucleus with an odd atomic number or odd mass number) can be studied, such as ^{19}F, ^{17}O, ^{14}N, ^{15}N, or ^{31}P.

B. ^{1}H NMR

Most ^{1}H nuclei come into resonance between 0 and 10 δ downfield from TMS. Each distinct set of nuclei gives rise to a separate peak. The compound dichloromethyl methyl ether has two distinct sets of ^{1}H nuclei. The single proton attached to the dichloromethyl group is in a different magnetic environment than are the three protons on the methyl group, and the two classes resonate at different frequencies. The three protons

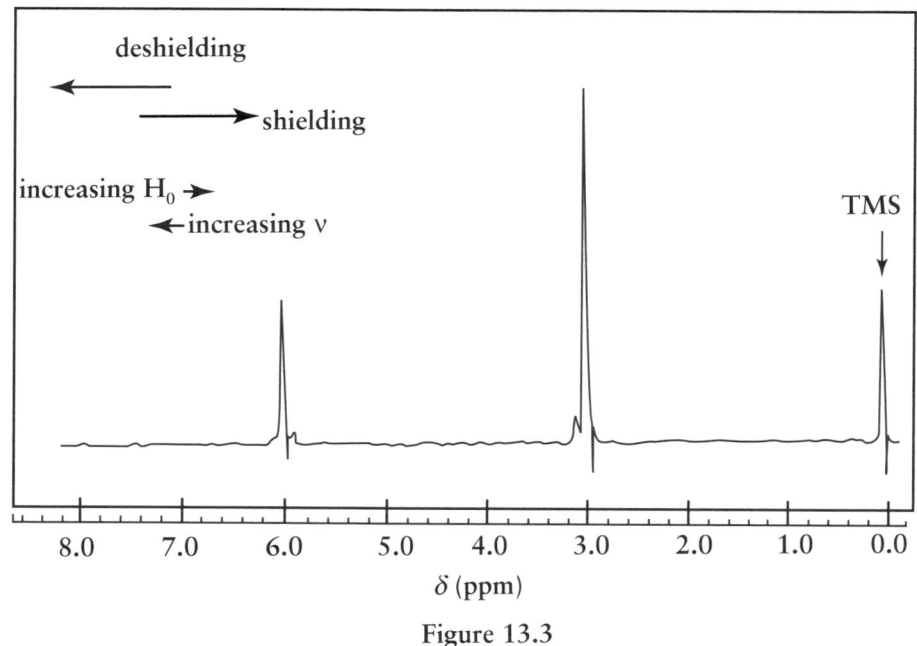

deshielding

shielding

increasing H_0

increasing ν

TMS

Figure 13.3

on the methyl group are magnetically equivalent, due to rotation about the oxygen-carbon single bond, and resonate at the same frequency. Thus, two separate peaks are expected, as shown in Figure 13.3.

The left-hand peak corresponds to the single dichloromethyl proton and the middle peak to the three methyl protons (the one on the far right is the TMS reference peak). Notice that if the areas under the peaks are integrated, the ratio between them is 3:1, corresponding to the number of protons producing each peak.

The single proton comes into resonance downfield from the methyl protons. This phenomenon is due to the electron-withdrawing effect of the chlorine atoms. The electron cloud that surrounds the ^{1}H nucleus ordinarily screens the nucleus somewhat from the applied magnetic field. The chlorine atoms pull away the electron cloud and **deshield** the nucleus. Thus, the nucleus resonates in a lower field than it would otherwise. By the same rationale, electron-donating atoms, such as the silicon atoms in TMS, **shield** the ^{1}H nuclei, causing them to come into resonance at a higher field.

If two magnetically different protons are within three bonds of each other, a phenomenon known as **coupling**, or **splitting** occurs. Consider two protons, H_a and H_b, on the molecule 1,1-dibromo-2,2-dichloroethane (Figure 13.4).

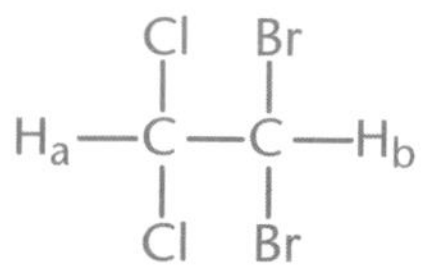

Figure 13.4

MCAT Synopsis

The splitting of the peak represents the number of adjacent hydrogens. A peak will be split into n + 1 peaks where n is the number of adjacent hydrogens.

At any given time, H_a can experience two different magnetic environments, since H_b can be in either the α or the β state. These different states of H_b influence nucleus H_a (if the two H atoms are within three bonds of each other), causing slight upfield and downfield shifts. Since there is approximately a 50 percent chance that H_b will be in either state, this results in a **doublet**, two peaks of equal intensity equally spaced around the true chemical shift of H_a. H_b experiences the two different states of H_a and is likewise coupled. The magnitude of the splitting, usually denoted in Hz, is called the **coupling constant, J**.

In 1,1-dibromo-2-chloroethane (Figure 13.5), the H_a nucleus is affected by two nearby H_b nuclei, and can experience four different states: αα, αβ, βα, or ββ.

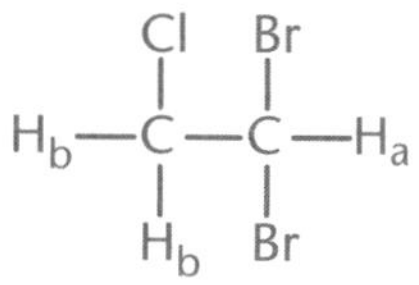

Figure 13.5

The αβ and βα states have the same net effect on the H_a nucleus, and the resonances occur at the same frequency. The αα and ββ states resonate at frequencies different from each other and from the αβ/βα frequency. The result is three peaks that are centered around the true chemical shift, with an area ratio of 1:2:1. In general, n hydrogen atoms couple to give n + 1 peaks, whose area ratios are given by Pascal's triangle, shown in Table 13.2.

Table 13.2. Pascal's Triangle

Number of Adjacent Hydrogens	Total Number of Peaks	Area Ratios
0	1	1
1	2	1:1
2	3	1:2:1
3	4	1:3:3:1
4	5	1:4:6:4:1
5	6	1:5:10:10:5:1
6	7	1:6:15:20:15:6:1
7	8	1:7:21:35:35:21:7:1

The following table indicates the chemical shift ranges of several different types of protons:

Table 13.2. Chemical Shifts

Type of Proton	Approximate Chemical Shift δ (ppm) Downfield from TMS
RCH_3	0.9
RCH_2	1.25
R_3CH	1.5
$-CH=CH$	4.6–6.0
$-C≡CH$	2.0–3.0
Ar–H	6.0–8.5
–CHX	2.0–4.5
–CHOH/–CHOR	3.4–4.0
RCHO	9.0–10.0
RCHCO–	2.0–2.5
–CHCOOH/–CHCOOR	2.0–2.6
$-CHOH–CH_2OH$	1.0–5.5
ArOH	4.0–12.0
–COOH	10.5–12.0
$-NH_2$	1.0–5.0

C. ^{13}C NMR

^{13}C NMR is very similar to ^1H NMR. Most ^{13}C NMR signals, however, occur 0–200 δ downfield from the carbon peak of TMS. Another significant difference is that only 1.1 percent of carbon atoms are ^{13}C atoms. This has two effects: first, a much larger sample is needed to run a ^{13}C spectrum (about 50 mg compared with 1 mg for ^1H NMR), and second, coupling between carbon atoms is generally not observed.

Coupling *is* observed, however, between carbon atoms and the protons directly attached to them. This one-bond coupling is analogous to the three-bond coupling in ^1H NMR. For example, if a carbon atom is attached to two protons, it can experience four different states of those protons (αα, αβ, βα, and ββ), and the carbon signal is split into a triplet with the area ratio 1:2:1.

An additional feature of ^{13}C NMR is the ability to record a spectrum *without* the coupling of adjacent protons. This is called **spin decoupling**, and produces a spectrum of **singlets**, each corresponding to a separate, magnetically equivalent, carbon atoms. For example, compare the following spectra of 1,1,2-trichloropropane. One (Figure 13.6) is a typical **spin-decoupled spectrum**, and the other (Figure 13.7) is spin-coupled.

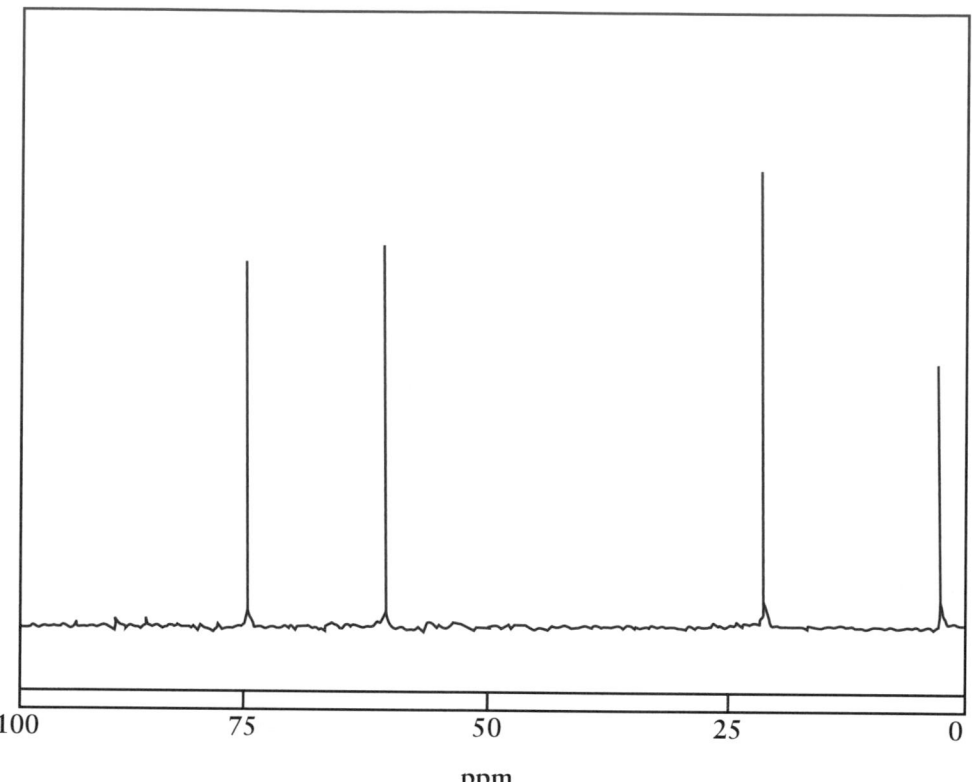

ppm

Figure 13.6. Spin-Decoupled Spectrum of 1,1,2-Trichloropropane

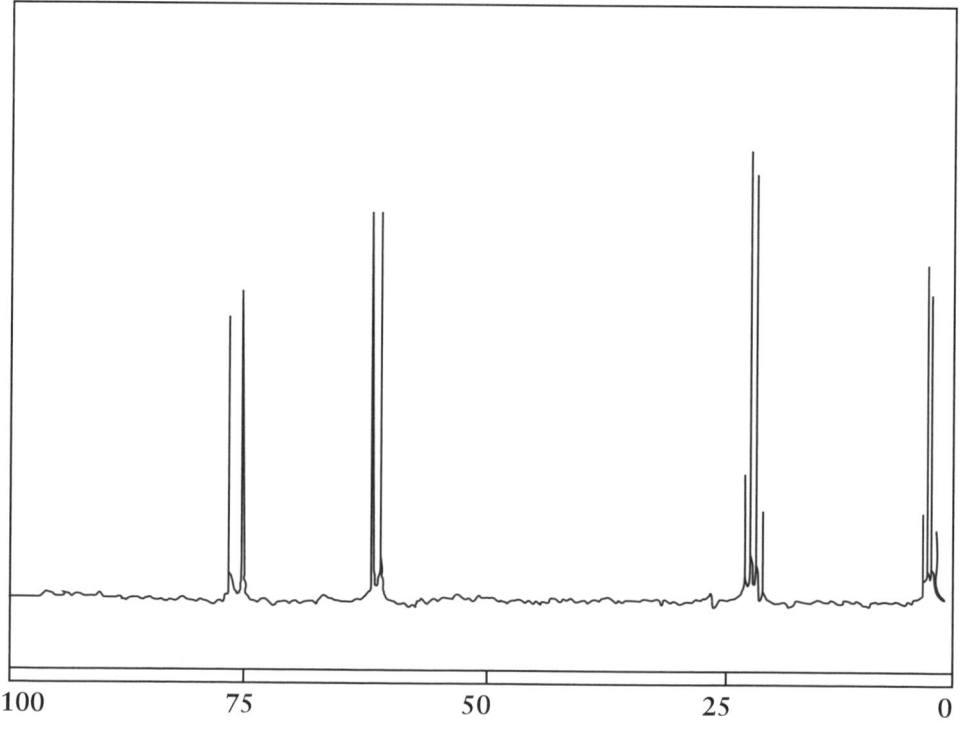

Figure 13.7. Spin-Coupled Spectrum of 1,1,2-Trichloropropane

In general, NMR spectroscopy provides information about the carbon skeleton of a compound, along with some suggestion of its functional groups. Specifically, NMR can provide the following types of information:

1. The number of nonequivalent nuclei, determined from the number of peaks.
2. The magnetic environment of a nucleus, determined by the chemical shift.
3. The relative numbers of nuclei, determined by integrating the peak areas.
4. The number of neighboring nuclei, determined by the splitting pattern observed (except for ^{13}C in the spin-decoupled mode).

ULTRAVIOLET SPECTROSCOPY

A. BASIC THEORY

Ultraviolet spectra are obtained by passing ultraviolet light through a chemical sample (usually dissolved in an inert, nonabsorbing solvent) and plotting absorbance versus wavelength. The wavelength of maximum absorbance provides information on the extent of the conjugated system as well as other structural and compositional information.

> **MCAT Synopsis**
>
> UV spectroscopy is most useful for studying compounds containing double bonds, and/or hetero atoms with lone pairs.

MASS SPECTROMETRY

A. BASIC THEORY

Mass spectrometry differs from the methods thus far discussed in that it is not true spectroscopy, i.e., no absorption of electromagnetic radiation is involved, and, in that it is a destructive technique, mass spectrometry, does not allow for reuse of the sample once the analysis is complete. Most commonly used mass spectrometers use a high-speed beam of electrons to ionize the sample to be analyzed, a particle accelerator to put the charged particles in flight, a magnetic field to deflect the accelerated cationic fragments, and a detector that records the number of particles of each mass exiting the deflector area. The initially formed ion is the molecular cation-radical (M^+) resulting from a single electron being removed from a molecule of the sample. This unstable species usually decomposes rapidly into a cationic fragment and a radical fragment. Since there are many molecules in the sample and (usually) more than one way for the initially formed cation-radical to decompose into fragments, a typical mass spectrum is composed of many lines, each corresponding to a specific mass/charge ratio (m/e). The spectrum itself plots mass/charge on the horizontal axis and relative abundance of the various cationic fragments on the vertical axis (see Fig. 13.8).

> **MCAT Synopsis**
>
> UV spectroscopy can be applied quantitatively by using Beer's law:
>
> $$A = \varepsilon bc$$
>
> where A is absorbance (measured by UV spectroscopy), ε is a constant for the substance at a given wavelength, and c is concentration.

B. CHARACTERISTICS

The tallest peak, belonging to the most common ion, is called the **base peak**, and is assigned the relative abundance value of 100 percent. The peak with the highest m/e ratio (see Figure 13.8) is generally the **molecular ion peak (parent ion peak)**, M^+, from which the molecular weight, M, can be obtained. The charge value is usually 1; hence the m/e ratio can usually be read as the mass of the fragment.

C. APPLICATION

Fragmentation patterns often provide information that helps identify or distinguish certain compounds. In particular, the fragmentation pattern provides clues to the compound's structure. For example, while IR spectroscopy would be of little use in distinguishing between propionaldehyde and butyraldehyde, a mass spectrum would allow unambiguous identification.

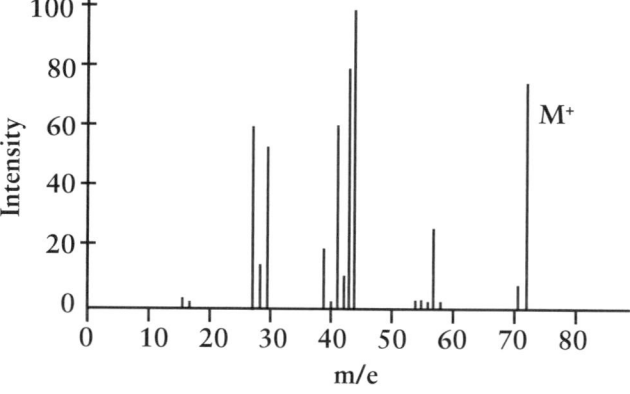

Figure 13.8

Figure 13.8 shows the mass spectrum of butyraldehyde. The peak at m/e = 72 corresponds to the molecular cation-radical, M^+, while the base peak at m/e = 44 corresponds to the cationic fragment resulting from the loss of a C_2H_4 neutral fragment (M − 28 = 44). Other peaks of note include those at 57 (M − 15, loss of CH_3 radical), 43 (M − 29, loss of C_2H_5 radical), and at 29 (M − 43, loss of C_3H_7 radical). The small peak at m/e = 15 can be attributed to the unstabled (and therefore not abundant) methyl cation.

14

CARBOHYDRATES

Carbohydrates are compounds containing carbon, hydrogen, and oxygen in the form of polyhydroxylated aldehydes or ketones. They have the general formula $C_n(H_2O)_n$ and serve many functions in biological systems, most notably as the chemical energy source for most organisms. A single carbohydrate unit is a **monosaccharide** (simple sugar), and a molecule with two sugars is a **disaccharide**. **Oligosaccharides** are short carbohydrate chains, while **polysaccharides** are long carbohydrate chains.

MONOSACCHARIDES

Monosaccharides, the simplest carbohydrate units, are classified according to the number of carbons they possess. For example, **trioses**, **tetroses**, **pentoses**, and **hexoses** have 3, 4, 5, and 6 carbons, respectively. The basic structure of monosaccharides is exemplified by the simplest, glyceraldehyde.

> **MCAT Synopsis**
>
> Monosaccharides are the simplest units and are classified by the number of carbons.

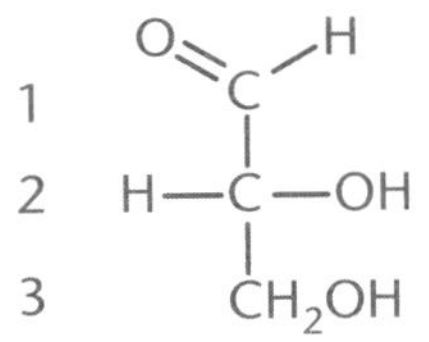

Glyceraldehyde

Figure 14.1

Glyceraldehyde is a polyhydroxylated aldehyde or **aldose** (aldehyde sugar). A polyhydroxylated ketone is called a **ketose** (ketone sugar). The numbering of the carbon atoms in a monosaccharide begins with the end closest to the carbonyl group.

A. STEREOCHEMISTRY

The stereochemistry of monosaccharides can be understood by studying the enantiomeric configurations of glyceraldehyde.

mirror

CHO		CHO
H——OH		HO——H
CH₂OH		CH₂OH

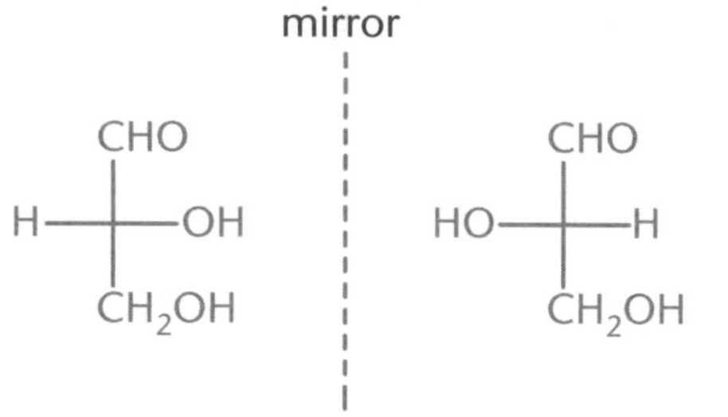

D-Glyceraldehyde   *L*-Glyceraldehyde

Figure 14.2

The D and L configurations of glyceraldehyde were assigned early in this century (before the *R* and *S* configurations were used) to designate the optical rotation of each enantiomer. D-glyceraldehyde was later determined to exhibit a positive rotation (designated as D-(+)-glyceraldehyde) and L-glyceraldehyde a negative rotation (designated as L-(–)-glyceraldehyde. However, other monosaccharides are assigned the D or L configuration depending on their relationship to glyceraldehyde: a molecule whose highest numbered chiral center (the chiral center farthest from the carbonyl) has the same configuration as D-(+)-glyceraldehyde is classed as a D sugar. A molecule that has its highest numbered chiral center in the same configuration as L-(–)-glyceraldehyde is classed as an L sugar. This is illustrated below:

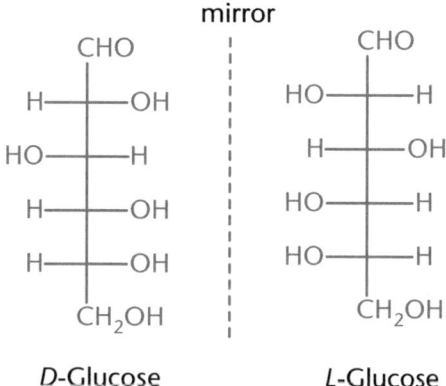

D-Glucose   *L*-Glucose

Figure 14.3

Monosaccharide stereoisomers are divided into two optical families, D and L; the stereoisomers within one family are known as **diastereomers**. Aldose diastereomers which differ only about the configuration of one carbon are known as **epimers**. For instance, D-ribose and D-arabinose are pentose epimers. They differ in configuration only at C–2.

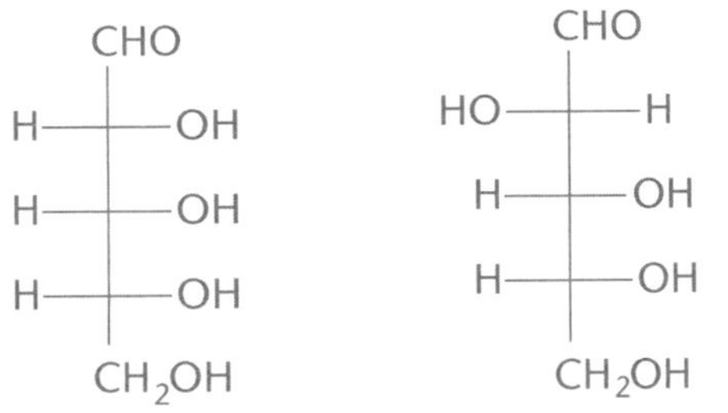

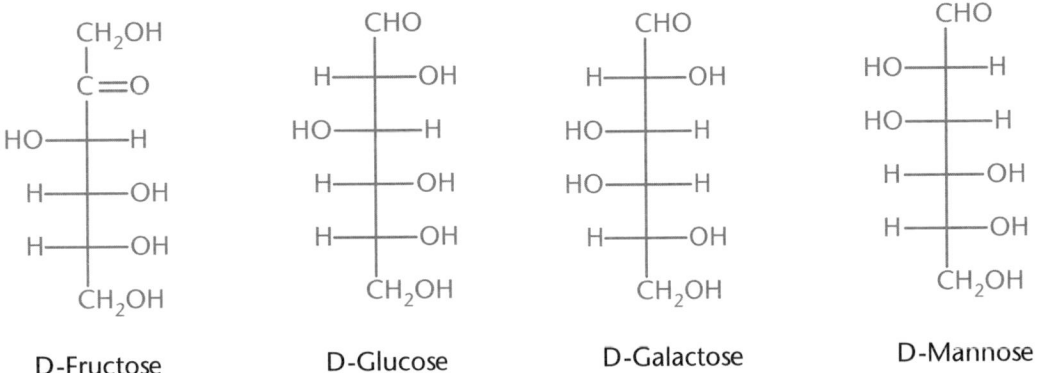

D-Ribose   D-Arabinose

Figure 14.4

Some important monosaccharides are shown in Figure 14.5.

D-Fructose   D-Glucose   D-Galactose   D-Mannose

Figure 14.5

B. RING PROPERTIES

Because monosaccharides contain both a hydroxyl group and a carbonyl group, they can undergo intramolecular reactions to form cyclic hemiacetals (or hemiketals, in the case of ketoses). These cyclic molecules are stable in solution and may exist as six-membered **pyranose** rings (as in glucose) or five-membered **furanose** rings. Like cyclohexane, the pyranose rings adopt a chairlike configuration, and the substituents assume axial or equatorial positions so as to minimize steric hindrance. When converting the monosaccharide from its straight-chain Fischer projection to the Haworth projection (shown in Figure 14.6), it is important to remember that any group on the right of the Fischer projection will be pointing down, while any group on the left side of the Fischer projection will be pointing up. The following reaction scheme depicts the formation of a cyclic hemiacetal from D-glucose.

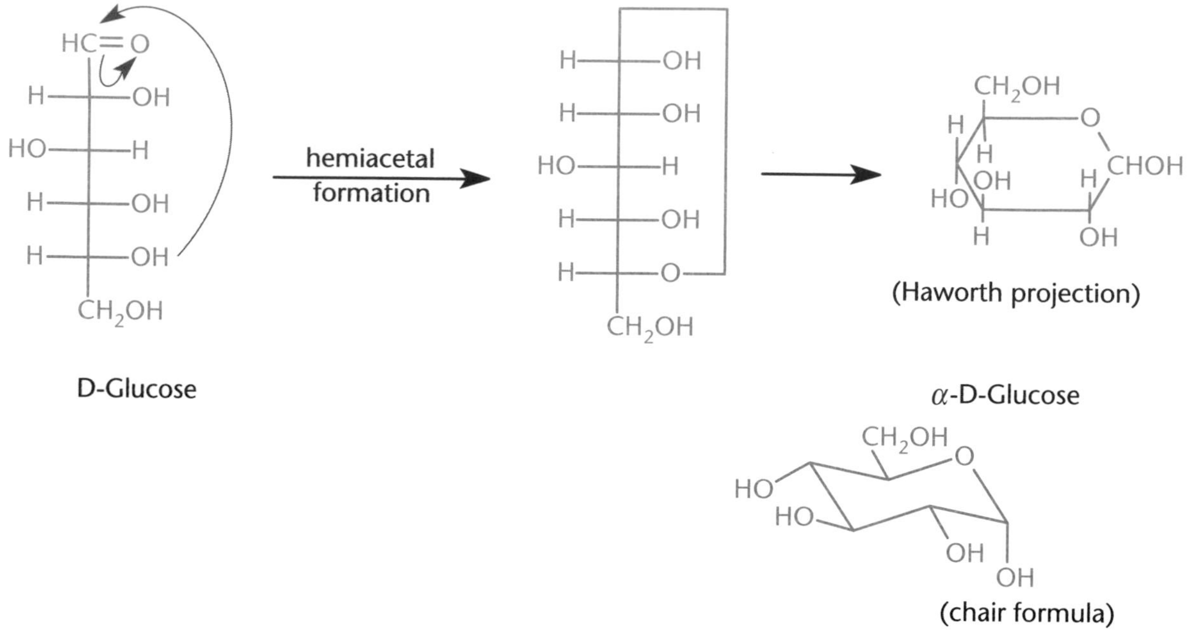

Figure 14.6

MCAT Synopsis

Anomers differ in configuration only at the newly formed chiral center. α = down. β = up.

When a straight-chain monosaccharide is converted to its cyclic form, the carbonyl carbon (C–1 for glucose) becomes chiral. Cyclic stereoisomers differing about the new chiral carbon are known as **anomers**. In glucose, the alpha anomer has the –OH group of C–1 *trans* to the CH_2OH substituent (down), while the beta anomer has the –OH group of C–1 *cis* to the CH_2OH substituent (up).

When exposed to water, hemiacetal rings spontaneously open and then reform. Because of bond rotation between C–1 and C–2, either the alpha or beta anomer may be formed. The reaction is more rapid when catalyzed by acid or base. The spontaneous change of configuration about C–1 is known as **mutarotation,** and results in a mixture containing both anomers in their equilibrium concentrations (for glucose, 36 percent alpha:64 percent beta). The alpha configuration is less favored because the hydroxyl group of C–1 is axial, making the molecule more sterically strained.

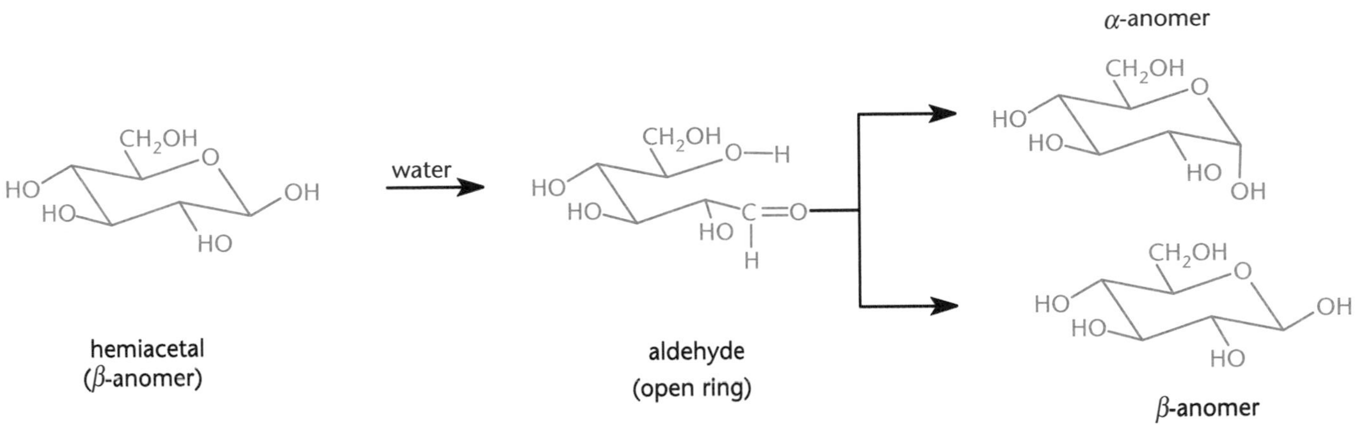

Figure 14.7

C. MONOSACCHARIDE REACTIONS

1. Ester Formation

Monosaccharides contain hydroxyl groups and can undergo many of the same reactions as simple alcohols. Therefore, they may be converted to either esters or ethers. In the presence of acid anhydride and base, all of the hydroxyl groups will be esterified. The following reaction is an example of glucose esterification.

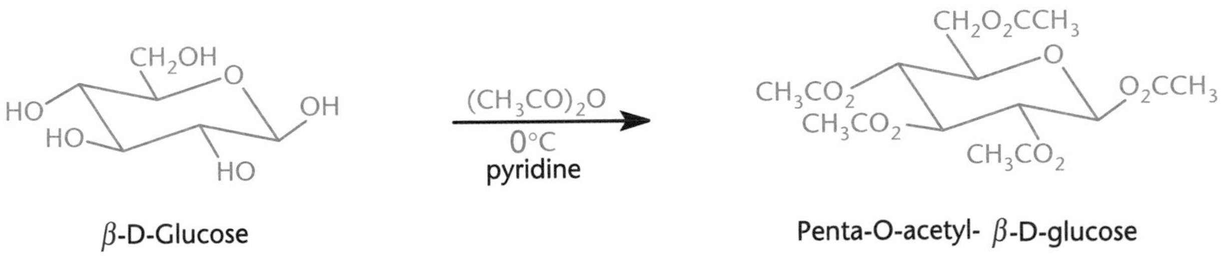

β-D-Glucose   Penta-O-acetyl- β-D-glucose

Figure 14.8

2. Oxidation of Monosaccharides

As they switch between anomeric configurations, the hemiacetal rings spend a short period of time in the open-chain aldehyde form. Like all aldehydes, these can be oxidized to carboxylic acids called **aldonic acids**. Thus, the aldoses are reducing agents. Any monosaccharide with a hemiacetal ring (–OH on C–1) is considered a **reducing sugar** and can be oxidized. Both Tollens reagent and Benedict reagent can be used to detect the presence of reducing sugars. A positive Tollens test involves the reduction of Ag^+ to form metallic silver. When Benedict reagent is used, a red precipitate of Cu_2O indicates the presence of a reducing sugar. Ketose sugars are also reducing sugars and give positive Tollens and Benedict tests, because they can isomerize to aldoses via keto-enol shifts.

> **MCAT Synopsis**
>
> Key reactions of monosaccharides include:
>
> - ester formation
> - oxidation
> - glycosidic reactions

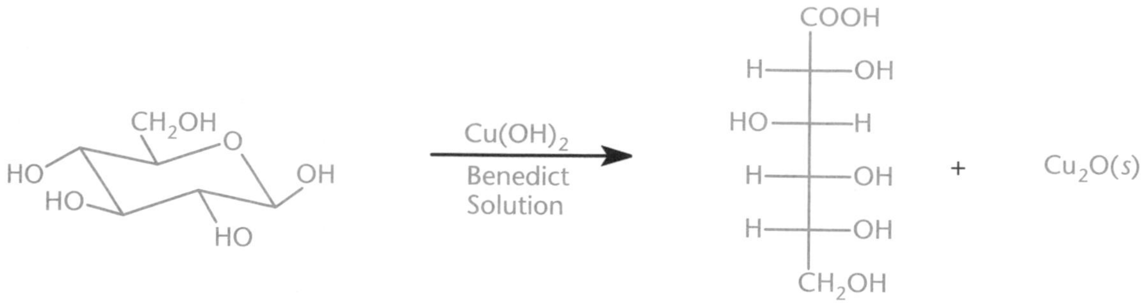

β-D-Glucose

D-Gluconic Acid
(an aldonic acid)

(red solid)

Figure 14.9

3. **Glycosidic Reactions**
Hemiacetal monosaccharides will react with alcohols under acidic conditions. The anomeric hydroxyl group is transformed into an alkoxy group, yielding a mixture of the alpha and beta acetals. The resulting bond is called a **glycosidic linkage**, and the acetal is known as a **glycoside**. An example is the reaction of glucose with ethanol.

Glycosides do not mutarotate and are stable in water.

Ethyl-α-D-glucoside
(an acetal)

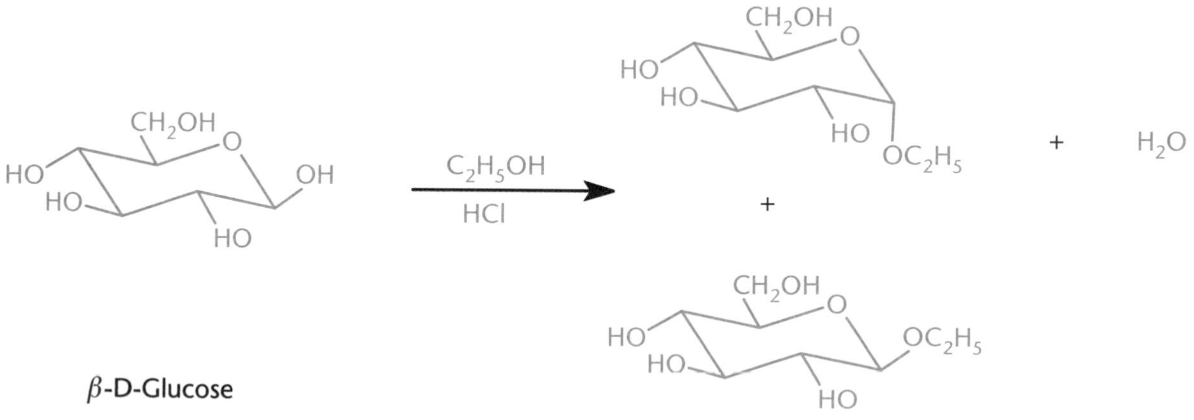

β-D-Glucose

Ethyl-β-D-glucoside
(an acetal)

Figure 14.10

DISACCHARIDES

As discussed above, a monosaccharide may react with alcohols to give acetals. When that alcohol is another monosaccharide, the product is called a **disaccharide**. The formation of a disaccharide is shown below.

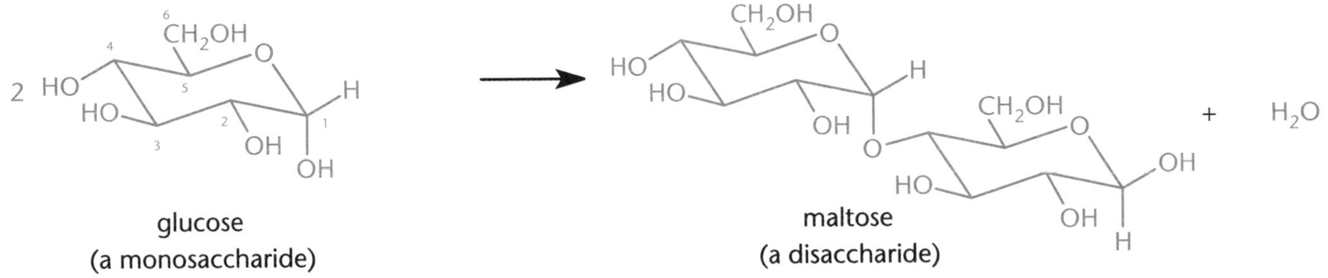

Figure 14.11

The most common glycosidic linkage occurs between C–1 of the first sugar and C–4 of the second, and is designated as a 1,4' link. 1,6' and 1,2' bonds are also observed. The glycosidic bonds may be either alpha or beta, depending on the orientation of the hydroxyl group on the anomeric carbon.

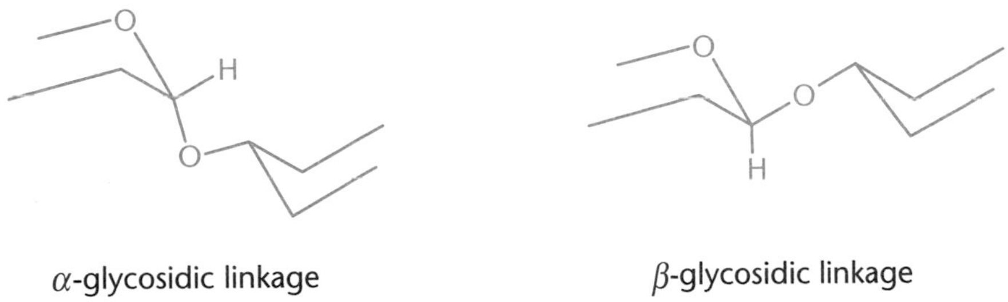

α-glycosidic linkage β-glycosidic linkage

Figure 14.12

These glycosidic linkages can often be cleaved in the presence of aqueous acid. For example, the glycosidic linkage of maltose, a disaccharide, can be cleaved to yield two molecules of glucose.

POLYSACCHARIDES

Polysaccharides are formed via linkage of monosaccharide units with glycosidic bonds. The three most important biological polysaccharides are **cellulose**, **starch**, and **glycogen**. Cellulose is comprised of D-glucose linked by 1,4'-beta-glycosidic bonds. Cellulose is the structural component of plants. Starch stores energy in plants and glycogen stores energy in animals; both are formed by linking glucose units in 1,4'-alpha-glycosidic bonds, with occasional 1,6'-alpha-glycosidic bonds creating branches. While all three are composed of glucose subunits, the orientation about the anomeric carbon gives them biological differences. Cellulose cannot be digested by humans, while starch and glycogen can, and are important energy sources for living organisms.

> **MCAT Synopsis**
>
> Key biological polysaccharides:
>
> cellulose (1,4' beta);
>
> starch and glycogen (mostly 1,4' alpha; some 1,6' alpha).

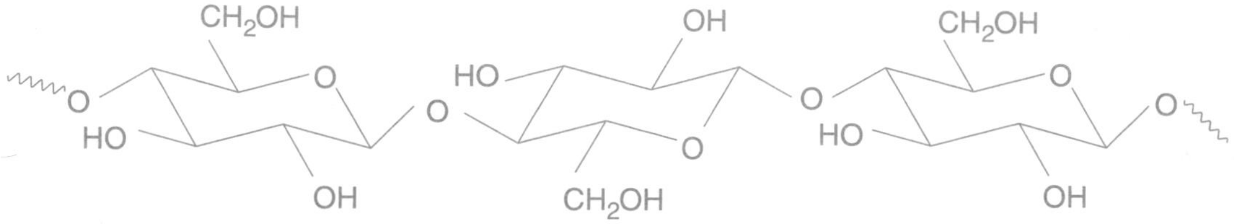

Cellulose, a 1,4′, -β-D-Glucose polymer

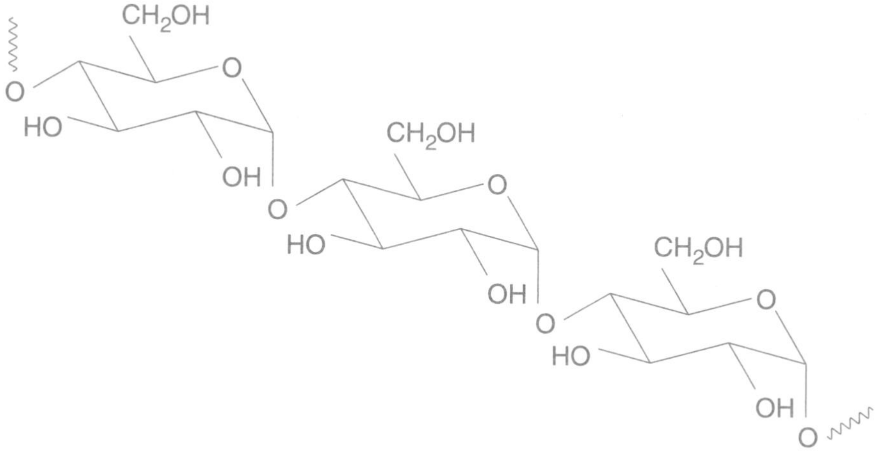

Starch, a 1,4′, -α-D-Glucose polymer

Figure 14.13

15

AMINO ACIDS, PEPTIDES, AND PROTEINS

Proteins are large polymers composed of many amino acid subunits. Proteins have diverse biological roles; for example, they provide structure (keratin, collagen), regulate body metabolism via hormonal control (insulin), and serve as catalysts (enzymes). (Protein function is discussed further in the Biology section.)

AMINO ACIDS

Amino acids contain an amine group and a carboxyl group attached to a single carbon atom (the alpha carbon atom). The other two substituents of the alpha carbon are usually a hydrogen atom and a variable side-chain referred to as the **R-group**.

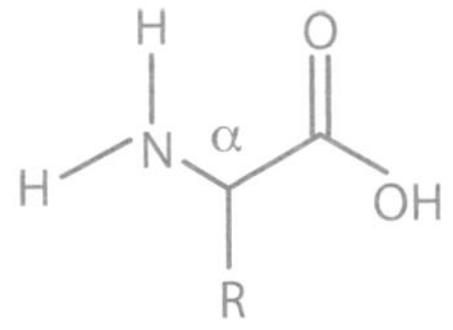

Figure 15.1

The alpha carbon is a chiral center (except in glycine, the simplest amino acid, where R=H), and thus all amino acids (except for glycine) are optically active. Naturally-occurring amino acids (of which there are 20) are L-enantiomers (see chapters 2 and 14).

By convention, the Fischer projection for an amino acid is drawn with the amino group on the left.

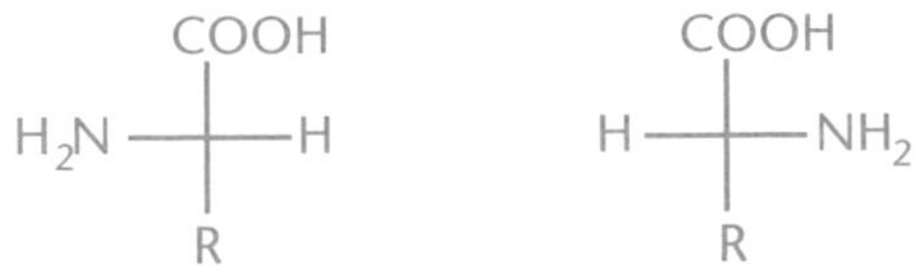

L-amino acid   D-amino acid

Figure 15.2

> ### MCAT Synopsis
> Except for glycine, all amino acids are chiral.

A. ACID-BASE CHARACTERISTICS

Amino acids have an acidic carboxyl group and a basic amino group on the same molecule (see General Chemistry, chapter 10 for a discussion of acids and bases). As a result, when they are in solution, amino acids sometimes take the form of dipolar ions, or **zwitterions** (from German *zwitter*, "hybrid"). The two halves of the molecules neutralize each other, so that at neutral pH they exist in the form of internal salts.

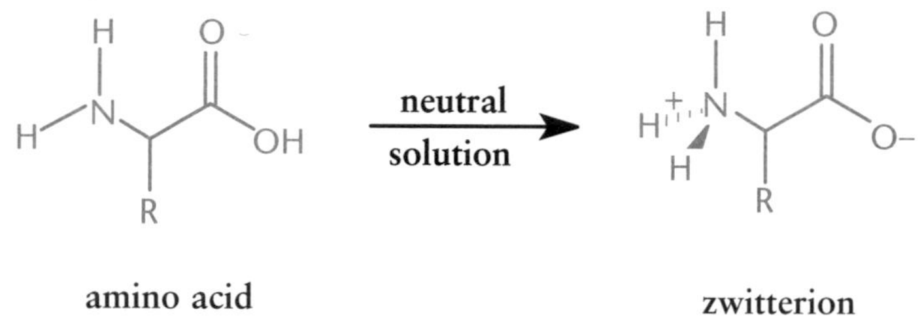

amino acid   zwitterion

Figure 15.3

Amino acids are **amphoteric**; i.e., they may act as either acids or bases, depending on their environment. Amino acids in acidic solution are fully protonated. Since they have two protons that can dissociate—one from the carboxyl group and one from the amino group—amino acids have at least two dissociation constants, K_{a_1} and K_{a_2}.

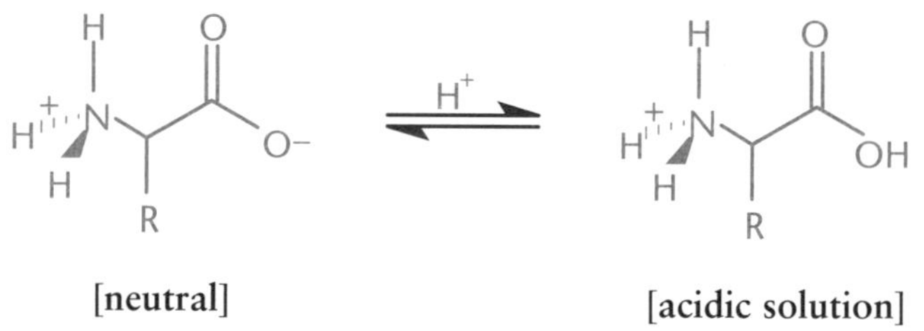

[neutral]   [acidic solution]

Figure 15.4

Amino acids in basic solution are deprotonated. They have two proton-accepting groups and, therefore, at least two dissociation constants, K_{b_1} and K_{b_2}.

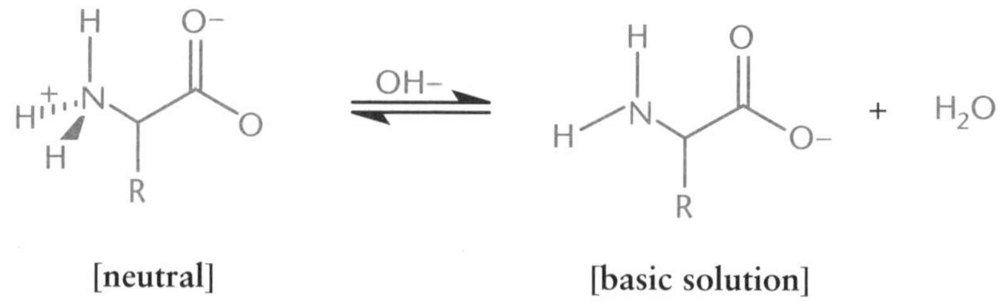

[neutral]   [basic solution]

Figure 15.5

> **MCAT Synopsis**
> ....
> At the isoelectric point, an amino acid is uncharged.

At low pH, the amino acid carries an excess positive charge, and at high pH, the amino acid carries an excess negative charge. The intermediate pH, at which the amino acid is electrically neutral and exists as a zwitterion, is the **isoelectric point (pI)**, or **isoelectric pH**, of the amino acid.

The isoelectric pH lies between pK_{a1} and pK_{a2}.

B. TITRATION OF AMINO ACIDS

Because of their acidic and basic properties, amino acids can be titrated. The titration of each proton occurs as a distinct step resembling that of a simple monoprotic acid. The titration curve of glycine is shown in Figure 15.7.

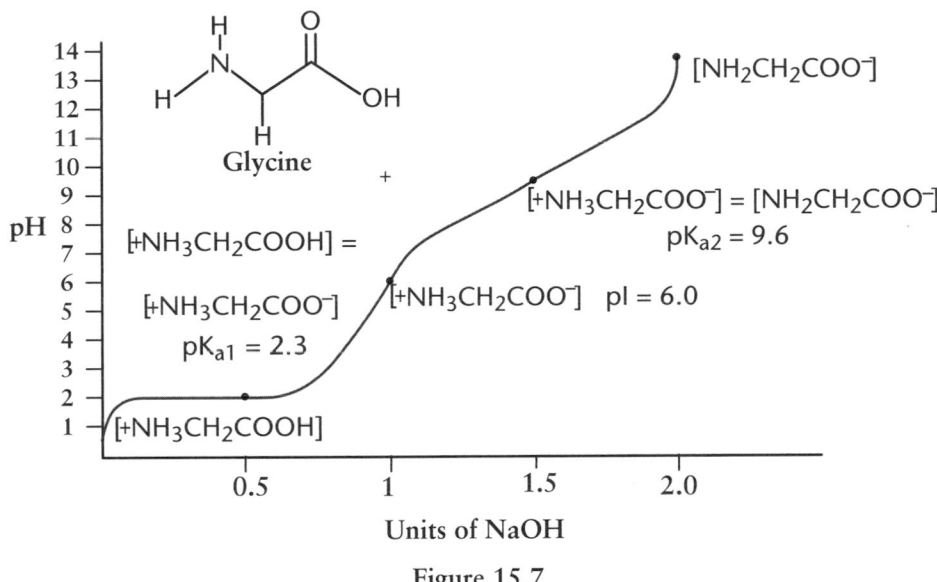

Figure 15.7

A 1M glycine solution is acidic; the glycine exists predominantly as $^+NH_3CH_2COOH$. The amino acid is fully protonated and carries a positive charge. As the solution is titrated with NaOH, carboxyl groups lose a proton. During this stage, the amino acid acts as a buffer and the pH changes very slowly. When 0.5 mol of base has been added to the amino acid solution, the concentrations of $^+NH_3CH_2COOH$ and $^+NH_3CH_2COO^-$ (its zwitterion) are equimolar. At this point the pH is equal to the pK_{a1}, and the solution is buffered against pH changes.

As more base is added, all of the carboxyl groups are deprotonated. The amino acid loses buffering capacity, and thus the pH rises more rapidly. When 1 mol of base has been added, glycine exists predominantly as $^+NH_3CH_2COO^-$. The amino acid is now electrically neutral; the pH is equal to glycine's pI.

Glycine passes through a second buffering stage during which pH change is slow because continued titration deprotonates amino groups. When 1.5 mol of base have been added, the concentrations of $^+NH_3CH_2COO^-$ and $NH_2CH_2COO^-$ are equimolar, and the pH is equal to pK_{a_2}.

As another 0.5 mol of base is added, all of the amino groups are deprotonated to $NH_2CH_2COO^-$; glycine is now completely deprotonated.

Certain things should be noted about the titration of amino acids:

1. When adding base, the carboxyl group loses its proton first; after all of the carboxyl groups are fully deprotonated, the amino group loses its acidic proton.

2. Two moles of base must be added in order to deprotonate one mole of most amino acids. The first mole deprotonates the carboxyl group, while the second mole deprotonates the amino group.

3. The buffering capacity of the amino acid is greatest at or near the two dissociation constants, K_{a_1} and K_{a_2}. At the isoelectric point, its buffering capacity is minimal.

4. It is possible to perform the titration in reverse, from alkaline pH to acidic pH, with the addition of acid; the sequence of events is reversed.

C. HENDERSON-HASSELBALCH EQUATION

The ratio of an amino acid's ions are dependent on pH. The **Henderson-Hasselbalch equation** defines the relationship between pH and the ratio of conjugate acid to conjugate base, and provides a mathematical expression for the dissociation constants of amino acids.

$$pH = pK_a + \log \frac{[\text{conjugate base}]}{[\text{conjugate acid}]}$$

When the pK_{a_1} of glycine is known, the ratio of conjugate acid to conjugate base for a particular pH can be determined. For example, at pH 3.3, glycine which has a pK_a of 2.3, will have the ratios:

$$3.3 = 2.3 + \log \frac{[^+H_3NCH_2COO^-]}{[H_3N^+CH_2COH]}$$

$$\text{By subtraction: } \log \frac{[H_3N^+CH_2COO^-]}{[H_3N^+CH_2COOH]} = 1$$

The antilog of 1 = 10, thus: $\dfrac{[H_3N^+CH_2COO^-]}{[H_3N^+CH_2COOH]} = \dfrac{10}{1}$

So, in this example, there are 10 times as many zwitterions as there are of the fully protonated form.

The Henderson-Hasselbach equation can be used experimentally to prepare buffer solutions of amino acids. The best buffering regions of amino acids occur within one pH unit of the pK_a or pK_b. For example, the carboxyl group of glycine, which has a pK_a of 2.6, shows high buffering capacity between pH 1.6 and 3.6.

D. AMINO ACID SIDE-CHAINS

Amino acid side-chains (R-groups) give chemical diversity to the backbone of the amino acid molecule. They also give proteins some distinguishing features. The twenty amino acids are classified according to whether their side chains are **nonpolar**, **polar** (but uncharged), **acidic**, or **basic**.

1. **Nonpolar Amino Acids**

   Nonpolar amino acids have R-groups that are saturated hydrocarbons. The R-groups are hydrophobic and decrease the solubility of the amino acid in water. Amino acids with nonpolar side-chains are usually found buried within protein molecules, away from the aqueous cellular environment.

> **MCAT Synopsis**
>
> Nonpolar amino acids are often found at the core of globular proteins or in transmembrane regions of proteins that are in contact with the hydrophobic portion of the phospholipid membrane.

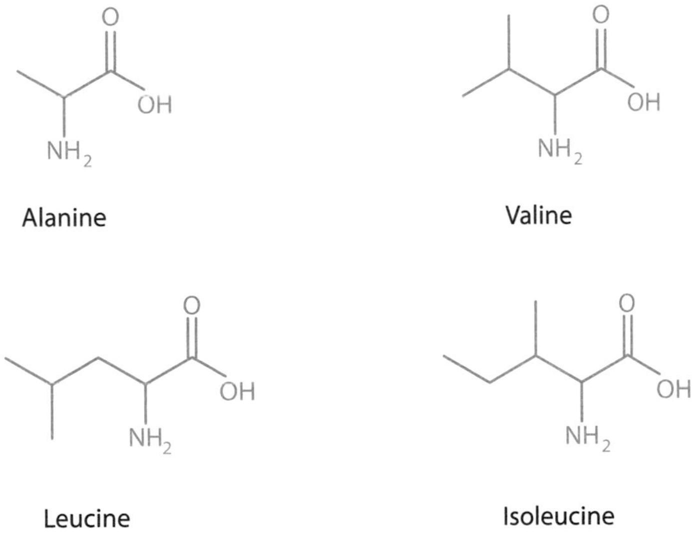

Alanine

Valine

Leucine

Isoleucine

Figure 15.8a

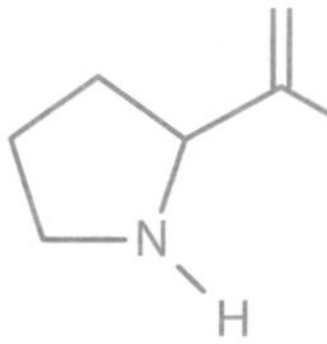

Proline

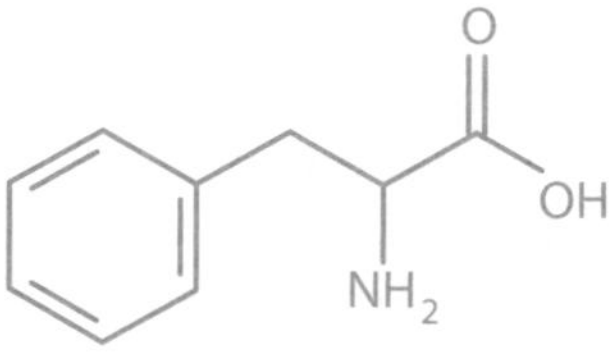

Phenylalanine

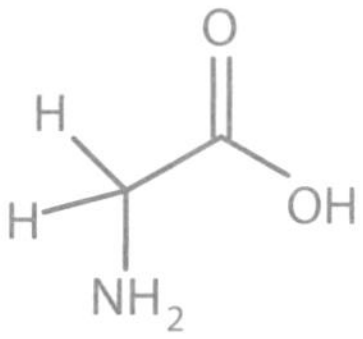

Glycine

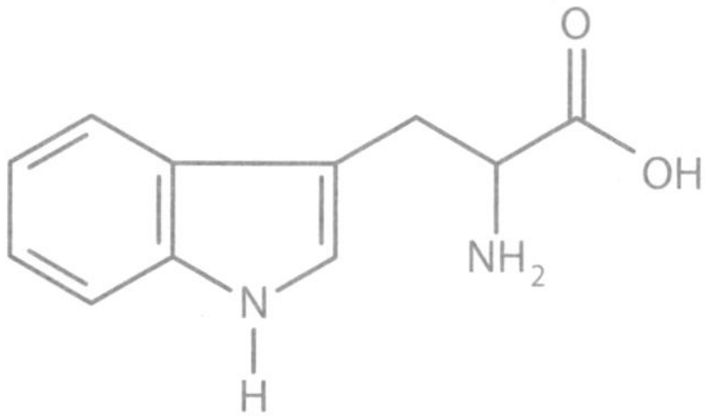

Tryptophan

Figure 15.8b

> **MCAT Synopsis**
>
> The other types of amino acids (polar, acidic and basic) are found in regions of proteins that are exposed to the aqueous, polar environment.

2. **Polar Amino Acids**

   Polar amino acids have polar, uncharged R-groups that are hydrophilic, increasing the solubility of the amino acid in water. They are usually found on protein surfaces.

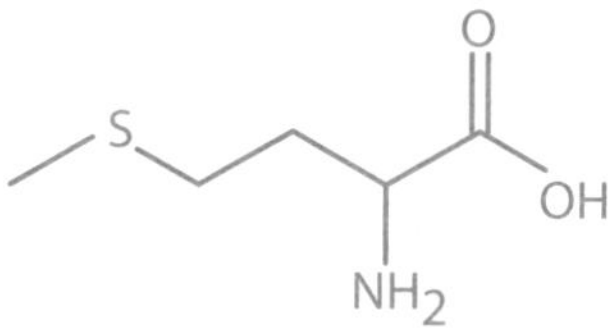

Methionine

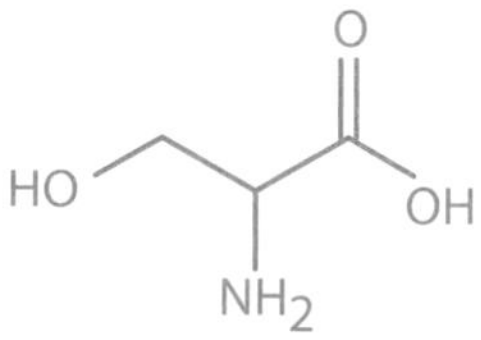

Serine

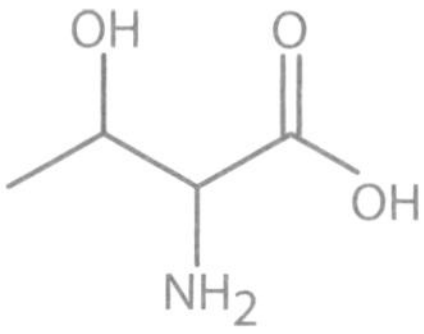

Threonine

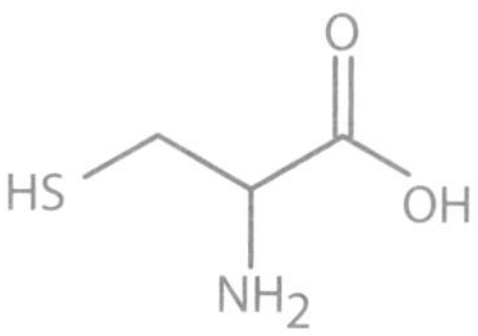

Cysteine

Figure 15.9a

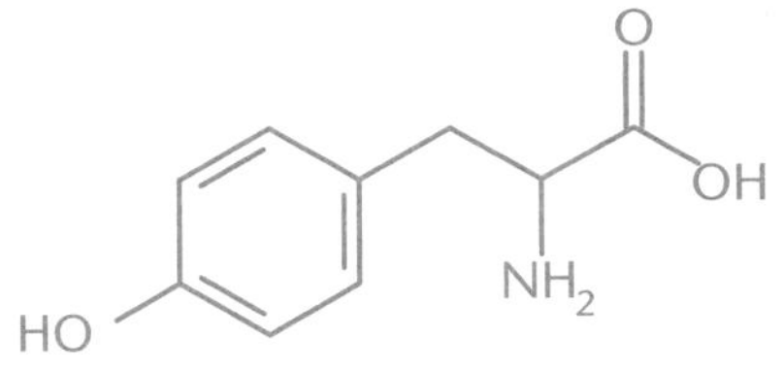

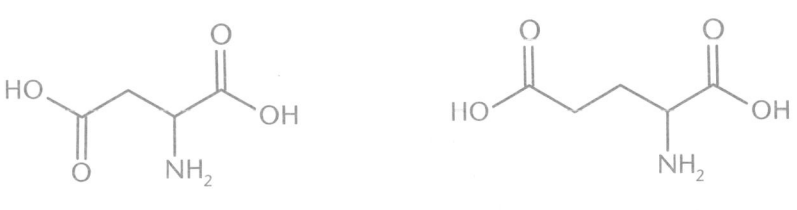

Tyrosine

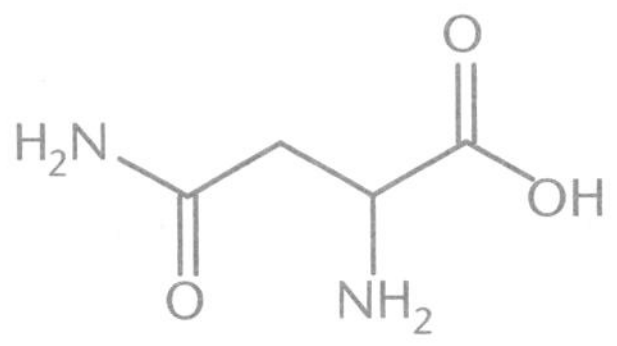

Asparagine

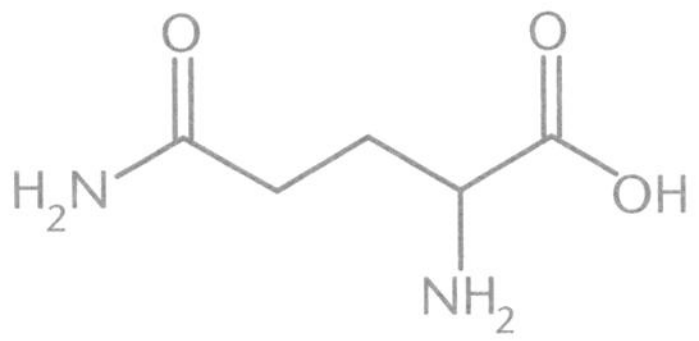

Glutamine

Figure 15.9b

3. **Acidic Amino Acids**

   Amino acids whose R-group contains a carboxyl group are called acidic amino acids. They have a net negative charge at physiological pH (pH 7.4),

> **MCAT Synopsis**
>
> Acidic amino acids have a negative charge at physiologic pH (pH 7.4). They have three distinct pK_a's.

Aspartic Acid

Glutamic Acid

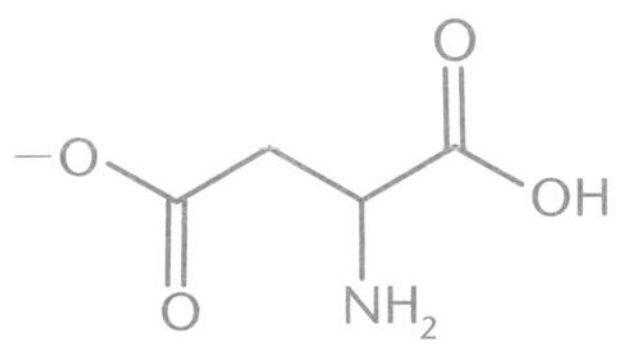

(Salt is Aspartate)

(Salt is Glutamate)

Figure 15.10

Aspartic acid and glutamic acid each have three groups that must be neutralized during titration (two –COOH and one $-NH_3^+$). Therefore, their titration curve is different from the standard curve for amino acids (exemplified by glycine). The molecule has three distinct dissociation constants (pK_{a1}, pK_{a2}, and pK_{a3}) although the neutralization curves of the two carboxyl groups overlap to a certain extent.

Because of the additional carboxyl group, the isoelectric point is shifted toward an acidic pH. Three moles of base are needed to deprotonate one mole of an acidic amino acid.

4. **Basic Amino Acids**

Amino acids whose R-group contains an amino group are called basic amino acids and carry a net positive charge at physiological pH.

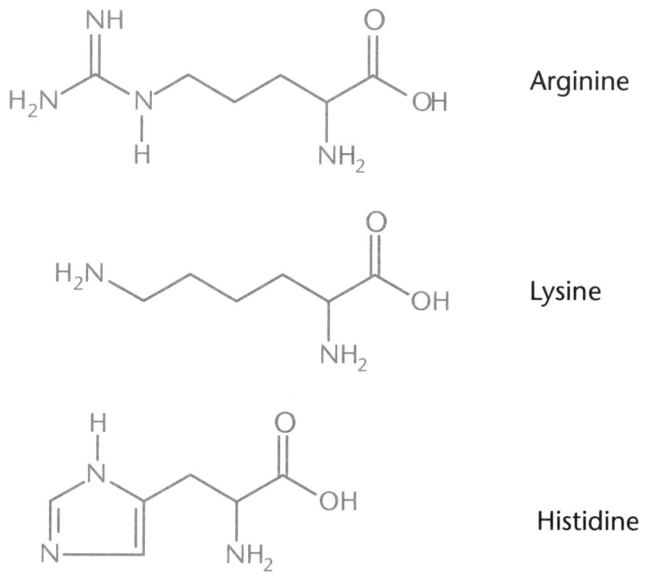

Arginine

Lysine

Histidine

Figure 15.11

The titration curve of amino acids with basic R-groups is modified by the additional amino group that must be neutralized. Although basic amino acids have three dissociation constants, the neutralization curves for the two amino groups overlap. The isoelectric point is shifted toward an alkaline pH. Three moles of acid are needed to neutralize one mole of a basic amino acid.

Understanding titration curves and isoelectric points helps predict the charge of particular amino acids at a given pH. For example, in a mixture of glycine, glutamic acid, and lysine at pH 6.0, glycine will be neutral, glutamic acid will be negatively charged, and lysine will be positively charged.

PEPTIDES

Peptides are composed of amino acid subunits, sometimes called **residues**, linked by **peptide bonds**. Peptides are small proteins (the distinction between a peptide and protein is vague). Two amino acids joined together form a **dipeptide**, three form a **tripeptide**, and many amino acids linked together form a **polypeptide.**

A. REACTIONS

Amino acids are joined by **peptide bonds** (amide bonds) between the carboxyl group of one amino acid and the amino group of another. This bond is formed via a condensation reaction (a reaction in which water is lost). The reverse reaction, hydrolysis (cleavage with the addition of water) of the peptide bond, is catalyzed by an acid or base.

Certain enzymes digest the chain at specific peptide linkages. For example, **trypsin** cleaves at the carboxyl end of arginine and lysine; chymotrypsin cleaves at the carboxyl end of phenylalanine, tyrosine, and tryptophan.

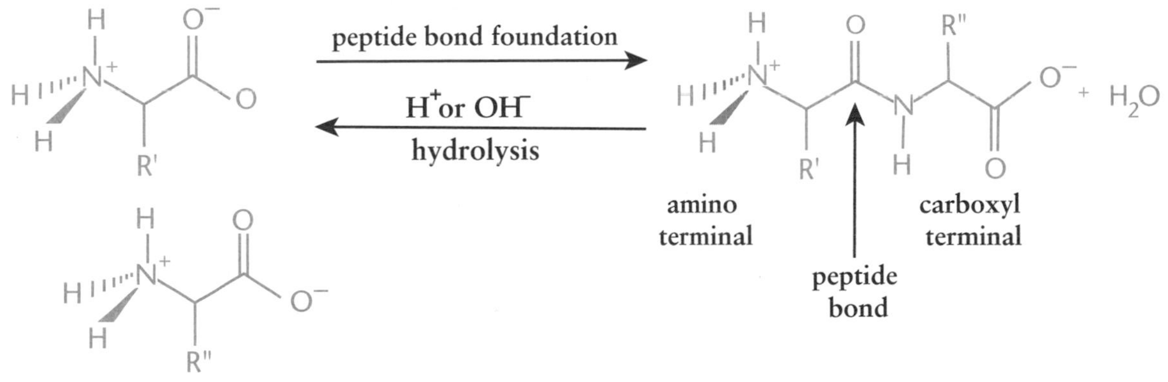

Figure 15.12

B. PROPERTIES

The terminal amino acid with a free alpha-amino group is known as the **amino-terminal** or **N-terminal** residue, while the terminal residue with a free carboxyl group is called the **carboxy-terminal** or **C-terminal** residue. By convention, peptides are drawn with the N-terminal end on the left and the C-terminal end on the right.

Amides have two resonance structures, and the true structure is a hybrid with partial double-bond character. As a result, rotation about the C–N bond is restricted. The bonds on either side of the peptide unit, however, have a great deal of rotational freedom.

> **MCAT Synopsis**
>
> Rotation is limited around the peptide bond because resonance gives the C–N bond partial double bond character.

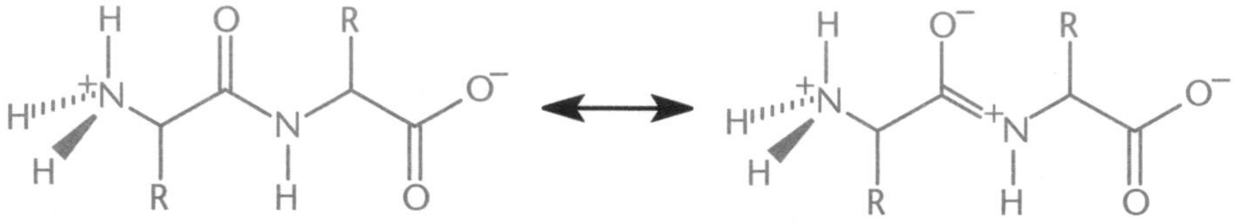

Figure 15.13

PROTEINS

Proteins are polypeptides that can range from only a few to more than a thousand amino acids in length. Proteins serve many diverse functions in biological systems, acting as enzymes, hormones, membrane pores, receptors, and elements of cell structure. Four structural levels of protein structure—**primary, secondary, tertiary,** and **quaternary**—are described below.

A. PRIMARY STRUCTURE

The primary structure of the protein refers to the sequence of amino acids, listed from the N-terminal to the C-terminal, and covalent bonds between residues in the chain. The most common of these bonds is a disulfide bond; two **cysteine** molecules become oxidized to form **cystine**, which has a disulfide bond. Disulfide bonds create loops in the protein chain.

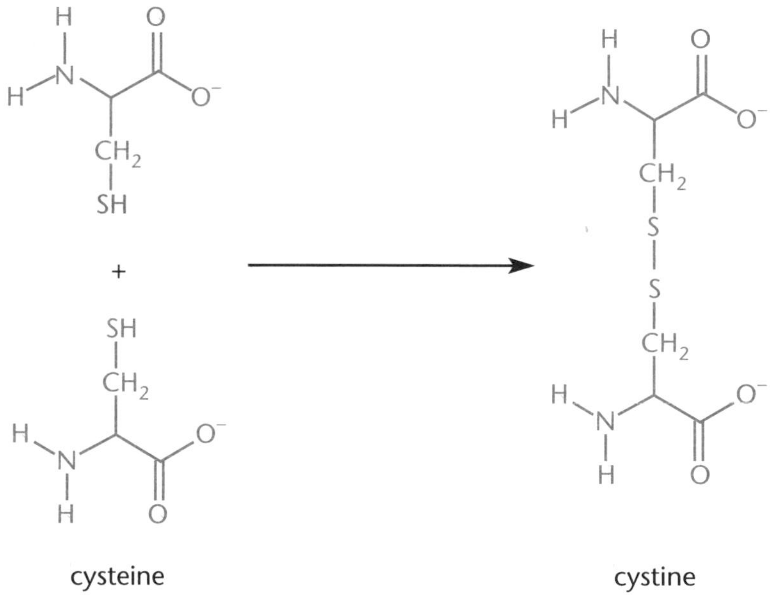

cysteine   cystine

Figure 15.14

The higher-level structures of a protein are dependent on the primary sequence; in other words, a protein will assume whatever secondary, tertiary, and quaternary structures are most energetically favorable given its primary structure and environment. The primary structure of a protein can be determined using a laboratory procedure called **sequencing**.

B. SECONDARY STRUCTURE

The secondary structure of a protein refers to the local structure of neighboring amino acids, governed mostly by hydrogen bond interactions within and between peptide chains. The two most common types of secondary structures are the **α-helix** and the **β-pleated sheet**.

1. **α-Helix**

   α-helix is a rodlike structure in which the peptide chain coils clockwise about a central axis. The helix is stabilized by intramolecular hydrogen bonds between carbonyl oxygen atoms and amine hydrogen atoms four residues away. The side-chains point away from the structure's core and interact with the cellular environment. A typical protein with this structure is **keratin**, which is found in feathers and hair.

2. **β-Pleated Sheet**

   In β-pleated sheets, the peptide chains lie alongside each other in rows. The chains are held together by intramolecular hydrogen bonds between carbonyl oxygen atoms on one peptide chain and amine hydrogen atoms on another. In order to accommodate the maximum number of hydrogen bonds, the β-pleated sheet assumes a rippled, or pleated, shape. The R-groups of the amino residues point above and below the plane of the β-pleated sheet. Silk fibers are composed of β-pleated sheets.

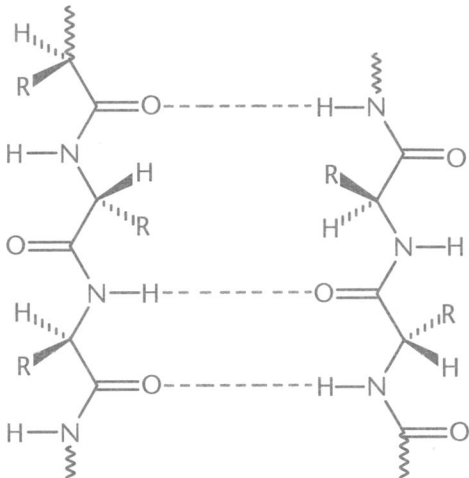

Figure 15.15: β-Pleated Sheet

C. TERTIARY STRUCTURE

Tertiary structure refers to the three-dimensional shape of the protein, as determined by hydrophilic and hydrophobic interactions between the R-groups of amino acids that are far apart on the chain.

Certain individual amino acids have significant effects on tertiary structure. For instance, disulfide bonds will cause loops and twists. Proline, because of its shape, cannot fit into an α-helix, and its presence causes a kink in the chain.

Amino acids with hydrophilic (polar and charged) R-groups tend to arrange themselves toward the outside of the protein, where they interact with the aqueous cellular environment. Amino acids with hydrophobic R-groups tend to be found close together, protected from the aqueous environment by polar amino and carboxyl groups.

Proteins are divided into two major classifications on the basis of tertiary structure. **Fibrous proteins**, such as **collagen**, are found as sheets or long strands, while **globular proteins**, such as **myoglobin**, are spherical in shape.

D. QUATERNARY STRUCTURE

Some proteins contain more than one polypeptide subunit. The quaternary structure refers to the way in which these subunits arrange themselves to yield a functional protein molecule. **Hemoglobin**, which is composed of four polypeptide chains, possesses quaternary structure.

E. CONJUGATED PROTEINS

Some proteins, known as **conjugated proteins**, derive part of their function from covalently attached molecules called **prosthetic groups**. Prosthetic groups may be organic molecules or metal ions. Many vitamins are prosthetic groups. Proteins with lipid, carbohydrate, and nucleic acid prosthetic groups are called **lipoproteins**, **glycoproteins**, and **nucleoproteins**, respectively. Prosthetic groups play major roles in determining the function of the proteins with which they are associated. For example, the **heme group** carries oxygen in both myoglobin and hemoglobin. The heme is composed of an organic porphyrin ring with an iron atom bound in the center. Hemoglobin is inactive without the heme group.

F. DENATURATION OF PROTEINS

Denaturation, or **melting**, is a process in which proteins lose their three-dimensional structure and revert to a **random-coil** state. Denaturation can be caused by detergent, or by changes in pH, temperature, or solute concentration. The weak intermolecular forces keeping the protein stable and functional are disrupted. When a protein denatures, the damage is usually permanent. However, certain gentle denaturing agents do not permanently disrupt the protein. Removing the reagent might allow the protein to **renature** (regain its structure and function).

> **MCAT Synopsis**
>
> Denaturation is the loss of three-dimensional structure.

Organic Chemistry
Practice Set

Use this practice set to evaluate your mastery
of the Organic Chemistry section of the test.

Read the explanations to all the practice
problems, and revisit the chapters that relate to
weak areas.

Good luck.

Organic Chemistry Practice Set

Passage I (Questions 1-8)

In organic synthesis reactions, functional groups are reacted to produce other functional groups. When a molecule contains two or more functional groups with similar reactivities, but only one needs to be changed, the other group must be "protected." Aldehydes and ketones can be protected from many unwanted reactions by conversion into acetals and ketals (or, better, cyclic ketals). Ketals, which are stable in basic solution, are formed by the reaction:

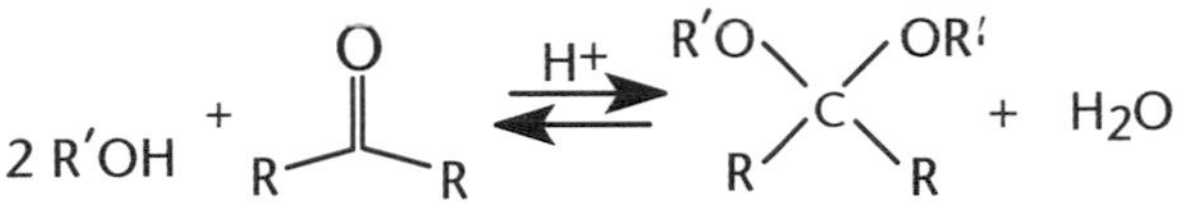

Reaction 1

This reaction is useful in a number of cases, one of which is illustrated below.

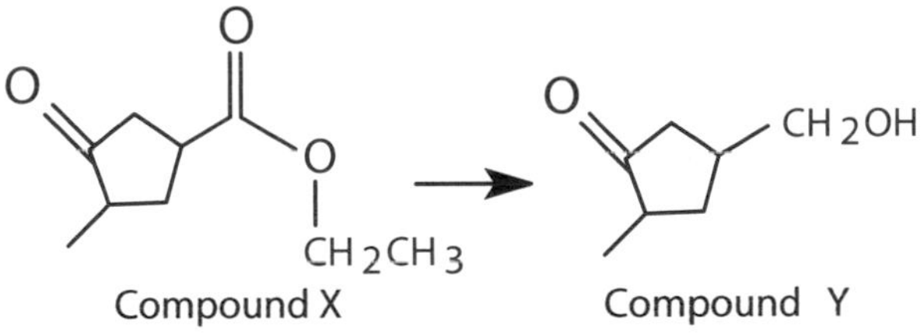

Reaction 2

The ester group of Compound X could be reduced to the desired alcohol by treatment with a reducing agent, such as lithium aluminum hydride (LAH). However, LAH would also react with the ketone group of Compound Y, since ketones are even more reactive than esters. To avoid this, the ketone is reacted with a diol to convert it to a cyclic ketal. Reaction of the ketal with a reducing agent, followed by removal of the diol with aqueous acid, gives Compound Y.

Protection of amino acid functional groups is an absolute requirement for polypeptide synthesis in the laboratory. For instance, consider the synthesis of the alanine-leucine dipeptide below. Activating the carboxyl group of alanine to react with leucine's amino group poses a problem, because the activated amino acid will also react with itself. Phenylacetyl chloride is used to protect the amino group; this substance can easily be removed with HBr in acetic acid. The carboxyl group of alanine is activated by normal means and can then be reacted with leucine.

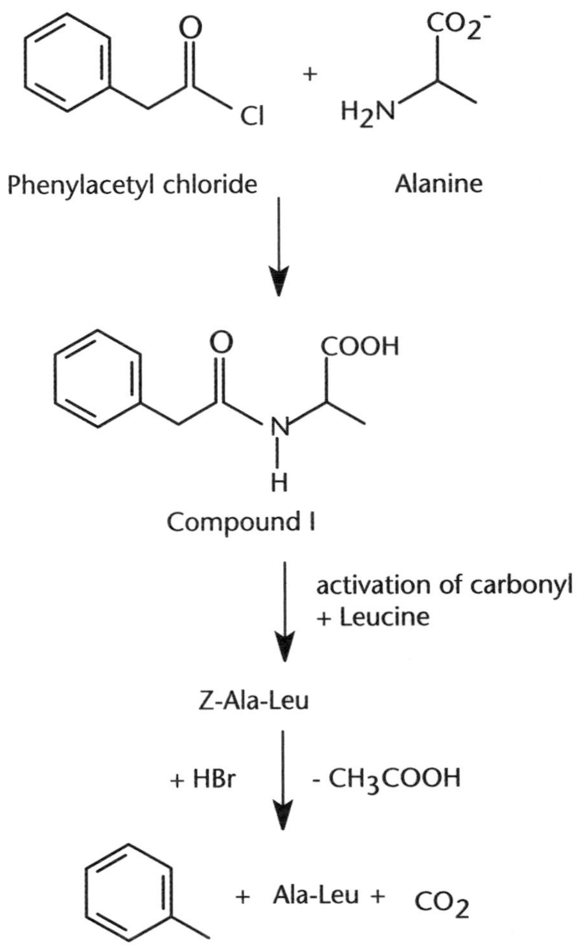

Figure 1

1. Which of the following compounds would best protect the ketone carbonyl group in Compound X?

A.

OH OH
(CH₃)₂CH   CH(CH₃)₂

(CH₃)₂CH   CH(CH₃)₂

C.

CH₃
   ⟩— CH₂OH
CH₃

B.

HOH₂C ⟍⟋⟍ CH₂OH

D.

HOH₂C — CH₂OH

2. Which of the following products would be formed if Compound X were reacted with LiAlH₄ without first being converted to a cyclic ketal?

A. H₃CH₂CO   O
    O═⟍⟍⟋   CH₂

C.
    HO⟍⟍   CO₂⁻

B.
    OH
    CH₂
HO⟍⟍

D.
    OH
    CH₂

3. Based on the information in the passage, which of the following reagents would be most likely to accomplish the reactions below?

S
⟍⟋⟍N   S   S   O
   ⟍N   →   ⟍⟋⟍N   →   ⟍⟋⟍N
   N   N   N

Compound I   Compound II   Compound III

A. C₃H₅CH₂SH followed by HCl
B. CH₃CH₂SH followed by dilute NaOH
C. HSCH₂CH₂SH followed by HCl
D. HSCH₂CH₂SH followed by dilute NaOH

4. In the reaction of alanine with phenylacetyl chloride shown in the passage, the amino group of alanine most likely acts as:

A. a nucleophile, attacking the electrophilic carbonyl carbon of phenylacetyl chloride.
B. an electrophile, being attacked by the carbonyl carbon of phenylacetyl chloride.
C. a nucleophile, attacking the electrophilic carbonyl oxygen atom of phenylacetyl chloride.
D. an oxidizing agent.

5. Once alanine's amino group is protected, its carboxyl group could be activated, thereby promoting its reaction with leucine to form a peptide bond, by:

A. converting it to an acyl chloride with SOCl₂.
B. heating the solution.
C. adding aqueous base.
D. esterifying the acid functionality by adding excess alcohol and HCl.

6. Chemists prefer to protect carbonyl groups by converting them to ketals or acetals rather than ethers. This is because, compared with acetals and ketals, ether groups are:

A. more susceptible to acidic cleavage.
B. less susceptible to acidic cleavage.
C. more susceptible to basic cleavage.
D. less susceptible to basic cleavage.

7. Which of the following pH values is likely to favor the form of the alanine molecule shown in the passage?

A. 3.0
B. 7.0
C. 9.0
D. Cannot be determined

8. What is the IUPAC name of Compound X?

A. 3-Methyl-2-oxocyclopentyl ethanoate
B. Ethoxy 3-methyl-2-oxocyclopentyl ester
C. 3-Ethoxy-5-methylcyclopentanone
D. Ethyl (4-methyl-3-oxocyclopentane) carboxylate

Passage II (Questions 9–12)

Coke is an essential hydrocarbon in the industrial conversion of iron to steel. Heating coal in the absence of air, followed by distillation, results in the formation of coke and a liquid known as coal tar. Among the components of these two substances are many polycyclic organic compounds, such as naphthalene, benzo[a]pyrene, anthracene, phenanthrene, and cholanthrene (shown in Figure 1), many of which are known to pose health hazards to humans.

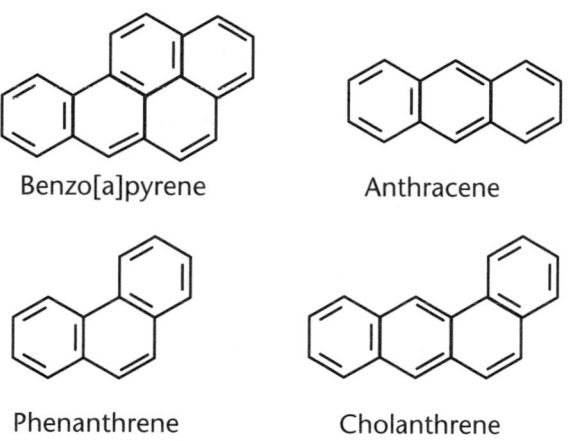

Benzo[a]pyrene   Anthracene

Phenanthrene   Cholanthrene

Figure 1

The effects of benzo[a]pyrene, which is also produced in significant quantities by other industrial processes including internal combustion, have been studied extensively. Benzo[a]pyrene is biotransformed, or metabolized, in the liver by the series of reactions shown in Figure 2. An oxidase enzyme adds an epoxide group to the molecule at C_7 and C_8. Another enzyme, an epoxide hydroxylase, cleaves the epoxide ring creating a trans diol. A second epoxidation at C_9 and C_{10} creates the final biotransformation product, which is a potent carcinogen.

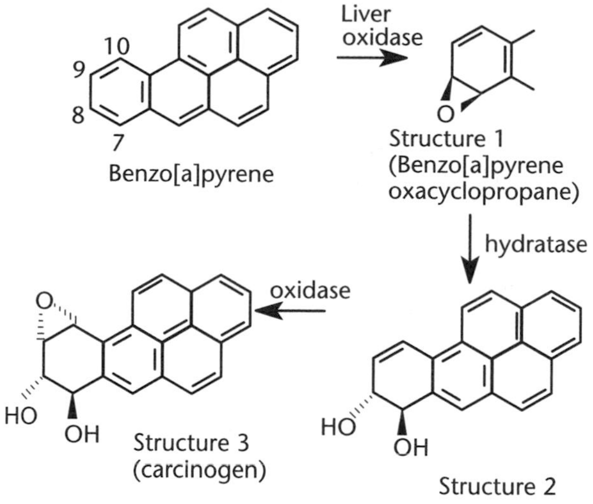

Benzo[a]pyrene

Structure 1
(Benzo[a]pyrene
oxacyclopropane)

Structure 3
(carcinogen)

Structure 2

Figure 2

The carcinogenic effect of this compound is due to its interaction with DNA. When the compound comes into contact with a DNA strand, it can bind covalently to a guanine nucleotide as shown in Figure 3. During DNA replication, the resulting adduct structure may bind to the wrong complementary nucleotide, thereby producing a mutation.

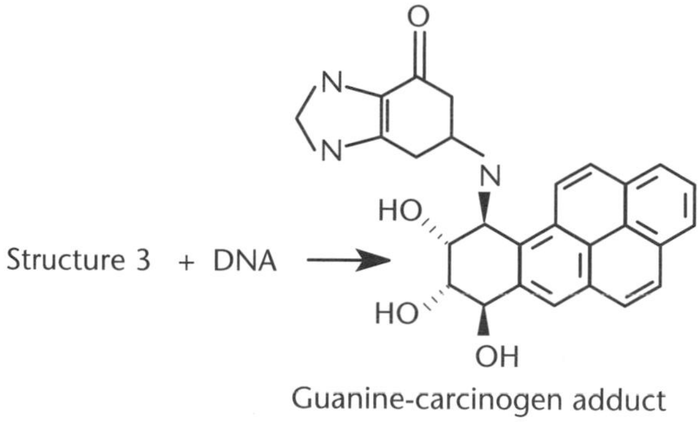

Structure 3 + DNA →

Guanine-carcinogen adduct

Figure 3

597

9. If the intermediate metabolite Structure 1 were isolated, what reagents and conditions could be used to convert it into Structure 2 in the laboratory?

    A. $KMnO_4$, H_2O, 0°C
    B. OsO_4, THF, 25°C
    C. H_2SO_4, H_2O
    D. HNO_3, H_2SO_4

10. What is the most likely explanation for the evolution of the liver biotransformation pathway described in Figure 2?

    A. The pathway transforms a number of different compounds, making some more toxic and some less toxic, with the overall effect of increasing an organism's survival ability.
    B. The pathway increases the rate of frameshift mutations and thereby enhances an individual organism's ability to adapt to its environment.
    C. The pathway increases an organism's survival ability in a polluted environment by detoxifying benzo[a]pyrene and related polycyclic organic compounds.
    D. The pathway's transformation of benzo[a]pyrene served an important function in an ancestral species and has not yet undergone enough selection to disappear.

11. The carcinogen's physiological activity is facilitated by its water solubility, which is far greater than that of benzo[a]pyrene. Which of the following statements correctly explains this solubility difference?

    A. The higher the molecular weight of a compound, the greater its solubility in water.
    B. The greater the number of ring substituents on an aromatic compound, the greater its solubility in water.
    C. The more polar a compound, the greater its solubility in water.
    D. The more saturated an organic compound, the greater its solubility in water.

12. Given the stereochemistry of the opening of Structure 1's epoxide ring by the hydratase enzyme, how is the new oxygen atom added to the substrate?

    A. At C–7, from the same side of the six-membered ring as the epoxide oxygen.
    B. At C–8, from the same side of the six-membered ring as the epoxide oxygen.
    C. At C–7, from the side of the six-membered ring opposite to the epoxide oxygen.
    D. At C–8, from the side of the six-membered ring opposite to the epoxide oxygen.

Questions 13 through 15 are NOT based on a descriptive passage.

13. If chlorobenzene is treated with sulfur trioxide (SO_3) and concentrated sulfuric acid, what will be the major product(s)?

    A. benzenesulfonic acid
    B. *m*-chlorobenzenesulfonic acid
    C. *o*- and *p*-chlorobenzenesulfonic acid
    D. benzene

14. Which of the following occurs during the reaction below?

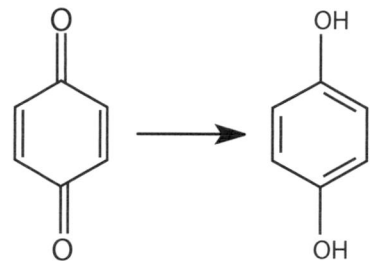

Quinone   Hydroquinone

    A. Quinone loses two electrons and gains two protons.
    B. Quinone gains two electrons and two protons.
    C. Quinone loses four electrons and gains two protons.
    D. Quinone gains four electrons and two protons.

15. Which of the following compounds can most easily undergo both E1 and S_N2 reactions?

    A. $(CH_3CH_2)_2CHCN$
    B. $(CH_3CH_2)_3CBr$
    C. $(CH_3CH_2)_3CCH_2Cl$
    D. $(CH_3CH_2)_2CHBr$

Passage III (Questions 16–20)

Ion-exchange chromatography (IEC) is a powerful laboratory tool that effectively separates compounds according to their net charges. An experimenter decides to use an IEC device to separate, identify, and measure the concentrations of different amino acids in a mixture. The device consists of a vertical column rifled with beads made of a special resin; each bead has a large number of carboxylate groups on its surface.

The procedure for analyzing the amino acid mixtures has three main steps:

In the first step, a mixture is added to the column at pH 3. This makes the amino acids bind to the negatively charged carboxylate groups on the bead surfaces.

In the second step, a specially programmed device washes the beads with a buffer made from sodium acetate (a carboxylate salt). The concentration of the buffer is kept constant, but the pH is gradually increased by the IEC device. The pH gradient eventually causes the sodium cations to displace the amino acid molecules from the beads. The device collects the eluted fractions in a series of tubes. For each fraction, the instrument measures the elution volume, which is the amount of solution that has passed through the column before the point at which that fraction is eluted. As shown in Figure 1, the buffer solution elutes several different amino acids as distinct fractions; and the individual fractions can be identified by comparing their elution volumes with those of known amino acid standards.

In the third step, the fractions are treated with ninhydrin, which reacts with primary amino groups to form a product with a characteristic blue color. The colored fractions are then analyzed by a spectrophotometer, which measures the amino acid concentrations as a function of optical absorbance.

16. Concentrations of which of the following amino acids could NOT be measured using the method described in the passage?

A. Phenylalanine

B. Proline

C. Tyrosine

D. Tryptophan

17. It can be inferred from the passage that an amino acid will be eluted most efficiently if its pI is:

A. lower than the pH of a sodium acetate solution.
B. equal to the pH of a sodium acetate solution.
C. higher than the pH of a sodium acetate solution.
D. higher than its pK_{a1}.

18. Which of the following graphs best represents the titration curve of Fraction F?

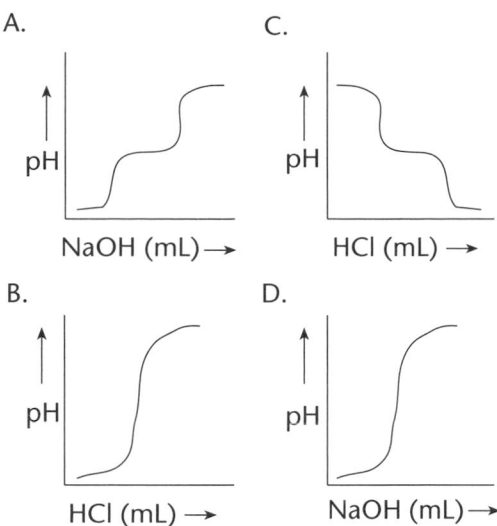

A.

pH | NaOH (mL) →

B.

pH | HCl (mL) →

C.

pH | HCl (mL) →

D.

pH | NaOH (mL) →

19. If a mixture of fractions B, D, and E were placed in a gel and subjected to isoelectric focusing, which of the following patterns of bands would be observed?

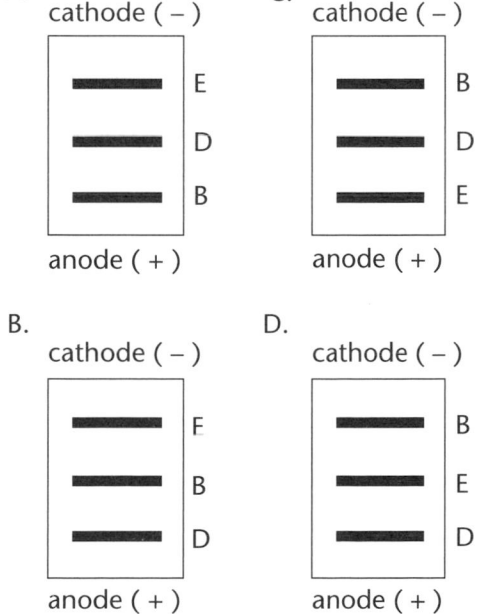

A.

cathode (–)

E
D
B

anode (+)

B.

cathode (–)

F
B
D

anode (+)

C.

cathode (–)

B
D
E

anode (+)

D.

cathode (–)

B
E
D

anode (+)

20. If a larger sample of the same mixture were separated on the IEC column, how would the results differ from those described in the passage?

A. The elution volume would be larger for each fraction.
B. The elution volume would be smaller for each fraction.
C. The separation of the fractions would be more distinct.
D. The separation of the fractions would be less distinct.

Passage IV (Questions 21–25)

Triglyceride molecules, the major components of fat deposits in animals, are composed of three fatty acid subunits attached to a glycerol molecule. Glycerol (1,2,3-propanetriol) is produced as a side-product in various metabolic pathways. Fatty acids are synthesized from 2-carbon acetyl groups by repetitions of a series of five steps, with each repetition using up one acetyl group and adding two carbons to the growing molecule. Figure 1 gives a slightly simplified version of this pathway, starting with acetyl CoA and showing the first repetition of the five reaction steps.

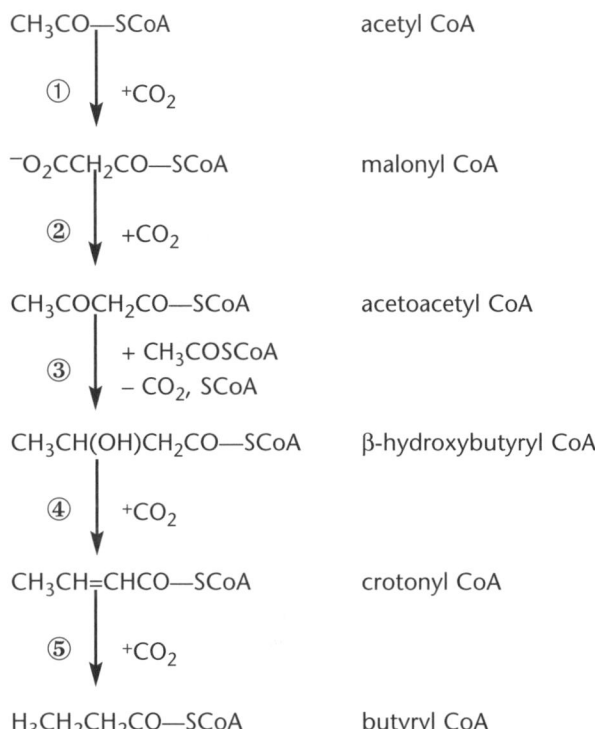

Figure 1

Butyryl CoA subsequently reacts with another acetyl CoA molecule to form β-ketocaproyl CoA ($CH_3CH_2CH_2COCH_2CO–SCoA$), and the cycle repeats several times until stearyl CoA [$CH_3(CH_2)_{16}COSCoA)$] is produced.

The fatty acid-CoA thioester molecules used by the pathway are formed from carboxylic acids; this process is known as activation of the carboxylic acids, and can occur by two different mechanisms.

In the heart, liver, and kidney, fatty acids react with CoA and ATP as follows:

$$RCH_2COOH + HSCoA + ATP \rightarrow RCH_2COSCoA + AMP$$

In peripheral tissues, fatty acids obtain CoA moieties through reversible reactions with other acyl CoA compounds, such as acetyl CoA or succinyl CoA, that have been imported into the cell.

21. In which two reactions of fatty acid biosynthesis does the α-carbon of the initial acetyl CoA molecule undergo a change in hybridization state?

    A. 1 and 3
    B. 2 and 3
    C. 3 and 4
    D. 4 and 5

22. Which of the following would be the most descriptive name for the enzyme that catalyzes reaction 3?

    A. β-carboxyisomerase
    B. β-ketoreductase
    C. β-acyltransferase
    D. β-ketooxidase

23. In the absence of crotonase, which catalyzes reaction 4, which of the following compounds could be most easily dehydrated by heating in acid?

    A. $(CH_3)_2COHCH_2CO–SCoA$
    B. $CH_3CHOHCH(CH_3)CO–SCoA$
    C. $CH_3CHOHCH_2CO–SCoA$
    D. $HOCH_2CH_2CO–SCoA$

24. A researcher has developed an in vitro system for carrying out the enzymatic fatty acid synthesis process in the laboratory. As substrate for this system, he uses acetyl CoA in which one carbon atom has been labeled with radioactive ^{14}C. His results show that all of the compounds in the pathway have become radioactive. What can he conclude?

    I. The labeled carbon atom could have been the carbon atom in the $^-CH_3$ group.

    II. The CO_2 released in Step 2 will be radioactive.

    III. The labeled carbon atom could not have been part of the CoA moiety.

    A. I only
    B. II only
    C. I and III only
    D. I, II, and III

25. In which of the following ways will the predominant β-enol form of acetoacetyl CoA be unlike the β-hydroxybutyryl molecule?

    A. The number of bonds to the β-carbon
    B. The number of hydrogen atoms attached to the α- and β-carbons
    C. The number of hydroxyl groups attached to the β-carbon
    D. The number of hydrogen atoms attached to the γ-carbon

Questions 26 and 27 are NOT based on a descriptive passage.

26. Which of the following acids is likely to have the weakest conjugate base?

    A. $H_2NCH_2CO_2H$
    B. $(CH_3)_3CCO_2H$
    C. $CH_3CH_2CO_2H$
    D. Cl_2CHCO_2H

27. For the reaction below, what is the most likely structure of Intermediate X?

$$(CH_3)_3CCH_2C=OCH_3 + H_2O + H^+ \rightleftharpoons X$$

$$\rightleftharpoons (CH_3)_3CCH_2C(OH)_2CH_3$$

A.

B.

C.

D.

Organic Chemistry Practice Set:
Answers and Explanations

ANSWER KEY

1. D	8. D	15. D	22. B
2. B	9. C	16. B	23. A
3. C	10. A	17. A	24. A
4. A	11. C	18. C	25. B
5. A	12. D	19. A	26. D
6. B	13. C	20. D	27. D
7. C	14. B	21. D	

EXPLANATIONS

Passage I (Questions 1–8)

1. D The method of protecting carbonyl groups given in the passage is to convert them to ketals by reacting them with alcohols; the structure of a ketal can be seen in Reaction 1. All four choices are alcohols, so you need to figure out which one will form the best ketal. The passage states, in the first paragraph, that carbonyls are protected more effectively by conversion to cyclic ketals. As you can see from Reaction 1, a noncyclic ketal is formed when a carbonyl group reacts with the hydroxyl groups of two alcohol molecules. Therefore, it is reasonable to suppose that a cyclic ketal can be formed by the reaction between a carbonyl group and a diol. So, choice (C), which contains just one hydroxyl group, would form a non-cyclic ketal and can be rejected right away. All the other choices are diols—choice (B) is a *trans* unsaturated 1,4-diol, and choices (A) and (D) are 1,2-diols. In choice (B), the hydroxyl groups are not adjacent, and the mobility of the carbon skeleton is quite limited due to the presence of the trans double bond; therefore, it would be impossible to form a cyclic ketal. Both remaining choices are 1,2-diols, but choice (A) has four isopropyl substituents—it is more sterically hindered, and therefore less reactive.

2. B The passage states that lithium aluminum hydride will reduce the ester group to an alcohol and would also react with the ketone if left unprotected. Therefore, choice (A), which shows the ketone group still intact, is wrong. You should also be able to eliminate choice (C). The passage and the diagram of Compound Y both indicate that the ester group is reduced to a CH_2OH alcohol group. So choice (C), which has it converted to a carboxyl group, is wrong. Finally, to choose between choices (B) and (D), you have to think about the effect of the reducing agent on the ketone group. You should know that lithium aluminum hydride is NOT a strong enough reagent to completely remove the oxygen atom and reduce the compound to the alkane form. Therefore, choice (D) is wrong, and choice (B) is the correct answer.

3. C The phrase "based on the information in the passage" in the question stem indicates that you need to look for analogies between the reaction shown in this question and the passage material. You should be aware that thiols react with carbonyl groups in much the same way as alcohols. In addition, given that oxygen and sulfur occupy adjacent positions in Group 6 of the Periodic Table, it is reasonable to assume that a sulfide group will react similarly to a ketone group. You can see that compound II is a cyclic thioketal, so just as a diol was used to form a cyclic ketal, a dithiol would be needed to produce a cyclic thioketal. Thus, choices (A) and (B) can be rejected right away. Choice (D) is also wrong, because the passage says that ketals are stable under basic conditions, but are hydrolyzed under acidic conditions. Therefore, assuming that thioketals behave similarly, compound II wouldn't be affected by base but would be hydrolyzed by acid to produce compound III. Therefore, choice (C) is the correct answer.

4. A The amino group nitrogen, which has a lone electron pair, is nucleophilic. Since oxygen is strongly electronegative, the C-O double bond on phenylacetyl chloride is polarized, giving the oxygen a partial negative charge, and the carbon a partial positive charge. As a result of this charge distribution, the carbon is attacked by the nitrogen atom, resulting in displacement of the chloride and the formation of an amide link. So choice (A) is correct. Choice (B) is wrong because, as we've just seen, the amino group is electron-rich and therefore nucleophilic, so it can't be an electrophile. Likewise, choice (C) is wrong because the carbonyl oxygen is nucleophilic, not electrophilic. Finally, the replacement of the chloride by the amino group is a simple nucleophilic substitution; there's no oxidation, or for that matter reduction, involved in the process at all. So choice (D) is wrong.

5. A You're looking for a way to make the carboxyl group more reactive in order to facilitate peptide bond formation. Peptide bonds form by the nucleophilic attack of the amino group of an amino acid on the carboxyl group of another. The reaction of thionyl chloride with a carboxylic acid substitutes a chlorine atom for the carboxyl hydroxyl group, producing an acyl chloride. An acyl chloride is the most reactive of the various kinds of carboxylic acid derivatives, and certainly more so than the corresponding carboxylic acid. This is because the chloride ion is a much better leaving group than the hydroxide anion and is therefore more easily displaced by the nucleophilic attack of the amino group. Thus, choice (A) is correct. Choice (B) is wrong because heating the solution will have no effect on the structure of the carboxyl group. Increasing the temperature may or may not promote the reaction, depending on the thermodynamics of the reaction, but NOT by activating the carboxyl, which requires some kind of chemical modification. Choice (C) is also wrong, because adding aqueous base to compound I would result in the formation of a carboxylate anion. This would be even less reactive towards an amino nucleophile than the acid. Finally, esterification of the acid, choice (D), would replace the hydroxyl group by an alkoxide group (RO). This alkoxide group would be a poor leaving group, and therefore the ester would not be reac-

tive enough to form the peptide bond, so choice (D) is also wrong.

6. B The passage states that ketals are stable in basic solution and are hydrolyzed in an acidic solution. Because of this pH dependence, other functional groups in the molecule can be transformed in basic solution, leaving the ketal untouched; the ketal can then be removed, using a dilute acid solution, to give the original ketone. Ketals are preferred as protecting groups over ethers because ethers are particularly unreactive compounds—they're pretty stable in both basic and acidic solution. Consequently, while ketals can be cleaved by adding dilute acid, cleavage of ethers would require higher temperatures and a more concentrated acid.

7. C As with any nonpolar amino acid, the acidic, neutral, and basic forms of alanine roughly correspond to acidic, neutral, and basic values of pH. At their isoelectric point, amino acids exist predominantly in the zwitterion form: positively charged ammonium groups and negatively charged carboxylate groups. As the pH falls, the carboxylate groups gain hydrogen ions and become neutral, while the ammonium groups retain their positive charges, so the molecules exist predominantly as cations. In contrast, as the pH rises above the isoelectric point, the ammonium groups lose their extra hydrogens to form neutral amino groups, whereas the carboxylate groups remain negatively charged, so that the molecules become anions. The form of alanine shown in the passage is an anion, and since the highest pH value is represented by choice (C), it is the correct answer.

8. D Compound X is a complicated polyfunctional molecule which you have to name according to IUPAC rules. The highest priority group in compound X is the ester. The first part of the name of an ester is the alcohol part of the molecule. In this case, the alcohol from which the ester is formed is ethanol, so the first word in the name should be "Ethyl." Next we have to decide the name of the acid part of the molecule. Well, the main carbon chain of the acid is a cyclopentane ring. The ring has two substituents, the ketone oxygen and the methyl group. Of these two, the oxygen takes priority, and so the carbons of the ring are numbered counter-clockwise, with the one attached to the ester group being number one. This makes the ketone carbon number three, and the methyl carbon number four. Therefore, the acid from which the ester is formed is "4-methyl-3-oxocyclopentane carboxylic acid." So, putting these two parts of the molecule together, the full name of the ester is ethyl (4-methyl-3-oxocyclopentane) carboxylate, which is choice (D).

Passage II (Questions 9–12)

9. C The reaction in question is the conversion of the epoxide group into a *trans*-1,2-diol—that is, a ring opening. The chemical method that's commonly used to open an epoxide ring is treatment with acid and water. This causes the epoxide oxygen to become protonated making one of the adjacent carbons susceptible to nucleophilic attack. If that nucleophile is water, the result is the formation of a *trans*-1,2-diol—just as with the enzymatic reaction, so choice (C) is correct. None of the other choices will open the ring. Choices (A) and (B), potassium permanganate and osmium tetroxide, are both used to create diols from alkene functional groups by adding two hydroxyl groups simultaneously. The products of these reactions are actually *cis* diols, because both hydroxyl groups are added from the same side of the double bond. But, more importantly, neither one would convert an epoxide into a diol, so (A) and (B) are both wrong. Choice (D), a mixture of nitric and sulfuric acids, forms the highly electrophilic nitronium ion and is used for the nitration of benzene or other aromatic rings. It would probably add NO_2 groups in various places on the conjugated ring system, producing a mixture of products, none of which would be what you're looking for.

10. A This is a biology question stuck into the middle of this organic chemistry passage and because the question asks for the most LIKELY explanation, you have to think through each answer choice carefully and figure out the right answer by elimination. First, consider what you know about the pathway shown in Figure 2. According to the passage, the net result of this series of reactions is to produce a carcinogen from benzo[a]pyrene. It's not clear from the passage whether benzo[a]pyrene is carcinogenic before the transformation; however, the molecule clearly doesn't have all the functional groups that are present in the carcinogen, and based on Figure 3, this means that it can't bind to DNA and cause mutations by the same mechanism. So, it seems likely that benzo[a]pyrene is actually LESS carcinogenic, meaning that the biotransformation process actually makes the compound MORE deleterious. Choice (A) suggests that the pathway toxifies some compounds and detoxifies others, with the net effect being beneficial, presumably meaning that detoxification predominates. This theory is consistent with the fact that the pathway apparently makes benzo[a]pyrene more carcinogenic; and it also provides a justification for the pathway's existence. Also, this theory is consistent with the general properties of enzymes and with the function of the liver: Many enzymes can act on a variety of related compounds, and this seems particularly likely for those in the liver, since the liver processes a wide variety of substances. So, choice (A) is a likely answer. Choice (B) is wrong on a technicality: The mutation mechanism described at the end of the passage—substitution of an incorrect base for the correct base during the formation of a new DNA strand—is NOT frameshift mutation, but point substitution. Moreover, due to the redundancy of the genetic code, it is possible for a point substitution to yield the same amino acid; at worst, one amino acid will be substituted for another, leaving the rest of the amino acids intact. Choice (C), which says that the pathway detoxifies benzo[a]pyrene, must be incorrect since benzo[a]pyrene which is mutagenic and carcinogenic is definitely a toxin. Choice (D) is not completely implausible: The biotransformation of benzo[a]pyrene could once have served some useful function that no longer exists, and the negative effects might not yet have selected against it to the point of inactivating the pathway. However, since DNA structure has been the same since very early in evolutionary time, the negative effects of benzo[a]pyrene biotransformation, which are based on its attacking guanine residues, must always have been considerable. So, since the passage gives no evidence that there were ever any positive effects, choice (D) is an outside chance at best. Choice (A) is the most likely choice, and therefore the correct answer.

11. C Here you simply need to remember the general rules for solubility. If you look at the two compounds you're comparing, you will see that they have almost the same ring structure, but the carcinogen has additional functional groups that benzo[a]pyrene lacks—two hydroxyl groups and one epoxide group, both located at the same end of the molecule. Since oxygen atoms are extremely electronegative, the electron density will be pulled towards them making the molecule polar. On the other hand, benzo[a]pyrene has no electronegative groups; and since it is conjugated, its pi electrons are evenly distributed throughout the molecule, making it nonpolar. You should remember that as a general rule, polarized or ionizable molecules are more soluble than nonpolar molecules in a polar solvent like water—in other words, "like dissolves in like." Therefore, choice (C) correctly explains why structure three is more soluble in water than benzo[a]pyrene. Choices (A), (B), and (D) are all wrong. Each of these choices defines a relationship between solubility and some other property of a compound. While it is true that the molecular weight, the number of substituents, and the amount of saturation can all influence solubility, it is not a direct correlation. By far the most important factor determining solubility is the structure of the molecule and whether or not it is similar to the structure of the solvent.

12. D To answer this question, you have to look at the stereochemistry of the ring opening and think about the mechanism involved. After the reaction, one of the hydroxyl groups is oriented above the ring, and one of them is below. This is due to the fact that the epoxide is protonated and then one of its carbon atoms is attacked by water. When the water molecule attacks, it displaces the epoxide oxygen from the carbon it attacks and leaves that oxygen bonded to the other carbon. In other words, there is an S_N2 reaction and so the configuration of that carbon is inverted, forming a *trans*-diol. Getting back to the question; in Figure 2 the epoxide ring is shown as being above the plane of the main, flat, conjugated part of the molecule, so you should be able to see from Figure 3 that the OH group on carbon 7, which is still above the six-membered ring, is the one that's derived from the old epoxide oxygen. Thus, the OH group at carbon 8 must be the one derived from the

attacking water molecule—that is, the one containing the new oxygen atom, which must have attacked from below the six-membered ring.

Discrete Questions

13. C To answer this question, you must first recall that a mixture of sulfur trioxide and concentrated sulfuric acid is used to sulfonate aromatic compounds. This means that an SO_3H group is substituted onto the ring in place of one of the hydrogens. So, you can immediately eliminate choice (D), since you will definitely get some form of substituted ring. In addition, the SO_3H group will not REPLACE the chlorine of chlorobenzene, so choice (A) is also wrong. To decide between the remaining two choices, you have to think about the directing effects of the chloro substituent. All the halogen elements are *ortho-para* directing deactivators, therefore, the final product will be a mixture of *para-* and *ortho*-chlorobenzenesulfonic acid, choice (C).

14. B There are far more electrons than protons, so instead of counting all the electrons, look at the protons first. All four choices say that quinone gains two protons in the reaction. You can verify this: The ring has four protons, which don't change, and both ketone groups become hydroxyls, so they must gain one proton each. This means two positive charges have been added; however, both the quinone and the hydroquinone molecules are neutral, so in order for the charges to balance, quinone must also gain two negative charges.

15. D This question requires you to know the structural factors that favor E1 and S_N2 reactions. Generally speaking, E1, or unimolecular elimination, which proceeds in two steps via a carbocation intermediate, is favored by highly branched carbon chains, since more substituted carbons form more stable carbocations. In contrast, S_N2, or bimolecular nucleophilic substitution, which proceeds via a one-step displacement of a leaving group by a nucleophile, is favored by unbranched carbon chains, because the nucleophilic attack is strongly affected by steric hindrance. Therefore, choice (B)—which is a tertiary alkyl halide—and choice (C)—which is a primary alkyl halide—can be rejected right away, since choice (B) couldn't react by S_N2, and choice (C) couldn't react by E1. In the remaining choices, the leaving groups, namely the cyanide group in choice (A) and the bromide group in choice (D), are bonded to secondary carbons—that is, to the carbons with an intermediate degree of branching. Therefore, from a purely structural point of view, both choices could undergo both E1 and S_N2 to some extent. To choose between them, you have to think about the leaving group. The cyanide group is a very poor leaving group and is therefore unlikely to be displaced via either E1 or S_N2; therefore, choice (A) can be rejected. On the other hand, the bromide group can easily be displaced via either E1 and S_N2; therefore, the correct answer is choice (D).

Passage III (Questions 16–20)

16. B You should note from reading the passage that ninhydrin, with which the amino acid fractions are treated prior to the photometric analysis, reacts only with primary amino groups. In this question, choices (A), (C), and (D) are all primary amines, but proline, choice (B), has a secondary amino group, in which the nitrogen atom is a constituent of a five-atom heterocyclic ring. Therefore, proline will not react with ninhydrin, and so its concentration can't be measured by the method described in the passage.

17. A This question tests your familiarity with the concept of pI, or isoelectric point. The pI is the pH value, specific for any given amino acid, at which it contains equal amounts of the positively and negatively charged forms, so that overall the amino acid is neutral. At pHs lower than the isoelectric point, the neutral amino acid molecule will be protonated and thus acquire an overall net positive charge, while at pHs higher than the isoelectric point, they will lose hydrogens and gain a net negative charge. Since the fractioning in IEC is based on different degrees of binding to negatively charged beads, positively charged molecules will bind to the greatest extent, neutral molecules will not bind, and negatively charged molecules will actually be repelled by the beads. In terms of the pI, this means that pHs that are lower than the pI will favor binding, since the majority of molecules will be positive, while pHs that are close to or higher than the pI will discourage binding, since the molecules will be neutral or negative. Therefore, amino acids whose pI is lower than the pH will be eluted best.

18. C To answer this question, you need to think about what type of amino acid makes up fraction F. As the passage says, positively charged molecules bind to the negatively charged beads in the column. Then, as the column is washed with buffer, the pH rises. Thus, the amino acids lose protons, their positive charge decreases, and eventually they elute from the column. So, those amino acids that start out with a low net positive charge—that is, acidic amino acids—will elute first, and those with a high net positive charge—basic amino acids—will elute last. As you can see from the graph, fraction F is eluted at high pH. This implies that fraction F is likely to be a basic amino acid. This allows you to reject choices (A) and (D) right off the bat, since basic amino acids can't be titrated by bases. Choice (B) is wrong as well, because titration with an acid will lower the pH, rather than raise it. However, the remaining choice, (C), shows a multistep titration curve, such as is typical of a basic amino acid, and so this is the correct answer.

19. A Amino acids with lower net positive charges are eluted at lower pHs, while those with higher net positive charges are eluted at higher pHs. Based on Figure 1, you can see that this means that the order of increasing positive charge for the three fractions in this question is B, D, E. Since the cathode is at negative potential, the amino acid in fraction E will be most strongly attracted to it, while fraction B will be least attracted. Hence, isoelectric focusing is likely to distribute these fractions in such a way that the band corresponding to fraction B will be closest to the anode, that of fraction E closest to the cathode, and that of fraction D somewhere in between—so choice (A) is the correct answer.

20. D The amount of amino acid that is placed in the column at the beginning of the experiment will not affect the elution volume at all, so choices (A) and (B) are wrong. The elution volume of a particular amino acid corresponds to a point on the pH gradient where the pH is high enough to cause a change in the charge on the molecules. This pH value depends on the pK_a values of the amino acid, not the amount of acid present. Therefore, a larger sample would elute from the column after the same volume of buffer solution had been collected. However, the elution volume attributed to the amino acid is only the average volume of buffer required to elute the fraction. As you can see in Figure 1, the whole fraction is not collected at one precise volume. Rather, the concentration of amino acid collected, as measured by the optical absorbance of the solution, rises to a peak and then drops. The position of the peak, that is, the volume at which most of the fraction is eluted, is the elution volume just discussed. This is unaffected by the size of the sample. However, the width of the peak is affected by the amount of compound placed onto the column. If a larger sample is used, the fraction will spread out over a wider range of elution volume. So the edges of the peaks will be closer together, giving a less distinct separation of the fractions.

Passage IV (Questions 21–25)

21. D For several of the questions on this passage, including this one, you need to be aware of the convention for naming carbons according to their positions relative to a functional group. The carbon that is directly bonded to the functional group in question (in this case a carbonyl group) is called the α-carbon. For example, the methyl carbon of acetyl coenzyme A (ACoA) is an α-carbon. A carbon adjacent to an α-carbon in the chain is called a β-carbon (as with the carbon containing the keto group in the β-ketocaproyl coenzyme A), and the carbon two over is γ, and so on. For this question, you also need to remember that the hybridization state of a carbon atom directly corresponds to the order of carbon-carbon bonds. Single-bonded carbons are sp^3-hybridized, double-bonded carbons are sp^2-hybridized, and triple-bonded carbons are sp-hybridized. Based on this information, you should trace the fate of the α-carbon of the first molecule of acetyl coenzyme A through the fatty acid biosynthesis pathway to find out which reactions change the character of its bonds. You can immediately see that the bonding order of the α-carbon changes in only two reactions: Reaction 4,

in which the single α-β bond becomes a double bond, and reaction 5, in which that double bond is converted back into a single bond. This corresponds to a change in the α-carbon's hybridization state from sp^3 to sp^2, and then back to sp^3. Therefore, choice (D) is the correct answer.

22. B Enzymes are generally named according to what they do; therefore, the first thing you need to figure out in order to answer this question is what type of process is going on in reaction 3. The diagram shows that reaction 3 reduces the beta carbonyl group of acetoacetyl coenzyme A to a hydroxyl group, forming beta-hydroxybutyryl coenzyme A; so the enzyme catalyzing this reaction could logically be called a reductase. Thus, choice (B) is correct. The other three answer choices all suggest other reactions, none of which is happening here. An isomerase, choice (A), would catalyze the conversion of one molecule into another molecule that has the same empirical formula but a different structure. Acetoacetyl CoA and β-hydroxybutyryl CoA have different molecular formulas, therefore, this can't be an example of an isomerization reaction. A transferase, choice (C), would catalyze the transfer of some group from one molecule to another, but as we can see in the reaction, no groups are being transferred, and so this choice is also incorrect. Finally, an oxidase, choice (D), would catalyze oxidation, but this reaction is an example of a reduction.

23. A Reaction 4 is a dehydration reaction, in which an alcohol is converted into an alkene. If no enzyme is present, such a reaction can be accomplished by heating the alcohol in an acid solution. In the reaction, the alcohol group is protonated forming an oxonium ion. The oxonium ion then loses water forming a carbocation. The presence of this carbocation facilitates the release of a proton from an adjacent carbon—producing a double bond. Alcohols that contain more substituted hydroxyl carbons form alkenes more easily as they are stabilized by their electron-donating alkyl groups. Thus, tertiary alcohols are most susceptible to dehydration, while primary alcohols are least susceptible. Among the four choices, (D) has a primary hydroxyl group, (B) and (C) have secondary hydroxyl groups, and (A) has a tertiary hydroxyl group. Therefore, choice (A) will be most susceptible to dehydration, so this is the correct answer.

24. A The fact that all the intermediates became radioactive implies that the radioactive carbon was incorporated into a part of the acetyl coenzyme A molecule that remained intact throughout the whole series of reactions. You can see from the diagram that the carbon atom in the CH_3 group of each acetyl coenzyme A remains bonded to the growing molecule; so if this were labeled with carbon 14, all the compounds would become radioactive. Thus, Statement I is correct. On the other hand, Statement II is wrong. If the CO_2 released in step two were radioactive, then the carbon 14 atom would be removed from the system at that point, and none of the succeeding compounds would be radioactive. Statement III is also wrong. The coenzyme A moiety of the original acetyl coenzyme A molecule remains attached to the growing molecule throughout all the compounds of the pathway. Therefore, one of its carbons could indeed have been the labeled one. Hence, the only correct statement is Statement I, and choice (A) is the correct answer.

25. B For the enol form of acetoacetyl coenzyme A to be produced, the carbonyl oxygen of the keto form must become a hydroxyl group by removing a hydrogen ion from one of the adjacent carbons. Of the two adjacent carbons, the one that is more substituted is the one located between the carbonyl carbons; therefore, the most acidic hydrogens available will be those attached to this carbon. So, one of these hydrogens will be abstracted by the keto oxygen, thereby forming a double bond between the former carbonyl carbon and this more highly substituted neighboring carbon. Since, in acetoacetyl coenzyme A, the more substituted neighbor of the β-carbon is the α-carbon, the β-enol form would contain the hydroxylated β-carbon doubly-bonded to the α-carbon. In this form, the α- and β- carbons carry, respectively, one hydrogen and no hydrogens. So the difference between the β-enol form of acetoacetyl coenzyme A and α-hydroxybutyryl coenzyme A lies in the number of hydrogen atoms attached to the α- and β-carbons, and choice (B) is correct.

Discrete Questions

26. D This question deals with the factors that affect the acidity of organic acids and with the Brønsted concept of conjugate acids and bases. Remember, the stronger the acid, the weaker its conjugate base. Therefore, what the question is asking, in a round-about way, is which of the compounds is the strongest acid. Generally speaking, acids that contain an electron-withdrawing substituent on the alpha carbon (that is, the carbon adjacent to the carboxyl carbon) tend to be stronger, since the dissipation of electron density has a stabilizing effect on the carboxylate anion that will be formed if a proton dissociates. Likewise, acids with electron-donating a substituents tend to be weaker. So, looking at the answer choices: choice (A) has an amino α-substituent, which is strongly electron-donating; choice (B) has a tertiary butyl substituent, which is also electron-donating; choice (C) has only hydrogens and a methyl group in the alpha position; and choice (D) has two chlorine substituents, which are electron-withdrawing. Therefore, choice (D) will give the most stable carboxylate anion when the proton is lost, and so is the strongest acid. This means it will have the weakest conjugate base, and so choice (D) is the correct answer.

27. D This question requires you to understand the mechanism of nucleophilic addition to carbonyl compounds. You should remember that aldehydes and ketones react slowly with water to form gem diols—that is, diols in which both hydroxyl groups are attached to the same carbon atom. Like any nucleophilic addition, the reaction between a carbonyl group and water proceeds in two principal steps. In the first step, which is accelerated by adding a small amount of acid, oxygen gains a proton, so that it acquires a strong positive charge. However, this form of the intermediate, with the charge located on the oxygen, is not the most stable, and therefore doesn't last for very long. Instead, the electrons of the carbon-oxygen pi bond migrate to the oxygen, neutralizing the positive charge. This produces a hydroxyl group and leaves behind a new positive charge on the former carbonyl carbon. Hence, the correct structure of Intermediate X is the one shown in choice (D). In the second step of the reaction, the positively-charged carbon of Intermediate X reacts with a water molecule and then loses a proton to form the gem diol. If you weren't sure of this mechanism, an inspection of the other choices should have led you to the correct answer. In choice (A), the carbonyl oxygen has gained a proton and is positively charged, but the carbon is negatively charged. However, nothing has happened to the carbon that could produce this charge; it is still bonded to four atoms, so it should still be uncharged. Also, since the molecule has gained a proton, it should have an overall positive charge, whereas choice (A) has one positive and one negative charge. So, for all these reasons, choice (A) is wrong. In choice (B), the β-carbon has a positive charge, and has one less hydrogen than the reactant. This could only be the case if this carbon had lost a hydride ion (H-), which is very unlikely. In any case, the α-carbon is shown as being uncharged but only has three bonds, and this is impossible. So, choice (B) is wrong as well. Choice (C) also shows an uncharged carbon with three bonds, so that's wrong too.

PHYSICS

UNITS AND KINEMATICS

In this first chapter we will review some of the basic mathematics necessary for the study of MCAT physics, such as scientific notation, basic trigonometric functions, and vectors. In addition, the topic of units is presented with emphasis on the three systems of units that you need to be familiar with, i.e., MKS, CGS, and FPS. Finally, the topic of kinematics, which is the study of motion, is discussed. Here, a review is given of the basic quantities of displacement, speed, velocity, and acceleration. These basic quantities are then applied to the study of motion with constant acceleration. The case of one-dimensional motion is discussed, including an example of free-fall. The case of projectile motion, which is motion in two dimensions, is also covered in a detailed example.

UNITS

A. FUNDAMENTAL MEASUREMENTS AND DIMENSIONS

Physics is the most basic of all the sciences. Everything in the world around us is subject to the laws of physics. In order to describe nature, physicists use the language of mathematics, in the form of equations, to make their quantitative descriptions.

These descriptions, however, mean nothing if they are not expressed in some kind of units. While explaining how you were pulled over on the highway doing seventy might mean something amongst friends, a scientist would ask whether your speed was 70 miles per hour or 70 kilometers per hour or some other speed. Scientists have developed systems of units that give meaning to all the numbers in the formulas. The British, or **FPS**, system is commonly used in America but virtually nowhere else in the world (not even in Britain). Basic units for length, weight, and time are the foot (ft), the pound (lb), and the second (s), respectively. The most common system of units is the metric system, the basic units of which include length, mass (instead of weight like in FPS), and time. The metric

MCAT Synopsis

Don't mix units! An answer with the correct number of *incorrect* units may be one of the choices.

system comes in two main variations. One metric system uses meter (m), kilogram (kg), and second (s) as its base, and is referred to as **MKS** and also **SI** (SI being the initials of the French abbreviation for the International System of Units). The other metric system uses centimeter (cm), gram (g), second (s) and is referred to as **CGS**. The SI system is becoming the standard.

The following chart lists some important units in the three systems:

Some Important Units

Quantity	CGS	SI	FPS
Length	centimeter (cm)	meter (m)	foot (ft)
Mass	gram (g)	kilogram (kg)	slug (sl)
Force	dyne (dyn)	Newton (N)	pound (lb)
Time	second (s)	second (s)	second (s)
Work & Energy	erg	Joule (J)	foot-pound (ft•lb)
Power	erg/second	Watt (W)	foot-pound/sec

In atomic sized systems, because of the extremely small scale of the interactions, some different scales are used that make the numbers a little easier to handle. Useful length units on the atomic scale include the angstrom (Å where $1 \text{ Å} = 10^{-10}$ m) and the nanometer (nm), where $1 \text{ nm} = 10^{-9}$ m. Also important at this level is the unit of energy called the electron–volt (eV), which is the energy acquired by an electron accelerating through a potential difference of one volt. Compared with the SI unit of energy, the Joule, the electron–volt is very small ($1 \text{ eV} = 1.6 \times 10^{-19}$ J).

Metric system prefixes are often added to units to make numbers easier to handle. The chart below lists prefixes sometimes encountered.

Multiples		
factor	prefix	prefix abbreviation
10^9	giga	G (or B)
10^6	mega	M
10^3	kilo	k

Submultiples		
factor	prefix	prefix abbreviation
10^{-2}	centi	c
10^{-3}	milli	m
10^{-6}	micro	μ
10^{-9}	nano	n
10^{-12}	pico	p

B. SCIENTIFIC NOTATION

Scientific notation is a convention for expressing numbers that simplifies computation and standardizes results. To express a number in scientific notation, convert it into a number between one and ten, then multiply it by ten to the appropriate power.

Example:　$123 = 1.23 \times 10^2$

1.23 is the **mantissa** and 2 is the **exponent** (power of ten).

Example:　$0.042 = 4.2 \times 10^{-2}$

One can easily obtain products and quotients of numbers expressed in scientific notation. When multiplying, one simply multiplies the mantissas and adds the exponents to find the new mantissa and exponent of the answer. Some additional conversion may be necessary so that the new mantissa is again between one and ten as in the third example on this page.

Example:　$(1.1 \times 10^6)(5.0 \times 10^{17}) = ?$

Solution:　Multiply the mantissas 1.1 and 5.0, and add the exponents 6 and 17.

The answer is 5.5×10^{23}.

The quotient of two numbers expressed in scientific notation is obtained by dividing the mantissa in the numerator by the mantissa in the denominator, and subtracting the power of ten in the denominator from the power of ten in the numerator.

Example:　$\dfrac{6.2 \times 10^5}{2.0 \times 10^{-7}}$

Solution:　Divide 6.2 by 2.0 and subtract −7 from 5 (note that 5 − (−7) = 5 + 7 = 12).

The answer is 3.1×10^{12}.

When a number expressed in scientific notation is raised to a power, the mantissa is raised to that power, and the exponent is multiplied by that number.

Example: $(6.0 \times 10^4)^2$

Solution: Square the 6.0 and multiply the exponent by 2.

$(6.0)^2 \times 10^{4 \times 2} = 36.0 \times 10^8 = 3.6 \times 10^9$

(Note that when we move the decimal point one place to the left we must increase the power of ten by one, from 8 to 9.)

When adding or subtracting numbers expressed in scientific notation they must have the **same** power of ten; when they do not, the appropriate conversion must be made first.

Example: $3.7 \times 10^4 + 1.5 \times 10^3 = ?$

Solution: First convert 1.5×10^3 to 0.15×10^4 so both numbers have the same exponent. Then $3.7 \times 10^4 + 0.15 \times 10^4 = 3.85 \times 10^4$ rounded to 3.9×10^4.

C. TRIGONOMETRIC RELATIONS

For the right triangle, the trigonometric functions for angle θ are:

$$\sin \theta = \frac{y}{h} = \frac{\text{opposite side}}{\text{hypotenuse}}$$

$$\cos \theta = \frac{x}{h} = \frac{\text{adjacent side}}{\text{hypotenuse}}$$

$$\tan \theta = \frac{y}{x} = \frac{\text{opposite side}}{\text{adjacent side}}$$

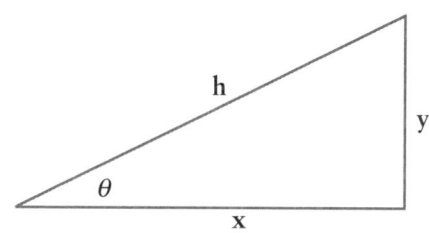

Some important values of the trigonometric functions:

θ	sin θ	cos θ
0°	0°	1
30°	$\frac{1}{2}$	$\frac{\sqrt{3}}{2}$
45°	$\frac{\sqrt{2}}{2}$	$\frac{\sqrt{2}}{2}$
60°	$\frac{\sqrt{3}}{2}$	$\frac{1}{2}$
90°	1°	0
180°	0°	−1

D. VECTORS AND SCALARS

Scalars are those numerical quantities that have **magnitude** but no direction, such as distance, speed and mass. **Vector** quantities have **both magnitude and direction.** Some vector quantities are displacement, velocity, and force.

1. **Vector Representation**

    We can represent a vector by an arrow. The direction of the arrow corresponds to the direction of the vector. The length of the arrow **may or may not** be proportional to the magnitude of the vector. Common notations for a vector quantity are either an arrow or **bold-face.** For example, vector A can be written as $\vec{A}$ or **A.** The magnitude of vector A can be represented as $|\vec{A}|$, $|\mathbf{A}|$, or simply, A (no arrow or boldface).

2. **Vector Addition**

    The **sum** of two or more vectors is called the **resultant** of the vectors. The terms vector sum and resultant are interchangeable.

    One method of finding the resultant **A + B** of the two vectors **A** and **B** is to place the tail of **B** at the tip of **A** (without changing the length or direction of either arrow). In this method of vector addition the lengths of the arrows **must** be proportional to the magnitudes of the vector. The vector sum **A + B** is the vector joining the tail of **A** to the tip of **B** and pointing towards the tip of **B.** For three or more vectors, proceed similarly (see Figure 1.1 below).

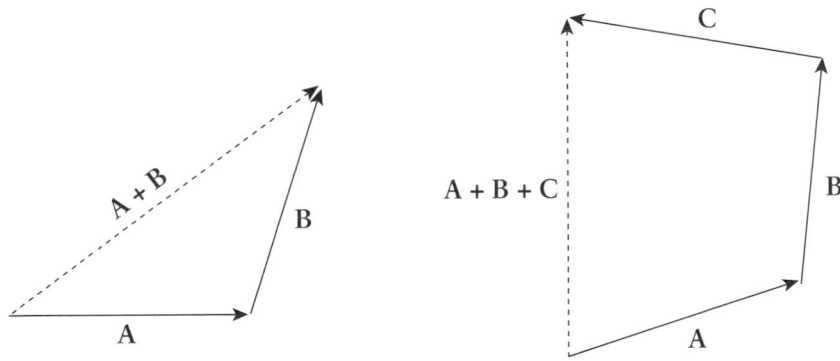

Figure 1.1

Another method more commonly used for finding the resultant of several vectors involves breaking each vector into perpendicular (X and Y) components. These components are often, but not always, horizontal and vertical.

Given any vector **V**, we can find the X component and the Y component by drawing a right triangle with **V** as the hypotenuse (see Figure 1.2 below). If θ is the angle between **V** and the x direction, then $\cos \theta = X/V$ and $\sin \theta = Y/V$. In other words:

$$X = V \cos \theta$$
$$Y = V \sin \theta$$

Example: V = 10 m/s
$\theta = 30°$

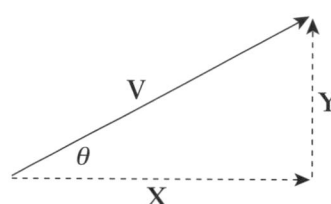

$$X = 10 \cos 30° = \frac{10\sqrt{3}}{2}$$
$$= 5\sqrt{3} \ \text{m/s}$$

$$Y = 10 \sin 30° = \frac{10}{2} = 5 \ \text{m/s}$$

Figure 1.2

Conversely, if we know X and Y, we can find V by using the Pythagorean theorem: $X^2 + Y^2 = V^2$; or $V = \sqrt{X^2 + Y^2}$.

Example: X = 3 m/s
Y = 4 m/s

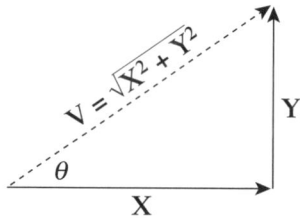

$$V = \sqrt{3^2 + 4^2} = \sqrt{25}$$
$$= 5 \ \text{m/s}$$

(Also note that we can find θ from $\tan \theta = Y/X$. In this example $\tan \theta = 4/3$, so $\theta = 53°$.)

Figure 1.3

The X component of the resultant vector is the sum of the X components of the vectors being added. Similarly, the Y component of the resultant vector is the sum of the Y components of the vectors being added.

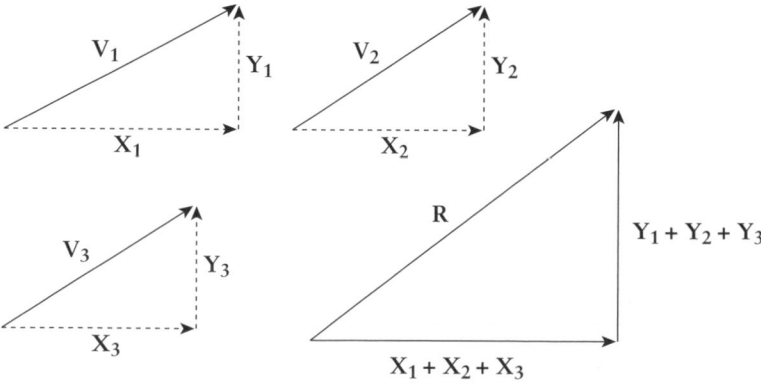

Figure 1.4

To find the resultant (**R**) using the components method:

1. Resolve the vectors to be summed into their X and Y components.
2. Add together the X components to get the X component of the resultant (R_x). In the same way, add the Y components to get the Y component of the resultant (R_y).
3. Find the magnitude of the resultant by using the Pythagorean theorem. If R_x and R_y are the components of the resultant then:

$$R = \sqrt{R_x{}^2 + R_y{}^2}$$

4. Find the direction (θ) of the resultant by using the relation $\tan \theta = \dfrac{R_y}{R_x}$. From the value of $\tan \theta$ you can find θ, the angle R makes with the x direction.

Example: Find the horizontal and vertical components of **V**.

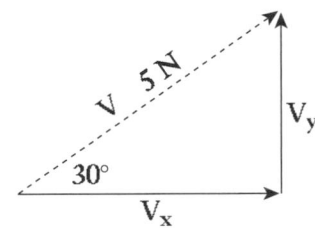

Figure 1.5

Solution: Let x be the horizontal direction and y be the vertical direction. Then:

$$V_x = V \cos \theta = 5 \cos 30° = \frac{5\sqrt{3}}{2} = 2.5\sqrt{3}\,N \approx 4.3\,N$$

$$V_y = V \sin \theta = 5 \sin 30° = \frac{5}{2} = 2.5\,N$$

Example: Find the resultant of **A**, **B**, **C**, and **D**.

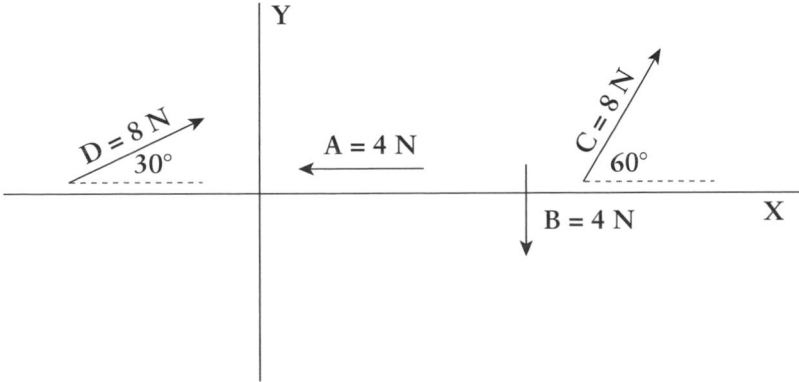

Figure 1.6

621

Solution: Resolve the vectors into their horizontal (x) and vertical (y) components. Note that we have x components going both left and right, and y components going both up and down. **In each case choose one direction as the positive direction. The other direction is then automatically the negative direction.** In this example we chose going to the right as the positive x direction (so to the left is negative), and up as the positive y direction (so down is negative). **A component in the positive direction is then positive and a component in the negative direction is then negative.**

a. $A_x = -4$ N

$B_x = 0$

$C_x = 8 \cos 60° = \dfrac{8}{2} = 4$ N

$D_x = 8 \cos 30° = \dfrac{8\sqrt{3}}{2} = 4\sqrt{3}$ N

b. $A_y = 0$

$B_y = -4$ N

$C_y = 8 \sin 60° = \dfrac{8\sqrt{3}}{2} = 4\sqrt{3}$ N

$D_y = 8 \sin 30° = \dfrac{8}{2} = 4$ N

Add together the components of **A**, **B**, **C**, and **D** to get the components of the resultant R:

a. $R_x = (-4) + 0 + 4 + 4\sqrt{3} = 4\sqrt{3}$ N

b. $R_y = 0 + (-4) + 4\sqrt{3} + 4 = 4\sqrt{3}$ N

Find the magnitude of the resultant:

$$R = \sqrt{R_x{}^2 + R_y{}^2}$$

$$R = \sqrt{(4\sqrt{3})^2 + (4\sqrt{3})^2} = \sqrt{96} = 4\sqrt{6}\ \text{N}$$

Find the angle the resultant makes with the horizontal:

$$\tan \theta = \dfrac{4\sqrt{3}}{4\sqrt{3}} = 1;\ \theta = 45°$$

Thus, we have found that **R** is a vector of magnitude of $4\sqrt{6}$ N, making an angle of 45° with the horizontal. (In general, $\tan \theta = |R_y|/|R_x|$ where θ is the smallest angle with the x-axis.)

3. **Vector Subtraction**

Subtracting two vectors is exactly the same as adding the negative of the vector being subtracted. When expressed in a mathematical formula, the idea looks like this:

$$\mathbf{A} - \mathbf{B} = \mathbf{A} + (-\mathbf{B})$$

By $-\mathbf{B}$ we mean a vector with the same magnitude as $\mathbf{B}$, but pointing in the opposite direction.

Example: What is the resultant of $\mathbf{A} - \mathbf{B}$ as pictured below?

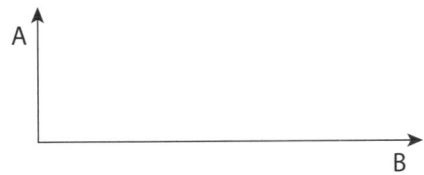

Figure 1.7

Solution: The first thing to do is make the vector $-\mathbf{B}$. This is done by erasing the arrow head at the tip of $\mathbf{B}$, and redrawing it where the tail used to be (see Figure 1.8(a)). Now, add this to $\mathbf{A}$. To do this move the tip of $\mathbf{A}$ to the tail of $-\mathbf{B}$, and join the tail of $\mathbf{A}$ to the tip of $-\mathbf{B}$ (see Figure 1.8(b)).

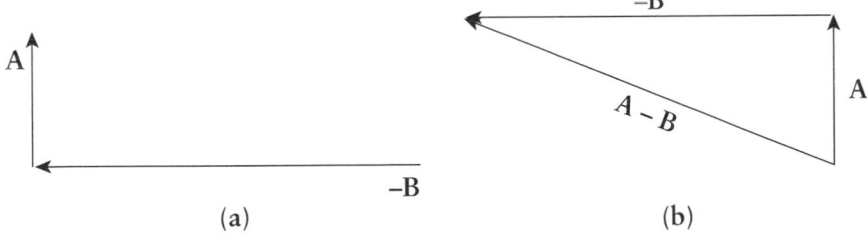

(a)   (b)

Figure 1.8

To find $-\mathbf{B}$ using the method whereby the vectors are broken up into their horizontal and vertical components, each vector component is multiplied by -1 before adding.

Example: If $\mathbf{A}$ has components $A_x = 3$ and $A_y = 4$ and $\mathbf{B}$ has components $B_x = 2$ and $B_y = 1$, then what is $\mathbf{A} - \mathbf{B}$?

Solution: First, remember $\mathbf{A} - \mathbf{B} = \mathbf{A} + (-\mathbf{B})$. Since $\mathbf{B}$ has components B_x and B_y, $-\mathbf{B}$ has components $-B_x$ and $-B_y$.

$$R_x = A_x - B_x = 3 - 2 = 1$$
$$R_y = A_y - B_y = 4 - 1 = 3$$

To get the magnitude of the final resultant vector **R**:

$$R = \sqrt{(3^2 + 1^2)}$$

$$= \sqrt{(9+1)} = \sqrt{10}$$

To get the direction:

$$\tan \theta = \frac{R_y}{R_x} = 3$$

$$\theta = 72°$$

4. **Multiplying a Vector by a Scalar**

   Now consider the case where a vector is multiplied by a scalar, **B** = n**A**. To find the magnitude of **B** simply multiply the magnitude of **A** by the absolute value of n, **B** = |n|**A**. If n is a positive number, then **B** and **A** are in the same direction. However, if n is a negative number, then **B** and **A** are in opposite directions. For example, if vector **A** is multiplied by +3, the resultant vector **B** will be three times as long as **A** and point in the same direction. However, if **A** is multiplied by –3, then **B** would again be three times as long as **A**, but it would point in the opposite direction.

KINEMATICS

Kinematics is that branch of mechanics dealing with the description of motion. In physics, the **position** of an object or particle is defined on a three-dimensional coordinate axis. Most problems you will have to deal with concerning motion will involve only one or two dimensions.

A. DISPLACEMENT

The **displacement** (Δx) of an object is a vector quantity that describes the change in position. It goes (in a straight line) from the initial position to the final position without regard to the actual path taken. Since this is a vector quantity, displacement has both direction and magnitude.

Example: A man walks 2 km east, then 2 km north, then 2 km west, and then 2 km south. His actual total distance traveled is 8 km, since distance is a scalar. But his displacement is a vector quantity that is the change in position. In this case his displacement is zero, since the man ends up in the same place he started (see Figure 1.9).

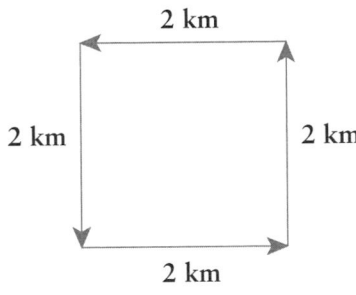

Figure 1.9

B. VELOCITY

1. Average Velocity

The **average velocity** of a particle is the ratio of the displacement vector over the change in time. It is a vector quantity.

$$\bar{v} = \Delta x / \Delta t$$

$\bar{v}$ has the same direction as Δx.

2. Instantaneous Velocity

The **instantaneous velocity** or **velocity** refers to a single instant of time. It is the average velocity as Δt approaches 0. This can be represented as:

$$v = \lim_{\Delta t \longrightarrow 0} \Delta x / \Delta t$$

Graphically, this corresponds to the slope of the graph of the object's position with respect to time at the particular time t.

3. Speed

The **average speed** is given by:

$$\bar{s} = d / \Delta t$$

where d is the actual distance traveled. It is a scalar. Since actual distance traveled is not always the same as the magnitude of the displacement vector, average speed is not always the same as the magnitude of the average velocity.

The **instantaneous speed** or **speed** is the magnitude of the instantaneous velocity vector. It is also a scalar.

> **Real World Analogy**
>
> If a car goes 10 miles to the north and then drives 10 miles to the south, it will end it up where it started.
>
> The $\Delta x = 0$
> The distance = 20 miles
>
> In addition, if the car drives the 20 miles in 1 hour, then the speed is 20 m/hr, but the velocity is 0 m/hr.

C. ACCELERATION

1. ### Average Acceleration

    Acceleration is the rate of change of an object's velocity. It is a vector quantity. **Average acceleration** $\bar{a}$ is the change in instantaneous velocity over the time period Δt:

    $$\bar{a} = \Delta v / \Delta t$$

2. ### Instantaneous Acceleration

    The **instantaneous acceleration**—the acceleration at one point of a particle's path—is defined the same way as instantaneous velocity, i.e., it is the average acceleration as Δt approaches 0.

    $$a = \lim_{\Delta t \longrightarrow 0} \Delta v / \Delta t$$

    Graphically, this corresponds to the slope of the graph of the object's velocity with respect to time at the particular time t. The direction of the acceleration vector is not always along the direction of the velocity vector. The direction of **a** is the same as the direction of $\Delta \mathbf{v}$.

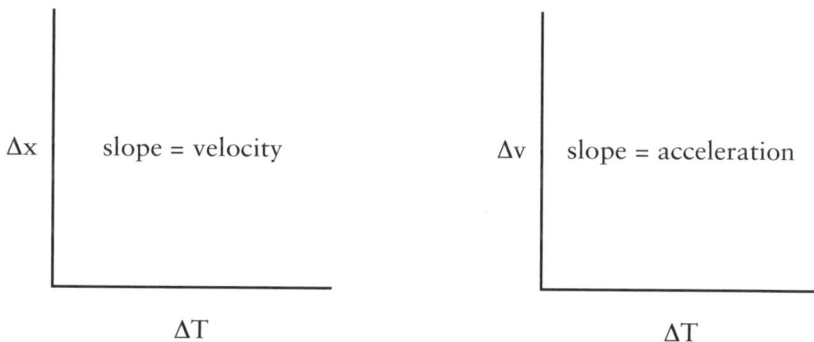

Figure 1.10

MOTION WITH CONSTANT ACCELERATION

The acceleration of a body is proportional to the force (see chapter 2) applied to that body. When a body is under the influence of a constant force, the acceleration is also constant. In the following sections it is assumed that the acceleration is constant.

A. LINEAR MOTION

In linear motion the acceleration and velocity vectors are along the line of motion. Note that the linear motion need not be in the horizontal direction. One-dimensional motion of this kind can be fully described by the following equations:

Notes:

$$v = v_0 + at$$

1. v_0, x_0 are v and x at t = 0.

$$x - x_0 = v_0t + \frac{at^2}{2}$$

2. When the motion is vertical, we use y instead of x.

$$v^2 = v_0^2 + 2a(x - x_0)$$

$$\bar{v} = \frac{(v_0 + v)}{2}$$

3. As illustrated below, in using these equations, we must remember that velocity and acceleration are vector quantities.

$$x - x_0 = \bar{v}t = \left(\frac{v_0 + v}{2}\right)t$$

By way of an example let's examine free-falling bodies. *Free-fall* means that the only force acting on a body is its own weight (gravity) and it neglects, for example, any force of air resistance. All objects in free-fall have the same acceleration called **the acceleration due to gravity (g)**, which in SI units is 9.8 m/s². The following example demonstrates the use of the above equations in the analysis of free falling bodies.

Example: A ball is thrown vertically up into the air with an initial velocity of 10 m/s.

    a. Find the position and velocity of the ball after 2 seconds.

    b. Find the distance and time at which the ball reaches its maximum height.

Solution: a. Remember that velocity and acceleration are vector quantities. Taking the initial position of the ball $y_0 = 0$, and taking "up" as positive, the initial velocity is $v_0 = +10$ m/s and the acceleration is $g = -9.8$ m/s². Notice g is negative because its direction is down, and we are taking "up" to be the positive direction. Velocity after two seconds can be found using the equation:

$$v = v_0 + at$$
$$= (+10) + (-9.8)(2)$$
$$= -9.6 \text{ m/s}$$

(Minus sign for v means that the ball is coming down).

After two seconds, the position of the ball is found using the equation:

$$y = v_0 t + \frac{at^2}{2} \quad (y_0 = 0)$$

$$= 10(2) + \frac{(-9.8)(2)^2}{2}$$

$$= 20 - 19.6$$

$$= +0.4 \text{ m}$$

b. When the ball is at its maximum height, the velocity, v, which has been decreasing on the way up, is zero. Using the following equation and plugging in values, we can find the maximum height the ball reaches above the ground:

$$v^2 = v_0^2 + 2ay$$

$$0 = (10)^2 + 2(-9.8)y$$

$$y = 5.1 \text{ m}$$

The time at which the ball reaches its maximum height can be found from the equation:

$$v = v_0 + at$$

$$0 = 10 + (-9.8)t$$

$$t = 1.0 \text{ s}$$

B. PROJECTILE MOTION

Note again that we have been considering only linear motion in the above example. In the case of **projectile motion**, however, the object has velocity and position components in both the vertical and horizontal directions. The two components of the velocity vector v_x and v_y are independent, so the change in the vertical velocity v_y due to gravity does not affect and is not affected by the constant horizontal velocity v_x. The following example demonstrates how projectile motion is analyzed.

Example: A projectile is fired from ground level with an initial velocity of 50 m/s and an initial angle of elevation of 37°. Assuming g = 10 m/s^2, find:

a. the projectile's total time in flight.
b. the maximum height attained.
c. the total horizontal distance traveled.
d. the final horizontal and vertical velocities just before it hits the ground.

(sin 37° = 0.6; cos 37° = 0.8)

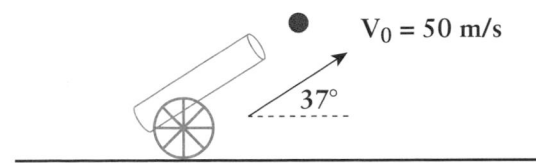

Figure 1.11

Solution: a. Let y equal the vertical height; let up be the positive direction.

$$a = -10 \text{ m/s}^2$$

$$y = v_{0_y}t + \frac{1}{2}at^2 \qquad (y_0 = 0)$$

$$v_{0_y} = v_0 \sin 37°$$
$$v_{0_y} = 50(0.6) = 30 \text{ m/s}$$
$$y = 30t - 5t^2$$

y = 0 both when the projectile is first fired and also when it hits the ground later. Its time in flight will be the difference between the values of t at the two points when y = 0.

$$30t - 5t^2 = 0$$
$$5t(6 - t) = 0$$
$$t = 0 \text{ (first fired)}, \ t = 6 \text{ (hits the ground)}$$

Time in flight = 6 − 0 = 6 s

b. To find the maximum height attained:

$$v_y^2 = v_{0_y}^2 + 2ay$$

$$0 = 30^2 + 2(-10)(y) \ (v_y = 0 \text{ at highest point})$$

$$y = \frac{900}{20}$$

$$y = 45 \text{ m}$$

c. To find the horizontal distance traveled:

$$x = v_x t \quad (a_x = 0)$$
$$v_x = 50 \cos 37° = 40 \text{ m/s}$$
$$x = 40(6) = 240 \text{ m}$$

d. The horizontal velocity remains constant, so $v_x = 40$ m/s.
To find the vertical velocity at impact:

$$v_y = v_{0_y} + at$$
$$v_y = 30 - 10(6)$$
$$v_y = 30 - 60$$
$$v_y = -30 \text{ m/s}$$

Since we chose up as positive, the minus sign means the
vertical component of the velocity is directed down.

2

NEWTONIAN MECHANICS

This chapter covers the most important area of MCAT physics, namely Newton's laws of motion. Basic to the study of Newton's laws are the fundamental concepts of force and mass, which are discussed along with the distinction between mass and weight and a detailed example of obtaining the resultant of two or more forces. The classic example of a block sliding down a frictionless incline is presented as an exercise for applying Newton's second law in a situation where there are forces in two directions. Translational and rotational equilibrium are discussed as examples of cases where the net force or net torque respectively vanishes. The real world problem of motion in the presence of friction is briefly discussed qualitatively, followed by a detailed numerical example. Lastly, the topic of circular motion is discussed along with the associated concepts of tangential and centripetal acceleration, and centripetal force.

NEWTON'S THREE LAWS

A. FORCE

Force is a vector quantity. Forces are observed as the push or pull on an object. Forces can either be exerted between bodies in contact (such as the force a person exerts to push a box across the floor), or between bodies not in contact (such as the force of gravity holding the earth in its orbit around the sun). The unit for force in SI is the Newton (N), and is equivalent to kilogram•meter/second^2.

B. MASS AND WEIGHT

The mass of an object should not be mistaken for the weight of an object. **Mass (m)** is a scalar quantity that measures a body's inertia, while **weight (W)** is a force vector that measures a body's gravitational attraction to the earth. The two are related by the equation:

$$W = mg$$

> **MCAT Favorite**
>
> g decreases with height above the earth. Near the earth's surface, use g = 10 m/s^2.

where **g** is the acceleration due to gravity. The unit for weight is the same as for any other force, the Newton (N).

When one of the forces acting on a body is its own weight, the entire force due to gravity can be thought of as applied at a single point, called the center of gravity. For a homogeneous body the center of gravity is at its geometric center.

C. NEWTON'S LAWS OF MOTION STATED

Mechanics is the study of bodies in motion and at rest. Newtonian mechanics is a way of describing the effect forces have on macroscopic bodies. In order to carry out such a description, it is first necessary to have an understanding of Newton's three laws of motion and how to apply them to various situations. Newton's three laws are:

1. A body either at rest or in motion with constant velocity will remain that way unless a net force acts upon it.

2. A net force applied to a body of mass m will result in that body undergoing an acceleration in the same direction as the net force. The magnitude of the body's acceleration is directly proportional to the magnitude of the net force and inversely proportional to the body's mass. This can be expressed in general terms as:

$$\mathbf{F}_{net} = \Sigma\mathbf{F} = m\mathbf{a}$$

or in components as:

$$\Sigma\mathbf{F}_x = ma_x$$

$$\Sigma\mathbf{F}_y = ma_y$$

Note that the acceleration in the x-direction depends only on the forces (or components of forces) in the x-direction (and the same is true for the y-direction).

3. If body A exerts a force **F** on body B, then B exerts a force −**F** back on A (equal in magnitude and opposite in direction). In Newton's words, "to every action there is always an opposed but equal reaction."

$$\mathbf{F}_B = -\mathbf{F}_A$$

D. FREE-BODY DIAGRAM

Another concept useful in force problems is the **free-body diagram**, which helps to clarify what forces are acting and what their directions are. The examples below demonstrate the use of this technique.

Example: Three people are pulling on ropes tied to a tire with forces of 100 N, 150 N, and 200 N, as shown in Figure 2.1. Find the magnitude and direction of the resultant force.

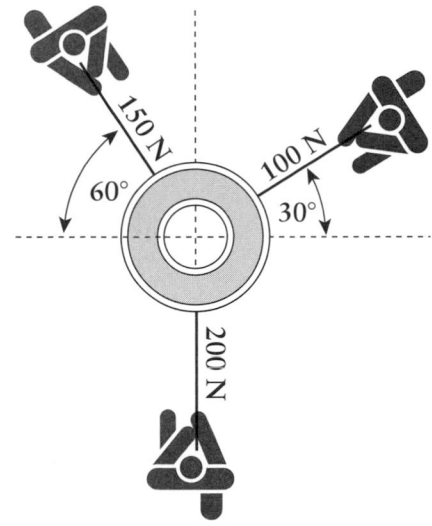

Figure 2.1

Solution: First we draw a free-body diagram that shows the forces acting on the tire. Its purpose is to identify and better visualize the acting forces.

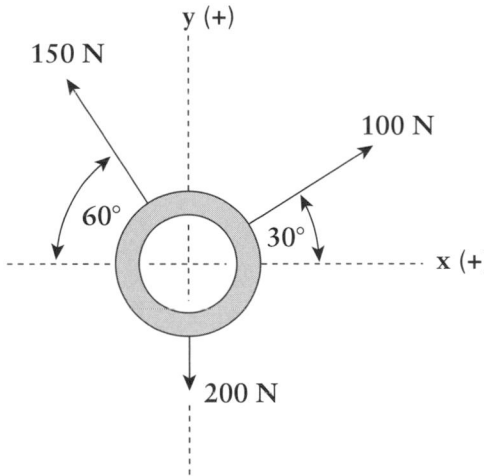

Figure 2.2

The resultant force is simply the sum of the forces. To find the resultant force vector, first we need the sum of the force components:

$$R_x = \Sigma F_x = 100 \cos 30° - 150 \cos 60°$$

$$= 86.6 - 75$$

$$= 11.6 \text{ N (positive x direction, to the right)}$$

$$R_y = \Sigma F_y = 100 \sin 30° + 150 \sin 60° - 200$$

$$= 50 + 129.9 - 200$$

$$= -20.1 \text{ N (negative y direction, down)}$$

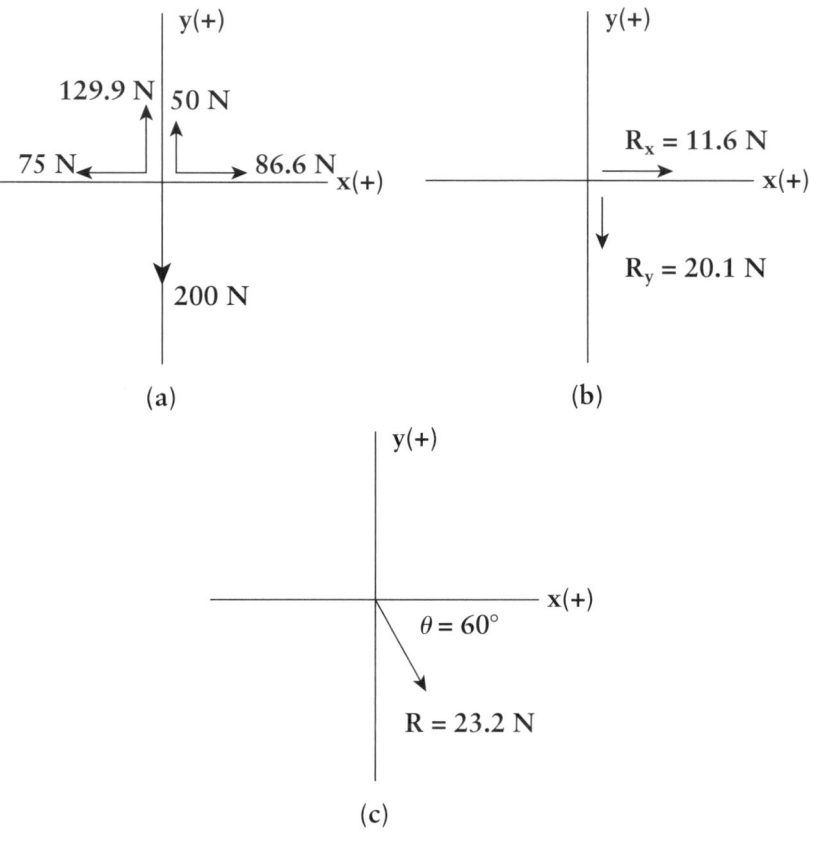

(a)   (b)

(c)

Figure 2.3

$$R = \sqrt{(11.6)^2 + (-20.1)^2}$$

$$= 23.2 \text{ N}$$

$$\tan \theta = \frac{-20.1}{11.6}$$

$$\theta = -60° \text{ (R is in the 4th quadrant)}$$

Example: Starting from rest, a 5 kg block takes 4 s to slide down a frictionless incline. Find the normal force, the acceleration of the block, and the vertical height h the block starts from, if the plane is at an angle of 30°.

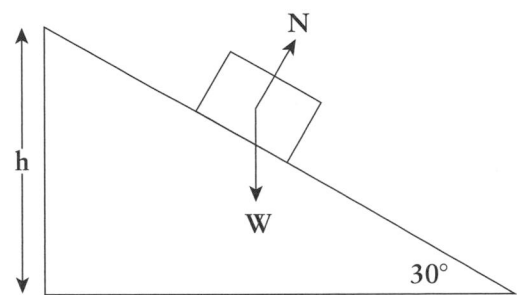

Figure 2.4

Solution: It is usually best to choose the x-and y-axes such that one of the axes is parallel to the surface, even when the surface is not horizontal. This is what we will do here. The force that the surface exerts on the block is broken up into two components, one perpendicular to the surface called the **normal force (N)**, and the other parallel to the surface, called the **friction force (f)**. In this problem the incline is frictionless (i.e., no **f**), so we have only the normal force **N**. The block's weight **W** is, of course, vertically down. We need to find the components of **W** parallel and perpendicular to the inclined surface (i.e., the components of **W** in the x and y directions, W_x and W_y).

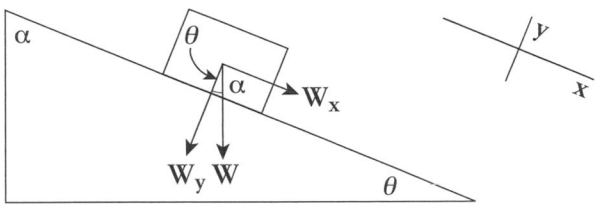

Figure 2.5

Note that in Figure 2.5 the angle **W** makes with the x-axis is α, and we would normally use this angle in expressing the components of **W**; $W_x = W \cos \alpha$ and $W_y = W \sin \alpha$. However, it is more useful to express the components of **W** in terms of the angle θ which the inclined surface makes with the horizontal. In terms of θ the components of **W** are:

$$W_x = W \sin \theta = mg \sin \theta \quad (W = mg)$$

$$W_y = W \cos \theta = mg \cos \theta$$

So let the *x*-axis be parallel to the inclined surface, and let the *y*-axis be perpendicular to it. The motion is along the inclined surface, in other words, along the *x*-axis. Therefore, any acceleration is only in the x direction, and a_y is automatically zero.

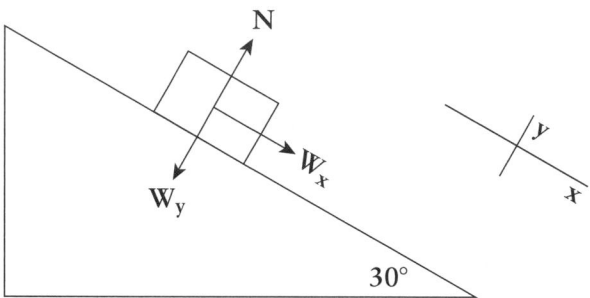

Figure 2.6

Only the forces in the x direction affect the motion of the block. Since there is no acceleration in the y direction, the sum of those forces equals zero.

$$\Sigma F_x = W_x = (5)(9.8) \sin 30° = 24.5 \text{ N} = ma_x$$

$$\Sigma F_y = ma_y = N - W_y = 0$$

From the second equation we can solve for N:

$$N = (5)(9.8) \cos 30° = 42.4 \text{ N}$$

From the first equation we can solve for a_x: (Note that $a_x = a$ since $a_y = 0$.)

$$a = \frac{F}{m}$$

$$= \frac{245}{5}$$

$$= 4.9 \text{ m/s}^2$$

The length d of the incline from where the block started can now be found using:

$$d = \frac{at^2}{2} \qquad (V_0 = 0)$$

$$= \frac{(4.9)(4)^2}{2}$$

$$= 39.2 \text{ m}$$

From trigonometry, the vertical height h is readily available:

$$\sin 30° = \frac{h}{d}$$

$$h = 39.2 \sin 30°$$

$$= 19.6 \text{ m}$$

E. GRAVITY

Gravity is an attractive force that is felt by all forms of matter. The magnitude of the **gravitational force (F)** is given as:

$$F = \frac{Gm_1m_2}{r^2}$$

where G is the gravitational constant (6.67×10^{-11} N•m^2/kg^2), m_1 and m_2 are the masses of the two objects, and r is the distance between their centers.

Example: Find the gravitational attraction between an electron and a proton at a distance of 10^{-11} m. (Proton mass $= 10^{-27}$ kg; electron mass $= 10^{-30}$ kg)

Solution: Using Newton's law of gravitation:

$$F = \frac{Gm_1m_2}{r^2}$$

$$= \frac{(6.67 \times 10^{-11})(10^{-27})(10^{-30})}{(10^{-11})^2}$$

$$= 6.67 \times 10^{-46} \text{ N}$$

EQUILIBRIUM

If several forces act on an object simultaneously, their vector sum may cancel, leaving the motion of the body unchanged. This balancing phenomenon is called **equilibrium.**

A. TRANSLATIONAL EQUILIBRIUM

An unbalanced force acting on an object accelerates the object in the direction of the force. For an object to be in **translational equilibrium,** the sum of the forces pushing the object through space in one direction must be counterbalanced by the sum of the forces acting in the opposite direction. This is called the first condition of equilibrium and can be written as:

$$\Sigma \textbf{F} = 0 \text{ (vector sum)}$$

> **MCAT Synopsis**
>
> Translational equilibrium implies two equations: $\Sigma F_x = 0$ and $\Sigma F_y = 0$.

or, if the vectors are resolved into their x and y components:

$$\Sigma F_x = 0 \qquad \Sigma F_y = 0$$

Example: A block of mass 20 kg is supported as shown in the diagram. Find the tensions T_1 and T_2.

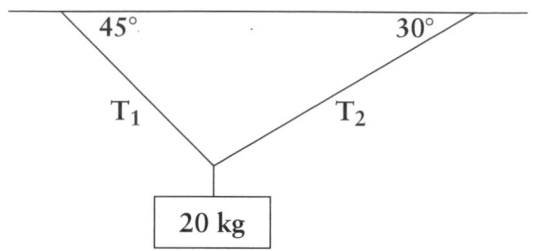

Figure 2.7

Solution: A free-body diagram at the point of intersection of the three cords will help solve this problem. Cords, strings, and the like can only exert pulling forces, and these are in the direction of each cord. Note also that the tension in the vertical cord is equal to the weight of the 20 kg mass, as shown in the other free-body diagram on the right.

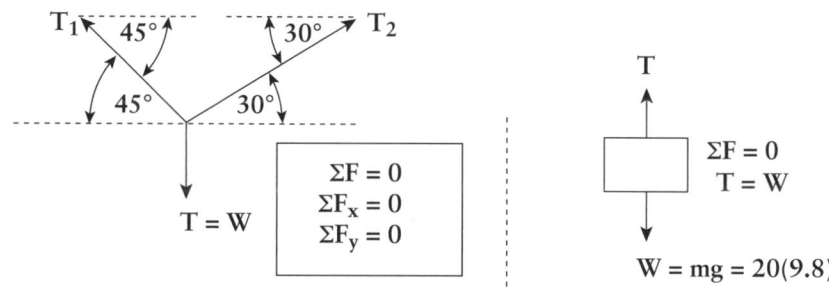

Figure 2.8

The force components are:

$$\Sigma F_x = 0 = T_2 \cos 30° - T_1 \cos 45°$$

$$\Sigma F_y = 0 = T_1 \sin 45° + T_2 \sin 30° - 20(9.8)$$

Solve the second equation for T_1:

$$T_1 = \frac{20(9.8) - T_2 \sin 30°}{\sin 45°}$$

$$= \frac{20(9.8) - T_2/2}{\sqrt{2}/2}$$

$$= \frac{196(2) - (T_2/2)2}{\sqrt{2}}$$

$$= \frac{392 - T_2}{\sqrt{2}}$$

Substitute this into the first equation:

$$\frac{T_2\sqrt{3}}{2} - \frac{\sqrt{2}}{2}\left(\frac{196 - T_2}{\sqrt{2}}\right) = 0$$

$$T_2(\sqrt{3} + 1) = 196$$

$$T_2 = \frac{196}{\sqrt{3} + 1}$$

$$= 71.7 \text{ N}$$

And now T_1 follows from this:

$$T_1 = \frac{196 - 71.7}{\sqrt{2}}$$

$$= 87.9 \text{ N}$$

B. ROTATIONAL EQUILIBRIUM

Unlike translational motion, rotational motion depends not only on the magnitude and direction of the force, but also on the distance from the force to the axis of rotation. The greater the distance, the greater the change in rotational motion that will be produced by a given force. (As an example, try closing a door first by pushing on it a few inches from the hinge, then by pushing far from the hinge. You'll find it's much easier to close the door when you push farther from the hinge because the distance between the axis and the force is greater.)

The quantity that causes rotation is called the **moment of the force** or the **torque** τ, and is given by:

$$\tau = rF \sin \theta$$

where F is the magnitude of the force, r is the distance between the axis and the force (also called the lever arm), and θ is the angle between **F** and **r**.

Torque can act in two directions about a pivot point, clockwise and counterclockwise. Counterclockwise is the positive direction and clockwise the negative direction. For **rotational equilibrium** to occur, the sum of the torques in both these directions must be equal. Since torques causing a rotation in the clockwise direction are negative and torques causing counterclockwise rotations are positive, we can also say that the sum of all the torques must be zero:

$$\Sigma \tau = 0$$

> MCAT Synopsis
>
> Maximum torque when $\theta = 90°$ ($\tau_{max} = rF$), minimum torque when $\theta = 0°$ ($\tau_{min} = 0$).

> MCAT Synopsis
>
> Clockwise torques are negative, while counterclockwise torques are positive.

This is called the second condition of equilibrium.

Example: A seesaw with a mass of 5 kg has one block of mass 10 kg two meters to the left of the fulcrum and another block 0.5 m to the right of the fulcrum. If the seesaw is in equilibrium,

a. find the mass of the second block.
b. find the force exerted by the fulcrum.

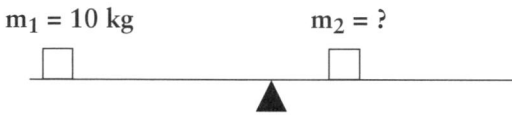

$m_1 = 10$ kg $m_2 = ?$

Figure 2.9

Solution: a. To find τ take the point of the fulcrum as the pivot point. This way, both the normal force and the weight of the seesaw will be eliminated from the equation ($r = 0$). Let's call the 10 kg mass object 1 and the block whose mass we are trying to find object 2.

$$\Sigma\tau = 0 = m_1 g d_1 - m_2 g d_2$$

$$m_2 = \frac{m_1 d_1}{d_2}$$

$$= \frac{10(2)}{0.5}$$

$$= 40 \text{ kg}$$

b. To find the normal force, N, exerted by the fulcrum, $\Sigma F_y = 0$. There is the upward force exerted by the fulcrum and the downward weights of the seesaw and the two masses. Don't forget that $W = mg$. Taking up as positive:

$$N - 5(9.8) - 10(9.8) - 40(9.8) = 0$$
$$N = 49 + 98 + 392 = 539 \text{ N}$$

MOTION

A. TRANSLATIONAL MOTION

Translational motion is defined as motion in which there is no rotation. An example of translational motion is a block sliding on an inclined plane. With Newton's three laws and enough initial conditions, any translational motion problem can be solved.

B. FRICTION

Whenever two objects are in contact, their surfaces rub together creating a friction force. **Static friction** f_s is the force that must be overcome to set an object in motion. Its equation is:

$$0 \le f_s \le \mu_s N$$

where μ_s is the **coefficient of static friction** and **N** is the normal force. Note that static friction can have any value up to some maximum $\mu_s N$. For example, to send a book that is at rest sliding across a table, a force greater than the maximum static friction force is required. Once the book starts to slide, though, the friction force is not quite as strong. This new friction force is called **kinetic friction** f_k, and its equation is:

$$f_k = \mu_k N$$

where μ_k is the **coefficient of kinetic friction** and **N** is the normal force. Remember that friction always acts to oppose motion.

Example: Two blocks are in static equilibrium as shown in Figure 2.10.

a. If block A has a mass of 15 kg and the coefficient of static friction μ_s equals 0.20, then find the maximum mass of block B.

b. If an extra 5 kg are added to B find the acceleration of A and the tension T in the rope. (μ_k equals 0.14)

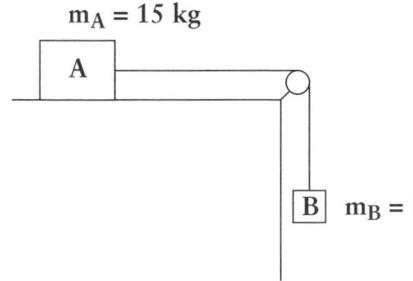

$m_A = 15$ kg

A

B $m_B = ?$

Figure 2.10

Solution: a.

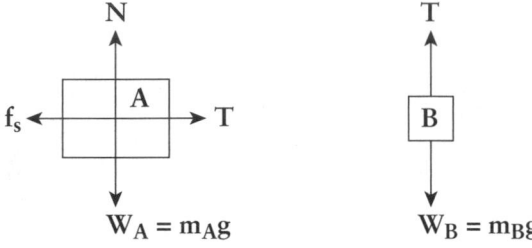

Figure 2.11

For block B:

$$\Sigma F_y = 0 = T - W_B$$
$$T = W_B = m_B g$$

For block A:

Asking for the maximum mass of block B means that the coefficient of static friction holding block A is at its maximum, $f_s = \mu_s N$.

$$\Sigma F_y = 0 = N - W_A$$
$$N = W_A = m_A g$$
$$\Sigma F_x = 0 = T - \mu_s N$$
$$T = \mu_s\, m_A g$$
$$T = (0.2)(15)(9.8)$$
$$T = 29.4\ N$$

Since block B is in static equilibrium, the tension in the rope must equal the weight of the block, so we have:

$$m_B g = 29.4$$
$$m_B = 3\ kg$$

b.

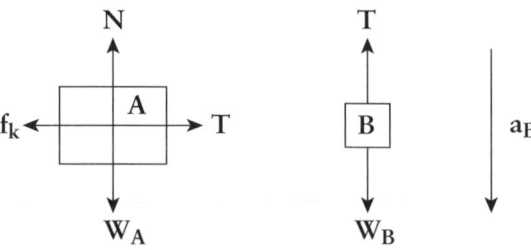

Figure 2.12

We found the maximum mass of B for the system to be in static equilibrium. Adding an extra 5 kg to B means that the system is now in motion.

For block B:

$$\Sigma F_y = m_B g - T = m_B a_B$$

For block A:

$$\Sigma F_x = T - \mu_k N$$
$$- T - \mu_k m_A g$$
$$= m_A a_A$$

Since the blocks are connected by the string, the magnitude of the acceleration for both of them is the same:

$$a_A = a_B = a$$

and

$$m_B g - T = m_B a$$
$$T - \mu_k m_A g = m_A a$$

Adding the two equations gives:

$$m_B g - T + T - \mu_k m_A g = (m_A + m_B)a$$

Solving for a:

$$a = \frac{(m_B - \mu_k m_A)g}{(m_A + m_B)}$$

$$= \frac{(8 - (0.14)(15))9.8}{(15 + 8)}$$

$$= 2.5 \text{ m/s}^2$$

Substituting this value into the equation $m_A a = T - \mu_k m_A g$ and solving for the tension gives:

$$T = m_A(\mu_k g + a)$$
$$= 15(0.14(9.8) + 2.5)$$
$$= 58.1 \text{ N}$$

CIRCULAR MOTION

The velocity vector is always tangent to the circular path. In general, the acceleration vector can be broken into radial and tangential components as shown in Figure 2.13.

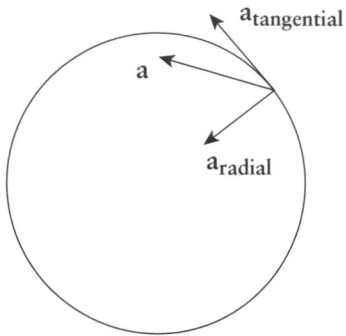

Figure 2.13

In uniform circular motion, the speed of the object remains constant. When uniform circular motion is assumed, there is no tangential acceleration. The radial component of the acceleration is always directed towards the center of the circle and is called **centripetal acceleration.** Its magnitude is given by:

$$a = \frac{v^2}{r}$$

The centripetal acceleration towards the center of the circle must be the result of some force also directed towards the center. Whatever the particular force happens to be, it is called the **centripetal force.** Using the relationship $a = v^2/r$ for the centripetal acceleration, the magnitude of the centripetal force on a particle in circular motion is given by:

$$F = ma = \frac{mv^2}{r}$$

In nonuniform circular motion, the speed of the object changes. In this case there is a tangential component of acceleration, and therefore the resultant acceleration is not directed towards the center of the circle. Instead its direction is given by the resultant of the radial component of the acceleration and the tangential component of the acceleration.

Consider a mass tied to a string, moving with circular motion. To keep the mass moving in a circular path, the string must constantly pull the object towards the center. In this case, the force exerted by the string is the centripetal force. If at some point the string breaks, the inward force no longer acts, and the mass flies off along a path tangential to the circle.

There is always some force that causes circular motion. As another example, consider a planet in orbit around the sun. In this case, the centripetal force is the force of gravity.

3

WORK, ENERGY, AND MOMENTUM

In this chapter we will review the fundamental concepts of energy and momentum and the associated concepts of work and impulse. Essentially, you can think of work as responsible for changing the energy of an object and impulse as responsible for changing the momentum of an object. Regarding energy and momentum, the great laws of conservation of energy and conservation of momentum are discussed along with concrete examples of problems that make use of these laws for their solution. The topic of collisions is discussed in detail as the most common example on the MCAT of the application of conservation of momentum. The concept of work is applied to the problem of pulley systems resulting in the definition of the efficiency of a simple machine. The chapter closes with a review of the equivalent concepts of center of mass and center of gravity.

WORK

A. WORK DEFINED

As was shown in chapter 2, solving mechanics problems using Newtonian methods involves analyzing the forces acting on a system. In this chapter, energy and momentum considerations, rather than forces, will be used to solve problems. Before we undertake a discussion of energy, though, it is important that we first talk about work. For a constant force **F** acting on an object which moves through a distance d, the **work** W is:

$$W = Fd \cos \theta$$

where θ is the angle between **F** and **d.** Units for work (and energy) are the Joule (J) in SI (1 Joule = 1 Newton•meter) and the foot•pound in FPS. Only the component of the force parallel to the path, F cos θ, is relevant. For a force perpendicular to the motion, W = 0 ($\theta = 90°$, thus cos 90° = 0). Note that for a force opposite to the motion ($\theta > 90°$), the work will be negative (cos $\theta < 0$).

> **MCAT Synopsis**
>
> When force and displacement are perpendicular, the work done is zero, therefore the centripetal force does no work.

Example: A block weighing 100 N is pushed up a frictionless incline over a distance of 20 m to a height of 10 m. Find:

a. the minimum force required to push the block;
b. the work done by the force;
c. the force required and the work done by the force if the block were simply lifted vertically 10 m.

Solution:

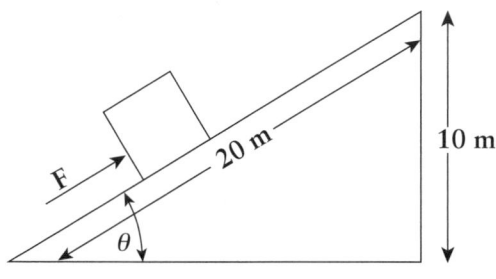

Figure 3.1

a. A free-body diagram of the forces acting on the block:

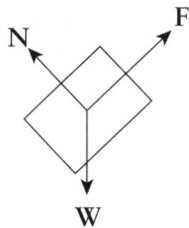

Figure 3.2

The minimum force needed is a force parallel to the plane that will push the block with no acceleration. Since a = 0, $\sum F = 0$:

$$\sum F = 0 = F - mg \sin \theta$$
$$F = mg \sin \theta$$

$mg = 100$ N; $\sin \theta = 10/20$. Therefore:

$$F = 100 \, \frac{10}{20}$$
$$= 50 \text{ N}$$

b. The work done by F is:

$$W = Fd \cos \theta$$

In this case θ is the angle between the force vector and the displacement vector. Since they are parallel, $\theta = 0$, therefore $\cos \theta = 1$. Substituting the numbers into the equation:

$$W = 50(20)(1)$$
$$= 1,000 \text{ J}$$

c. To raise the block vertically, the force should also be vertical and equal to the object's weight.

$$F = mg$$
$$= 100 \text{ N}$$

The work done by the lifting force is:

$$W = Fd \cos \theta$$
$$= 100(10)(1)$$
$$= 1,000 \text{ J}$$

The same amount of work is required in both cases, but twice the force is needed to raise the block vertically compared with pushing it up the incline.

> **MCAT Synopsis**
>
> The force needed to lift an object equals the weight of the object.

B. POWER

Often, the amount of work required to perform an operation is less important than the amount of time required to do the work. The rate at which work is done is called **power** (P), and is given as:

$$P = \frac{W}{t}$$

Units of power are the Watt (W) in SI (1 Watt = 1 Joule/sec) and foot•pound/sec in FPS.

> **Pavlov's Dog**
>
> When you see "rate of work" or "rate of change of energy," think power!

Example: Find the power required to raise the block (of the previous example) in four seconds in each case.

Solution: When lifted up the incline, power is:

$$P = \frac{W}{t}$$

$$= \frac{1,000}{4}$$

$$= 250 \text{ W}$$

When lifted straight up, the power equals:

$$P = \frac{1,000}{4}$$

$$= 250 \text{ W}$$

ENERGY

A. KINETIC ENERGY

A body in motion possesses energy. This energy of motion is called **kinetic energy,** and is defined for a body of mass m and velocity v as:

$$K = \frac{mv^2}{2}$$

Units for kinetic energy are Joules (J) in SI.

Example: A 15 kg block, initially at rest, slides down a frictionless incline and comes to the bottom with a velocity of 7 m/s. What is the kinetic energy at the top and at the bottom?

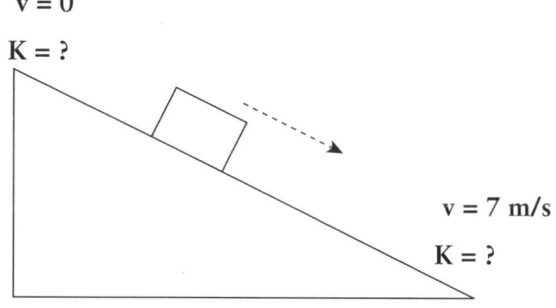

$v = 0$

$K = ?$

$v = 7 \text{ m/s}$

$K = ?$

Figure 3.3

Solution: At the top v = 0, so kinetic energy is:

$$K = \frac{mv^2}{2}$$

$$= \frac{15(0)}{2}$$

$$= 0$$

At the bottom:

$$K = \frac{15(7)^2}{2}$$

$$= 367.5 \text{ J}$$

B. POTENTIAL ENERGY

Another form of energy a body can possess is **potential energy.** Unlike kinetic energy, which depends upon a body's motion, potential energy depends upon a body's **position.** One example of potential energy is the gravitational potential energy an object has when it is raised to a height h. Objects on the earth possess greater potential energy the higher they are from the surface. Gravitational potential energy (U) is given as:

$$U = mgh$$

where m is the mass of the body, g is the acceleration due to gravity, and h is the height of the body. Just as for work and kinetic energy, potential energy's units are Joules (J).

MCAT Synopsis

The equation mgh for potential energy means the ground (h = 0) is the zero of potential energy.

MCAT Synopsis

Potential energy in a stretched or compressed spring is $1/2kx^2$. (See chapter 9.)

Example: An 80 kg diver leaps from a 10 m cliff into the sea. Find the diver's potential energy at the top of the cliff and just as he hits the water (set height equal to zero at sea level).

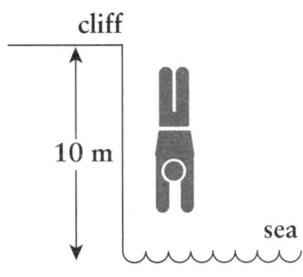

Figure 3.4

Solution: At the top of the cliff:

$$\begin{aligned} U &= mgh \\ &= 80(9.8)(10) \\ &= 7{,}840 \text{ J} \end{aligned}$$

At the water's surface:

$$\begin{aligned} U &= 80(9.8)(0) \\ &= 0 \end{aligned}$$

C. TOTAL MECHANICAL ENERGY

Kinetic and potential energy are both forms of mechanical energy. The total mechanical energy (E) is the sum of the kinetic and the potential energies:

$$E = K + U$$

where K is the kinetic energy of a system and U is the potential energy. Mechanical energy is conserved when the sum of the potential and kinetic energies remains constant. Mechanical energy is not always conserved, though. For example, when friction is present, mechanical energy is drained away in the form of heat.

CONSERVATION OF ENERGY

A. WORK-ENERGY THEOREM

The work-energy theorem relates the work performed by **all** the forces acting on a body in a certain time interval to the change in kinetic energy during that time. In equation form, the theorem is:

$$W = \Delta K$$

Example: A baseball of mass 0.25 kg is thrown straight up in the air with an initial velocity of 30 m/s. Assuming no air resistance, find the work done by the force of gravity when the ball is at its maximum height.

Solution: Neglecting air resistance, the only force acting on the ball is gravity. Since the ball's speed is 0 at its maximum height, using the work-energy theorem:

$$W = \Delta K$$
$$= 0 - \frac{mv^2}{2}$$
$$= \frac{-(0.25)(30)^2}{2}$$
$$= -112.5 \text{ J}$$

B. CONSERVATIVE AND NONCONSERVATIVE FORCES

Conservative forces have associated potential energies (e.g., gravity). There are two equivalent tests that are used to determine whether a force is conservative or not:

1. If the work done to move a particle in any round trip path is zero, the force is conservative.
2. If the work needed to move a particle between two points is the same regardless of the path taken, then the force is conservative.

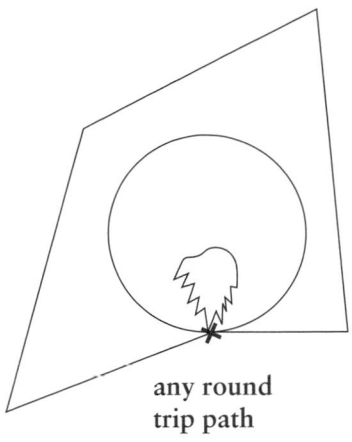 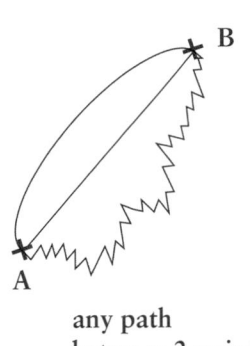

any round
trip path

any path
between 2 points

Figure 3.5

For our purposes we will simply use the following rule of thumb: A force that has an associated potential energy (e.g., gravity) is conservative. An object's weight is just another name for the gravitational force on the object, so an object's weight is a conservative force.

C. CONSERVATION OF ENERGY

When the work done by the nonconservative forces is 0 (or when there are no nonconservative forces, for example, an object falling without air resistance), the total mechanical energy remains constant, and we have **conservation of energy:**

$$E = K + U = \text{constant}$$

or equivalently:

$$\Delta E = \Delta K + \Delta U = 0$$

However, when nonconservative forces such as friction or air resistance are present, mechanical energy is **not** conserved. The equation for a nonconservative system is:

$$W' = \Delta E = \Delta K + \Delta U$$

where **W' is the work done by the nonconservative forces only.** Note that if the work done by the nonconservative forces is zero (which is automatically true if there aren't any such forces), $W' = 0 = \Delta E = \Delta K + \Delta U$ and we have conservation of energy.

> Example: A baseball of mass 0.25 kg is thrown in the air with an initial speed of 30 m/s, but because of air resistance the ball returns to the ground with a speed of 27 m/s. Find the work done by air resistance.

> **MCAT Favorite**
>
> Conservation of energy means $E_{initial} = E_{final}$, so $\Delta E = E_{final} - E_{initial} = 0$.

> **MCAT Synopsis**
>
> In the presence of friction: $E_{initial} > E_{final}$, and the lost energy goes into heat.

Solution: Air resistance is a nonconservative force. To do this problem, the energy equation for a nonconservative system is needed. The work done by air resistance is W'.

$$W' = \Delta E = \Delta K + \Delta U$$

Since $\Delta U = 0$ (final height = initial height):

$$W' = \Delta K$$

$$= \frac{mv_f^2}{2} - \frac{mv_i^2}{2}$$

$$= \frac{1}{2}(0.25)[(27)^2 - (30)^2]$$

$$= -21.4 \text{ J}$$

PULLEYS

Pulley systems allow heavy weights to be lifted using a much smaller force. Consider first the heavy block in Figure 3.6, suspended from two ropes. The force that the block exerts downwards is equaled by the sum of the tensions in the two ropes. For a symmetrical system, the tensions in the two ropes are the same and are equal to half the weight of the block.

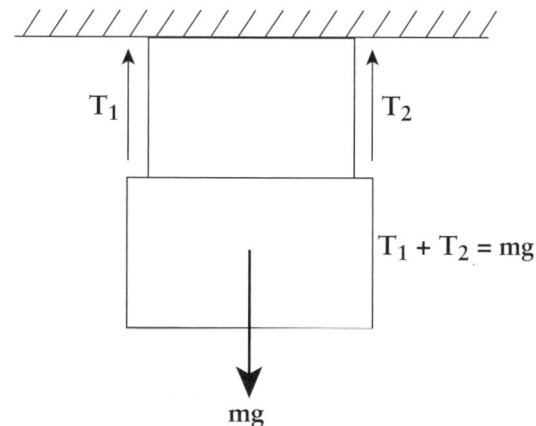

Figure 3.6

Now consider the pulley setup in Figure 3.7, with the block being held stationary. The tension in both vertical ropes will be equal; if they were different, then the pulleys would turn until the tensions on both sides were equal. Since the tensions are equal, each rope supports half the total weight of the block. This means that the force required to raise the block is now only half the total weight of the block. Though only half the force is now required to lift the block, the length of rope that must be pulled through is twice the distance that the block moves upwards. This can be visualized more clearly in considering a case when a block is raised 5 meters. For this to happen, both sides of the supporting rope have to shorten 5 meters, and the only way to accomplish this is by pulling through 10 meters of rope.

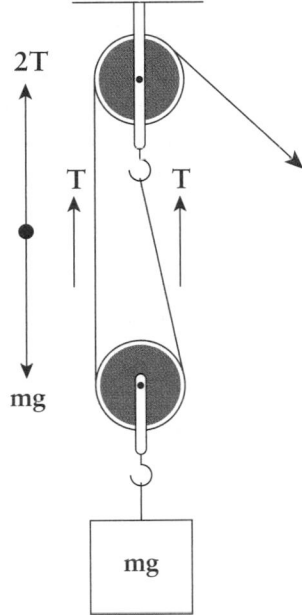

Figure 3.7

In a frictionless pulley system in which the pulleys themselves have no mass, the work expended pulling the rope and the potential energy gained by the mass would be equal. However, no pulley system has these properties, since the pulleys do have mass and are not frictionless. This implies that no real pulley system is 100 percent efficient. At this point it is worth defining some terms. The weight of the object being lifted is the **load,** and the distance it rises is the **load distance.** The force exerted on the rope when lifting the load is known as the **effort,** and the distance through which the effort is exerted is the **effort distance.** It has been mentioned previously that work is force multiplied by the distance that the force moves an object through. Work input is, therefore, the product of the effort and the effort distance, and work output is the product of the load and the distance the load moves through. A measure of the **efficiency** of the system is given by the ratio of the work output to the work input, and is given by

$$\text{Efficiency} = \frac{W_{out}}{W_{in}}$$

$$= \frac{\text{Load} \times \text{Load distance}}{\text{Effort} \times \text{Effort distance}}$$

Efficiencies are often spoken of as percentages (multiply decimal by 100 to get percent), but in doing calculations efficiencies have to be decimals or fractions (divide percentage by 100 to get a decimal). The efficiency gives a measure of the amount of work a person puts into a machine that comes out as useful work.

Consider the pulley system in Figure 3.8. By increasing the number of pulleys, it is possible to reduce the effort still further. In this case, the load has been divided among six strands of the rope, so the effort required is now only one sixth the load. However, it is important to note that, generally speaking, as the number of pulleys increases, the efficiency decreases. This decrease in efficiency is caused by the added weight of each pulley as well as the increase in frictional forces.

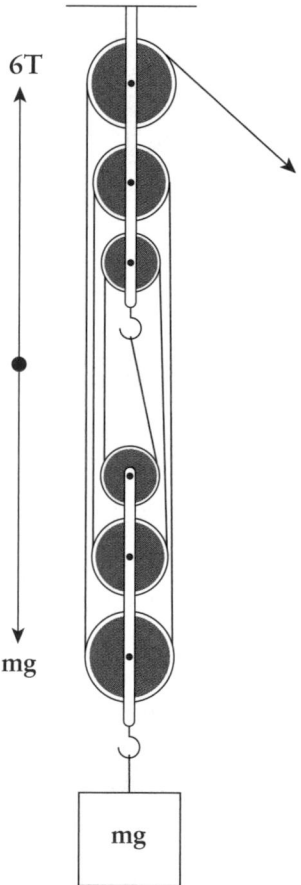

6T

mg

mg

Figure 3.8

Example: The pulley system of Figure 3.8 has an efficiency of 80% and a person is required to lift 200 kg. Find:

    a. the distance through which the effort must move to raise the load a distance of 4 m.

b. the effort required to lift the load.

c. the work done by the person lifting the load through a height of 4 m.

Solution: a. For the load to move through a vertical distance of 4 m, all 6 of the supporting ropes must shorten 4 m also. This may only be accomplished by pulling $6 \times 4 = 24$ m of rope through. So the effort must move through a distance of 24 m.

b. To calculate the effort required, the equation for efficiency must be used. The load is the weight of the object being lifted and is equal to the mass times the acceleration due to gravity g. Since g is approximately 10 m/s² and all the other parameters except the effort are known, it is possible to substitute into this equation to calculate the effort:

$$\text{Efficiency} = \frac{\text{Load} \times \text{Load distance}}{\text{Effort} \times \text{Effort distance}}$$

$$0.80 = \frac{(200)(10)(4)}{(\text{Effort})(24)}$$

$$\text{Effort} = \frac{(2,000)(4)}{(0.80)(24)}$$

$$= 417 \text{ N}$$

c. The work done is given by:

$$\text{Work done} = \text{Effort} \times \text{Effort distance}$$

$$= 417 \times 24$$

$$= 10,000 \text{ J}$$

CONSERVATION OF MOMENTUM

A. MOMENTUM

In nonrelativistic physics, **momentum p** means the product of mass and velocity. Momentum, like velocity, is a vector quantity. In equation form it is given as:

$$\mathbf{p} = m\mathbf{v}$$

For two or more objects, the total momentum is the vector sum of the individual momentums.

> **MCAT Favorite**
>
> Total momentum is vector sum of individual momenta. Keep track of velocity directions!

B. IMPULSE

Applying a force to an object over time will cause that object's momentum to change. The product of the force applied **F** and the time it was applied for t is a vector quantity, and is given the name **impulse J**. For constant forces, impulse and momentum are related by the equation:

$$J = Ft = mv - mv_0 = \Delta p$$

In one-dimensional problems the forces and velocities are either in the positive or the negative direction, and the equation becomes a single scalar equation:

$$J = Ft = mv - mv_0$$

(In this equation, J, F, v, and v_0 are positive or negative depending on whether the corresponding vectors are in the positive or the negative direction.)

Example: A 7 kg bowling ball initially at rest is acted on by a 110 N force for 3.5 s. Find the final speed of the ball.

Solution: From the equation for impulse:

$$Ft = mv - mv_0$$

$$v = v_0 + \frac{Ft}{m}$$

$$= 0 + \frac{110(3.5)}{7}$$

$$= 55 \text{ m/s}$$

C. CONSERVATION OF MOMENTUM

Those forces that one part of a system exerts on another are called **internal forces**. Those forces that are exerted on any part of a system from outside the system are called **external forces**. The principle of **conservation of momentum** states that when the net impulse of the external forces acting on a system is zero, the total momentum of the system remains constant. This condition is automatically satisfied when there are no external forces, or when their vector sum is zero.

> **MCAT Synopsis**
>
> Conservation of momentum means $P_{initial} = P_{final}$ (p's are total initial and final momentum).

D. COLLISIONS

One of the most common applications of conservation of momentum occurs when two objects collide in an idealized collision: one that occurs instantaneously at a specific location. Because there are no external forces, conservation of momentum applies. Conservation of momentum means that the total momentum before the collision equals the total momentum after the collision. For a collision between two objects a, and b, this is given by:

$$\mathbf{p}_{ai} + \mathbf{p}_{bi} = \mathbf{p}_{af} + \mathbf{p}_{bf}$$

where $\mathbf{p}_{ai}$, $\mathbf{p}_{bi}$ are the momenta before the collision, and $\mathbf{p}_{af}$, $\mathbf{p}_{bf}$ are the momenta after the collision. Since momentum has been defined previously as $\mathbf{p} = m\mathbf{v}$, the conservation of momentum equation may be written as:

$$m_a\mathbf{v}_{ai} + m_b\mathbf{v}_{bi} = m_a\mathbf{v}_{af} + m_b\mathbf{v}_{bf}$$

where $\mathbf{v}_{ai}$, $\mathbf{v}_{bi}$ are the velocities before the collision, and $\mathbf{v}_{af}$, $\mathbf{v}_{bf}$ are the velocities after the collision.

In one-dimensional problems, velocities are either in the positive direction or in the negative direction, and the conservation of momentum equation becomes a simple scalar equation:

$$m_av_{ai} + m_bv_{bi} = m_av_{af} + m_bv_{bf}$$

v_{ai}, v_{bi}, v_{af}, and v_{bf} are the magnitudes of the respective velocity vectors. They have positive signs if the velocities are in the positive direction, and negative signs if the velocities are in the negative direction. The positive direction is chosen arbitrarily.

Example: Figure 3.9 shows two bodies moving towards each other on a frictionless air track. Body A has a mass of 2 kg and a speed of 4 m/s, body B has a mass of 3 kg and has a speed of 1 m/s. After the bodies collide, body A moves away with a velocity of 2 m/s to the left. What is the final velocity of body B?

4 m/s   1 m/s

A   B

$m_a = 2$ kg $m_b = 3$ kg

Figure 3.9

Solution: This problem may be solved by equating the total momentum before the collision with the total momentum after the collision. Let the final velocity of body B be v_{bf}. Taking the right as positive (and therefore the left as negative):

$$m_av_{ai} + m_bv_{bi} = m_av_{af} + m_bv_{bf}$$
$$2(4) + 3(-1) = 2(-2) + 3(v_{bf})$$
$$v_{bf} = \frac{8 - 3 + 4}{3}$$
$$v_{bf} = 3 \text{ m/s}$$

The fact that the solution is positive means that body B is moving to the right after the collision.

In many typical one-dimensional problems the velocities before the collision are known, and **both** velocities after the collision are unknown. The two most common types of such problems are **completely inelastic collisions** and **completely elastic collisions**.

1. **Completely Inelastic Collisions**

    A completely inelastic collision is one in which the colliding bodies stick together after the collision. This means that the final velocities of the two bodies are equal, and hence:

$$v_{af} = v_{bf} = v_f$$

Thus, there is only one unknown final velocity. This can be combined with the principle of the conservation of momentum to give:

$$m_a v_{ai} + m_b v_{bi} = (m_a + m_b)\, v_f$$

Example: Two rail freight cars are being hitched together. The first car has a mass of 15,750 kg and is moving at a speed of 4 m/s toward the second car which is stationary and which has a mass of 19,250 kg. Calculate the final velocity of the two cars.

Solution: Using the modified equation above for the conservation of momentum:

$$m_a v_{ai} + m_b v_{bi} = (m_a + m_b)\, v_f$$

$$v_f = \frac{m_a v_{ai} + m_b v_{bi}}{m_a + m_b}$$

Taking the direction of the initial velocity of the car as the positive direction:

$$v_f = \frac{15,750(4) + 19,250(0)}{(15,750 + 19,250)}$$

$$v_f = 1.8 \text{ m/s}$$

The fact that v_f is positive means that after the collision, the two cars together are moving in the direction that the first car was moving initially.

2. **Completely Elastic Collisions**

    A completely elastic collision is one in which kinetic energy is conserved. The final velocities are not necessarily equal. If neither is given, then from the conservation of momentum equation there is one equation and two unknowns. However, in a completely elastic collision, the kinetic energy is conserved. That is to say, the sum of the kinetic energies just after the collision equals the sum of the kinetic energies just before the collision. This provides the needed second equation.

Conservation of momentum:

$$m_a v_{ai} + m_b v_{bi} = m_a v_{af} + m_b v_{bf}$$

Conservation of kinetic energy:

$$\frac{1}{2} m_a v_{ai}^2 + \frac{1}{2} m_b v_{bi}^2 = \frac{1}{2} m_a v_{af}^2 + \frac{1}{2} m_b v_{bf}^2$$

> **MCAT Synopsis**
>
> Use conservation of energy and conservation of momentum in elastic collisions.

Example: Using the results obtained from the example accompanying Figure 3.9, establish whether the collision was completely elastic.

Solution: For the collision to be completely elastic, both the kinetic energy and the momentum must be conserved. The second condition has already been satisfied. Now the kinetic energy before the collision and the kinetic energy after the collision must be calculated, and only if these values are equal can it be said that the collision was completely elastic.

The kinetic energy before the collision is:

$$\frac{1}{2} m_a v_{ai}^2 + \frac{1}{2} m_b v_{bi}^2$$

$$= \frac{1}{2}(2)(4)^2 + \frac{1}{2}(3)(-1)^2$$

$$= 17.5 \text{ J}$$

> **MCAT Favorite**
>
> In elastic collisions: (total kinetic energy before collision) = (total kinetic energy after collision).

The kinetic energy after the collision is:

$$\frac{1}{2} m_a v_{af}^2 + \frac{1}{2} m_b v_{bf}^2$$

$$= \frac{1}{2}(2)(-2)^2 + \frac{1}{2}(3)(3)^2$$

$$= 17.5 \text{ J}$$

Since the kinetic energy is not changed by the collision, it can be said that the collision was completely elastic.

CENTER OF MASS

Every object has a special point known as the **center of mass**. Consider a tennis racket being thrown into the air. Each part of the racket moves in its own way, so it's not possible to represent the motion of the racket as a single particle. However, there will be one point along the axis of the racket that moves in a simple parabolic path, very similar to the flight of a tennis ball. It is this point that is known as the center of mass. This is shown more clearly in Figure 3.10.

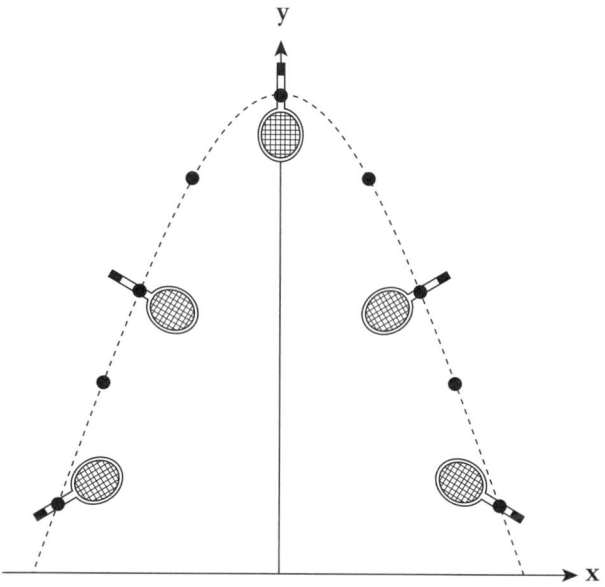

Figure 3.10

For a system of two masses m_1, m_2 lying along the x-axis at points x_1 and x_2 respectively, the center of mass is:

$$X = \frac{m_1x_1 + m_2x_2}{m_1 + m_2}$$

For a system with several masses strung out along the x-axis, the center of mass is given by

$$X = \frac{m_1x_1 + m_2x_2 + m_3x_3 + \ldots}{m_1 + m_2 + m_3 + \ldots}$$

For a system in which the particles are distributed in all three dimensions, the center of mass is defined by the three coordinates:

$$X = \frac{m_1x_1 + m_2x_2 + m_3x_3 + \ldots}{m_1 + m_2 + m_3 + \ldots}$$

$$Y = \frac{m_1y_1 + m_2y_2 + m_3y_3 + \ldots}{m_1 + m_2 + m_3 + \ldots}$$

$$Z = \frac{m_1z_1 + m_2z_2 + m_3z_3 + \ldots}{m_1 + m_2 + m_3 + \ldots}$$

The **center of gravity** is the point at which the entire force due to gravity can be thought of as acting. It is found from similar formulas:

$$X = \frac{W_1x_1 + W_2x_2 + W_3x_3 + \ldots}{W_1 + W_2 + W_3 + \ldots}$$

$$Y = \frac{W_1y_1 + W_2y_2 + W_3y_3 + \ldots}{W_1 + W_2 + W_3 + \ldots}$$

$$Z = \frac{W_1z_1 + W_2z_2 + W_3z_3 + \ldots}{W_1 + W_2 + W_3 + \ldots}$$

Since $W = mg$, the center of gravity and the center of mass will be the same point as long as g is constant.

Example: Find the center of mass with respect to the *x*- and *y*-axes of two uniform metal cubes that are attached to each other as shown in the figure below. One cube has a mass of 2 kg and is 0.4 m on its side, the other has a mass of 0.5 kg and is 0.2 m on its side.

MCAT Synopsis

The force of gravity on an object acts through the center of gravity.

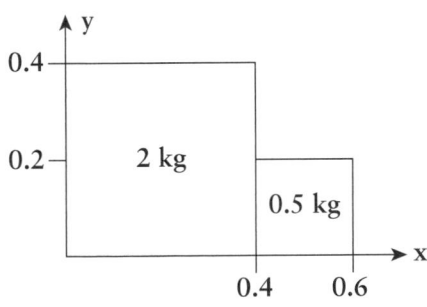

Figure 3.11

Solution: The fact that the cubes are uniform implies that the center of mass for each cube is located at the center of that cube. Therefore, the problem becomes finding the center of mass of two point masses; one is a 2 kg mass located at 0.2 m along the *x*-axis and 0.2 m along the *y*-axis, and the other is a 0.5 kg mass located at 0.5 m along the *x*-axis and 0.1 m along the *y*-axis.

Let's consider the x-coordinate first. The x component of the center of mass can be determined by the following formula:

$$X = \frac{m_1x_1 + m_2x_2 + m_3x_3 + \ldots}{m_1 + m_2 + m_3 + \ldots}$$

Taking m_1 as 2 kg, x_1 as 0.2 m, m_2 as 0.5 kg, and x_2 as 0.5 m:

$$X = \frac{m_1x_1 + m_2x_2}{m_1 + m_2}$$

$$= \frac{2(0.2) + 0.5(0.5)}{2 + 0.5}$$

$$= \frac{0.65}{2.5}$$

$$= 0.26 \text{ m}$$

The y component of the center of mass can be determined by the following formula:

$$Y = \frac{m_1y_1 + m_2y_2 + m_3y_3 + \ldots}{m_1 + m_2 + m_3 + \ldots}$$

Taking m_1 as 2 kg, y_1 as 0.2 m, m_2 as 0.5 kg, and y_2 as 0.1 m:

$$Y = \frac{m_1y_1 + m_2y_2}{m_1 + m_2}$$

$$= \frac{2(0.2) + 0.5(0.1)}{2 + 0.5}$$

$$= \frac{0.45}{2.5}$$

$$= 0.18 \text{ m}$$

4

THERMODYNAMICS

Thermodynamics is the study of heat and its effects. Primary to this study are the concepts of temperature, heat, pressure, volume, work, internal energy, and entropy. As applications of these concepts, we will review thermal expansion, heat transfer processes, the notion of specific heat, heat of transformation (latent heat), and p-v diagrams, including the relationship between work, pressure, and volume. The first law of thermodynamics, or conservation of energy in the presence of heat transfer, is reviewed as is the second law of thermodynamics along with the associated concept of entropy.

TEMPERATURE

A. TEMPERATURE

All bodies possess a property called **temperature.** In common usage, temperature is the relative measure of how hot or cold something is. In the study of thermodynamics, however, temperature must be measured quantitatively on a defined scale. There are three scales used to make these measurements of temperature on a thermometer: the **Fahrenheit** (°F), the **Celsius** (°C), and the **Kelvin** (K) scales. Absolute zero and the boiling and freezing points of water for the three scales are listed in the table below.

> **MCAT Synopsis**
>
> Temperature is a measure of the random kinetic energy of the molecules of a substance.

Temperature Scales

Situation	K	°C	°F
absolute zero	0	−273	−460
freezing point of water	273	0	32
boiling point of water	373	100	212

The Kelvin scale is most commonly used for scientific measurements and is a base unit in SI. The Celsius scale is convenient for everyday usage because of its phase change points for water. The Kelvin degree and

Celsius degree are the same size. The following formulas are used to convert from one scale to another:

$$T_C = T_K - 273$$

$$T_F = \frac{9}{5}T_C + 32$$

where T_C stands for degrees Celsius, T_K stands for degrees Kelvin, and T_F stands for degrees Fahrenheit.

Example: If the weatherperson says that the temperature will reach a high of 303 K today, what will be the temperature in °C and in °F?

Solution: To convert from Kelvin to Celsius use:

$$T_C = T_K - 273$$
$$= 303 - 273$$
$$= 30°C$$

Now to convert from Celsius to Fahrenheit use:

$$T_F = \frac{9}{5}T_C + 32$$

$$= \frac{9}{5}(30) + 32$$

$$= 86°F$$

B. THERMAL EXPANSION

Rising temperatures cause most solids to increase in length. The amount of expansion, known as **thermal expansion**, is proportional to the length of the solid and the increase in temperature:

$$\Delta L = \alpha L \Delta T$$

where ΔL is the change in length, L is the original length, and ΔT is the change in temperature. The **coefficient of linear expansion** α is a constant that characterizes how a specific material's length changes as the temperature changes. This usually has units of K^{-1}, though it may sometimes be quoted as $°C^{-1}$. Note that since a change of 1 K is the same as a change of 1°C, α quoted in units of K^{-1} is absolutely equal to α quoted in units of $°C^{-1}$.

Example: A metal rod of length 2 m and a coefficient of expansion of 11×10^{-6} K^{-1} is heated from 30°C to 1,080°C. By what amount does the rod expand?

Solution: By using the information given in the problem, we can substitute directly into the thermal expansion formula:

$$\Delta L = \alpha L \Delta T$$
$$= (11 \times 10^{-6})(2)(1{,}080 - 30)$$
$$= 0.023 \text{ m}$$

Liquids also expand when heated, but in their case the only meaningful parameter of expansion is **volume expansion**. The formula that governs this expansion for both solids and liquids is:

$$\Delta V = \beta V \, \Delta T$$

where $\beta = 3\alpha$.

Example: Assume that a thermometer with 1 ml of mercury is taken from a freezer with a temperature of –25°C and placed near an oven at 225°C. If the coefficient of volume expansion of mercury is 1.8×10^{-4} K^{-1}, by how much will the liquid expand?

Solution: Using the information given:

$$\Delta V = \beta V \, \Delta T$$
$$= (1.8 \times 10^{-4})(1)(225 - (-25))$$
$$= 0.045 \text{ ml}$$

HEAT

As was stated in the earlier section, all macroscopic objects have a property called temperature. What exactly does a body's temperature say about that body? The answer is that a body's temperature is related to the internal energy of that body. At constant volume, an increase in temperature indicates an increase in internal energy, and a decrease in temperature indicates a decrease in internal energy.

When two objects that are at different temperatures are brought into contact, the object with a higher temperature will give off **heat** energy to the cooler body until both objects have the same temperature. Heat can be defined as the energy transferred between two objects as a result of a difference in temperature. Note that heat can never be transferred from a cooler body to a warmer body without doing work on the system.

A. HEAT TRANSFER

Heat energy can be transferred by conduction, convection, or radiation (or any combination of these processes). **Conduction** is the direct transfer of energy from molecule to molecule through molecular collisions.

Metals are the best heat conductors, since mobile electrons play a role in heat transfer from one molecule to the next. Gases tend to be the poorest heat conductors. An example of heat transfer through conduction is the heat that is rapidly conducted to your finger when you touch a hot stove.

Convection is the transfer of heat by the physical motion of the heated material. Since convection involves a flow of material, it can take place only in fluids (liquids and gases). During convection, heated portions of fluid rise from the source of heat, while colder portions sink. Thus, convection involves the transfer of heat through a flow of material.

Radiation is the transfer of energy by electromagnetic waves, which can travel through a vacuum. An example of this form of heat transfer is the warming effect the sun has on the earth.

B. UNITS

Units of heat are either the **calorie** (cal) for SI, or the **British thermal unit** (Btu) for English units. Note that the calorie defined here (lowercase c) and the term **Calorie** used in nutrition (uppercase C) are not the same. One food Calorie is equal to one thousand calories.

Since heat is equivalent to energy, the **Joule** is also suitable.

The conversion factors among the heat units are as follows:

$$1 \text{ Cal} = 10^3 \text{ cal} = 3.97 \text{ Btu} = 4,184 \text{ J}$$

C. SPECIFIC HEAT

The heat Q gained or lost by an object and the change in temperature of that object ΔT are related by the equation:

$$Q = mc\, \Delta T = mc(T_f - T_i)$$

where m is the mass of the object and c is a proportionality constant called the **specific heat.** The specific heat can be defined as the amount of heat required to raise 1 kg of a substance 1 K or 1°C, and depends solely on the material of the object. This formula applies provided that the phase of the object—solid, liquid, or gas—does not change.

D. HEAT OF TRANSFORMATION

The formula discussed above, $Q = mc\, \Delta T$, applies only when there is no change of phase. During a phase change the temperature remains constant and the heat gained or lost is related to the amount of material which changes phase. The amount of heat needed to change the phase of 1 kg of a substance is the **heat of transformation** L. The total amount of heat gained or lost by a substance during a phase change is given by:

$$Q = mL$$

where Q is the heat gained or lost, m is the mass of the substance, and L is the heat of transformation of the substance.

The phase change from liquid to solid, or solid to liquid, occurs at the melting point temperature. The corresponding heat of transformation is often referred to as the **heat of fusion.** On the other hand, the phase change from liquid to gas, or gas to liquid, occurs at the boiling point temperature. Here the heat of transformation is often referred to as the **heat of vaporization.**

MCAT Synopsis

Temperature is constant during a phase transition, i.e., when melting ice at 0°C, all of the ice must melt before the temperature increases. For more on phase transitions, see chapter 8 of the General Chemistry section.

Example: Silver has a melting point of roughly 1,000°C and a heat of fusion of 1×10^5 J/kg. The specific heat of silver is roughly 250 J/kg•°C. Approximately how much heat is required to completely melt a 1 kg silver chain, whose initial temperature is 20°C?

Solution: Before melting the chain, we must first get the temperature of the chain to the melting point. To figure out how much heat is required, we use the formula:

$$Q = mc(T_f - T_i)$$
$$= 1(250)(1,000 - 20)$$
$$= 245,000 \text{ J}$$
$$= 245 \text{ kJ}$$

This tells us we have to add 245 kJ of heat to the chain just to get the chain's temperature to the melting point. The chain is still in the solid phase. To melt it (change its phase to liquid), we must continue to add heat in accordance with the formula:

$$Q = mL$$
$$= 1(1 \times 10^5)$$
$$= 100,000 \text{ J}$$
$$= 100 \text{ kJ}$$

The total heat needed to melt the solid silver chain is 245 kJ + 100 kJ = 345 kJ.

FIRST LAW OF THERMODYNAMICS

A. PRESSURE

Consider a gas contained in a box. The gas particles move in random direction and some of them hit the wall of the box. As the gas particles hit the wall of the box, they impart a force to the wall. If many particles hit the wall, the net force on the wall increases. The force per unit area is the **pressure** of the gas:

$$P = \frac{F}{A}$$

The SI unit of pressure is the Pascal (Pa). The Pascal is equivalent to a Newton/meter^2. Since this unit is a relatively low pressure, you will often see the pressure quoted in kilopascals (kPa) where 1 kPa = 10^3 Pa. The pressure at sea level can also be used as a unit. This is called an atmosphere (atm), and one atm is equal to 1.013×10^5 Pa.

B. WORK

When dealing with the various problems of thermodynamics, the concept of a system is used. To describe a physical process there are two things to take into account: the system whose behavior is being observed and everything else (the environment).

A good example of a system is a gas contained in a cylinder with a piston that is able to move up when the gas expands and down when the gas is compressed. When the piston moves up, a force is exerted by the gas inside the cylinder to physically expand the system. Since the volume of the system has increased because of a pressure applied by it, work is said to have been done **by** the system. When the piston is compressed, causing the system's volume to decrease, work is done **on** the system by the environment. This implies that work, in thermodynamics problems, depends on pressure and volume.

During any thermodynamic process, a system goes from some initial state with an initial pressure and volume to some other state with a different pressure or volume. These thermodynamic processes are often represented in graphical form with volume on the x-axis and pressure on the y-axis [see Figure 4.1(a)–4.1(d)]. There are an infinite number of paths between an initial and final state. Different paths require different amounts of work. You can calculate the work done on or by a system by finding the area under the pressure-volume curve. Note that if volume doesn't change, then there can be no work done because there is no area to calculate. On the other hand, if pressure remains constant, the area under the curve is a rectangle of length P and width ($V_f - V_i$) or ΔV. Thus, for processes in which the pressure remains constant,

$$W = P \, \Delta V$$

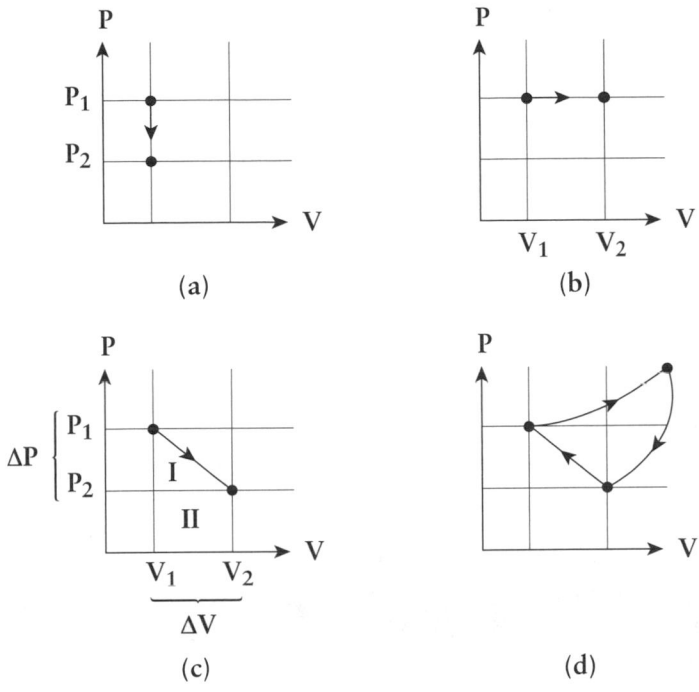

Figure 4.1

Figure 4.1(a) shows that the system undergoes a decrease in pressure from P_1 to P_2. The work done in this process is zero, because volume is constant. In Figure 4.1(b) the system expands from V_1 to V_2 at constant pressure. When the pressure remains constant, the process is called **isobaric.** Here the work done is found using the formula shown above. The work in this case is positive. Figure 4.1(c) shows a case in which neither pressure nor volume is held constant. The total area under the graph (Regions I and II) gives the work done. Region I is a triangle whose base is ΔV and whose height is ΔP and so the area is:

$$A_I = \frac{1}{2}\Delta V \Delta P$$

Region II is a rectangle with base ΔV and height P_2 so its area is:

$$A_{II} = P_2 \Delta V$$

Work now is the sum of region I and II:

$$W = A_I + A_{II}$$

Figure 4.1(d) shows a closed cycle in which, after certain interchanges of work and heat, the system returns to its initial state. Here, the work done is the area enclosed by the curve.

C. FIRST LAW OF THERMODYNAMICS

Internal energy (U) is the measure of all the energy, potential and kinetic, possessed by molecules in a system. The internal energy of a system can be increased by doing work on it or by adding heat to it. This change in internal energy ΔU is calculated from the **First Law of Thermodynamics:**

$$\Delta U = Q - W$$

where Q is the heat energy transferred to the body and W is the work done by the system. Note, we have chosen to use the more common letter U to represent internal energy; however, you may see it also represented by E. Also, note the following **sign convention:** Work done by the system is positive, but work done on the system is negative; heat flow into the system is positive, but heat flow out of the system is negative. The table below gives some special cases of the First Law:

Some Special Cases of the First Law of Thermodynamics

Process	First Law Becomes
Adiabatic (Q = 0)	$\Delta U = -W$
Constant Volume (W = 0)	$\Delta U = Q$
Closed Cycle ($\Delta U = 0$)	$Q = W$

Example: A gas in a cylinder is kept at a constant pressure of 3.5×10^5 Pa while 300 kJ of heat are added to it, causing the gas to expand from 0.9 m^3 to 1.5 m^3. Find:
a. the work done by the gas.
b. the change in internal energy of the gas.

Solution: a. The pressure is held constant through the entire process so the work can be found using the equation:

$$W = P\Delta V$$
$$= (3.5 \times 10^5)(1.5 - 0.9)$$
$$= 2.1 \times 10^5 \text{ J}$$

b. The change in internal energy can be found from the First Law of Thermodynamics:

$$\Delta U = Q - W$$
$$= 3 \times 10^5 - 2.1 \times 10^5$$
$$= 0.9 \times 10^5$$
$$= 9 \times 10^4 \text{ J}$$

ENTROPY AND THE SECOND LAW OF THERMODYNAMICS

Entropy can be defined as the measure of disorder of a system. One way to picture entropy is to imagine a pool divided in two by an impermeable barrier; one side is filled with water, and the other with ink. This system is highly ordered because the ink molecules and water molecules are physically separated. The position of a particular ink molecule is limited to one half of the pool; therefore, there is some degree of certainty as to where a given ink molecule can be found. If someone were to remove the barrier, however, the water and ink would mix until there was no discernible difference between them. The position of a particular ink molecule is less certain now because it has access to the entire pool, as opposed to half of it. Therefore, the order of the system has decreased and its entropy has increased.

The Second Law of Thermodynamics states that in any thermodynamic process that moves from one equilibrium state to another, the entropy of the system and environment together will either increase or remain unchanged. The entropy of the system and environment together will not change during a totally reversible process, but the entropy will increase in an irreversible process. (For a complete discussion of reversible and irreversible processes, see chapter 5 of the General Chemistry section.) Reexamination of the pool described above shows that it is perfectly acceptable for the ink and water to diffuse and mix together, but it is a violation of the Second Law for the mixture to spontaneously separate into two distinct sections of water and ink.

> **MCAT Synopsis**
>
> The entropy of an isolated system increases for all real (irreversible) processes. The entropy of a system (not isolated) can decrease as long as the entropy of its surroundings increases by at least as much (refrigerators are examples of such a system).

Isothermal processes are processes in which the temperature remains constant throughout. For reversible isothermal processes, the change in entropy of the system or of the environment can be found from:

$$\Delta S = \frac{Q}{T}$$

where T is the constant temperature of the system or environment in Kelvins.

Example: If, in a reversible process, 6.66×10^4 J of heat is used to change a 200 g block of ice to water at a temperature of 273 K, what is the change in the entropy of the system? (The heat of fusion of ice = 333 kJ/kg.)

Solution: We know that during a change of phase the temperature is constant, in this case 273 K. From the information given,

$$\Delta S = \frac{Q}{T}$$

$$= \frac{6.66 \times 10^4}{273}$$

$$= 244 \text{ J/K}$$

Note that we did not need to know the mass.

5

FLUIDS AND SOLIDS

In this chapter we review the physics of both fluids and solids. The basic concepts of density and pressure are covered as well as the applied concept of the pressure as a function of depth in a fluid. Hydrostatics, or the study of fluids at rest, is presented from the point of view of the two dominant concepts of hydrostatics: Pascal's principle and Archimedes' principle. Hydrodynamics, or the study of fluids in motion, takes us into a discussion of the continuity equation and Bernoulli's equation, as well as a brief discussion of the viscosity and behavior of real fluids. Finally, the elastic properties of solids are discussed along with the associated concepts of stress, strain, Young's Modulus, Shear Modulus, and the Bulk Modulus.

A. FLUIDS AND SOLIDS

Both liquids and gases are classified as fluids; solids are not. Fluids are characterized by their ability to flow and to conform to the boundaries of any container they are put in. Solids, however, are characterized by their rigidity. While both fluids and solids can exert forces perpendicular to their surfaces, only solids can withstand shear (tangential) forces.

> **MCAT Synopsis**
>
> Different materials have different densities. Density is independent of the size of an object.

B. DENSITY AND PRESSURE

Density ρ is a scalar quantity that is defined as mass m per unit volume V. In equation form:

$$\rho = \frac{m}{V}$$

The units of density are kg/m³ (SI). From the definition of density, the weight of an object can be expressed as the product of its density, volume, and the acceleration due to gravity:

$$W = mg$$
$$m = \rho V$$
$$W = \rho Vg$$

The density of water is 10^3 kg/m³ (= 1 gm/cm³). The ratio of the density of a substance to the density of water is called **specific gravity.** Since it is a ratio, specific gravity has no units.

Example: Find the specific gravity of benzene, given that the density of benzene is 879 kg/m^3.

Solution: The ratio of the density of benzene to the density of water is the specific gravity.

$$\text{specific gravity} = \frac{\rho_{benzene}}{\rho_{water}}$$

$$= \frac{879}{1,000}$$

$$= 0.879$$

Pressure P is also a scalar quantity. It is defined as the magnitude of the normal force F per unit area A. As an equation it reads:

$$P = \frac{F}{A}$$

The SI unit of pressure is the Newton per square meter, also called the Pascal (1 Pa = 1 N/m^2). Another commonly used unit of pressure is the atmosphere, which is the average atmospheric pressure at sea level. It is related to the SI unit of pressure by:

$$1 \text{ atm} = 1.013 \times 10^5 \text{ Pa}$$

Example: The window of a skyscraper measures 2.0 m by 3.5 m. If a storm passes by and lowers the pressure outside the window to 0.997 atm while the pressure inside the building remains at 1 atm, what net force is pushing the window out?

Solution: The forces acting inside and outside the building are needed. However, before the forces may be calculated, the values of the pressure both inside and outside the building must be converted from atmospheres to Pascals.

$$1 \text{ atm} = 1.013 \times 10^5 \text{ Pa}$$
$$0.997 \text{ atm} = (0.997)(1.013 \times 10^5)$$
$$= 1.010 \times 10^5 \text{ Pa}$$

Using the equation for pressure, the force inside pushing out is:

$$F_i = P_i A$$
$$F_i = (1.013 \times 10^5)(7.0)$$
$$= 7.091 \times 10^5 \text{ N}$$

and the force outside pushing in is:

$$F_o = P_o A$$
$$F_o = (1.010 \times 10^5)(7.0)$$
$$= 7.070 \times 10^5 \text{ N}$$

The net force is the difference of these two:

$$F_{net} = 7.091 \times 10^5 - 7.070 \times 10^5$$
$$= 2,100 \text{ N}$$

To find the **absolute pressure P** in a fluid due to gravity somewhere below the surface use the equation:

$$P = P_0 + \rho g h$$

where P_0 is the pressure at the surface, ρ is the density of the fluid, g is the acceleration due to gravity, and h is the depth. In many applications the pressure at the surface is atmospheric pressure, $P_0 = P_{atm} = 1.013 \times 10^5$ Pa. More common in everyday usage than the absolute pressure is what is called the **gauge pressure**. Automobile tire pressure is, for example, reported as gauge pressure. Gauge pressure P_g, is simply the difference between the absolute and atmospheric pressure. The equation for gauge pressure is:

$$P_g = P - P_{atm}$$

Note that if $P_0 = P_{atm}$, then $P_g = \rho g h$ at a depth h.

Example: A diver in the ocean is 20 m below the surface.
   a. What is the absolute pressure he experiences? (density of sea water = 1,025 kg/m³)
   b. What is the gauge pressure?

Solution: a. Using the equation for absolute pressure in a liquid:

$$P = P_{atm} + \rho g h$$
$$= 1.013 \times 10^5 + (1,025)(9.8)(20)$$
$$= 3.02 \times 10^5 \text{ Pa}$$

b. Using the equation for gauge pressure:

$$P_g = P - P_{atm}$$
$$= (3.02 - 1.013) \times 10^5$$
$$= 2.01 \times 10^5 \text{ Pa}$$

HYDROSTATICS

A. PASCAL'S PRINCIPLE

Pascal's principle deals with the transmission of pressures in enclosed fluids. The principle states:

> A change in the pressure applied to an enclosed fluid is transmitted undiminished to every portion of the fluid and to the walls of the containing vessel.

For example, a fluid in a tube exerts pressure on an object at any depth below the surface of the fluid. When the pressure on the fluid is increased, pressure will be increased throughout the fluid and on any submerged object in the fluid.

Pascal's principle is the basis of the hydraulic lever (see Figure 5.1). Consider the case when an external force of magnitude F_1 is applied to the left-hand piston of area A_1. To keep the system in equilibrium, a force of magnitude F_2 must be applied to the right-hand piston of area A_2.

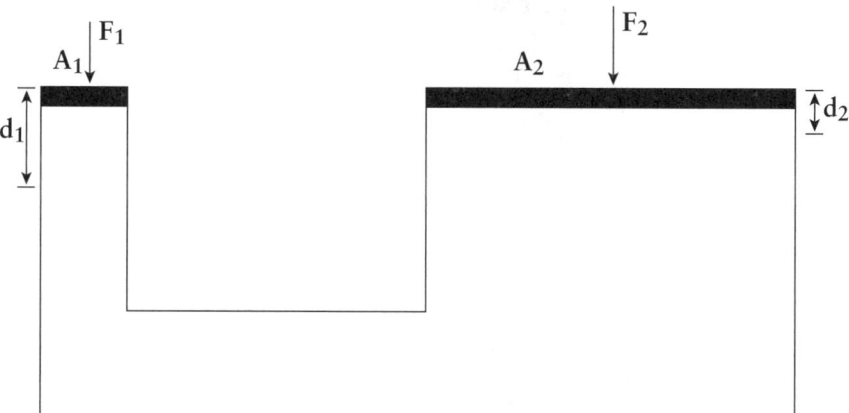

Figure 5.1

Pascal's principle states that a change in pressure is transmitted to every portion of the fluid. Since the system remains in equilibrium as the pressure changes, the change in pressure in both pistons must be equal and is given by:

$$\Delta P = \frac{F_1}{A_1} = \frac{F_2}{A_2}$$

$$F_2 = \frac{F_1 A_2}{A_1}$$

This equation shows that F_2 can be made larger if $A_2 > A_1$.

When piston 1 is moved down a distance d_1, piston 2 moves up a distance d_2. If the fluid is incompressible, then the volume in the system must remain constant. This implies that:

$$V = A_1 d_1 = A_2 d_2$$

$$d_2 = d_1 \frac{A_1}{A_2}$$

By combining the above two equations the expression below is obtained:

$$F_1 d_1 = F_2 d_2 = W$$

where work W is the product of force and distance. This shows that no additional work is being done by the greater force; the greater force is moving through a smaller distance.

Example: A hydraulic press has a piston of radius 5 cm, which pushes down on an enclosed fluid. A 45 kg weight rests on this piston. The other piston has a radius of 20 cm. Taking g = 10 m/s², what force is needed on the larger piston to keep the press in equilibrium?

Solution: Using Pascal's principle:

$$\frac{F_2}{A_2} = \frac{F_1}{A_1}$$

$$F_2 = \frac{F_1 A_2}{A_1}$$

Since $F_1 = mg$, and $A = \pi r^2$, it is possible to solve for F_2:

$$F_2 = \frac{45(10)\pi(0.2)^2}{\pi(0.05)^2}$$

$$= 7{,}200 \text{ N}$$

B. ARCHIMEDES' PRINCIPLE

Archimedes' principle deals with the buoyancy of objects when placed in a fluid. It explains why ships float and why objects seem lighter when underwater. The principle states:

> A body wholly or partially immersed in a fluid will be buoyed up by a force equal to the weight of the fluid that it displaces.

In other words, when any object is placed in a fluid, it displaces some of that fluid, and the weight of the displaced fluid equals the magnitude of the upward buoyant force which the fluid exerts on the object. If the volume of fluid displaced by the object has a weight greater than the object's weight, then the object will float. If the weight of fluid displaced is less than the object's weight, then the object will sink deeper until the weight of the displaced fluid exceeds its own weight. If the weight of the displaced fluid is less than the object's weight even when fully submerged, then the object will sink. In terms of density, if the average density of the object is less than that of the surrounding fluid, then the object will float. However, if the average density of the object is greater than that of the surrounding fluid, then the object will sink.

Example: A wooden block floats in the ocean with half its volume submerged. Find the density of the wood ρ_b. (The density of seawater is 1,024 kg/m³.)

Solution: The weight of the block of total volume V_b is:

$$W_b = m_b g = \rho_b V_b g$$

The weight of the displaced seawater is the buoyant force and is given by:

$$W_w = F_{buoy} = m_w g = \rho_w V_w g$$

where ρ_w is the density of seawater (1,024 kg/m³) and V_w is the volume of displaced water, which is also the volume of that part of the block which is submerged. Since the block is floating, the buoyant force equals the block's weight:

$$W_b = F_{buoy}$$

$$\rho_b V_b g = \rho_w V_w g$$

We are given that half the block is submerged, so $V_w = V_b/2$.

$$\rho_b V_b g = \frac{1}{2} \rho_w V_b g$$

$$\rho_b = \frac{1}{2} \rho_w$$

$$\rho_b = \frac{1}{2} (1,024)$$

$$= 512 \text{ kg/m}^3$$

C. SURFACE TENSION

There are two types of forces that the molecules of a liquid experience. The first type is **adhesion,** which is the attractive force that a molecule of the liquid feels toward the molecules of some other substance. For example, the adhesive force causes water droplets to stick to the windshield of a car even though gravity is pulling them downward.

The second type of force experienced by the molecules in a liquid is **cohesion.** Cohesion is the attractive force that a molecule of the liquid feels toward the other molecules of the liquid. Below the surface of the liquid, the cohesive forces cancel out since any one molecule is surrounded on all sides by the other molecules of the liquid. However, on the surface, the molecules feel an unbalanced force pulling them back toward the liquid. This causes the surface to behave like a skin and results in what is known as the **surface tension.** An example of the force of the surface tension is the fact that an insect can float on water even though its density is greater than that of water.

HYDRODYNAMICS

A. STREAMLINES

When talking about the steady, nonturbulent flow of fluids, it is helpful to use streamlines. Streamlines are the paths followed by tiny fluid elements (sometimes called fluid particles) as they move. The velocity of a fluid particle will always be tangent to the streamline at that point. It is important to note that streamlines may never cross.

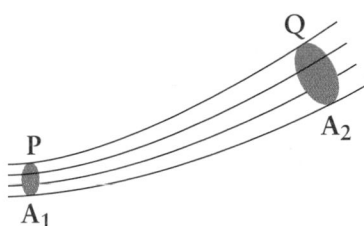

Figure 5.2

Figure 5.2 shows a tube of flow defined by streamlines that form its boundary. Mass flows from cross sectional area A_1 to A_2. The mass of fluid flowing per second through cross sectional area A is given by $Av\rho$, where v is the velocity and ρ is the density. Since matter is conserved, the mass flow rate of fluid must remain constant from one cross-section to another. It is also assumed that the fluid is incompressible, which implies that the densities are equal. Therefore, canceling the density, we find that the volume flow rate is given by:

$$v_1 A_1 = v_2 A_2 = \text{constant}$$

which is known as the **continuity equation.** This equation states that in narrow passages the flow is faster than in wide passages.

B. BERNOULLI'S EQUATION

The continuity equation, stated previously, results from the conservation of the mass of the fluid. This equation is a statement of the fluid's incompressibility as it flows from one point to another. Energy is also conserved as the fluid flows, and Bernoulli formulated this fact into the following equation that bears his name:

$$P_1 + \frac{\rho v_1^2}{2} + \rho g y_1 = P_2 + \frac{\rho v_2^2}{2} + \rho g y_2 = \text{a constant}$$

where P is the absolute pressure of the fluid, ρ is the density of the fluid, v is the velocity of the fluid, g is the acceleration due to gravity, and y is the height of the fluid relative to some reference height. Like the continuity equation, the Bernoulli equation also refers to two distinct points along the fluid flow labeled by subscripts 1 and 2, respectively. An important relation is derived for the case in which the height of the fluid doesn't change from point 1 to point 2 ($y_1 = y_2$). The pressure of the fluid then decreases as the velocity of the fluid increases and vice versa.

Example: An office building with a bathroom 40 m above ground has its water enter the building through a pipe at ground level with an inner diameter of 4 cm. If the flow velocity when entering is 3 m/s and at the top is 8 m/s, find the cross-sectional area of the pipe at the top and the pressure needed at the bottom so that pressure in the bathroom is 3×10^5 Pa.

Solution: The cross-sectional area of the pipe in the bathroom is calculated using the continuity equation, where point 1 is the ground level and point 2 is the bathroom:

$$A_2 = A_1 \frac{v_1}{v_2}$$

$$= \pi (0.02)^2 \, \frac{3}{8}$$

$$= \pi (1.5 \times 10^{-4})$$

$$= 4.71 \times 10^{-4} \text{ m}^2$$

The pressure can be found from Bernoulli's equation:

$$P_1 + \frac{1}{2} \rho v_1^2 + \rho g y_1 = P_2 + \frac{1}{2} \rho v_2^2 + \rho g y_2$$

$$P_1 = P_2 + \frac{1}{2}\rho(v_2{}^2 - v_1{}^2) + \rho g(y_2 - y_1)$$

$$= 3 \times 10^5 + \frac{1}{2}(1 \times 10^3)((8)^2 - (3)^2) + (1 \times 10^3)(9.8)(40)$$

$$= 7.2 \times 10^5 \text{ Pa}$$

C. VISCOSITY

Viscosity η is a measure of the internal friction of a fluid. Because of viscosity, a force must be exerted to cause one layer of fluid to slide past another. Both liquids and gases have viscosity, though the viscosity of gases is much lower than that of liquids since a gas has a much lower density. Consider a person moving a hand through air. Little effort is required to move the air out of the way. Hence the viscosity of air is very low. However, for the same person to move the same hand through a tub of water is much more difficult. This is because water has a much higher viscosity than air, and so a greater force is required to move the water out of the way.

The SI unit of viscosity is the Newton•second/meter^2 (N•s/m^2). The CGS unit is the dyne•second/centimeter^2 (dyn•s/cm^2), also called the poise. 1 N•s/m^2 = 10 poise.

D. LAMINAR AND TURBULENT FLOW

The simplest type of flow in a tube is **laminar flow**: thin layers of liquid sliding over one another. However, when the velocity of a fluid flowing in a tube exceeds a certain critical velocity v_c (dependent on the properties of the fluid and the diameter of the tube), the nature of the flow becomes very complex. In this case laminar flow occurs only in a very thin layer adjacent to the walls, called the boundary layer. The flow velocity is zero at the tube walls and increases uniformly throughout the layer. Beyond the boundary layer, the motion is highly irregular. Here, random local circular currents called vortices develop within the fluid, and this results in a large increase in resistance to flow. This type of flow is known as **turbulent flow**.

For a fluid flowing through a tube of diameter D, a critical velocity v_c exists below which the flow is laminar and above which it is turbulent. This critical velocity can be calculated from the properties of the fluid flow and is given by:

$$v_c = \frac{N_R \eta}{\rho D}$$

where N_R is a dimensionless constant called the Reynolds number, η is the viscosity of the fluid, ρ is the density of the fluid, and D is the diameter of the tube.

ELASTIC PROPERTIES OF SOLIDS

A. YOUNG'S MODULUS

The elasticity of a solid is characterized by a number of different quantities called **moduli.** When subjected to a stretching or tensile force F, a material will stretch a length ΔL. Defining a modulus in terms of F and ΔL is difficult because two bodies made of the same substance might require differing forces to yield the same ΔL. This ambiguity is eliminated by defining the tensile stress as the force per unit area, where the force is perpendicular to the area. Similarly, the change in length ΔL may vary for identical materials of different starting lengths L. This ambiguity is also eliminated by defining a quantity called the **strain,** which is the elongation per unit length ΔL/L. It is assumed that upon termination of the stress, the material returns to its original length. **Young's modulus** Y is then defined as the quotient of stress over strain and is given by:

$$Y = \frac{(F/A)}{(\Delta L/L)}$$

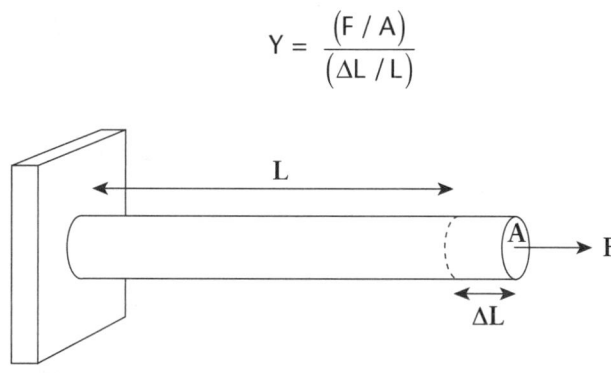

Figure 5.3

Yield strength is the point beyond which a material will not return to its original dimensions once the force is removed. If more stress is applied, eventually the ultimate strength is reached. Beyond that point, rupture occurs.

B. SHEAR MODULUS

Another type of deforming stress is **shearing,** which is measured in units of force per unit area. However, in this case the force vector lies parallel to the area as shown in Figure 5.4. The corresponding deformation or strain is x, the movement in the direction of the force, divided by h. The **shear modulus** is defined as the ratio of the stress to the strain and is given by:

$$S = \frac{(F/A)}{(x/h)}$$

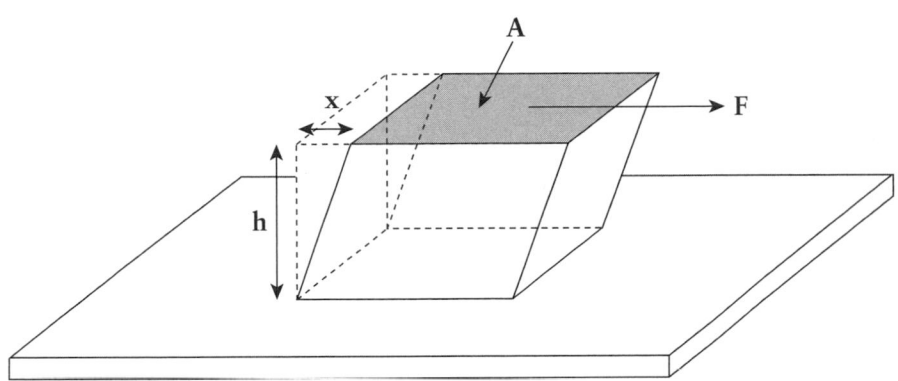

Figure 5.4

C. BULK MODULUS

The **bulk modulus** relates the change in pressure acting on the surfaces of a solid or fluid to the change in volume that is produced. The stress is the change in pressure ΔP and the strain is $\Delta V/V$, where V is the original volume and ΔV is the decrease in volume. This leads to the following equation for the bulk modulus:

$$B = \frac{\Delta P}{\Delta V / V}$$

6

ELECTROSTATICS

Electrostatics is the study of stationary or static charges and the forces between them. In this chapter we will review Coulomb's law, which gives the electrostatic force between two charges and then discuss the concept of the electric field, which gives the electrostatic force per unit charge. The topic of electric potential energy is discussed along with the related topic of the electric potential, which is electric potential energy per unit charge. One can think of the electric potential being related to the electric potential energy in the same way as the electric field is related to the electric force. Associated with the electric field and electric potential are the concepts of field lines and equipotential lines which are reviewed separately. Finally, a detailed discussion of the electric dipole is presented with a worked example of a real life dipole, the H_2O molecule.

CHARGES

Charge may be either positive or negative. A positive charge and a negative charge attract one another; positive repels positive; and negative repels negative. To summarize: **unlike charges attract, like charges repel.** The force that exists between stationary charges is known as the **electrostatic** force.

Net charge can appear on a macroscopic object due to friction. If a glass rod is rubbed on a piece of silk, electrons, which are negatively charged, flow from the glass rod to the silk cloth. This results in the glass rod being positively charged and the silk cloth being negatively charged. The rod and cloth then attract each other; this is known as static cling.

The SI unit of charge is the **Coulomb** and the **fundamental unit of charge** is:

$$e = 1.60 \times 10^{-19} \text{ C}$$

Both protons and electrons have this amount of charge, though protons are positively charged (q = +e), and electrons are negatively charged (q = −e).

COULOMB'S LAW

Coulomb's law gives the magnitude of the electrostatic force F between two charges, q_1 and q_2, whose centers are separated by a distance r:

$$F = k\frac{q_1 q_2}{r^2}$$

where k is called **Coulomb's constant** or the **electrostatic constant,** and is a number that depends on the units used in the equation. In SI units $k = 1/4\pi\varepsilon_0 = 8.99 \times 10^9 \ N\bullet m^2/C^2$, where $\varepsilon_0 = 8.85 \times 10^{-12} C^2/N\bullet m^2$ and is called the **permittivity of free space.**

Coulomb's law in SI units is therefore:

$$F = k\frac{q_1 q_2}{r^2} = \frac{1}{4\pi\varepsilon_0}\frac{q_1 q_2}{r^2} = 8.99 \times 10^9 \frac{q_1 q_2}{r^2}$$

where the force F is in Newtons, the charges q_1 and q_2 are in Coulombs, and the distance r is in meters. The direction of the force may be obtained by remembering that unlike charges attract and like charges repel. The force always points along the line connecting the centers of the two charges.

Example: A positive charge is attracted to a negative charge a certain distance away. The charges are then moved so that they are separated by twice the distance. How has the force of attraction changed between them?

Solution: Coulomb's law states that the force between two charges varies as the inverse of the square of the distance between them. Therefore, if the distance is doubled, the square of the distance is quadrupled and the force is reduced to 1/4 of what it was originally. Note that it was not necessary to know the distance or the units being used, but only the fact that the distance was doubled and that the relation was an inverse square law.

Example: Negatively charged electrons are electrostatically attracted to positively charged protons (together they form hydrogen atoms). Because electrons and protons have mass, they will be gravitationally attracted to each other as well. Compare the two forces using Coulomb's law and Newton's law of gravitation. (Use $m_p = 1.67 \times 10^{-27}$ kg, $m_e = 9.11 \times 10^{-31}$ kg, and a Bohr radius separation between the electron and proton so that r = 5.29×10^{-11}m.)

Solution: Both Coulomb's law and Newton's law state that the attractive forces between the electron and proton vary as the inverse of the square of the distance between them. As calculated in chapter 2, the gravitational attractive force is:

$$F_N = \frac{Gm_pm_e}{r^2}$$

$$= \frac{(6.67 \times 10^{-11})(1.67 \times 10^{-27})(9.11 \times 10^{-31})}{(5.29 \times 10^{-11})^2} F$$

$$= 3.63 \times 10^{-47} \text{ N} \approx 10^{-47} \text{ N}$$

On the other hand, the magnitude of the electrostatic attractive force is:

$$F_c = \frac{1}{4\pi\varepsilon_0} \frac{q_pq_e}{r^2}$$

$$= \frac{(8.99 \times 10^9)(1.60 \times 10^{-19})(1.60 \times 10^{-19})}{(5.29 \times 10^{-11})^2}$$

$$= 8.22 \times 10^{-8} \text{ N} \approx 10^{-7} \text{ N}$$

Note that the electrostatic attraction between the electron and proton is stronger than the gravitational attraction by a factor of approximately 10^{40}.

ELECTRIC FIELD

Every electric charge sets up a surrounding **electric field**. The electric field can be detected by the force it exerts on other electric charges. It is defined as the force on a stationary positive test charge q_0 divided by the charge. It is therefore a vector quantity given by:

$$E = \frac{F}{q_0}$$

The electric field **E** points in the direction of the force **F** on the positive test charge q_0. In SI units, **E** is measured in Newtons/Coulomb, which equals Volts/meter. The Volt will be defined in the next section where the electric potential is discussed.

Given an electric field **E** in some region of space, any charge q placed in the field experiences a force **F** given by:

$$F = qE$$

MCAT Synopsis

The Electric field is a vector with units given by $E = \dfrac{F}{q_0} =$ Newtons/Coulomb.

MCAT Synopsis

A positive charge in an electric field feels a force in the direction of the field. A negative charge in an electric field feels a force in the direction opposite the field.

In this vector equation we keep the sign of the charge, so that the force **F** is in the direction of q**E**: that is, in the same direction as **E** itself if q is positive, but in the opposite direction to **E** if q is negative.

The force on a positive test charge q_0 placed a distance r from a charge q is given by Coulomb's Law:

$$F = k\frac{qq_0}{r^2}$$

Using this equation and the fact that the electric field $E = F/q_0$, we get an equation for the electric field at any distance r from a charge q:

$$E = k\frac{q}{r^2}$$

The **direction** of the electric field vector is such that it points away from q if q is a positive charge, but it points towards q if q is a negative charge. In order to visualize the direction and magnitude of the electric field vector over a wide number of points, it is helpful to think of **field lines.** Field lines, or **lines of force,** as they are sometimes called, are imaginary lines that represent how a positive test charge would be accelerated in the electric field. For example, the field lines for a negatively charged particle such as an electron would point radially toward the charge, since the positive test charge would be attracted toward a negative charge. Similarly, the field lines point radially away from a positive charge, such as a proton, since the positive test charge would be repelled away from another positive charge.

The direction of the electric field, at a given point, is always tangent to the field line at that point and in the same direction. Field lines also indicate the relative strength of the electric field. Where the field lines are closer together the electric field is stronger; where the field lines are farther apart the electric field is weaker.

For a collection of charges, the total electric field at a point in space is the **vector sum** of the electric field due to each charge:

$$\mathbf{E}_{total} = \mathbf{E}_{q_1} + \mathbf{E}_{q_2} + \mathbf{E}_{q_3} + \cdots \text{ (vector sum)}$$

The vector sum must be carried out using the rules of vector addition, as shown in the following example.

Example: A positive charge of $+1 \times 10^{-5}$ C is located one meter away from another positive charge of $+2 \times 10^{-5}$ C. At what point along the line between the two charges is the electric field equal to zero?

MCAT Synopsis

The electric field of a positive charge points radially outward from the charge. The electric field of a negative charge points radially inward towards the charge.

MCAT Synopsis

The electric field strength is stronger where the field lines are closer together and weaker where the field lines are farther apart.

MCAT Synopsis

Electric fields of separate charges add as vectors.

Solution: In order for the sum of two vectors to be zero, they must be equal in magnitude and opposite in direction. Because both of the charges are positive, the electric field vector of each charge points away from the charge. Along the line between the two charges the two electric field vectors point in opposite directions. If the charges were equal in magnitude, the point at which the two fields have the same magnitude (and therefore where the resultant field is zero) would be exactly halfway between them. However, the charges are not equal, since one charge is half the charge of the other. Let x be the distance from the $+1 \times 10^{-5}$ C charge. The distance from the other charge is the total distance of one meter minus x, or $(1 - x)$.

Setting the magnitudes of the two fields equal to each other to find the distance x that will make them equal, we have:

$$k\frac{(1 \times 10^{-5})}{x^2} = k\frac{(2 \times 10^{-5})}{(1-x)^2}$$

$$\frac{1}{x^2} = \frac{2}{(1-x)^2}$$

$$2x^2 = (1-x)^2$$

$$\sqrt{2}\,x = 1 - x$$

$$x(1 + \sqrt{2}) = 1$$

$$x = \frac{1}{\sqrt{2}+1}$$

$$x = 0.41 \text{ m}$$

As might be expected, this point is closer to the smaller charge since the field of the larger charge is stronger.

ELECTRIC POTENTIAL

Just as work is required to lift an object against the earth's gravitational field, work must be done to move an electric charge in an electric field. The **electric potential** at a point is defined as the amount of work needed to move a positive test charge q_0 from infinity to that point divided by the test charge q_0:

$$V = \frac{W}{q_0}$$

In SI units electric potential is measured in **Volts** (V) where 1 Volt = 1 Joule/Coulomb.

The electric potential at a distance r from a point charge q is:

$$V = k\,\frac{q}{r}$$

V is a scalar quantity whose sign is determined by the sign of the charge q. For a positive charge V is positive, but for a negative charge V is negative. For a collection of charges, the total electric potential at a point in space is the **scalar sum** of the electric potential due to each charge:

$$V_{total} = V_{q_1} + V_{q_2} + V_{q_3} + \ldots \text{ (scalar sum)}$$

Potential difference (voltage) is the difference in potential between two points. If V_a and V_b are the electric potentials at points a and b, then the potential difference between a and b is $V_b - V_a$. From the definition of electric potential, it follows that the potential difference between a and b can be expressed as:

$$V_b - V_a = \frac{W_{ab}}{q_0}$$

where W_{ab} is the work needed to move a test charge q_0 through an electric field from a to b. The work depends only on the potentials at the two points a and b, and is independent of the path. This means that like the gravitational force in chapter 3, the electrostatic force is a conservative force.

Typical voltages encountered in medical research range from the millivolt (e.g., the 70 to 90 millivolt potential across a cell membrane), to 10 volts (the approximate pulse voltage of a pacemaker), to the tens of billions of volts (gigavolts or GV) used to accelerate protons for nuclear medicine purposes (as in the preparation of radioisotopes).

EQUIPOTENTIAL LINES

An **equipotential line** is one for which the potential at every point is the same. The potential difference between any two points on an equipotential line is zero. From the above equation it follows that no work is done when moving a test charge q_0 from one point to another on an equipotential line. Work will be done in going from one line to another, but the **work depends only on the potential difference of the two lines and not on the path.**

Example: In Figure 6.1 an electron goes from point a to point b in the vicinity of a very large positive charge. The electron could be made to follow any of the paths shown. Which path requires the least work to get the electron charge from a to b?

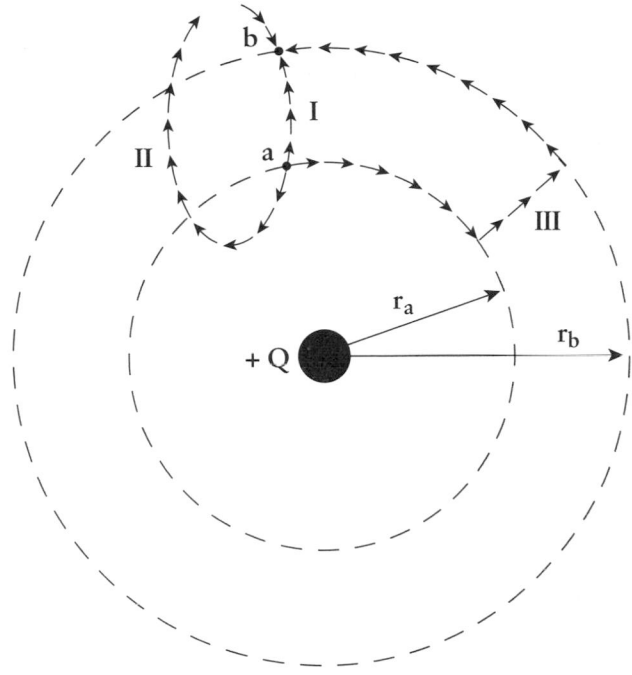

Figure 6.1

Solution: As stated, the **work depends only on the potential difference and not on the path**, so any of the paths shown would require the same amount of work in moving the electron from a to b, namely:

$$W_{ab} = q_e(V_b - V_a)$$

$$= q_e(k\frac{Q}{r_b} - k\frac{Q}{r_a})$$

So paths I, II, and III all require the same amount of work to move the electron. (Note that W_{ab} is positive in this example since $r_a < r_b$ and $q_e = -e$).

ELECTRIC POTENTIAL ENERGY

We have already defined the electric potential V at a point in space as the amount of work W required to move a positive test charge q_0 from infinity to that point divided by q_0. We now define the electric potential energy U of an arbitrary charge q at that point in space to be the amount of work needed to move it from infinity to the point. Using the definition of the electric potential we get:

$$U = W = qV$$

> ### MCAT Favorite
>
> The amount of work necessary to move a charge in an electric field depends only on the potential difference. Recall that in the case of gravity, the work required to move a mass depends only on the difference in height.

> ### MCAT Synopsis
>
> Electric potential energy, U, equals charge times electric potential: U = qV. Change in electric potential energy equals charge times change in electric potential: $\Delta U = q\Delta V$.

where V is the electric potential due to the other charges. Note that the sign of U depends on the signs of q and V. Since U = qV, it may be said that V = U/q; electric potential can also be thought of as electric potential energy per unit charge. When V is due to just one other charge Q, V is given by kQ/r, and U may be rewritten as:

$$U = k\frac{qQ}{r}$$

$$= \left(\frac{1}{4\pi\varepsilon_0}\right)\frac{qQ}{r}$$

If the charges are both positive or both negative (in other words, like charges), U will be positive, but if one charge is positive and the other negative (that is, unlike charges), U will be negative.

Example: If a charge of +2e and a charge of –3e are separated by a distance of 3 nm, what is the potential energy of the system? (e is the fundamental unit of charge equal to 1.6×10^{-19} C.)

Solution:

$$U = k\frac{qQ}{r}$$

From the question stem we know that q = +2e, Q = –3e, and r = 3nm = 3×10^{-9}m. So, putting these numbers into the equation, and approximating k as 9.0×10^9:

$$U = (9 \times 10^9)\frac{(2)(1.6 \times 10^{-19})(-3)(1.6 \times 10^{-19})}{3 \times 10^{-9}}$$

$$= -4.6 \times 10^{-19}\ J$$

THE ELECTRIC DIPOLE

Two equal and opposite charges a small distance d away from each other form what is called an **electric dipole**. Suppose there is a dipole with charges +q and –q, as shown in Figure 6.2.

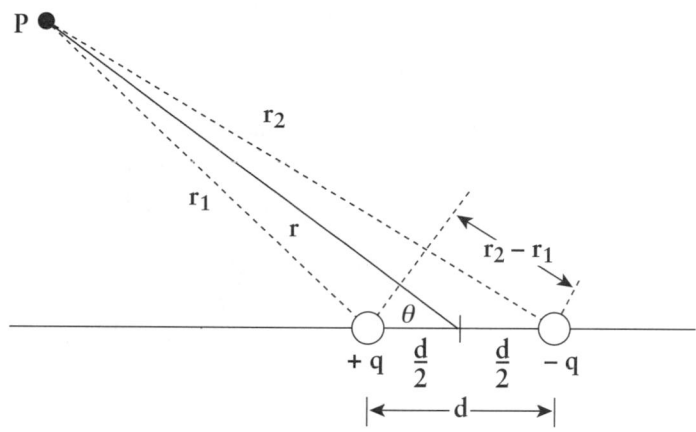

Figure 6.2

The potential at any point P is given by the sum of the two potentials:

$$V = k\frac{q}{r_1} - k\frac{q}{r_2}$$

$$= kq(\frac{r_2 - r_1}{r_1 r_2})$$

For points relatively far from the dipole (compared to d), $r_1 r_2 \cong r^2$ and $r_2 - r_1 \cong d\cos\theta$. With these approximations the potential becomes:

$$V = k\frac{qd}{r^2}\cos\theta$$

The product of qd is defined as the **dipole moment p** with SI units of C•m. This is a vector quantity. Its magnitude is equal to the product qd, and its direction lies along the line connecting the charges (dipole axis) and points from the negative charge toward the positive charge. (Beware! Chemists often reverse this convention, having **p** point from the positive toward the negative charge.) In terms of dipole moment, one can rewrite the dipole potential as:

$$V = k\frac{p}{r^2}\cos\theta$$

Note that the potential is zero for $\theta = 90°$ and that this is the plane that lies halfway between +q and –q (called the perpendicular bisector of the dipole).

The electric field produced by the dipole at any point is the vector sum of each of the individual fields due to each of the two charges. Along the perpendicular bisector of the dipole the magnitude of the electric field can be approximated as:

$$E = \frac{1}{4\pi\varepsilon_0} \frac{p}{r^3}$$

The field will point in the opposite direction to **p**.

Example: The H_2O molecule has a dipole moment of 1.85 D, where D = Debye unit = 3.34×10^{-30} C•m. Calculate the electric potential due to an H_2O molecule at a point 89 nm away along the axis of the dipole. (Use k = 9×10^9 N•m^2/C^2.)

Solution: Since the question asks for the potential along the axis of the dipole, the angle θ is given by 0°. Substituting the values into the equation for the dipole potential and multiplying 1.85 D by 3.34×10^{-30} to convert it to C•m:

$$V = k\frac{p}{r^2} \cos \theta$$

$$= 9 \times 10^9 \frac{(1.85)(3.34 \times 10^{-30})(\cos\ 0°)}{(89 \times 10^{-9})^2}$$

$$= 7 \times 10^{-6} \text{ V}$$

Now consider the case when an electric dipole is placed in a uniform external electric field. If there is no field present, the dipole moment will assume any random orientation. With a uniform external electric field present, however, each of the equal but opposite charges that make up the dipole will feel a force exerted on it by the external electric field. The net force will be zero, since the force on each charge is equal in magnitude but opposite in direction. The dipole therefore feels no translational force. However, there will be a nonzero torque about the center:

$$\tau = F\frac{d}{2} \sin \theta + F\frac{d}{2} \sin \theta$$
$$= Fd \sin \theta$$
$$= qEd \sin \theta$$
$$= (qd)E \sin \theta$$
$$= pE \sin \theta$$

where p is the magnitude of the dipole moment (p = qd), E is the magnitude of the uniform external electric field, and θ is the angle the dipole moment makes with the electric field. This torque will cause the dipole to reorient itself by rotating, so that its dipole moment, **p**, aligns with the electric field **E**. This is shown in Figure 6.3.

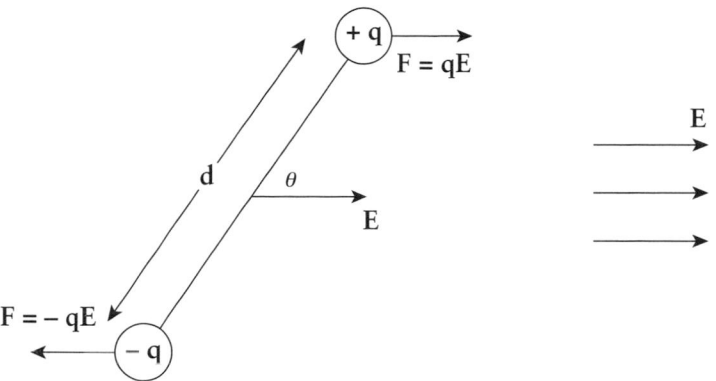

Figure 6.3

For more information on dipole moments, see chapter 3 of the General Chemistry section.

7

Magnetism

In this chapter we will review the subject of magnetism. Unlike with electrostatics, where electric charges create electric fields that exert forces on other electric charges, magnetism has no fundamental magnetic charges. Instead, magnetic fields are created by moving charges, currents in wires, and permanent magnets. These magnetic fields, in turn, exert magnetic forces on the very things that create them, i.e., moving charges, currents in wires, and permanent magnets.

The first half of the chapter is concerned with the determination of the magnetic force due to a given magnetic field. Since force is a vector, both the magnitude and direction of the magnetic force are considered. The second half of the chapter then examines sources of magnetic fields, including a brief review of magnetic materials, and also a discussion of the two most common current configurations, the straight wire and the loop of wire.

MCAT Synopsis
....

Magnetic fields are created by moving charges and permanent magnets, and in turn exert forces on moving charges and permanent magnets.

THE MAGNETIC FIELD

In discussing the magnetic force on moving charges and on current-carrying wires, we will assume the presence of a fixed and uniform magnetic field **B**. Of course, this field must be produced by some external source such as a magnet or arrangement of current-carrying wires, but for our purposes we are concerned only with the strength and direction of this field.

Like all physical quantities, magnetic fields have units. The SI unit of the magnetic field is the Tesla (T) where $1\ T = 1\dfrac{N \bullet s}{m \bullet C}$. Small magnetic fields are sometimes measured in Gauss where 1 Tesla $= 10^4$ Gauss.

MCAT Favorite
....

When a charge moves parallel to (θ = 0°) or antiparallel to (θ = 180°) a magnetic field, the magnetic force is zero.

A. FORCE ON A MOVING CHARGE

When a charge moves in a magnetic field, a magnetic force is exerted on it. This force, like all forces, is a vector. The **magnitude** of F is given by:

$$F = qvB \sin \theta$$

In this formula, θ is the smallest angle between the vectors q**v** and **B** (more on q**v** below), q is the charge of the moving particle, v is the particle's speed, and B = $|\mathbf{B}|$ is the magnitude of the magnetic field vector.

Right-Hand Rule for the direction of the magnetic force on a moving charge. Turning our attention to the **direction** of the magnetic force, we should first note that q**v** is a vector that depends on the velocity vector **v** and the sign of the charge q. If q is nonzero and positive (positive charge), then q**v** points in the same direction as **v**. If q is nonzero and negative (negative charge), then q**v** points in the opposite direction as **v**. (If q or **v** is zero, then the magnetic force will be zero.) The direction of the magnetic force will be **perpendicular** to the plane defined by q**v** and **B**, but this could be either of two directions. To find the correct direction, let the thumb of the **right hand** (left-handed people must be careful to use the correct hand) point in the direction of the vector q**v** (that is, parallel to **v** if q is positive and antiparallel to **v** if q is negative). Let the remaining fingers of the **right hand** point in the direction of **B**. Your **palm** now points in the direction of **F**, the magnetic force on q.

(Note: The right-hand rule as stated above may differ from what you have previously learned. A different version would have the right index finger in the direction of q**v** and right middle finger in the direction of **B** and, holding the thumb perpendicular to these two fingers, the right thumb points in the direction of **F**. It is important only to get the direction correct no matter which rule you use. **If you have committed to memory another version of the rule, and it works, then feel free to use it.**)

Because of the three-dimensional nature of problems involving magnetic fields, scientists have chosen the following conventions to denote magnetic fields going into the page, or coming out of the page. The symbol x represents a field going into the page. The x represents the tail end of an arrow travelling into the page. The symbol • represents a field coming out of the page. The • represents the tip of an arrow coming out of the page.

> ### MCAT Synopsis
>
> The symbol 'x' means the magnetic field direction is into the page, and the symbol '•' means the magnetic field direction is out of the page.

Example: Suppose a proton, whose charge is +1.6 × 10⁻¹⁹ C, is moving with a speed of 15 m/s in a direction parallel to a uniform magnetic field of 3.0 T. What is the magnitude and direction of the magnetic force on the proton?

Solution: Because the proton is positively charged, the vector q**v** is in the same direction as **v**, which is the same direction as **B** as stated in the problem. Since q**v** and **B** are pointing in the same direction, the angle between the vectors is zero. Since sin 0° = 0 and F = qvB sin θ, the magnetic force on the proton is zero, too. Note that if the charge had been negative (an electron, for example), the angle between **qv** and **B** would have been 180° and since sin 180° = 0, the magnetic force on a negative charge moving parallel to a uniform magnetic field would be zero as well. In general, the magnetic force on a moving charge will be zero if the charge is moving parallel or antiparallel to the magnetic field.

Example: Suppose a proton whose charge equals $+1.6 \times 10^{-19}$ C is moving with a speed of 15 m/s toward the top of the page and through a uniform magnetic field of 3.0 T directed into the page [see Figure 7.1(a)]. What is the magnitude and direction of the magnetic force on the proton?

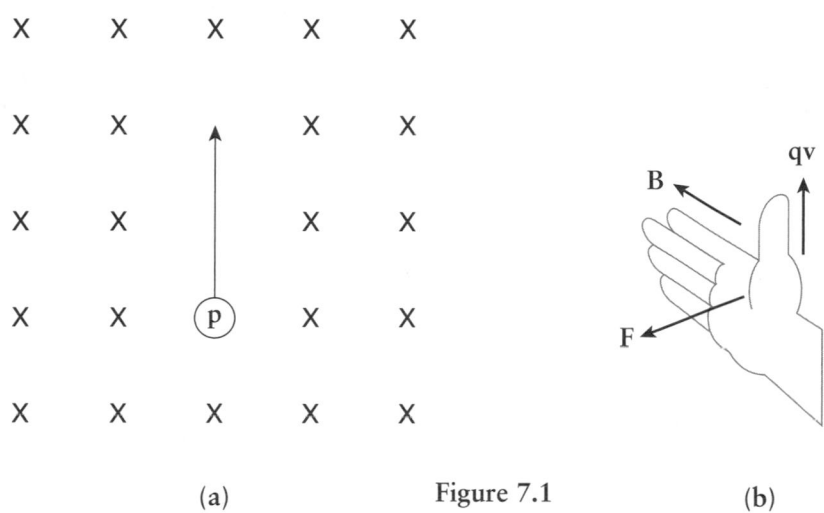

(a)   Figure 7.1   (b)

Solution: Because the proton is positively charged, the vector **qv** is in the same direction as **v**, which is perpendicular to **B** as stated in the problem. (**B** is perpendicular to the plane of the page.) Because qv and **B** are perpendicular, the angle between the vectors is $\theta = 90°$, and since sin 90° = 1, the magnetic force on the proton is:

$$F = qvB \sin \theta$$
$$= qvB$$
$$= (1.6 \times 10^{-19})(15)(3.0)$$
$$= 7.2 \times 10^{-18} \text{ N}$$

By holding the thumb of the **right hand** so that it is directed toward the top of the page, then holding the remaining fingers of the **right hand** so that they point towards (into) the page, one's **right hand** palm points to the left [see Figure 7.1(b)]. Hence, the proton is deflected to the left on its upward journey. As the velocity of the proton changes, so does the magnetic force that it experiences. Note that if the charge had been negative (an electron, for example), the angle between **qv** and **B** still would have been 90°, but the right-hand rule would have required that **qv** point toward the bottom of the page, meaning that one's right-hand palm would point to the right. Hence, an electron is deflected to the right on its upward journey. One can readily see that the direction of the magnetic force on a negative charge moving through a magnetic field is opposite to the direction of the magnetic force acting on a positive charge moving in the same direction.

When a charged particle moves **perpendicular** to a **constant, uniform magnetic field,** the resulting motion is circular motion with constant speed in the plane perpendicular to the magnetic field. A centripetal force is always associated with circular motion. In this case, the centripetal force is the magnetic force (F = qvB). Since the centripetal force equals mv^2/r, we get:

$$F = qvB = \frac{mv^2}{r}$$

From this equation one can solve for the orbit radius, the magnetic field, and so on:

$$r = \frac{mv}{qB} \qquad B = \frac{mv}{qr}$$

Example: Suppose the proton of the previous example is allowed to circle (counterclockwise) in the same perpendicular magnetic field of 3.0 T with the same speed of 15 m/s [as in Figure 7.2(a)]. What is the orbit radius r? (The mass of a proton is 1.67×10^{-27} kg.)

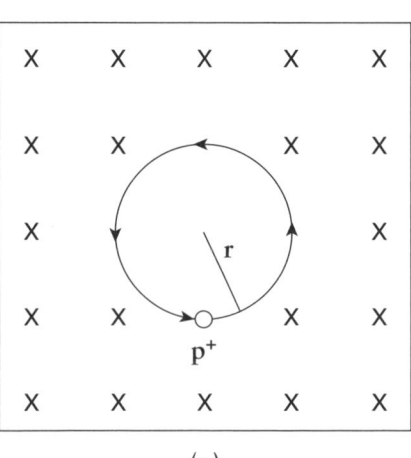

(a)

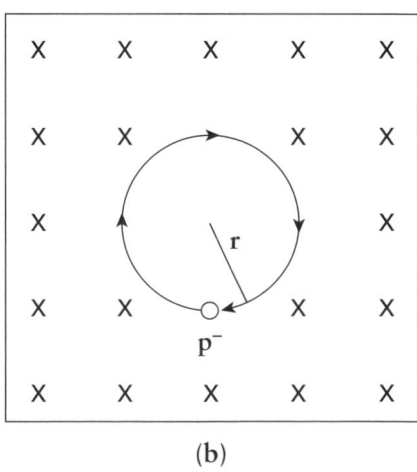

(b)

Figure 7.2

Solution: By equating the centripetal force to the magnetic force and solving for the orbit radius as shown above:

$$r = \frac{mv}{qB}$$

$$= \frac{(1.67 \times 10^{-27})(15)}{(1.6 \times 10^{-19})(3)}$$

$$= 5.2 \times 10^{-8} \text{ m}$$

Note that the direction of the magnetic force on a negative charge moving through a uniform magnetic field is opposite to the direction of the magnetic force acting on a positive charge moving in the same direction. Therefore, if the charge had been negative (an antiproton, for example, which has the mass of the proton but is negatively charged), it would have circled in the **clockwise** direction with the same orbit radius. [See Figure 7.2 (b).]

B. CURRENT

Electric current will be discussed more completely in chapter 8. However, it is important to realize that when two points at different electric potentials are connected with a conductor (such as a metal wire), charge flows between the two points. The flow of charge is called an **electric current.** The magnitude of the current i is the amount of charge Δq passing through the conductor per unit time Δt, or in the form of an equation:

$$i = \frac{\Delta q}{\Delta t}$$

The SI unit of current is the Ampere (1 A = 1 Coulomb/second).

Charge is transmitted by a flow of electrons in a conductor. Since electrons are negatively charged, they go from lower potentials to higher potentials. But, **by convention,** the direction of **current** is the direction in which **positive charge** would flow, or from high to low potential. **Thus the direction of current is opposite to the direction of electron flow.**

C. FORCE ON A CURRENT-CARRYING WIRE

Since moving charge is subject to magnetic forces and electric current is a flow of charge, it is no surprise that magnetic forces can act on a current-carrying wire. For a straight wire of length L carrying a current i in a direction that makes an angle θ with a uniform magnetic field **B**, the magnitude of the magnetic force on the current-carrying wire is:

$$F = iLB \sin \theta$$

MCAT Synopsis

Current is in the direction that positive charges would flow.

MCAT Synopsis

A current in a magnetic field behaves similarly to a positive charge moving in a magnetic field since current is a collection of moving positive charges.

The direction of the force is given by a simple right hand rule, the **Right-Hand Rule for the magnetic force on currents.** The force will be **perpendicular** to the plane defined by **B** and the direction of the current flow, but this could be either of two directions. To find the correct direction, let the thumb of the **right hand** (left-handed people must be careful to use the correct hand) point in the direction of the current i. Now let the remaining fingers of the **right hand** point in the direction of **B.** The palm of the **right hand** now points in the direction of **F,** the magnetic force on the current-carrying wire. (Note: This rule is virtually the same as the rule given above for moving charges. Again, you should feel free to use any right-hand rule that you have committed to memory and that gives the correct direction.)

Example: Suppose a wire of length 2.0 m is conducting a current of 5.0 A toward the top of the page and through a 30 Gauss uniform magnetic field directed into the page [see Figure 7.3(a)]. What is the magnitude and direction of the magnetic force on the wire?

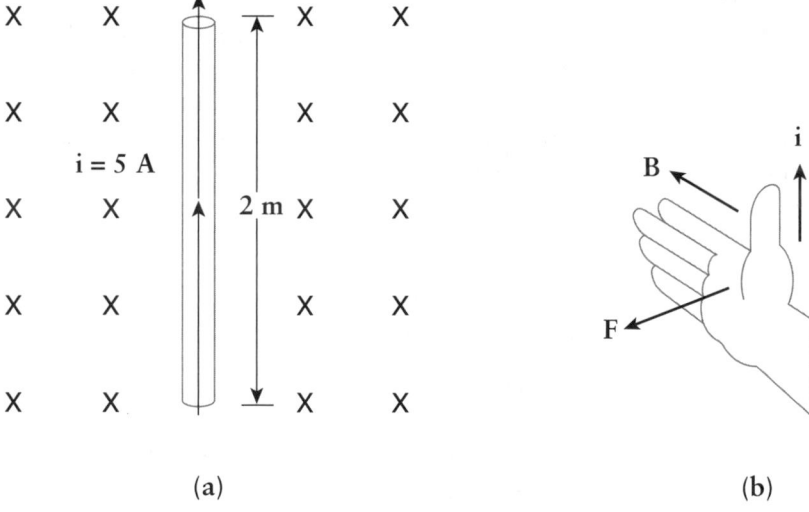

(a)

(b)

Figure 7.3

<table>
</table>

MCAT Synopsis

For direction of magnetic force on a current, use same right hand rule as for charges, but replace velocity direction with current direction.

MCAT Synopsis

Wires are electrically neutral, so there's no magnetic force if the wire simply moves through a magnetic field with no current in the wire.

Solution: Since 1 T = 10^4 Gauss, 1 Gauss = 10^{-4} T, 30 Gauss = 30×10^{-4} T = 3×10^{-3} T. The wire is conducting current toward the top of the page, and the magnetic field points into the page; therefore, the current is perpendicular to **B.** The angle between them is $\theta = 90°$, and since $\sin 90° = 1$, the magnetic force on the wire is:

$$F = iLB \sin \theta = iLB$$
$$= 5.0(2.0)(3.0 \times 10^{-3})$$
$$= 3.0 \times 10^{-2} \text{ N} = 0.03 \text{ N}$$

By holding the thumb of the **right hand** so that it is directed toward the top of the page, then holding the remaining fingers towards (into) the page, the palm of the **right hand** points to the left. Hence the force on the wire is to the left.

SOURCES OF MAGNETIC FIELD

The previous section dealt with the magnetic force on a moving charge and a current-carrying wire, but it did not discuss how the field was generated. Any moving charge creates a magnetic field. Magnetic fields may be set up by the "flow" of charge in permanent magnets, or electric currents, or simply by individual moving charges (e.g., an electron moving through space). This section deals only with permanent magnets and current-carrying wires, but it is important to realize that each of these sources of magnetic field has, in one sense or another, a flow of charge or a current—it is the movement of charge that gives rise to the magnetic field.

As with electric fields, magnetic **field lines** can be used to visualize the magnetic field. At any point along a field line the magnetic field itself is in the tangential direction.

A. MAGNETIC MATERIALS

Materials are classified as diamagnetic, paramagnetic, and ferromagnetic. In a **diamagnetic material** the individual atoms have no net magnetic field. Diamagnetic materials will be repelled from the pole of a strong bar magnet, so they are sometimes called weakly antimagnetic. In **paramagnetic** and **ferromagnetic** materials the individual atoms do have a net magnetic field, but normally these individual atomic fields are randomly oriented so the material itself exhibits no net magnetic field. In a paramagnetic material under certain conditions, some degree of alignment of the individual atomic magnetic fields can occur. Paramagnetic materials will be attracted towards the pole of a strong bar magnet, so they are sometimes called weakly magnetic. In a ferromagnetic material a special effect takes place when the temperature drops below a critical value that allows a high degree of alignment of the magnetic fields of the individual atoms to occur. Above this critical temperature, called the Curie temperature, the material is paramagnetic. Ferromagnetic materials are sometimes called strongly magnetic and include iron, nickel, and cobalt. When the Curie temperature is above room temperature, ferromagnetic materials are permanently magnetized at room temperature (for example, the familiar bar magnet).

When a paper with iron filings is placed on top of a permanent bar magnet, the iron filings tend to form lines connecting the top of the magnet

Flashback

Magnetic field lines are analogous to electric field lines, i.e., the magnetic field is tangent to the magnetic field line at any point. (See chapter 6.)

MCAT Synopsis

Magnetic field lines come out of north poles and go into south poles. Opposite magnetic poles attract and like poles repel.

to the bottom of the magnet. The iron filings are showing the **magnetic field lines.** All bar magnets have a **north** and **south** pole. The north pole is the place where the magnetic field lines emerge; the south pole is where they enter. Given two bar magnets, opposite poles attract each other, like poles repel.

B. CURRENT-CARRYING WIRES

A current-carrying wire will produce a magnetic field in its vicinity. The magnetic field of a current carrying wire is the vector sum of the magnetic fields due to the individual moving charges that comprise the current. The final result depends on the shape of the wire. Special cases include a **long straight wire** and the **center of a circular loop of wire.**

At a perpendicular distance r from an infinitely long and straight current-carrying wire the magnitude of the magnetic field produced by the current i in the wire is given by:

$$B = \frac{\mu_0 i}{2\pi r}$$

where μ_0 is the **permeability of free space** = $4\pi \times 10^{-7}$ Tesla • meter/Ampere = 1.26×10^{-6} T•m/A. The above equation shows that for a long straight wire, the field strength drops off with distance.

The magnetic field lines are concentric perpendicular circles about the wire. You can use a **Right-Hand Rule to find the direction of the magnetic field produced by a long straight wire.** This rule differs from the previous ones. In this rule your **right thumb** points in the direction of the current. Your remaining **right fingers** mimic the circular magnetic field lines and curl around the wire. Your fingers now show you the direction of the magnetic field lines and the direction of B itself at any point. Note that this rule differs from the previous two in that it gives the direction of the field lines produced by the current instead of starting with a given direction of **B** to find the direction of a force. Also note that, as shown in a later example, this rule may be applied to current loops as well as straight wires.

Example: A straight wire carries a current of 5 A toward the top of the page (see Figure 7.4(a)). What is the magnitude and direction of the magnetic field at point P, which is 10 cm to the left of the wire? What is the magnitude and direction of the magnetic field at point Q, which is 2 cm to the right of the wire?

MCAT Synopsis

Magnetic field lines encircle currents. Use the right hand rule (different than the rule for magnetic force on a moving charge) to find the field direction.

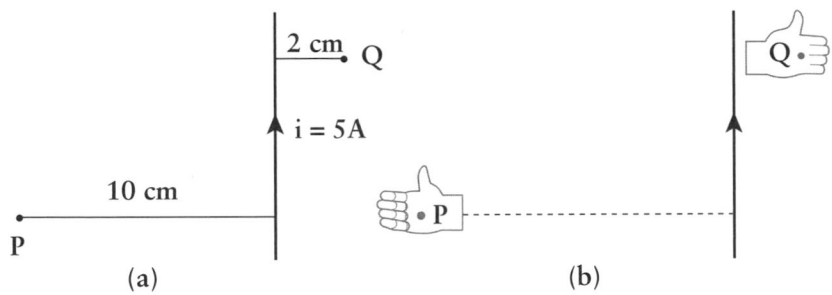

Figure 7.4

Solution: To find the magnitude at point P:

$$B = \frac{\mu_0 i}{2\pi r}$$

$$= \frac{(4\pi \times 10^{-7})(5)}{2\pi(0.1)}$$

$$= 10^{-5} \text{ T} = 0.1 \text{ Gauss}$$

To find the magnitude at point Q:

$$B = \frac{(4\pi \times 10^{-7})(5)}{2\pi(0.02)}$$

$$= 5 \times 10^{-5} \text{ T} = 0.5 \text{ Gauss}$$

Now to get the direction of the field for each of these points, we use the Right-Hand Rule. Hold your **right thumb** towards the top of the page. Now curl your fingers around the wire. At Q your fingers should point into the page. Keep curling around and you notice that at point P your fingers come out of the page. [See Figure 7.4 (b).] So your answer should be: **B** (at P) = 0.1 Gauss, pointing out of the page, and **B** (at Q) = 0.5 Gauss, pointing into the page. Note that as we move farther from the wire the magnitude of magnetic field decreases.

The magnitude of the magnetic field at the center of a circular loop of current-carrying wire of radius r is:

$$B = \frac{\mu_0 i}{2r}$$

Notice that these two laws for magnetic fields look similar. For the long straight wire, r refers to the perpendicular distance from the wire and gives B for any point away from the wire. However, r in the second case is the radius of the loop and the expression gives the magnetic field at the loop's center point only. The following example illustrates how to find directions.

Example: Suppose a wire is formed into a loop that carries current clockwise (that is, electrons flow counterclockwise) as in Figure 7.5(a). Find the direction of the magnetic field produced by this loop:
    a. within the loop.
    b. outside of the loop.

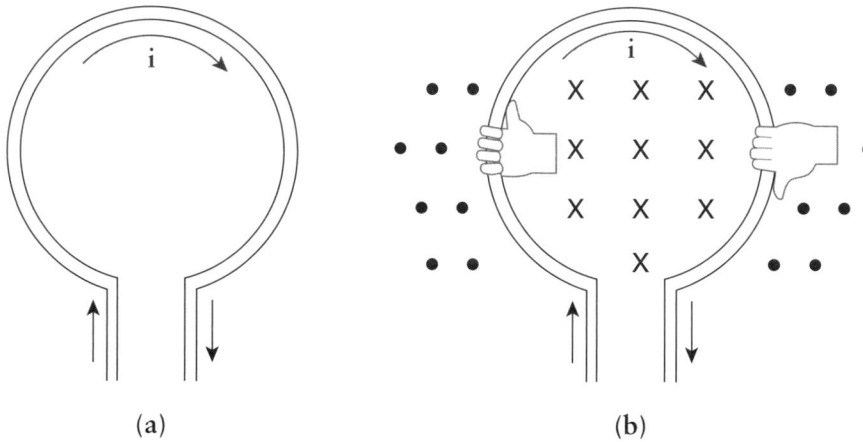

(a)   (b)

Figure 7.5

Solution: Look at Figure 7.5(b). By holding your **right thumb** anywhere around the loop in the direction of current flow (clockwise) and encircling the wire with the remaining fingers of the **right hand,** your **right fingers** should point:
    a. into the page. Thus the magnetic field within the loop points into the page.
    b. out of the page. Thus the magnetic field outside the loop points out of the page.

8

DC AND AC CIRCUITS

Electric circuits pervade our everyday world, existing in myriad forms in the various necessities of modern day living, most notably, televisions, VCRs, and stereos. In this chapter we will review the essentials of DC circuits, touching only briefly and qualitatively on the subject of AC circuits. Included are the usual topics of DC circuit theory: emf, resistance, power dissipated by resistors, Kirchhoff's laws, parallel and series resistor circuits, capacitors, parallel and series capacitor circuits, and a brief discussion of dielectrics. Although the topic of DC circuits can be a place to encounter a substantial amount of algebra when solving complicated circuits, the emphasis on the MCAT and in this chapter is on the essential concepts involved and on applying those concepts in simple situations. Let's begin with a short review of conductors and insulators, the essential materials of the wires of any circuit.

Some materials allow electric charge to move freely within the material. These materials are called electrical **conductors**. Metal atoms can easily lose one or more of their outer electrons, which are then free to move around in the metal. This makes most metals good electrical conductors. In most conductors, the positive ions remain fixed and the liberated electrons are free to move.

In other materials electric charge is bound to the constituent atoms and is not free to move. These materials severely retard the flow of electricity and are called **insulators.** Most nonmetals are good insulators.

The wires to most appliances have a conducting core of copper wire perhaps, with an insulating sheath of some plastic. The copper wire conducts the electricity to the appliance from the wall socket. The insulating sheath protects you from touching the wire and getting an electric shock.

DIRECT CURRENT

A. CURRENT AND CIRCUIT VOLTAGE

The flow of charge is called an **electric current**. The magnitude of the current i is the amount of charge Δq passing a given point per unit time Δt, and is given by:

$$i = \frac{\Delta q}{\Delta t}$$

The SI unit of current is the **Ampere** (1 A = 1 Coulomb/second). The two basic types of current flow are **direct current** (DC), where the charge flows in one direction only, and **alternating current** (AC), where the flow changes direction periodically. AC current will be discussed later.

When two points at different electric potentials are connected by a conductor (such as a metal wire), charge flows between the two points. In a conductor, only negatively charged electrons are free to move. These act as the charge carriers, and move from low to high potentials. By convention, however, the direction of the **current** is taken as the direction in which **positive charge** would flow, from high to low potential. **Thus the direction of current is opposite to the direction of electron flow.**

A voltage (potential difference) can be produced by an electric generator, a voltaic cell, or by a group of cells wired into a battery. **Electromotive force** (emf or ε) is the name given to the voltage across the terminals of a cell when no current is flowing. Electromotive force should not be confused with a force or an electric field; it is a potential difference and is measured in Volts.

Because cells typically have a small internal resistance r_{int} of their own, the voltage they actually furnish to a circuit is reduced by ir_{int}, where i is the current supplied by the cell. The voltage V across the terminals of the cell when current is flowing out, is given in terms of the cell's emf and internal resistance by:

$$V = \varepsilon - ir_{int}$$

Note: If the cell is supplying no current (i = 0), or if the cell has no internal resistance ($r_{int} = 0$), then $V = \varepsilon$. For cases in which the current supplied is greater than zero and the internal resistance is not negligible, then $V < \varepsilon$. When a cell is supplying current (discharging), the current flows out of the positive terminal and into the negative terminal. When a cell is being recharged, current from another source is sent into the positive terminal.

MCAT Synopsis

Current flows from higher potential (positive terminal), to lower potential (negative terminal), analogous to masses which naturally fall (flow) from higher potential energy to lower potential energy.

B. RESISTANCE

1. Resistance and Ohm's Law

Resistance R can be thought of as the opposition within a conductor to the flow of an electric current. This opposition takes the form of an energy loss or drop in potential. **Ohm's law** states that the voltage drop across a resistor is proportional to the current it carries, with R being the proportionality constant:

$$V = iR$$

This equation applies to a single resistor within a circuit, to any part of a circuit, or to an entire circuit (provided one knows how to add resistances in series and parallel). Note that the current is unchanged as it passes through the resistor. This is because no charge is lost inside the resistor. Therefore, the current that is supplied to several resistors wired in series must all flow through each resistor. The SI derived unit of electrical resistance is the **Ohm** (Ω).

2. Resistance of a Conductor

The resistance of an object depends on its size, the type of material from which it is made, and its temperature. Specifically the resistance depends on:

a. Length (L)

Resistance is directly proportional to length. A longer conductor means greater resistance, because there is a longer path that current-carrying electrons must travel. For example, two wires, identical in every respect except that one is twice as long as the other, will have different resistances. The longer one will have twice the resistance of the shorter one.

> **MCAT Synopsis**
>
> - The resistance of a wire increases with increased length.
> - The resistance of a wire decreases with increased cross-sectional area.

b. Cross-sectional area (A)

The resistance of a conductor is inversely proportional to its cross-sectional area. An increase in cross-sectional area causes a decrease in resistance. This is because there is an increase in the number of conduction paths electrons can follow. For example, two wires, identical in every respect except that one has twice the cross-sectional area of the other, will have different resistances. The thinner wire will have twice the resistance of the thicker wire.

c. Resistivity of the conductor (ρ)

Some materials are intrinsically better conductors of electricity than others. For example, copper conducts electricity much better than does glass. The number that characterizes the intrinsic resistance to current flow in a material is called the **resistivity** (ρ), where the SI unit of resistivity is the Ohm•meter. The resistivity is therefore

> **MCAT Synopsis**
>
> Resistivity, ρ, is a measure of the intrinsic resistance of a type of material, independent of length and cross-sectional area.

defined as the proportionality constant relating a conductor's resistance to the ratio of its length over its cross-sectional area:

$$R = \rho \frac{L}{A}$$

d. **Temperature**

Most conductors have greater resistance at higher temperatures. This is due to increased thermal oscillations of atoms in the conductor which produce a greater resistance to electron flow. The resistivity can then be thought of as a function of temperature. A few materials, such as glass, pure silicon, and most semiconductors are exceptions to this general rule.

3. **Power Dissipated By a Resistor**

Electric potential is electric potential energy per unit positive charge. Since current is a flow of charge, it should come as no surprise that through a current-carrying resistor there is a **flow of energy**. In a resistor, this electric energy is converted into heat. The **rate** at which the energy loss occurs is equal to the power dissipated by the resistor and is given by:

$$P = iV$$

where i is the current flowing through the resistor and V is the potential drop across the resistor. Using Ohm's law this expression can be rewritten as:

$$P = i^2R = V^2/R$$

C. CIRCUIT LAWS

An electric circuit is a conducting path that usually has one or more voltage sources (such as a cell) connected to one or more **passive circuit elements** (such as resistors). This subsection deals primarily with voltages, resistances, and currents in DC circuits.

1. **Kirchhoff's Laws**

a. **At any point or junction in a circuit the sum of currents directed into that point equals the sum of currents directed away from that point.** This is a consequence of the **conservation of electric charge.**

Example: Three wires (a, b, and c) meet at a junction point P, as in Figure 8.1. A current of 5 A flows into P along wire a, and a current of 3 A flows away from P along wire b. What is the magnitude and direction of the current along wire c?

> ### MCAT Synopsis
>
> $P = iV$ means $P = $ (charge/second) $\times$ (energy/charge). So $P = $ energy/second, as power always does.

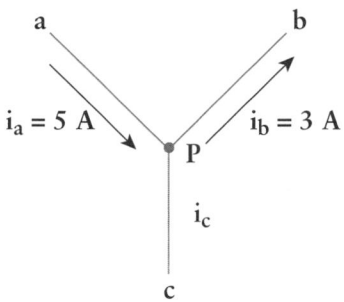

Figure 8.1

Solution: The sum of currents entering P must equal the sum of the currents leaving P. Assume for now that i_c flows out of P. If we find that it is negative, then we know that it flows into P.

$$i_a = i_b + i_c$$
$$i_c = 5 - 3$$
$$i_c = 2 \text{ A}$$

Thus a current of 2 A flows out of P along wire c. Note that the total current into and out of P is then zero.

b. **The sum of voltage sources is equal to the sum of voltage (potential) drops around a closed circuit loop.** This is a consequence of the conservation of energy: All the electrical energy supplied by a source gets fully used up by the rest of the circuit. No excess energy appears or disappears. (But remember that voltage is energy per unit charge not just energy.)

2. Resistors in Series

It has already been mentioned that the same current flows through all the resistors in series and from the above laws we can deduce that voltage drops add in series. Therefore, using Ohm's law we find that resistances add in series (see Figure 8.2). That is:

$$R_s = R_1 + R_2 + R_3 + \cdots + R_n$$

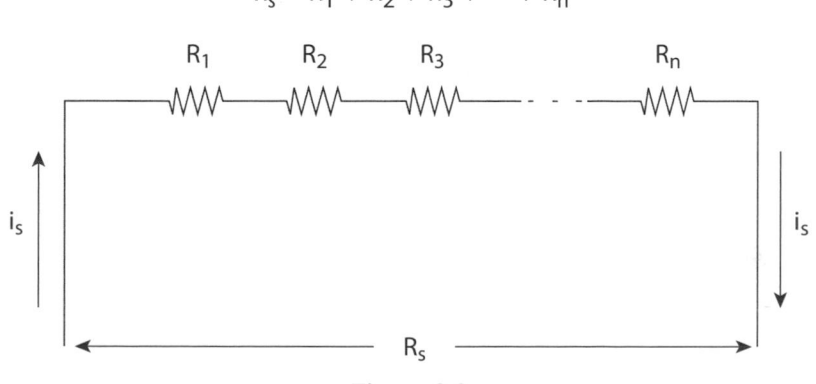

Figure 8.2

> **MCAT Synopsis**
>
> Energy is conserved in one complete loop of a circuit. Energy lost in the resistors is gained back in the battery.

> **MCAT Synopsis**
>
> Each additional resistor in a series of resistors increases the total resistance and thus decreases the total current.

Example: A circuit is wired with one cell supplying 5 V (neglect the internal resistance of the cell) in series together with three resistors of 3 Ω, 5 Ω, and 7 Ω also wired in series as shown in Figure 8.3. What is the resulting voltage across, and current through, each resistor of this circuit, as well as the entire circuit?

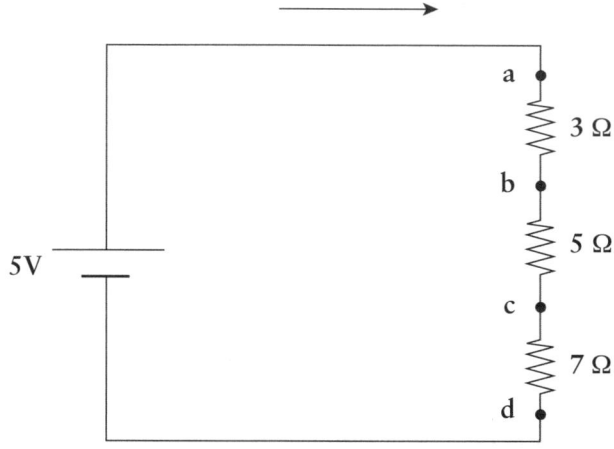

Figure 8.3

Solution: The total resistance of the resistors is:

$$R_s = R_1 + R_2 + R_3$$
$$= 3 + 5 + 7$$
$$= 15 \ \Omega$$

Now use Ohm's law to get the current through the entire circuit (since everything is in series this is also the current through each element):

$$i_s = \frac{V_s}{R_s} = \frac{5}{15} = \frac{1}{3} A$$

Now use Ohm's law for each of the resistors in turn. From a to b the voltage drop across R_1 is:

$$iR_1 = (1/3)(3)$$
$$= 1.0 \ V$$

From b to c the voltage drop across R_2 is:

$$iR_2 = (1/3)(5)$$
$$= 1.67 \ V$$

From c to d the voltage drop across R_3 is:

$$iR_3 = (1/3)(7)$$
$$= 2.33 \ V$$

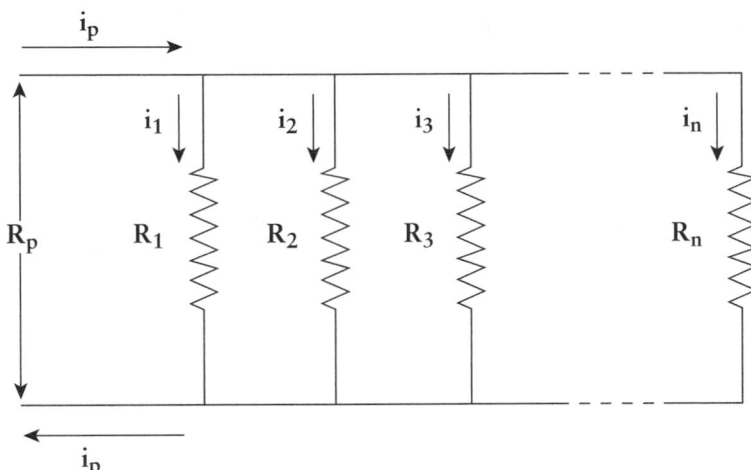

Figure 8.4

3. Resistors in Parallel

When resistors are wired in parallel, they are all wired with a common high potential terminal and a common low potential terminal (see Figure 8.4). The effect of **adding resistors in parallel** is the same as that of increasing the cross-sectional area of a conductor. It increases the paths by which current can flow and thereby **decreases resistance** (there is also the analogy to viscous blood flow through capillaries—flow resistance is reduced when several capillaries are arranged in parallel). The rule for combining resistances in parallel is a bit more complicated than the previous rules. It states that the reciprocal of the equivalent resistance equals the sum of the reciprocals of their individual resistances. In equation form this may be written as:

$$\frac{1}{R_p} = \frac{1}{R_1} + \frac{1}{R_2} + \frac{1}{R_3} + \cdots + \frac{1}{R_n}$$

> **MCAT Synopsis**
>
> Each additional resistor added in parallel acts to decrease the total resistance and thus increase the current.

When resistors are in parallel, the voltage drop across each is the same and is equal to the voltage drop across the entire combination:

$$V_p = V_1 = V_2 = V_3 = \cdots V_n$$

Example: Consider two equal resistors wired in parallel. What is the equivalent resistance of the two?

Solution: The equation for summing resistors in parallel is:

$$\frac{1}{R_p} = \frac{1}{R_1} + \frac{1}{R_2}$$

> **MCAT Synopsis**
>
> Parallel resistors experience the same voltage drop.

Find the common denominator of the right-hand side and take the inverse to find:

$$R_p = \frac{R_1 R_2}{(R_1 + R_2)}$$

Since $R_1 = R_2$ in this special case, let $R = R_1 = R_2$:

$$R_p = \frac{R^2}{2R} = \frac{R}{2}$$

In the above example, it is seen that the total resistance is **halved** by wiring two identical resistors in parallel. More generally, when n identical resistors are wired in parallel, the total resistance is given by R/n. Note that the voltage across each of the parallel resistors is equal and, that for equal resistances, the current flowing through each of the resistors is also equal.

Example: Consider two resistors wired in parallel with $R_1 = 5\ \Omega$ and $R_2 = 10\ \Omega$. If the voltage across them is 10 V, what is the current through each of the two resistors?

Solution: First the current flowing through the whole circuit must be found. To do this, the combined resistance must be determined:

$$\frac{1}{R_p} = \frac{1}{R_1} + \frac{1}{R_2}$$

$$= \frac{1}{10} + \frac{1}{5}$$

$$= \frac{3}{10}$$

$$R_p = \frac{10}{3}\ \Omega$$

Using Ohm's law to calculate the current flowing through the circuit gives:

$$i_p = \frac{V_p}{R_p}$$

$$= \frac{10}{(10/3)}$$

$$= 3\ A$$

Three Amps flow through the combination R_1 and R_2. Since the resistors are in parallel $V_p = V_1 = V_2 = 10$ V. Apply Ohm's law to each resistor individually:

$$i_1 = \frac{V_p}{R_1} = \frac{10}{5} = 2A$$

$$i_2 = \frac{V_p}{R_2} = \frac{10}{10} = 1A$$

As a check, note that $i_p = 3$ A $= i_1 + i_2 = 2 + 1 = 3$ A. More current flows through the smaller resistance. In particular note that R_1 with half the resistance of R_2 has twice the current. Once i_p was found to be 3 A, the problem could have been solved by noting that because R_1 is half of R_2, $i_1 = 2i_2$, and $i_1 + i_2 = 3$ A.

D. CAPACITORS AND DIELECTRICS

1. **Capacitors and Capacitance**

When two electrically neutral plates of metal are connected to a voltage source, positive charge builds up on the plate connected to the positive terminal, and an equal amount of negative charge builds up on the plate connected to the negative terminal. The two plate system stores charge and is called a **capacitor.** It is important to remember that charge collects on a capacitor any time there is a potential difference between the plates. The **capacitance** C of a capacitor is defined as the ratio of charge stored (meaning the absolute value of the charge on one plate) to the total potential difference across the capacitor. So, if a voltage difference V is applied across the plates of the capacitor and a charge Q collects on it (with +Q on the positive plate and –Q on the negative plate), then the capacitance is given by:

$$C = \frac{Q}{V}$$

The SI unit of capacitance is the **Farad** (where 1 F = 1 Coulomb/Volt). Because one Coulomb is such a large amount of charge, one Farad is a very large capacitance. Capacitances are therefore quoted in submultiples of the Farad such as microfarads (1 μF = 10^{-6} F), or nanofarads (1) nF = 10^{-9} F), or picofarads (1 pF = 10^{-12} F). Note also that the Farad should not be confused with the Faraday, the unit of charge equal to the charge on a mole of elementary charges (= 9.65×10^4 Coulombs).

The capacitance of a capacitor is dependent on the geometry of the two conducting surfaces. For the simple case of the parallel plate capacitor, the capacitance is given by:

$$C = \varepsilon_0 \frac{A}{d}$$

> **MCAT Synopsis**
>
> The total charge on a capacitor is zero, +Q on one plate, and –Q on the other.

where ε_0 is the **permittivity of free space** ($\varepsilon_0 = 8.85 \times 10^{-12}$ F/m), A is the area of overlap of the two plates, and d is the separation of the two plates. The separation of charges sets up an electric field between the plates of the capacitor. The electric field between the plates of a parallel plate capacitor is a uniform field whose magnitude at any point is given by:

$$E = \frac{V}{d}$$

The direction of the electric field at any point between the plates is toward the negative plate and away from the positive plate.

2. Dielectric Materials

When an insulating material (such as glass, plastic, or certain metal oxides) is placed between the plates of a charged-up capacitor, the voltage across the capacitor decreases. Such insulating materials are called **dielectrics.** By lowering the voltage across the charged-up capacitor the dielectric has "made room for" even more charge, hence, the capacitance of the capacitor is increased. Dielectric materials are characterized by a dimensionless number called the **dielectric constant K**, which tells by what factor the capacitance of a capacitor is increased:

$$C' = KC$$

where C' is the new capacitance with the dielectric, and C is the original capacitance.

Example: The voltage across the terminals of an isolated 3 μF capacitor is 4 V. If a piece of ceramic having dielectric constant K = 2 is placed between the plates, find:

a. the new charge on the capacitor.
b. the new capacitance of the capacitor.
c. the new voltage across the capacitor.

Solution: a. The introduction of a dielectric by itself has no effect on the charge stored on the isolated capacitor. There is no new charge, so the charge is the same as before. The charge stored is therefore given by:

$$
\begin{aligned}
Q' &= Q \\
&= CV \\
&= (3 \times 10^{-6})(4) \\
&= 12 \times 10^{-6} \text{ C} \\
&= 12 \ \mu\text{C}
\end{aligned}
$$

b. By introducing a dielectric with a value of 2, the capacitance of the capacitor is doubled (C' = KC). Hence the new capacitance is 6 μF.

c. Using the relationship V' = Q'/C', the new voltage across the capacitor may be determined. Putting numbers into the equation gives:

$$V' = \frac{12 \times 10^{-6}}{6 \times 10^{-6}}$$

$$= 2 \text{ V}$$

Example: The voltage across the terminals of a 3 μF capacitor is 4 V. Now suppose a piece of ceramic having dielectric constant K = 2 is placed between the plates **and the voltage is held constant** (e.g., by a battery). What is the new charge on the capacitor?

Solution: By introducing the dielectric ceramic the capacitance of the capacitor has been altered. But because the voltage was held constant, the charge on the capacitor plates must have been altered. From the definition of dielectric constant and the above example it is clear that the new capacitance is:

$$C' = KC$$
$$= 6 \ \mu F$$

But the new voltage is still 4 V, so the new charge must be:

$$Q' = C'V'$$
$$= (6 \times 10^{-6})(4)$$
$$= 24 \times 10^{-6} \text{ C}$$
$$= 24 \ \mu C$$

Since the original charge was Q = CV = (3 × 10^{-6})(4) = 12 μC, by keeping the voltage constant the battery had to supply an additional +12 μC of charge to the positive plate and −12 μC to the negative plate.

3. **Capacitors in Parallel**

When wired in parallel, capacitors can be added directly. The capacitors wired in parallel can be thought of as combining to form a single capacitor with increased capacitance. Since the wire from one capacitor to the next is a conductor and an equipotential surface, the potential of all plates on one side are the same (see Figure 8.5).

$$C_p = C_1 + C_2 + C_3 + \ldots + C_n$$

> **MCAT Synopsis**
>
> Each capacitor added in parallel acts to increase the total capacitance of the combination.

The voltage across each parallel capacitor is the same, and is equal to the voltage across the entire combination:

$$V_p = V_1 = V_2 = V_3 = \dots = V_n$$

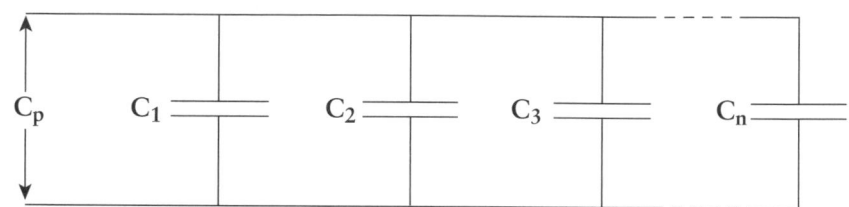

Figure 8.5

4. **Capacitors in Series**

Each additional capacitor added in series decreases the total capacitance of the circuit, so just as for resistors in parallel, the reciprocal of the total capacitance in series is equal to the sum of the reciprocals of the individual capacitances (see Figure 8.6).

$$\frac{1}{C_s} = \frac{1}{C_1} + \frac{1}{C_2} + \frac{1}{C_3} + \dots + \frac{1}{C_n}$$

For capacitors in series, the total voltage is the sum of the individual voltages:

$$V_s = V_1 + V_2 + V_3 + \dots + V_n$$

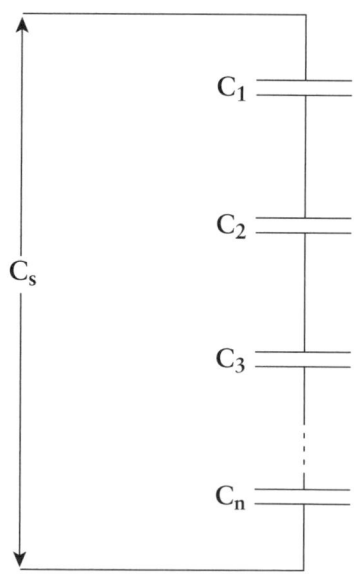

Figure 8.6

E. A SUMMARY OF CIRCUIT ELEMENT ADDITION

SERIES

$$R_s = R_1 + R_2 + R_3 + \ldots + R_n$$

$$\frac{1}{C_s} = \frac{1}{C_1} + \frac{1}{C_2} + \frac{1}{C_3} + \cdots + \frac{1}{C_n}$$

PARALLEL

$$\frac{1}{R_p} = \frac{1}{R_1} + \frac{1}{R_2} + \frac{1}{R_3} + \cdots + \frac{1}{R_n}$$

$$C_p = C_1 + C_2 + C_3 + \ldots + C_n$$

ALTERNATING CURRENT

A. ALTERNATING CURRENT

Alternating current (AC) changes its direction of flow periodically. The most common form of AC current oscillates in a sinusoidal way as shown in Figure 8.7. Note that for half of the cycle the current flows in one direction, and for the other half of the cycle the current flows in the opposite direction. Such a current can be described by the equation

$$i = I_{max} \sin (2\pi ft)$$
$$= I_{max} \sin \omega t$$

where i is the instantaneous current at the time t, I_{max} is the maximum current, f is the frequency, and $\omega = 2\pi f$ is the angular frequency.

The most common sinusoidal current is the ordinary AC house current that oscillates with a frequency f of 60 Hz. In some countries, such as England, the frequency is 50 Hz.

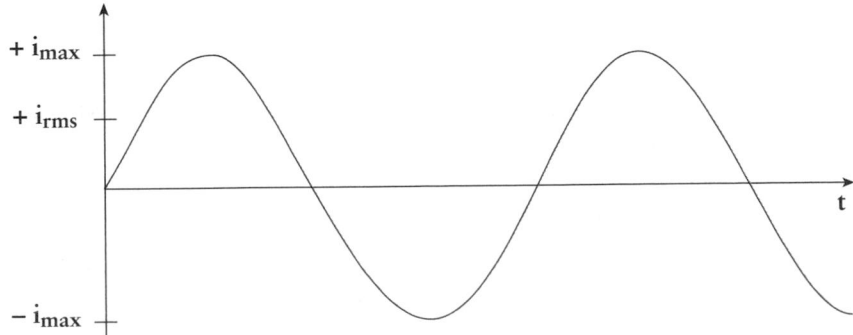

Figure 8.7

B. RMS CURRENT

In alternating current circuits the magnitude of the current varies from a maximum positive value to a minimum negative value. A problem arises when one tries to calculate the average current for sinusoidal AC currents: for one cycle, the sum of the positive current flowing in one direction is exactly canceled by the sum of the negative current that flows in the other direction. Yet there is AC current; it delivers power. Consider the power dissipated in a resistor R that carries an AC current i. It is given by the equation $P = i^2R$. Therefore, in order to find the average power dissipated we must find the average of i^2 over one period. This is equal to I_{rms}^2, where I_{rms} is the root-mean-square (rms) current given by:

$$I_{rms} = \frac{I_{max}}{\sqrt{2}}$$

Example: What is the rms current of an AC signal that will produce a maximum current of 1.00 A?

Solution:

$$I_{rms} = \frac{I_{max}}{\sqrt{2}}$$

$$= \frac{1.00}{\sqrt{2}}$$

$$= \frac{1.00}{1.41}$$

$$= 0.71 \text{ A}$$

C. RMS VOLTAGE

Voltage in AC circuits, like current, is sinusoidal and changes sign back and forth over time. It can be described by an equation similar to the equation for sinusoidal current. So just as for current, one can calculate an **rms voltage:**

$$V_{rms} = \frac{V_{max}}{\sqrt{2}}$$

Example: The AC current used in a home is frequently called "120 V AC." Assuming that this refers to the rms voltage, what is the maximum voltage?

Solution: Using the above equation gives:

$$V_{max} = \sqrt{2}\, V_{rms}$$

$$= \sqrt{2}\,(120)$$

$$= 170 \text{ V}$$

9

PERIODIC MOTION, WAVES, AND SOUND

OSCILLATIONS

Oscillating systems are those that continuously show repetitive movement of some kind. There are many different examples of oscillatory motion in the natural world, from the waves in the ocean to the waves of light that illuminate our world to the waves of sound that literally bring music to our ears. In this chapter, we will first lay the foundation for understanding wave phenomena by reviewing the subject of simple harmonic motion. General properties of waves are then introduced including the concepts of amplitude, wavelength, frequency, wave speed, and resonance. The superposition of two waves is discussed along with the related concepts of constructive versus destructive interference and the production of standing waves, both in strings and open and closed pipes. The subject of sound is reviewed as a subject that is rich in wave-related phenomena, such as beats and the Doppler effect. A brief summary is also given of sound production by musical instruments.

A. SIMPLE HARMONIC MOTION

A very important type of oscillation, or periodic motion, is **simple harmonic motion** (SHM). In SHM, a particle or mass oscillates about an equilibrium point subject to a linear restoring force. A linear restoring force has two characteristics: (i) it is always directed back towards the equilibrium position, and (ii) its magnitude is directly proportional to the displacement from the equilibrium position. By Newton's second law, the particle's acceleration is also proportional to the displacement from equilibrium:

$$F = -kx$$
$$a = -\omega^2 x$$

where the angular frequency ω is given by:

$$\omega = \sqrt{k/m}$$

A mass attached to a spring, and a simple pendulum (provided the angle of swing is not too large) are two examples of simple harmonic oscillators. A stretched or compressed spring exerts a linear restoring force, where the constant k is called the **spring constant** (or force constant), and the equation $F = -kx$ is called **Hooke's Law**. k is a measure of the stiffness of the spring. Figure 9.1(a) shows a spring-mass system with the mass at the equilibrium position. Figure 9.1(b) shows the same system with the mass displaced a distance x from the equilibrium position.

For other systems that execute SHM, k may be related to other properties of the system. In the case of a simple pendulum, $k = mg/L$ where m is the mass, and L is the length of the pendulum. Figure 9.1(c) shows a simple pendulum displaced at an angle θ with the vertical.

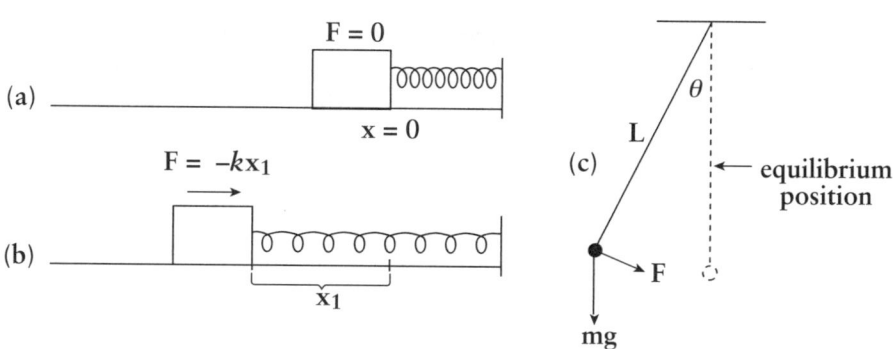

Figure 9.1

Let X be the particle's amplitude (maximum displacement x from the equilibrium position). Then assuming the particle has a maximum displacement at $t = 0$, the equation that describes the particle's displacement x is:

$$x = X \cos(\omega t)$$

where t is the time and ω is the angular frequency. ($\omega = 2\pi f = 2\pi/T$, where f is the frequency and T is the period.)

One final consideration in simple harmonic motion is energy. If the forces are conservative and the system is frictionless, by the conservation of energy:

$$E = K + U = \text{constant}$$

where K is the kinetic energy and U is the potential energy. Kinetic energy for both the mass attached to the spring and the pendulum mass is given by:

$$K = \frac{1}{2}mv^2$$

For the pendulum, the potential energy is the gravitational potential energy (mgh) as it swings up. For the spring, the potential energy is given by:

$$U(\text{spring}) = \frac{1}{2}kx^2$$

When the mass is at the equilibrium position, the potential energy is zero and the kinetic energy is a maximum given by $E = K_{max}$. However, when the oscillation reaches its maximum displacement the mass has zero speed. At this point the kinetic energy is zero and the potential energy is a maximum given by $E = U_{max}$.

The chart below gives important information on both the mass-spring system and the simple pendulum and shows the similarities between them. Note that when talking about a simple pendulum we commonly refer to the angle θ which it makes with the vertical.

NOTE: Period (T) is the time to complete 1 cycle, frequency (f) is the number of cycles completed in 1 second, and angular frequency $\omega = 2\pi f = 2\pi/T$. In SHM the frequency and period are independent of the amplitude.

	mass-spring	simple pendulum
force constant k	spring constant k	mg/L
period T	$2\pi\sqrt{m/k}$	$2\pi\sqrt{L/g}$
ang. freq. ω	$\sqrt{k/m}$	$\sqrt{g/L}$
frequency f	1/T or $\omega/2\pi$	1/T or $\omega/2\pi$
kinetic energy K	$\frac{1}{2}mv^2$	$\frac{1}{2}mv^2$
K_{max} occurs at	x = 0	$\theta = 0$ (vertical position)
potential energy U	$\frac{1}{2}kx^2$	mgh
U_{max} occurs at	x = ±X	max value of θ
max acceleration at	x = ±X	max value of θ

Example: What is the length of a pendulum that has a period of one second?

Solution: Using our equation for the period of a simple pendulum we can find the length:

$$T = 2\pi\sqrt{L/g}$$
$$L = T^2g/4\pi^2$$
$$= g/4\pi^2$$
$$= 0.25 \text{ m}$$

B. UNIFORM CIRCULAR MOTION AND SHM

Consider a particle moving around a circular path at constant angular frequency ω. If the path were projected onto a line adjacent to the circle (Figure 9.2), it is obvious that the particle is oscillating back and forth between +X and −X and obeying the laws of SHM. This fact helps give some insight as to where the idea of angular frequency comes from.

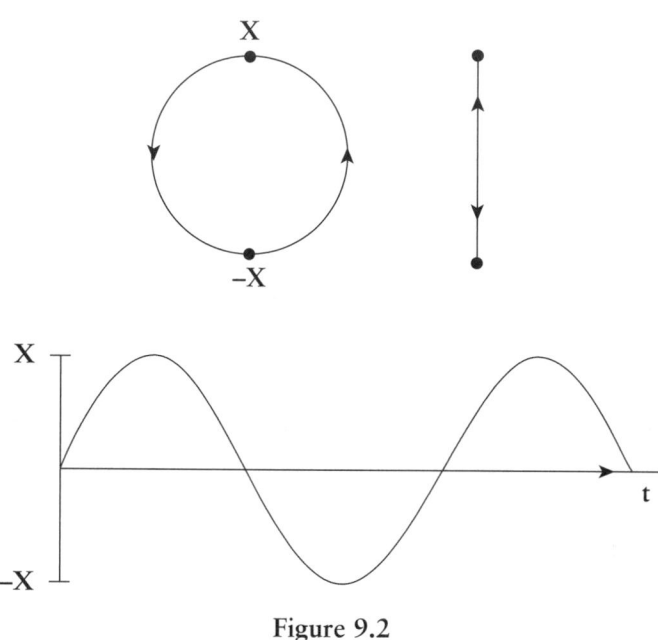

Figure 9.2

GENERAL WAVE CHARACTERISTICS

A. TRANSVERSE AND LONGITUDINAL WAVES

This chapter will be primarily concerned with sinusoidal waves. In such waves the individual particles oscillate back and forth with simple harmonic motion. In the case of **transverse waves** the particles oscillate perpendicular to the direction of the wave motion as shown in Figure 9.3(a). The oscillating string elements are moving at right angles to the direction of travel of the wave. In the case of **longitudinal waves** the particles oscillate along the direction of the wave motion, and this is illustrated in Figure 9.3(b). In this case, the longitudinal wave created by the person moving the piston back and forth consists of oscillating air molecules that move parallel to the direction of motion of the wave.

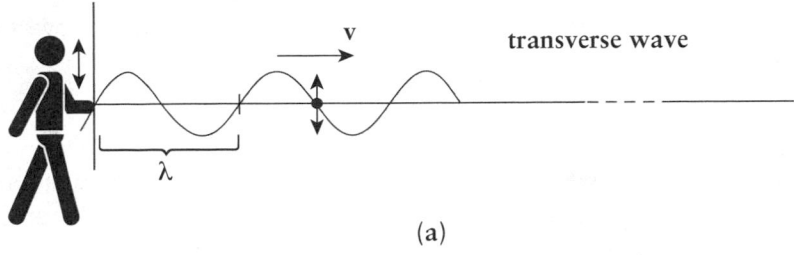

(a)

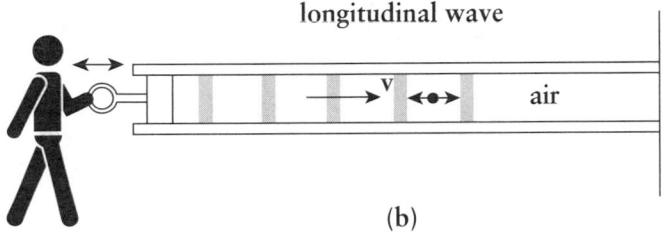

(b)

Figure 9.3

B. DESCRIBING WAVES

The displacement y of a particle may be plotted at each point x along the direction of the wave's motion. It is given mathematically by:

$$y = Y \sin (kx - \omega t)$$

where Y is the amplitude (maximum displacement), k is the wave number (not to be mistaken with the *k* of Hooke's Law), ω is the angular frequency, and t is the time.

The distance from one maximum (crest) of the wave to the next is the wavelength λ. The frequency f is the number of wavelengths passing a fixed point per second (cycles per second (cps) or Hertz (Hz)). The speed of the wave v is related to the frequency and wavelength by the very important equation:

$$v = f\lambda$$

The following relations define k and ω:

$$k = \frac{2\pi}{\lambda}$$

$$\omega = 2\pi f = \frac{2\pi}{T}$$

> **MCAT Synopsis**
>
> The maximum displacement or amplitude is Y, since the maximum of the sin function is 1.

> **MCAT Favorite**
>
> Frequency and period are reciprocals of one another:
>
> $f = 1/T$, $T = 1/f$.

where the period T is the time for the wave to move one wavelength (f = 1/T). The following relationships for the velocity of the wave follow from the above definitions:

$$v = f\lambda = \frac{\omega}{k} = \frac{\lambda}{T}$$

Example: If a wave on a string were described by the equation y = (0.01) sin (2x − 10t), find the frequency, wavelength, and speed of the wave. (Assume units of meters and seconds.)

Solution: Everything that is needed to find the frequency, wavelength, and speed is given in the wave's equation, y = Y sin (kx − ωt) = (0.01) sin (2x − 10t). Remembering that frequency is given by f = 1/T and that T = 2π/ω:

$$f = \omega/2\pi$$
$$= 5/\pi$$
$$= 1.59 \text{ Hz}$$

The wavelength is given by:

$$\lambda = 2\pi/k$$
$$= 2\pi/2$$
$$= \pi$$
$$= 3.14 \text{ m}$$

and the speed:

$$v = f\lambda$$
$$= (5/\pi)\pi$$
$$= 5 \text{ m/s}$$

> **MCAT Synopsis**
>
> A phase difference between two waves means that the crests (or troughs) don't occur at the same points in space.

C. PHASE

When comparing two waves, we often speak about a **phase difference.** This phase difference describes how "in step" two waves are with each other. Let's take two separate waves that have the same frequency, amplitude, and wavelength. If the waves are perfectly in phase, the maxima and minima of each wave coincide, i.e., they occur at the same point. In this case, the phase difference is zero. However, if the two waves are out of phase, then one wave is shifted with respect to the other by some definite fraction of a cycle. This phase difference is usually expressed as an angle. In Figure 9.4(a), waves y_1 and y_2 are nearly in phase; their phase difference is approximately 0°. In Figure 9.4(b), wave y_2 is shifted nearly one-half wavelength with respect to y_1. The phase difference in this case is almost 180°.

> **MCAT Synopsis**
>
> When two waves are in phase and interfere, the resultant amplitude is the sum of the two separate amplitudes.

D. PRINCIPLE OF SUPERPOSITION

The principle of superposition states simply that when waves interact with each other the result is a sum of the waves. When the waves are in phase, the amplitudes add together (**constructive interference**), but when waves are 180° out of phase, the resultant amplitude is the difference between interacting amplitudes (**destructive interference**). Figures 9.4(a) and (b) show the interference between two waves when they are nearly in phase and when they are nearly 180° out of phase.

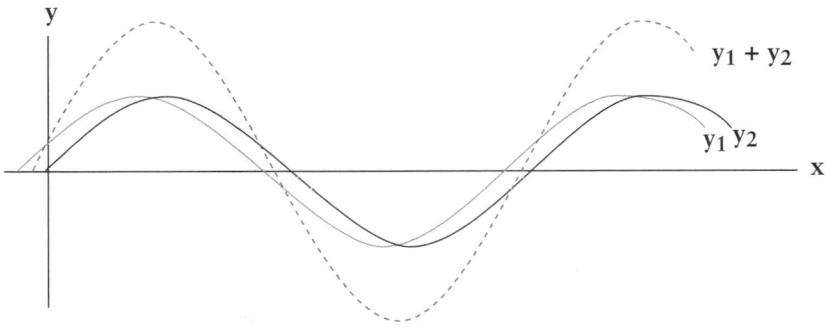

Figure 9.4(a)

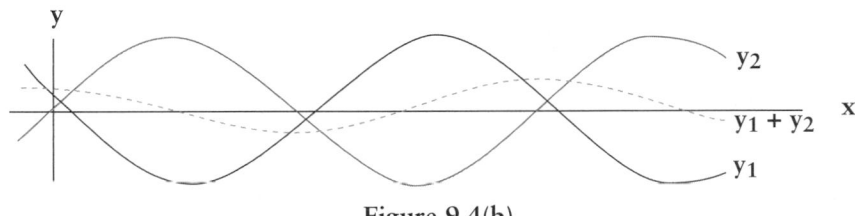

Figure 9.4(b)

E. TRAVELING AND STANDING WAVES

If a string fixed at one end is moved from side to side, it is seen that a wave travels or propagates down the string. Such a wave is known as a **traveling wave.** When the wave reaches the fixed boundary it is reflected and inverted (see Figure 9.5). If the free end of the string is continuously moved from side to side, there will then be two waves: the original wave moving down the string and the reflected wave moving the other way. These waves will then interfere with each other.

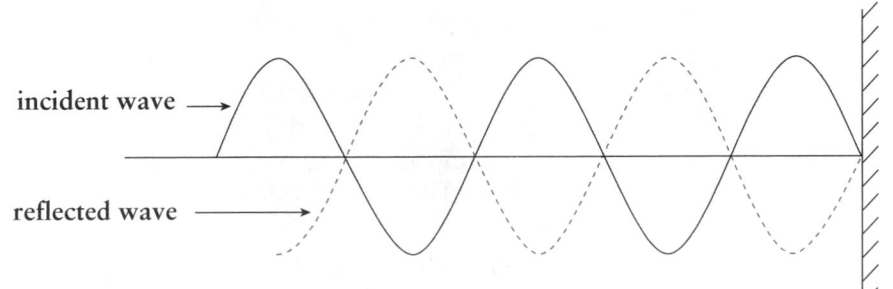

Figure 9.5

Consider now the case when both ends of the string are fixed and traveling waves are excited in the string. Certain wave frequencies can result in a waveform remaining in a stationary position, while the amplitude fluctuates. These waves are known as **standing waves.** Points in the wave that remain at rest are known as **nodes,** and points that are midway between these nodes are known as **antinodes.** Antinodes are points that fluctuate with maximum amplitude.

It is also possible to set up standing waves in pipes in much the same way as in a string. Standing waves in strings and pipes are discussed in more detail under SOUND, E. STANDING WAVES.

F. RESONANCE

In any oscillatory system there will be one or more **natural frequencies** (normal modes) of vibration; that is to say that the system will oscillate at one of these natural frequencies if there are no external forces involved (in the case of the free swinging pendulum there is only one natural frequency, whereas a stretched string will have an infinite number of natural frequencies).

If a periodically varying force is applied to the system, the system will then be driven at a frequency equal to the frequency of the force. This is known as a **forced oscillation.** The amplitude of this motion will generally be small. However, if the frequency of the applied force is close to that of the natural frequency of the system, then the amplitude becomes much larger.

If the frequency of the periodically varying force is equal to a natural frequency of the system, then the system is said to be **resonating,** and the amplitude of the oscillation is a maximum. If the oscillating system were frictionless, then the periodically varying force would continually add energy to the system, and the amplitude would increase indefinitely. However, since no system is completely frictionless, there is always some damping that results in a finite amplitude of oscillation.

SOUND

Sound is transmitted by oscillation of particles along the direction of motion of the sound wave. It is therefore a longitudinal wave. More generally, sound is a mechanical disturbance propagated through a deformable medium, and so it can be transmitted through solids, liquids, and gases, but NOT through a vacuum. The relative speed of sound in a medium is determined by the spacing of adjacent particles. The smaller the spacing between the particles, the faster sound will travel in that medium. For this reason, sound travels faster in a solid than in a liquid, and faster in a liquid than in a gas.

This section will be primarily concerned with waves that, when they strike the ear, produce the sensation we call sound. For humans, such waves are called **audible waves** and have frequencies ranging from 20 Hz to 20,000 Hz. Waves whose frequencies are below 20 Hz are called **infrasonic waves,** and those whose frequencies are above 20,000 Hz are called **ultrasonic waves.** For sound waves in air at 0°C, the speed of sound is 331 m/s.

A. CHARACTERISTICS OF SOUND

Intensity is defined as the average rate per unit area at which energy is transported across a perpendicular surface by the wave. In other words, the intensity is the power transported per unit area. In SI it has units of W/m^2. The amplitude of the sound wave is a measure of its energy. The total power P carried across a surface area (such as an eardrum) equals the product of the intensity I and the surface area A, when the intensity is uniformly distributed. Mathematically, one can write:

$$P = IA$$

The **sound level,** β, is measured in decibels and is defined as:

$$\beta = 10 \log \frac{I}{I_0}$$

where I_0 is a reference intensity of 10^{-12} W/m^2, corresponding to the faintest sound that can be heard by humans.

> **MCAT Synopsis**
>
> Intensity is always power/area and is simply energy per unit time per unit area.

Example: A detector with a surface area of one square meter is placed one meter from an operating jackhammer. It measures the power of the jackhammer's sound to be 10^{-3} W. Find:

a. the intensity and the sound level of the jackhammer.
b. the ratio of the intensities of the jackhammer and a jet engine (assume β_{jet} = 130 dB).

Solution: a. Intensity is equal to power divided by area.

$$I = \frac{P}{A}$$

$$= \frac{10^{-3}}{1}$$

$$= 10^{-3} \text{ W/m}^2$$

The sound level is given by:

$$\beta = 10 \log \frac{I}{I_0}$$

$$= 10 \log \left(\frac{10^{-3}}{10^{-12}} \right)$$

$$= 10 \log 10^9$$

$$= 90 \text{ dB}$$

b. The ratio of 2 intensities of sound can be found from the difference of their sound levels:

$$\beta_{jet} - \beta_{jack} = 10 \log \left(\frac{I_{jet}}{I_{jack}} \right)$$

$$130 - 90 = 10 \log \left(\frac{I_{jet}}{I_{jack}} \right)$$

$$4 = \log \left(\frac{I_{jet}}{I_{jack}} \right)$$

$$10,000 = \left(\frac{I_{jet}}{I_{jack}} \right)$$

Thus the jet engine's sound is 10,000 times more intense than the jackhammer's.

Another characteristic of sound is **pitch.** This refers to the sensation of sound that enables one to classify the frequency of a note.

B. PRODUCTION OF SOUND

For sound to be produced, there must be a longitudinal oscillation of air molecules. This oscillation can be produced by the vibration of a solid object that sets adjacent air molecules into motion, or by means of an acoustic vibration in an enclosed space.

Sound produced by the vibration of a solid object includes sound that is created by string and percussion instruments such as the guitar, violin, and piano. In this case, a string or several strings are set into motion and vibrate at their normal mode frequencies. Since the strings are very thin, it makes them ineffective in transmitting their vibration to the surrounding air. For this reason a solid body is employed to provide a better coupling to the air. In the case of a guitar, the vibration is transmitted through the bridge to the body of the instrument, which vibrates at the same frequency as the string.

Sound created by acoustic vibration includes sound from instruments such as organ pipes, the flute, and the recorder. There are no moving parts, and sound is produced by a vibrating motion of air within the instrument. In the case of an organ pipe, the pitch is determined by the length of the pipe. However, instruments such as the recorder and the flute are able to generate more than one pitch by the opening and closing of holes.

In the case of the human voice, sound is created by passing air between the vocal cords. The pitch is controlled by varying the tension of the cords. This is very similar to the production of sound in wind instruments such as the oboe and the clarinet, but these use a reed instead of vocal cords. Pitch in this case is controlled both by the opening and closing of holes and by varying the tension across the reed.

C. BEATS

Beats are heard when two waves that have nearly equal frequencies are superimposed. By the principle of superposition, the two waves add together, and what results is a periodic variation in loudness called beats. The beat frequency is:

$$f_{beat} = f_1 - f_2$$

Example: Two tuning forks are sounded. One has a frequency of 250 Hz while the other has a frequency of 245 Hz. What is the frequency of the beats?

Solution: The frequency of the beats is the difference of the frequencies of the interacting waves:

$$f_{beat} = f_1 - f_2$$
$$= 250 - 245$$
$$= 5 \text{ Hz}$$

D. DOPPLER EFFECT

A qualitative description of the **Doppler Effect** is that when a source emitting sound and the detector of that sound are moving relative to each other along the line joining them, the perceived frequency of the sound received f' differs from the actual frequency emitted f. If the source and detector are moving towards each other, the observed frequency increases, and if the source and detector are moving away from each other, the observed frequency decreases. This can be seen from the following equation:

$$f' = f \frac{(v \pm V_D)}{(v \pm V_S)}$$

where v is the speed of sound in the medium, V_D is the speed of the detector relative to the medium, and V_S is the speed of the source relative to the medium. The upper sign on V_D (V_S) is used when the detector (source) moves toward the source (detector), while the lower sign is used when it moves away.

Example: The siren of a police car cruising at 144 km/hr is sounding while the car is in pursuit of a speeding motorist. Assume that the speed of sound is 330 m/s. The siren emits sound at a frequency of 1450 Hz. What is the frequency heard by a stationary observer when:

a. the police car is moving towards the observer?
b. the police car has passed the observer?

Solution: a. To do this problem the speed of the police car must first be converted to m/s.

$$\frac{144 \text{ km}}{hr} \cdot \frac{10^3 \text{ m}}{km} \cdot \frac{hr}{3,600 \text{ s}} = 40 \text{ m/s}$$

Since the police car is moving toward the stationary observer, the denominator is $v - V_S$, and the numerator is simply v (since $V_D = 0$). This gives:

$$f' = f \frac{v}{v - V_S}$$

$$= \frac{1,450(330)}{330 - 40}$$

$$= 1,650 \text{ Hz}$$

b. In this part of the question the police car is now moving away from the observer, so the denominator is $v + V_S$. The numerator remains unchanged since the observer is still stationary.

$$f' = f \frac{v}{v + V_s}$$

$$= \frac{1,450(330)}{330 + 40}$$

$$= 1,293 \text{ Hz}$$

This example shows precisely why the pitch of a siren changes when an ambulance or police car passes you on the street. In this case, when the police car is moving towards the observer the perceived frequency is 1,650 Hz, whereas when the car has passed the observer the perceived frequency has decreased to 1,293 Hz.

E. STANDING WAVES

1. Strings

Consider a string fixed rigidly at both ends. Since the string is fixed at both ends, each end must be a node (a point in a wave that remains at rest). This implies that if the string is to support a standing wave, the string's length L must be equal to some integer multiple of half a wavelength (e.g., $\lambda/2$, $2\lambda/2$, $3\lambda/2$, and so on). This string will be able to support standing waves with wavelengths:

$$\lambda = 2L, \frac{2L}{2}, \frac{2L}{3}, \dots \frac{2L}{n} \qquad (n = 1,2,3,\dots)$$

From the relationship that $f = v/l$, where v is the speed of the wave, the possible frequencies are:

$$f = \frac{v}{2L}, \frac{2v}{2L}, \frac{3v}{2L} \dots = \frac{nv}{2L} \qquad (n = 1,2,3,\dots)$$

The lowest frequency that the string can support is given by $v/2L$ and is known as the **fundamental frequency (first harmonic)**. The frequency given by $n = 2$ is known as the first overtone (second harmonic) and so on. All the possible frequencies that the string can support are said to form a **harmonic series**. The waveforms of the first three harmonics are shown in Figure 9.6 below. (Note: N stands for node and A for antinode.)

> **MCAT Synopsis**
>
> Higher harmonics have shorter wavelengths and higher frequencies, but the same wave speed.

> **MCAT Synopsis**
>
> For the nth harmonic on a string, n half wavelengths exactly fit along the length of the string.

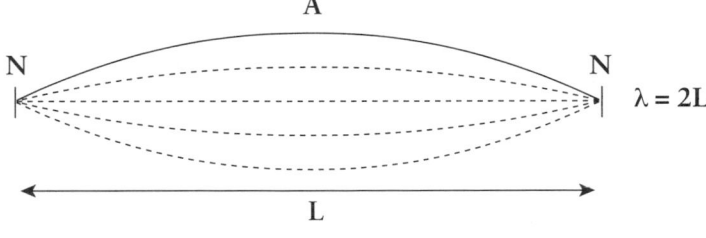

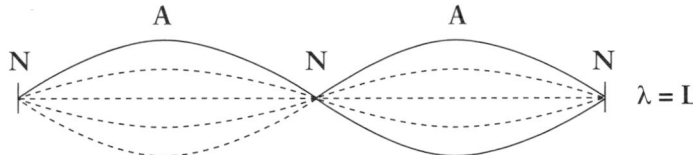

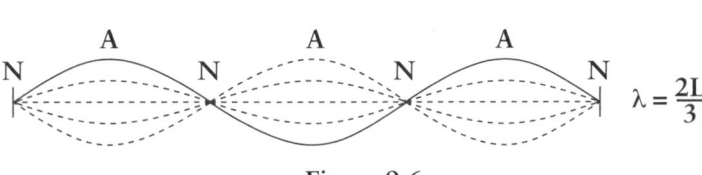

Figure 9.6

2. **Pipes**

Whereas strings are typically fixed at both ends, pipes may be open or closed at each end. In pipes the standing waves (if they occur) are sound waves originating in the air column. A closed end of a pipe corresponds to a fixed end of a string, and if standing waves occur a node will be at a closed end. On the other hand, at an open end of a pipe there will be an antinode. One end of the pipe will typically be open to allow air to enter. The pipe is then called open or closed depending on whether the other end is open or closed. The rules for the wavelengths and frequencies of the possible standing waves in a pipe of length L depend on whether the pipe is open (both ends are open) or closed (one end is open and the other end is closed).

Open pipes

An open pipe supports standing waves with antinodes at both ends. It is more difficult to illustrate the standing wave patterns in a pipe, since a sound wave is longitudinal. However, Figure 9.7 gives a symbolic representation, and it can be seen that this produces the same rule as for the string:

$$\lambda = \frac{2L}{n} \qquad (n = 1,2,3,\ldots)$$

$$f = \frac{nv}{2L} \qquad (n = 1,2,3,\ldots)$$

where v is the speed of the waves.

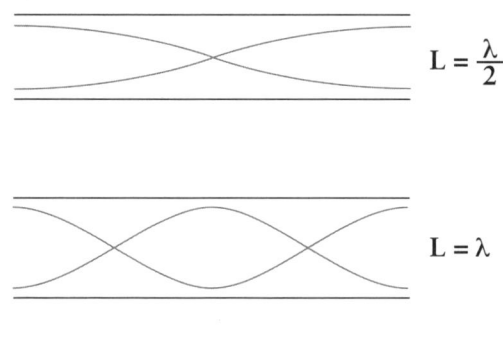

$L = \frac{\lambda}{2}$

$L = \lambda$

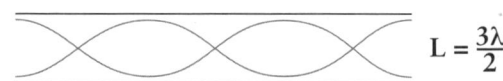

$L = \frac{3\lambda}{2}$

Figure 9.7

Closed pipes

In the case of a pipe open at one end but closed at the other, there is a node at the closed end. As in the case of the open pipe, the open end has an antinode. A symbolic representation of the standing wave patterns for a closed pipe is shown in Figure 9.8.

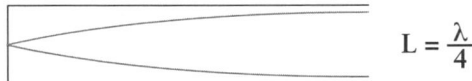

$$L = \frac{\lambda}{4}$$

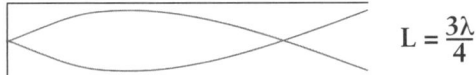

$$L = \frac{3\lambda}{4}$$

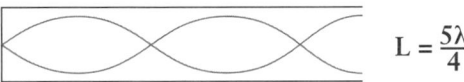

$$L = \frac{5\lambda}{4}$$

Figure 9.8

It can be seen that in this case, because the wave goes from a node to an antinode, the length of the pipe needed to produce the fundamental frequency needs to be a quarter-wavelength long. The first overtone occurs when the pipe is $3/4\lambda$; the next at $5/4\lambda$; etc. This can be represented by the general expression:

$$\lambda = \frac{4L}{n} \quad (n = 1, 3, 5, \ldots \text{odd integers only})$$

$$f = \frac{nv}{4L} \quad (n = 1, 3, 5, \ldots \text{odd integers only})$$

10

LIGHT AND OPTICS

In this chapter we will review the basics of optics, which is the study of the reflection and transmission of light through material media and through constrictions such as apertures and slits. Our review will cover the two main areas of optics. The first is termed geometrical optics because we treat light as moving in a straight-line path and can apply simple geometry to determine its behavior. Geometrical optics pertains to the study of mirrors and lenses along with the concepts of reflection and refraction. The second topic is concerned with the wave nature of light and particularly how light behaves when it is passed through apertures and slits. In these instances the light doesn't simply travel in straight-line paths to the wave; concepts of superposition and interference are needed to understand the behavior. A brief review is also provided of the physical nature of light itself, i.e., the electromagnetic wave.

ELECTROMAGNETIC SPECTRUM

A. ELECTROMAGNETIC WAVES

A changing magnetic field can cause a change in the electric field, and a changing electric field can cause a change in the magnetic field. Since changing electric fields affect changing magnetic fields which affect changing electric fields (and so on and so on), we can begin to see how **electromagnetic waves** occur in nature. One field affects the other, totally independent of matter, and electromagnetic waves can travel through a vacuum.

Electromagnetic waves are transverse waves because the oscillating electric and magnetic field vectors are perpendicular to the direction of propagation. Furthermore, the electric field and the magnetic field are perpendicular to each other. This is illustrated in Figure 10.1.

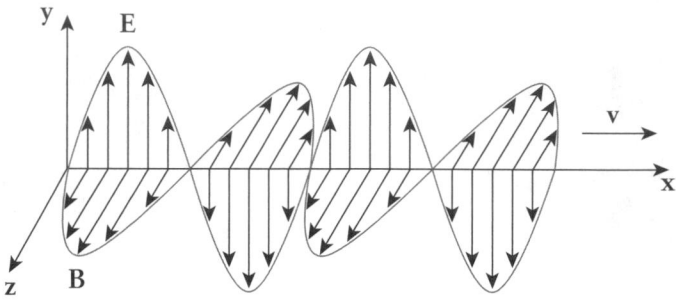

Figure 10.1

The **electromagnetic spectrum** is a term used to describe the full range in frequency and wavelength of electromagnetic waves. The following prefixes are often used when quoting wavelength: 1 mm = 10^{-3} m, 1 μm = 10^{-6} m, 1 nm = 10^{-9} m, and 1 Å = 10^{-10}m. The full spectrum is broken into many regions which, in descending order of wavelength, are: radio (10^9 m to 1 mm), infrared (1 mm to 700 nm), visible light (700 nm to 400 nm), ultraviolet (400 nm to 50 nm), X ray (50 nm to 10^{-2} nm), and gamma ray (smaller than 10^{-2} nm). These regions have arbitrary boundaries, and some authors quote slightly different values. For example, one person will call 50 nm "short wavelength ultraviolet," while another may call it "long wavelength X ray."

Electromagnetic waves can vary in frequency or wavelength, but in a vacuum all electromagnetic waves travel at the same speed, called the **speed of light.** This constant is represented by the letter c and is equal to: 3.00×10^8 m/s. To a first approximation, electromagnetic waves also travel in air with this velocity. Now the familiar equation $v = f\lambda$ becomes:

$$c = f\lambda$$

for all electromagnetic waves in a vacuum and, to a first approximation, in air.

B. COLOR AND THE VISIBLE SPECTRUM

We just mentioned that the electromagnetic spectrum is broken up into many regions. The visible part of the spectrum is the only part that is perceived as light by the human eye. Within this region different wavelengths induce sensations of different colors, with violet at one end of the visible spectrum (400 nm) and red at the other end of the visible spectrum (700 nm).

Light that contains all the colors in equal intensity is seen as white. The color of an object that does not emit its own light is dependent on the color of light that it reflects. So an object that appears red is one that absorbs all light except red. This implies that a red object receiving green light will appear black, since it absorbs the green light and has no light to reflect.

GEOMETRICAL OPTICS

When light travels through a single homogeneous medium it travels in a straight line. This is known as rectilinear propagation. The behavior of light at the boundary of a medium or interface between two media is described by the theory of geometrical optics.

A. REFLECTION

Reflection is the rebounding of incident light waves at the boundary of a medium.

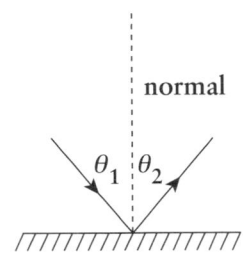

Figure 10.2

The law of reflection is:

$$\theta_1 = \theta_2$$

Important note: In optics, angles are always measured from a line drawn perpendicular to the boundary of a medium, often referred to as the **normal.**

1. Plane Mirrors

    Parallel incident rays remain parallel after reflection from a plane mirror. In general, images created by a mirror can be either real or virtual. An image is said to be **real** if the light actually converges at the position of the image. An image is **virtual** if the light only *appears* to be coming from the position of the image but does not converge there.

    Plane mirrors always create virtual images. In a plane mirror the image appears to be the same distance behind the mirror as the object's distance in front of it. Because the reflected light remains in front of the mirror but the image is behind the mirror, the image is virtual.

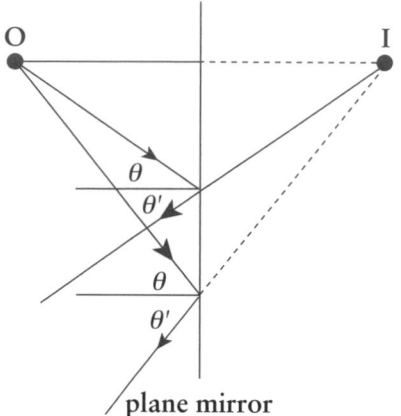

Figure 10.3

2. Spherical Mirrors

Spherical mirrors come in two varieties, **concave** and **convex**. The word *spherical* implies that the surface of the mirror has the shape of a sphere. In other words, if you had a sphere made out of a mirror-like material, a spherical mirror would be a small portion cut out of that sphere. Therefore, spherical mirrors have a **center of curvature** C and a **radius of curvature** r associated with them.

If you were to look from the inside of a sphere to its surface, you would see a concave surface. However, if you were to look from outside the sphere you would see a convex surface. The **focal length** f is the distance between the focal point and the mirror. For all spherical mirrors $f = r/2$. For a convex surface the center of curvature and the focal point are behind the mirror. Concave mirrors are called **converging mirrors** and convex mirrors are called **diverging mirrors**.

There are several important distances associated with mirrors. The focal length f is the distance between the focal point F and the mirror; the radius of curvature r is the distance between C and the mirror (remember that $r = 2f$); the distance of the object from the mirror is o; the distance of the image from the mirror is i. There is a simple relation satisfied by these distances:

$$\frac{1}{o} + \frac{1}{i} = \frac{1}{f} = \frac{2}{r}$$

While it is not important which units of distance are used in this equation, it is important that all values used have the same units, be they centimeters, meters, or whatever.

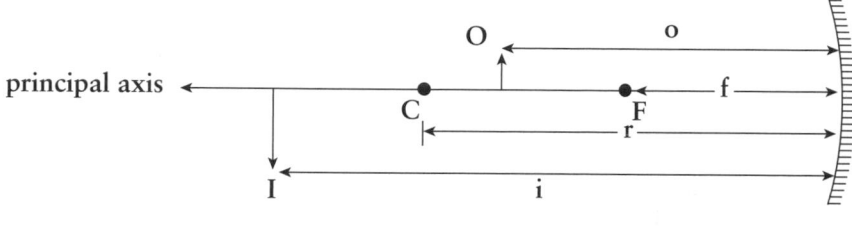

Figure 10.4

Often you will use this equation to calculate the image distance. If the image has a positive distance, it is a real image, which implies that the image is in front of the mirror. If the image has a negative distance, it is virtual and thus located behind the mirror. Note also that for a plane mirror $r = f = \infty$, and the equation becomes $1/o + 1/i = 0$ or $i = -o$ (virtual image).

The **magnification** (m) is a dimensionless value that is the ratio of the image's height to the object's height. Following the sign convention given below, the orientation of the image compared with the object can also be determined. A negative magnification signifies an inverted image, while a positive value means the image is upright.

$$m = -\frac{i}{o}$$

If $|m| < 1$ the image is reduced, if $|m| > 1$ the image is enlarged, and if $|m| = 1$ the image is the same size as the object.

Figure 10.5 shows ray diagrams for a concave spherical mirror with the object at three different points. A ray diagram is useful for getting an approximation of where the image is. In general, there are three important rays to draw. For a concave mirror, a ray that strikes the mirror parallel to the horizontal is reflected back through the focal point. A ray that passes through the focal point before reaching the mirror is reflected back parallel to the horizontal. A ray that strikes the mirror right where the normal intersects it gets reflected back with the same angle (measured from the normal).

A single diverging mirror forms only a virtual erect image, regardless of the position of the object. The image formed by a single converging mirror depends on the position of the object, demonstrated by Figure 10.5. When the object is farther away from the mirror than the focal point, the image is real and inverted. By moving the object to the focal point, the image disappears as the light rays reflect off the mirror parallel to each other and never converge. Moving the object closer to the mirror than the focal length makes an image that is virtual and erect.

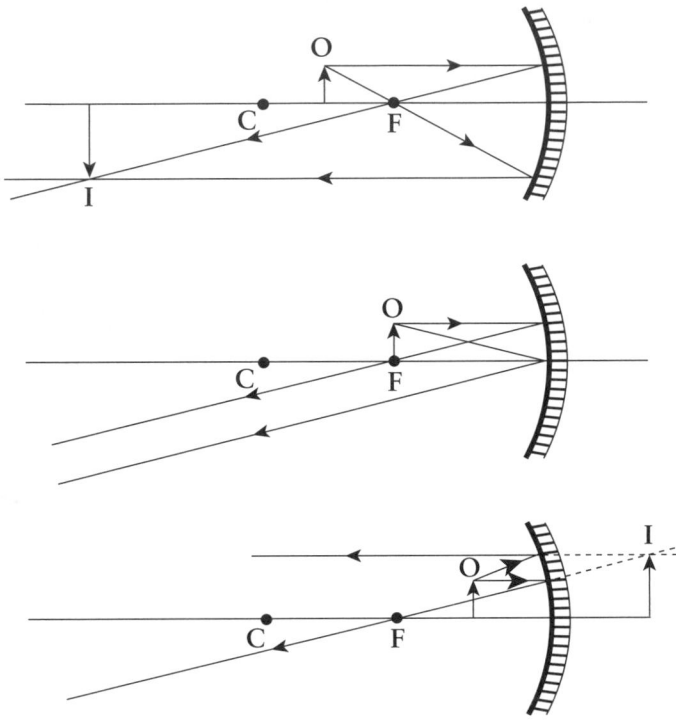

Figure 10.5

3. **Sign Convention**

The following chart gives the proper signs for various instances when dealing with single mirrors. Note that R side is used to denote Real side, which for mirrors is in front of the mirror. Similarly, V side stands for Virtual side, which is behind the mirror.

SIGN CHART FOR SINGLE MIRRORS

symbol	positive	negative
o	object is in front of mirror (R side)	object is behind mirror (V side)
i	image is in front of mirror (R side)	image is behind mirror (V side)
r	concave mirrors	convex mirrors
f	concave mirrors	convex mirrors
m	image is upright (erect)	image is inverted

Note that in almost all problems the object will be in front of the mirror, and thus the object distance o will be positive.

Example: An object is placed 7 cm in front of a concave mirror that has a 10 cm radius of curvature. Determine the image distance, the magnification, whether the image is real or virtual, and whether it is inverted or upright.

Solution: Using the mirror equation:

$$\frac{1}{i} + \frac{1}{o} = \frac{2}{r}$$

$$\frac{1}{i} = \frac{2}{r} - \frac{1}{o}$$

$$\frac{1}{i} = \frac{2}{10} - \frac{1}{7}$$

$$i = +17.5 \text{ cm}$$

The magnification m is:

$$m = -\frac{i}{o}$$

$$= -\frac{17.5}{7}$$

$$= -2.5$$

The image is in front of the mirror (i is positive) and therefore real. The image is inverted (m is negative) and 2.5 times larger ($|m| = 2.5$).

B. REFRACTION

1. **Snell's Law**
   When light is not in a vacuum, its speed is less than c. (As previously noted, when light is in air, $v \cong c$.) For a given medium:

$$n = \frac{c}{v}$$

where c is the speed of light in a vacuum, v is the speed of light in the medium, and n is a dimensionless quantity called the **index of refraction** of the medium. Because $v < c$, $n > 1$. For air, to a first approximation, $v = c$ and $n = 1$.

> **MCAT Synopsis**
>
> Light travels more slowly in material media (like glass) than in a vacuum. The wavelength changes accordingly while the frequency remains constant.

Refracted rays of light obey **Snell's law** as they pass from one medium to another:

$$n_1 \sin \theta_1 = n_2 \sin \theta_2$$

n_1 and θ_1 are for the medium the light is coming from, and n_2 and θ_2 are for the medium the light is going into. Note that θ is measured with respect to the perpendicular (normal) to the boundary.

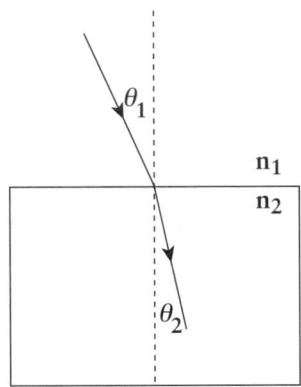

Figure 10.6

In general, when light enters a medium with a higher index of refraction ($n_2 > n_1$) it bends towards the normal so that $\theta_2 < \theta_1$. Conversely, if the light travels into a medium where the index of refraction is smaller ($n_2 < n_1$), the light will bend away from the normal so that $\theta_2 > \theta_1$.

Example: A penny sits at the bottom of a pool of water ($n = 1.33$) at a depth of 3.0 m. If an observer 1.8 m tall stands 30 cm away from the ledge, how close to the side can the penny be and still be visible?

Solution: First draw a picture of the situation as in Figure 10.7. Note that the light is coming from the water ($n_1 = 1.33$) and going into the air ($n_2 = 1$), so the light is bent away from the normal ($\theta_2 > \theta_1$).

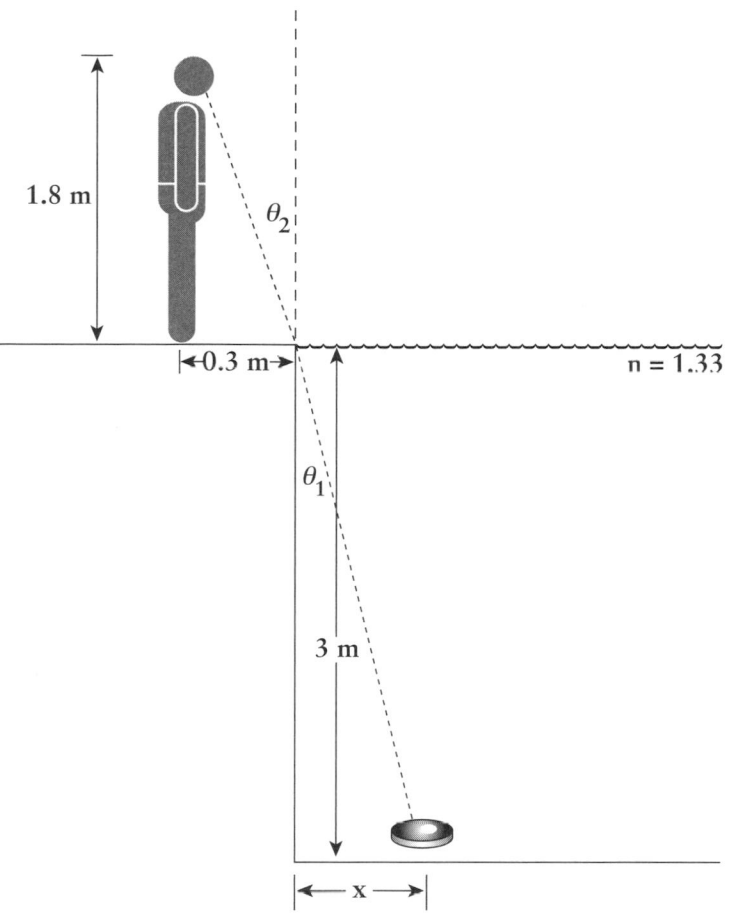

MCAT Synopsis

Refraction (bending of light) can cause optical illusions.

Figure 10.7

We need to find the angles that the light rays make with the normal to the water's surface:

$$\tan \theta_2 = \frac{0.3}{1.8}$$

$$\theta_2 = 9.5°$$

Using Snell's law we can solve for θ_1:

$$\sin \theta_1 = \frac{n_2}{n_1} \sin \theta_2$$

$$= \frac{0.165}{1.33}$$

$$\theta_1 = 7.1°$$

We can find x using trigonometry:

$$x = 3 \tan \theta_1$$
$$= 0.37 \text{ m}$$
$$= 37 \text{ cm}$$

2. **Total Internal Reflection**

When light travels from a medium with a higher index of refraction to a medium with a lower index of refraction, the refracted angle is larger than the angle of incidence ($\theta_2 > \theta_1$). As the angle of incidence is increased, a special angle is reached, called the **critical angle** (θ_c), where for this value of θ_1 the refracted angle θ_2 equals 90°. The critical angle can be found from Snell's Law:

$$n_1 \sin \theta_1 = n_2 \sin \theta_2$$
$$n_1 \sin \theta_c = n_2 \sin 90° = n_2$$
$$\sin \theta_c = \frac{n_2}{n_1}$$

Total **internal reflection,** a condition in which all the light incident on a boundary is reflected back into the original material, results for any angle of incidence greater than θ_c.

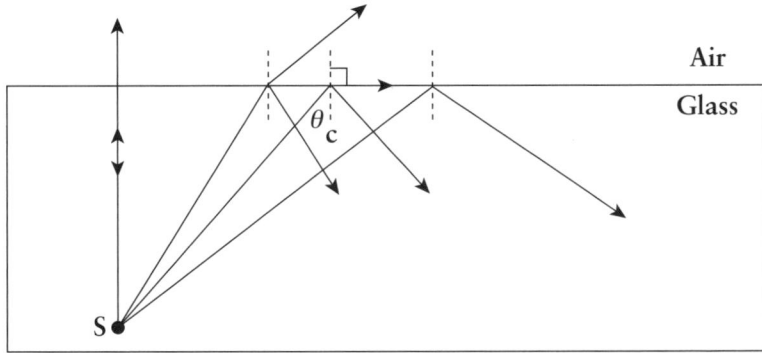

Figure 10.8

Example: From the previous example, suppose another penny is 10 times farther out than the first one. Will a light ray going from this penny to the top edge of the pool emerge from the water?

Solution: First find the critical angle:

$$\sin \theta_c = \frac{n_2}{n_1}$$

$$= \frac{1}{1.33}$$

$$\theta_c = 48.8°$$

The angle made by the second penny's light ray is:

$$\tan \theta_1 = \frac{0.37 \times 10}{3} = 1.23$$

$$\theta_1 = 51°$$

$\theta_1 > \theta_c$, therefore the light ray will be totally internally reflected and will not emerge.

3. **Thin Spherical Lenses**

There is an important difference between lenses and mirrors aside from the obvious fact that lenses refract light while mirrors reflect it. When working with lenses, you are dealing with *two* surfaces that affect the light path. For example, a person wearing glasses sees light that travels from an object through the air into the glass lens (first surface). Then the light travels through the glass until it reaches the other side, where again it travels out of the glass into the air (second surface).

A thin lens is a lens whose thickness can be neglected. Since light can be coming from either side of a lens, a lens has two focal points (one on each side of the lens) and two focal lengths (see Figure 10.9). For thin spherical lenses the focal lengths are equal, and so we speak of the focal length.

Figure 10.9(a) also illustrates that a **converging lens** is always thicker at the center, while Figure 10.9(b) illustrates that a **diverging lens** is always thinner at the center.

> **MCAT Synopsis**
>
> Mirrors reflect light, whereas lenses refract light. The refraction occurs at both surfaces of the lens.

> **MCAT Synopsis**
>
> Converging lenses cause parallel rays to converge at the focal point and rays from the focal point to emerge parallel.

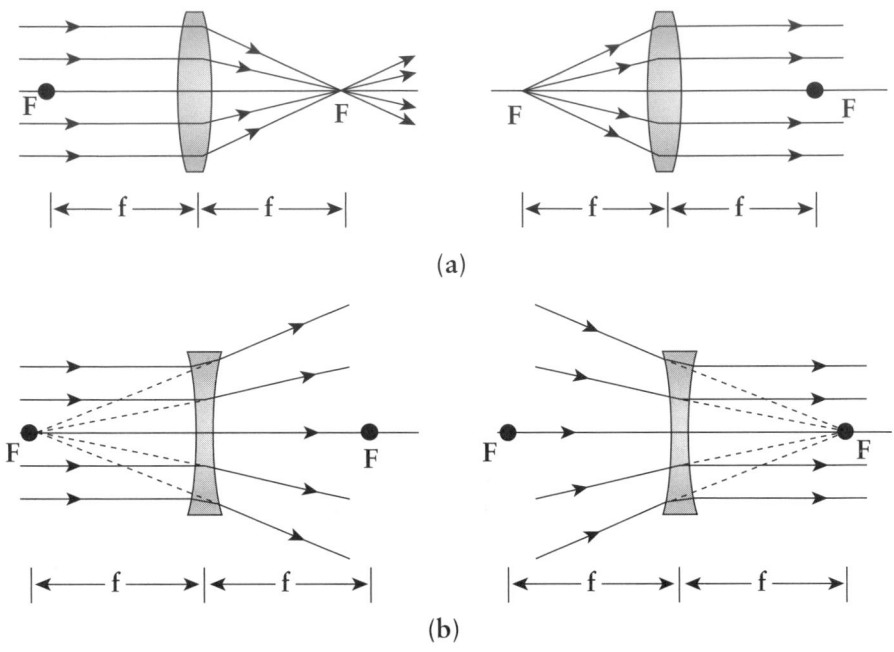

(a)

(b)

Figure 10.9

The basic formulas for finding image distance and magnification for spherical mirrors (except $r = 2f$,) also apply to lenses. The object distance o, image distance i, focal length f, and magnification m, are related by:

$$\frac{1}{o} + \frac{1}{i} = \frac{1}{f}$$

$$m = -\frac{i}{o}$$

For lenses whose thicknesses cannot be neglected, the focal length is related to the curvature of the lens surfaces and the index of refraction of the lens by the **Lensmaker's equation:**

$$\frac{1}{f} = (n - 1)\left(\frac{1}{r_1} - \frac{1}{r_2}\right)$$

where r_1 is the radius of curvature of the first lens surface and r_2 is the radius of curvature of the second lens surface.

Note that sign conventions change slightly for lenses. (Sign conventions are the trickiest part to optics.) For both lenses and mirrors, positive magnification means upright images and negative magnification means inverted images. Also, for both lenses and mirrors, a positive image distance means that the image is real and is located on the R side, whereas a negative image distance means that the image is virtual and located on the V side.

However, where to place the R side and V side confuses most people because it is different for mirrors and lenses. To place the R side, remember that the R side is where the light really goes after interacting with the mirror or lens. For mirrors, light is reflected and therefore stays in front of the mirror. The image may either appear in front of or behind the mirror, but the light rays always remain in front of the mirror. Since the R side is in front of the mirror, the V side is behind the mirror. For lenses, it is different: Light travels through the lens and comes out on the other side. The light really travels to the other side of the lens, and therefore, for lenses, the R side is on the opposite side of the lens from where the light came from. Thus the V side must be the side of the lens that the light came from. Although the object of a single lens is on the V side, this does not make the object virtual. Objects are real, with a positive object distance, unless they are in certain multiple lens systems.

Focal lengths have a simple sign convention. For both mirrors and lenses, converging lenses and mirrors have positive focal lengths and diverging mirrors and lenses have negative focal lengths. For radii of curvature you have to remember that a lens has two surfaces, each with its own radius of curvature (r_1 and r_2, where the surfaces are numbered in the order that they are encountered by the traveling light). For both mirrors and lenses, a radius of curvature is positive if the center of curvature is on the R side and negative if the center of curvature is on the V side.

SIGN CHART FOR SINGLE LENSES

symbol	positive	negative
o	object on side of lens light is coming from	object on side of lens light is going to
i	image on side of lens light is going to (R side)	image on side of lens light is coming from (V side)
f	converging lens	diverging lens
m	image erect	image inverted
r	when on R side (convex surface as seen from side the light is coming from)	when on V side (concave surface as seen from side the light is coming from)

Optometrists often describe a lens in terms of its **power** (P). This is measured in **diopters** when f is in meters and is given by the equation:

$$P = \frac{1}{f}$$

P has the same sign as f and is therefore positive for a converging lens and negative for a diverging lens.

4. Multiple Lens Systems

Lenses in contact are a series of lenses with negligible distances between them. These systems behave as a single lens with equivalent focal length given by:

$$\frac{1}{f} = \frac{1}{f_1} + \frac{1}{f_2} + \ldots$$

$$(P = P_1 + P_2 + \ldots)$$

A good example is the eye.

For **lenses not in contact** the image of one lens is used to make the object of another lens. The image from the last lens is the image of the system. Microscopes and telescopes are good examples. The magnification for the system is $M = m_1 \times m_2 \times m_3 \times \ldots$

Example: An object is 15 cm to the left of a thin diverging lens with a 45 cm focal length as shown below. Find:

a. where the image is formed, if it is upright or inverted, and if it is real or virtual.
b. the radii of curvature assuming the lens is symmetrical and made of glass (n = 1.50).

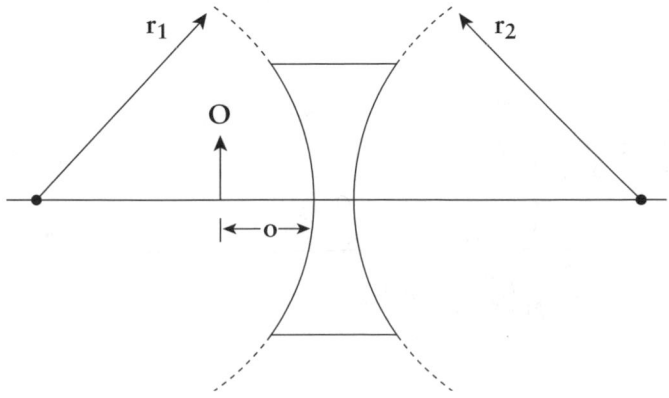

Figure 10.10

Solution: a. The image distance (i) is found using the equation:

$$\frac{1}{i} + \frac{1}{o} = \frac{1}{f}$$

$$\frac{1}{i} = \frac{1}{f} - \frac{1}{o}$$

Since the lens is diverging the focal length takes a negative sign, f = –45 cm. The object (like all objects in a single lens system) has a positive sign, o = 15 cm. Solving for i:

$$\frac{1}{i} = \frac{-1}{45} - \frac{1}{15}$$

$$= \frac{-1}{45} - \frac{3}{45}$$

$$= \frac{-4}{45}$$

$$i = -11.25 \text{ cm}$$

The negative sign indicates that the image is on the left side of the lens and therefore virtual (the light went through the lens and is on the right side). To find out whether the image is upright or inverted we need to calculate the magnification:

$$m = -\frac{i}{o}$$

$$= -\frac{-11.25}{15}$$

$$= \frac{11.25}{15}$$

$$= 0.75$$

Since the magnification is positive, the image is upright. Furthermore, since $|m| < 1$, the image is smaller than the object.

b. Since the lens is symmetrical, the radii are equal but opposite in sign. They can be found from the Lensmaker's equation:

$$\frac{1}{f} = (n - 1)\left(\frac{1}{r_1} - \frac{1}{r_2}\right)$$

As the light progresses from left to right, the first surface of the lens is concave (r_1 negative) and the second surface of the lens is convex (r positive). So:

$$\frac{1}{f} = (n - 1)\left(\frac{1}{-r} - \frac{1}{r}\right)$$

$$= (n - 1)\left(-\frac{2}{r}\right)$$

We know that f = –45 cm (diverging lens). Therefore:

$$-\frac{1}{45} = (1.5 - 1)\left(-\frac{2}{r}\right)$$

$$= \frac{-1}{r}$$

$$r = 45 \text{ cm}$$

C. DISPERSION

As noted earlier, the speed of light for all wavelengths in a vacuum is the same. However, when light travels through a medium, different wavelengths travel at different velocities. This fact also implies that the index of refraction of a medium is a function of the wavelength, since the index of refraction is related to the velocity of the wave by n = c/v. When the speed of the wave varies with wavelength a material exhibits **dispersion**. The most common example of dispersion is the splitting of white light into its component colors using a prism.

If a source of white light is incident on one of the faces of a prism, the light emerging from the prism is spread out into a fan shaped beam, as shown in Figure 10.11. The light has been dispersed into a spectrum. This occurs because violet light "sees" a greater index of refraction than red does and so is bent to a greater extent.

MCAT Synopsis

A prism splits white light into its component colors (wavelengths) because each wavelength has a different index of refraction.

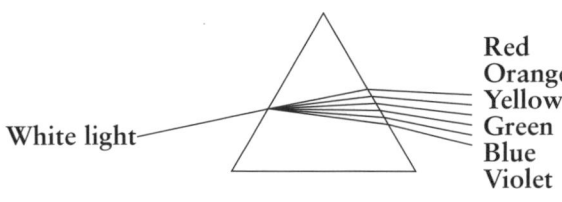

Figure 10.11

DIFFRACTION

When we first began discussing geometrical optics, we asserted that light travels in straight lines. But there are situations in which this is not strictly true. For example, when light passes through a narrow opening (an opening whose size is on the order of wavelengths), the light waves seem to spread out as is seen in Figure 10.12. As the slit narrows, the light is spread out more. This spreading out of light as it passes through a narrow opening is called **diffraction**.

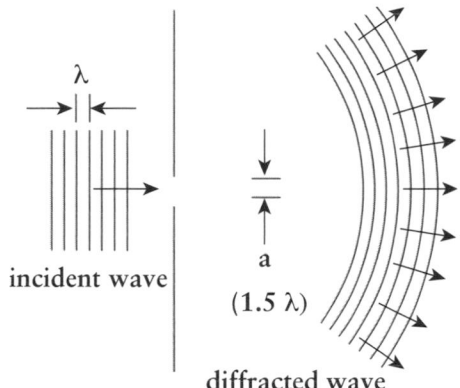

Figure 10.12

If a lens is placed between a narrow slit and a screen, a pattern is observed consisting of a bright central fringe with alternating dark and bright fringes on each side (see Figure 10.13). The central bright fringe is twice as wide as the bright fringes on the sides, and as the slit becomes narrower the central maximum becomes wider. The location of the dark fringes is given by the following formula:

$$a \sin \theta = n\lambda \quad (n = 1, 2, 3, \ldots)$$

where a is the width of the slit, λ is the wavelength of the incident wave, and θ is the angle made by the line drawn from the center of the lens to the dark fringe and the line perpendicular to the screen. Note that bright fringes are halfway between dark fringes.

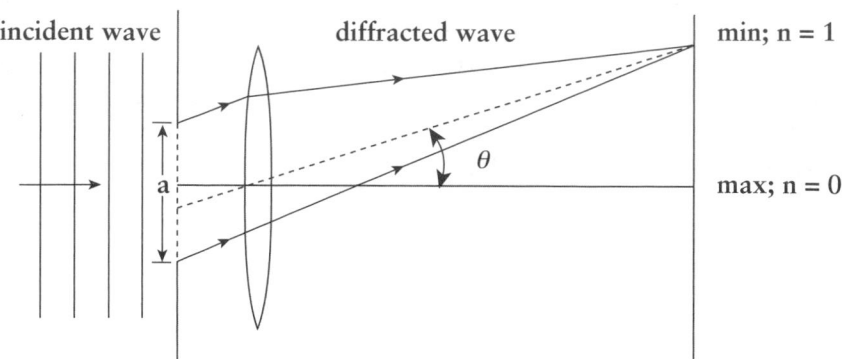

Figure 10.13

INTERFERENCE

By the superposition principle, when waves interact with each other, the amplitudes of the waves add together in a process called **interference** (see chapter 9). Young's experiment showed that two light waves can interfere with one another, and this contributed to the wave theory of light. Figure 10.14(a) shows the typical setup for Young's double slit experiment. When monochromatic light illuminates the slits, an interference pattern is observed on a screen placed behind the slits. Monochromatic light is light that consists of just one wavelength, and coherent light consists of light waves whose phase difference does not change with time. Regions of constructive interference between the two light waves appear as regions of maximum light intensity on the screen. Conversely, in regions where the light waves interfere destructively, the light is at a minimum intensity and the screen is dark. An interference pattern produced by a double slit setup is shown in Figure 10.14(b).

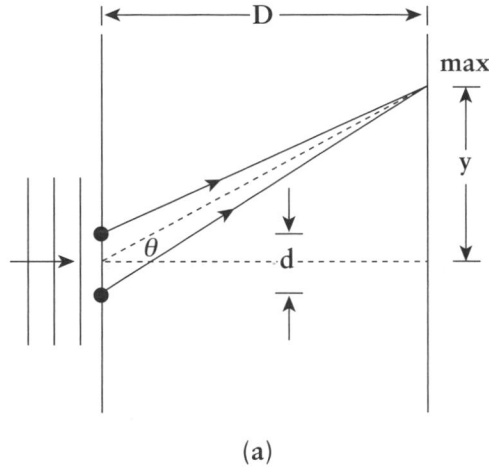

(a)

Zeroth fringe

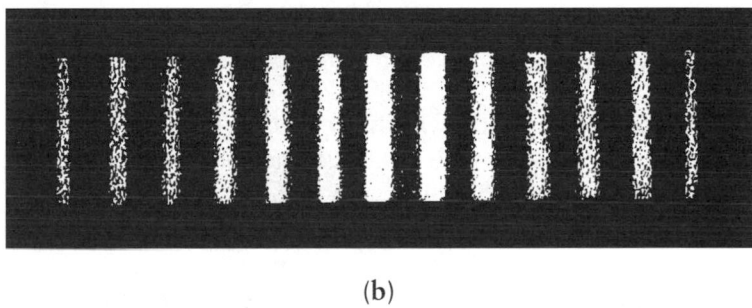

(b)

Figure 10.14

The position of maxima and minima on the screen can be found from the following equations:

(maxima) $d \sin \theta = m\lambda$ $m = 0, 1, 2, \ldots$

(minima) $d \sin \theta = (m + \frac{1}{2})\lambda$ $m = 0, 1, 2, \ldots$

where d is the distance between the slits, θ is the angle between the dashed lines shown in Figure 10.14a, λ is the wavelength of the light, and m is an integer representing the order.

> Example: What is the linear distance y, between the sixth and eighth maxima on the screen? The wavelength λ is 550 nm, the slits are separated by 0.14 mm, and the screen is 70 cm from the slits.

> Solution: Using the small angle approximation $\sin \theta \approx \tan \theta \approx \theta$, the equation for the distance between maxima is derived as follows:

$$\sin \theta = \frac{m\lambda}{d}$$

$$\tan \theta = \frac{y}{D} \approx \frac{m\lambda}{d}$$

$$\Delta y \approx \frac{\Delta m \lambda D}{d}$$

where Δm is the difference between fringe numbers. Substituting the numbers gives:

$$y = \frac{2(550 \times 10^{-9})(0.70)}{0.14 \times 10^{-3}}$$

$$= 5.5 \text{ mm}$$

POLARIZATION

Plane-polarized light is light in which the electric fields of all the waves are oriented in the same direction, i.e., their electric field vectors are parallel. It is true that their magnetic fields vectors are also parallel, but convention dictates that the plane of the electric field identifies the plane of polarization.

Unpolarized light corresponds to a random orientation of the electric field vectors. Sunlight is a prime example. However, there are filters called polarizers, often used in cameras and sunglasses, which allow only light whose electric field is pointing in a particular direction to pass. If you hold one polarizer out the window, it will let through only that portion of the daylight that has a given E vector orientation. If you now hold up another polarizer and slowly turn it, you will see the light transmitted through the two polarizers vary from total darkness to the level of the original polarizer alone. When both the first and second polarizer are polarizing in the same direction, all the light that passed through the first also passes through the second. When the second polarizer is turned so that it polarizes in a direction perpendicular to the first, no light gets through at all.

11

ATOMIC PHENOMENA

Toward the end of the 19th century and throughout the 20th, research has shown that different sets of laws take effect at short distances, due to the wave nature of the discrete bits of matter. The theory that was developed to explain such phenomena is known as quantum mechanics. This chapter will primarily cover particular applications of quantum mechanical ideas to atomic physics but will not cover the formal theory of quantum mechanics. The first two topics covered here, blackbody radiation and the photoelectric effect, provided a first look at the quantum or discrete aspects of nature at the atomic level, particularly the discrete or particle nature of light. The quantum theory was later applied to the structure of the hydrogen atom, thus uncovering the discrete nature of the electron energies in hydrogen. This theory of the hydrogen atom, Bohr's theory, is reviewed along with a discussion (also due to Bohr) of the interaction of electromagnetic quanta (photons) with atoms. The application of quantum mechanics to nuclear physics is discussed in chapter 12.

> **MCAT Synopsis**
>
> Since all matter has temperature above absolute zero, all matter emits electromagnetic radiation.

THERMAL BLACKBODY RADIATION

At any temperature above absolute zero, matter will emit electromagnetic radiation. The amount of radiant energy emitted at a given wavelength depends on the temperature of the emitter. In addition, different materials may emit different amounts of radiant energy at a particular wavelength due to the differences in their atomic structure. Because of these complications, physicists at the turn of the century turned their attention to an **ideal radiator** known as a **blackbody** (because of the fact that any ideal radiator is also an ideal absorber and would appear totally black if it were at a lower temperature than its surroundings). In practice, a blackbody radiator can be approximated rather closely by radiation produced in a cavity within a hot object. Hence blackbody radiation is approximated by what is called **cavity radiation**.

Physicist Max Planck developed the theoretical derivation of the blackbody spectrum. His radiant spectrum for two blackbodies at different temperatures is shown in Figure 11.1. In the derivation Planck had to use a number called **Planck's constant** (h) whose value is given by:

$$h = 6.63 \times 10^{-34} \text{ J} \cdot \text{s} = 4.14 \times 10^{-15} \text{ eV} \cdot \text{s}$$

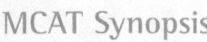

MCAT Synopsis

The blackbody curve or spectrum shows the amount of energy radiated as a function of wavelength.

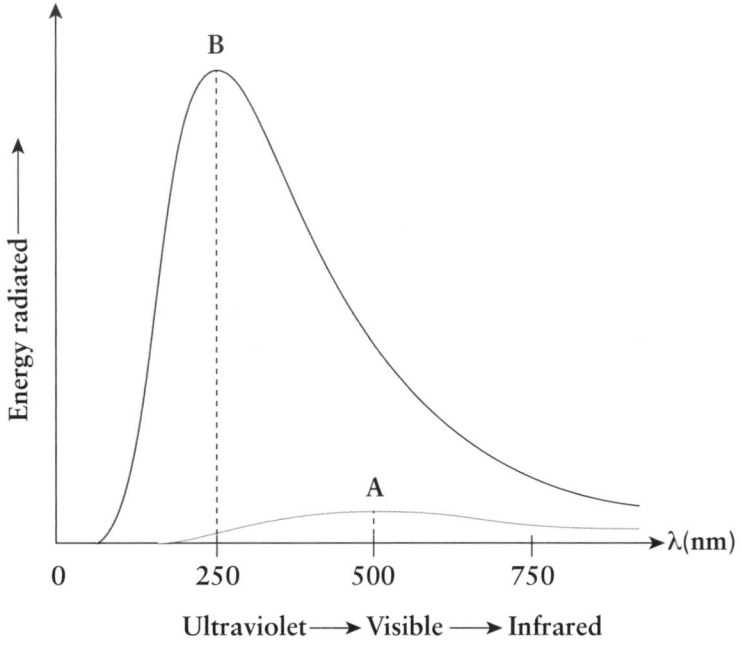

Figure 11.1

An analysis of Planck's formula for the blackbody spectrum shows that for a blackbody there is one wavelength at which the maximum amount of energy is emitted (λ_{peak}). This wavelength depends on the absolute temperature of the blackbody in a relation known as **Wien's displacement law,** which is expressed mathematically as:

$$\lambda_{peak} T = \text{constant}$$

The value of the constant is 2.90×10^{-3} m•K. Note that λ_{peak} is the wavelength at which more energy is emitted than any other wavelength. λ_{peak} **does not** refer to the maximum wavelength emitted.

Also, according to the **Stefan-Boltzmann law,** the total energy being emitted per unit area per second is proportional to the fourth power of the absolute temperature:

$$E_T = \sigma T^4$$

where σ is the Stefan-Boltzmann constant (5.67×10^{-8} J•s•m^2•K^4).

Example: In Figure 11.1 the radiant spectrum for two blackbodies is plotted. The first body is at temperature T_a, and the second body is at temperature T_b. How do the temperatures of the two blackbodies compare?

Solution: From the plots we find that $\lambda_{peak-a} = 2\lambda_{peak-b}$, and from Wien's law we know that $T_b = 2T_a$. [By the Stefan-Boltzmann law the emitted energy per unit area per second of blackbody b is $2^4 = 16$ times greater than that of blackbody a.]

PHOTOELECTRIC EFFECT

When light of a sufficiently high frequency (typically, blue or ultraviolet light) is incident on a metal in a vacuum, the metal emits electrons. This phenomenon, first discovered by Heinrich Hertz in 1887, is called the **photoelectric effect.** The minimum frequency of light that accomplishes this ejection of electrons is known as the **threshold frequency** f_T. The threshold frequency depends on the type of metal being exposed to the light. Einstein's explanation of these results was that the light beam consists of an integral number of light quanta, called photons, with the energy of each photon proportional to the frequency f of the light:

$$E = hf$$

The constant of proportionality h is Planck's constant.

It should also be noted that by knowing the frequency of the light you can easily find the wavelength λ via the relation:

$$\lambda = \frac{c}{f}$$

where c is the speed of light (3.00×10^8 m/s). These relations predict that shorter wavelength means higher frequency and therefore higher energy photons (toward the blue and ultraviolet end of the spectrum). Longer wavelength means lower frequency and therefore lower energy photons (toward the red and infrared end of the spectrum). Common units used for wavelength include nanometers (1 nm = 10^{-9} m) and Angstroms (1 Å = 10^{-10} m).

In the photoelectric effect, if the frequency of a photon incident on a metal is at the threshold frequency for the metal, the electron barely escapes from the metal. However, if the frequency of an incident photon is above the threshold frequency of the metal, the photon will have more than enough energy to eject a single electron, and the excess energy will be converted to kinetic energy of the ejected electron. The maximum kinetic energy can be calculated from the formula:

$$K = hf - W$$

> **MCAT Favorite**
>
> The energy, E, of a quantum of light (photon) of frequency f is: $E = hf$.

> **MCAT Synopsis**
>
> Wavelength and frequency of light in vacuum are related to speed of light by $c = \lambda f$, just as wavelength, frequency, and velocity of any wave are related by $v = \lambda f$.

> **MCAT Synopsis**
>
> $E = hf = hc/\lambda$, which says that higher frequency or shorter wavelength light has higher energy, and lower frequency or longer wavelength light has lower energy.

where W is the **work function** of the metal in question (the minimum energy required to eject an electron) which is related to the threshold frequency of that metal by:

$$W = hf_T$$

So for $f > f_T$ the photon will eject electrons with the excess energy appearing as kinetic energy (K). For $f < f_T$ the photon does not carry enough energy to eject an electron from the metal.

We can think of all of the electrons liberated from the metal by the photoelectric effect as producing a net charge flow per unit time, or a current. Provided that a light beam's frequency is above the threshold frequency of the metal, light beams of greater intensity produce greater current. This is because the higher the intensity of the beam, the greater the number of photons per unit time that fall on an electrode, producing a greater number of electrons per unit time liberated from the metal. When the light's frequency is above threshold frequency, the current is directly proportional to the intensity of the light beam.

Example: If the work function of a metal is 2.00 eV and blue light of frequency 6.00×10^{14} Hz is incident on the metal, will there be photo ejection of electrons? If so, how much kinetic energy will an electron carry away?

Solution: If the photons have a frequency of 6.00×10^{14} Hz, each photon has an energy given by:

$$E = hf$$
$$= (4.14 \times 10^{-15})(6.00 \times 10^{14})$$
$$= 2.48 \text{ eV}$$

Clearly then, any given photon has more than enough energy to get an electron in the metal to overcome the 2.00 eV barrier. In fact, the excess kinetic energy carried away by the electron turns out to be:

$$K = hf - W$$
$$= 2.48 - 2.00$$
$$= 0.48 \text{ eV}$$

MCAT Synopsis

A photon can liberate an electron from a metal surface (photoelectric effect) only if the energy of the photon, $E = hf$, is greater than or equal to the work function, W, of the metal.

THE BOHR MODEL OF THE HYDROGEN ATOM

A. ENERGY LEVELS

The hydrogen atom consists of an electron in orbit about a single, more massive, proton. As such, it is the simplest atom to describe and is a proving ground for any atomic theory. Before a more complete quantum mechanical description was developed, Niels Bohr proposed a model of the hydrogen atom consisting of the single electron in discrete circular orbits about the proton. It was necessary for Bohr to resort to new quantum ideas, since a classical model of hydrogen would require the electron to continuously radiate electromagnetic waves, thereby losing energy and spiraling into the proton. Bohr postulated that there were **specific stable, or allowed, orbits** of quantized (discrete) energy in which electrons did not radiate energy. This led him to deduce an **energy level formula.**

The Bohr energy corresponding to the closest allowed orbit to the nucleus or the **ground state** (n = 1), is –13.6 eV. The energies corresponding to orbits farther away from the nucleus (n = 2,3,4,...) are less negative and therefore greater, until the electron is given so much energy that it is free from the electrostatic (Coulomb) pull of the nucleus and can have any positive energy (**ionization**). An electron occupying one of these higher energy orbits or energy levels, but still bound to the proton, is said to be in an **excited state.** The quantum energy levels in the Bohr model of the hydrogen atom can be arranged from lowest to highest, each with an associated **principal quantum number** (n) that is a positive integer from n = 1 to n = ∞. The energy levels for hydrogen are given in electron-volts by the formula:

$$E_n = \frac{-13.6}{n^2} \quad \text{(hydrogen)}$$

MCAT Synopsis

The lowest energy (ground state) of an electron in hydrogen is negative. Higher energy bound states are also negative in energy but progressively smaller in magnitude.

MCAT Synopsis

Ionization means the electron ends up with an energy of at least 0 eV and is unbound (free).

ELECTRON ENERGY LEVELS IN HYDROGEN

Principal quantum number n	Energy level E_n
1	$\frac{-13.6}{1}$ eV = –13.6 eV
2	$\frac{-13.6}{4}$ eV = –3.40 eV
3	$\frac{-13.6}{9}$ eV = –1.51 eV

$$4 \qquad \frac{-13.6}{16} \text{ eV} = -0.85 \text{ eV}$$

$$\cdot \qquad\qquad\qquad \cdot \qquad\qquad \cdot$$
$$\cdot \qquad\qquad\qquad \cdot \qquad\qquad \cdot$$
$$\cdot \qquad\qquad\qquad \cdot \qquad\qquad \cdot$$

$$\infty \qquad \frac{-13.6}{\infty} \text{ eV} = 0 \text{ eV}$$

Positive energy states have no principal quantum number, since the electron is not bound to the proton. It is in a free electron state and can have any positive energy.

B. EMISSION AND ABSORPTION OF LIGHT

It was found from experiments that hydrogen atoms radiate light only at particular frequencies. Bohr put forward a set of postulates that form the basis of his model. The postulates are:

1. Energy levels of the electron are stable and discrete. They correspond to specific orbits.
2. An electron emits or absorbs radiation **only** when making a transition from one energy level to another (from one allowed orbit to another).
3. To jump from a lower energy (inner orbit) to a higher energy (outer orbit), an electron must **absorb** a photon of precisely the right frequency such that the photon's energy (hf) equals the energy difference between the two orbits.
4. When jumping from a higher energy (outer orbit) to a lower energy (inner orbit), an electron **emits** a photon of a frequency such that the photon's energy (hf) is exactly the energy difference between the two orbits.

Bohr's initial ideas were replaced with the advent of full quantum mechanical theories of atomic structure. In contemporary theories, the electron is not envisioned as following a circular or elliptical path like the planets do in orbiting the sun. However, the Bohr model is still useful for certain calculations.

An electron in the lowest allowed energy level (n = 1 or ground state) cannot emit any more energy (though it could absorb radiation and jump up to a higher energy level). An electron occupying an **excited state** can either emit radiation when it jumps down to a lower energy level or absorb radiation when it jumps up to a higher energy level.

Bohr's third and fourth postulates can be used to find the frequency of radiation emitted or absorbed by an electron in going from energy level E_i to energy level E_f. The change in the electron's energy is $\Delta E = E_f - E_i$. Since

---

MCAT Synopsis

Conservation of energy applies to absorption and emission. For absorption, energy of photon absorbed equals increase in energy of electron. For emission, loss of electron energy equals energy of photon emitted.

MCAT Favorite

Absorption yields color. Emission yields fluorescence.

---

bound state energy levels are negative, if ΔE is negative then the electron has jumped from a higher, less negative energy state (less tightly bound state) to a lower, more negative energy state (more tightly bound state). There is then an **emission** of a photon of frequency f where:

$$\Delta E < 0$$
$$hf = - \Delta E \text{ (emission)}$$

On the other hand, if ΔE is positive, then the electron has **absorbed** a photon and jumped from a lower, more negative energy state to a higher, less negative energy state. The absorbed photon has a frequency f where:

$$\Delta E > 0$$

$$hf = \Delta E \text{ (absorption)}$$

Example: What wavelength of light is emitted by a hydrogen electron going from the n = 5 to the n = 2 energy levels?

Solution: For hydrogen, the energy for a given principle quantum number n is given in electron-volts by

$$E = \frac{-13.6}{n^2}$$

Since the electron goes **from** n = 5 **to** n = 2, the initial energy level is:

$$E_i = E_5 = \frac{-13.6}{25} = -0.544 \text{ eV}$$

The final energy level is:

$$E_f = E_2 = \frac{-13.6}{4} = -3.40 \text{ eV}$$

Therefore:

$$\Delta E = E_f - E_i$$
$$= -3.40 + 0.544$$
$$= -2.856 \text{ eV}$$

The negative value of ΔE confirms that the light is emitted. The frequency is found by:

$$f = \frac{|\Delta E|}{h}$$

$$= \frac{2.856}{4.14 \times 10^{-15}}$$

$$= 6.90 \times 10^{14} \text{ Hz}$$

> **MCAT Synopsis**
>
> Use E = hf to find frequency of photon given energy of photon.

Now we can easily find the wavelength (and convert to different units for comparison):

$$\lambda = \frac{c}{f}$$

$$= \frac{3.00 \times 10^8}{6.90 \times 10^{14}}$$

$$= 4.35 \times 10^{-7} \text{ m}$$

$$= 435 \text{ nm}$$

$$= 4350 \text{ Å}$$

Example: What wavelength of light is needed to free an electron from the ground state of hydrogen?

Solution: As previously mentioned, the electron in the ground state ($n = 1$) of hydrogen has an energy of -13.6 eV. Negative energies mean a bound state; positive energies mean a free state. It would take a photon of at least $+13.6$ eV to free the electron. Find the frequency:

$$f = \frac{E}{h}$$

$$= \frac{13.6}{4.14 \times 10^{-15}}$$

$$= 3.29 \times 10^{15} \text{ Hz}$$

Now the wavelength is given by:

$$\lambda = \frac{c}{f}$$

$$= \frac{3.00 \times 10^8}{3.29 \times 10^{15}}$$

$$= 9.12 \times 10^{-8} \text{ m}$$

$$= 91.2 \text{ nm}$$

$$= 912 \text{ Å}$$

FLUORESCENCE

Fluorescence refers to the process in which certain substances emit visible light when excited by other radiation, usually ultraviolet radiation. Photons corresponding to ultraviolet radiation have relatively high frequencies (short wavelengths). After being excited to a higher energy state by the ultraviolet radiation, the electron returns to its original state in two or more steps. By returning in two or more steps, each step involves less energy. In each step a lower frequency (longer wavelength) photon is emitted, whose wavelength may fall in the visible portion of the spectrum. This is the principle of the fluorescent light.

12

NUCLEAR PHENOMENA

The subject of this final chapter is the nucleus and nuclear phenomena, and it begins with a review of some of the standard terminology used in nuclear physics. The concept of binding energy and the equivalent concept of the mass defect are then introduced. Briefly, an amount of energy, called the binding energy, is required to break up a given nucleus into its constituent protons and neutrons. That energy is converted to mass via Einstein's $E = mc^2$, resulting in a larger mass for the constituent protons and neutrons than that of the original nucleus, the difference being called the mass defect. The remainder, and bulk, of the chapter is concerned with a brief discussion of nuclear reactions (fission and fusion) and an extended treatment of radioactive decay, which itself is presented in two distinct parts. The first deals with the four different types of radioactive decay and a discussion of the reaction equations that describe them. The second covers the general problem of determining the number of nuclei that have not decayed as a function of time, along with the associated concept of the half-life of a decay process.

NUCLEI

At the center of an atom lies its nucleus, consisting of one or more **nucleons** (protons or neutrons) held together with considerably more energy than the energy needed to hold electrons in orbit around the nucleus. The radius of the nucleus is about 100,000 times smaller than the radius of the atom. Some common nuclear properties are:

A. ATOMIC NUMBER (Z)

Z is always an integer, and is equal to the **number of protons** in the nucleus. Each element has a unique number of protons; therefore the atomic number Z identifies the element. Z is used as a presubscript to the chemical symbol in **isotopic notation.** The chemical symbols and the atomic numbers of all the elements are given in the periodic table.

MCAT Synopsis

Each element is defined by its atomic number Z (number of protons in the nucleus).

ATOMIC NUMBERS OF THE CHEMICAL ELEMENTS

Atomic number Z	Chemical symbol	Element name
1	H	hydrogen
2	He	helium
3	Li	lithium
.	.	.
.	.	.
92	U	uranium
.	.	.
.	.	.
.	.	.

B. MASS NUMBER (A)

A is an integer equal to the total **number of nucleons** (neutrons and protons) in a nucleus. Let N represent the number of neutrons in a nucleus. The equation relating A, N, and Z is simply:

$$A = N + Z$$

In isotopic notation, A is a presuperscript to the chemical symbol.

Examples: $_{1}^{1}H$ —a single proton; the nucleus of ordinary hydrogen.

$_{2}^{4}He$ —the nucleus of ordinary helium, consisting of 2 protons and 2 neutrons. It is also known as an alpha particle (α-particle).

$_{92}^{235}U$ —a fissionable form of uranium, consisting of 92 protons and 143 neutrons.

C. ISOTOPE

The nucleus of a given element can have different numbers of neutrons and hence different mass numbers. For a nucleus of a given element with a given number of protons (atomic number Z), the various nuclei with different numbers of neutrons are called **isotopes** of that element. The term *isotope* is also used in a generic sense to refer to any nucleus. The term **radionuclide** is another generic term used to refer to any radioactive isotope, especially those used in **nuclear medicine.**

Example: The three isotopes of hydrogen are:

$_{1}^{1}H$ —a single proton; the nucleus of ordinary hydrogen.

$^{2}_{1}H$ —a proton and a neutron together often called a **deuteron;** the nucleus of one type of heavy hydrogen called **deuterium.**

$^{3}_{1}H$ —a proton and two neutrons together often called a **triton;** the nucleus of a heavier type of heavy hydrogen called **tritium.**

D. ATOMIC MASS AND ATOMIC MASS UNIT

Atomic mass is most commonly measured in **atomic mass units** (abbreviated amu or simply u). By definition, 1 amu is exactly one-twelfth the mass of the neutral carbon-12 atom (not just the nucleus—the atom includes the nucleus and all 6 electrons). In terms of more familiar mass units:

$$1 \text{ amu} = 1.66 \times 10^{-27} \text{ kg} = 1.66 \times 10^{-24} \text{ g}$$

E. ATOMIC WEIGHT

Because isotopes exist, atoms of a given element can have different masses. The atomic weight refers to a weighted average of the **masses** (not the weights) of an element. The average is weighted according to the natural abundances of the various isotopic species of an element. The atomic weight can be measured in amu.

Example: 99.985499% of hydrogen occurs in the common ^{1}H isotope with a mass of 1.00782504 u. About 0.0142972% occurs as deuterium with a mass (including the electron) of 2.01410 u, and about 0.0003027% occurs as tritium with a mass of 3.01605 u. The atomic weight of hydrogen $A_r(H)$ is the sum of the mass of each isotope multiplied by its natural abundance (x):

$$A_r(H) = m_{1H}x_{1H} + m_{2H}x_{2H} + m_{3H}x_{3H}$$
$$= (1.00782504)(0.99985499)$$
$$+ (2.01410)(0.000142972)$$
$$+ (3.01605)(0.000003027)$$
$$= 1.00797 \text{ amu}$$

NUCLEAR BINDING ENERGY AND MASS DEFECT

Every nucleus (other than $^{1}_{1}H$) has a smaller mass than the combined mass of its constituent protons and neutrons. The difference is called the **mass defect.** Scientists had difficulty explaining why this mass defect occurred until Einstein discovered the equivalence of matter and energy, embodied by the equation $E = mc^2$. The mass defect is a result of matter that has been converted to energy. This energy, called **binding energy,** holds the nucleons

> **MCAT Synopsis**
>
> The mass of a nucleus is always less than the combined masses of its constituent protons and neutrons.

together in the nucleus. (Note: The binding energy per nucleon peaks at iron, which implies that iron is the most stable atom. In general, intermediate-sized nuclei are more stable than large and small nuclei.)

The mass defect and binding energy of ^{4}He are calculated in the following example.

Example: Measurements of the atomic mass of a neutron and a proton yield these results:

$$\text{proton} = 1.00728 \text{ amu}$$
$$\text{neutron} = 1.00867 \text{ amu}$$

A measurement of the atomic mass of a ^{4}He nucleus yields:

$$^4\text{He} = 4.00260 \text{ amu}$$

^{4}He consists of 2 protons and 2 neutrons which should theoretically give a ^{4}He mass of:

$$Z(m_p) + N(m_n) = 2(1.00728) + 2(1.00867)$$
$$= 4.03190 \text{ amu}$$

What is the mass defect and binding energy of this nucleus?

Solution: The difference 4.03190 − 4.00260 = 0.02930 amu is the mass defect for ^{4}He, and is interpreted as the conversion of mass into the binding energy of the nucleus. The rest energy of 1 amu is 932 MeV, so using $E = mc^2$ we find that $c^2 = 932$ MeV/amu. Therefore the binding energy of ^{4}He is:

$$\text{B.E.} = \Delta m \, c^2$$
$$= (0.02930)(932)$$
$$= 27.3 \text{ MeV}$$

NUCLEAR REACTIONS AND DECAY

Nuclear reactions such as fusion, fission, and radioactive decay involve either combining or splitting the nuclei of atoms. Since the binding energy per nucleon is greatest for intermediate-sized atoms, when small atoms combine or large atoms split a great amount of energy is released.

A. FUSION

Fusion occurs when small nuclei combine into a larger nucleus. As an example, many stars, including the Sun, power themselves by fusing four hydrogen nuclei to make one helium nucleus. By this method, the sun produces 4×10^{26} J every second. Here on Earth, researchers are trying to find ways to use fusion as an alternative energy source.

B. FISSION

Fission is a process by which a large nucleus splits into smaller nuclei. Spontaneous fission rarely occurs. However, by the absorption of a low energy neutron, fission can be induced in certain nuclei. Of special interest are those fission reactions that release more neutrons, since these other neutrons will cause other atoms to undergo fission. This, in turn, releases more neutrons, creating a chain reaction. Such induced fission reactions power commercial nuclear electric-generating plants.

Example: A fission reaction occurs when uranium-235 (U-235) absorbs a low energy neutron, briefly forming an excited state of U-236 which then splits into xenon-140, strontium-94, and x more neutrons. In isotopic notation form the reactions are:

$$^{235}_{92}U + {}^{1}_{0}n \longrightarrow {}^{236}_{92}U \longrightarrow {}^{140}_{54}Xe + {}^{94}_{38}Sr + x{}^{1}_{0}n$$

How many neutrons are produced in the last reaction?

Solution: The question is asking "What is x?" By treating each arrow as an equal sign, the problem is simply asking to balance the last "equation." The mass numbers (A) on either side of each arrow must be equal. This is an application of **nucleon** or **baryon number conservation**, which says that the total number of neutrons plus protons remains the same, even if neutrons are converted to protons and vice versa, as they are in some decays. Since $235 + 1 = 236$, the first arrow is indeed balanced. To find the number of neutrons solve for x in the last equation (arrow):

$$236 = 140 + 94 + x$$
$$x = 236 - 140 - 94$$
$$= 2$$

So there are two neutrons produced in this reaction. These neutrons are free to go on and be absorbed by more ^{235}U and cause more fissioning, and the process continues in a chain reaction. Note that it really was not necessary to know that the intermediate state $^{236}_{92}U$ was formed.

Some radioactive nuclei may be induced to fission via more than one **decay channel** or **decay mode.** For example, a different fission reaction may occur when uranium-235 absorbs a slow neutron and then immediately splits into barium-139, krypton-94, and three more neutrons with no intermediate state:

$$^{235}_{92}U + {}^{1}_{0}n \longrightarrow {}^{139}_{56}Ba + {}^{94}_{36}Kr + 3{}^{1}_{0}n$$

> **MCAT Synopsis**
>
> Total mass number, A, remains unchanged in nuclear reactions.

C. RADIOACTIVE DECAY

Radioactive decay is a naturally occurring spontaneous decay of certain nuclei accompanied by the emission of specific particles. It could be classified as a certain type of fission. Radioactive decay problems are of three general types:

- The integer arithmetic of particle and isotope species
- Radioactive half-life problems
- The use of exponential decay curves and decay constants

1. **Isotope Decay Arithmetic and Nucleon Conservation**

   Let the letters X and Y represent nuclear isotopes, and let us further consider the three types of decay particles and how they affect the mass number and atomic number of the **parent isotope** $_{Z}^{A}X$ and the resulting **daughter isotope** $_{Z'}^{A'}Y$ in the decay:

$$_{Z}^{A}X \longrightarrow {}_{Z'}^{A'}Y + \text{emitted decay particle}$$

   a. **Alpha decay** is the emission of an α-particle, which is a ^{4}He nucleus that consists of two protons and two neutrons. The alpha particle is very massive (compared to a beta particle) and doubly charged. Alpha particles interact with matter very easily; hence they do not penetrate shielding (such as lead sheets) very far.

   The emission of an α-particle means that the daughter's atomic number Z will be 2 less than the parent's atomic number and the daughter's mass number will be 4 less than the parent's mass number. This can be expressed in two simple equations:

α decay

$$Z_{daughter} = Z_{parent} - 2$$
$$A_{daughter} = A_{parent} - 4$$

   The generic alpha decay reaction is then:

$$_{Z}^{A}X \longrightarrow {}_{Z-2}^{A-4}Y + \alpha$$

Example: Suppose a parent X alpha decays into a daughter Y such that:

$$_{92}^{238}X \longrightarrow {}_{Z'}^{A'}Y + \alpha$$

What are the mass number (A') and atomic number (Z') of the daughter isotope Y?

Solution: Since $\alpha = {}_{2}^{4}He$, balancing the mass numbers and atomic numbers is all that needs to be done:

$$238 = A' + 4$$
$$A' = 234$$
$$92 = Z' + 2$$
$$Z' = 90$$

So $A' = 234$ and $Z' = 90$. Note that it was not necessary to know the chemical species of the isotopes to do this problem. However, it would have been possible to look at the periodic table and see that $Z = 92$ means X is uranium-238 ($^{238}_{92}U$) and that $Z = 90$ means Y is thorium-234 ($^{234}_{90}Th$).

b. **Beta decay** is the emission of a β-particle, which is an electron given the symbol e^- or $β^-$. Electrons do not reside in the nucleus, but are emitted by the nucleus when a neutron in the nucleus decays into a proton and a β– (and an antineutrino). Since an electron is singly charged, and about 1,836 times lighter than a proton, the beta radiation from radioactive decay is more penetrating than alpha radiation. In some cases of induced decay, a positively charged anti-electron known as a **positron** is emitted. The positron is given the symbol e^+ or $β^+$.

β– decay means that a neutron disappears and a proton takes its place. Hence, the parent's mass number is unchanged and the parent's atomic number is increased by 1. In other words, the daughter's A is the same as the parent's, and the daughter's Z is one more than the parent's.

In positron decay, a proton (instead of a neutron as in β– decay) splits into a positron and a neutron. Therefore, a β+ decay means that the parent's mass number is unchanged and the parent's atomic number is decreased by 1. In other words, the daughter's A is the same as the parent's, and the daughter's Z is one less than the parent's. In equation form:

β⁻ decay

$$Z_{daughter} = Z_{parent} + 1$$
$$A_{daughter} = A_{parent}$$

β⁺ decay

$$Z_{daughter} = Z_{parent} - 1$$
$$A_{daughter} = A_{parent}$$

The generic negative beta decay reaction is:

$$^A_Z X \longrightarrow\ ^A_{Z+1}Y + β^-$$

The generic positive beta decay reaction is:

$$^A_Z X \longrightarrow ^{\ A}_{Z-1} Y + \beta^+$$

Example: Suppose a cobalt-60 nucleus beta-decays:

$$^{60}Co \longrightarrow ^{A'}_{Z'}Y + e^-$$

What is the element Y and what are A′ and Z′?

Solution: Again, balance mass numbers:

$$60 = A' + 0$$
$$A' = 60$$

Now balance the atomic numbers, taking into account that cobalt has 27 protons (you learn this by consulting the periodic table) and that there is one more proton on the right-hand side:

$$27 = Z' - 1$$
$$Z' = 28$$

Look at the periodic table to find that Z′ = 28 is nickel:

$$Y = ^{60}_{28}Ni$$

c. **Gamma decay** is the emission of γ–particles, which are high energy photons. They carry no charge and simply lower the energy of the emitting (parent) nucleus without changing the mass number or the atomic number. In other words, the daughter's A is the same as the parent's, and the daughter's Z is the same as the parent's.

γ decay

$$Z_{parent} = Z_{daughter}$$
$$A_{parent} = A_{daughter}$$

The generic gamma decay reaction is thus:

$$^A_Z X \ast \longrightarrow ^A_Z X + \gamma$$

MCAT Synopsis

γ-particles are high energy photons. γ-decay releases energy but doesn't change A or Z.

Example: Suppose a parent isotope $^A_Z X$ emits a β^+ and turns into an excited state of the isotope $^{A'}_{Z'} Y^*$, which then γ decays to $^{A''}_{Z''} Y$, which in turn α decays to $^{A'''}_{Z'''} W$. If W is ^{60}Fe, what is $^A_Z X$?

Solution: Since the final daughter in this chain of decay is given, it will be necessary to work backward through the reactions. By looking at the periodic table one finds that W = Fe means $Z''' = 26$; hence the last reaction is the following α decay:

$$^{A''}_{Z''} Y \longrightarrow {}^{60}_{26}\text{Fe} + {}^4_2\text{He}$$

By balancing the atomic numbers you find:

$$Z'' = 26 + 2 = 28$$

A balancing of the mass numbers implies:

$$A'' = 60 + 4 = 64$$

The second-to-last reaction is a γ decay that simply releases energy from the nucleus but does not alter the atomic number or the mass number of the parent. That is: $Z' = Z'' = 28$ and $A' = A'' = 64$. So the second reaction is:

$$^{64}_{28} Y^* \longrightarrow {}^{64}_{28} Y + \gamma$$

The first reaction was a β^+ decay that must have looked like:

$$^A_Z X \longrightarrow {}^{64}_{28} Y^* + e^+$$

Again, balance the atomic numbers:

$$Z = 28 + 1 = 29$$

You carry out a balancing of mass numbers by taking into account that a proton has disappeared on the left and reappeared as a neutron on the right, leaving mass number unchanged:

$$A = 64 + 0 = 64$$

By looking at the periodic table, you find that $Z = 29$ means that X is Cu. $A = 64$, so that means that the solution is:

$$^A_Z X = {}^{64}_{29} Cu$$

Even though the problem did not ask for it, it is possible again to look at the periodic table to find that $Z' = Z'' = 28$ means $Y^* = Y = Ni$. The total chain of decays can be written as:

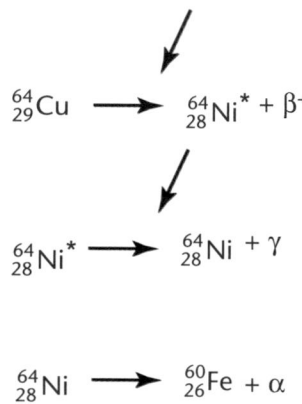

$$^{64}_{29} Cu \longrightarrow {}^{64}_{28} Ni^* + \beta^+$$

$$^{64}_{28} Ni^* \longrightarrow {}^{64}_{28} Ni + \gamma$$

$$^{64}_{28} Ni \longrightarrow {}^{60}_{26} Fe + \alpha$$

d. Electron capture

Certain unstable radionuclides are capable of capturing an inner (K or L shell) electron that combines with a proton to form a neutron. The atomic number is now one less than the original, but the mass number remains the same. Electron capture is a rare process that is perhaps best thought of as an inverse β^- decay.

> **MCAT Synopsis**
>
> (fraction of original nuclei remaining after n half-lives) $= (1/2)^n$.

2. Radioactive Decay Half-Life ($T_{1/2}$)

In a collection of a great many identical radioactive isotopes, the **half-life** ($T_{1/2}$) of the sample is the time it takes for half of the sample to decay.

Example: If the half-life of a certain isotope is 4 years, what fraction of a sample of that isotope will remain after 12 years?

Solution: If 4 years is 1 half-life, then 12 years is 3 half-lives. During the first half-life—the first 4 years—half of the sample will have decayed. During the second half-life (years 4 to 8), half of the remaining half will decay, leaving one-fourth of the original. During the third and final period (years 8 to 12), half of the remaining fourth will decay, leaving one-eighth of the original sample. Thus the fraction remaining after 3 half-lives is $(1/2)^3$ or $(1/8)$.

3. **Exponential Decay**

Let n be the number of radioactive nuclei that have not yet decayed in a sample. It turns out that the **rate** at which the nuclei decay ($\Delta n/\Delta t$) is proportional to the number that remain (n). This suggests the equation:

$$\frac{\Delta n}{\Delta t} = -\lambda n$$

where λ is known as the **decay constant**. The solution of this equation tells us how the number of radioactive nuclei changes with time. The solution is known as an **exponential decay**:

$$n = n_0 e^{-\lambda t}$$

where n_0 is the number of undecayed nuclei at time t = 0. (The decay constant is related to the half-life by $\lambda = \dfrac{\ln 2}{T_{1/2}} = \dfrac{0.693}{T_{1/2}}$).

> ···
> **MCAT Synopsis**
> ···
> (number of nuclei that have decayed in time t) = (n_0– n), where $n = n_0 e^{-\lambda t}$.
> ···

Example: If at time t = 0 there is a 2 mole sample of radioactive isotopes of decay constant 2 (hour)$^{-1}$, how many nuclei remain after 45 minutes?

Solution: Since 45 minutes is 3/4 of an hour, the exponent is:

$$\lambda t = 2\left(\frac{3}{4}\right) = \frac{6}{4} = \frac{3}{2}$$

The exponential factor will be a number smaller than 1:

$$e^{-\lambda t} = e^{-3/2} = 0.22$$

So only 0.22 or 22% of the original 2-mole sample will remain. To find n_0 multiply the number of moles we have by the number of particles per mole (Avogadro's number):

$$n_0 = 2(6.02 \times 10^{23}) = 1.2 \times 10^{24}$$

From the equation that describes exponential decay, you can calculate the number that remain after 45 minutes:

$$
\begin{aligned}
n &= n_0 e^{-\lambda t} \\
&= (1.2 \times 10^{24})(0.22) \\
&= 2.6 \times 10^{23} \text{ particles}
\end{aligned}
$$

Physics Practice Set

Use this practice set to evaluate your mastery of the physics section of the test.

Read the explanations to all the practice problems, and revisit the chapters that relate to weak areas.

Good luck.

Physics Practice Set

Passage I (Questions 1–8)

A children's playground contains a swing, a slide, and a merry-go-round. Padded safety tiles, designed to be less dangerous to fall on than the surrounding concrete, are laid beneath each playground ride.

The swing has a seat that hangs on two 3.25 m chains which pivot from the cross-piece of a frame 4 m above the ground. Safety tiles cover the ground beneath the swing in such a way that, if the swing breaks, a person riding on it will fall on the tiles rather than on the concrete.

The slide consists of a flat, 6 m-long piece of metal inclined at an angle of 30° to the horizontal, ending in a 1 m-long horizontal section at the foot that is 50 cm above the ground. The horizontal and inclined sections of the slide are made from the same type of metal. The padded safety tiles beneath the slide extend 15 m beyond the point directly below the end of the slide.

The merry-go-round is a disk of radius 2.0 m set in a horizontal plane 90 cm above the ground. It spins about a vertical axle that runs through its center and is fixed to the ground in the center of a square of safety tiles. When the merry-go-round is in motion, a constant frictional torque opposes the resultant applied torque. (Note: A body travelling at a constant speed around a circle is subject to an acceleration towards the center of the circle of v^2/r where v is the speed of the body and r is the radius of the circle.)

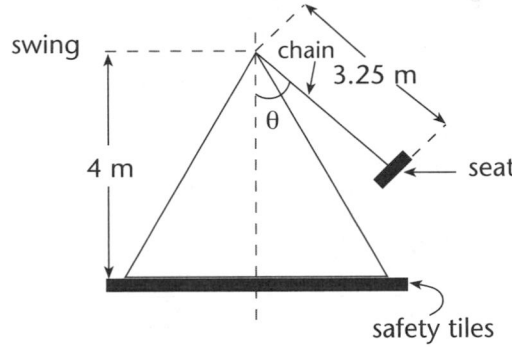

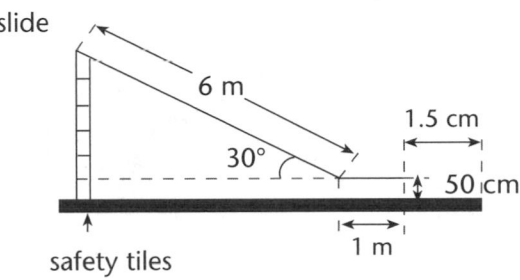

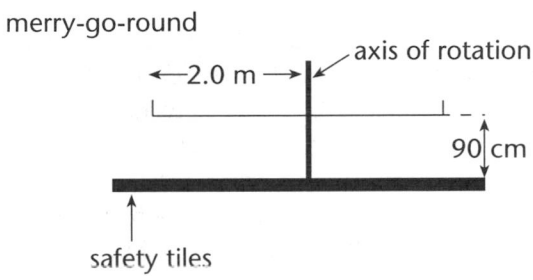

1. A child swinging on the swing reaches a maximum angle of $\theta = 35°$. At what value for θ does the child have the greatest gravitational potential energy?

   A. −10°
   B.   0°
   C. 20°
   D. 35°

2. Which of the following graphs best describes how v, the speed of a child sitting on the swing, varies as a function of h, the height of the seat above its lowest point?

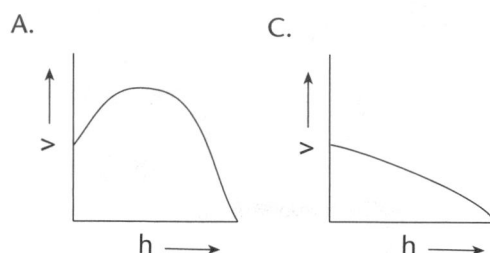

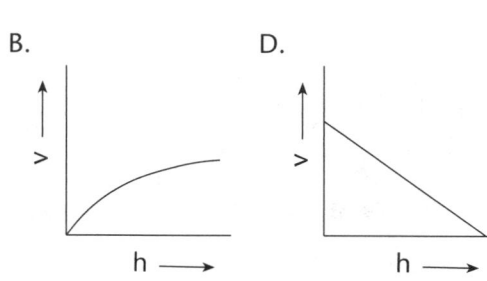

3. Instead of sliding down the slide, the children play a game in which they send different blocks down the slide. If block A has twice the mass of block B, and if both blocks start from rest, what is the ratio of the distance travelled by block A to the distance travelled by block B after leaving the slide? (Note: Ignore friction and air resistance.)

A. 4:1
B. 2:1
C. 1:1
D. 1:2

4. A 25 kg child begins at the top of the slide with no initial speed and slides all the way to the bottom, stopping just as she reaches the end. What is the work done by friction?

A.   0 J
B.   −735 J
C.   −980 J
D. −1485 J

5. A child originally sitting at rest at the top of the slide starts moving down the slide. Based on this information, which of the following must be true of μ_s, the coefficient of static friction between the slide and the child?

A. $(\mu_s \sin 30° + \cos 30°) \cos 30° > 1$
B. $\mu_s \cos 30° < 1$
C. $\mu_s < \sin 30°$
D. $\mu_s < \tan 30°$

6. What is the ratio of the force required to push a child up the slide at a constant speed of 1 m/s to the force required to push the child up at a constant speed of 2 m/s?

A. 1:4
B. 1:2
C. 1:$\sqrt{2}$
D. 1:1

7. A 30 kg child sits on the edge of the merry-go-round holding onto a handle. If he can hold on with a force of 60 N, what is the maximum frequency at which the merry-go-round can revolve without throwing the child off?

   A. $\dfrac{2}{\pi}s^{-1}$

   B. $\dfrac{1}{\pi}s^{-1}$

   C. $\dfrac{1}{2\pi}s^{-1}$

   D. $\dfrac{1}{4\pi}s^{-1}$

8. Which of the following best explains why falling on the safety tiles is less dangerous than falling on concrete?

   A. The time over which the impact force acts is greater for a fall on the safety tiles, and therefore the average impact force is less.
   B. The safety tiles absorb all the kinetic energy of a falling person very quickly, whereas concrete absorbs the kinetic energy more slowly.
   C. A person who falls on the tiles will bounce slightly, reducing the average impact force.
   D. The safety tiles are softer than concrete, so the impulse is smaller on the tiles.

Passage II (Questions 9–12)

The power per unit area reaching the Earth's surface from the Sun, averaged over 24 hours, is 0.2 kW/m². This solar energy can be converted directly into electrical energy via the photoelectric effect. For example, in the photoelectric cell shown in Figure 1, a cathode emits electrons when illuminated by light of a high enough frequency. The ejected electrons travel to the anode, and a small electric current flows.

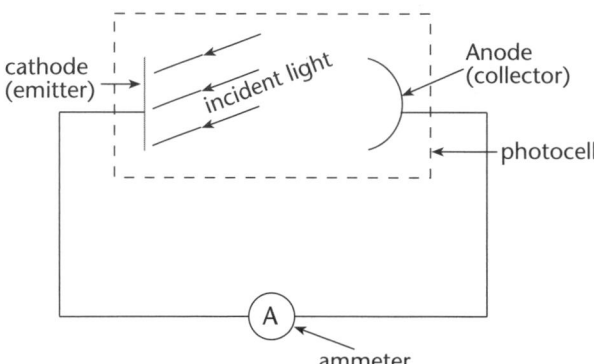

Figure 1

An electron within the cathode requires a minimum energy to break free from the cathode surface. This minimum energy is known as the work function, W, and is a constant intrinsic to the material of which the cathode is composed. An individual photon incident on the cathode collides with an electron and is absorbed, transferring all of its energy to the electron. The energy of each incident photon is given by $E_p = hf$, where f is the frequency of incident light and h is Planck's constant. If E_p is less than W, then no electrons will be ejected from the cathode at all. The maximum kinetic energy, E_{max}, of an electron liberated from the cathode is given by

$$E_{max} = E_p - W$$

A voltage source can be connected across the photoelectric cell to oppose the current flow. At a critical applied voltage, called the stopping voltage, even an electron ejected from the cathode with a kinetic energy of E_{max} will not be able to reach the anode; therefore, the current will stop altogether. The value of this stopping voltage is dependent only on E_{max}.

9. The most efficient modern photovoltaic cells can convert the Sun's energy into electrical energy with an efficiency of 35 percent. Approximately what area would have to be covered by such cells in order to supply a household with 20 kW-hours of electrical energy per day?

   A.   0.5 m²
   B.   12 m²
   C.   285 m²
   D. 6850 m²

10. Light intensity is defined as the energy flowing per unit area per unit time for an area perpendicular to the direction of energy flow. In an experiment, the frequency of light incident on the cathode of a photoelectric cell is held constant, but the intensity is varied. As the intensity of the incident light is increased, the stopping voltage:

   A. increases, because more electrons are ejected from the cathode as the number of photons striking it increases.
   B. remains the same, because the energy supplied to one electron depends only on the energy of an individual photon.
   C. increases, because the electrons in the cathode absorb more energy per unit time.
   D. remains the same, because each incident photon shares its energy between several electrons in the cathode.

11. The behavior of light is sometimes explained in terms of particles and sometimes in terms of waves. Which of the following CANNOT be explained by a theory that refers to light in terms of waves alone?

 A. Current flow in a photoelectric cell can be stopped by reducing the intensity of the incident light while maintaining the same frequency.

 B. An electron requires energy to escape from the surface of a photosensitive cathode.

 C. Current flow in a photoelectric cell can be stopped by reducing the frequency of the incident light while maintaining the same intensity.

 D. The angle through which light is refracted when it moves from one medium to another is a function of frequency, rather than intensity.

12. Under which of the following conditions will the stopping voltage across a photoelectric cell be greatest?

 A. The wavelength of the incident light is short, and the work function of the cathode material is low.

 B. The wavelength of the incident light is short, and the work function of the cathode material is high.

 C. The wavelength of the incident light is long, and the work function of the cathode material is low.

 D. The wavelength of the incident light is long, and the work function of the cathode material is high.

Questions 13 and 14 are NOT based on a descriptive passage.

13. An electron is moving parallel to a long, straight, current-carrying wire in the same direction as the current flow. In what direction does the force on the electron point?

   A. Parallel to the wire and in the same direction as the current.
   B. Parallel to the wire and in the opposite direction to the current.
   C. Perpendicular to the wire and towards the wire.
   D. Perpendicular to the wire and away from the wire.

14. A bubble of warm air rises within a thunder cloud during a storm. Which of the following factors will reduce the rate at which the air inside this bubble cools?

   A. Water vapor in the bubble condenses as it rises.
   B. Pressure on the bubble decreases, and it expands as it rises.
   C. Air from the surrounding environment is drawn into the bubble as it rises.
   D. Pressure on the bubble increases, and it contracts as it rises.

Passage III (Questions 15–21)

Mercury is the only metallic element that is normally liquid at room temperature. It possesses the properties usually associated with metals, such as high electrical and thermal conductivity. Since it remains liquid over a wide range of temperatures, it can be put to many practical uses. Thermometers, manometers, and sealed electrical switches and relays all commonly utilize mercury. Table 1 compares some of the properties of mercury with those of water and iron.

Table 1

	Freezing point (°C)	Boiling point (°C)	Density (g/cm^3)	Specific heat (J/kg•K)
Mercury	−38.87	357	13.6	138
Water	0.0	100	1.00	4190
Iron	1535.0	3000	7.8	470

An experiment is performed to measure the relative densities of water and mercury. An iron cube with sides 2 cm long is lowered into a "Eureka Can," shown in the figure below, that has been filled with water to the level of the bottom of the spout. A test tube labeled W is used to collect the displaced water. This procedure is now repeated a second time, using mercury instead of water, and the displaced mercury is collected in a test tube labelled M.

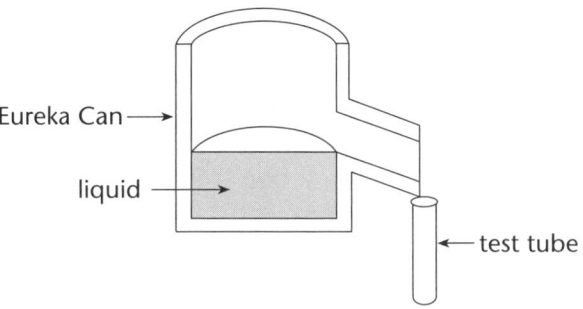

15. A solid object is placed in a fluid. Archimedes' principle states that:

    A. the volume of fluid displaced equals the volume of the object.
    B. the upward (buoyant) force on the object equals the weight of the object.
    C. if the object is more dense than the fluid, it will sink; otherwise, it will float.
    D. the upward (buoyant) force on the object equals the weight of fluid displaced.

16. Which test tube contains the largest volume of liquid after the iron cube is lowered into the can?

    A. Tube W contains a larger volume of liquid, because although the same mass of liquid is displaced in each case, 1 g of water occupies a larger volume than 1 g of mercury.
    B. Tube W contains a larger volume of liquid, because the cube sinks in water but floats in mercury.
    C. Tube M contains a larger volume of liquid, because a greater mass of mercury than water is displaced.
    D. Tube M contains a larger volume of liquid, because mercury is more dense than water and is therefore able to exert a greater upward force on the cube.

17. If the iron cube used in the experiment is replaced with a cube of the same size made of a wood that is less dense than water, and the experiment is repeated, which test tube will collect a larger volume of liquid?

    A. Tube W collects more liquid, because the weight of liquid displaced is the same in each case, but 1 g of water occupies more volume than 1 g of mercury.
    B. Tube W collects more liquid, because water is less dense than mercury, and therefore water must exert a greater upward thrust to keep the wood afloat.
    C. Tube M collects more liquid, because the weight of mercury displaced equals the weight of water displaced, but 1 g of mercury occupies more volume than 1g of water.
    D. Tubes W and M collect the same volume of liquid, because the wooden cube floats in both water and mercury.

18. Why can a ship made from iron float in the ocean?

    A. Seawater is more dense than pure water.
    B. The ship is shaped so that its volume is mostly filled with air, making its overall density low.
    C. The ship has a large surface area, and therefore the force exerted by the sea on the ship is great enough to keep it afloat.
    D. The hub of the ship is shaped so as not to break the surface tension of the ocean.

19. A cube of metal sinks in water. Which of the following describes the change that will occur if a cube made of the same metal, but with sides twice as long, is lowered into water?

    A. The buoyant force will increase by a factor of 8, and the cube's downward acceleration will be reduced.
    B. The buoyant force will increase by a factor of 4, and the cube's downward acceleration will be reduced.
    C. The buoyant force will remain the same, and the cube's downward acceleration will also remain the same.
    D. The buoyant force will increase by a factor of 8, and the cube's downward acceleration will remain the same.

20. A 10 cm³ sample of water is collected and heated at a constant rate. The following graph shows the temperature as a function of time.

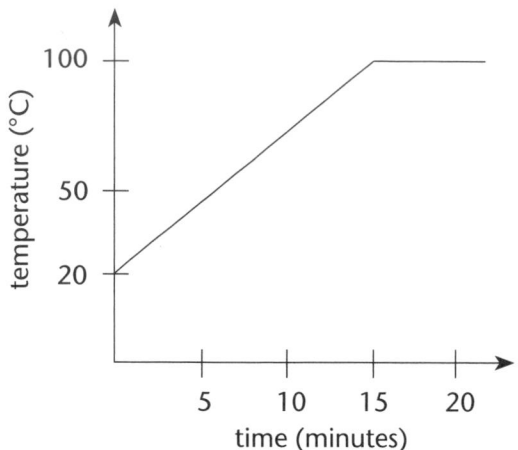

If 10 cm³ of mercury were heated at the same rate, which of the following graphs might represent the results? (Note: The energy, Q, required to raise the temperature by ΔT is given by $Q = mc\Delta T$, where m is the mass and c is the specific heat.)

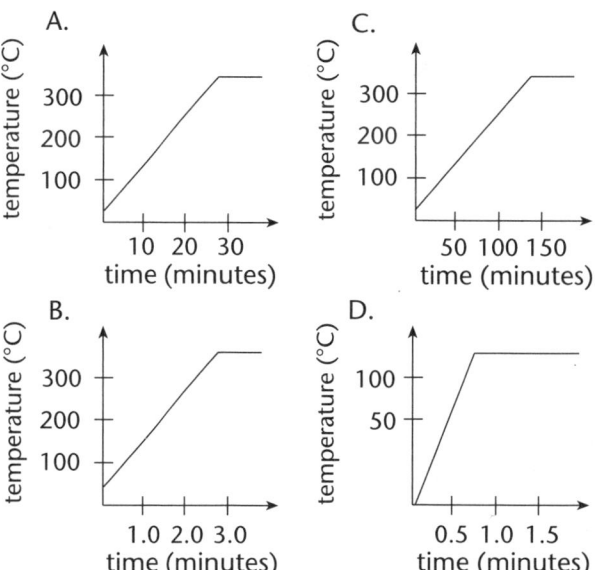

21. If an iron cube were lowered into water on the moon, where the acceleration due to gravity is approximately one-sixth of that on Earth, how would the results change?

A. The iron cube would float in water.
B. The volume of water displaced would be greater.
C. The iron cube would sink at exactly the same rate as on Earth.
D. The iron cube would sink more slowly than on Earth.

Questions 22 through 24 are NOT based on a descriptive passage.

22. Heat is supplied to a gas that is constrained within a rigid container. The work done by the gas is:

    A. negative, because the internal energy of the gas increases.
    B. zero, because the pressure remains constant.
    C. zero, because the volume remains constant.
    D. positive, because the gas is an isolated system.

23. The wavelengths of the sound emitted by 2 consecutive harmonic vibrations of a string that is fixed at both ends are 25 cm and 20 cm respectively. How long is the string? (Note: The wavelength, λ, of the nth harmonic on a string of length L is given by: $\lambda = 2L/n$.)

    A. 20 cm
    B. 25 cm
    C. 50 cm
    D. 100 cm

24. A sound meter gives a reading which is equal to the sound level in dB PLUS the relative response of the meter itself. The relative response of the meter is shown as a function of frequency in the graph below.

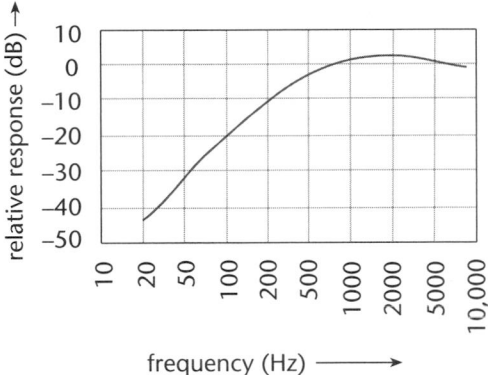

What will the reading of the sound meter be if it is placed near an airplane that is emitting a 100 dB sound at a frequency of 50 Hz?

    A.   50 dB
    B.   70 dB
    C. 100 dB
    D. 130 dB

Passage IV (Questions 25–30)

The centrifuge shown in Figure 1 is being used to separate solid particles from a liquid. The particles suspended in the liquid are all more dense than the liquid itself, and hence would eventually settle to the bottom of the liquid if the suspension were left alone. Spinning the suspension around inside the centrifuge increases the rate at which the solid particles settle to the bottom of the liquid—that is, the rate of sedimentation.

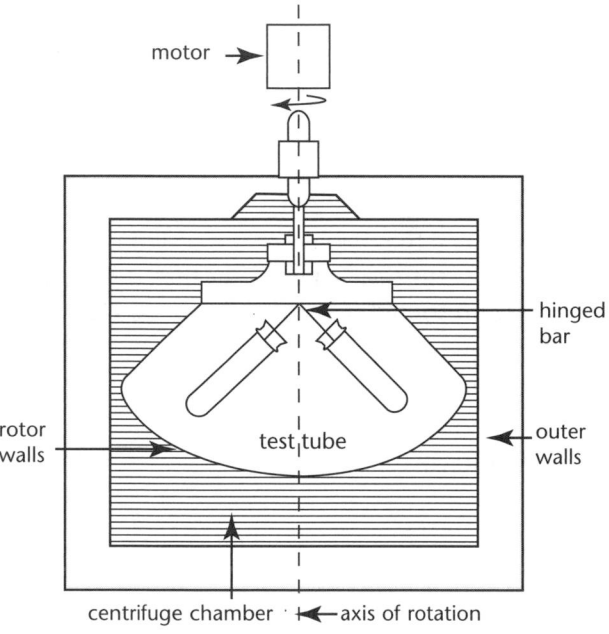

motor

hinged bar

rotor walls

test tube

outer walls

centrifuge chamber · ←—axis of rotation

Figure 1

Special test tubes containing the suspension to be separated are placed inside a bowl-shaped rotor, which turns on oiled bearings within the centrifuge chamber. The test tubes are mounted on hinged bars that can swing freely in the vertical plane. The motor exerts a torque on the rotor axle, causing the rotor to rotate about a vertical axle through its center. The rotor rotates at a frequency that increases at a rate that is directly proportional to the net torque about the axis of rotation. The extent to which the centrifuge increases the sedimentation rate depends on the frequency of rotation and the length of the hinged bar and test tube, as well as the conditions within the suspension.

The efficiency with which a centrifuge separates sediment from a liquid can be drastically reduced by convection currents within the centrifuge. These currents disturb the settling out of the sediment and cause some remixing. The temperature variation inside the centrifuge, which causes convection currents, is primarily due to the rotor wall being heated by friction with the gas in the centrifuge chamber. The part of the rotor wall that is farthest from the axis moves fastest, and therefore the frictional heating is greatest there, and least near the axis of rotation. The result is a thermal gradient (temperature variation) within the rotor, with the periphery at a higher temperature than the axis. This temperature variation causes the undesirable convection currents just described. (Note: The centripetal force on a body of mass m moving in a circle of radius r is mv^2/r, where v is the speed of the body.)

25. Which of the following best describes the effect that causes the sediment to settle more rapidly inside the working centrifuge than outside?

   A. As the rotor spins, the gravitational field inside the centrifuge increases.
   B. As the rotor spins, a force arises on each sedimentary particle, accelerating it away from the axis of rotation.
   C. As the rotor spins, the force acting on each sedimentary particle is not great enough to keep it moving in a circle.
   D. As the rotor spins, convection currents inside the liquid carry the sediment away from the axis of rotation.

26. When the centrifuge in Figure 1 is started, the temperature of the rotor wall begins to rise. The temperature will STOP rising when:

    A. the rate of heat flow by conduction from the rotor wall equals the rate of heat flow by convection to the rotor wall.

    B. the rate of heat flow by conduction and convection from the rotor wall equals the rate of heat generation by friction.

    C. the temperature of the outside walls of the centrifuge equals the temperature of the rotor wall.

    D. the temperature of the gas reaches boiling point, and the heating due to gaseous friction therefore falls dramatically.

27. Which of the following would best help reduce the convection currents set up in the centrifuge?

    A. Blowing hotter air toward cooler areas of the centrifuge

    B. Increasing the rate of rotation to make the rotation smoother

    C. Cooling the test tubes before they are inserted into the rotor

    D. Reducing the gas pressure inside the centrifuge chamber

28. Which of the particles in the suspension settle most quickly in the centrifuge?

    A. Small particles with large mass

    B. Large particles with large mass

    C. Small particles with small mass

    D. Large particles with small mass

29. In the centrifuge shown in Figure 1, the angle of the test tubes to the vertical will be largest if:

    A. the acceleration due to gravity is high, and the rotor rotates at a high frequency.

    B. the acceleration due to gravity is high, and the rotor rotates at a low frequency.

    C. tile acceleration due to gravity is low, and the rotor rotates at a high frequency.

    D. the acceleration due to gravity is low, and the rotor rotates at a low frequency.

30. As soon as the motor is turned on, the frequency of rotation of the rotor will increase until:

    A. the motor can no longer apply any torque to the rotor.

    B. the magnitude of the frictional torque on the rotor equals the magnitude of the torque applied by the motor.

    C. the gas in the centrifuge chamber is stirred up, and a frictional torque begins to act on the rotor.

    D. the net torque required to increase the frequency of rotation of the rotor increases beyond the maximum torque the motor can supply.

In the laboratory, the voltage across a particular circuit element can be measured by a voltmeter. A voltmeter has a very high resistance and should be connected in parallel to the circuit element whose voltage is being measured. Connected improperly, the voltmeter will affect the circuit, interrupting it and preventing current from flowing through the circuit element that it is meant to measure.

An experiment is conducted in which a voltmeter is used to investigate voltages in a circuit containing a capacitor and a light bulb. The bulb and the capacitor are connected in series with a battery, and the voltmeter is placed in different positions: in the first case across the capacitor, in the second case across the light bulb, and in the third case across the battery (see Figure 1). The voltmeter reading is recorded every 10 seconds. The voltage for Case 1 as a function of time is shown in Figure 2.

Figure 1

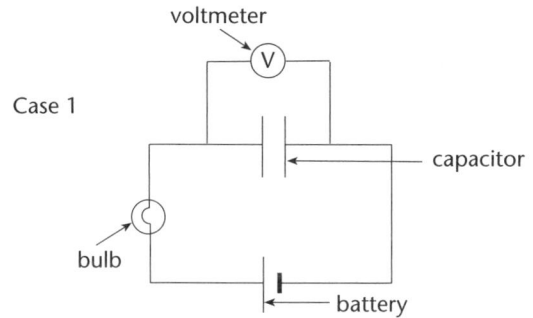

Case 1

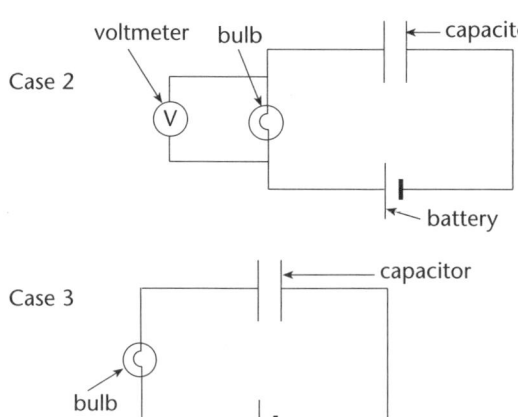

Case 2

Case 3

Figure 2

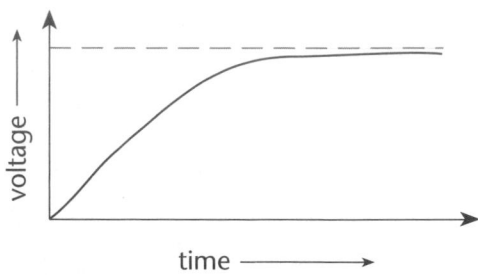

A capacitor consists of two conducting plates separated by a nonconducting material. When a battery is connected to a circuit containing a capacitor and a light bulb in series, a current will flow, causing positive charge to accumulate on one capacitor plate and an equal amount of negative charge to accumulate on the other. After the current has flowed for a finite time, the capacitor will be fully charged. The ratio of the absolute amount of charge on one plate to the voltage across the plates is defined as the capacitance; this is constant for a given capacitor. A light bulb is a resistor that, when enough current flows through it, becomes hot enough to emit energy in the form of light. (Note: Assume that the battery has no internal resistance and that the resistance of the light bulb is constant.)

31. In the circuit shown in Figure 1, which of the following conditions would indicate that the capacitor was fully charged?

    I. A voltmeter connected across the capacitor reads a constant voltage.
    II. The light bulb in the circuit stops shining.
    III. The voltage across the bulb equals the voltage across the battery.

    A. I only
    B. III only
    C. I and II only
    D. I, II, and III

32. Which one of the following graphs could correctly represent the voltage across the battery as a function of time during the experiment described in the passage?

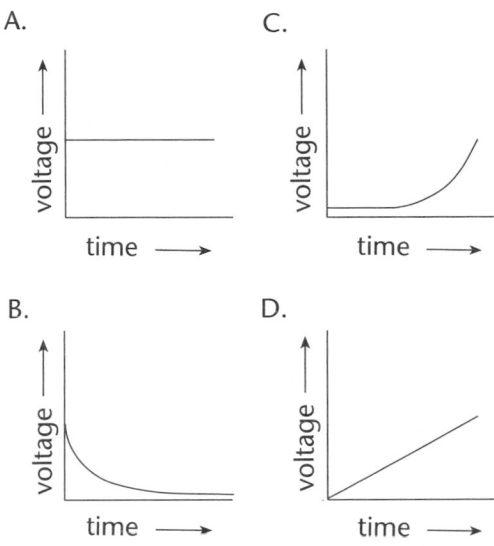

A.

C.

B.

D.

33. After the experiment described in the passage is completed, the battery is taken out of the circuit and the wires are reconnected. Which of the following graphs represents the voltage across the capacitor as a function of time?

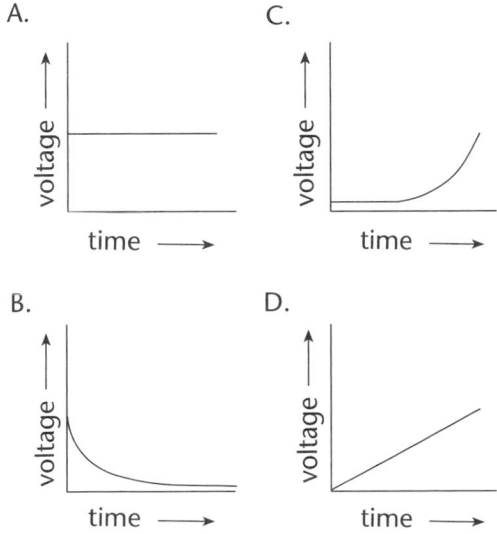

A.

C.

B.

D.

34. How will the voltage across the light bulb vary with time as the capacitor is charging?

   A. It will decrease, because as the capacitor plates fill with charge, they will impede further charge, which will decrease the current and the voltage across the bulb.

   B. It will remain the same, because as the capacitor plates fill with charge and impede the current, the voltage output of the battery will increase to keep the current constant.

   C. It will increase, because as the capacitor plates fill with charge, they will induce further charge, which will create a greater voltage across the bulb.

   D. It will increase, because as the capacitor plates fill with charge, the voltage across the capacitor will decrease, and therefore the voltage across the light bulb will increase.

35. The light bulb shown in Figure 1 is replaced first with two identical resistors in series, and then with the same two resistors in parallel. The total time taken for the capacitor to charge is measured in both cases, and found to be longer for the first case. It can be deduced that:

   A. when the resistance of the circuit is increased, the capacitance of the capacitor increases.

   B. the presence of resistors affects the final voltage across the capacitor plates.

   C. more charge is absorbed by the resistors as the resistance of the circuit increases.

   D. the presence of resistors hinders the flow of charge, thus reducing the current in the circuit.

36. In the diagram below, a voltmeter is connected in series to a circuit that includes a battery and two bulbs in series. The bulbs, which had been shining in the absence of the voltmeter, immediately stop shining. How might the circuit be modified in order to make the bulbs shine steadily again with their former brilliance without removing the voltmeter?

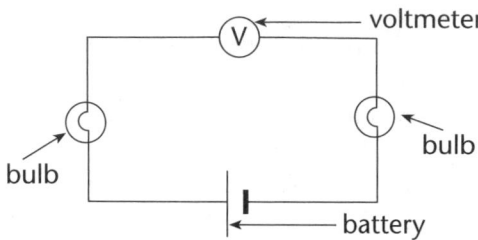

A.

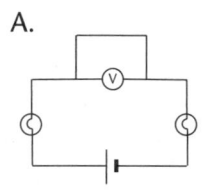

B.

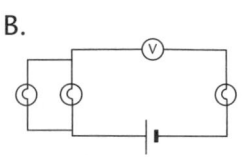

C.

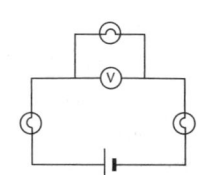

D.

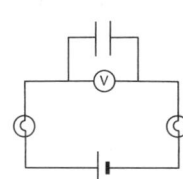

Questions 37 and 38 are NOT based on a descriptive passage.

37. In the following decay, which quantity is NOT conserved?

$$^{238}U \rightarrow {}^{234}Th + \alpha$$

A. Momentum
B. Charge
C. Total energy
D. Mass

38. Which of the following situations would produce no net force on a test particle of charge
of +q?

I.

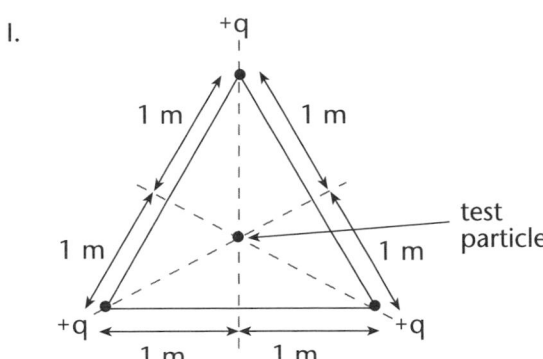

II.

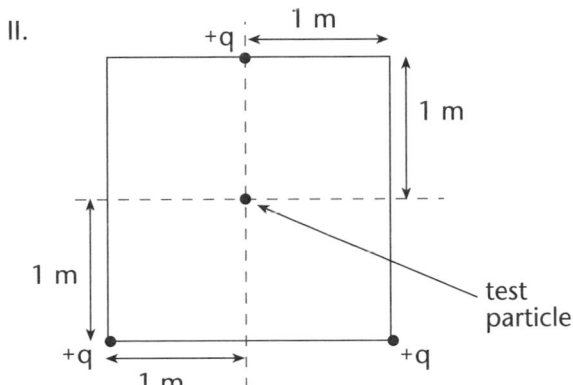

III.

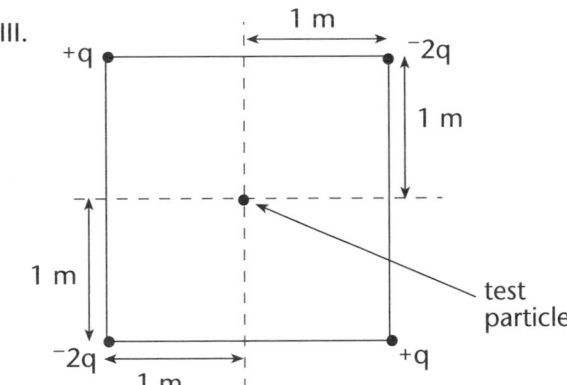

A. I only
B. II only
C. I and III only
D. II and III only

Physics Practice Set: Answers and Explanations

ANSWER KEY

1. D	11. C	21. D	31. C
2. C	12. A	22. C	32. A
3. C	13. D	23. C	33. B
4. B	14. A	24. B	34. A
5. D	15. D	25. C	35. D
6. D	16. B	26. B	36. A
7. C	17. A	27. D	37. D
8. A	18. B	28. A	38. C
9. B	19. D	29. C	
10. B	20. A	30. B	

EXPLANATIONS

Passage I (Questions 1–8)

1. D Gravitational potential energy near the surface of the Earth is given by Wh or mgh, where W is the weight, m is the mass, g is the acceleration due to gravity, and h is height. The greatest gravitational potential energy of the child corresponds to the greatest height that the child reaches. From the geometry of the swing in the figure, we see that the height increases as the angle increases. The maximum height will therefore be for the maximum angle.

2. C The swing momentarily stops moving when it reaches its maximum height. From this one fact, you can eliminate choice (B). There is a maximum height at which the speed of the swing is zero.

To have a more precise idea of how the speed of the swing varies with the height above ground, look at the law of energy conservation. This says that the total kinetic energy plus the total gravitational energy is a constant. This is an idealization, since some energy will be lost due to air resistance and friction. However, you can assume that these energy losses are small for one swing since you expect the swing to keep moving for some time. Another approximation that is useful to make is to assume that the chains holding the swing up are

relatively light compared to the child on the swing. Let the potential energy at the swing's lowest height be zero. Then the potential energy of the child on the swing is mgh, where g is the acceleration due to gravity. So as the swing rises, h increases, and therefore the potential energy goes up. The kinetic energy plus the potential energy is a constant. So, as the potential energy goes up, the kinetic energy goes down. The kinetic energy of the child on the swing is $(1/2)mv^2$, where m is the mass of the child and the seat. So, as the kinetic energy decreases, the speed decreases too. So, as the height of the swing increases, the speed decreases. But incorrect choice (A) initially shows the speed increasing as the height increases.

Since kinetic energy contains a v^2, you can expect a graph showing speed against height to be a curve rather than a straight line. Thus choice (D) is wrong, and answer choice (C) is correct. Here's why: Potential energy plus kinetic energy is constant. Thus $mgh + (1/2)mv^2$ is equal to a constant. Dividing by m and multiplying by 2, you get $2gh + v^2$ equals another constant. Solving for v^2, we find that v^2 equals a constant minus $2gh$. So, v equals the square root of the quantity "constant minus $2gh$." The graph given in choice (C) describes this relationship correctly.

3. C The distance the block will travel after leaving the slide depends upon its speed when it leaves the slide and the time it takes to hit the ground after leaving the slide. To solve this, begin with the speed when the block leaves the slide. The total energy of the block initially is $mv_i^2/2 + mgh_i$ where v_i is the initial velocity and h_i is the height of the top of the slide. Since $v_i = 0$, the total energy is just mgh_i. This must equal the total energy when the block leaves the end of the slide since there is no friction or air resistance. If v_f is the velocity of the block at the end of the slide, then the total energy can be written as $mv_f^2/2 + mgh_f$, where h_f is the height of the bottom of the slide. From conservation of energy, $mgh_i = mv_f^2/2 + mgh_f$. The masses all cancel, and therefore

v_f is independent of the block's mass. In other words, v_f is the same for both blocks.

After leaving the slide, the blocks are projectiles executing projectile motion. When they leave the slide, both blocks have the same initial horizontal velocity and fall the same 50 cm to the ground. The horizontal distance that a projectile travels is just equal to its horizontal velocity times the time it takes the projectile to fall to the ground. So, $d = vt$. Since for both blocks the initial horizontal velocity when they leave the slide is the same, the distances they travel depend upon the times.

A projectile's falling motion in the vertical direction is independent of its horizontal motion. Both blocks start with no vertical velocity when they leave the slide and fall the same 50 cm to the ground. In the vertical direction, the falling motion of a projectile is given by $h = v_i t + 1/2\ gt^2$, where h is the height, v_i is the initial vertical velocity, g is the acceleration due to gravity, and t is the time. For both blocks the initial vertical velocity is zero. So $h = 1/2\ gt^2$ or t equals $(2h/g)^{1/2}$. Since h is the same for both blocks, t will be the same for both blocks. We previously saw that the horizontal distances the two blocks traveled depended upon the time. Since the times are the same, the distances are the same.

4. B The crucial point to notice is that the child comes to a complete stop just as she reaches the end of the slide. If there had been no friction, then the child would have reached the end of the slide with a kinetic energy equal to the difference between her initial and final potential energy.

The friction, acting opposite to the direction of motion of the child on the slide, does negative work on the child. This means that the result of the action of the force of friction is to take energy away from the child. Because you know that the child is at rest when she reaches the end of the slide, you know that she has zero kinetic energy. Therefore, you may conclude that the friction force has done enough work to take away all the kinetic energy that the child would have had at the end of the

slide, had there been no friction. Had there been no friction, this kinetic energy would have been equal to the initial potential energy, mgh.

So, the work done by friction is equal to –mgh, where m is the mass of the child, g is the acceleration due to gravity, and h is the vertical height through which the child falls. From the diagram of the slide, you can see that h is 6 meters times the sine of 30 degrees. So, the work done by friction is equal to –25(g)(6)sin30°. The sine of 30 degrees is 0.5, and g is approximately 10, so you see that choice (B) is correct: –735 joules.

Note that you are not given the coefficient of friction, so you cannot actually work out the value of the force of friction. Therefore, it is impossible to determine the work done by friction by using the formula work done = force times distance. Instead, you've used the fact that the work done by friction is equal to the decrease in total mechanical energy. Kinetic energy does not change overall, since it starts and ends at zero, and therefore the work done by friction is the negative of the initial gravitational potential energy, which is –mgh.

5. D Draw a free body diagram of the child at the top of the slide. You can use the picture of the slide shown in the passage and represent the child by drawing a block. The forces on the child are the weight, acting vertically downwards, the normal force, acting perpendicular to the slide's surface, and the force of friction. To attempt to prevent the child from going down the slide, the force of friction must be directed up the slide. The weight is equal to mg, where m is the mass of the child, and g is the acceleration due to gravity. Call the normal force N, and the force of friction F.

You are told that the child is initially at rest when she starts to move down the slide. Newton's first law says that a body will remain at rest unless it is acted upon by a net force. Thus, in order for the child to begin sliding, a net force down the slide must act on the child. According to the diagram, there are two forces acting parallel to the slide.

There is the component of the weight parallel to the slide, which is mg sin 30° and is directed down the slide, and the force of friction F parallel to the slide and directed up the slide. The component of the weight down the slide must be greater than the force of friction directed up the slide, otherwise the child would not begin to move down the slide. Thus, the quantity mg sin 30° is greater than F. The force of static friction is a variable force having a maximum value equal to the normal force times the coefficient of static friction. In other words, $F_{max} = \mu_s N$. You know that the person does not lift off the slide, and therefore there is zero resultant force perpendicular to the slide's surface. Therefore the normal force N is equal to the component of the weight that is perpendicular to the slide's surface, which is mg cos 30°. So, N equals mg cos 30°, and therefore, $F_{max} = \mu_s$ mg cos 30°.

Substituting this value for F in the inequality you previously arrived at, you find that mg sin 30° is greater than μ_s mg cos 30°. Canceling the mg's, you get sin 30° is greater than m_s cos 30°, and therefore the tan 30° is greater than μ_s, or μ_s is less than tan 30°, answer choice (D).

6. D The question askes the ratio of forces reqired to push a child up a slide at a **constant speed** of 1 m/s to the force required to push the same child up a slide at a **constant speed** of 2 m/s. The key is to realize that constant speed implies an acceleration of zero. From Newton's second law (F = ma), you know that if acceleration equals zero, then the net force equals zero. This means that the net force on the child in both cases is zero. If it were not, then the child would be accelerating or decelerating, and the speed would not be constant. So, the upward force on the child along the slide is equal to the downward force along the slide in both cases.

If the child is moving up the slide, then the downward force along the slide is equal to the component of the child's weight along the slide, plus the force of friction. Remember that kinetic friction is always opposite to the motion. Now, both the weight of the child and the friction force are independent of the speed. Therefore, the upward

force is the same in the case when the child is moving at a constant speed of 1 meter per second, as when she is moving at a constant speed of 2 meters per second. The force that makes the child move at a constant speed does not depend on the value of the speed. This makes choice (D) correct.

7. C The frequency can be calculated from the velocity of the child because the velocity v equals 2πr times the frequency f. The child must hold on to the merry-go-round with a force equal to the centripetal force, mv^2/r. Since the mass of the child is 30 kg and the radius of the merry-go-round is 2.0 m, you get $30v^2/2$ or $15v^2$ newtons for the centripetal force. Setting this equal to the maximum gripping force of the child, which equals 60 N, gives $60 = 15v^2$, so $v^2 = 4$, and v = 2 m/s. Since v = 2πrf, then the frequency equals v/2πr. v = 2 m/s and r = 2m, so f = 2/(4π), or f = 1/(2π), which is choice (C).

8. A Think about what happens to the person as he hits the ground. There will be a force acting on the person when he hits the ground, and the greater this force is, the more dangerous the fall will be.

Considering the impulse is often a good way to begin impact questions. What is the impulse on the person as he hits the ground? The impulse of a force acting on a body equals the change in its momentum due to that force. Ignoring the possibility of bouncing for the time being; the person's momentum is initially downward and is zero after colliding with the ground. The impulse is the change in momentum, which, in this case is equal in magnitude to the initial momentum minus zero or simply the initial momentum. So, regardless of what the person falls on, provided there is no bouncing, the impulse on the person is the same as long as the initial momentum is the same.

Impulse is also equal to average force times time over which the force acts. This tells us that average force equals impulse or change in momentum divided by time. So, the longer the time over which the force acts, the smaller the average force. Think of the change of momentum being spread out over a longer time. In this case, the change of momentum will be more gradual and the average force is smaller. The safety tiles which give slightly as somebody falls on them increase the impact time. As a result, the time taken for the person to come to rest on the tiles is greater than on concrete. Thus, the average force is lower on the safety tiles, and choice (A) is correct.

Choice (B) talks of the safety tiles absorbing the kinetic energy of the person quickly. You know that kinetic energy is associated with motion. If the kinetic energy is absorbed quickly, the person must come to a halt quickly, but this means that the time of impact is short. Thus, the average force on the person upon impact, which is equal to the impulse divided by the time, is large.

Choice (C) suggests that bouncing on the tiles will make a fall less dangerous. What will happen to the impulse felt by a person if he bounces? The momentum after the impact is upward instead of being zero. So the change in momentum is actually greater than it would be if the final momentum were zero. Thus, if a person bounces on impact with the tiles, he must have felt a greater impulse than he would have felt if he didn't bounce. This would be more, not less dangerous.

As you've already seen, the impulse on a person falling onto the tiles is just the change in his momentum. The softness of the tiles may change the time over which the impulse acts, but it cannot reduce the impulse itself, so choice (D) is wrong.

Passage II (Questions 9–12)

9. B You may notice straight away that the question is about photovoltaic cells, whereas the passage talks mostly about photoelectric cells. But you don't actually need to know how a photovoltaic cell works. You just need to know about its efficiency and about the power of the Sun.

The passage talks of the power of the Sun. The question stem talks of the energy supply to a household. So, effectively you have a choice; you can think in terms of power or in terms of energy. Choose energy, since it is the more basic concept.

So, how do you get 20 kilowatt hours of energy out of a photovoltaic cell?

Averaged over 24 hours, the power reaching the Earth's surface from the Sun is 0.2 kilowatts per square meter. Since kilowatts are units of power, relate power to energy. Power is equal to energy divided by time, or, rearranging this, energy is equal to power times time. Thus, the total solar energy reaching the Earth's surface in 24 hours is the power averaged over 24 hours multiplied by 24 hours.

Now you can work out the amount of solar energy reaching a photovoltaic cell. Call the area in square meters to be covered by the photovoltaic cells A. Averaged over 24 hours, solar power at the Earth's surface per square meter is 0.2 kilowatts. So, the total solar energy reaching these cells in 24 hours is the power, 0.2 kilowatts per square meter x A square meters x 24 hours, or 0.2 x A x 24 kilowatt hours. The question tells you that the efficiency of the cells is 35%. So the energy output of the cells over the period of a day is 35 over 100 times the energy reaching the cells.

It's always a good idea to write something down for calculation questions. If you follow the steps we've just been through, you might have written down; "solar power at cell equals 0.2 x A; energy reaching cell in a day equals 0.2 x A x 24; energy output by cell in a day equals (0.2 x A x 24 x 35)/100." You equate this last value to the energy needed, 20 kilowatt hours. Thus: (0.2 x A x 24 x 35)/100 = 20. Solving for A, you get A = 12 m² which is choice (B). (Note: Always try simplifying arithmetic by cancelling and approximating.)

10. B Note that the rate at which photons hit the cathode is not the frequency. Frequency is a wavelike property of light. When talking about photons, it's easiest to think in terms of the energy of a photon, and to remember that photon energy, E, is related to the frequency of the light, f, by $E = hf$, where h is Planck's constant.

You are told in the last sentence of the passage that the stopping voltage depends only on the maximum kinetic energy of an individual electron ejected from the cathode. What about the kinetic energy of the electrons then? Well, you're told in the second paragraph that the energy given to an electron breaking free from the cathode comes from an individual photon. But, the energy of an individual photon is given by $E_p = hf$, where h is Planck's constant, and f is frequency, and is thus constant if the frequency is held constant.

Putting these facts together is enough to indicate that B is the correct answer: The stopping voltage will not change as the intensity of light is varied, because it is the energy of individual photons which provides the kinetic energy of electrons ejected from the cathode, and this does not change if the frequency of the light is held constant.

11. C The question asks you to decide which answer choice cannot be explained by the wave theory of light, so consider each answer choice and see if you can explain it using this theory. If you can't, and you have to talk about particles of light, or photons, then you've found the correct answer choice.

Choice (A) is wrong because, you can explain it in terms of waves. The intensity of a wave is energy flow per unit area per unit time. So, if you reduce the intensity, you reduce the rate that energy strikes the cell. The current in the photocell is electrical energy. So reducing the rate at which energy strikes the cell causes the current to fall. You can understand this in terms of waves because the intensity (energy per unit time, per unit area) is being varied, and intensity is a property you can apply to waves. Actually, unless the intensity of light incident on the photocell falls to zero, there will be some current. So, the statement in choice (A) isn't even strictly correct.

Choice (B) has nothing to do with the incident light at all, so it doesn't matter whether light is referred to as particles or waves. The passage tells you that the amount of energy that is required is the work function, W. But W is a property of the material of the cathode. In order to break free from the coulomb forces of attraction within the cathode material, an electron that is escaping from the

cathode must have some energy. This explanation doesn't depend on the use of either the "light-as-waves" theory, or the "light-as-particles" theory.

You cannot explain answer choice (C) if you only refer to light as a wave, so it's the correct answer choice. What's the problem with the wave theory here? The intensity of the incident light is kept constant; only the frequency is varied. If you use only wave terminology, the frequency of light, f, is related to wavelength, λ, and speed, v, by v equals $f\lambda$, but changing the frequency does not limit the energy supplied to the electrons in the cathode. Indeed, you are told that the intensity of the incident light is being held constant. So, the total energy delivered to the photocell per unit time is being held constant. Given just these wavelike properties of light, you cannot explain how the current stops when the frequency changes. So choice (C) is correct. This very problem led Einstein to refer to light in terms of photons. When an electron absorbs a photon, all the photon's energy is given to the electron. The energy of an individual photon, E, is related to the frequency of light, f, by $E = hf$, where h is Planck's constant. So, using the photon theory of light, you see that changing the frequency of incident light does affect the energy that can be given to an electron. Because the intensity is constant, the total energy per unit time isn't changed, but the energy of each individual photon is changed when the frequency changes. If the frequency of light goes down, the energy of each individual photon goes down; and eventually the energy of an individual photon is too small to knock an electron out of the cathode, and the current in the photocell stops altogether.

Choice (D) is wrong because the refraction of light as it passes from one medium to another is dependent on frequency rather than intensity and can thus be explained solely in terms of the wavelike properties of light.

12. A What makes the stopping voltage across a photoelectric cell increase? The stopping voltage is the voltage needed to stop current flowing in the cell. You are told in the last paragraph that the maximum kinetic energy of electrons ejected from the cathode determines the stopping voltage. How does the stopping voltage depend on the kinetic energy of the electrons liberated from the cathode? The voltage connected across the cell to oppose the current flow sets up an electric force against which the electrons have to struggle. The electric force decelerates the electrons so that they are slower, and therefore have a smaller kinetic energy by the time they reach the anode. If the maximum kinetic energy of the electrons is high, then the voltage needed to stop them reaching the anode will also be high.

What makes the maximum kinetic energy of the electrons high? The formula in the passage, $E_{max} = E_p - W$, tells you that E_{max}, the maximum kinetic energy of the electrons ejected from the cathode, is high when E_p is high and W is low. So you want W, the work function of the cathode material, to be low. This eliminates answer choices (B) and (D).

What makes E_p, the energy of the incident photons, high? $E_p = hf$, where h is Planck's constant, and f is the frequency of incident light. So high frequency light means each photon has a high energy. Frequency is inversely proportional to wavelength. In fact the formula that relates the frequency of a wave, f, to its wavelength, λ, is $v = f\lambda$, where v is the speed of the wave. This means that if the frequency is high, the wavelength is short. You want high frequency light since you want photons with a high energy, therefore you want short wavelength light. Answer choice (A) is correct, and (C) is wrong.

Discrete Questions

13. D   You're asked about the force on a moving electron. The electron is charged, and there is a current-carrying wire nearby which must generate a magnetic field. So, the force you need to know about is the magnetic force, the one where you have to use the right-hand rule to find the direction. The right-hand rule will tell the direction of the force on the electron provided you know the direction in which the charge is moving, and the direction of the magnetic field.

Imagine the long, straight, current-carrying wire. You can use your pen as a visual aid. Place the pen vertically in front of you, and imagine the current flowing upward along it. First, find the direction of the magnetic field generated. To do this, point the thumb of your right hand in the direction of current flow in the wire, curling your fingers toward your palm. The magnetic field lines are circles around the wire pointing in the direction of your curled fingers. So in this case, as seen from above, the magnetic field lines are circles, pointing counter-clockwise. Imagine the electron as traveling along a line parallel to the long, straight wire. The question tells you that the electron is traveling in the same direction as the current flow, so it is also going vertically upward. You know that on the right-hand side of the wire the magnetic field lines go away from you, and on the left side they come toward you. If you imagine the line along which the electron is moving to be to the right of the wire, you can use the right-hand rule to find the direction of the force. Hold your right hand out flat, with your thumb at a right angle to your fingers. If the electron were a positive charge, you would point your thumb along its direction of motion. However, since the charge on an electron is negative, point your thumb in the opposite direction of the motion, vertically downwards. The direction of the magnetic field is away from you on the right-hand side of the wire, so point your fingers directly away from you. The direction your palm is pointing indicates the direction of the force. Here, your palm will be pointing to the right, away from the wire.

If you had imagined the electron to the left of the wire, or imagined the current going downward, you would have reached the same conclusion. The force is perpendicular to, and away from, the wire. Answer choice (D) is correct.

14. A   You don't actually need to know any of the complex dynamics of a thunder cloud to answer this question. You're asked to choose something that would reduce the rate of cooling. All you know about the bubble of air is that it is rising and cooling. Any water vapor inside the bubble will also be cooling. If the water vapor cools enough, it will start to condense into moisture, as answer choice (A) suggests. It takes energy to boil water, turning it into vapor. So, energy is given off when water vapor condenses into water. The energy will be given off in the form of heat, and so we expect the rate at which the air loses heat to be reduced. So answer choice (A) is correct.

(B) says that the pressure on the bubble will decrease as it rises, and so it will expand. Atmospheric pressure decreases as we go higher; the air gets thinner. So the pressure exerted on the bubble of rising air does indeed decrease. To see why the bubble cools as it expands, consider the first law of thermodynamics. The change in internal energy of the air bubble, ΔU, is equal to the heat supplied, Q, minus the work done by the bubble, W. As the bubble expands, it is doing work, pushing against the surrounding atmosphere. This means that ΔU is negative, and therefore that the internal energy goes down as the bubble expands. Choice (B) is wrong because the reduction in pressure actually increases the rate of cooling.

Air from the environment that surrounds the bubble of warm air is going to be colder than the air in the bubble. Generally, the atmosphere gets colder the higher you go because the Sun warms the ground more than the air. So, if air from the surrounding atmosphere is drawn into the bubble, it will be cooled more quickly, so choice (C) is wrong. And since atmospheric pressure decreases the higher you go, choice (D) is wrong.

Passage III (Questions 15–21)

15. D   Choice (A) says that the volume of fluid displaced equals the volume of the object. This is true only if the object is entirely immersed in the liquid. In such cases, the object takes up a space in the fluid equal to its own volume, and therefore displaces its own volume of fluid. If the object were only partially immersed, it would occupy a space in

the fluid smaller than its own volume, and thus displace a volume of liquid smaller than its own volume. So, floating objects do not displace their own volume of liquid. The special thing about Archimedes' principle is that it applies to all objects placed in fluids, those that float as well as those that sink. Choice (A) applies only to objects that sink, and therefore cannot be Archimedes' principle.

Choice (B) says that the buoyant force is equal to the weight of the object. If this is true, then the vertical forces on the object balance out and therefore the object will float. So, choice (B) is true only when the object is afloat. Archimedes' principle applies to objects in fluids in all circumstances, not just floating objects, and not just sunken objects.

Choice (C) says that if an object is more dense than a fluid it will sink in it; otherwise it will float. This is certainly true, and it is this rule that allows us to decide whether iron floats in mercury and water. Iron is less dense than mercury and thus floats in it. Iron is more dense than water and thus sinks in it. So choice (C) is true—it just isn't Archimedes' principle.

Choice (D) is correct. The upward (buoyant) force on a body placed in a fluid is equal to the weight of fluid displaced.

16. B   This is two-part question. Both parts must be true in order for a given choice to be the correct answer. Not only must you know whether Tube W or Tube M contains a larger volume of liquid, but you must also know which of the explanations are correct. A strategy for handling this type of question is to evaluate the first part of each answer choice first and then to eliminate the answer choices that contain an incorrect first part.

First, this question is asking whether a larger volume of water or mercury is displaced by the iron cube. Decide whether the iron cube sinks or floats in the two liquids. If an object is more dense than a fluid, it will sink in that fluid; otherwise it will float. From the information given in Table 1, you learn that iron is more dense than water and therefore sinks in it. Iron is less dense than mercury and therefore floats in it.

When the iron cube is lowered into the water, it will sink and therefore be completely submerged underneath the surface of the water. It will occupy a space in the water equal to its own volume. So the volume of water displaced will be equal to the volume of the iron cube. When the iron cube is lowered into the mercury, it will float. If you picture the floating cube, you can see that it will be only partially submerged in the mercury. Therefore, the cube will displace a volume of mercury smaller than its total volume. So the volume of mercury displaced will be less than the volume of the iron cube. Therefore, test tube W, the test tube collecting the displaced water, will collect more liquid than test tube M, the test tube collecting the displaced mercury.

Only choices (A) and (B) state that Tube W collects more liquid. So you can eliminate choices (C) and (D). Choice (B) also gives the correct explanation which coincides with the previous analysis. Therefore, choice (B) is the correct answer choice. If this were the actual MCAT, you would now go on to the next question. However, for purposes of review, here's why choice (A) is wrong. The second part of choice (A) states that the same mass of liquid is displaced in each case. If the masses of liquid displaced were the same in each case, then the buoyant force of the liquid on the iron cube would be the same in each case. This is not so. The cube sinks in water, but floats in mercury. Therefore, the buoyant forces are not the same. So the mass of water displaced is not the same as the mass of mercury displaced. This proves that answer choice (A) is incorrect.

17. A This question asks you to consider what will happen if a cube of wood is used instead of iron. The first thing to notice is that the wood is less dense than water. (You are told this in the question.) Immediately, this tells you that wood floats in water. Since mercury is more dense than water, anything that floats in water will also float in mercury. Thus, the cube of wood floats in both mercury and water. This means that in both mercury and water the buoyant force equals the weight of the wooden cube which is a fixed num-

ber (the mass of the cube multiplied by the acceleration due to gravity). Thus, the buoyant (upward) force on the cube must be the same whether it is floating in mercury or in water.

Applying Archimedes' principle, which states that the buoyant force on an object equals the weight of displaced fluid, you now know that that the weight of liquid displaced in each case is identical. But mercury is more dense than water. Therefore, a given volume of mercury weighs more than that same volume of water. Equivalently, if equal masses of mercury and water are considered, then the water will occupy a larger volume. So, since equal weights (and thus masses) of liquid are displaced in each case, a larger volume of water is displaced than mercury.

18. B The ship is shaped so that its volume is mostly filled with air. Thus, its overall density is low. This question should be straightforward to answer. Remember that whether an object sinks or not depends only upon whether it is more or less dense than the fluid it is placed in. A dense object will sink whatever shape and size it is. This should be enough to eliminate choices (C) and (D), since they do not even mention the densities of the seawater or of the ship.

The fact that large ships float in the sea tells you that the overall density of those ships is less than the density of seawater. This must be true, since otherwise ships would sink, whatever shape or size they were. Choice (B) explains how it is that the overall density of an iron ship is lower than that of iron itself. Think of the total volume a ship occupies. Some of that space is filled with dense material like iron. However, between the solid walls of a ship, in between the hull and the deck, for instance, is a lot of air. So, the overall density of the ship is much lower than the density of iron. Of course, if the hull of a ship were filled with water instead of air, the overall density would be much higher, and it would sink. A submarine changes its overall density by letting in water into ballast tanks and then pumping it out again. This enables the submarine to dive and to surface.

Choice (A) tells you that sea water is denser than pure water. This is true. Indeed, if it were very dense, then solid lumps of iron could float around on it. However, sea water is not much more dense than pure water. Reject this choice on the grounds that seawater cannot possibly be as dense as iron.

19. D A cube of metal sinks in water. You are asked what would change if a cube of the same metal, but with sides twice as long, were lowered into water. Looking at the answer choices, you see that you need to decide what will happen to the buoyant force on the cube and its rate of acceleration.

Archimedes' principle tells you about buoyant forces. You should immediately think about using this principle when you realize that the question is asking about buoyant forces. What happens to the buoyant force when the sides of the cube are doubled? Archimedes' principle tells you that the buoyant force equals the weight of liquid displaced, so whatever happens to the weight of water displaced, also happens to the buoyant force. You need to find out what happens to the weight of water displaced.

The original cube sinks in water, and since the larger cube is made of the same metal, it too must sink. Because both cubes sink, they occupy a space in the water equal to their own volume, and therefore displace that volume of liquid. The larger cube has sides twice as long, and therefore a volume 8 times as big. (This follows from the fact that the volume of a cube is the length of its sides cubed, and therefore that doubling the length of the sides of a cube means multiplying its volume by 2 x 2 x 2, or 8). So, the volume of water displaced by the larger cube is eight times that displaced by the smaller cube. Archimedes' principle therefore, tells you that the buoyant force will increase by a factor of eight.

You can now eliminate choices (B) and (C). Next, decide how the acceleration of the cube will change. This is a bit harder. It's easiest to figure out what's going on if you draw a free-body diagram. The weight of the cube acts downwards, and the buoyant force acts upwards.

Call the weight of the smaller cube mg. Call the upward buoyant force on the smaller cube U. Thus, the overall downward force on the smaller cube is mg – U. Use Newton's second law, F = ma, to calculate the acceleration of the cube. The mass of the smaller cube is m, and therefore its downward acceleration is (mg – U)/m.

The larger cube has a mass eight times that of the smaller one. This follows from your calculation that its volume is eight times greater, and from your knowledge that the densities of each cube are the same. So, the weight of the larger cube is eight times that of the smaller cube. The weight of the larger cube is 8 mg. The upward buoyant force on the larger cube is eight times that on the smaller cube. So, the overall downwards force on the larger cube is 8 mg – 8 U. Using Newton's second law to calculate the acceleration, you find that the downward acceleration of the larger cube is 8 mg – 8 U over the mass of the larger cube, 8 m. So the acceleration of the larger cube turns out to be (mg – U)/m, the same value as the acceleration of the smaller cube.

The acceleration of both cubes turns out to be the same. This makes a good deal of sense, since you know that it is only the densities of object and fluid that determines whether an object floats or sinks. If you could decrease the rate of acceleration of an object, that is, the rate at which it sinks, by altering its size, then it would seem strange that you could not reduce that acceleration to zero and thus stop it sinking altogether. You have already seen that changing the size of an object without changing its density does not alter whether it sinks or floats. Changing the size and shape of an object without changing its density cannot alter the rate at which it sinks. So, answer choice (D) is correct. The buoyant force will increase by a factor of eight, and the cube will accelerate downwards at the same rate as before.

20. A To answer this question, you need to be able to interpret the graph given in the question stem, which shows the rate at which the temperature of water increases as it is heated. For the first

15 minutes during which heat is supplied to the water, its temperature rises at a constant rate. The formula you are given in the question tells you that $\Delta T = Q/mc$. In other words, the change in temperature of a substance is equal to the heat supplied to it divided by mc. From this you can deduce that the rate at which the temperature of a substance increases equals the rate at which heat is supplied to it divided by mc. The slope of the graph is equal to the rate at which the temperature of the substance increases. A steep line indicates a large change in temperature for a small change in time. This is the most important point: the slope of the graph, that is, the rate of temperature increase, is equal to the rate at which heat is supplied divided by mc.

After 15 minutes, the graph tells you that the temperature of the water has reached 100°C, the boiling point of water. After this point, the energy supplied to the water does not raise the temperature, but instead is used to boil the water, and so, although the rate at which heat is supplied remains constant, the temperature stops increasing. Therefore, the graph becomes a horizontal line when the temperature reaches boiling point of water.

Back to the question: consider what would happen to 10 centimeters cubed of mercury if it is heated at the same rate as the water. Again, the temperature should rise at a constant rate for some time. When the mercury reaches its boiling point, the heat supplied will no longer make the temperature rise but will instead be used to boil the mercury. Therefore the graph should level off at 357°C, which is the boiling point of mercury given in the passage. This allows you to eliminate choice (D), which shows the mercury boiling at 100°C. Now consider what happens before the mercury boils. During this interval, a graph of temperature against time, like those given in the question, will display a straight line whose slope is equal to the rate at which heat is supplied divided by mc.

If you examine the answer choices (A), (B) and (C), you find that the only difference between them is the slope of the line before the mercury reaches its boiling point. Be very careful to look at the scales on the diagrams. Each one is different. Graph B is steepest, then graph A. Graph C is the least steep.

So you want to know the rate at which the temperature of mercury will increase, so that you may decide how steep the graph of temperature against time should be. You know from the passage that the specific heat of mercury is 138 joules per kilogram per Kelvin. This value is approximately 30 times smaller than the specific heat of water, and thus you might expect the value of mc to be 30 times smaller for mercury than for water. This would lead you to expect that the slope of the graph for mercury should be 30 times steeper than that for water since, as you have seen, the slope is inversely proportional to mc. Such a graph is shown in choice (B). However, you have also to consider the difference in the mass of mercury heated from the mass of water heated. So choice (B) is wrong.

Mercury is approximately 14 times more dense than water, and therefore 10 centimeters cubed of it has approximately 14 times more mass than the same volume of water. So, if you consider the change in the mass as well as the change in the specific heat of mercury compared to water, you find that the mc value for mercury is approximately 14 over 30, times as large as the mc value for water. 14 over 30 is about one half. So, the rate of increase of temperature for mercury should be about twice the rate for water. (Remember the rate of temperature increase is inversely proportional to mc, and the rate at which heat is supplied to the mercury is the same as the rate at which it is supplied to the water.) So the graph for mercury should show a line approximately twice as steep as that for water. Such a graph is shown in correct choice (A).

21. D The iron cube would sink more slowly than on Earth. You can answer this question quickly by eliminating the wrong choices, but it is actually quite complicated if you want to work out the details. Choice (A) is wrong. You know that whether or not an object floats in water depends upon its density. Taking the water and the iron to the moon will not alter their densities. Because iron is more dense than water, it will sink in water, whatever the acceleration due to gravity is.

You've decided that the iron cube will sink in water. This is true both on the moon and on Earth. If the iron cube sinks, it will occupy a space in the water equal to its own volume. Thus, the volume of water displaced by the cube will be equal to its own volume. So the iron cube sinks in the water, displacing the same volume of water whether on the moon or on Earth. Therefore, choice (B) is wrong.

Choice (C) is also wrong. However, this may not be so obvious. Call the weight of the cube on the Earth W and the buoyant force on the cube when it's on the Earth U. The downward force on the cube when it's on the Earth is W – U. Newton's second law, F = ma, tells you that the downward acceleration, a, is equal to the downward force divided by the mass of the cube. On Earth, the downward acceleration is W – U, all divided by m.

What happens on the moon? The weight of the iron cube is its mass times the acceleration due to gravity. The mass will be the same on the moon as on the Earth, but the acceleration due to gravity is 6 times lower on the moon. So the weight of the iron cube on the moon is $\frac{1}{6}$ what it is on the Earth, or W/6.

The buoyant force is equal to the weight of water displaced. Because the volume of water displaced is the same on the moon as on the Earth, the mass of water displaced is the same in both cases. Therefore, the weight of water displaced on the moon will be $\frac{1}{6}$ of the weight of water displaced on the Earth. So, on the moon, the buoyant force is U/6. The downward acceleration is just net force divided by mass. So, on the moon, the downward acceleration is (W/6 – U/6)/m, which is $\frac{1}{6}$ of the acceleration on Earth.

Discrete Questions

22. C   A gas can only do work by expanding and pushing. If the gas is compressed, then work is done on it, which is the same as saying that the gas does negative work. Since the gas in this question is contained within a constant volume, it cannot expand, and therefore it does zero work.

The first law of thermodynamics states that ΔU = Q – W, where ΔU is the change in internal energy of a system, Q is equal to the heat supplied to the system, and W is the work done by the system. So, if Q is zero, then positive ΔU means negative W, which makes answer choice (A) tempting. But in this case, there is a heat transferal, Q is not zero, and this is why ΔU is positive. The work done, W, is zero. So choice (A) is wrong.

The pressure of this gas will not remain constant. Heat is supplied to it, so its temperature will rise. You know the volume is constant, so the pressure must change. The gas molecules will be moving around faster, because they have collectively acquired heat energy. So they will be hitting the walls of the container more often. Since the pressure will rise, choice (B) is wrong.

An isolated system can exchange neither matter nor energy with its surroundings. So, for an isolated system, Q is zero. However, here the gas is not an isolated system, and so Q is not zero. The heat supplied to the gas changes the internal energy of the gas, but because of the constraints of the rigid container, the gas does zero work.

23. C   You are given the general equation you need in the note at the end of the question. You are told about two harmonic vibrations of the string; so you have two equations. It's best if you write down the equation for each case, substituting in all the numbers you know.

You know the wavelengths in both cases. The length of the string is the unknown we're trying to find. What about n, the harmonic number? You're told that the vibrations are consecutive harmonics. So, if the first vibration is the nth harmonic, the other vibration is the $(n + 1)^{th}$ harmonic. The two equations are simultaneous equations, with two unknowns: the length of the string, L, and n, the harmonic number. The first equation reads: 25 = 2L/n, and the second equation is 20 = 2L/(n + 1).

To solve this simultaneous equation problem, you need to eliminate one of the unknowns. L is easy to eliminate by dividing the first equation by the second. You get: 25/20 on the left hand side, and this equals the (n + 1)/n. The 2 L's have canceled out. Now 25/20 = 5/4. So, multiplying both sides of the equation by 4n, you get that 5n = 4n + 4. Therefore 5n – 4n = 4, or n = 4.

You've found n, so there's only one more step to go to find L. Take either one of the original equations, and substitute n = 4. So, using the first equation, you get 25 = 2L/4. Solving this, and bearing in mind that you've been using units of centimeters, you find that L = 50 centimeters. Answer choice (C) is correct. If, after all this, you still have time, you can check your answer quickly by substituting L = 50 into the second equation: 20 = 2 x 50, over the quantity 4 + 1. This is consistent, so you know that you've gotten it right.

24. B   You are asked what the sound meter will read, when it is placed near a 100 decibel sound with a frequency of 50 Hz. The first part of the question tells you that the reading on the meter will be equal to the sound level in decibels plus the relative response of the meter.

The sound level is easy—100 decibels near the plane. What about the relative response of the meter? Find this out from the graph. Notice that the frequency scale on the graph is a log scale. So, as you look along the x-axis to find 50 hertz, be careful—weird things happen on log scales. Because of the log scale, 50 hertz is closer on the graph to 100 hertz than it is to 10 hertz. Checking along the curve at 50 hertz, you find a relative

response of –30 decibels. So the relative response of the meter when it's placed near the plane is –30 decibels.

The meter will therefore give a reading of 100 decibels plus a quantity which is –30 decibels, so you have 100 – 30 decibels, which is 70 decibels, making answer choice (B) correct.

If you chose (D), you may not have realized that the relative response of the meter is negative. Meters like this one are used to measure levels of noise pollution. The reading that the meter gives is

a measure of the noise pollution level, taking into account the fact that high frequency sound is more polluting than low frequency sound. Since low frequency sound is less obtrusive than high frequency sound, the meter has a negative relative response for low frequency sound.

Passage IV (Questions 25–30)

25. C   Think about the motion of each particle of sediment. Each particle is kept inside the test tube which is whirling round the axis of rotation of the rotor. You know from Newton's second law that in order to keep a particle moving in a circle, it must be constantly accelerated towards the center of that circle. So there must be some force on each particle of sediment towards the axis of rotation, called the centripetal force. If this were not so, then the particle would move off in a straight line, tangential to the circle in which the test tube is spinning. So you see that there is a natural tendency for the particles to move off at a tangent to the circle, in other words, to move away from the axis of rotation.

Unless there is a sufficient centripetal force on a sedimentary particle, it will tend to drift away from the axis of rotation. If a particle is drifting away from the axis of rotation, it is settling toward the bottom of the test tube. Thus, answer choice (C) is correct.

26. B   The passage tells you that the rotor wall heats up because of friction with the gas in the centrifuge chamber. That explains why the temperature increases. Why, then, does the temperature of the rotor wall stop increasing? Heat must be flowing away from the rotor walls. Choice (B) is the only possible explanation. Heat flow away from the rotor wall balances heat generation by friction at the rotor wall.

Here's a more detailed look at what you can deduce about the heat flow in the centrifuge. You're told that the primary cause of convection currents is the heating of the rotor wall by friction with the gas in the centrifuge chamber. From this you can reason that the heating of the other parts of the centrifuge is less than the heating of the rotor wall. Therefore, the rotor walls are hotter than other parts of the centrifuge. A basic rule of thermodynamics is that there will be heat flow from hotter places to colder places if possible. Both convection and conduction are possible here, since there are gases inside the centrifuge chamber and since conduction will occur through the material of the rotor wall.

27. D The third paragraph of the passage tells you that the rotor walls are heated by friction with the gases in the centrifuge chamber. The friction is the primary cause of temperature variations in the centrifuge, and the temperature variations cause the convection currents. To take away the primary cause of the convection currents, you need to take measures to reduce the frictional heating of the rotor walls.

Reducing the pressure of the gas inside the centrifuge means that there are less gas particles around, and therefore means that there will be less friction of gas with the rotor walls. This will reduce the friction heating of all parts of the centrifuge, in turn reducing the temperature gradient, and thus reducing the convection currents inside the centrifuge.

28. A To tackle this question, you need a grip on what is going on within the centrifuge. Consider a particle of sediment within a suspension held in a test tube that is being whirled around in a circle. At any one instant in time, the velocity of this particle is tangential to the circle in which the test tube is traveling. If there were no forces on this particle, it would continue to move along this straight line, tangential to the circle. A particle moving off at a tangent to the circle around which the centrifuge is turning will be moving away from the axis of rotation. The bottom of a test tube spinning in the centrifuge will be farther away from the axis than the top, and therefore, an outward motion with respect to the axis of rotation is a downward, sinking motion with respect to the liquid in the test tube.

Now that you understand how particles sink in a centrifuge, you need to think about which particles sink most quickly. To maintain a circular motion, a particle must be constantly accelerated towards the center of that circle by a centripetal force. Looking at the note at the end of the passage, you see that the centripetal force on a particle moving in a circle is directly proportional to the mass of the particle, m. So, the more massive an object is, the larger the centripetal force needed to make it move in a circle. This means that a centripetal force which is sufficient to make a particle with a small mass move in a circle, is too small to make a more massive particle move in a circle. So, for a given centripetal force, particles with a large mass, will settle most quickly in a centrifuge. Thus you want to choose choices (A) and (B) in preference to choices (C) and (D).

To decide whether smaller or larger particles settle most quickly, you need to think about what provides the centripetal force on a sedimentary particle in the centrifuge. Actually, the centripetal force is due to the buoyancy of the particles in the liquid. The buoyant force pushes up from the bottom of the liquid to the top, which in this case makes it an inward force. Archimedes' principle tells you about the buoyant force; the buoyant force on a body immersed in a liquid is equal to the weight of the displaced liquid. A small particle will displace less liquid than a large particle of the same mass, and so will experience a smaller buoyant force. So the centripetal force on a particle will be lower, the smaller it is. You can infer that small particles settle more quickly than large particles of the same mass. Thus, choice (A) is correct.

In fact, you might have predicted this result using common sense. The passage tells you that the centrifuge simply speeds up the pace of sedimentation. But you know that more dense things sink faster than less dense things. Small, massive particles are dense particles, and so sink more quickly than less dense particles. The centrifuge simply speeds up the rate at which particles settle out; it does not change which particles settle out most quickly.

29. C You need to know what happens to the test tubes when the frequency of rotation of the rotor and the acceleration due to gravity are changed. If the acceleration due to gravity is low, then the downward force on the test tubes must be small. You know that the tubes would fly off at a tangent were they not being held at their top ends. So, if the downward force on the test tubes is small, they will more easily swing upward on their hinges. Indeed, if there were no gravitational force at all, then the test tubes would swing right up into the horizontal plane. Conversely, if the acceleration due to gravity is high, then the downward force on the test tubes is high. So the tubes get pulled downward, and swing towards the vertical.

So you've decided that the angle that the test tubes make with the vertical will be greater when the acceleration due to gravity is low than the angle will be when the acceleration due to gravity is high. So, you can eliminate answer choices (A) and (B).
If the frequency of rotation is high, then there will be more of a tendency for the test tubes to fly off at a tangent than if the frequency is low. It seems intuitively true that the tubes will swing up when the frequency is high, and so choice (C) is correct. If you are pressed for time, then acting on an intuition like this may be the best thing to do; Newtonian physics usually does make intuitive sense. However if you'd like to confirm your intuition, consider the forces on the test tube. There are only two forces acting on each test tube: gravity and the tension in the bar from which the test tube hangs. What's the centripetal force on the tubes? The circle that the test tubes move in is horizontal—around the vertical rotor axis, so the centripetal force must also be horizontal. This can't be gravity, because gravity is vertical. The horizontal component of the tension in the bar is the centripetal force pulling on the test tubes.

The equation in the note at the end of the passage relates the centripetal force to speed. When the speed of the test tubes is high, the centripetal force required to make them move in a circle is also high. So, if the speed of the test tubes is high, then the horizontal component of the tension in the bars that hold the test tubes up is high too. If you call the tension T, and the angle that a test tube makes with the vertical θ, then the horizontal component of the tension is $T \sin \theta$.

When the centrifuge is going around at a constant frequency, the test tubes will be at a constant angle to the vertical; they won't be swinging up and down. Because there is no vertical motion, you know that the upward force on a test tube, which is the vertical component of the tension in the bar, must equal the downward force, which is just the weight. But the weight doesn't change when the frequency of rotation changes. So, the vertical component of the tension, which is $T \cos \theta$ must still equal the weight whether the frequency at which the rotor rotates is low or high.

We've said that $T \sin \theta$ is high when the frequency of rotation is high and that $\cos \theta$ is the same for high or low frequency. Dividing the first by the last tells you that $\tan \theta$ is high, and therefore that θ itself is high if the frequency at which the rotor turns is high.

30. B The question asks when the frequency at which the rotor rotates stops increasing. In other words, when is the rate of increase of the frequency at which the rotor rotates zero? The second paragraph of the passage tells you that the rate of increase of the frequency of rotation is proportional to the net torque. So, when the resultant torque is zero, the rate at which the frequency increases is also zero.

The frictional torque on the rotor acts to oppose the rotation, in the same way as kinetic friction opposes the linear motion of a body. Therefore the frictional torque acts in the opposite direction as the torque applied by the motor. So, if the motor makes the rotor rotate clockwise, the frictional torque will be counter-clockwise, and visa versa. Therefore, if the magnitude of the frictional torque equals the magnitude of the torque applied by the motor, then the net torque is zero, and so the frequency at which the rotor rotates does not change.

Passage V (Questions 31–36)

31. C In this question you need to understand what happens when the capacitor is fully charged. Capacitors are described in paragraph 3. When a battery is connected to a circuit containing a resistor and a capacitor in series, a current will flow; positive charge will accumulate on one plate, and an equal amount of negative charge on the other. You are also told that after a finite time the capacitor becomes fully charged. In other words, when the capacitor is fully charged, the flow of charge stops, which is the same as saying that the current is zero.

Notice that statement I appears in three out of four answer choices. If you decided it was true, it wouldn't help you very much. Look at statement II first. Statement II says that the light bulb in the circuit stops shining when the capacitor is fully charged. You've already established that a fully charged capacitor can accept no more charge on its plates, and so no more current can flow through the circuit. No current through the circuit means no current through the bulb, and therefore the bulb will not shine. Statement II is correct. So you can eliminate choices (A) and (B) since they do not contain statement II.

Statement III suggests that when the capacitor is fully charged, the voltage across the bulb equals the voltage across the battery. The current in the circuit is zero, so Ohm's law, V = IR, tells you that the voltage across the bulb will be zero too. But the voltage across the battery will definitely not be zero. You should know that the voltage across the terminals of a battery is used as a voltage source for many applications and is fairly steady. So statement III is false. Therefore, choice (C), I and II only, is correct.

By using the strategy for Roman numeral questions, you didn't even need to consider statement I, which is correct. It suggests that a voltmeter connected across the capacitor would read a constant voltage. Look again at Figure 2, which graphs voltage versus time for the charging of the capacitor. Notice that starting from zero, as time goes on the voltage increases and plateaus at some final value. Compare this with the statement in the passage which tells you that after the current has been flowing for a finite time, the capacitor becomes fully charged. Putting these two ideas together, as the capacitor is being charged, the voltage increases and reaches some final constant value when finally charged.

32. A Here you're asked to predict the voltage versus time graph when the voltmeter is placed across the battery. In most of the circuits you've seen, the battery is an element with a given voltage. In fact, it is probably the voltage source of most of the fundamental circuits you've seen. When you buy batteries for your radio, they have a voltage of, say, 9 Volts. This should point you to (A), the correct answer. Actually the voltage of a real battery may not remain completely steady during its operation. Like in most real-life situations, there are hidden complexities that you hope to avoid by looking at idealized situations. A battery typically has an internal resistance which will cause a significant drop in the output voltage if there is a large current in the circuit. You know that this won't matter to you when you answer this question, however, because there is a parenthetical note at the end of the passage that tells you that you can ignore the battery's internal resistance.

33. B Without the battery, you just have the capacitor connected to the bulb. What will happen? It was the battery that was maintaining the charge on the capacitor plates. There is now nothing preventing the positive charges built up on one plate from repelling each other, and the same is true for the negative charges built up on the other plate. This is exactly what happens; the charges on the plates repel each other, and charge flows around the circuit until everything is even again and there is no net charge on either plate of the capacitor.

When you remove the battery, the charge will leave the capacitor plates, and the capacitor will discharge. While this is happening, the moving charge will again produce a current in the circuit. This question is asking you to infer how the voltage across the capacitor varies with time as the capacitor is discharging. One way to think about this problem is to use Figure 2. It shows how the voltage varies with time as the capacitor charges. You can see that, at the beginning of the charging process, there is no voltage across the capacitor, and at the end the voltage has reached some final, constant value. In this question, exactly the opposite process is going on; you are removing charge from the capacitor's plates. So you might infer that the discharging graph would be the opposite of the charging graph in Figure 2. Indeed, initially, when the capacitor is fully charged, you know there is a potential difference across it. As the charge on the capacitor plates falls, the voltage across the capacitor falls too, and when the capacitor has been completely discharged, you know that there is no potential difference across it. From this alone you should pick choice (B).

34. A   Here you are asked to determine how the voltage across the light bulb would vary with time and why. In a series circuit, the sum of the individual voltages equals the total voltage. So, in this case, the voltage across the bulb plus the voltage across the capacitor equals the voltage of the battery. From this you know that the voltage across the bulb equals the voltage across the battery minus the voltage across the capacitor. As discussed earlier, you can assume the battery voltage to be constant. The voltage across the capacitor is shown in Figure 2. As the capacitor charges, the voltage across it increases. Therefore, the voltage across the bulb decreases as the capacitor charges. This alone tells you that answer choice (A) is correct.

You can also think of what's going on in terms of the current. As the charge on the plates increases, the capacitor resists more charge being deposited on the plates. This is because the negative charge on the negative plate repels more negative charge that is flowing to the plate, and similarly, the positive charge that is on the positive plate repels positive charge. This slows down the flow of charge around the circuit as the capacitor charges. Current is equal to rate of flow of charge. Therefore, the current through the light bulb decreases as the capacitor charges.

Ohm's law, $V = IR$, relates the voltage across the bulb, V, to the current through the bulb, I, and the resistance of the bulb, R. The note at the end of the passage tells you that you may treat the bulb's resistance as a constant. So, since the current through the bulb decreases, the voltage across the bulb also decreases.

35. D   Here you are asked to interpret the results of a slightly changed experiment. The light bulb is replaced by two identical resistors which are first in series with each other, then in parallel with each

other. What you are measuring is the total time it takes to charge the capacitor in both cases. The capacitor took less time to charge when the resistors were in parallel.

Changing the configuration of resistors changes their total resistance. In going from the series to the parallel configurations, you need to find out if you are increasing or decreasing the total resistance. Call the resistance of each bulb R. Resistors in series add directly, so $R_{total} = R + R$, which equals 2R. However, for resistors in parallel, you have to use the reciprocal formula: $1/R_{total} = 1/R + 1/R$, which equals $2/R$. So $1/R_{total} = 2/R$. Taking the inverse of this, you find that for the resistors in parallel, $R_{total} = R/2$. In series the total resistance is 2R, but in parallel it's R/2. So you've decreased the resistance in going from the series connection to the parallel connection. The question tells you that the charging time was longest for the first case, when the resistors were in series. Now you can see that as the resistance increased so did the time it took to charge the capacitor.

With this in mind, look at the answer choices. Choice (A) suggests that increasing the resistance increases the capacitance of the capacitor. If the capacitance did increase, it would explain the results you have. A capacitor with a large capacitance would take a longer time to charge up, and you do see an increase in the time it takes to charge up as the resistance of the circuit is increased. However, it's only the resistance that's getting changed in this question. How could this affect the capacitance? In the third paragraph of the passage you are told that the capacitance of a particular capacitor is constant. You couldn't change the capacitance of a capacitor by changing the circuit it was placed in; you would have to change the capacitor itself. So choice (A) is wrong.

Choice (B) says that the experiment implies that resistors affect the final voltage across the capacitor plates. Does the data in the question really imply this? All that the data in the question says is that the charging time varies; you can't deduce anything about the final voltage. So choice (B) must be wrong. In fact, the capacitor charges to the same voltage whatever the resistance of the other part of the circuit.

Choice (C) suggests that charge is absorbed by the resistors. Resistors don't absorb charge. Some of the energy of the flowing charge is certainly taken out of the circuit and converted to heat, but the charge itself is not absorbed by the resistor. Choice (C) must therefore be wrong.

Answer choice (D) suggests that resistors act to hinder the flow of charge, thus reducing the current in the circuit. As the resistance increases, the charging time increases. This means that it takes a longer time for the maximum amount of charge to be deposited on the capacitor plates. Since current is the amount of charge flowing past a given point per unit time, the current decreases as the resistance increases. So you can say that resistors do hinder the flow of charge.

36. A Here you have a circuit with two bulbs and a voltmeter connected in series. From the first paragraph of the passage, you know that this is not the proper way to connect a voltmeter. Now, instead of just measuring the voltage of a circuit element, the voltmeter will affect the circuit itself. The bulbs stop shining because the voltmeter's high resistance makes the current in the circuit small. Without enough current flowing through them, the bulbs can't shine. In a series circuit the current going through each circuit element is the same and is equal, by Ohm's law, to the voltage of the battery divided by the total resistance of the circuit. Since resistors in series add directly and the resistance of the voltmeter is so high, the total resistance of the circuit is high. Ohm's law tells you that current is inversely proportional to resistance, and so the current going through each circuit element is very low. That's why the bulbs stop shining.

Your task is to find a way to remedy that without completely removing the voltmeter. Choice (A) puts a plain wire across the voltmeter. Now the current has two paths that it can follow: it can either travel through the high resistance voltmeter or through the wire, which has little, if any, resistance. Since current tends to go down the path of least resistance, almost all of the current will flow through the wire and ignore the voltmeter. The wire bypasses the voltmeter, and in fact it's almost as if there is no voltmeter there at all; the bulbs will shine with their former brilliance. This is the correct answer.

Choice (B) shows an extra bulb placed across one of the other light bulbs. You know that the voltmeter is the circuit element that's stopping the bulbs shining. This new bulb does not even affect the voltmeter. On those grounds alone, it can be discarded.

Choice (C) shows a bulb being put over the voltmeter. Since the bulb has much less resistance than the voltmeter, it also nullifies the effect of the voltmeter. However, you want the bulbs to shine with their former brilliance. Now, instead of having a circuit with two bulbs, you have a circuit with three bulbs. Each bulb, therefore, will be somewhat dimmer than each bulb in a circuit with only two bulbs. This answer is close, but not quite right.

In choice (D), you see a circuit with a capacitor across the voltmeter. As in choices (A) and (C) when the current comes to the capacitor and voltmeter junction, it will see the capacitor as the path of least resistance and so will follow that path. Since the capacitor is initially uncharged, charge will accumulate on the plates. The flowing current will initially cause the bulbs to brighten. However, very quickly the charge on the capacitor plates will reach its maximum value and will not allow any more current to flow that way. At this point the bulbs will again stop shining.

Discrete Questions

37. D If a quantity is conserved in a reaction, the quantity has the same value before the reaction occurs as it does after the reaction. So the question is really asking: which quantity is not the same before the reaction as it is after?

The first thing to notice about the decay given in the question stem is that it is a nuclear reaction. Nuclear reactions involve the combination or splitting of nuclei. In this particular reaction, a uranium-238 nucleus splits up into a thorium-234 nucleus and an alpha particle. We know that energy is given off in nuclear reactions; here the alpha- particle carries away some kinetic energy. Where does the energy come from? Einstein's mass-energy equivalence formula, $E = mc^2$, where E is energy, m is mass, and c is the speed of light in a vacuum, tells us that mass can be converted to energy. So, in this decay, some of the mass of the uranium nucleus is converted to energy. This means that the mass on the right-hand side of the equation is less than the mass on the left, and therefore mass is not conserved. Therefore, answer choice (D) is correct.

Mass is converted to energy. Doesn't that mean that the total energy changes? No: Energy is being converted from one form to another, but the total energy remains the same. When we say mass is converted to energy in a nuclear reaction, we really mean that energy in the form of mass is converted to energy in some other form, usually kinetic energy. So the total energy remains constant. Energy conservation is a fundamental principle of physics that you should know. A familiar way of expressing the principle of energy conservation is to say: energy cannot be created or destroyed. Energy can be converted from one form to another, but total energy is always conserved. So, answer choice (C) is wrong.

Choice (A) is wrong because the total momentum of the product particles in a reaction must equal the total momentum of the reactant particles; total momentum is always conserved. Choice (B) is wrong because charge conservation is also a principle that never fails. There must always be the same net charge on the right-hand side of an equation as there is on the left. An example of how this happens is ordinary beta decay. A negatively charged electron, and a positively charged proton are created from a neutral neutron. So the total charge before equals the charge afterwards.

38. C   Each test particle will experience electrostatic forces due to the attraction or repulsion of the other charged particles. The net force on the test particle will be the vector sum of these forces. You should know that the electrostatic force between two charged particles is given by Coulomb's law: $F = kq_1q_2/r^2$, where F is the force, k is a constant, q_1 and q_2 are the absolute values of the charges on the particles, and r is the distance between the particles. Notice that this means that the electrostatic force between two charged particles depends only on the charge on the particles and the distance between

them. The direction of the force lies along a line connecting the two particles and is attractive if the charges have opposite signs and repulsive if they have the same sign.

The symmetry of the first figure means that there is zero net force on the test particle. The test particle has a charge of +q so it will be repelled by each of the three other particles. The center of an equilateral triangle is equidistant from each of the triangle's vertices so the magnitude of the force due to each particle will be the same. Again, the symmetry of the situation should make it clear that the upward pull is balanced by the downward pull and that the leftward pull is balanced by the rightward pull. Suppose that there was a net upward force on the test particle. If you rotate the triangle through 120 degrees, the direction of this net force will also be rotated with the triangle. But, because the triangle is equilateral, the diagram will be exactly the same as it was before. So, if there was a net upward force on the test particle before, there would be a net upward force now too. Therefore, there cannot have been a net upward force on the test particle to begin with. Thus, statement I is correct. Answer choices (B) and (D) must be wrong, since they don't include statement I.

To choose between answer choices (A) and (C), look at the third figure. Again the symmetry tells you that there is no net force. To see this clearly, look at the forces along the two diagonals which go through opposite corners of the square and cross in the middle, where the test particle is. First, look at the forces along the diagonal which goes from the bottom left of the square to the top right. Now, the test particle is midway between two equal charges of −2q that lie at the ends of this diagonal. So, the attractive force toward the top right is exactly balanced by the attractive force toward the bottom left, and their resultant is zero.

The forces along the diagonal that goes from the bottom right of the square to the top left balance in the same way. The positively charged test particle is midway between two particles of charge +q. So, the repulsive force due to the particle at the top left of the square is exactly balanced by the repulsive force due to the particle at the bottom right. So these two forces also add up to zero. So, the forces on the test particle in Figure 3 completely balance, and therefore there is no net force. Statement III is correct, and as is choice (C).

Even though you know choice (C) is the correct answer, take a look at statement II. It does not have the same symmetry as statement I. The distance between the test particle and the particle at the top of the square is 1 meter. But the distance of the test particle from the particles at the bottom corners of the square is greater. This lack of symmetry means that the downward force on the test particle due to repulsion by the particle at the top of the square is greater than the total upward force on the test particle due to repulsion by the bottom two particles. So the net force is not zero, and statement II is wrong.

VERBAL REASONING

The following sample Verbal Reasoning tests will help you acquire the specialized reading skills required by the MCAT. You may wish to review the MCAT Strategies section on Verbal Reasoning before taking these practice tests.

Verbal Reasoning Test One

Time—60 minutes

DIRECTIONS: Each of the passages in this test is followed by a set of questions based on the passage's content. After reading each passage decide on the one **best** response to each question. If you are unsure of an answer, eliminate the choices you know are wrong and choose from the remaining choices. You may refer to the passages while answering the questions.

Passage I

The theory of moral reasoning advanced by Lawrence Kohlberg holds that the thought processes of an individual contemplating a moral dilemma are more revealing than the person's
5 actual behavior in a real situation. On the basis of thousands of interviews attempting to probe such thought processes, Kohlberg concluded that every person passes through three distinct stages of moral reasoning—each divided into two sub-
10 stages. According to Kohlberg, the evidence shows that more persons at "higher" stages of moral reasoning are found in older age groups and that persons observed over a period of years typically advance to a higher level. Having studied subjects
15 in the United States and many other countries, Kohlberg claims cross-cultural validity for his findings.

Within Kohlberg's most basic stage of moral reasoning, the "preconventional" stage, the first sub-
20 stage is that of "punishment-obedience." An individual at this substage will justify a course of action on the basis of tangible consequences such as incurring or avoiding trouble or punishment. A more advanced but still preconventional attitude,
25 the "instrumental relativist orientation," involves reasoning on the basis of satisfying one's own desires and needs. Preconventional reasoning is most commonly observed among young children and preteens.

30 The next, or "conventional," stage is initially marked by an "interpersonal concordance" orientation, and later by an orientation toward law and order. The former is characterized by a comprehension of "good" or "bad" motives for a particu-
35 lar action; the latter is concerned not with intent but with authority as an absolute—the law must be respected at all times. Adolescents and young adults are usually conventional reasoners.

Kohlberg's final, "postconventional," stage is more
40 independent of prevailing social mores and stresses the individual's personal values. In the "social contract orientation" substage, a person takes social standards into account but not as absolutes: They are valid because agreed on by society, but
45 they apply only within a pertinent sphere and may be disregarded in appropriate circumstances. In the higher substage of "universal ethical principle orientation," abstract ideals such as human rights, justice, or equality are invoked to justify behavior;
50 deviation from socially accepted standards—even breaking one's own rules—is justifiable if one remains true to one's own underlying ethical ideals. Kohlberg asserts that most adults reason at one of the two postconventional substages.

55 There appears to be some correlation between the level of moral reasoning attained by an individual and that person's level of cognitive development; Kohlberg's theory is thus regarded as an extension of Piaget's views, which regard cognitive develop-
60 ment as occurring in successive stages from the earliest sensorimotor coordination through mastery of "concrete operations" and finally "formal operations." Piaget believed age and external stimuli pushed an individual to higher levels of cogni-
65 tive development; Kohlberg similarly claims that individuals are capable of such longitudinal movement, although he attributes advances to social development. It is important to realize, however, that Kohlberg's stages are not directly correlative
70 to behavior; what develops is not the degree to which one engages in acts one considers "right" or "wrong" but is the kind of justification offered for doing so.

GO TO THE NEXT PAGE.

1. Which of the following most accurately describes the passage?

   A. An analysis of the ways in which moral reasoning differs from behavior in real life situations
   B. A critique faulting Kohlberg's theory for not accurately predicting real behaviors
   C. A description of Kohlberg's theory of the stages of moral reasoning
   D. A consideration of that which distinguishes moral thought from immoral behavior

2. The passage suggests that an individual displaying an "interpersonal concordance" orientation would reason on the basis of:

   A. an understanding of law and order.
   B. comprehension of good and bad.
   C. respect for the concept of the social contract.
   D. consideration of the values of justice and equality.

3. Which of the following best describes Kohlberg's conception of the development of moral reasoning, as implied by the passage?

   A. Moral reasoning usually moves from concrete justifications to more abstract and personal ideals.
   B. Human behavior generally becomes increasingly moral in older age groups.
   C. People are increasingly guided by their own personal needs and desires as they mature.
   D. In general, human beings become more conservative in their moral judgments with the passing of time.

4. According to the passage, a difference between Kohlberg's views and those of Piaget is that:

   A. Kohlberg describes moral behavior while Piaget catalogues cognitive development.
   B. Piaget's stages regard actual behavior while Kohlberg's regard thought processes.
   C. Kohlberg's theory concerns cognitive development through adulthood while Piaget focuses on the development of children.
   D. Kohlberg attributes development of thought processes to social development, whereas Piaget attributes it to age and external stimuli.

5. Which of the following would most seriously weaken Kohlberg's theory?

   A. A study that shows "postconventional" reasoners sometimes decide to act against socially accepted norms
   B. A study that concludes that infants and toddlers are not capable of grasping the concept of altruism
   C. An experiment that reveals individuals reason at all three levels of Kohlberg's typology throughout life
   D. A study that strongly suggests that the development of moral reasoning and cognitive development coincide

6. The author most likely uses the phrase *longitudinal movement* (lines 66–67) to mean:

   A. advancement to progressively higher levels of reasoning.
   B. lateral motion between different substages.
   C. exhibition of increasingly moral behavior.
   D. alternation between moral and cognitive development.

GO TO THE NEXT PAGE.

7. Which of the following might be indicative of a person in the "conventional" stage of moral reasoning?

   A. A driver who runs a red light in order to reach an appointment in good time
   B. A clerk who witnesses but doesn't report an impoverished woman's shoplifting
   C. A person who believes that police should use whatever means necessary to maintain order
   D. A counterfeiter who flees the country when his scheme is brought to light

8. The last sentence of the passage (lines 68–73) implies that Kohlberg's theory:

   A. helps only in understanding the motives behind moral behavior.
   B. is flawed by its inability to predict specific behavior.
   C. is most concerned with the rationalization of behavior.
   D. is ultimately inferior to the developmental theories of Piaget.

Passage II

Cloud-to-ground lightning occurs when a discrepancy in electric charge develops between a cloud and the Earth. When this discrepancy reaches a certain breakdown potential, a surge of electric
5　charge, known as lightning, rushes suddenly between the negative and positive charge centers. By preventing the requisite charge polarization, scientists hope someday to discourage the creation of cloud-to-ground lightning.

10　Many authorities theorize that the charging process occurs when a supercooled water droplet (a droplet whose temperature has fallen below 0°C but has not yet frozen) collides with an ice particle of precipitation size (a hailstone). At the moment of
15　contact, a large portion of the droplet freezes, while a smaller portion, still in its supercooled state, breaks away. As a result, a negative charge is left on the hailstone and a positive charge on the supercooled droplet. Responding to gravity, the relative-
20　ly heavy hailstone then falls, while updrafts carry the extremely light, supercooled droplet to higher regions of the cloud. Assuming the veracity of this account of charge separation, scientists speculate

that they will be able to discourage polarization by
25　reducing the quantity of supercooled water in a cloud. Many scientists have conducted preliminary seeding experiments. These experiments attempt to freeze excess water by dropping large quantities of dry ice and silver iodide into potential thunder-
30　clouds. The results of these experiments, however, are still inconclusive.

Bernard Vonnegut and Charles B. Moore offer a different account of the polarization process. They contend that the primary cause of electrical charge
35　formation in clouds is the capture of ionized (electrically charged) gas molecules by water droplets. According to the theory, the droplets absorb the ionized gas molecules and are then transported by updrafts and downdrafts to various portions of the
40　cloud. In support of their explanation of cloud polarization, they conducted a series of space charge experiments. After suspending a high-voltage wire above nine miles of Illinois countryside, they released large quantities of ions into the
45　atmosphere below forming clouds. Airplanes specially equipped for electrical measurements determined that the ions were actually distributed to different regions of the clouds. Vonnegut and Moore suggest that, in order to combat the effects
50　of this transport of ions, it would be necessary to modify the properties of ions beneath accumulating clouds.

9. Which of the following best summarizes the main point of the passage?

   A. Several recent breakthroughs have increased our understanding of the causes of lightning.
   B. Charge polarization in clouds can result both from the freezing of supercooled droplets and from modifying the properties of ions.
   C. The standard explanation of the causes of lightning is inaccurate and should be modified.
   D. Scientists have not yet agreed on the causes of cloud-to-ground lightning or the methods of controlling it.

GO TO THE NEXT PAGE.

10. It can be inferred that the term *breakdown potential* (line 4) refers to:

   A. a charge polarity sufficient to cause lightning.
   B. the intensity of the lightning bolt.
   C. the distance between the negatively charged earth and the positively charged cloud.
   D. the duration of the lightning event.

11. Scientists agree that lightning can occur when:

   A. ions are transported by updrafts to higher regions of a thundercloud.
   B. supercooled droplets collide with hailstones in clouds.
   C. a difference in charge exists between a cloud and the ground.
   D. dry ice is released into a potential thundercloud.

12. The accounts of cloud polarization in paragraphs two and three differ with respect to:

   I. the role of gas ions in causing polarization.
   II. the ability of water droplets to carry an electrical charge.
   III. whether air currents play a part in the process of polarization.

   A. I only
   B. III only
   C. I and II only
   D. II and III only

13. All of the following statements are consistent with the account of cloud polarization offered by Vonnegut and Moore EXCEPT:

   A. Ions are the major cause of electrification in clouds.
   B. Charge is transported within clouds via updrafts and downdrafts.
   C. Lightning is caused by a discrepancy in electric charge between a cloud and the ground.
   D. Lightning occurs when positively and negatively charged droplets are absorbed by hailstones.

14. It can be inferred that in relation to their theory of charge polarization in clouds, Vonnegut and Moore's space charge experiments:

   A. provided supporting but not conclusive evidence for the theory.
   B. definitively proved the theory.
   C. greatly weakened the theory.
   D. disproved a competing theory and thus indirectly strengthened Vonnegut and Moore's theory.

Passage III

The generation of British writers who participated in the First World War are often considered a group, united as they were by university educations and upper class backgrounds, as well as their
5   shared sense of the horror and absurdity of the world's first thoroughly mechanized war. The "Great War" combined nearly unimaginable destruction (in the quietest intervals, 7,000 British soldiers were killed or wounded daily) with sheer
10 inanity or seemingly interminable trench stalemate. The writer/officer was in an ideal position to witness the farcical polarities of such a war: the idealism of the newly enlisted soldier and the cynicism of the veteran; the peaceful French countryside
15 and the nightmare of bombardment; the earnest battle strategies and the stagnation of perpetual conflict. Paul Fussell, in *The Great War and Modern Memory,* asserts that to these writers "the great tragic satire which was the war [was] seen to con-
20 sist of its own smaller constituent satires, or ironic actions."

Irony was the formal strategy chosen by each author as he confronted the war on paper. Fussell notes that this device, unprecedented in the litera-
25 ture of war, allowed the "trench writers" to avoid both sentimentality and understatement—either of which would have diminished the tragic absurdity of the situation. Ironic detachment provided the psychological distance necessary to commit to
30 paper what was almost beyond description.

Frequently, the ironic mode was used to intensify the horror rather than to offset it. One reads of saturation bombing, bayonetting, and gassing within a world incongruously filled with poppies, gardens,

GO TO THE NEXT PAGE.

sheep, and shepherds. By casting modern carnage
in the pastoral imagery familiar from a long English
poetic tradition, these authors deepened the sense
of brutal paradox. Thus, as Fussell notes, Wilfred
Owen's metaphor of "the shrill, demented choirs
40 of wailing shells" both "gauges the obscenity of
industrialized murder and returns us for a fleeting
instant to the pastoral world where the choirs consist of benign insects and birds." Where Owen suggested this pastoral tradition only through allusion,
45 Edmund Blunden, in *Understones of War,* describes
the havoc wreaked on an actual pastoral setting:
"The greensward, suited by nature for the raising
of sheep, was all holes, and new ones appeared
with a great uproar as we passed."

50 The imprint of the Great War on literary sensibility
proved indelible; in different ways, the writers of
the Second World War, and even of Korea and
Vietnam, drew on the ironic tradition forged in the
trenches of France.

15. The author is primarily concerned with:

    A. synthesizing divergent interpretations of a
       school of writing.
    B. debunking a currently fashionable
       interpretation of a group of writers.
    C. describing a literary response to a histori-
       cal event.
    D. proposing a methodology for literary
       investigation.

16. The author would most probably assert that:

    A. the use of nature imagery to describe vio-
       lence was a novel approach to an artistic
       problem.
    B. the use of traditional imagery by the war
       writers expressed their sentimentality.
    C. irony was an inappropriate device for
       portraying the destruction of war.
    D. the upper class backgrounds of the
       "trench writers" strongly influenced their
       reaction to the war.

17. The author quotes Paul Fussell in paragraph
one in order to:

    A. present evidence of the tremendous
       destructiveness of the war.
    B. distinguish between two aspects of the
       war experience.
    C. show that World War I was a tragic satire.
    D. introduce the point that irony was central
       to the literary response to the war.

18. The author suggests that Wilfred Owen's
description of a shelling (lines 39–40):

    A. employed completely unfamiliar
       techniques and imagery.
    B. failed to express the violence of war.
    C. was successful primarily because of its use
       of naturalistic description.
    D. fused distinct elements into an effective
       description of violence.

19. The author would probably characterize
Edmund Blunden's technique, in comparison
to Wilfred Owen's, as more:

    A. direct.
    B. passionate.
    C. innovative.
    D. startling.

20. According to the passage, the literature of the
Second World War, Korea, and Vietnam
demonstrate the:

    A. uniqueness of the literature of each histor-
       ical period.
    B. radical changes in literary tone that fol-
       lowed World War I.
    C. continuity of the ironic sensibility.
    D. imitativeness of later war literature.

GO TO THE NEXT PAGE.

21. According to the passage, all of the following stimulated the "trench writers" to adopt the ironic mode EXCEPT their:

   A. experience of the war as a series of sharp contrasts.
   B. involvement in a war of unprecedented death and destruction.
   C. need to detach themselves from the battle conditions.
   D. refusal to take the tragic aspects of the war seriously.

22. The author of this passage would probably find most value in a study of a writer's work that:

   A. related the work to the writer's childhood experience.
   B. analyzed the writer's use of formal literary devices.
   C. stressed the work's impact on the public events of the time.
   D. showed how the writer responded artistically to important events of the time.

Passage IV

Until recently, most scientists believed that memory inevitably deteriorates with age. One commonly cited example of this deterioration is the fact that elderly people often cannot remember recent
5 events, even though they may recall details from the distant past. But contemporary research into how the mind stores and retrieves information refutes the notion of the inevitable decline in memory. New studies suggest that we have more
10 than one kind of memory, and imply that elderly people who suffer from forgetfulness can utilize other types of memory to compensate for the decline.

This new conception of memory stems from a shift
15 in methodology of memory research. While older studies of memory and aging involved comparisons among different age groups, recent investigations tested the same group of people over a number of years. Such longitudinal data more
20 clearly establishes the relationship between memory and aging. Through these studies of older adults, researchers concluded that there exist three major kinds of memory, only one of which declines in old age.

25 Previous investigations into the workings of memory usually tested "episodic" memory, which describes the recall of specific events as well as the ability to remember names and the whereabouts of items like car keys. This ability usually remains
30 intact until the mid-sixties, when people often become forgetful of things like recent events and minor details. While some researchers suggest that this well known decline in episodic memory in the elderly stems from degeneration of the frontal
35 lobes of the brain, many scientists believe that such memory loss is largely due to retirement: After the demands of work stop, most people no longer exercise their mental faculties as strenuously. Thus, regular mental exercise might curtail memory loss.

40 But episodic memory comprises only part of this intricate brain function. Memory researchers have identified two other types of memory, neither of which seems to deteriorate with age. "Semantic" memory, which describes our ability to recall
45 knowledge and facts as well as events in the distant past, does not seem to lessen over the course of a lifetime. In fact, such memory may be even sharper in elderly people than in the young or middle-aged. When a group of men and women in their
50 sixties were tested on a specific vocabulary list and retested on the same list a decade later, the group had improved their scores by an average of six words—an increase researchers consider substantial. Such studies suggest that by taking notes or
55 mulling over events, elderly people who suffer from forgetfulness can store more information in the semantic memory, thus compensating for episodic memory loss.

A third type of memory, "implicit" memory, deals
60 with the tremendous variety of mental activities we perform without making any intentional effort. Examples of these include actions like driving a car, touch-typing, or riding a bicycle. Scientists have learned through observations of amnesiacs that
65 this type of memory is distinct from both episodic and semantic memory. In one such study, an amnesiac patient who had been an avid golfer before developing a memory problem remembered which club to use for each stroke; however,

GO TO THE NEXT PAGE.

he forgot that he had played a hole within minutes of having done so. In addition, further studies of amnesiacs have shown that people with these disorders can learn new facts but cannot remember when and where they had learned them. Studies of people in their sixties and seventies showed similar results: Like amnesiacs, older people are able to learn from new experience as well as younger people, but often have difficulty remembering the source of their knowledge or skill.

Such studies into the structure of memory shed new light on the problems of memory loss in the aged. While the findings are encouraging, it must be noted that such studies do not deal with memory problems associated with illness, disease, or injury to the brain.

23. The passage implies that advanced age might adversely affect which of the following?

   I. Memory of details of a recent conversation
   II. Recollection of childhood memories
   III. Ability to perform routine tasks

   A. I only
   B. II only
   C. III only
   D. I and II only

24. The primary purpose of the passage is to:

   A. discuss the ways in which a new theory of memory challenges common assumptions regarding memory and aging.
   B. explain why past investigations into memory tested only episodic memory.
   C. describe recent research into the functioning of the brain.
   D. consider the reasons episodic memory diminishes in later years.

25. It can be inferred from the passage that recent developments in memory research can be attributed largely to:

   A. scientists' efforts to dismantle stereotypes regarding the abilities of elderly people.
   B. recent discoveries that distinguish age-related forgetfulness from disease and injury-related memory loss.
   C. the realization that mental exercise frequently diminishes memory loss.
   D. new methodologies that clarify the relationship between memory and aging.

26. According to the passage, older people often forget recent events but remember the distant past because:

   A. childhood events exist as part of implicit memory.
   B. episodic memory declines while implicit memory does not.
   C. episodic memory declines but semantic memory improves with age.
   D. retired elderly people make few demands on their semantic memory.

27. The passage suggests that an elderly person who cannot remember how to tie her shoes is most probably suffering from:

   A. amnesia.
   B. semantic memory loss.
   C. episodic memory loss.
   D. implicit memory loss.

28. Which of the following provides the best concluding sentence for the passage?

   A. Since many elderly people suffer from such organic dysfunctions, memory research remains more theoretical than practical.
   B. However, scientists hope that these studies will contribute to our understanding of these disorders as well.
   C. It is likely that researchers will turn toward these more critical problems in the near future.
   D. Since such disorders do not conform to the tripartite model of memory, most researchers are not interested in them.

GO TO THE NEXT PAGE.

Passage V

The harbor seal, *Phoca vitulina,* is a member of the order *Pinnepedia,* and lives amphibiously along the northern Atlantic and Pacific coasts. This extraordinary mammal, which does most of its fishing at
5 night when visibility is low and where noise levels are high, has developed several unique adaptations that have sharpened its visual and acoustic acuity. The need for such adaptations has been compounded by the varying behavior of sound
10 and light in each of the two habitats of the harbor seal—land and water.

While the seal is on land, its ear operates much like that of the human, with sound waves traveling through air and entering the inner ear through the
15 auditory canal. The directions from which sounds originate are distinguishable because the sound waves arrive at each inner ear at different times. In water, however, where sound waves travel faster than they do in air, the ability of the brain to dif-
20 ferentiate arrival times between each ear is severely reduced. Yet it is crucial for the seal to be able to pinpoint the exact origins of sound in order to locate both its offspring and prey. Therefore, through processes of adaptation to the demands
of its environment, the seal has developed an
25 extremely sensitive quadrophonic hearing system, composed of a specialized band of tissue that extends down from the ear to the inner ear. In water, sound is conducted to the seal's inner ear by this special band of tissue, making it possible for
30 the seal to identify the exact origins of sounds.

The eye of the seal is also uniquely adapted to operate in both air and water. The human eye, adapted to function primarily in air, is equipped with a cornea, which aids in the refraction and
35 focusing of light onto the retina. As a result, when a human eye is submerged in water, light rays are further refracted and the image is blurry. The seal's cornea, however, has a refractive index similar to that of water. Therefore, in water light rays are
40 transmitted by the cornea without distortion, and are clearly focused on the retina. In air, however, the cornea is astigmatic. The result is a distortion of incoming light rays. The seal compensates for this by having a stenopaic pupil, which constricts into

45 a vertical slit. Since the astigmatism is most pronounced in the horizontal plane of the eye, the vertical nature of the pupil serves to minimize its effect on the seal's vision.

Because the harbor seal procures its food under
50 conditions of low visibility, some scientists hypothesize that harbor seals have an echolocation system akin to the sensory capabilities of bats, porpoises, and dolphins. This kind of natural and instinctual radar involves the emission of high-
55 frequency sound pulses that reflect off obstacles such as predators, prey, or natural barriers. The reflections are received as sensory signals by the brain, which interp rets them and processes them into an image. The animal, blinded by unfavorable
60 surroundings or lighting conditions, is thus able to perceive its surroundings. Scientists believe that echolocation in the harbor seal is suggested by the fact that these seals emit clicks, high-frequency sounds produced in short, fast bursts that occur
65 mostly at night, when visual acuity is low.

Finally, there is speculation that the seal's vibrissae, or whiskers, act as sensory receptors. Evidence for this is found in the fact that vibrissae are unusually well developed in *Pinnepedia* and are highly sensi-
70 tive to movement. Scientists hypothesize that the vibrissae may be instrumental in catching prey and, because they are sensitive to vibrations, may sense wave disturbances produced by nearby moving fish, allowing the seal to home in on and
75 capture prey.

Having met the sensory demands of dual habitats, the harbor seal is one of the most interesting animals on Earth. Its amphibious existence has demanded a sensory acuity and flexibility matched
80 by few other mammals.

29. According to the passage, scientists think vibrissae help harbor seals to catch prey by:

   A. improving underwater vision.
   B. sensing aerial vibrations.
   C. camouflaging predator seals.
   D. detecting underwater movement.

GO TO THE NEXT PAGE.

30. The passage implies that a harbor seal's vision is:

    A. inferior to a human's vision in the water, but superior to it on land.
    B. superior to a human's vision in the water, but inferior to it on land.
    C. inferior to a human's vision both in the water and on land.
    D. equivalent to a human's vision both in the water and on land.

31. The passage supplies information for answering which of the following questions?

    A. Why does the harbor seal do most of its fishing at night?
    B. What proportion of the harbor seal's time is spent on land?
    C. Do all types of seals in the *Pinnepedia* order live amphibiously?
    D. How does the harbor seal's eye compensate for the distortion of light rays on land?

32. Which of the following would most strengthen the claim that harbor seals hunt down prey by echolocation?

    A. The harbor seal's eye has become increasingly efficient underwater over time.
    B. Harbor seals rely on their vibrissae to sense prey at close range and do most of their hunting within very limited areas.
    C. Other members of their order of species are known to possess the facility of echolocation.
    D. Harbor seals are not closely related to bats, porpoises, or dolphins.

33. The author compares harbor seal sensory organs with human sensory organs primarily in order to:

    A. point out similarities among mammals.
    B. explain how the seal's sensory organs function.
    C. show that seals are related to humans.
    D. prove that seals are more adaptively successful than humans.

34. The author of this passage is most likely a:

    A. paleontologist.
    B. zoologist.
    C. taxonomist.
    D. geneticist.

35. According to the passage, harbor seals are found in:

    A. many arctic regions.
    B. most areas with abundant fish populations.
    C. most island and coastal regions.
    D. some North American coastal regions.

GO TO THE NEXT PAGE.

Roman Italy was a world of small communities. Hundreds of small cities, towns, and villages dotted the Italian peninsula, each with a slightly different landscape, history, and social and economic structure, but all sharing certain political, social, and economic institutions, physical structures, and rituals of daily life.

Without this structure of rural communities, the Roman Empire could not have existed. Primitive communications and an underdeveloped bureaucracy made a highly centralized government impossible. The largely autonomous communities maintained civic order on the local level. The local community should therefore be seen as a key element in the success of the Roman system.

In spite of the ubiquity and importance of these local communities, they have been rather neglected in recent Roman historical research. The reasons for this are complex and tell us much about the development of Roman historical and archaeological studies. The neglect began with the ancient Romans themselves. Although many Roman writers were born in the small towns of Italy, most migrated at a relatively young age to the capital. They concentrated their attention on the society and events of the city of Rome and on the major political and military events that shaped the Republic and the Empire. Like urbanites the world over, they had little interest in the daily life of the small towns.

Modern students of ancient Rome have not treated this local society much more kindly . . . . The mainstream of ancient historical studies during the eighteenth, nineteenth, and twentieth centuries has been directed to the reconstruction of a national Roman history. This suited the predilections of increasingly professional scholars who viewed Roman history as elite, institutional, and legal history concerned with consuls, generals, and emperors, rather than decuriones and small-town shopkeepers. One important exception to this trend was the great Russian historian Michael Rostovtzeff. He was very much interested in the smaller Roman city with its local bourgeoisie and he tied closely the fate of the larger Empire to the rise and fall of that socioeconomic class. He appreciated the importance of the archaeological remains at a site like Pompeii for understanding aspects of Roman society little reflected written record. Yet Rostovtzeff had few true followers . . . .

Roman agricultural history, and especially the changes in rural social and economic structures that took place during the later Republic has, however, received considerable attention. This was a topic that happened to interest the ancient, and modern historians attended to their concerns. Such distinguished social scientists as Max Weber have done research on Roman agrarian history. The debate also included the related issues of Roman slavery and the development of a colonate during the later Empire. Marxist scholars were attracted to these topics, which highlighted class oppression and conflict. Partly as a result of this Marxist concern, we have an especially rich bibliography on such topics as Roman slavery, slave revolts, and the rise of the great estates. Although the Marxist models have sometimes distorted our reconstructions of Roman rural life, there is no question that the approach has stimulated much important research.

Recently, more scholarly attention has been focused on the Roman commercial economy. Research has centered on such questions as the nature of senatorial investment in commerce, the development of sea-borne trade, the rise of major trading center such as Puteoli and Ostia, and even the degree to which the Roman economy can be considered "modern." Less attention has been paid to the development of the regional and local economies and to the combined use of literary, epigraphical, and archaeological information to answer questions related to these local systems.

GO TO THE NEXT PAGE.

36. The author of this passage would most likely urge support for historical research involving:

   A. Marxist models of social and economic analysis.
   B. a synthesis of archaeological and other nonliterary evidence with literary evidence.
   C. investigations into the genealogies of eminent Roman families.
   D. a reconstruction of the operations of the central bureaucracies that collected taxes and administered justice.

37. The amount of modern scholarship on Roman agriculture suggests that:

   A. modern scholars often reflect the interests of ancient writers.
   B. modern scholars have actually had long-standing interests in the rural communities of Roman Italy.
   C. modern scholars have had little interest in the rural communities of Roman Italy.
   D. modern scholars have tended to have elitist interests.

38. "The neglect [that] began with the ancient Romans themselves" (lines 21–22) refers to the:

   A. Romans' inability to centralize political power.
   B. incompetence of historians and archaeologists.
   C. urban mind-set of the major Roman writers.
   D. proclivities of recent scholars of Roman history.

39. Suppose that a single, previously unknown artifact from ancient Roman Italy could be unearthed at whim. Which of the following would be most useful to the sort of study that the author seeks to undertake?

   A. A well preserved plough.
   B The records of an ancient town council.
   C. A trading ship that had been sunk with a full cargo.
   D. A cache of swords and spears.

40. In the context of the passage, the word *decuriones* (line 40) refers to:

   A. important military officers.
   B. slaves and impoverished peasants.
   C. local political leaders.
   D. powerful noblemen.

STOP. IF YOU FINISH BEFORE TIME HAS EXPIRED, CHECK YOUR WORK. YOU MAY GO BACK TO ANY QUESTION IN THIS PART ONLY.

Verbal Reasoning Test One: Answers and Explanations

ANSWER KEY

1. C	16. A	31. D
2. B	17. D	32. C
3. A	18. D	33. B
4. D	19. A	34. B
5. C	20. C	35. D
6. A	21. D	36. B
7. C	22. D	37. A
8. C	23. A	38. D
9. D	24. A	39. B
10. A	25. D	40. C
11. C	26. C	
12. A	27. D	
13. D	28. B	
14. A	29. D	
15. C	30. B	

Passage I (Questions 1–8): KOHLBERG

1. C This question asks about the primary purpose of the passage. The author's tone is merely descriptive, and his topic is the stages of Kohlberg's theory of the stages of moral reasoning, so (C) answers this question. The last paragraph of the passage cautions that Kohlberg's theory concerns the justifications behind behaviors but does not describe the behaviors themselves; since the author never compares moral reasoning and behavior in real life situations, neither (A) nor (D) accurately describes the main purpose of the passage. Choice (B) is incorrect because it suggests the author criticizes Kohlberg's theory, whereas he merely describes the theory without judging it.

2. B In paragraph three, "interpersonal concordance" is characterized by comprehension of "good" and "bad" motives (B); it is the first of the two substages of Kohlberg's "conventional" stage of moral reasoning. An understanding of law and order (A) is the second substage of the conventional orientation, which an individual in the interperson-

al concordance orientation would not yet comprehend. Similarly, respect for the concept of the social contract (C) and consideration of the values of justice and equality (D) are the two substages of Kohlberg's most advanced orientation—the postconventional stage; since this follows the conventional stage, the individual displaying an interpersonal concordance orientation would not reason on a postconventional basis.

3. A To answer this question, which asks about the overall pattern of the development of moral reasoning, you need to make an inference based upon the specific stages Kohlberg creates. Paragraph two describes the preconventional stage as based on tangible consequences; paragraph three sketches the conventional stage as characterized by a comprehension of simple concepts; and paragraph four describes the postconventional stage as one based on principles, values and abstract ideals. Therefore, (A) correctly describes a progression from concrete justifications to abstract and personal ideals. (B) concerns human behavior, whereas the last paragraph clearly states that Kohlberg's theory concerns justifications for behavior, not actual behaviors themselves. (C), suggests that people are increasingly guided by their own needs as they mature, but Kohlberg characterizes such an orientation in paragraph two as common to young children and preteens, not adults. (D) is wrong because Kohlberg's theory does not discuss conservative or liberal moral judgements; again, his theory concerns patterns of moral reasoning.

4. D The fifth paragraph compares Kohlberg's views to those of Piaget. Since Kohlberg's views regard moral development and thought processes rather than behavior, (A) is wrong in suggesting that Kohlberg's theory has to do with moral behavior. (B) suggests that Piaget's theory regards actual behavior, which the passage neither states nor implies in its discussion of cognitive development. Nor does the author suggest that Piaget focuses on the development of children, while Kohlberg studies adults (C): The passage implies that both theorists are concerned with cognitive development throughout life. Only (D) correctly contrasts the theories of Kohlberg and Piaget—the author clearly states in paragraph five that Piaget considers age and external stimuli as factors leading to cognitive development, while Kohlberg claims that social development is responsible for the development of thought processes.

5. C This application question asks you to consider statements that might weaken Kohlberg's theory. Paragraph four discusses the postconventional stage of reasoning, which stresses personal values and abstract ideals; (A), then, describes reasoning in accordance with Kohlberg's depiction of this stage. Kohlberg claims in paragraph two that young children reason on the basis of their own needs and desires, so a study concluding that infants and toddlers cannot grasp the concept of altruism jibes with the description of this early stage of reasoning (B). The first sentence of the fifth paragraph states that there seems to be a correlation between the development of moral reasoning and cognitive development. Therefore, (D) would merely emphasize the similarities between Kohlberg's and Piaget's views and would not have the effect of weakening Kohlberg's theory. But since the author states in the first paragraph that we pass through three distinct stages of moral reasoning as we age, (C) would weaken Kohlberg's theory because it suggests that individuals do not progress according to Kohlberg's—or any particular—pattern.

6. A The author mentions longitudinal movement in the last paragraph. The very sentence containing this phrase suggests that longitudinal movement refers to the advancement through progressively higher levels of reasoning. (B) is incorrect because "longitudinal" suggests vertical motion, not lateral, horizontal, motion; furthermore, this paragraph concerns advancement up and through more advanced stages, not movements across and between substages. The first and last sentences of the passage emphasize that Kohlberg's theory concerns not actual behavior, but justifications for behavior, so (C) is wrong. The first sentence of paragraph five does suggest a "correlation" between

one's level of moral development as related to cognitive development, but the author never suggests any alternating pattern of development, so (D) is wrong. See paragraph three, which discusses Kohlberg's conventional stage as marked by a basic understanding of "good" and "bad," and later by a concept of law and order.

7. C (C) correctly describes a person in this stage, who would conceivably support any police action because of an unwavering belief in the need for lawful order. A driver who runs a red light (A) is likely considering his or her own needs, which is indicative of preconventional, not conventional reasoning. (D) also describes preconventional reasoning, based on an even more basic desire to avoid punishment. (B) describes postconventional reasoning in that it indicates a deviation from socially acceptable standards, justified by underlying ethical codes.

8. C To answer this question you need to consider the author's tone as well as the information contained in the last sentence of the passage. The author notes that Kohlberg's theory does not concern behavior but the justifications behind behavior. He does this not to criticize the theory but to clarify the theory's focus on the rationalization of behavior, choice (C). Both choices (B) and (D) imply that the author is criticizing Kohlberg's theory, and are therefore incorrect. Choice (A) is wrong because it incorrectly suggests that Kohlberg's theory is only concerned with the motivations leading to moral behavior, whereas the author is interested in the motivations behind behavior in general.

Passage II (Questions 9–14):
LIGHTNING

9. D Paragraph one introduces the topic: Charge polarization and its application to controlling cloud-to-ground lightning. Each of the next two paragraphs sums up a competing theory about charge potential and its possible application to controlling lightning. Neither theory gains the author's endorsement. All this leads to choice (D). While the author doesn't directly state this idea, (D) sums up the content of the passage. None of the other choices is quite accurate, and none hits the main point. In (A), there are no "recent breakthroughs"; neither theory has been confirmed, and only one has experimental support. We have *not* come closer to understanding the causes of lightning. (Also—minor point—the passage discusses only cloud-to-ground lightning.) Choice (B) is a detail (charge polarization is only part of the topic), and it's inaccurate: The supercooled droplets (in paragraph two) collide with hailstones, and the gas molecules (in paragraph three) are already ionized when they are absorbed by water droplets. (C) is wrong because neither theory is standard; the background material in paragraph one *may* be a standard theory, but it's never questioned.

10. A See sentences two and three. Lightning occurs when the "breakdown potential," later referred to as the "requisite charge polarization," is reached. Breakdown potential is the condition for lightning to occur, rather than a characteristic of the lightning (B, D). Distance between the cloud and the earth (C) is not mentioned.

11. C Scientists do not agree on what causes the difference in charge, but they do agree that lightning occurs when charge differences of the requisite magnitude exist between a cloud and the ground. All of the other answer choices refer to the various theories put forward to explain charge polarization—on which there is no agreement. (A) and (B) sum up the theories delineated in paragraphs three and two, respectively. (D) is even further from the mark, as it refers to a phase of the experiments designed to test the contested theories. Absolutely no one proposes that lightning occurs under the circumstances described in this choice.

12. A Gas ions (I) are involved only in the Vonnegut-Moore theory (paragraph three); paragraph two proposes that the electrical charges are carried by water droplets and hailstones, with no mention of gas ions. Hence, option I identifies a difference between the theories. Both theories, however, involve charged water droplets, the charge occurring in paragraph two through the interaction with hailstones and in paragraph three through the capture of ions. Both also involve air currents—updrafts in paragraph two, updrafts and downdrafts in paragraph three. Options II and III are therefore not matters of controversy.

13. D See paragraph three. Choices (A) and (B) paraphrase information in the first and second sentences of that paragraph, respectively. (C) is the underlying fact that is the basis for all theories of cloud polarization—and is specifically mentioned in the first paragraph. (D), however, is incorrect. Hailstones figure only in the theory summarized in paragraph two; moreover, (D) gets even that theory wrong—the droplets have no net charge until they dissociate from the hailstones and become positively charged.

14. A Relate detail questions to the main idea! If you simply remember that two competing theories are presented but neither is proved, choices (B), (C), and (D) can be discarded immediately. More specifically, Vonnegut and Moore theorized (sentence two of paragraph three) that ions are absorbed by water droplets and then transported within the clouds by updrafts and downdrafts. The space charge experiments are said to have shown that "the ions were being distributed to differing regions of the clouds." Clearly this supports their theory rather than weakens it (C). It has no bearing on the competing "supercooled droplets" theory (D), since that theory doesn't deal with ion transport at all. But, the experimental result shows only that ions are moving, not that they have been captured by water droplets, or that this is the prime cause of charge polarization, so the experienced result is not definitive proof of Vonnegut and Moore's theory but only supporting evidence. Use the process of elimination to get to the correct answer, choice (A).

Passage III (Questions 15–22): WAR POETS

15. C   Since the passage examines a group of writers in terms of their common literary responses to World War I, (C) is the correct choice. Choice (A) is wrong because no divergent interpretations are given (only Fussell's views are presented) and the author makes no attempt to synthesize different views. In (B), even if Fussell's interpretation is now in fashion (and we don't know), the author doesn't debunk it; in general, loaded words like this one are usually wrong in MCAT reading. The author does not propose any methodology (D), or even describe Fussell's methodology except to note that Fussell describes the writers' use of irony.

16. A   The "artistic problem" in this choice is the one raised by the "farcical polarities," the "tragic satire" of war (paragraph one). Nature imagery that describes violence is part of the ironic approach to this dilemma (paragraph three), and this approach as a whole is described as "unprecedented in the literature of war" (paragraph two) and hence new, or novel. The author seems to admire the "trench writers," both as a school and as individuals, and to feel, with Fussell, that their use of irony is justified by its effectiveness in conveying the tragedy. This eliminates choice (C). The upper-class backgrounds of the writers (D) are referred to only in passing (first paragraph), not described as a strong influence on their work. If we take the "traditional imagery" of (B) to mean the pastoral imagery of Owen and others, then its use as an ironic counterpoint to scenes of violence frees it from sentimental overtones; the author describes this technique as an alternative to sentimentality.

17. D   The Fussell quote in paragraph one contains the first mention of irony in the passage; it introduces the idea of irony as a literary approach to tragic events, a theme developed in the rest of the passage. Paragraph one does present evidence of the destructiveness of the war (A), but not in the Fussell quote—the evidence is factual and comes in the second and third sentences. Paragraph one also talks about the "farcical polarities" of the war; these are not quite the same as the "two aspects" in choice (B), and in any case, the Fussell quote

doesn't distinguish between them—it comments on the ironic character of the polarities. Choice (C) is too flatfooted; yes, Fussell comments that the war was a tragic satire, but this isn't the real point even of his own statement (Fussell's point is that the big satire consisted of many smaller satires) and it's not the author's point in quoting Fussell.

18. D   The "distinct elements" in this choice are the "obscenity of industrialized murder" and the benignity of the pastoral world evoked by the references to "choirs." The author, following Fussell, shows that Owen fused these elements in one image, which the author implies was an effective one. Of the wrong choices, (A) is tempting because the passage does stress that the trench writers' use of irony was novel but the imagery was not unfamiliar—part of Owen's irony lay in using very familiar imagery in a new way. The author implies that Owen's "shrill, demented choirs of wailing shells" expressed violence very effectively (B). (C) might apply more to Blunden than to Owen, whose effectiveness, the author suggests, lies mainly in his metaphors.

19. A   We're told that Owen suggests the pastoral tradition through allusion—which is an indirect reference to something familiar to the reader that is not mentioned directly. Blunden, on the other hand, "describes...an actual pastoral setting." Blunden's contrast between the pastoral and the violent, then, is a direct one, while Owen's is indirect (A). The author says nothing to imply that he or she considers Blunden's approach more impassioned, original, or surprising choices (B), (C) and (D).

20. C The short final paragraph says that the imprint of the Great War (an ironic imprint, as we've seen) was "indelible" and that later writers "drew on the ironic tradition" forged in the trenches. Clearly, the ironic sensibility of the trench writers reappeared in the work of these later writers. This eliminates (A) and (B); each literary period may be unique in some ways, and no doubt changes did follow World War I, but the author is stressing continuity here. The author doesn't, however, suggest that later writers were merely "imitative," (D)—they drew on the ironic tradition in different ways.

21. D Choice (A) refers to the "polarities" set up in paragraph one. (B) only slightly paraphrases the second sentence of that paragraph. The necessity for psychological distance (C) and its achievement through ironic detachment are summarized in the final sentence of paragraph two. (D) is the correct choice—their "shared sense of horror and absurdity" in the first paragraph becomes the "indelible imprint" of the last. Throughout the passage, it is evident that the writers' ironic treatment came about not because they didn't feel pain, but on the contrary, because they did.

22. D You should assume that the author would find value in a study that approached a writer's work in the same way that the author has already done in the passage. The author's basic concern is to show how certain writers reflected a key event of the time—World War I—in their works. Only two choices mention public events, (C) and (D). (C) is something the author never tries to do in this passage; there is no indication of what impact the trench writers' works had on public events, or even that they had any. (In reality, their works did affect English views of the war, about 10 years after the event; our author does not mention this.) (D), on the other hand, is exactly the angle the author has chosen to explore in the passage; presumably, another study that did the same for another writer would seem similarly valuable to this passage's author. Of the other wrong choices, (B) has something going for it because of the author's stress on the use of irony; overall, though, this passage is not one that concentrates on the trench writers' formal techniques, so (B) is not a good choice. Choice (A) is easy to get rid of—the author says nothing about these writers' childhood experiences.

Passage IV (Questions 23–28): MEMORY

23. A The third paragraph of the passage states that only episodic memory deteriorates with age. The first sentence of this paragraph says that episodic memory contains memory of recent events and minor details; therefore, option I does describe the sort of memory that might be affected in old age. Recollection of childhood events (II) is related to semantic memory, which is described in the fourth paragraph as positively affected by age, not adversely affected. The ability to perform routine tasks (III) is based in the implicit memory, which the author describes in the fifth paragraph as unaffected by age. Therefore, according to the passage, advanced age could adversely affect only that aspect of memory offered in option I and the answer to this question is choice (A), I only.

24. A This question addresses the primary purpose of the passage: How contemporary research into memory suggests that we have three kinds of memory, only one of which deteriorates with age. In suggesting this, this research refutes established ideas about memory and aging (A). (B) correctly states that past investigations into memory only tested episodic memory; however, the passage does not explain exactly why this was the case: its purpose is not to explain such background information. (C) is too general; this passage has to do with just one aspect of the brain's functioning—memory. While the third paragraph discusses the reasons why episodic memory diminishes with age (D), this is just a detail supporting the passage's main thrust regarding new research.

25. D The answer to this inference question regarding developments in memory research can be found in the second paragraph, which suggests that recent developments in memory research stem from methodological changes that clarify the relationship between memory and aging (D). Although the first and second sentences of the first paragraph say that it is commonly known that older people are often forgetful, the passage does not imply that such stereotypes have limited scientific research, and you cannot infer that scientists have attempted to dismantle such stereotypes or that such effort has changed our conceptions of the elderly (A).

Not until the last paragraph does the author mention disease and injury-related memory loss, and since the author does not imply that scientists have confused disease-related problems with age related memory problems, (B) is incorrect. Choice (C) confuses a detail of the passage. The idea that mental exercise might diminish memory loss (see paragraph three) has *resulted from* the new developments in memory research; such an idea has not *led to* innovations in memory research.

26. C See paragraphs two and three. Older people forget recent events but remember the distant past because recent events are stored in episodic memory, which declines with age, while distant memories reside in the semantic memory, which actually improves with age (C). You may have realized immediately that (A) is wrong in saying that childhood events exist as part of the implicit memory. (B) incorrectly attributes memory of the distant past to the implicit memory. There are a couple of things wrong with choice (D). This choice suggests that semantic memory is the aspect of memory for recollection of recent events and that it is this aspect of memory that seems to degenerate from lack of use after retirement. In fact, we know from the third paragraph that it is episodic memory that stores recent events, and it is this aspect of memory that may falter from lack of use.

27. D The ability to remember how to tie shoelaces is an example of the kind of activity we perform without any intentional effort—stored in the implicit memory and discussed in the beginning of the fifth paragraph (D). Although amnesia (A) is mentioned in the middle of the fifth paragraph, the author suggests this disorder affects recent memory, while semantic memory (B), discussed in paragraph four, concerns facts and events in the distant past, and therefore would not be involved in an inability to tie shoes. Episodic memory (C) is discussed in paragraph three, and concerns recall of specific events, not habitual activities.

28. B Although the body of the passage optimistically relates developments in memory research, the last paragraph notes that such findings do not consider memory problems associated with illness or disease. (B) picks up on this concluding comment while also accurately reflecting the author's generally optimistic tone. (A) asserts that memory research is "more theoretical than practical" and, in doing so, seems to fault the character of the research in a way that is not suggested previously in the passage and does not jibe with the author's generally approving and optimistic tone. (C) calls problems of disease and illness "more critical" than other memory disorders, while this opinion is not suggested anywhere in the passage. (D) suggests that illnesses or diseases of memory do not conform to the tripartite model of memory described in this passage and, therefore, are not of interest to researchers; however, the author neither implies that they do not fit the model, nor that researchers would not be interested in them for that reason. Readers should steer clear of any answer choices that require such assumptions.

Passage V (Questions 29–35):
HARBOR SEAL

29. D   This is a detail question about the seal's vibrissae. The last two sentences of the fifth paragraph tell us that vibrissae sense underwater movement, allowing harbor seals to locate and capture prey, so choice (D) is our answer. Vibrissae are whiskers and they have *nothing* to do with improving underwater vision (A). Choice (B) is wrong because vibrissae detect *underwater* vibrations, not aerial vibrations. The passage doesn't say anything about vibrissae being used for camouflage purposes (C).

30. B   This is a question comparing a harbor seal's vision to a human's vision. The seal's eye is discussed in relation to the human eye in the third paragraph of the passage. There we learn that in the water a harbor seal's vision is clear, while a human's vision is blurry. There we also learn that on land a human's vision is clear, while a harbor seal's vision is slightly astigmatic. In other words, a harbor seal's vision is *superior* to a human's vision in the water, but *inferior* to a human's vision on land (B). Choices (A), (C), and (D) all *contradict* this information.

31. D   This is a detail question asking you to determine which one of four questions can be answered on the basis of information in the passage. The last two sentences of the third paragraph tell us *how* the harbor seal's eye compensates for the distortion of light rays on land, choice (D). The passage tells us that the harbor seal does most of its fishing at night, but we are not told *why* the harbor seal fishes at night, so choice (A) is wrong. Information throughout the passage indicates that the harbor seal spends time on land, but nowhere are we told *how much* time the harbor seal spends on land, so choice (B) is wrong. Choice (C) is wrong because the passage discusses only the harbor seal, not other seals or other members of the *Pinnepedia* order.

32. C   This is a question that asks you to decide which statement would most strengthen the claim that harbor seals catch prey through echolocation. If the harbor seal's eye has become more efficient underwater over the course of time (A), it would be reasonable to think that the harbor seal's vision may provide the seal with its means to hunt, and the claim that harbor seals hunt down prey by echolocation would be weakened. If harbor seals were known to do most of their hunting in a limited area and rely on their vibrissae to sense prey at close range (B), then vibrissae would provide the seal with its means to hunt, and the claim that harbor seals hunt down prey by echolocation would be weakened again. If other members of the *Pinnepedia* order—animals genetically similar to the harbor seal—were known to possess echolocation systems, it would be reasonable to think harbor seals might also possess echolocation to help them hunt at night, so choice (C) is our answer. According to the passage, bats, porpoises, and dolphins all have echolocation systems which they use to catch prey. The fact that harbor seals are not closely related to these species (D), then, would either not affect the claim that harbor seals use echolocation to hunt down prey or, at most, would tend to weaken the claim.

33. B   This question asks about the author's reason for comparing the sensory organs of harbor seals and humans. These comparisons are made in the second and third paragraphs. In these paragraphs the author illustrates the differences between a harbor seal's ear and eye and a human's ear and eye in order to explain to readers how the seal's sensory organs function (B). He refers to human sensory organs only in order to clarify his points by relating them to something very familiar to readers. Choice (A) is wrong because the author discusses the ways a particular mammal, the harbor seal, has adapted to its environment and only mentions humans by way of comparison. It is true that both humans and seals are mammals, but the author compares the differences between these two mammals. He does not point out similarities. (C) is wrong because nowhere in the passage does the author suggest that seals are related to humans. And the author neither suggests nor argues that seals are more adaptatively successful than humans (D).

34. B In order to answer this question it is important to consider the passage as a whole. Of the choices listed, (B), a zoologist, is most likely to have authored the passage because zoologists study individual animal species in depth. A paleontologist (A) is not likely to have written this passage because paleontologists primarily study fossils and this passage is not about fossils. (C) is wrong because taxonomists classify various animals in relation to other species and according to their traits. While this passage briefly touches on the relationship between the harbor seal and other species, these comparisons certainly are not the main thrust of the passage. A geneticist (D) deals with issues at the level of the cell and chromosome. Since the passage doesn't discuss cells or chromosomes, a geneticist is not likely to have written this passage.

35. D This is a detail question about the harbor seal's habitat. According to the first sentence of the first paragraph, the harbor seal lives along the northern Atlantic and Pacific coasts, so choice (D) is our answer. Choice (A) is wrong because the passage says nothing about harbor seals living in arctic regions. Since the passage mentions only two regions where the harbor seal lives and doesn't say whether these regions have abundant fish populations, (B) is wrong. (C) is wrong because the passage tells us that harbor seals live only along coastal regions, but doesn't say anything about island regions.

Passage VI (Questions 36–40): ROMAN ITALY

36. B   The author's main purpose in this passage is to point out a deficiency in modern scholarship. The sort of research he would want to see done would remedy this deficiency. The correct choice emphasizes the author's view that a new sort of scholarship is needed. At the end of paragraphs four and six the author expresses his belief that nonliterary evidence should be used in a more sophisticated manner. (A) is wrong because the author describes the work of Marxist historians as useful only in a limited number of specific instances (on matters regarding slavery, slave revolts, great estates) and as having a distorting effect to boot. (C) is wrong because it involves the sort of elitist research that he attributes to the "predilections of increasingly professional scholars." (D) is wrong because the author emphasizes the impossibility of centralized bureaucracy in the second paragraph.

37. A   The amount of modern scholarship on Roman agriculture refers to the great amount of scholarship on this particular topic. (A) is correct. Even though the author states the answer explicitly, you may be lead astray. The author, having spent four paragraphs on the lack of scholarly interest in rural communities, devotes a paragraph to the great amount of scholarly interest in agriculture. A subtle difference, a subtle shift that must nevertheless be taken into account! (B) contradicts everything the author says on the matter. (C) is wrong even though taken by itself it is true; it just doesn't jibe with the stem. Though scholars have indeed had little interest in the rural communities, there nevertheless exists a great amount of scholarship on agriculture. (D) is wrong for the same reason as (C): Though scholars have indeed tended to have elitist interests, there nevertheless exists a great amount of scholarship on agriculture.

38. D   In paragraph three, "the neglect [that] began with the ancient Romans themselves" refers to the first sentence of the paragraph: "In spite of the ubiquity and importance of these local communities, they have been rather *neglected in recent Roman historical research.*" The correct choice identifies the group with whom the neglect lies. (A) is wrong because it has nothing to do with recent historical research. (B) is wrong because the word incompetence is, as the student should expect, too negative. A deficiency in the scholarship does not indicate incompetence on the part of the scholars. (C) is wrong because, even though it tells why this neglect began with the ancient Roman writers, it does not refer to the "recent Roman historical research" of modern scholars.

39. B   Remember that the author's main purpose is to discuss remedying a deficiency in modern scholarship. (B) is correct because "the records of an ancient town council" would seem to be most useful to a scholar who wants to investigate local communities. (A) is wrong because the author notes that there is no lack of scholarship on agricultural matters in the beginning of paragraph five. (C) is wrong because the author specifically refers to an increase in scholarship on Roman commerce—sea trade. (D) is wrong because the author specifically refers to the military interests of both ancient writers and modern scholars in paragraphs three and four.

40. C You do not need to know technical terminology but rather you should be able to figure it out according to its context. To do so here you must note how the author juxtaposes a group consisting of "consul, general, and emperor" with a group consisting of "*decuriones* and small-town shopkeepers." Whatever *decuriones* are, they must be of the same relative social rank as shopkeepers. (C) is correct because the key word in the answer is *local,* for it accords with the author's interest in local communities. (A) is wrong because important military officers would belong in the first group along with generals. (B) is wrong because slaves and impoverished peasants do not fit into this context; they are too humble to be paired with shopkeepers. Moreover, the author notes that scholars have shown great interest in Roman slavery. (D) is wrong for the same reason as (A): Powerful noblemen belong in the group with generals and emperors.

Verbal Reasoning Test Two
Time—60 minutes

DIRECTIONS: Each of the passages in this test is followed by a set of questions based on the passage's content. After reading each passage decide on the one **best** response to each question. If you are unsure of an answer, eliminate the choices you know are wrong and choose from the remaining choices. You may refer to the passages while answering the questions.

Passage I

In 1855, excavations at the site of the ancient city of Larsa, in present-day Iraq, unearthed a large number of tablets traceable to Sumero-Babylonian times, approximately 1900–1500 b.c. The materials
5 appeared to be receipts, accounts, and tables. Interpretation revealed that the number system of this ancient civilization was sexagesimal (counting was by 10s and 60s). The symbols used were quasi-positional; the symbol for "1" could also signify the
10 powers of 60 and even 10 times the powers of 60, depending upon the specific nature of the transaction.

It is now known that not only the number system but also the system of linear measure used by the
15 Sumero-Babylonian society was based on 60. A clay tablet recovered at Larsa some time after the initial findings, believed to be a standard text copied as part of the school curriculum, shows a systematic and progressive sequence of linear mea-
20 sure utilizing units that represented specific quantities of barley, the society's food staple and currency. Six she (grains) were equal to 1 shu-si (finger), 30 shu-si equaled 1 kush (cubit), 12 kush equaled 1 nindan, 60 nindan equaled 1 USH, and
25 30 USH added up to 1 beru. The factors used to convert from one unit to another—6, 30, 12, 60, and 30—are multiples of 6, and each is a factor of 60, the base in the sexagesimal number system.

Later excavations revealed that the Sumero-
30 Babylonian mathematical system was a successor of sexagesimal systems that had appeared both in earlier eras and in other geographical locations. Tablet fragments discovered in the 1920s at Jemdet Nasr in Iraq disclosed that the numerical
35 and linear systems first noted in 1855 probably had been in use as early as 2900–2800 b.c. The pic

tographic inscriptions appeared to be a precursor of a Sumerian form of writing known as cuneiform, while the numerical symbols—circles, cuplike
40 shapes, and slashes—were similar to those on the tablets found at Larsa. In both, the notations reflected computation in multiples of 10 and 60 while the basic unit of measure was the she or grain. The Jemdet Nasr findings are thus consid-
45 ered proto-Sumerian.

Research at Susa, the ancient Elamite city located in present-day Iran, has revealed that even this separate culture probably used the mathematical system noted at the various Sumerian sites. Initial
50 excavations at Susa uncovered tablets inscribed with both the cuneiform writings and numerals of Sumero-Babylonia. Later excavations there revealed evidence of a society in existence at least a millennium before that of the Elamites. This proto-Elamite
55 culture, which was roughly contemporary with that of the proto-Sumerians, used numbers and linear measures virtually identical to theirs, despite a completely different style of writing.

1. This passage was most likely taken from:
   A. a newspaper feature about ancient market transactions.
   B. a journal article regarding ancient numerical systems.
   C. a lecture on archeological discoveries in the Near East.
   D. an encyclopedia entry on Sumero-Babylonian forms of writing.

GO TO THE NEXT PAGE.

2. Based on the information in the passage, which of the following archeological findings is LEAST likely?

   A. A tablet or pictographic writing dating from 2700 B.C. using the units she and shu-si
   B. A tablet containing sexagesimal numbers and cuneiform writing, dating from 3200 B.C.
   C. A tablet inscribed with cups and slashes describing a transaction involving measurement in terms of fingers and cubits
   D. A tablet dating from 1300 B.C. showing a table of measurements with conversion factors of 6, 30, 12, 60, and 30

3. Which of the following characteristics could be common to both a Sumerian and a proto-Sumerian tablet?

   A. Slashes and circles
   B. Cuneiform inscriptions
   C. Positional notation using the number 0
   D. A system of measure based on the finger as the smallest unit

4. The proto-Elamite society existed approximately:

   A. 2,500–3,000 years ago.
   B. 3,500–4,000 years ago.
   C. 4,500–5,000 years ago.
   D. 5,500–6,000 years ago.

5. Which of the following most probably is the sequence in which the societies mentioned in the passage flourished?

   A. Proto-Elamite, Elamite, Proto-Sumerian, Sumero-Babylonian
   B. Proto-Elamite, Elamite, Sumero-Babylonian, Proto-Sumerian
   C. Elamite, Proto-Sumerian, Sumero-Babylonian, Proto-Elamite
   D. Proto-Sumerian, Proto-Elamite, Elamite, Sumero-Babylonian

6. The author mentions excavations at Susa in order to:

   A. prove that the proto-Sumerian culture was dominant in the ancient Middle East.
   B. explain the ways in which an aspect of proto-Sumerian culture spread to other areas of the ancient Middle East.
   C. support the notion that sexagesimal mathematical systems were used by several ancient Middle Eastern societies.
   D. indicate that the mathematical system used in Sumero-Babylonian times was heavily influenced by proto-Elamite culture.

GO TO THE NEXT PAGE.

Passage II

The big bang, the spontaneous explosion that created the universe some 10 to 20 billion years ago,
initiated developmental processes that have led to
an uneven distribution of luminous matter
5 throughout the universe and spurred a continual
expansion of the universe. The study of these
developmental processes is a relatively young discipline. Before the 20th century, astronomers knew
little about space beyond our own galaxy, the
10 Milky Way, and could only speculate about the
existence of "external" galaxies. In the 20th century, the development of sophisticated observation
technology, including the radio telescope, has
made it possible for astronomers to study the com-
15 ponents and properties of the universe and to for-
mulate their own theories about its development.

One popular theory of the universe's development,
introduced in 1972 by Soviet astronomers
Zel'dovich and Sunyaev, proposes that gases pres-
20 ent in the early universe became quite dense and
unevenly distributed in response to gravitational
forces. Over time, dense pockets of gas formed
vast sheets of luminous material that astronomers
refer to as "pancakes." Because these gaseous pan-
25 cakes were located in regions of the universe
where multiple clusters of galaxies now exist,
Zel'dovich and Sunyaev reasoned that early in the
universe's development the pancakes must have
fragmented into galactic clusters and individual
30 galaxies. In other regions of the universe, the
astronomers reasoned, limited quantities of gas
prevented the development of luminous matter,
leaving much of space empty.

Zel'dovich and Sunyaev's attempt to explain the
35 development of the universe has its origin in their
observations of the distribution of galaxies.
Galaxies are grouped in structures called "clusters." Clusters vary in size; small clusters may contain only a few galaxies while the largest clusters
40 may contain many thousands of them. Clusters, in
turn, form structures known as "superclusters."
Superclusters are so large that any individual member galaxy, in motion for billions of years, will have
traversed only a fraction of its supercluster's diam-
45 eter. Four superclusters have been identified by
astronomers thus far, but astronomers disagree
about their precise boundaries.

Whatever the exact boundaries of superclusters,
scientists believe that even these huge structures
50 occupy only a small part of the total area of the
universe. Most of space consists of vast empty
regions devoid of luminous matter known as
"voids." The existence of voids has been confirmed
only in the last few years. Astronomers are still
55 unsure of the exact composition of voids, but speculate that voids are made up of nonluminous matter. This dark matter cannot be seen and appears,
in observation from Earth, as nothing more than
vast areas of nothingness.

60 Thus, the Zel'dovich-Sunyaev theory has shed considerable light on the workings of the universe and
has significantly contributed to our understanding
of celestial structures. However, while their theory
describes and explains the uneven distribution of
65 luminous matter it still only partially accounts for
the conditions of the universe today. Zel'dovich
and Sunyaev failed to address the continual expansion of the universe. To understand this aspect of
the universe's development, astronomers have had
70 to refer to the work of Edwin Hubble, a prominent
astronomer of the 1920s and '30s. By using a technique known as "red shift analysis," Hubble was
able to develop the notion of diverging galaxies. In
astronomical observation, the more distant a
75 celestial body from the Milky Way, the more its
light shifts to the red end of the spectrum. Hubble
observed that the light emitted from galaxies
moved farther to the red end of the spectrum over
time.

80 Consequently, he concluded that other galaxies
must be moving away from our own. His discovery
of the divergence of galaxies was later codified as
Hubble's Law. From this, astronomers today have
been able to infer that, in a continuing response to
85 the huge initial release of energy that occurred at
the time of the big bang explosion, celestial bodies—including galactic clusters, superclusters, and
voids—are expanding, resulting in a general
expansion of the universe.

GO TO THE NEXT PAGE.

7. The passage implies that galaxies move:

   A. in a random fashion.
   B. toward the Milky Way.
   C. out of their original clusters.
   D. as a consequence of a massive energy discharge.

8. According to the passage, which of the following is true of the composition and properties of the universe?

   A. There are no more than four superclusters in our universe.
   B. Gravitational forces have no effect on concentrations of gas.
   C. Galaxies will eventually assume fixed positions in the universe.
   D. The distribution of galaxies today reflects the effects of gravity on gaseous formations.

9. The author considers the Zel'dovich-Sunyaev theory to be:

   A. illuminating, but incomplete.
   B. enlightening and comprehensive.
   C. uninformed, but original.
   D. insightful, but lacking evidence.

10. While observing the movement of galaxies, an astronomer on Earth notices that light emitted from galaxy A is farther to the red end of the spectrum than light coming from galaxy B. Based on this astronomer's observations, it can be inferred from the passage that:

    A. galaxy B is farther from the Milky Way than galaxy A.
    B. galaxy B is traveling away from the Milky Way at a faster pace than galaxy A.
    C. galaxy B is diverging at a faster rate than galaxy A.
    D. galaxy B is closer to the Milky Way than galaxy A.

11. According to the passage, astronomers today disagree about the:

    A. utility of red shift analysis.
    B. existence of external galaxies.
    C. effects of gravity on pancakes.
    D. dimensions of superclusters.

12. The author introduces Hubble's Law in order to:

    A. contradict the theory of diverging galaxies.
    B. explain the technique of red shift analysis.
    C. prove the existence of dark matter.
    D. supplement the Zel'dovich-Sunyaev theory.

GO TO THE NEXT PAGE.

13. According to the passage, prior to the 20th century astronomers:

A. used radio telescopes to observe other galaxies.
B. were only able to study the Milky Way.
C. knew of the existence of clusters and superclusters.
D. formulated the idea of the big bang.

14. It can be inferred from the passage that at some time in the future:

I. the huge amount of energy released by the big bang explosion will be exhausted.
II. the Milky Way will be larger than its present size.
III. the configuration of the universe will remain constant.

A. I only
B. II only
C. I and II only
D. I, II, and III only

GO TO THE NEXT PAGE.

The two essays in which Virginia Woolf explores women's role in art and politics have traditionally been seen as problematic adjuncts to her novels. While *A Room of One's Own,* with its acerbic wit,
5 has been given grudging respect, the outspokenly programmatic *Three Guineas* has been dismissed as a pacifist-feminist tract. No doubt these essays lack the subtlety and superb control of the novels, but to a recent generation of critics they remain signif-
10 icant because of their anticipation of many of the concerns of contemporary feminism.

A Room of One's Own (1929) is written in the form of a lecture delivered at a fictitious women's college. Woolf begins by contrasting the paltry luncheon
15 given at the college with the luxurious fare offered at a nearby men's university. The difference symbolizes more profound disparities which—Woolf now comes to her main point—bear directly on the fortunes of women artists. For the woman
20 author, financial independence, opportunities for education, tranquility, and privacy are necessary preconditions, without which women are unlikely to produce works of genius. Great art can never be expected from "labouring, servile, or uneducated
25 people." (Among modern feminists, Tillie Olsen makes a similar point in *Silences,* though without Woolf's undertone of class condescension.) When a woman obtains a room of her own, in all its senses, she may, according to Woolf, develop what
30 Coleridge termed "the androgynous mind," one that, having united its male and female sides, "transcends and comprehends the feelings of both sexes."

In *Three Guineas* (1938), Woolf's central argument,
35 again foreshadowing a key contention of later feminism, is that the process of changing gender restrictions in the public world and in the private individual are interdependent. Such issues as childrearing (which she felt should be a shared respon-
40 sibility) and professional equality between the sexes are not separate considerations, but rather different aspects of the same problem. Woolf also attempts to define women's responsibilities in the larger political world. Discussing the probability of
45 another world war, she argues that women with jobs in manufacturing should refuse to produce

arms for use in a male-instigated debacle. Both at that time and since then, many readers have found this argument naive. One working-class reader,
50 Agnes Smith, wrote, to Woolf that the book was decidedly class-bound; working women could hardly afford to jeopardize their employment for a pacifist ideal. Current feminist critics accept the validity of Smith's point—indeed they acknowledge that
55 it exposes a limitation of Woolf's feminism generally—but they also note that the mild derision which greeted *Three Guineas* from the male establishment was typical of the reception often given a female thinker's ideas.

15. As used by Woolf, the phrase *a room of one's own* apparently refers to all of the following EXCEPT:

    A. freedom from economic insecurity.
    B. separation of the male and female sides of consciousness.
    C. educational opportunities for women equal to that available to men.
    D. personal autonomy.

16. Judging from the second paragraph, which of the following assumptions did Woolf make in her discussion of women writers?

    A. The mind can be characterized as having masculine and feminine aspects.
    B. All great authors have come from economically privileged backgrounds.
    C. There have been no truly great women writers in the past.
    D. Artistic development is independent of formal education.

GO TO THE NEXT PAGE.

17. The passage provides information to answer which of the following questions?

    A. Why did Woolf write *A Room Of One's Own* as a lecture when in fact it was not?

    B. Why did Woolf's tone shift in *Three Guineas* as compared to *A Room Of One's Own*?

    C. How did Woolf struggle against male prejudice in her writing career?

    D. What conditions foster the development of the "androgynous mind"?

18. The author would state that, in comparison to her novels, Woolf's essays on feminist themes could be regarded as more:

    A. original.

    B. familiar to the public.

    C. accepted by critics.

    D. blunt and direct.

19. It can be inferred from the passage that *A Room Of One's Own* and *Three Guineas* are similar in which of the following respects?

    I. Both discuss social issues in terms of artistic development.

    II. Neither presents specific ways in which women can fight a male-dominated society.

    III. Both deal implicitly with the concerns of economically advantaged women.

    A. I only

    B. III only

    C. II and III only

    D. I, II, and III

20. By "different aspects of the same problem" (line 42), the author is most probably referring to the problem of:

    A. assigning social roles according to gender.

    B. increasing hostilities among nations.

    C. equalizing the domestic responsibilites of men and women.

    D. discrimination against women in the workplace.

GO TO THE NEXT PAGE.

Passage IV

For more than a century, there has been a dispute among scholars over the authorship of the heroic poem *Beowulf.* Was *Beowulf* the work of one author or of several? Can the author or authors be identi-
5 fied as pagan or Christian? Of the theories that have attempted to come to grips with these questions, three have been especially prominent.

The earliest of the three, the tribal-lay theory, stresses that *Beowulf* is an amalgam of older
10 Germanic and Nordic tribal myths. Proponents of this theory argue that the poem in its final form is the work of several authors whose earlier works were joined together by a number of later editors. This conclusion is based on the poem's numerous
15 digressions from the main theme. These digressions, including Sigemund's battle with the dragon, are only tenuously linked to the hero Beowulf's struggles with monsters and men. Interestingly, while many critics see the poem as a Christian alle-
20 gory with Beowulf as the champion of goodness battling the forces of evil, tribal-lay theorists seem to ignore the poem's obvious Christian overtones and consider its ethical tone to be a reflection of lay Germanic and Nordic codes of loyalty to tribe
25 and vengeance to enemies.

Like the tribal-lay theory, the growth by accretion theory supports the notion of multiple authorship. But according to the accretion view, *Beowulf* began as a short, simple work of mythology by a single
30 author and was gradually transformed into a long, intricate poem as later authors added to it over a period of several centuries. As evidence in support of this view, scholars point to the mixture of pagan rituals and themes with Christian values. This
35 strange combination of conflicting motifs, some believe, could only have been the result of multiple authorship.

A third theory originates from a paper by J.R.R. Tolkien, entitled "*Beowulf:* The Monsters and the
40 Critics." In his paper, Tolkien argued that *Beowulf* was the work of a single Christian author, probably a member of a royal court, who used pagan material as the basis of his poem. Scholars who believe this Christian authorship theory argue that it is not

45 at all surprising that a Christian would have written such a poem. At the time of *Beowulf*'s writing, some time between the years A.D. 650 and 850, the bulk of the population of England—including much of the literate strata—was only nominally
50 Christian and still clung to pagan beliefs and practices. Although Christianity had gained a foothold in England, it had yet to displace pagan culture. Christian authorship theorists reason that a nominal Christian would have been perfectly comfort-
55 able incorporating both pagan and Christian elements into the same work. These scholars further argue that since the Anglo-Saxons were engaged in constant warfare with the Vikings, Scots, and Picts at the time of *Beowulf*'s writing, its author may
60 have deliberately emphasized certain pagan motifs, particularly the cult of the warrior, for the political purpose of bolstering morale among both the aristocracy and the masses at a time when they were under constant military pressure.

65 Although it is not possible to conclusively prove that one theory is correct and the other two wrong, most scholars favor the Tolkien view. The tribal-lay and the growth by accretion theories are generally dismissed because of the epic's essential
70 unity despite disparate references and seemingly conflicting motifs. Most scholars find historical analyses of the context of the author's writing provide the best resolutions to the poem's apparent contradictions.

21. The author mentions Sigemund's battle with the dragon (lines 16–17) in order to:

    A. show that the Christian theme of good versus evil is central to *Beowulf.*
    B. provide support for the notion that *Beowulf* is an incorporation of more ancient tribal myths.
    C. prove that *Beowulf* is the work of a single pagan author.
    D. provide an allegorical representation of the Anglo-Saxon struggle with Vikings, Scots, and Picts.

GO TO THE NEXT PAGE.

22. According to the Christian authorship theory, the emphasis on the pagan cult of the warrior in *Beowulf* is a reflection of:

    A. major themes in Germanic and Norse culture.
    B. the author's position as a military official in a royal court.
    C. political upheavals in England at the time of the epic's writing.
    D. an 8th-century decline in Christian faith among Anglo-Saxons.

23. Which of the following statements are compatible with the ideas of the growth by accretion theorists?

    I. *Beowulf* represents the result of contributions made by multiple authors.
    II. Conflicting motifs in *Beowulf* indicate that the poem is not the work of a single author.
    III. The essential unity of *Beowulf* defies the constant turmoil and warfare of the period in which its author wrote.

    A. I and II only
    B. I and III only
    C. II and III only
    D. I, II, and III

24. According to the passage, a major distinction between the tribal-lay and growth by accretion theorists is:

    A. the degree of emphasis each group places on the epic's historical context.
    B. the different ways in which the theorists interpret the poem's allegorical references.
    C. their varied conceptions of the multiple authorship of *Beowulf.*
    D. the way in which each group accounts for *Beowulf*'s Christian elements.

25. Which of the following would most seriously weaken the Christian authorship theory?

    A. During an excavation of an 11th century Norwegian church, archaeologist find a partially translated manuscript of *Beowulf.*
    B. Historians now believe that Anglo-Saxon conflicts with the Vikings, Scots, and Picts were much more intense and long lasting than previously thought.
    C. Recently discovered documents indicate that *Beowulf* is an English translation of a Germanic myth of earlier origin.
    D. Some linguists have concluded that *Beowulf* was written by a literate peasant because the poem contains phrases and terms used by peasants but not found in the language of aristocrats.

26. The passage suggests that most scholars favor the Christian authorship theory because:

    A. it is able to locate many of the obscure references made in *Beowulf* in Germanic and Norse mythology.
    B. other theories fail to appreciate the significance of Christian elements in *Beowulf.*
    C. it is able to resolve inconsistencies in *Beowulf* by referring to the context in which it was written.
    D. no other theory attempts to explain the epic's disparate references and varied motifs.

27. The author mentions a paper written by J.R.R. Tolkien (lines 38–40) in order to:

    A. lend authoritative support to multiple authorship theories.
    B. discredit the notion that *Beowulf* was written by a Christian.
    C. disprove previous theories regarding *Beowulf*'s authorship.
    D. introduce a contextual analysis of the writing of *Beowulf.*

GO TO THE NEXT PAGE.

Passage V

The idea that every human has certain inalienable rights first emerged in the 17th and 18th centuries. Human rights initially meant simply the right to representative government, as conveyed in the
5   aims of the American and French revolutions of the 1700s, but subsequently was enlarged to encompass freedom of speech, religion, and assembly; an unrestricted press; protection against enslavement and torture or freedom from coercion; and due
10 process or equal protection under the law. A largely 20th-century concern for economic or welfare issues has resulted in the expansion of the definition to include the right to be employed, to own property, and to receive at least minimal levels of
15 food, shelter, health care, and education.

Sovereign governments are responsible for the translation of human rights theory into concrete policies, often a difficult and controversial task. There may be occasions when the safeguarding of
20 personal rights impinges upon equally important societal goals. In times of war, for instance, the right to free speech and press has been restrained in the name of national security. The rationale is that the dissemination of certain information or
25 opinions would endanger all human rights by creating a situation wherein the survival of the government itself is threatened. Another problem is defining the extent of a particular guarantee. For example, the amount of education to which every
30 citizen supposedly is entitled has meant basic literacy to some and university instruction to others. Still another view holds that education is not a right at all but is instead a privilege; it may be bestowed or rescinded at society's will. The pro-
35 tection of human rights also implies the existence of an elaborate network of courts, police, schools, hospitals, and employment opportunities, but providing these is not always practical, especially in developing countries.

40 Many governments have attempted to guarantee rights not only to their own citizens but also to citizens of foreign nations. However, the issues are even more complex at the international level. First, different governments may have varying interpre-
45 tations of what constitutes a basic right. Second, even if it is assumed that all political, civil, and economic rights are applicable to all times and places, one nation does not necessarily have the authority to pass judgment on another's domestic
50 policies; international legal agreements usually preclude intervention in the internal affairs of other nations. A third problem is that human rights and "humanitarian interests" may be used as a facade for selfish geopolitical goals. Fourth, intercession in
55 another nation's internal affairs in the name of human rights may transgress domestic laws specifically prohibiting foreign intervention, thereby violating citizens' rights to a responsive and representative government.

60 Although occasionally amorphous, mechanisms do exist at the domestic and international levels for ensuring the protection of human rights. Most nations have adopted constitutions or other binding documents that specifically enumerate the
65 rights to which their citizens are entitled. In the international realm, direct intervention is one means of safeguarding human rights, although generally undesirable and illegal. A more palatable option is diplomacy; one or more governments fre-
70 quently can impel another nation to respect human rights through persuasive tactics, trade agreements, and other quiet techniques. A third alternative is the creation of formal international organizations, such as the United Nations, to pro-
75 vide a global forum for discussion of human rights policies. Finally, extra-governmental organizations can draw attention to possible abuses of individual rights by conducting media and public information campaigns.

GO TO THE NEXT PAGE.

28. The author suggests that a political thinker of the 18th century and a 20th-century counterpart would most likely differ on which of the following?

    A. Proper methods of ensuring international human rights
    B. The amount of education to which every citizen is entitled
    C. The definition of basic human rights
    D. The importance of representative government

29. According to the passage, direct intervention by one government in another's domestic affairs is likely to involve which of the following?

    I. A violation of citizens' rights
    II. Civil unrest in the intervening country
    III. A violation of international legal agreements

    A. I only
    B. II only
    C. I and III only
    D. II and III only

30. With which of the following statements concerning the guarantee of human rights would the author be most likely to agree?

    A. Translating human rights theory into policies is impossible because no consensus exists concerning the extent of basic rights.
    B. Many rights can be considered privileges and need not be guaranteed by sovereign governments.
    C. The enforcement of human rights on the international level does not conflict with other geopolitical goals.
    D. Governments lacking sufficient resources may be unable to safeguard their citizens' basic rights.

31. In the second paragraph, the author mentions national security considerations as evidence that:

    A. governments often violate the rights of their citizens for selfish geopolitical goals.
    B. the interests of a government may sometimes conflict with the rights of its citizens.
    C. safeguarding the right to free speech and press is an impossible endeavor.
    D. agreeing on the extent of a particular right is always problematic.

32. The author provides support for which of the following assertions?

    A. The concept of human rights should not be expanded to include the right to an education.
    B. Governments should never attempt to influence the human rights practices of other countries.
    C. Diplomacy is the only rational means of safeguarding human rights on the international level.
    D. Difficulties can arise when putting the concept of human rights into practice.

33. The author mentions all of the following as possible mechanisms for ensuring the protection of human rights EXCEPT:

    A. the creation of constitutions outlining citizens' rights.
    B. the existence of nongovernment groups devoted to publicizing rights violations.
    C. development of a universal definition of human rights.
    D. imposition of diplomatic measures to persuade nations to respect human rights.

GO TO THE NEXT PAGE.

34. It can be inferred from the passage that the author considers direct intervention by one country in the internal human rights practices of another to be:

A. undesirable, and generally in breach of international law.
B. undesirable, but justifiable if all other methods of intervention have first been applied.
C. undesirable, but necessary as long as violations of basic human rights continue to occur.
D. desirable, because everything must be done to ensure human rights for all people.

35. The author organizes the passage by:

A. making distinctions between two levels of human rights, domestic and international.
B. explaining what is meant by human rights and then discussing the difficulties and methods involved in safeguarding them.
C. gradually refining the definition of basic human rights through a series of observations.
D. presenting an argument in favor of broad human rights and then suggesting techniques to guarantee them.

GO TO THE NEXT PAGE.

Passage VI

The earliest telescopes were refractors, in that they used lenses to bend incoming light. By using refractive lenses, early astronomers were able to gather light and view images with greater resolu-
5   tion and magnification than possible with the naked eye. But because pioneer telescope makers knew relatively little about optics, their lenses exhibited two serious defects. The first problem, spherical aberration, is a distortion that occurs
10 when a lens with round surfaces fails to focus light from a point object to a point image. The second problem, chromatic aberration, stems from the fact that an ordinary lens refracts different wavelengths of light to slightly different degrees, result-
15 ing in a different focal length for each color, and therefore, an out-of-focus image with a colorful halo.

A number of scientists, among them Johannes Kepler, realized that spherical aberration could be
20 corrected simply by using a differently shaped lens. A solution to chromatic aberration, however, proved more difficult. When Sir Isaac Newton announced that it seemed impossible to correct chromatic aberration, scientists turned their atten-
25 tion to reflecting telescopes. Like refractors, these telescopes also increased light, resolution, and magnification of an image. But reflectors use curved mirrors in lieu of clear lenses in order to avoid the chromatic distortion of refraction.
30 However, early reflecting telescopes had their problems too: the mirrors they utilized were made of metal alloys, which absorbed light and thus obscured images. One solution to this problem was to build larger telescopes, since bigger mirrors
35 mean greater light reception and brighter images. Unfortunately, the opticians and foundries of the day were not yet up to the challenge. Mirror technology progressed slowly, as did the development of better reflector telescopes.

40 Chromatic aberration remained a problem in refractors, until Englishman Peter Hall discovered that a compound lens (i.e., one that combined different surfaces) could compensate for the dispersion of different colors by focusing them back
45 together. Unfortunately, his findings were little known. Later, mathematician Leonhard Euler hit upon a similar solution using two lenses with water between them. Soon after, noted optician John Dolland followed Euler's lead and sandwiched a
50 piece of flint glass between two pieces of crown glass, an arrangement that corrected both chromatic and spherical aberration. As a result of this advancement and subsequent modifications, the refractor once again became the telescopic instru-
55 ment of choice and remained so for about 100 years.

But the refractor continued to have one inescapable limitation—a constraint on the maximum effective lens diameter, which limits the light-
60 gathering property of the telescope. For this reason, as well as because of technical advances in mirror making, the reflector would once again assume prominence. At the Great Exposition of 1851, Varnish and Mellish presented the first
65 chemical technique for layering silver onto glass. The mirrors that ultimately resulted from this breakthrough were silvered on the front and represented a double advantage. First, the silver surface (financially feasible because of the small amount of silver required) increased reflectivity of
70 mirrors some 50 percent. Second, using glass in place of metal eliminated problems of shrinkage and cracking.

The refractor never again surpassed the reflector.
75 With further advances in the development of heat-resistant glass and casting techniques, larger and larger mirrors became possible, and astronomers saw farther and farther into the universe.

36. Of the following, the author is most interested in discussing:

   A. how different shapes of lenses influence resolution and magnification in telescopes.
   B. why refractors have become more popular than reflectors.
   C. how two basic telescope designs alternately succeeded each other in importance and popularity.
   D. the ways in which technological constraints have shaped the course of science.

37. The author mentions the views of Sir Isaac Newton (lines 22–24) in order to:

   A. explain why scientists initially turned toward reflecting telescopes.
   B. emphasize the severity of the problem of spherical aberration.
   C. show that early scientists often reached erroneous conclusions.
   D. tacitly challenge the view that Sir Isaac Newton was a brilliant scientist.

38. According to the passage, chromatic aberration can be corrected by:

   A. a lens with rounded surfaces.
   B. using glass in place of metal alloys.
   C. building larger telescopes for greater light reception.
   D. an arrangement of two lenses separated by water.

39. The author mentions all of the following as problems associated with refractors EXCEPT:

   A. chromatic aberration.
   B. limited lens diameter.
   C. spherical aberration.
   D. overabsorption of light.

40. The passage implies that the development of better telescopes was primarily hindered by:

   A. technological constraints.
   B. imprecise methodologies.
   C. disinterest among scientists.
   D. inavailability of materials.

STOP. IF YOU FINISH BEFORE TIME HAS EXPIRED, CHECK YOUR WORK. YOU MAY GO BACK TO ANY QUESTION IN THIS PART ONLY.

Verbal Reasoning Test Two: Answers and Explanations

ANSWER KEY

1. B	16. A	31. B
2. B	17. D	32. D
3. A	18. D	33. C
4. C	19. B	34. A
5. D	20. A	35. B
6. C	21. B	36. C
7. D	22. C	37. A
8. D	23. A	38. D
9. A	24. C	39. D
10. D	25. C	40. A
11. D	26. C	
12. D	27. D	
13. B	28. C	
14. B	29. C	
15. B	30. D	

EXPLANATIONS

Passage I (Questions 1–6): SUMERO-BABYLONIA

1. B In order to answer a question about the source of a passage, it is vital to consider the passage as a whole. The detached tone, highly specialized subject matter (ancient numerical systems), and detailed historical material used to support the author's points suggest this passage is both academic and, most probably, geared to a rather specialized circle of scholars who study ancient numerical systems. Therefore, this passage most likely comes from a journal article on ancient numerical systems (B). If the passage had come from a newspaper feature on ancient market transactions (A), we would expect a more popular writing style and a greater focus on the details of ancient markets. This passage is not likely to have come from a lecture on archeological discoveries in the Near East (C) because the passage only discusses archeological discoveries to help support and shed light on ancient numerical systems. A lecture on archeological finds in the Near East would probably have been broader, touching on more sites and other kinds of discoveries. And this passage is not likely to have come from an encyclopedia entry on Sumero-Babylonian forms of writing (D) because the passage only briefly mentions Sumero-Babylonian writing (cuneiform) in the course of its discussion of ancient numerical systems.

2. B According to paragraphs three and four, the societies flourishing at approximately 2900–2800 B.C.—the proto-Sumerians and proto-Elamites—utilized sexagesimal number systems but not cuneiform inscriptions. Apparently cuneiform writing did not appear until after 2900–2800 B.C.; such inscriptions would not have appeared in 3200 B.C. The date and style of writing in (A) are appropriate to the types of tablets unearthed at Jemdet Nasr (paragraph three). The mathematical symbols and inscriptions in (C) are appropriate to any of the societies mentioned (except possibly Susa—the passage is not explicit). (D) essentially describes findings like those at Larsa, as discussed in paragraphs one and two; although the date is a little late, you should not assume that the use of the sexagesimal system (or conversion factors characteristic of it) died out immediately following the Sumero-Babylonian period.

3. A These characteristics would have been common to tablets unearthed from both Sumerian and proto-Sumerian sites. Although the societies used different styles of writing—Sumerians employing cuneiform and proto-Sumerians utilizing pictographic inscriptions (B)—each culture used similar mathematical symbols. As stated in sentence three of paragraph three, the numerical symbols of the proto-Sumerians, "circles, cuplike shapes, and slashes," were quite similar to those noted on the tablets earlier unearthed at the Sumerian city of Larsa. All number systems mentioned in the passage were *quasi*-positional, and the use of 0 is never mentioned (C). The she (grain), not the shu-si or finger, is the smallest unit mentioned (D).

4.   C   According to paragraph four, the proto-Elamite culture was "roughly contemporary with that of the proto-Sumerians." The proto-Sumerian culture, as exemplified by the Jemdet Nasr archeological findings discussed in paragraph three, was in existence at approximately 2900–2800 B.C. Therefore, the proto-Elamite society also may be traced to 2900–2800 B.C., approximately 4800–4900 years ago. If you selected (A), you probably failed to add 2,000 years to 2900–2800 B.C. to account for the modern "A.D." Choice (B) is more appropriate to the Sumero-Babylonian and Elamite societies, which can be dated to about 2000–1500 B.C. Finally, you may have chosen (D) if you thought the proto-Sumerians were contemporaries of the Elamites rather than the proto-Elamites. Adding another 1,000 years to account for the gap between the Elamites and proto-Elamites would have led to this choice.

5.   D   Of the four societies described in the passage, only two are assigned specific historical dates: the Sumero-Babylonians are said to have flourished in the years 1900–1500 B.C., while the proto-Sumerians existed in the years 2900–2800 B.C. Paragraph four places the proto-Elamites contemporary with the proto-Sumerians; the Elamites were at least 1,000 years later, although there is not enough detail to determine their actual date. Thus, in the final sequence, the proto-Elamites and proto-Sumerians should be placed in immediate proximity to one another, followed by the Elamites and the Sumero-Babylonians (or vice versa). Only (D) fulfills this requirement. Choice (A), while it may sound plausible at first, is inconsistent with the information given. (B) and (C) place proto societies later than their successors and are thus easy to reject.

6.   C   Excavations at Susa are discussed in the last paragraph of the passage, where the author tells us that, in addition to the proto-Sumerian and Sumero-Babylonian societies the proto-Elamite and Elamite societies also used sexagesimal mathematical systems, supporting the notion that sexagesimal mathematical systems were used by several ancient Middle Eastern societies (C). The author doesn't *prove* that proto-Sumerian culture was dominant in the ancient Middle East (A). In fact, in the last paragraph the author seems to *undermine* the notion of proto-Sumerian cultural dominance by saying that a completely different style of writing was found at Susa in later excavations, revealing a proto-Elamite culture contemporary to proto-Sumerian culture, yet differing from it. The author does not discuss or explain the ways in which aspects of culture spread (B). He merely suggests that they did so, somehow, without detailing the *ways* in which that occurred. And the author *never* indicates that the mathematical system used in Sumero-Babylonian times was heavily influenced by proto-Elamite culture (D). On the contrary, throughout the passage, the author suggests that it was Sumerian and proto-Sumerian cultures that exerted influence upon neighboring cultures, including those of the Elamites and their predecessors. That is probably why the mathematical system is referred to as "Sumero-Babylonian" and not "Elamite."

Passage II (Questions 7–14): ZEL'DOVICH-SUNYAEV

7. D This is an implied detail question concerning the movement of galaxies. The first sentence of the first paragraph says that the big bang, the massive energy discharge that gave birth to the universe, has resulted in a continuing expansion of the universe. The last sentence of the final paragraph adds that galaxies are diverging as part of the continuing expansion of the universe. So, galaxies are moving as a result of a massive energy discharge (D). Choice (A) is wrong because the fifth through eighth sentences of the final paragraph tell us that galaxies diverge, moving away from each other. Thus, they are not moving in random ways. The eighth sentence of the final paragraph says that other galaxies are moving away from our own galaxy, the Milky Way, so choice (B) is incorrect. There is no suggestion that galaxies are moving out of their original clusters (C). We are told in the final paragraph that celestial bodies, including galactic clusters, are expanding; consequently, galaxies are not leaving their original clusters, but remaining within the boundaries of expanded clusters.

8. D This is a detail question concerning the composition and properties of the universe. The first few sentences of the second paragraph state that gravitational forces in the early universe determined the current distribution of galaxies by concentrating gas in certain regions of the universe, so choice (D) correctly describes an aspect of the universe. Choice (A) is wrong because, according to the sixth sentence of the third paragraph, four superclusters have been identified by astronomers so far. This is very different from saying that there are no more than four superclusters in the universe. Choice (B) is incorrect because the first sentence of the second paragraph tells us that gravitational forces have an effect on gaseous "pancakes." Nowhere in the passage is there any indication that galaxies will eventually stop moving, so choice (C) is wrong.

9. A This question asks you about the author's view of the Zel'dovich-Sunyaev theory. At the beginning of the final paragraph, the author notes that the Zel'dovich-Sunyaev theory has contributed greatly to our understanding of the universe. But, he goes on to say that this theory cannot explain the universe's continual expansion. Choice (A)—illuminating, but incomplete—conveys this author's attitude and is our correct answer. Choice (B) is wrong because the author believes the theory is not complete—not comprehensive. And the author does not criticize the theory for being "uninformed," so (C) is wrong. Paragraphs two, three, and four summarize evidence that supports the Zel'dovich-Sunyaev theory, so (D) is incorrect in saying that the author considers it lacking in evidence.

10. D This is a question that asks you to apply your understanding of red shift analysis. Red shift analysis is discussed in the middle of the last paragraph. According to this technique, the more distant a celestial body from the point of observation, the more its light shifts to the red end of the spectrum. Thus, since the problem tells us that light emitted from galaxy A is further to the red end of the spectrum than light emitted from galaxy B, we can infer that galaxy B is closer to Earth and the Milky Way than galaxy A (D). Choice (A) misinterprets and contradicts the principles behind red shift analysis. And, as far as we know from the information in the passage, red shift analysis tells us something about the relative distance, not the speed, of galaxies A and B; consequently, we cannot infer anything about speed, and choices (B) and (C) are incorrect.

11. D This is a detail question concerning a current disagreement among astronomers. The last sentence of the third paragraph states explicitly that astronomers disagree about the dimensions of superclusters, so choice (D) is our correct answer. Choice (A) is wrong because the final paragraph—the one that discusses red shift analysis—implies that astronomers agree that this technique is very useful. Paragraphs two through five imply that astronomers agree that our galaxy, the Milky Way, is only one among an enormous number of galaxies distributed throughout the universe (B). The influence of gravity on "pancakes" is a central part of the Zel'dovich-Sunyaev theory, which is popular among astronomers, so it's unlikely that they disagree on the issue of gravity and pancakes (C).

12. D This question asks about the author's purpose in introducing "Hubble's Law." This law and its relevance are discussed in the final paragraph. There the author notes that the Zel'dovich-Sunyaev theory fails to account for the continuing expansion of the universe, but Hubble's Law fills this gap. Thus, the author introduces this law to complement or supplement the Zel'dovich-Sunyaev theory, choice (D). Choice (A) is wrong because Hubble's Law is the theory of diverging galaxies. (B) is wrong because the author introduces red shift analysis to explain Hubble's Law, not the other way around. Hubble's Law deals with the movement of galaxies and has little to do with dark matter, so the author hardly introduces this law to prove the existence of dark matter (C).

13. B This is a detail question about astronomy prior to the 20th century. The third sentence of the first paragraph tells us that little about space beyond our own galaxy was known prior to the 20th century, implying that astronomers were restricted to studying the Milky Way, choice (B). The fourth sentence of the first paragraph tells us that radio telescopes were not used until the 20th century, so choice (A) cannot be right. Since the third sentence of the first paragraph informs us that astronomers could only speculate about the existence of "external" galaxies prior to the 20th century, they could not have discovered the existence of galactic clusters and superclusters (C) until the 20th century. Finally, we cannot assume that the big bang was formulated prior to the 20th century (D) because the passage tells us nothing about when the big bang idea was formulated.

14. B This question in Roman numeral format tests your ability to understand the passage's inferences about the future through its discussion of present conditions and trends. The passage never mentions or suggests that the huge amount of energy released by the big bang explosion will be exhausted (I). However, the last sentence of the passage does indicate that, as a result of the huge energy release at the time of the big bang, today's celestial bodies and bounds of the entire universe continue to expand. On this basis, it makes sense to infer that the Milky Way, our galaxy, will continue to grow in size over time, so option II is a valid inference. Option III suggests that the configuration of the universe will remain constant in the future. But this is contrary to the notion of the expanding universe which we just referred to from the last paragraph of the passage. Thus, only option II can be inferred from the passage, making choice (B) correct.

Passage III (Questions 15–20): WOOLF

15. B Paragraph three lists the preconditions needed for women to produce works of genius, which are then figuratively summed up as "a room of [one's] own, in all its senses." These preconditions provide our wrong answers. Choices (A) and (C) are virtual paraphrases of "financial independence" and "opportunities for education," respectively. If a writer is no longer "labouring and servile," she is then relatively autonomous (D). Choice (B), the correct choice, is something to be *overcome* when one obtains a "room of one's own."

16. A According to paragraph two, one goal of a woman writer is to develop an "androgynous mind," one that has united male and female characteristics. Thus, Woolf's assumption is that there is an *a priori* division of mental processes according to gender that is transcended by genius. The assumption in choice (A) is required for Woolf's discussion to make sense. (B) makes an all-inclusive generalization that distorts Woolf's emphasis on financial security; it implies that *no* great artists have come from lower class backgrounds—a distortion of the idea that women writers must *gain* financial security. Similarly, (C) goes way overboard. That Woolf would think there has *never* been a great woman writer is implausible; paragraph two says merely that without financial independence, women are *unlikely* (not unable) to produce great art. (D) is contrary to Woolf's argument—she is saying that education is needed for women to become great writers. True, she does not directly deny (D), but it certainly is not one of her assumptions.

17. D The conditions for the development mentioned in choice (D) are discussed in paragraph three. If a woman author obtains a room of her own in all its meanings (education, financial independence), she may then go on to develop an "androgynous" mind. No information is given on why Woolf used the lecture format in *A Room of One's Own* (A). Although a tone shift between *A Room of One's Own* and *Three Guineas* is implied by the terms used to describe them (paragraph one), the cause of the change is not specified (B). The passage gives only one example of apparent male prejudice against Woolf (C)—the response to *Three Guineas* (paragraph three); and we don't learn what Woolf's reaction was.

18. D The novels are mentioned only in the first paragraph, which makes this question easy. In the last sentence of the paragraph, the author concedes that the essays "no doubt . . . lack the subtlety" of the novels; the essays, then, are "unsubtle," and this idea is expressed in (D). Originality (A) and comparative familiarity to the public (B) are not mentioned. The essays have traditionally been seen as "problematical," so they are *not* more accepted than the novels (C)—even the reference to recent critics in the last sentence of the paragraph doesn't say that these critics value the essays *more* than the novels.

19. B Statement III is correct. As paragraph two makes clear, *A Room of One's Own* discusses the achievement of financial independence by women who already possess some education and freedom from poverty; the fictitious setting of the college underlines this point. *Three Guineas,* as demonstrated by the criticism of Agnes Smith (endorsed by the author), was "class-bound"—relevant mainly to nonworking-class women. The author refers to this as a "limitation of Woolf's feminism generally," further strengthening (III). Social issues (I) are analyzed in both works, but only *A Room Of One's Own* discusses artistic development. Specific ways of fighting male domination are brought up in *Three Guineas* (pacifist action against a "male-instigated" war), ruling out (II).

20. A   Woolf's contention (see paragraph four) is that the equalizing of women's rights in the public sphere is necessarily linked to the equalizing of responsibilities in the private sphere. Thus, child-rearing, a private issue, and job equality, a public concern, are intertwined. The problem of which these are aspects is, by inference, that of assigning roles by gender in the two spheres (A). (B) is a misplaced reference, as it refers to "the probability of another war" which introduces a new topic *following* the quote specified in the question stem. (C) and (D) focus on the "different aspects" rather than on the problems as a whole—(C) refers to changes in the home, (D) refers by implication to changes in the workplace, whereas Woolf feels these issues are necessarily connected.

Passage IV (Questions 21–27): BEOWULF

21. B The author mentions Sigemund's battle with the dragon in his discussion of the tribal-lay theory in paragraph two. This theory considers *Beowulf* an amalgam of older myths and the work of many authors or editors. Sigemund's battle is mentioned to support this theory (B) because his battle with the dragon is seen as an inconsistency or digression that would characterize such an amalgamation. While the author mentions Sigemund as an example of the digressions suggested by the tribal-lay theory, he also mentions a failure to recognize Christian themes as a source of criticism of the theory. So the author's discussions of Sigemund's battle and Christian themes are for completely different and unrelated purposes, making choice (A) wrong. As discussed above, Sigemund's battle with the dragon is mentioned to support the theory that *Beowulf* is the product of many authors, not a single author (C). Finally, the battles between the Anglo-Saxons and the Vikings, Scots, and Picts are discussed in regard to the Christian authorship theory in the fourth paragraph; the author treats these conflicts and Sigemund's battle with the dragon as completely different issues, so (D) is incorrect.

22. C The Christian authorship theory, discussed in paragraph four, holds that *Beowulf*'s author might have emphasized pagan motifs—like the cult of the warrior—to boost morale for political purposes during a time of military upheavals. Therefore, the cult of the warrior is a reflection of political upheavals in England at the time of its writing (C). The idea that *Beowulf* illustrates major themes in Germanic and Norse culture is stressed in the tribal-lay theory, not the Christian authorship theory, so (A) is wrong. While the author mentions that Tolkien argues the Christian author of *Beowulf* was probably a member of a royal court (B), he does not say that the writer was a military official and accounts for the emphasis on the role of the warrior by referring to the historical context rather than the author's background. The Christian authorship theory holds that from A.D. 650 to 850, Christian and pagan beliefs coexisted, and implies that Christianity was gradually replacing pagan beliefs, even if some people continued to cling to them. So there is no basis for inferring that *Beowulf*'s emphasis on the pagan cult of the warrior exhibits a decline in Christian faith (D).

23. A The growth by accretion theory (see paragraph three) states that *Beowulf* is the product of a number of authors over a period of centuries. Considering that, option I is true, and is part of our answer. Proponents of this theory point to conflicting pagan and Christian themes as evidence of *Beowulf*'s multiple authorship, so option II is also true, and is also part of the answer to this question. However, option III plays upon the Christian authorship theory's emphasis upon unity, while also attempting to relate the poem's literary qualities to its historical context. All of this has nothing to do with the growth by accretion theory. Therefore, only options I and II are true of growth by accretion theorists, making choice (A) correct.

24. C Both the tribal-lay and growth by accretion theories hold that *Beowulf* was written by multiple authors. Tribal-lay theorists believe that the poem began as works of several authors, later combined by editors (paragraph two). Growth by accretion theorists, however, propose that *Beowulf* began as the short work of a single author, later contributed to by numerous authors. Therefore, these two theories agree on multiple authorship, but differ in their conceptions of what it entailed (C). (A) is incorrect because it wrongly attributes historical analysis to the multiple authorship theories when it is the Christian authorship theory that emphasizes the epic's historical context. Paragraph two mentions the poem's allegorical references in relation to criticism of the tribal-lay theory. But the passage provides no details of the growth by accretion theorists' interpretations or perspectives regarding these allegories. Since the passage provides us with no basis for comparing interpretations of the poem's references, (B) is wrong. (D) is wrong in suggesting differences in the ways theorists account for the poem's Christian elements. In fact, the author stresses that tribal-lay theorists tend to ignore the poem's "obvious Christian overtones" entirely (paragraph two). They would hardly "account for" or explain references they do not recognize in the first place. So there is no basis for comparing explanations of Christian elements among theorists.

25. C The Christian authorship theory rests on the belief that *Beowulf* had a single Christian author who wrote the poem, based on pagan material, sometime between the years 650 and 850. It is perfectly consistent to think that a partially translated (presumably into Norwegian) manuscript of *Beowulf* may have existed in an 11th-century Norwegian church (A). This would not affect the Christian authorship theory, which places *Beowulf*'s birthplace in England around the time of the 8th century. The Christian authorship theory argues that the Anglo-Saxons were involved in constant warfare with the Vikings, Scots, and Picts, so the discovery of even more intense or long-lasting conflict among the groups would not weaken this theory (B). The Christian authorship theorists speculate that *Beowulf* may have been written by an aristocratic Christian author, but this kind of speculation is not central to the theory. The fact that Tolkien felt *Beowulf* was "probably" written by a member of the royal court suggests that it also might not have been. Therefore, the suggestion that the poem was written by a literate peasant (D) would not weaken the theory significantly. However, if it were discovered that *Beowulf* is an English translation of an earlier Germanic myth (C), the Christian authorship theory that *Beowulf* originated in England between 650 and 850 would be severely weakened. Since the theory relies heavily upon and is specific to the epic's historical context, the realization that its origins were other than those suggested by Tolkien would erode the very foundations of the Christian authorship theory.

26. C The passage's last paragraph explains why most scholars favor the Christian authorship theory: Historical analyses of the context in which *Beowulf* was written provide the best resolution to the poem's contradictions or inconsistencies (C). The author does not claim that the Christian authorship theory locates references in *Beowulf* in Norse and Germanic mythology (A). It is the tribal-lay theory that emphasizes Nordic and Germanic sources. And while the tribal-lay theory does not consider the epic's Christian overtones, the growth by accretion theory does, so it would be incorrect to say that scholars favor the Christian authorship theory because it it is the only one that appreciates the significance of *Beowulf*'s Christian elements (B). Finally, all three of the theories discussed in the passage attempt to explain the epic's disparate references and varied motifs (D); in fact, all of the theories discussed in the passage attempt such an explanation.

27. D The author mentions a work written by J.R.R. Tolkien, originator of the Christian authorship theory, in order to introduce a contextual analysis of the writing of *Beowulf* (D). Although you may recognize Tolkien as the prominent author of *The Hobbit,* the passage's author does not mention Tolkien to lend support to multiple authorship theories (A). In fact, Tolkien's theory contradicts the notion of multiple authorship entirely. According to the second sentence of the forth paragraph, Tolkien argues that *Beowulf* was written by a single Christian author, eliminating choice (B). (C) is incorrect because the author of this passage does not attempt to *disprove* previous theories of *Beowulf*'s authorship. While it is true that the author's tone seems to favor the theory of "Christian authorship," he writes in the first sentence of the last paragraph that it would be impossible to conclusively prove or disprove any of the theories.

Passage V (Questions 28–35): HUMAN RIGHTS

28. C The first paragraph states that the basic meaning of human rights has changed considerably since the 18th century—what initially meant simply the right to representative government now encompasses the right to be employed, to own property, and to receive at least minimal levels of food, shelter, health care, and education. This information allows us to infer that an 18th-century political thinker's understanding of human rights would differ considerably from that of his 20th-century counterpart. Choices (A) and (B) involve unrelated details discussed in other parts of the passage—we're given no evidence to infer that our hypothetical political thinkers would disagree on the proper methods of ensuring international human rights or on the amount of education to which every citizen is entitled. No comparison between 18th- and 20th-century conceptions of these issues is mentioned or suggested. There is also no indication that the political thinkers would differ in their opinions of the importance of representative government (D)—that the 20th-century political thinker includes many more things in his concept of human rights does not mean he values representative government less than his 18th-century counterpart did.

29. C The author mentions the effects of direct intervention by one government in another's affairs in the third and fourth paragraphs. Option I is supported by the last sentence of the third paragraph, which states that intervention could transgress domestic laws, thereby "violating citizen's rights to a responsive and representative government." Support for option III comes in the fourth sentence of paragraph three ("international agreements usually preclude intervention") and in the third sentence of paragraph four (direct intervention is "generally undesirable and illegal"). Although the passage states that direct intervention could violate the rights of citizens in the intervening country, no evidence is given that the violation would necessarily lead to "civil unrest" (option II).

30. D The author discusses the difficulty of guaranteeing human rights in paragraph two. At the end of the paragraph, he mentions that certain economic and social resources are necessary to protect human rights—and indicates that providing them is not always practical. This evidence points to (D). Choice (A) goes too far—true, no consensus concerning the extent of basic rights exists, and the author indicates that putting theory into practice is sometimes difficult, but he never says it is *impossible*. Choice (B) distorts a detail in paragraph two. There the author just states that some people consider education a privilege rather than a right that must be guaranteed. He never goes so far as to say or suggest "many rights need not be guaranteed." The author mentions "geopolitical goals" in the third paragraph, but only to say that some countries interfere in the human rights actions of other countries in order to further their own interests. The author never suggests that such intervention does not conflict with other geopolitical goals. The very nature of such intervention suggests otherwise. So, there is no support for (C).

31. B The reference to national security considerations comes in the second paragraph, within the author's discussion of how "equally important societal goals" sometimes conflict with the rights of citizens—to ensure its survival during war, for example, a government may have to interfere with certain individual rights, like freedom of speech. Choice (A) involves an unrelated detail—the author does not make reference to "selfish geopolitical goals" until the next paragraph. (C) exaggerates to the point of distortion—the author only says that government interests may sometimes conflict with citizens' rights (like the right to free speech and press), *not* that safeguarding those rights is an "impossible endeavor." Choice (D) refers to an unrelated detail discussed a little later in the second paragraph—where the author uses the example of education. While both do concern the question of the extent and limits of rights, the author's discussion of national security is not specifically aimed at providing evidence that the extent of rights is problematic.

32. D The author uses the entire second paragraph to discuss the difficulties sovereign governments face when they try to, transform, human, rights, theories into, concrete policies; therefore, choice (D) is correct. Choices (A), (B), and (C) distort various details mentioned in the passage. The author mentions halfway through paragraph two that *some people* consider education a privilege rather than a right, but he does not argue that education should not be included among human rights (A). Paragraph three discusses the difficulties involved when a country interferes in the human rights practices of another, but the author never argues that governments should never try to influence one another (B). In fact, in paragraph four, he details a number of methods countries could use to influence human rights on the international level. Of these, the author feels that diplomacy is more "palatable" than direct intervention, but he never claims that it is the "only rational means" (C).

33. C The author discusses the various "mechanisms" for ensuring the protection of human rights in paragraph four. Choice (A) is mentioned in the second sentence, (B) in the last sentence, and (D) in the fourth sentence. Nowhere does the author mention the development of a "universal definition of human rights," making (C) the correct choice. In fact, the author's discussion of difficulties in translating human rights theory into policies suggests (C) would be highly improbable.

34. A The fourth sentence of the third paragraph states that "international legal agreements usually preclude intervention in the internal affairs of other nations," and the fourth sentence of paragraph four says direct intervention is "generally undesirable and illegal." Choices (B) and (C) are on the right track—the author does consider direct intervention "undesirable"—but he never indicates that it's nonetheless "justifiable" or "necessary" under certain conditions. Choice (D) is out right from the start—this contradicts parts of the passage cited above in the explanation of correct choice (A).

35. B The author outlines the general meaning of human rights and how it has evolved in the first paragraph, then goes on to discuss the difficulties of putting theory into practice on the domestic level (paragraph two), and on the international level (paragraph three). In the last paragraph, he mentions some ways to safeguard human rights on both levels. Choice (B) accurately summarizes this structure. The author does not organize his discussion around any "distinctions" between human rights on the domestic and international levels (A), nor does he refine the definition of human rights through a series of observations (C). Choice (D) is out because the author does not really argue a point. His tone is merely that of an objective presenter of information.

Passage VI (Questions 36–40): TELESCOPES

36. C This question addresses the primary purpose of the passage: How the refractor and reflector telescopes alternately developed in response to both scientific discovery and technical innovation. While the author does discuss different shapes of lenses throughout the passage, choice (A) is not the main topic of the passage; the effects of different lenses are considered only in support of the more general discussion of the development of telescope design. (B) contradicts the conclusion that reflectors are currently more popular, so it can't be right. This passage is about ways in which technological constraints have affected the development of the telescope, but that's just one example of how technological constraints have affected the course of science, so (D) is too broad to be the primary purpose.

37. A See the third sentence of paragraph two. Scientists turned to reflectors because Newton thought chromatic aberration in refractors was unsolvable. (B) is wrong because the passage says that spherical aberration is simply corrected. The thought that chromatic aberration was unsolvable was not mentioned for the purposes of deriding Newton or his ways of thinking. Nothing in the passage or in the author's tone suggests such a purpose, so both (C) and (D) are too judgmental to jibe with the author's intentions.

38. D A straightforward detail question. See paragraph three—Leonhard Euler provided a solution to chromatic aberration using two lenses with water between them. According to the passage, using a lens with rounded surfaces (A) may cause spherical aberration but solves nothing. (B) and (C) refer to improvements made in reflectors, which do not suffer from chromatic aberration.

39. D Problems associated with refractors are discussed in paragraphs one, three, and four. Chromatic aberration (A) and spherical aberration (C) are both mentioned in paragraph one. Limited lens diameter (B) is discussed in sentence one of paragraph four. Only choice (D) is not associated with refractors: over-absorption of light is a problem of reflectors, discussed in paragraph two.

40. A Various problems with materials and construction of telescopes are discussed throughout the passage, which implies that technological constraints hindered the development of telescopes. The passage never implies (B); it scarcely discusses methodology at all and does not suggest any problem with methods being imprecise. Contrary to choice (C), the author implies that scientists were extremely interested in developing better telescopes. There is no suggestion that materials were scarce or unavailable (D).

WRITING SAMPLE

INTRODUCTION

ABOUT THIS SECTION

The Writing Sample section introduces you to the seven-step approach to writing an essay and gives you a chance to practice your new skills. However, the skills involved in producing a good essay in thirty minutes cannot be learned instantly; it takes time and practice to assimilate our method.

Chapter 1 provides you with important information about the MCAT essay assignment as well as a general summary of the Kaplan approach to essay writing.

Chapter 2 takes you through Kaplan's seven-step method, one step at a time.

Chapter 3 provides you with practice essay assignments to give you the opportunity to become expert at the whole seven-step process. You can develop your critical skills by comparing your own essays with others written by students on the same topics.

ABOUT THE MCAT WRITING SAMPLE

The essay section of the MCAT that you take on test day will most likely contain two 30-minute timed essays. You will type your responses on the computer. After working on the first question for 30 minutes, you will be told to stop and go on to the second essay question, for which you will again be allowed 30 minutes. It will be up to you to pace yourself during each 30-minute period and not get bogged down.

You cannot choose to write on any other topic. You must write in English, not a foreign language, and you must try to accomplish everything the instructions require.

The Writing Sample's Purpose and Format

The writing sample tests your ability to:

1. Develop a central idea
2. Synthesize ideas
3. Express ideas logically and cohesively
4. Write clearly, using standard written English and proper punctuation

In other words, it tests your ability to write a good, brief essay. Of course, you are not expected to produce final-draft quality; the MCAT readers know you have only 30 minutes to write. But don't assume this means they have low standards. When you read the sample essays in the MCAT student manual, you will see that the test makers' expectation of a good essay really *is* a good essay.

Each essay question will have the same format: a statement followed by a set of instructions containing three distinct tasks. Each question will look something like this:

Consider this statement:

True leadership leads by example rather than by command.

Write a unified essay in which you perform the following tasks. Explain what you think the above statement means. Describe a specific situation in which true leaders lead by command rather than by example. Discuss what you think determines when a leader should lead by example or by command.

THE STATEMENT

On your test the statement may be an opinion, a widely shared belief, a philosophical dictum, or an assertion regarding general policy concerns in such areas as history, political science, business, ethics, or art. You can be sure that the statement will *not* concern scientific or technical topics (e.g., biology, physics, or chemistry), your reasons for entering the medical profession, emotionally charged religious or social issues (e.g., abortion), or obscure social or political issues that might require specialized knowledge. In fact, you will not need any specialized knowledge to do well on this part of the MCAT. Even so, you might want to start reading a good, national newspaper in order to become better acquainted with some of the current social concerns.

THE INSTRUCTIONS

Though worded slightly differently each time, the instructions that follow the statement will ask you to perform these **three tasks:**

1. Provide your interpretation or explanation of the statement.
2. Offer a concrete example (hypothetical or actual) that illustrates a point of view directly **opposite** to the one expressed in or implied by the statement.
3. Explain how the conflict between the viewpoint expressed in the statement and the viewpoint you described for the second task can be resolved.

These tasks give you quite a lot to complete in a scant 30 minutes. It's a good idea, therefore, to approach this section prepared for what you'll find. That's where this part of the *MCAT Premier Program* will help: It will familiarize you with the section and give you a firm sense of how to accomplish all necessary tasks. Actually, once you know what you're doing, the three tasks make your job somewhat easier since they "design" your essay for you (a good part of the battle!).

FREQUENTLY ASKED QUESTIONS ON SCORING AND RELATED TOPICS

Question: Is there a right or wrong answer to these essay questions?

Answer: No. Essays won't be judged on whether or not the reader agrees with your position or thinks your points true. Further, the essays' instructions will not ask you to take a position on the statements you discuss. If you feel that offering your position on the statement or a related issue will make a better essay, that's fine. But don't feel pressured to agree or disagree with the statement.

Question: Who grades my essays?

Answer: A reader reads the essays and scores them; your essays also are graded by computer.

Question: What kind of score will be reported?

Answer: Once the reader and the computer have graded your essays, the total scores for both essays will be added together. This combined score will then be converted into an alphabetic rating (ranging from J to T) and sent to you and to the medical schools that receive your other MCAT information. The medical schools will also get percentile information regarding how well you did compared with your peers.

Question: What's a good score?

Answer: Statistically speaking, there will be very few six-point essays. An essay of four or five places you at the upper range of those taking this exam. But a good score is a personal estimation. After all, if you have very weak writing skills and pump up your skills using the Kaplan materials, you may feel very good about getting a score of three—and you'd be right to feel that way.

Question: How are my essays graded?

Answer: Your reader and computer grader will use a holistic grading technique. That means that each supplies a single numeric score for the essay as a whole. (Organization, style, grammar, and so on are not graded separately.) Your graders will first of all determine how thoroughly and meaningfully you responded to the three writing tasks. They will note whether you offer appropriate illustrations or examples and how well you tie your thoughts together into a unified whole. In addition, they will pay attention to how well you organize your paragraphs individually and collectively. They will also look for varied sentence structure and word choice. This does not mean your graders want convoluted sentences or big "dictionary" words; they *do* want the kind of lively writing that comes with active *thinking*.

Question: I'm lousy at grammar and punctuation. Will those kinds of errors count for very much?

Answer: Your graders know you are writing under time pressure and expect you to make a certain number of mistakes in writing mechanics (grammar, spelling, etc.). A few scattered mistakes of this kind *do not* carry much weight. However, a series of such mistakes can mar your work's overall impression. So while we suggest that you not be overly concerned with mistakes of this nature, don't ignore this area if it is a particularly weak one.

Question: In writing my essays, do I have to follow a certain format?

Answer: Many students think they have to write a standard five-paragraph essay: an introductory paragraph, three body paragraphs, and a conclusion—the kind often taught in high schools. There is *no* set format. As long as you address all three writing tasks, you can do so in whatever order and form you choose. However, since you will be scored partly on your essay's unity, giving the reader a sense of a definite beginning, middle, and end will be an advantage.

Question: Do I need to throw around a lot of big, impressive sounding words in order to do well?

Answer: Some test-prep companies tell their students to memorize impressive sounding words and work them into the essay. That's cynical and silly. People who have to memorize impressive words probably don't have much practice using them—so the words stick out and look awkward. Besides, the best essays make their points simply, concisely, and straightforwardly. If you have a large vocabulary, this will help you make your points more convincingly since you'll be able to choose more precise words. If you're not comfortable using a large vocabulary, it's a poor idea to toss in fancy words for the sake of impressing a reader. What your readers want is *clarity.* You don't have to put on an act. Better to stick to the words you know than run the risk of a malapropism.

ABOUT THE KAPLAN APPROACH

To most writers, the process of essay writing is one filled with starts and stops. As a writer works on drafting an essay, he or she thinks about the topic from several angles and comes up with ideas that eventually must be refined, rephrased, or thrown out. The writer might compose several introductory paragraphs before finding the right tack or be halfway through writing when a better idea comes to mind, requiring a major revision. This is the natural way for most people to compose.

But there is nothing natural about a timed-essay test.

You simply don't have time to let your thoughts flow in their natural, cyclic way. Yet it is essential to hash out and refine your ideas if you are going to produce an essay of any substance. Therefore, what you need is a method to speed up the writing process and make it more efficient.

We suggest you use a proven method that will help you take good advantage of each one of those 30 minutes. The purpose of the method is to provide you with a clearly defined track on which to move through the writing process, performing what needs to be done in as little time as possible. It consists of seven steps:

THE SEVEN STEPS

Step 1. Read and Jot Down Notes on Scratch Paper
Step 2. Prewrite First Task on Scratch Paper
Step 3. Prewrite Second Task on Scratch Paper
Step 4. Prewrite Third Task on Scratch Paper
Step 5. Clarify Main Idea and Plan
Step 6. Write Essay
Step 7. Proofread

Though they represent only about one-sixth of your total work time (or approximately five minutes), the most important steps in this method are one through five. It is during this time, the *prewriting* time, that you will do the hashing out, refining, and organizing of ideas that a writer usually does during the whole of the first-draft process.

In the rest of this section, you'll have ample opportunity to practice the seven-step approach. You'll become familiar with how each step relates to the whole. In time, you'll find yourself going through the steps in your own way—making them a natural part of your essay writing. As you do so, you'll find they take less and less time. Follow Kaplan's seven-step method and you will be able to produce well reasoned essays on the toughest topics within the 30-minute time limit.

2

BUILDING YOUR ESSAY

PREWRITING: STEPS 1–5

Your ability to write is directly linked to your ability to think analytically and logically. You might have a wonderful command of the English language, but if you can't get your thoughts organized and your ideas clear in your mind, your essay will be a jumbled mess. So, since you don't have time to write a sloppy first draft and then revise it, you must do the basic part of refining your ideas *before* starting to write. In other words, you must *prewrite*.

The prewriting steps clarify what work you must get done before you are ready to write. Also, they help you get that work done efficiently. At first, you should practice these steps in sequence to familiarize yourself thoroughly with what prewriting involves. But as you get to know them, you'll probably find it more natural to jump around from one step to another rather than to work linearly.

For instance, you'll find that as you do Step 1 (reading and taking notes), ideas for any one of the other prewriting steps may well start popping into your mind right away. Step 3 (thinking of an opposing example) often helps to clarify your ideas about the statement's meaning (Step 2). Clarifying a main idea (Step 5) helps to focus all of your ideas for Steps 2 through 4, and so on. Once you learn the process, there is no need to feel that you must perfect each step before moving on to the next. Going back and refining your ideas as you move through the prewriting process will allow you to build a set of ideas that fit together into a coherent whole.

 Go Online

Take advantage of monthly essay practice.

Taking Notes

It is essential to take notes during the prewriting process. Only a very extraordinary person can keep straight all of the ideas generated during prewriting. But note taking is a difficult thing to teach since each person must develop his or her own style. No one but you is going to read your notes; they don't need to be clear or comprehensible to anyone else. The trick is to develop a style that you can read and understand but that lets you abbreviate your ideas as much as possible. You don't want to waste time writing out whole sentences, but you must be able to make sense of your notes when you work on your essay. This takes practice.

STRATEGY: *As you take your notes, categorize them according to the three tasks given in the essay instructions. Divide your note-taking page into three areas and number them, one for each task. Ideas that explain or illustrate the statement (the first task) get jotted down in area #1, ideas that explore the opposing view (the second task) go in area #2, etc. This method will automatically order your thoughts, even if you are not coming up with them in an orderly way.*

All Five Steps in Just Five Minutes?

As we discuss the prewriting process, it may seem as though it requires much too much time for a 30-minute essay. Don't worry. At first, the steps take explaining and practice, but once you understand the process, you'll be able to work efficiently. You'll discover that the five minutes you spend prewriting will speed up the writing process.

MOST COMMON PREWRITING MISTAKES

- The student fails to pay close attention to the meaning of the statement and/or the instructions.
- The student rushes into typing the essay, hoping to figure things out while composing the essay.
- The student is immediately struck by an idea that addresses the second or third task (the easier ones) and starts writing without prewriting the first task.

MOST COMMON SYMPTOMS OF POOR PREWRITING

- The essay does not thoroughly fulfill all of the tasks in the instructions.
- The essay has no clear main idea.
- The essay is poorly organized.
- The first paragraph or two are vague and pointless.
- All of the best ideas are jammed in at the end of the essay.
- The essay is incomplete: The student was cut short by the time limit and was unable to respond to all parts of the instructions.

Prewriting can be the single most important way of helping your final essay achieve clarity, order, and authority. Now let's look at the steps one by one.

STEP 1: READ AND JOT DOWN NOTES ON SCRATCH PAPER

PURPOSE: To clarify for yourself what the statement says and what the instructions require.

PROCESS: Read the statement and instructions carefully.

Jot down any words or phrases in the statement that:

- Are easy to miss but are crucial to a good understanding of the statement
- Are ambiguous or confusing
- Refer to vague or abstract concepts (e.g., *freedom*, *happiness*, etc.) that need clarification.

Jot down any words in the instructions that will help you remember exactly what it is you're supposed to do.

Good communication requires more than just speaking or writing clearly; it first requires paying attention to what you are being asked to communicate *about*. And that means paying attention to what the given statement and instructions say. An essay that does not relate clearly and directly to the idea expressed in the statement or that does not fulfill the specific tasks put forth in the instructions is unlikely to receive more than a grade of three.

Why bother taking notes?

Especially under pressure of a time limit, it is easy to waste the first few minutes with anxious worrying or nervous, unstructured thinking. Jotting down words puts your mind in gear. It helps you focus your attention on what needs to be done and forces you to concentrate on this important first step.

STEP 2: PREWRITE FIRST TASK ON SCRATCH PAPER

PURPOSE: To develop a clear interpretation of the statement.

PROCESS: • Think of one or more supporting examples.
- Clarify/define/interpret abstract, ambiguous, or confusing words.
- Ask yourself questions to get beyond the superficial meaning of the statement.

The MCAT test makers say that the statement in the essay assignment will not be simply factual or self-evident. This means that, in order to explain the meaning of the statement, you must develop some ideas of your own about its meaning or about the meaning of certain words or concepts within it. But often it is difficult to see exactly where or why a statement *needs* explaining. It may *seem* perfectly self-evident to you. The trick is to imagine that you must explain this statement to your intelligent 15-year-old sibling and you want this 15-year-old to understand the statement on more than just a superficial level.

Take, for instance, the statement: The United States is a free country. This statement is often used in many different contexts. Yet, if you asked 20 different people what they thought about this statement, you'd get 20 different responses. So how do you explain to your 15-year-old why this is not just a simple statement of fact or opinion? You try to give an explanation of its *deeper* meaning. For one thing, there's a good deal of *history* behind the statement. The belief that the people of this country should be "free" to pursue their individual goals began with the first European settlers who came here in search of freedom from religious and economic oppression. But there is also the *philosophical* question: What *is* freedom? Much *controversy* revolves around this question. In fact, many people feel this country is "free" only for a privileged few. Thus, what might seem like a simple cliché is actually a very complex tangle of ideas and implications.

Obviously, you can't go into depth on all these subjects in a 30-minute essay. (And your 15-year-old would fall asleep!) But to explain the statement with any clarity you must consider these issues, decide which you need to discuss, and put your ideas together to make the best interpretation you can. The MCAT essay readers are looking for a *thorough exploration* of the topic.

Here is a sampling of some of the many questions you can ask to get yourself started on an "exploration" of a statement:

- What are some situations (hypothetical or real) that illustrate what this statement is saying?
- Are there any specific words in the statement that need clarifying before you can discuss the meaning of the statement as a whole?
- What is the historical background of the idea(s) in the statement? (Have the ideas been around for a long or a short time? Why? Where did they come from?)
- What is the philosophical background of the statement? (Are there some basic beliefs or assumptions on which this statement depends?)
- What kinds of people are concerned with this statement today and why are they concerned with it?
- Does this statement mean different things to different people? If so, what are these different meanings? What meaning do *you* give it and why?

This is certainly a lot to think about!
With all these directions to go in, how do you keep your ideas from running all over the place? Here's one useful approach:

> **STRATEGY:** *Before trying to define the statement, think up one or two illustrations of it. This will give you something concrete to think about and will help you identify what areas you need to explore with this particular topic.*

All MCAT Writing Sample topics will most likely strike you as at least partly true. Even if you disagree with the statement in a general way, you'll probably be able to think of *some* situation that illustrates a way in which the statement is true. This kind of illustration will help you figure out the *meaning* of the statement. (And if you want, you can use the example in your essay.)

Warning! Don't let a strong personal reaction to the statement ruin your essay.

A strong reaction to a statement can fool a student into rushing headlong into writing. But your powerful feelings or your eagerness to say a lot about a topic does not release you from having to follow the instructions.

REMEMBER: The first task asks you to explain what you think the statement means. You can talk about ideas that oppose the statement when you address the second task.

You don't have to take a stand.
You are not being tested on your opinions or your morals. The purpose of the essay assignment is to test your ability to think and to write. The instructions will not ask you to agree or disagree with the statement. You may take a stand if you feel that to do so will help you write a clearer essay, but you don't have to.

EXAMPLE OF STEP 2
Below is an essay topic. A student's prewriting notes for Step 2 have been added. These notes are just one student's response—each student will respond in his or her own way.

> *Consider this statement:*
>
> *True leadership leads by* example *rather than by command.*

Write a unified essay in which you perform the following tasks. Explain what you think the above statement means. Describe a specific situation in which true leaders lead by command rather than by example. Discuss what you think determines when a leader should lead by example or by command.

① *By example—*
Alexander
Gandhi
Agassiz
Clara B.
—had a special gift ⟶ *people compelled to follow*

You can see in the notes above that this student first got down to business by thinking up several examples of leaders who lead by example. With these in mind, she could generalize more clearly about the kind of leader who leads by example. The circled number one shows that these ideas all apply to the first task.

(The essay for which these notes were written can be found as Essay #1 in the discussion of Step 6.)

STEP 3: PREWRITE SECOND TASK ON SCRATCH PAPER

PURPOSE: To further explore the meaning of the statement by examining a situation that represents an opposing point of view.

PROCESS: Think up one or more specific situations that demonstrate a way in which the statement is *not* true.

Of the three tasks, this one is the easiest for most students because it is so specific. Thinking up specific examples is a lot easier than defining abstract ideas. Further, it's almost always easier to find a flaw in something than it is to explain what's true about it.

Once they learn to handle the prewriting process, many students find that it helps to work a bit on the second task before tackling the first. In any case, working on the second task is very likely to help you develop and clarify your ideas about a statement.

That the second task is helpful in clarifying ideas is no coincidence. The three tasks provided for you by the MCAT test makers follow a standard method of argument. The tasks, if you follow them, actually *help* you write a good essay. So follow them.

> **STRATEGY:** *Don't try to write or outline the essay in your head while you're prewriting the three tasks. Do the tasks first. They will help you develop a set of ideas on which you can build an essay. If you try to compose your essay before you're ready, you will only waste time.*

Even if you agree completely with the statement, you can come up with an opposing example.

The creators of the MCAT Writing Sample purposely pick statements that are sufficiently complex to have more than one side. If you are having trouble thinking of a good illustration, imagine a person who actively disagrees with the statement—what illustrations would he or she provide?

> **STRATEGY:** *Don't waste time struggling to think of an example from history or current events. If you can't think of a real-life example, make up a hypothetical one. You are not being tested on your knowledge of history, politics, or any other area.*

If you disagree with the statement, the second task allows you to air your views.

It's difficult, if you have a strong reaction against a statement, not to launch right away into an explanation of that reaction. But your ideas will sound much more levelheaded if you take the time to clarify the meaning of the statement before talking about how that meaning is wrong. The second task (as well as the third) gives you a place to express an opposing opinion, so save your criticisms or revisions for your response to this task. The result will be a set of logical prewriting notes rather than a jumble of reactions.

It's OK to discuss more than one example, but don't spread yourself too thin.

Sometimes students find they can think of several different ways in which the statement is not true. Should this happen to you, focus on just one area. You may want to illustrate that the statement is untrue with a single example or with several examples—either way is fine. What's important is to make sure that all of the examples work together to illustrate the same general idea. You do not want to try to tackle more than one opposing idea. You don't have the time, and your essay is likely to lose focus.

EXAMPLE OF STEP 3

Below is the same essay topic shown in Step 2. Here the student's notes for Step 3 have been added.

> *Consider this statement:*
>
> *True leadership leads by* example *rather than by command.*

Write a unified essay in which you perform the following tasks. Explain what you think the above statement means. Describe a specific situation in which true leaders lead by command *rather than by example. Discuss what you think determines when a leader should lead by example or by command.*

① *By example—*
Alexander
Gandhi
Agassiz
Clara B.
—had a special gift ⟶ *people compelled to follow*

② *By command—*
When people confused/defeated/need a common goal
leader takes charge
nations, businesses, etc.

From the notes responding to the second task (those next to the circled number two), we can see that our student has developed the idea that leadership by command is appropriate in a certain kind of situation.

(The essay for which these notes were written can be found as Essay #1 in the discussion of Step 6.)

STEP 4: PREWRITE THIRD TASK ON SCRATCH PAPER

PURPOSE: To find a way to resolve the conflict between the statement given in the essay topic and the opposing situation(s) you thought of for the second task.

PROCESS: Read the instructions for the third task carefully. Look back at the ideas you generated for the first and second tasks. Develop your response based on these ideas.

The third task follows naturally from the first and second tasks. If you think of an idea and then think of an opposition to that idea, it's only natural to try to reach some kind of resolution of the conflict. In fact, many students find that a resolution to the conflict just comes to them, before they even really think about the third task. That's fine. You often have your best ideas when your thoughts get rolling like that. Nonetheless, do take the time to read carefully the instructions regarding the third task.

> **STRATEGY:** *The instructions for the third task are likely to give you quite a specific approach to resolving the conflict. This approach will, in turn, make your job more specific and therefore easier. Be sure to check back to the wording of the instructions for this task.*

What if you can't think of a good way to resolve the conflict?
This task tests your ability to look at a *general* problem (the conflict) and, using your powers of judgment and evaluation, come up with a way of handling the problem. If your good judgment tells you that there is no easy

or problem-free solution, then write what you think is the *best* solution. You are not expected to solve the problems of the world in this essay.

You don't have to resolve the conflict in support of, or in opposition to, the statement.
Remember, your readers don't care whether you agree or disagree with the statement. Use your own good judgment to resolve the conflict in any way that makes sense to you. Just be sure to explain your reasoning. Your reasoning is what counts, not your particular stance on the conflict.

EXAMPLE OF STEP 4
Below is the same essay topic shown in Steps 1 through 3. Here, the student's prewriting notes responding to the third task have been added.

> Consider this statement:
>
> *True leadership leads by* example *rather than by command.*

Write a unified essay in which you perform the following tasks. Explain what you think the above statement means. Describe a specific situation in which true leaders lead by command *rather than by example. Discuss what you think determines when a leader should lead by example or by command.*

① *By example—*
Alexander
Gandhi
Agassiz
Clara B.
—had a special gift ⟶ people compelled to follow

② *By command—*
When people confused/defeated/need a common goal
leader takes <u>charge</u>
nations, businesses, etc.

③ *Followers shared a common vision*
If no shared vision ⟶ command is needed

The notes responding to the third task (next to the circled number three) show that the student looked back over her notes and compared the kind of leadership she thought about in response to the first task with the kind of leadership she thought about in response to the second task. She apparently found a clear point of contrast between her two ideas of leadership. In one type of leadership, the followers share a common vision; in the other, they do not. As a result, she can clarify what determines when leadership should be by example or by command.

(The essay for which these notes were written can be found as Essay #1 in the discussion of Step 6.)

STEP 5: CLARIFY MAIN IDEA AND PLAN

PURPOSE: To do final organization and clarification of ideas. To take a mental "breath" before beginning to write.

PROCESS: Take a quick moment to look back over your notes in light of the ideas you have reached in prewriting the third task. Check to make sure your ideas are consistent with each other. Cross out those that no longer belong. Decide in what order your essay will address the three tasks.

Although it sounds like a lot to do, this step is actually the quickest of them all. If you have prewritten all three tasks, and have organized your notes so that you can clearly see which ideas pertain to which task, then most of your prewriting work is done. Having prewritten each of the tasks, you've now developed and refined your ideas in response to the essay topic.

You already have a main idea.

Many people find main ideas to be confusing things. But we don't need to bother with trying to define them. If you have prewritten the third task, then you have everything you need. You have reached a conclusion, an idea toward which all your other ideas lead. Treat this as your main idea.

Take a fast look over the rest of your notes to get rid of or clarify any ideas that don't relate to your main idea in a way that makes sense.

Then plan how you are going to order the ideas in your essay and you will be ready to write.

In fact, you already have a plan, too!

Although the MCAT people say that you can structure your essay any way you want, there is one very obvious and simple structure that helps make writing this essay quite a bit easier. The three tasks, in the order in which they are given, supply you with a straightforward structure that makes good sense.

> **STRATEGY:** *Use the basic essay format provided by the three tasks.*

First Part of Essay—Address the first task: This gives you the perfect opportunity to introduce the topic to be discussed and clarify its meaning. Establishing the basics in this way is essential for any argument to be clear.

Second Part of Essay—Provide an opposing idea to the one expressed in the statement: This lets you look at the statement from a different angle.

Doing this lets you further develop your essay, delving more deeply into the nature of the statement and expanding on your ideas.

Third Part of Essay—Resolve the conflict between the statement and the opposing idea: This lets you synthesize your ideas into a focused conclusion—a natural ending to your discussion.

What do the prewriting notes for Step 5 look like?

Usually they are invisible, as most of Step 5 is done simply by looking over your notes and clarifying how your main idea will be the focus of the essay. You might cross out a phrase, add a word or two, draw an arrow between two ideas—whatever you need for that final mental preparation before actually writing.

FINAL PREWRITING REMINDER

Keep your notes in order by categorizing them according to the task they address: three tasks, three bunches of notes. You don't have to *think* of them in order, just record them in the fashion we suggest, and you'll have an effective outline to help you through your essay.

STEP 6: WRITE

PURPOSE: Write a complete essay that addresses all three tasks in approximately 25 minutes (the total essay time, minus 5 minutes of prewriting).

PROCESS: Using your prewriting notes for guidance, compose a straightforward essay that thoroughly explains your response to each of the three tasks.

Writing an essay can truly be fun if you have sufficiently clarified your basic ideas beforehand. If you have a good general sense of what you want to say, you can let your mind roll along without fear of getting seriously off track or losing your focus. This is the time when you will get your best ideas—when you become creative.

But don't let the writing carry you away—stick to the tasks.

If the statement or some related idea inspires you to write an essay all your own, or only obliquely related to the topic, squelch that inspiration. You don't have time to fool around with experimental first drafts. If you want to produce a good essay *and* fulfill the three tasks, be conservative.

Does it seem boring, constraining, or babyish to follow the tasks?

Follow them anyway. That's the requirement of the MCAT Writing Sample.

You don't have to spend an equal amount of time responding to each task.

How much emphasis you give one task or another depends entirely on the ideas you develop. But don't be skimpy. The MCAT people expect you to take their instructions seriously. And they are looking for "depth of thought."

Does the length of the essay matter?

What matters is whether or not your essay is a good one, but good essays do tend to be on the long side. A well written essay means a well thought out essay in which ideas are explained, illustrated, and developed until the implications are clear. Yet just filling up space with blather, so it looks as if you are thinking, won't get you anywhere.

Following the tasks will help you produce a unified essay.

Unity in an essay means that all of the ideas focus on a common topic and that they all lead to a central idea. If you fulfill each of the three tasks, you will naturally achieve unity: The tasks all relate to each other, and they lead from first to second to third in a logical manner.

SOME COMMON TRANSITION WORDS AND PHRASES

Using transitions is an extremely important technique for achieving coherence and unity. Transitions provide the reader with signals about the structure of your essay's argument; the reader should be able to guess at your logical structure simply by looking at your transition words and phrases.

For contrast:

although
however, counterevidence suggests
still
however
nevertheless
on the one hand . . .
   on the other hand
despite
otherwise
but
yet
though
because . . .

For comparison:

likewise
similarly
just as . . . so

For continuing argument:

also
moreover
further(more)
besides
in addition
and
not just because, but also
this (argument)
that (attitude)
these (attempts)

For conclusion:
then
in conclusion
therefore
if this is true, then
hence
finally
in sum
thus
consequently

To introduce examples:
for instance
consider the case of
one reason for this is . . .
* another reason for this is . . .*
one example of this is . . .
* another example of this is . . .*

To introduce one idea and then suggest a better alternative:

certainly . . . yet
undoubtedly . . . but
obviously . . . nevertheless

granted . . . however
to be sure . . . nonetheless
admittedly . . . still

EXAMPLE OF STEP 6

Essay #1, just below, and Essay #2, following, are both responses to the essay topic shown in the Examples of Steps 2 through 4. The prewriting notes shown in those earlier examples were written in preparation for Essay #1.

ESSAY #1

Even though we might all disagree about the precise definition of <u>leadership</u>, we could probably agree that, as one Supreme Court justice once wrote of pornography, we can recognize it when we see it. Through the lens of history, leadership can often seem mysteriously compelling, a kind of divine gift. In the story of Alexander the Great, legend and history combine to hand down the image of the brave, determined young man who fought more fiercely than his troops, proving by his own example that a band of Macedonians could indeed endure great hardship and overcome better-equipped adversaries in their conquest of the known world.

But we must not assume that leadership is only seen on the battlefield. By example, Clara Barton inspired the young women who helped make nursing a respected profession. It was by humble but powerful example that Gandhi taught his people that passive resistance could drive out their British oppressors . . . by example that great researcher/teachers like Louis Agassiz led a generation of budding scientists . . . and by example that writers like James Joyce can cause the development of literature to swerve in a new direction. Thus, no matter what the field of endeavor, it is usually the case that great leaders seem to lead by setting an example. Brave actions compel others to follow.

Yet these famous instances of successful leadership all benefit from a circumstance that does not always apply when strong leadership is needed. Those who followed Alexander, Gandhi, Barton, and Agassiz were already united in purpose. In each case, as well, the followers probably shared roughly similar backgrounds and social attitudes. By contrast, when a group is so diverse that common ground cannot be easily found or when there is no shared goal, leadership can only succeed when the leader commands, using his authority and inspiration to bring people together.

Consider the familiar cliché that a leader "forges" a nation, particularly when its people have suffered defeat. Is this not often the case in sports, business, and the arts, as well? A team, company, or theater group threatens to fall apart because the common vision has been lost. Its members are depressed, say, and they forget what brought them together in the first place. In such instances, a leader must take charge, order them to work together and ensure that a shared goal can be attained. Only after the work begins to take shape and the group regains its sense of purpose can the leader relax his command and lead by example. To my mind, it is always preferable to have leaders who can inspire us by example, for we as followers can therefore choose whether or not to follow. I do think we must recognize, however, that disorganized or confusing situations sometimes cry out for a leader who can assume command for the greater good of the group.

Evaluation and Discussion of Essay #1
Holistic Score: 6

Each of the three writing tasks is addressed separately in a response that is unified by a strong personal voice and a steady focus on the topic. All three tasks are addressed in a thorough way, demonstrating complexity of thought.

Paragraphs one and two address the first task in some depth. Paragraph one opens with an attention-getting, yet relevant, comparison to a famous comment about pornography. The author then goes on to provide a number of examples that work together to clarify the meaning of the statement. Notice that these paragraphs refrain from saying anything about what the statement does not mean; they are unified around ideas that refer to the first task only.

Paragraph three takes the tasks out of turn and addresses the third task. This method of organization is successful in this case for two reasons: 1) The author uses the third task as a transition to move from her description of leadership by example to her description of leadership by command; 2) The author returns to the ideas related to the third task in the final sentences of paragraph four, and thus creates a unifying conclusion to the essay as a whole.

The first six sentences of paragraph four address the second task by describing a set of characteristics that make leading by command the best method. Although this discussion does not contain actual examples as in paragraphs one and two, the characteristics described are specific and thorough enough to make the author's point clear.

The author's effective use of transitions (e.g., yet, therefore, however) creates a smooth progression of ideas. The transitional sentences beginning paragraphs two and three establish a clear relationship between the paragraphs.

> **STRATEGY:** *Variety in sentence structure and length keeps your writing from sounding monotonous or mechanical; it also adds sophistication.*

The use of parallelism in paragraph two, as well as the variety in sentence length demonstrated by the short sentence concluding paragraph two, demonstrates a lively writing style. Variety of this sort shows energy—and it keeps the reader awake.

ESSAY #2

True leadership leads rather than commands. Where commands are given, followers do what they are told, but only what they are told, and only when they are told. When people are led by example they do as they are shown, not only when they are shown, but on their own as well. This is not to say that commanders do not get things done with their groups. Armies are run by commanders instead of leaders, because they want not soldiers who will work and think on their own, but who will do as they are told when they are told. But commanding is not the same as leadership.

True leaders lead by example rather than by command because leadership is different from command. In situations apart from the military, where it is preferable to have followers who think and act for themselves, leadership by example is a far more effective motivator and guiding force. Workers who are browbeaten into submission are far less motivated than workers encouraged to work steadily at their own pace, with their own ideas. Workers commanded to perform a duty a certain way are less productive than workers guided and trained to think cleverly and creatively about their tasks.

Commanding and leadership are two different things whose results are quite often similar, but also often not, depending on the situation. Leadership leads by example, not by command, because of its very nature. When leadership commands, it ceases to be leadership.

Evaluation and Discussion of Essay #2
Holistic Score: 3

This essay contains the beginnings of some interesting ideas and is written in language that is quite clear and straightforward. It does not focus, however, on providing a thorough explanation of the statement and its implications.

Nor does the paper fulfill all three tasks. In fact, only the first task is addressed, in a response that is poorly developed and organized. All three paragraphs work in some way to reinforce the statement that true leadership leads by example. Paragraphs one and two provide us with partial development of the idea by stating that people led by example can think for themselves and that workers who think for themselves perform better than those who do not. Although both of these ideas are interesting, they lack the necessary development. The author never clarifies why leading by example creates followers who can think for themselves. And he never pulls his ideas together into a coherent explanation of the meaning of the statement.

The author's main purpose in this essay seems to have been to establish that leadership and command are two different things. Yet he never makes clear what his purpose is in establishing this difference, nor does he use this difference to reach any conclusion. He simply restates the difference in each paragraph. The result is an excessive repetition of ideas.

It seems, therefore, that this author paid little attention to the tasks listed in the essay topic. Nonetheless, the paper receives a score of 3 rather than 2 for two reasons: 1) It succeeds in sustaining a focus on the topic provided without significant digression or distortion, and 2) the quality of language demonstrates adequate control of mechanics, sentence structure, and vocabulary.

In all likelihood, this author could have produced a significantly better essay had he paid closer attention to the precise requirements of the tasks. By prewriting, he would have had the chance to get himself on the right track before starting to write. By thinking about each task in turn, he would have had the opportunity to form a more fully developed sequence of ideas. By addressing each task in turn, he would have had the opportunity to produce paragraphs that had a single, logical purpose.

> **STRATEGY:** *To achieve unified paragraphs, address one task in each paragraph. This will help ensure that the ideas in each paragraph all share a common focus.*

STEP 7: PROOFREAD

This final step should be a quick one. You won't have much time at all to revise your essay substantially, so don't bother. What you should look for are blatant errors or significant omissions.

Here's a checklist of what to look for when proofing:

Problems in Meaning

1. Any missing words, transition phrases, or brief ideas?
2. Any sentence fragments or otherwise incomplete ideas?
3. Any confusing punctuation?
4. Any incorrect grammatical forms?

Problems in Mechanics

1. Did you misspell a word?
2. Did you always capitalize when necessary?
3. Did you make unnecessary abbreviations?

> **STRATEGY:** *Learn the types of mistakes you usually tend to make and look for them.*

Another important rule to follow in proofreading is to prioritize. For example, the problems in meaning are usually more important that those in mechanics. If your reader cannot follow your thinking, you stand to lose more ground than if he or she spots a misspelling.

Once again, if you write up until the 30-minute limit, you will miss being able to take Step 7. Plan to check your watch toward the end of the half hour and stick to the seven-step method. Even if you do not absolutely finish your thoughts, it is vital that you proofread. Be disciplined enough to leave yourself a minute or two to accomplish this step.

3

PRACTICE QUESTIONS AND RESPONSES

In this section you will have opportunities to practice writing essays of your own on topics that closely resemble the kind you are likely to get on test day. So this is a good place to hone your grasp of the seven-step method you learned in chapter two.

Practice is vital for this as well as other sections of the MCAT. There is simply no substitute for sitting down and taking a test question under test conditions. That means that you should be hard on yourself: Don't allow yourself any extra minutes to complete an essay; don't look at an essay topic in advance of taking a practice test. Being tough on yourself now will give you an edge on test day.

Two Sections

This chapter has two main sections. The first section offers you the chance to write on four essay topics; you should type your essays on the computer. The second section includes sample student essays responding to the same four topics. These sample essays have been evaluated using the MCAT-style holistic grading technique discussed in the Introduction to this section. As a special plus, we've included a "reactions" page after each essay. Here the student writer gives you his or her first reactions to the special problems encountered while taking this particular test.

Essay Questions Give You Important Practice

The first section, as stated, provides you with four practice essay questions. You should spend 30 minutes and only 30 minutes answering each essay question.

Since the actual MCAT will require you to write two essays back-to-back, you may want to take these practice topics in two one-hour sittings. In this way, you can test yourself under conditions as close as possible to those you'll encounter on test day, or you may may want to give yourself four single-topic practice tests. This method will give you more sustained practice as well as the chance to critique each essay before trying the next. Or you may want to combine the methods. Take the first two essay topics on separate occasions, and then take the last two together in a full one-hour test. It's up to you.

Sample Student Essays Help You Develop Your Critical Skills

After writing on an essay topic, or on a pair of topics, turn to the sample essays that correspond to the topics you chose, and see how other students responded.

Please do *not* look at a sample essay before writing on the topic yourself! Doing so would defeat the purpose of these practice test questions.

When you do look at a sample essay, try first to form your *own* opinion regarding the essay's merits. Pretend you are a professional MCAT reader and give the essay a grade based on the criteria the MCAT people care about. *Then* look at how our readers evaluated the essay. Doing this will help you develop your own critical skills, a crucial step to becoming a good writer.

By the way, we hope you're interested in reading comments from the writers themselves on how they assessed their own performances. These brief and informal comments are personal glimpses into the problems they encountered in writing on these topics, and we feel they offer good insights into how your peers cope with this demanding assignment.

Ask Someone Else to Critique Your Essay

Another way to critique your own work is to ask someone else's opinion. If you know someone else taking the MCAT, it might be a good idea to swap essays. Or you can give your work to someone whose writing skills you respect: a friend, teacher, or family member. If you do so, tell them about the nature of the assignment and about the time limit. If your readers are not knowledgeable about the MCAT essay section, you may find it a good idea to show them the student essays and evaluations found in the latter part of this section. In that way, your readers will become better critics of your work.

If you do find someone to comment on your work, do your best to take their criticism with a cool head. To get the most out of these practice essays, you must put aside your emotional attachment to your writing and try to achieve a certain degree of objectivity. Remember that your evaluators are not trying to tear you down when they point out certain areas that need further practice.

Remember the Seven Steps

When judging your own essays' merits, think about your performance in terms of the seven steps. Could your initial approach to the topic be better? Did you skip or skimp on any of the prewriting steps? If so, you may want to review the appropriate sections in chapter two. Did you do all the prewriting steps but fail to finish your essay or leave time to proofread? If so, you probably need to practice the prewriting steps a bit more in order to improve your ability to accomplish them in the five minutes we recommend.

Take the Practice Tests Seriously

Give yourself 30 minutes; don't allow yourself "extra" minutes to finish that last paragraph. You won't get extras on the day of the test.

Take each practice test under testlike conditions. You should have total peace and quiet in which to write. Take notes on scratch paper and type the final essay on the computer, just as you will do on test day.

Use the seven-step method. You can become comfortable with this efficient method only by practicing it. If you are not clear about any part of it, go back over chapter two to refresh your memory.

PRACTICE ESSAY QUESTIONS

Observe the time limit. Use the lined pages that follow each question for your prewriting notes. Type the essays on a computer.

Time Limit: Each essay should take no longer than 30 minutes.

QUESTION 1

Consider the following statement:

The best kind of education encourages students to question authority.

Write a unified essay in which you accomplish the following tasks. Explain what you think the above statement means. Describe a specific situation in which encouraging students to question authority is not the best kind of education. Discuss what you think determines when students should be encouraged to question authority.

Scratch paper

Scratch paper

Scratch paper

Scratch paper

Scratch paper

QUESTION 2

Consider this statement:

Violence is never a real solution to a political crisis.

Write a unified essay in which you accomplish the following tasks. Explain what you think the above statement means. Describe a specific situation in which violence could be considered a real solution to a political crisis. Discuss what you think determines when violence is justified in solving such a crisis.

Scratch paper

Scratch paper

Scratch paper

Scratch paper

Scratch paper

QUESTION 3

Consider this statement:

To be effective, government officials must have completely crime-free pasts.

Write a unified essay in which you accomplish the following tasks. Explain what you think the above statement means. Describe a specific situation in which a government official who once committed a crime could still perform effectively. Discuss what you believe determines when a criminal past would not interfere with a government official's effectiveness.

Scratch paper

Scratch paper

Scratch paper

Scratch paper

Scratch paper

QUESTION 4

Consider this statement:

The government should fund scientific research only when it has a direct application to societal problems.

Write a unified essay in which you accomplish the following tasks. Explain what you think the above statement means. Describe a specific situation in which the government should fund scientific research that does *not* have a direct application to societal problems. Discuss what you think determines whether or not the government should fund scientific research that has no direct application to societal problems.

Scratch paper

Scratch paper

Scratch paper

Scratch paper

Scratch paper

STUDENT
RESPONSES
AND
EVALUATIONS

The following pages contain student essays written in response to the questions provided in the previous section. Read each response only after you have first attempted to write on the question yourself.

Student's Essay in Response to Question 1

Education that consists of just memorizing details and facts is hardly education at all. True education demands active participation of both teacher and student. In true education, the roles of the student and the teacher are somewhat flexible: the teacher can learn from the student as well as the student learn from the teacher. By actively participating, instead of taking for granted the truth of everything the teacher says, the student thinks about the issues more thoroughly. Rather than just parroting the views of the teacher, the student by questioning authority develops views that are his own, and also learns a way to think critically about future issues. He learns how to think rather than what to think. This gives him intellectual freedom and a framework for thinking that he can use throughout his life.

But there are moments when the best kind of education does not encourage students to question authority. For instance, education in the hard sciences requires an acceptance of basic formulas and theorems if the student is to make any progress at all. A basic foundation must be laid before the challenges can begin. In other words, questioning authority must take place within the proper sequence. If the student is unable to accept the teacher's authority at least partially, then he will find himself unable to learn from the teacher at all. Questioning authority should develop out of a mutual trust and if such questioning comes about prior to the establishment of such a trust, a student will do his education a real injury. To begin by questioning the teacher's authority, without first having a solid foundation of knowledge, would be counterproductive and tend to impede learning.

In determining when education that encourages students to question authority is the best, we must consider two main factors. First, what type of education is in question? If we are dealing with the physical sciences, a basic groundwork must be agreed upon before questioning authority can begin. Second, to what degree is the authority being questioned? If the authority is seen as totally questionable, the validity of the authority as an authority will be destroyed.

It is important to remember that when a student is taught to question authority he must be also taught to question his <u>own</u> authority as well as that of a teacher or textbook. The purpose of questioning authority is not to teach the student to place himself in the role of the authority figure while totally disregarding the teacher. In such a situation the learning process will fail miserably. The purpose of questioning authority is to examine and analyze ideas before accepting them as true. When a student learns to do this with his own ideas as well as with others', he will truly have received the best education.

Student's Self-Evaluation

In general, I feel good about this essay. I managed my time well and stuck to my prewriting main idea and defense. I also benefited from keeping track of the time and pacing myself accordingly.

I felt a bit nervous about using the example of the hard sciences in paragraph two. Perhaps that wasn't specific enough. Perhaps I'd have done better to use just one of the sciences—like physics—and thus avoid potential problems of over-generalization.

Reader's Evaluation of Student's Response to Question 1
Holistic Score: 6

This paper presents a thorough and thoughtful response to all three writing tasks, focusing clearly on the issue defined by the given statement. Paragraphs one and two address the first and second tasks, respectively; paragraphs three and four address the third task.

Paragraph one introduces the topic with a straightforward clarification of the statement's meaning (sentences one through three), and then continues with some analysis of the statement's meaning as it relates to the benefits of an education that questions authority (sentences four through six). Paragraph two's first sentence is a clear topic sentence, leading to the counterexample of education in the hard sciences. The bulk of paragraph two explores the implications of a student's premature questioning. The discussion is abstract, since it quickly leaves the specifics of the example behind, but precisely argued. It amply satisfies the requirement of the second task; it also paves the way for paragraph three's examination of the two factors that should be taken into account in resolving the conflict between the ideas in the preceding two paragraphs. Paragraph four extends this discussion by introducing the related idea that students should question their own authority. These last two paragraphs amply discuss the third task: The author has explored the grounds for questioning authority, the problems associated with premature or unrestricted questioning, and the need for self-questioning.

The discussion in each of the paragraphs is organized around a unifying idea and is presented coherently and logically. Furthermore, the paragraphs relate well to each other. For example, the transitional phrase, "But there are moments" (paragraph two, sentence one), effectively guides the reader from the discussion in paragraph one to the new idea to be discussed in paragraph two. The use of such transitional phrases occurs throughout the essay, creating a smooth and coherent argument. General statements are given an appropriate amount of specific explanation and/or illustration (paragraph four, for instance).

The language is clear and effective throughout. The essay also provides variety in sentence structure (e.g., the fourth, fifth, and sixth sentences of paragraph one).

Student's Essay in Response to Question 2

In a political crisis, violence is often the first reaction in trying to reach a solution, much as a tantrum is the first reaction when a child fails to get his way. Yet if anything is to be resolved, violence in itself is not a solution. While violence may have an immediate effect on a crisis, it does not solve the crisis. It may control the situation temporarily, but the roots are still there and may flare up once the violence has passed.

Certainly there are situations where violence seems justified. Terrorists' acts of violence must sometimes be curtailed with violence when negotiations have failed. Similarly, defense from offensive military maneuvers. But violence in and of itself is not a full solution. The bombing of Hiroshima was seen by some as the only solution to a long and bloody war. Yet this act of violence in a violent political crisis has left terrible scars on all of humanity, and further development of nuclear weapons has led to deeper political crises, crises too dangerous to the entire planet to be resolved by violence.

Yet violence, like an occasional tantrum, does get attention and does often begin a series of events that lead to a solution. The storming of the Bastille did lead—after years of violence and terror in France—to freedom from the aristocracy. And storming the beaches at Normandy did save Europe from Nazi rule.

Violence in itself is not a real solution to a political crisis, but it can be an effective step in reaching a solution. On that ground alone, one can say that it is justifiable. Nonetheless, violence in itself can lead to a bigger crisis. But violence can play a vital part as an intermediate step toward a real resolution of hostilities.

Student's Self-Evaluation

I guess the main problem with this essay is that it got kind of repetitive. By the time I got around to really focussing on the third task, I felt I had said everything I had to say on the subject. As a result, I'm not happy with my final paragraph since it doesn't say much of substance. I wish I had focussed more directly on each task.

Reader's Evaluation of Student's Response to Question 2
Holistic Score: 4

This essay addresses the first and second tasks in paragraphs one, two, and three. In paragraph four, the third task is addressed as well.

The essay is confusingly organized and does not adequately respond to the third task; it is for these two reasons that it did not receive a score of 5. On the other hand, its use of relevant and interpreted examples raised it from a score of 3.

While paragraphs one and four are organized around central ideas, the remainder of the essay is confusingly put together. For example, paragraph two's first sentence seems as if it is introducing a paragraph that will take up the second task, but the rest of the paragraph reverts to a discussion of task 1.

The essay addresses the third task in the final paragraph—introducing the notion that violence can be an "intermediate step" in solving a political crisis—however, the essay presents no clear analysis of what constitutes justified use of violence in such circumstances. Instead, the author repeats the idea that violence can make bad things worse.

The essay's allusions to the Hiroshima catastrophe, the storming of the Bastille, and the invasion at Normandy create a solid sense of specificity. If the essay were better organized, such examples would gain more force. Furthermore, the essay lacks clear transitions between paragraphs (between paragraphs three and four, for example); the author could improve the overall flow of the argument by creating more substantive links between major groups of ideas.

Though generally clear, the language at times lacks vigor (the repeated use of the word *violence,* for instance). Sentence structure does show some variety (paragraph three, for example), though there are occasional problems in sentence construction (e.g., the third sentence in paragraph two is missing a verb and predicate, and therefore constitutes a sentence fragment).

Student's Essay in Response to Question 3

Of his own free will, no one would elect a known criminal to an important government post. In a free society, we like to have government leaders who honor and support the laws that we have made to protect the people and to keep the society smoothly running. When we find that a candidate or officeholder has not upheld the law in his earlier life, we doubt that he will do so in office. Hence, to be an effective politician, one must have a completely crime-free past.

Electing leaders with "clean records" must be kept in mind. We would not elect a known gangster or an individual with a long record of hideous or outrageous crimes or even a person accused of taking bribes because we fear that such individuals would continue such actions in office. Yet certainly one or two small spots on one's record in one's youth when for many years he has been "crime-free" cannot be considered reason enough not to elect an otherwise fine candidate. Certainly we would not want Al Capone or Charles Manson as our Senators, but even if John Kennedy had swiped an apple when he was ten years old or had a parking infraction at twenty, he would have still been one of our greatest leaders.

Having crime-free officials is a ideal, but there is a difference between <u>completely</u> crime-free and <u>generally</u> crime-free pasts. An effective official is more than merely one who has never committed a major crime. After all, Capone would probably be a more effective leader (in some ways) than many of the presidents we have had in the U.S. simply because he knew how to run a big organization and get things done quickly. Of course, his style of power is not how we would like to have things done in a free society, but it was effective.

The question of crime-free or not crime-free hinges on what we mean by "effective." In a free democracy, we like our leaders to be nearly crime-free, but we can see that it is nearly impossible to have officials who are completely crime-free.

Student's Self-Evaluation

I could have spent more time planning this essay. I started writing almost immediately because I felt I knew exactly what I wanted to say. But halfway in, I felt a bit lost. I also wondered whether my use of "we" to make general remarks about society was appropriate.

Reader's Evaluation of Student's Response to Question 3
Holistic Score: 4

This essay accomplished all three writing tasks: paragraph one discusses the first task, paragraph two discusses the second, and paragraphs three and four discuss the third. Despite this relatively clear organization, however, the discussion lacks the depth of a level five essay.

Paragraph one introduces the topic by examining the meaning of the statement. The paragraph's ideas are well organized, but the writer does not closely analyze certain key terms, such as *effective* or *completely*. Doing so would have improved the essay's general clarity and sharpened its argument. Paragraph one, in addition, ends somewhat too abruptly. Sentence three raises the issue of people doubting tainted candidates, but this is not linked to the next sentence's assertion that effectiveness requires a politician to have a completely crime-free past.

Paragraph two describes a counterexample—the case of people having a slightly tarnished record, such as a Kennedy—but spends too much time arguing that career criminals would not be trusted. Hence the paragraph does not elucidate the meaning of the counterexample as much as it could have. In addition, the writer's failure to specify what "completely crime-free" means causes a lack of depth in this paragraph.

This last conceptual weakness carries over into paragraphs three and four, which examine the grounds for effectiveness by discussing the difference between degrees of criminality. The example of Capone in paragraph three directly addresses the third task, but the discussion borders on the simplistic. The final paragraph's first sentence makes a good point, but the essay never clarifies what "effectiveness" entails. Hence, the conclusion lacks clarity.

This paper would be most improved by a clarification of the author's main ideas. The last paragraph is headed in a productive direction since its extension would logically take up the definition of *effective*. Yet this attempt is not enough and it comes too late to add direction to the preceding discussion.

The writing shows a basic control of vocabulary and sentence structure, but transitions could be more effectively used. The first sentence of paragraph two, for example, does not effectively lead into the main topic of paragraph two, nor does it link this paragraph to the preceding one. Similarly, paragraph three could be better tied to the discussion in paragraph two; the phrase "having crime-free officials is a great idea" does not adequately make the necessary transition.

Student's Essay in Response to Question 4

The statement "The government should restrict its funding of scientific research to programs with a direct application to societal problems" is defined by me as follows: no monies shall be allocated to commercial, military, or other programs not of benefit on some humanistic level.

In the case of space research, many would say that no funding should be given, in that this research is either pure adventurism or only of military or theoretical importance. But I believe that space research should be funded for two reasons: *1*) it represents a solution other than population control for the problem of global overcrowding and *2*) it advances many helpful technologies such as food preservation, fuel conservation, and computer applications.

The criteria used to determine whether or not government funds should be used for any individual research project are difficult to put boundaries on. But I will outline some parameters here.

Programs should not concern military issues. The funding of such programs is the responsibility of the Defense Department and are a different issue altogether. For nonmilitary research, researchers should be required to describe, in layman's terms, what their project is, what its history has been and what they think its future will be. There should be a board with as fair a cross-section of the people as possible to decide on funding. And there should be a set of regulations to add weight to research that does have a more direct application to immediate social problems.

Student's Self-Evaluation

I think that when tested I get too hung up on trying to use fancy language and then lose track of my own thoughts. I think my ideas would flow better if I could get them clearer before I jump into building a sentence, but the time pressure makes me too nervous.

Answering the third task seemed the hardest to me. I felt as if I had to start all over again and write a whole new essay.

Reader's Evaluation of Student's Response to Question 4
Holistic Score: 3

This paper addresses all three tasks, focuses consistently on the given topic, presents paragraphs that are unified around a central topic, and contains a clear organization of ideas. Furthermore, the ideas are all substantial enough to be appropriate for an assignment of this kind. None of the ideas is sufficiently developed, however, and as a result the paper is simplistic.

Paragraph one addresses the first task but merely rephrases the statement in different words. No attempt is made to expand our understanding of its meaning by explaining why or in what way it is valid.

Paragraph two addresses the second task by offering an example in which scientific research without direct application to societal problems deserves funding. The author provides a bit more explanation here than in paragraph one, but it is still insufficient. Vague phrases such as "pure adventurism" and "theoretical importance" are left unexplained. More importantly, the author's defense for why space research should be supported is one-sided. Since paragraph one gives us no insight into why someone would *oppose* such research, the argument in paragraph two for *supporting* the research lacks a relevant context.

Paragraph three responds to the third task, but the ideas presented have little relation to the ideas in paragraph two. Therefore, though the paper is unified in its focus on the statement provided, it lacks coherency—the ideas do not relate to each other.

The language of the essay is quite clear, on the whole, and the ideas are expressed without difficulty. In addition, variety in sentence length adds some energy to the style (see first two sentences of paragraph four).

The most significant improvements to be made in this essay involve a more thorough exploration of ideas and a greater emphasis on the relationship between those ideas. The first place to work on improving these weaknesses is in the prewriting process. Asking questions will help expand the explanation of a topic (the first task). Looking back over the first and second tasks' prewriting notes (the third task) will help develop a central idea that will create a coherent relationship between all the ideas in the essay.

FULL-LENGTH
PRACTICE MCAT

Instructions for Taking the Practice Test

Before taking the practice test, find a quiet place where you can work uninterrupted.

Use the answer grid on the following page to record your answers. You'll find the answer key and score conversion chart following the test. Keep in mind that you'll be taking the real test on the computer.

Good luck.

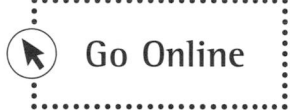 Go Online

To take a full-length practice test in computerized format, visit the Practice Test portion of your online syllabus, accessible by registering at kaptest.com/MCATbooksonline.

1	Ⓐ Ⓑ Ⓒ Ⓓ	41	Ⓐ Ⓑ Ⓒ Ⓓ	81	Ⓐ Ⓑ Ⓒ Ⓓ	121	Ⓐ Ⓑ Ⓒ Ⓓ
2	Ⓐ Ⓑ Ⓒ Ⓓ	42	Ⓐ Ⓑ Ⓒ Ⓓ	82	Ⓐ Ⓑ Ⓒ Ⓓ	122	Ⓐ Ⓑ Ⓒ Ⓓ
3	Ⓐ Ⓑ Ⓒ Ⓓ	43	Ⓐ Ⓑ Ⓒ Ⓓ	83	Ⓐ Ⓑ Ⓒ Ⓓ	123	Ⓐ Ⓑ Ⓒ Ⓓ
4	Ⓐ Ⓑ Ⓒ Ⓓ	44	Ⓐ Ⓑ Ⓒ Ⓓ	84	Ⓐ Ⓑ Ⓒ Ⓓ	124	Ⓐ Ⓑ Ⓒ Ⓓ
5	Ⓐ Ⓑ Ⓒ Ⓓ	45	Ⓐ Ⓑ Ⓒ Ⓓ	85	Ⓐ Ⓑ Ⓒ Ⓓ	125	Ⓐ Ⓑ Ⓒ Ⓓ
6	Ⓐ Ⓑ Ⓒ Ⓓ	46	Ⓐ Ⓑ Ⓒ Ⓓ	86	Ⓐ Ⓑ Ⓒ Ⓓ	126	Ⓐ Ⓑ Ⓒ Ⓓ
7	Ⓐ Ⓑ Ⓒ Ⓓ	47	Ⓐ Ⓑ Ⓒ Ⓓ	87	Ⓐ Ⓑ Ⓒ Ⓓ	127	Ⓐ Ⓑ Ⓒ Ⓓ
8	Ⓐ Ⓑ Ⓒ Ⓓ	48	Ⓐ Ⓑ Ⓒ Ⓓ	88	Ⓐ Ⓑ Ⓒ Ⓓ	128	Ⓐ Ⓑ Ⓒ Ⓓ
9	Ⓐ Ⓑ Ⓒ Ⓓ	49	Ⓐ Ⓑ Ⓒ Ⓓ	89	Ⓐ Ⓑ Ⓒ Ⓓ	129	Ⓐ Ⓑ Ⓒ Ⓓ
10	Ⓐ Ⓑ Ⓒ Ⓓ	50	Ⓐ Ⓑ Ⓒ Ⓓ	90	Ⓐ Ⓑ Ⓒ Ⓓ	130	Ⓐ Ⓑ Ⓒ Ⓓ
11	Ⓐ Ⓑ Ⓒ Ⓓ	51	Ⓐ Ⓑ Ⓒ Ⓓ	91	Ⓐ Ⓑ Ⓒ Ⓓ	131	Ⓐ Ⓑ Ⓒ Ⓓ
12	Ⓐ Ⓑ Ⓒ Ⓓ	52	Ⓐ Ⓑ Ⓒ Ⓓ	92	Ⓐ Ⓑ Ⓒ Ⓓ	132	Ⓐ Ⓑ Ⓒ Ⓓ
13	Ⓐ Ⓑ Ⓒ Ⓓ	53	Ⓐ Ⓑ Ⓒ Ⓓ	93	Ⓐ Ⓑ Ⓒ Ⓓ	133	Ⓐ Ⓑ Ⓒ Ⓓ
14	Ⓐ Ⓑ Ⓒ Ⓓ	54	Ⓐ Ⓑ Ⓒ Ⓓ	94	Ⓐ Ⓑ Ⓒ Ⓓ	134	Ⓐ Ⓑ Ⓒ Ⓓ
15	Ⓐ Ⓑ Ⓒ Ⓓ	55	Ⓐ Ⓑ Ⓒ Ⓓ	95	Ⓐ Ⓑ Ⓒ Ⓓ	135	Ⓐ Ⓑ Ⓒ Ⓓ
16	Ⓐ Ⓑ Ⓒ Ⓓ	56	Ⓐ Ⓑ Ⓒ Ⓓ	96	Ⓐ Ⓑ Ⓒ Ⓓ	136	Ⓐ Ⓑ Ⓒ Ⓓ
17	Ⓐ Ⓑ Ⓒ Ⓓ	57	Ⓐ Ⓑ Ⓒ Ⓓ	97	Ⓐ Ⓑ Ⓒ Ⓓ	137	Ⓐ Ⓑ Ⓒ Ⓓ
18	Ⓐ Ⓑ Ⓒ Ⓓ	58	Ⓐ Ⓑ Ⓒ Ⓓ	98	Ⓐ Ⓑ Ⓒ Ⓓ	138	Ⓐ Ⓑ Ⓒ Ⓓ
19	Ⓐ Ⓑ Ⓒ Ⓓ	59	Ⓐ Ⓑ Ⓒ Ⓓ	99	Ⓐ Ⓑ Ⓒ Ⓓ	139	Ⓐ Ⓑ Ⓒ Ⓓ
20	Ⓐ Ⓑ Ⓒ Ⓓ	60	Ⓐ Ⓑ Ⓒ Ⓓ	100	Ⓐ Ⓑ Ⓒ Ⓓ	140	Ⓐ Ⓑ Ⓒ Ⓓ
21	Ⓐ Ⓑ Ⓒ Ⓓ	61	Ⓐ Ⓑ Ⓒ Ⓓ	101	Ⓐ Ⓑ Ⓒ Ⓓ	141	Ⓐ Ⓑ Ⓒ Ⓓ
22	Ⓐ Ⓑ Ⓒ Ⓓ	62	Ⓐ Ⓑ Ⓒ Ⓓ	102	Ⓐ Ⓑ Ⓒ Ⓓ	142	Ⓐ Ⓑ Ⓒ Ⓓ
23	Ⓐ Ⓑ Ⓒ Ⓓ	63	Ⓐ Ⓑ Ⓒ Ⓓ	103	Ⓐ Ⓑ Ⓒ Ⓓ	143	Ⓐ Ⓑ Ⓒ Ⓓ
24	Ⓐ Ⓑ Ⓒ Ⓓ	64	Ⓐ Ⓑ Ⓒ Ⓓ	104	Ⓐ Ⓑ Ⓒ Ⓓ	144	Ⓐ Ⓑ Ⓒ Ⓓ
25	Ⓐ Ⓑ Ⓒ Ⓓ	65	Ⓐ Ⓑ Ⓒ Ⓓ	105	Ⓐ Ⓑ Ⓒ Ⓓ		
26	Ⓐ Ⓑ Ⓒ Ⓓ	66	Ⓐ Ⓑ Ⓒ Ⓓ	106	Ⓐ Ⓑ Ⓒ Ⓓ		
27	Ⓐ Ⓑ Ⓒ Ⓓ	67	Ⓐ Ⓑ Ⓒ Ⓓ	107	Ⓐ Ⓑ Ⓒ Ⓓ		
28	Ⓐ Ⓑ Ⓒ Ⓓ	68	Ⓐ Ⓑ Ⓒ Ⓓ	108	Ⓐ Ⓑ Ⓒ Ⓓ		
29	Ⓐ Ⓑ Ⓒ Ⓓ	69	Ⓐ Ⓑ Ⓒ Ⓓ	109	Ⓐ Ⓑ Ⓒ Ⓓ		
30	Ⓐ Ⓑ Ⓒ Ⓓ	70	Ⓐ Ⓑ Ⓒ Ⓓ	110	Ⓐ Ⓑ Ⓒ Ⓓ		
31	Ⓐ Ⓑ Ⓒ Ⓓ	71	Ⓐ Ⓑ Ⓒ Ⓓ	111	Ⓐ Ⓑ Ⓒ Ⓓ		
32	Ⓐ Ⓑ Ⓒ Ⓓ	72	Ⓐ Ⓑ Ⓒ Ⓓ	112	Ⓐ Ⓑ Ⓒ Ⓓ		
33	Ⓐ Ⓑ Ⓒ Ⓓ	73	Ⓐ Ⓑ Ⓒ Ⓓ	113	Ⓐ Ⓑ Ⓒ Ⓓ		
34	Ⓐ Ⓑ Ⓒ Ⓓ	74	Ⓐ Ⓑ Ⓒ Ⓓ	114	Ⓐ Ⓑ Ⓒ Ⓓ		
35	Ⓐ Ⓑ Ⓒ Ⓓ	75	Ⓐ Ⓑ Ⓒ Ⓓ	115	Ⓐ Ⓑ Ⓒ Ⓓ		
36	Ⓐ Ⓑ Ⓒ Ⓓ	76	Ⓐ Ⓑ Ⓒ Ⓓ	116	Ⓐ Ⓑ Ⓒ Ⓓ		
37	Ⓐ Ⓑ Ⓒ Ⓓ	77	Ⓐ Ⓑ Ⓒ Ⓓ	117	Ⓐ Ⓑ Ⓒ Ⓓ		
38	Ⓐ Ⓑ Ⓒ Ⓓ	78	Ⓐ Ⓑ Ⓒ Ⓓ	118	Ⓐ Ⓑ Ⓒ Ⓓ		
39	Ⓐ Ⓑ Ⓒ Ⓓ	79	Ⓐ Ⓑ Ⓒ Ⓓ	119	Ⓐ Ⓑ Ⓒ Ⓓ		
40	Ⓐ Ⓑ Ⓒ Ⓓ	80	Ⓐ Ⓑ Ⓒ Ⓓ	120	Ⓐ Ⓑ Ⓒ Ⓓ		

Remove this answer sheet and use it to complete the full-length practice MCAT.

Physical Sciences Test

Time—70 minutes

Questions 1–52

DIRECTIONS: Most of the questions in the following Physical Sciences test are organized into groups, with a descriptive passage preceding each group of questions. Study the passage, then select the single best answer to each question in the group. Some of the questions are not based on a descriptive passage; you must also select the best answer to these questions. If you are unsure of the best answer, eliminate the choices that you know are incorrect, then select an answer from the choices that remain. Indicate your selection by blackening the corresponding circle on your answer sheet. A periodic table is provided below for your use with the questions.

PERIODIC TABLE OF THE ELEMENTS

Period	1 IA 1A	2 IIA 2A	3 IIIB 3B	4 IVB 4B	5 VB 5B	6 VIB 6B	7 VIIB 7B	8 ---- VIII ---- -- ------ 8 ------	9	10	11 IB 1B	12 IIB 2B	13 IIIA 3A	14 IVA 4A	15 VA 5A	16 VIA 6A	17 VIIA 7A	18 vIIIA 8A
1	1 H 1.008																	2 He 4.003
2	3 Li 6.941	4 Be 9.012											5 B 10.81	6 C 12.01	7 N 14.01	8 O 16.00	9 F 19.00	10 Ne 20.18
3	11 Na 22.99	12 Mg 24.31											13 Al 26.98	14 Si 28.09	15 P 30.97	16 S 32.07	17 Cl 35.45	18 Ar 39.95
4	19 K 39.10	20 Ca 40.08	21 Sc 44.96	22 Ti 47.88	23 V 50.94	24 Cr 52.00	25 Mn 54.94	26 Fe 55.85	27 Co 58.47	28 Ni 58.69	29 Cu 63.55	30 Zn 65.39	31 Ga 69.72	32 Ge 72.59	33 As 74.92	34 Se 78.96	35 Br 79.90	36 Kr 83.80
5	37 Rb 85.47	38 Sr 87.62	39 Y 88.91	40 Zr 91.22	41 Nb 92.91	42 Mo 95.94	43 Tc (98)	44 Ru 101.1	45 Rh 102.9	46 Pd 106.4	47 Ag 107.9	48 Cd 112.4	49 In 114.8	50 Sn 118.7	51 Sb 121.8	52 Te 127.6	53 I 126.9	54 Xe 131.3
6	55 Cs 132.9	56 Ba 137.3	57 La* 138.9	72 Hf 178.5	73 Ta 180.9	74 W 183.9	75 Re 186.2	76 Os 190.2	77 Ir 190.2	78 Pt 195.1	79 Au 197.0	80 Hg 200.5	81 Tl 204.4	82 Pb 207.2	83 Bi 209.0	84 Po (210)	85 At (210)	86 Rn (222)
7	87 Fr (223)	88 Ra (226)	89 Ac~ (227)	104 Rf (257)	105 Db (260)	106 Sg (263)	107 Bh (262)	108 Hs (265)	109 Mt (266)	110 --- ()	111 --- ()	112 --- ()		114 --- ()		116 --- ()		118 --- ()

Lanthanide Series*	58 Ce 140.1	59 Pr 140.9	60 Nd 144.2	61 Pm (147)	62 Sm 150.4	63 Eu 152.0	64 Gd 157.3	65 Tb 158.9	66 Dy 162.5	67 Ho 164.9	68 Er 167.3	69 Tm 168.9	70 Yb 173.0	71 Lu 175.0
Actinide Series~	90 Th 232.0	91 Pa (231)	92 U (238)	93 Np (237)	94 Pu (242)	95 Am (243)	96 Cm (247)	97 Bk (247)	98 Cf (249)	99 Es (254)	100 Fm (253)	101 Md (256)	102 No (254)	103 Lr (257)

The equation of state of an ideal gas is given by the ideal gas law:

$$PV = nRT$$

where P is the pressure, V is the volume, n is the number of moles of gas, R is the ideal gas constant, and T is the temperature of the gas. The gas particles in a container are constantly moving at various speeds. These speeds are characterized by the Maxwell distribution, shown in the figure below.

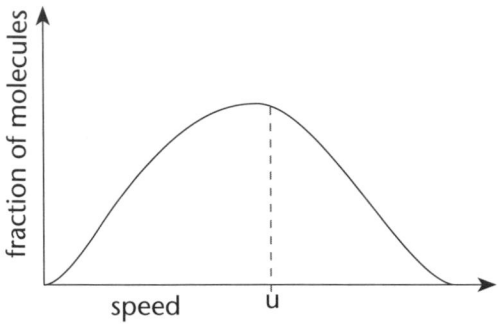

If two particles collide, their velocities change. However, if the gas is in thermal equilibrium, the velocity distribution of the gas as a whole will remain unchanged by the collision.

The average kinetic energy (E) of the gas is given by:

$$E = (1/2)mu^2$$

Equation 1

where m is the mass of one particle and u is the root-mean-square speed (rms speed) of the gas particles (i.e., $u = [1/n(v_1^2 + v_2^2 + \ldots + v_n^2)]^{1/2}$, where n is the number of gas particles; this is different from the average speed). For an ideal gas:

$$E = (3/2)\,nRT$$

Equation 2

where n is the number of moles of gas. Combining these equations gives:

$$u = (3rt/m)^{1/2}$$

Equation 3

where m is the molar mass of the gas particles.

The average distance a particle travels between collisions is known as the mean free path l. Intuitively, the mean free path (mfp) could be expected to be larger for gases at low pressure, since there is a lot of space between particles. Similarly, the mfp should be larger when the gas particles are small. The following expression for the mfp shows this to be correct.

$$l = kT/(2^{(1/2)}\pi s^2 P)$$

Equation 4

In this equation, s is the atomic diameter (typically on the order of 10^{-8}), k is the Boltzmann constant, and P is the pressure.

In addition to colliding with each other, gas particles also collide with the walls of their container. If the container wall has a pinhole that is small compared to the mfp of the gas, and a pressure differential exists across the wall, the particles will effuse (or escape) thorough this pinhole without disturbing the Maxwellian distribution of the particles. The rate of effusion can be described by:

$$dN_{ef}^{f}/dt = A(Pi - P_O)/(2\pi MRT)^{1/2}$$

Equation 5

where N_{eff} is the number of moles of effusing particles, A is the area of the pinhole, Pi and P_O are the pressures on the inside and outside of the container wall respectively, and $Pi > P_O$.

1. Which of the following gives values for both standard temperature and pressure?

    A. 273 K and 760 Torr
    B. 273 K and 1 atm
    C. 0°C and 760 mm Hg
    D. All of the above

GO TO THE NEXT PAGE.

2. If a pinhole were made in a container containing a mixture of equal amounts of H_2, O_2, N_2, and CO_2, which gas would have the fastest effusion rate?

   A. H_2
   B. O_2
   C. N_2
   D. CO_2

3. The mean free path (mfp) of a gas will be longer if the:

   A. pressure of the gas is increased.
   B. number of gas particles per unit volume is increased.
   C. distance between collisions is decreased.
   D. pressure of the gas is decreased.

4. What is the relative rate of effusion for a mixture of two noble gases, G_A and G_B, that escapes through the same pinhole?

   A. 1
   B. $A_B(M_B)^{1/2}/A_A(M_A)^{1/2}$
   C. $(M_B/M_A)^{1/2}$
   D. $P_B(M_B)^{1/2}/P_A(M_A)^{1/2}$

5. The average kinetic energy of an ideal gas can be directly related to the:

   A. rms speed.
   B. temperature.
   C. Boltzmann constant.
   D. universal gas constant.

6. Which of the following will have the smallest root mean square speed at 298 K?

   A. $Cl_2(g)$
   B. $O_2(g)$
   C. $CO_2(g)$
   D. $N_2(g)$

GO TO THE NEXT PAGE.

The periodic beating of the heart is controlled by electrical impulses that originate within the cardiac muscle itself. These pulses travel to the sinoatrial node and from there to the atria and the ventricles, causing the cardiac muscles to contract. If a current of a few hundred milliamperes passes through the heart, it will interfere with this natural system and may cause the heart to beat erratically. This condition is known as ventricular fibrillation, and is life-threatening. If, however, a larger current of about 5 to 6 amps is passed through the heart, a sustained ventricular contraction will occur. The cardiac muscle cannot relax, and the heart stops beating. If at this point the muscle is allowed to relax, a regular heartbeat will usually resume.

The large current required to stop the heart is supplied by a device known as a defibrillator. A schematic diagram of a defibrillator is shown below. This device is essentially a "heavy-duty" capacitor capable of storing large amounts of energy. To charge the capacitor quickly (in 1 to 3 seconds), a large DC voltage must be applied to the plates of the capacitor. This is achieved using a step-up transformer, which creates an output voltage that is much larger than the input voltage. The transformer used in this defibrillator has a step-up ratio of 1:50.

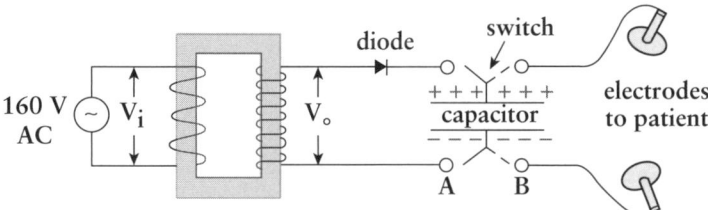

The AC voltage that is obtained from the transformer must then be converted to DC voltage in order to charge the capacitor. This is accomplished using a diode, which allows current flow in one direction only. Once the capacitor is fully charged, the charge remains stored until the switch is moved to position B and the plates are placed on the patient's chest. To cut down the resistance between the patient's body and the defibrillator, the electrodes are covered with a

wetting gel before use. Care must be taken to insure that the patient is not in electrical contact with the ground while the defibrillator is in use.

7. If the defibrillator has a capacitance of 10μF, how much charge will build up on the two plates?

    A. 0.08 C
    B. 1.6×10^{-3} C
    C. 6.25×10^{-8} C
    D. 1.25×10^{-9} C

8. The resistance between the two electrodes when placed apart on the patient's chest is 1,000 Ω when wetting gel is used. What is the initial current through the patient's heart, assuming that all the current takes this path?

    A. 0.16 A
    B.   4 A
    C. 6.25 A
    D.   8 A

9. The plates of the capacitor are originally separated by a vacuum. If a dielectric K > 1 is introduced between the plates of the capacitor, and the capacitor is allowed to charge up, which of the following statements are true?

    I.   The capacitance of the capacitor will increase.
    II. The voltage across the capacitor plates will increase.
    III. The charge stored on the capacitor will increase.

    A. I only
    B. I and II only
    C. II and III only
    D. I and III only

GO TO THE NEXT PAGE.

10. Why is it important to ensure that the patient is not in electrical contact with the ground while the defibrillator is in use?

A. Contact with the ground will decrease the resistance across the patient's body.

B. The doctor administering the treatment will be in greater danger of receiving an electric shock if the patient is in electrical contact with the ground.

C. Contact with the ground will cause a smaller current to pass through the patient's heart.

D. The patient receiving the treatment will be in greater danger of receiving burns due to the high current density if he is in electrical contact with the ground.

11. If a dielectric were inserted between the plates of the capacitor in the defibrillator when the switch is in position A:

A. the energy stored in the capacitor would increase.

B. the energy stored in the capacitor would decrease.

C. the electric field between the plates would increase.

D. the electric field between the plates would decrease.

GO TO THE NEXT PAGE.

12. Solution X boils at 100.26°C and Solution Y boils at 101.04°C. Both solutions are at atmospheric pressure and contain the same solute concentration. Which of the following conclusions can be drawn?

    A. The freezing point of Solution X is lower than that of Solution Y.
    B. The vapor pressure of Solution X is higher than that of Solution Y and 100.26°C.
    C. Solution X and Solution Y are immiscible.
    D. The vapor pressure of Solution X is lower than that of Solution Y at 100.26°C.

13. A converging lens has a focal length of 8 cm. If the object is 10 cm to the left of the lens, what are the position of the image formed and the magnification of the lens?

    A. 0.025 cm to the right of the lens and 0.0025x
    B. 4.4 cm to the right of the lens and 0.4x
    C. 40 cm to the right of the lens and 4x
    D. 40 cm to the left of the lens and 4x

14. If 29 grams of maleic acid ($C_4O_4H_4$) is dissolved in 500 grams of ammonia (NH_3), what is the molality of the resulting solution?

    A. 0.05 m
    B. 0.10 m
    C. 0.25 m
    D. 0.50 m

15. An electron travels in the plane of the page from left to right, perpendicular to a magnetic field that points into the page. The direction of the resulting magnetic force on the electron will be in the plane of the page and:

    A. upwards.
    B. downwards.
    C. to the left.
    D. to the right.

16. How much solid NaOH is required to neutralize 700 mL of 2 N HNO_3?

    A. 40 g
    B. 48 g
    C. 56 g
    D. 64 g

17. A body is dropped from a height of 30 m on Earth and hits the ground with a velocity v_e. The body is then taken to the moon, which has a gravitational acceleration 1/6 that of Earth. It is again dropped from a height of 30 m, hitting the moon with a velocity of v_m. What is the ratio of v_m/v_e?

    A. 1/6
    B. $\sqrt{1/6}$
    C. 6
    D. 36

GO TO THE NEXT PAGE.

Every atomic orbital contains plus and minus regions, defined by the value of the quantum mechanical function for electron density. When orbitals from different atoms overlap to form bonds, an equal number of new molecular orbitals results. These are of two types: σ or π bonding orbitals, formed by overlap between orbital regions with the same sign, and antibonding σ* or π* orbitals, formed by overlap between regions with opposite signs. Bonding orbitals have lower energy than their component atomic orbitals, and antibonding orbitals have higher energy. The electron pairs reside in the lower-energy bonding orbitals; the higher-energy, less stable orbitals remain empty when the molecule is in ground state.

A benzene ring has six unhybridized p_z electrons, which together form six molecular π orbitals, each one delocalized over the entire ring, and each consisting of a different combination of electron spins. Of the possible π orbital structures for benzene, the one with the lowest energy has the plus region of all six p orbital functions on one side of the ring. The six electrons fill the three most stable molecular orbitals, leaving the other three empty.

Molecular orbitals are filled from lowest to highest energy level. The number of bonds between atoms is determined by the number of filled bonding orbitals minus the number of filled antibonding orbitals; each antibonding orbital cancels out a filled bonding orbital. For a diatomic molecule, orbitals in the n = 2 energy level are filled as follows: σ_2s, σ^*_2s, σ_{2p_y}, π_{2p_x} and π_{2p_y}, (equal in energy), $\pi^*_{2p_x}$ and $\pi^*_{2p_y}$ (equal in energy), $\pi^*_{2p_z}$. (The designation of the three p orbitals as p_x, p_y, and p_z are interchangeable.)

Absorption of a photon can raise an electron to a higher-energy molecular orbital. The excited electron does not immediately change its spin, which is opposite to that of the electron with which it was previously paired. This singlet state is relatively unstable: The molecule may interact with another molecule, or fluoresce and return to its ground state. Alternatively, there may be a change in spin direction somewhere in the system; the molecule then enters the so-called triplet state, which generally has lower energy. The molecule now cannot return quickly to its ground state, since the excited electron no longer has a partner of opposite spin with which to pair. It also cannot return to the singlet state, because the singlet has greater energy. Consequently, the triplet state, which has two unpaired electrons in separate orbitals, is long-lived by atomic standards, with a lifetime that may be 10 seconds or more. During this period, the molecule is highly reactive.

18. Which of the following four depictions of molecular π orbitals represents the highest energy state for a 6-carbon polyene molecule? (The signs given are the signs for the mathematical functions defining the p orbitals on one side of the molecule.)

    A. − − − − − −
    B. + + + − − −
    C. + + − − + +
    D. + − + − + −

19. Among conjugated polyenes (molecules with alternating carbon-carbon double and single bonds), why are those that are longer able to absorb longer wavelengths of light?

    A. Larger molecular orbitals have a lower ground state.
    B. A longer wavelength is better able to interact with a longer molecular orbital.
    C. The larger number of molecular orbitals allows for smaller energy transitions.
    D. Larger molecular orbitals can absorb more energy.

20. Given the order in which orbitals are filled, which molecule is a triplet in its ground state?

    A. H_2
    B. O_2
    C. N_2
    D. F_2

GO TO THE NEXT PAGE.

21. Molecular orbitals in hydrocarbons are formed between the 1s atomic orbital of hydrogen and the *sp*, *sp*^{2}, or *sp*^{3} hybrid atomic orbitals of carbon. Which choice correctly lists the energy level of the C–H bonds, from lowest to highest?

 A. C_6H_6, HC≡CH, CH_4
 B. $H_2C=CH_2$, CH_4, C_6H_6
 C. C_6H_6, CH_4, $H_2C=CH_2$
 D. HC≡CH, C_6H_6, CH_4

22. Which of the following figures describes the shape of σ$^*_{2p_z}$ molecular orbital?

A.

C.

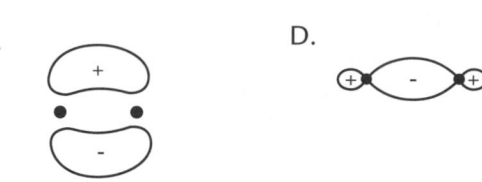

B.

D.

23. The quantum number that distinguishes the p_x orbital from the p_y orbital is called the:

 A. azimuthal quantum number.
 B. magnetic quantum number.
 C. principal quantum number.
 D. spin quantum number.

GO TO THE NEXT PAGE.

Passage IV (Questions 24–29)

A ski jump is an inclined track from which a ski jumper takes off through the air. After traveling down the track, the skier takes off from a ramp at the bottom of the track. The skier lands farther down on the slope.

Figure 1 shows a ski jump, in which the ramp at the lower end of the track makes an angle of 30° to the horizontal. The track is inclined at an angle of θ to the horizontal and the slope is inclined at an angle of 45° to the horizontal. A ski jumper is stationary at the top of the track. Once the skier pushes off, she accelerates down the track, and then takes off from the ramp. The vertical height difference between the top of the track and its lowest point is 50 m, and the vertical height difference between the top of the ramp and its lowest point is 10 m.

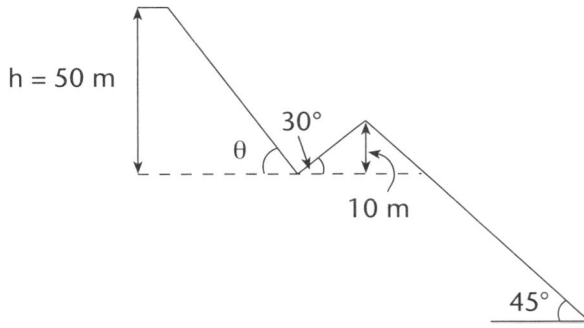

Figure 1

The distance traveled by the skier between leaving the ski jump ramp and making contact with the slope is called the jump distance. In some cases, in order to increase the jump distance a skier will jump slightly upon leaving the ramp, thereby increasing the vertical velocity.

Unless otherwise stated, assume that friction between the skis and the slope is negligible, and ignore the effects of air resistance. (Note: cos 30° = $\sqrt{3}$/2; sin 30° = 0.5; cos 45° = $\sqrt{2}$/2; acceleration due to gravity = 9.8 m/s².)

24. How would the speed of a skier leaving the jump ramp change if the vertical height of the jump ramp were increased from its original height of 10 meters?

   A. increase
   B. decrease
   C. remain the same
   D. The answer depends on the incline angle of the jump ramp.

25. Another ski jumper sets off from a point farther down the jump track, and leaves the ramp at a speed of 16 m/s. If the time in flight is 4 s, what is the total horizontal distance traveled by the ski jumper after leaving the ramp?

   A. 4 m
   B. $8\sqrt{3}$ m
   C. $32\sqrt{3}$ m
   D. 48 m

26. Which of the following would increase the jump distance?

   I.   Increasing the vertical height h of the jump track
   II. Increasing the angle of incline θ of the jump track
   III. Carrying extra weight to increase the total mass of the ski jumper

   A. I only
   B. I and II only
   C. II and III only
   D. I and III only

27. How would the work done by gravity on the skier when she skis down the track compare with the work done by gravity on the skier if she fell the same vertical height?

   A. Less work would be done on the skier when she skis down the track.
   B. More work would be done on the skier when she skis down the track.
   C. Equal amounts of work would be done.
   D. The answer depends on the angle of the track.

GO TO THE NEXT PAGE.

28. What is the acceleration of an 80 kg skier going down the track if $\theta = 45°$?

   A. 6.9 m/s^2
   B. 9.8 m/s^2
   C. 13.9 m/s^2
   D. 80.0 m/s^2

29. If a skier uses skis of greater surface area, which of the following would occur?

   A. The normal force of the slope on the skier would increase.
   B. The normal force of the slope on the skier would decrease.
   C. The pressure exerted on the slope by the skis would increase.
   D. The pressure exerted on the slope by the skis would decrease.

GO TO THE NEXT PAGE.

Questions 30 through 34 are NOT based on a descriptive passage.

30. Suppose an α-particle starting from rest is accelerated through a 5 megavolt potential difference. What is the final kinetic energy of the α-particle? (Note: Assume that e = 1.6×10^{-19} C.)

    A. 1.6×10^{-12} J
    B. 8.0×10^{-13} J
    C. 6.4×10^{-26} J
    D. 3.2×10^{-26} J

31. Based on the table below, what is the cell voltage for the following reaction?

Half-reaction	Standard Potential (V)
$Fe^{2+} + 2e^- \rightarrow Fe$	−0.44V
$Fe^{3+} + 3e^- \rightarrow Fe$	−0.037V
$2H_2O + 2e^- \rightarrow H_2 + 2OH^-$	−0.83V
$Al^{3+} + 3e^- \rightarrow Al$	−1.66V

$$Fe_2O_3 + 2Al \rightarrow 2\,Fe + Al_2O_3$$

    A. −1.33 V
    B. 1.99 V
    C. 1.33 V
    D. 1.62 V

32. A particle of mass m moves in a circle of radius r at a uniform speed and makes 1 revolution per second. What is the energy of the particle?

    A. $m^2r^2/4\pi^2$
    B. $2\pi^2mr^2$
    C. $4\pi^2mr^2$
    D. $mr^2/2$

33. Which titration curve would be produced by titrating 25 mL of a 0.1 N weak base with a 0.1 N strong acid?

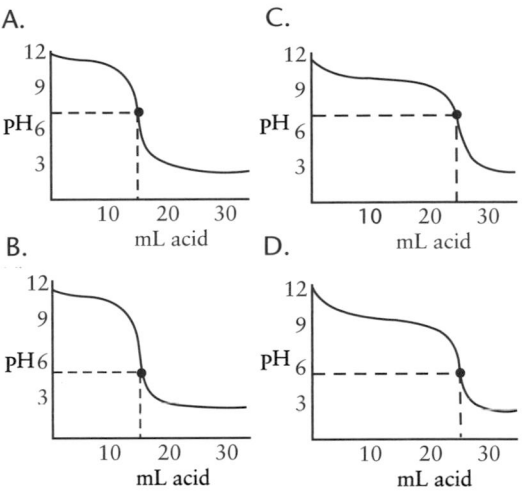

34. Four charges of equal magnitude but different sign are arranged in the four corners of a square, as shown below. What is the direction of the electric field in the center of the square?

    A. A
    B. B
    C. C
    D. D

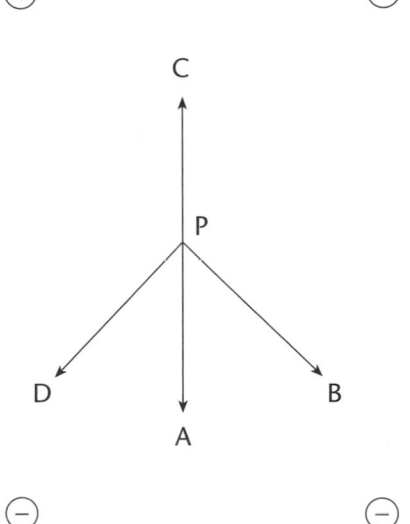

GO TO THE NEXT PAGE.

Passage V (Questions 35–41)

Several techniques have been developed to determine the order of a reaction. The rate of a reaction cannot be predicted on the basis of the overall equation, but it can be predicted on the basis of the rate-determining step. For instance, the following reaction can be broken down into three steps.

$$A + D \rightarrow F + G$$

Step 1	$A \rightarrow B + C$	(slow)
Step 2	$B + D \rightarrow E + F$	(fast)
Step 3	$E + C \rightarrow G$	(fast)

Reaction 1

In this case, the first step in the reaction pathway is the rate-determining step. Therefore, the overall rate of the reaction must equal the rate of the first step, $k_1[A]$ where k is the rate constant. (Rate constants of the different steps are denoted by k_x, where x is the step number.)

In some cases, it is desirable to measure the rate of a reaction in relation to only one species. In a second-order reaction, for instance, a large excess of one species is included in the reaction vessel. Since a relatively small amount of this large concentration is reacted, we assume that the concentration essentially remains unchanged. Such a reaction is called a *pseudo first-order reaction*. A new rate constant, k', is established, equal to the product of the rate constant of the original reaction, k, and the concentration of the species in excess. This approach is often used to analyze enzyme activity.

In some cases, the reaction rate may be dependent on the concentration of a short-lived intermediate. This can happen if the rate-determining step is not the first step. in this case, the concentration of the intermediate must be derived from the equilibrium constant of the preceding step.

For redox reactions, the reaction rate at equilibrium can be correlated with the voltage produced by two half-cells by means of the Nernst equation. This equation states that any given moment:

$$E = E^\circ_{tot} - (RT/nF)\ln([C]^c[D]^d/[A]^a[B]^b)$$

Equation 1

When

$$a\,A = b\,B \rightarrow c\,C + d\,D$$

Reaction 2

(**Note:** $R = 8.314$ J/K • mol; $F = 9.6485 \times 10^4$ C/mol.)

35. An enzyme, R, catalyzes the oxidation of A to B. Reacting various concentrations of A and B with a large excess of R produced the following results during the first few minutes of the reaction.

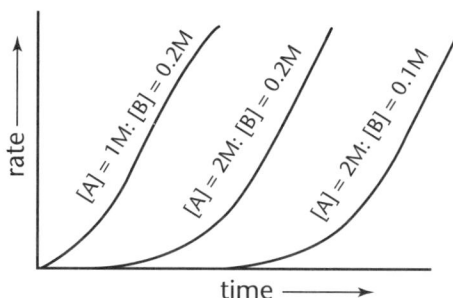

Which of the following is the best tentative rate equation?

A. Rate = $k'[A]^x$
B. Rate = $k'[B]^y$
C. Rate = $k'[A]^x[B]^y$
D. Rate = $k[A]^x[B]^y[R]^z$

GO TO THE NEXT PAGE.

36. In a test of the rate of Step 3 of Reaction 1, a solution is prepared containing a 0.1 Moles per liter concentration of E and a 50 Moles per liter concentration of C. The rate is calculated after the reaction has gone 50% to completion. By what percent will the calculated rate differ from the true rate if we treat the reaction as pseudo first-order?

    A. 0.02%
    B. 0.05%
    C. 0.1%
    D. 0.2%

37. If Step 2 above were the rate-determining step of Reaction 1, which of the following equations would correctly define the rate?

    A. Rate = $k_1 k_2 [D]/k_{-1}[C]$
    B. Rate = $k_1 k_2 [D]/k_{-1} k_{-2}[C]$
    C. Rate = $k_1 k_2 [A][D]/k_{-1}[C]$
    D. Rate = $k_1 k_2 [A][D]/k_{-1} k_{-2}[C]$

38. Which of the following is true of a reaction at equilibrium?

    I. $k_1/k_{-1} = 1$
    II. $E = E°$
    III. $\ln([C]^c[D]^d/[A]^a[B]^b) = nFE°/RT$

    A. I only
    B. III only
    C. I and II only
    D. I, II, and III

39. What is the effect of increasing the concentration of reactants in a voltaic cell?

    A. The voltage increases, while the spontaneity of the reaction remains the same.
    B. The spontaneity of the reaction increases, but the voltage remains the same.
    C. Both the voltage and the spontaneity of the reaction increase.
    D. The reaction rate increases, but the voltage and spontaneity of the reaction are unchanged.

40. What would be the cell emf of the following system at 298 K?

    $$Zn(s)|Zn^{2+}(0.2M)||Cu^{2+}(0.02M)|Cu(s)$$

    $$E°_{cell} = +1.10 \text{ V}$$

    A. 1.07 V
    B. 1.10 V
    C. 1.13 V
    D. 1.20 V

41. Catalysts are effective in increasing the rate of a reaction because they:

    A. increase the energy of the activated complex.
    B. increase the value of the equilibrium constant.
    C. decrease the number of collisions between reactant molecules.
    D. lower the activation energy.

GO TO THE NEXT PAGE.

A researcher in a molecular biology lab planned to carry out an extraction procedure known as an alkaline plasmid prep, which is designed to purify plasmids, small pieces of the hereditary material DNA, from bacterial cells. The bacteria are first placed into a test tube containing liquid nutrient medium and allowed to grow until they reach a high population density. The culture, which consists of solid cells suspended in the medium, is then centrifuged; a solid pellet is formed. The supernatant is poured out, leaving the pellet behind, and the cells are resuspended in 1 mL of lysis buffer solution (50 mM glucose, 25 mM Tris buffer and 10 mM ethylenediaminetetraacetic acid (EDTA), with 5 mg of the enzyme lysozyme added). They are then incubated for 30 minutes at 0°C, during which time the bacterial cell walls break down and the cell contents are released into the solution. After incubation, 1 mL of 0.4 N sodium hydroxide and 1 mL of 2% sodium dodecyl sulfate (SDS) are added, and the solution is again incubated on ice for 10 minutes. Two mL of 3 M sodium acetate are added and the mixture is incubated for 30 minutes at 0°C. The test tube is centrifuged once more, and the supernatant is decanted into a clean tube, leaving behind the protein and most other cell components in the pellet.

Finally, 10 mL of pure ethanol are added to the supernatant from the previous step to precipitate out the DNA, and the test tube is incubated at –20°C for 60 minutes, during which the mixture remains liquid. The mixture is centrifuged a final time, and the supernatant removed. The translucent precipitate that results is washed with 70% ethanol (70% ethanol and 30% water by volume), allowed to dry, and resuspended in 1 mL of TE buffer (10 mM Tris, 1 mM EDTA).

In preparation for this experiment, the researcher prepared stock solutions of the various chemicals that she would need in the experiment. Stock solutions are highly concentrated solutions of commonly used chemicals in water from which dilute solutions are prepared for daily use. Table 1 shows the chemicals, their molecular formulas and weights, and the composition of commonly used stock solutions.

Compound	Formula	MW	Stock
Tris	$(CH_2OH)_3CNH_2$	121	1 M (pH 8)
EDTA	$(HOOCCH_2)_4(CNH_2)_2$	292	0.5 M (pH 8)
Sodium hydroxide	NaOH	40	5 N
SDS	$C_{11}H_{23}CH_2OSO_3^-Na^+$	288	10%
Sodium acetate	$CH_3COO^-Na^+$	82	3 M (pH 5.2)
Ethanol	CH_3CH_2OH	46	95%

Table 1

42. EDTA is available commercially in the form of a hydrated sodium salt, $Na_2EDTA \cdot 2H_2O$. How much of this salt must be used to produce 1 L of a 0.5 M stock solution?

    A. 145 g
    B. 146 g
    C. 186 g
    D. 187 g

43. Tris (Tris(hydroxymethyl)aminomethane) is generally used as a buffer. If pH 8.0 is a good buffering region for Tris, then:

    I. the pK_a of Tris must be near pH 8.0.
    II. if Tris is titrated with acid, the titration curve will possess a steep region near pH 8.0.
    III. a great deal of NaOH would have to be added to pH 8.0 Tris in order to significantly affect the pH.

    A. I only
    B. III only
    C. I and II only
    D. I and III only

44. What is the molality of a stock solution that is 10% SDS by mass?

    A. 0.028 m
    B. 0.100 m
    C. 0.347 m
    D. 0.385 m

GO TO THE NEXT PAGE.

45. Pure ethanol (CH_3CH_2OH) is difficult to prepare and therefore expensive; 95% ethanol is much cheaper. Consequently, 95% ethanol is generally used in the preparation of dilute ethanol solutions. How much 95% ethanol would be needed to produce a 500 mL solution of 70% ethanol by volume in water?

   A. 333 mL
   B. 350 mL
   C. 368 mL
   D. 475 mL

46. Which of the following conclusions can be reached based on the fact that DNA precipitates in the last step of the plasmid prep procedure?

   A. DNA dissolves better in water at lower temperatures.
   B. DNA is polar and therefore dissolves better in water than in a mixture of water and ethanol.
   C. DNA is nonpolar and therefore dissolves better in ethanol than in water.
   D. DNA dissolves well in ethanol and precipitates only because the solution is centrifuged.

47. What would be the pH of 100 mL of the sodium acetate stock solution after the addition of 3.6 g of HCl? (pK_a of acetic acid = 4.74)

   A. 1.0
   B. 4.74
   C. 5.2
   D. 6.0

GO TO THE NEXT PAGE.

Passage VII (Questions 48–53)

The simple harmonic motion of a mass suspended from vertical springs is investigated in two experiments. The springs used in both experiments have a spring constant k and a natural length L_0. The material used to make the springs has a Young's modulus of 2×10^{11} Pa.

In the first experiment a mass m is suspended from a spring as shown in Figure 1 below. The mass stretches the spring to a new length L, called the equilibrium length.

In the second experiment the mass m is suspended from two identical springs as shown in Figure 2 below. When the mass m is in equilibrium, each spring is stretched from its natural length by the same amount x_e.

In both experiments the masses of the springs are negligible, and the elastic limits of the springs are never exceeded.

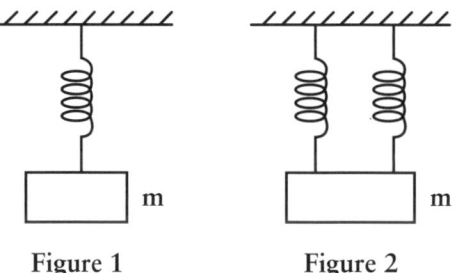

Figure 1   Figure 2

48. In the first experiment, what is the mass of the object hanging from the spring?

   A. kL/g
   B. kL_0/g
   C. $k(L - L_0)/g$
   D. k/g

49. The mass in the first experiment is pulled down a distance A from its equilibrium position and then released from rest. The mass then oscillates with simple harmonic motion. As the mass moves up and down, energy is dissipated due to factors such as air resistance and internal heating of the spring. The mass will no longer oscillate when the total energy dissipated equals:

   A. $kL^2/2$
   B. $kA^2/2$
   C. $k(L + A)^2/2$
   D. $kL_0^2/2$

50. In the first experiment the mass is pulled down and set into motion. The position of greatest speed is:

   A. at the equilibrium position.
   B. at the position where the spring's length is its natural length.
   C. at the lowest point in its motion.
   D. at the highest point in its motion.

GO TO THE NEXT PAGE.

51. In the first experiment, when a 5 kg mass is oscillating, the frequency of oscillation is 2 Hz. What is the value of the spring constant?

    A. $5/\pi^2$ N/m
    B. 20 N/m
    C. $40\pi^2$ N/m
    D. $80\pi^2$ N/m

52. The two springs in Experiment 2 are replaced by a single spring having a spring constant k′ such that the equilibrium length x_e does not change. What is the ratio of k′ to k?

    A. 1/2
    B. 1
    C. $\sqrt{2}$
    D. 2

STOP. IF YOU FINISH BEFORE TIME HAS EXPIRED, CHECK YOUR WORK. YOU MAY GO BACK TO ANY QUESTION IN THIS PART ONLY.

Verbal Reasoning Test

Time—60 minutes

Questions 53–92

DIRECTIONS: There are six passages in this Verbal Reasoning test. Each passage is followed by several questions. After reading a passage, select the one best answer to each question. If you are not certain of an answer, eliminate the alternatives that you know to be incorrect and then select an answer from the remaining alternatives. Indicate your selection by blackening the corresponding circle on your answer sheet.

Passage I (Questions 53–59)

In the early nineteenth century a large number of communal experiments, both secular and religious, sprang up in the northeastern United States. Perhaps the most famous secular commune was Brook Farm, founded by transcendentalists George Ripley and William H. Channing to promote the pursuit of leisure, and culture through the proper application of time and labor. Its members (among the more notable were Nathaniel Hawthorne and Margaret Fuller) pursued field labor by day, art and philosophy by night. For a time the system worked so well that two afternoons a week were set aside for leisure, and Brook Farm began outcompeting local farmers at the produce market. But by nature the farm's members were thinkers, not workers; despite their success they remained mainly interested in the theoretical and philosophical implications of the experiment. Thus, when a devastating fire brought the community considerable financial burdens in its fifth year, the members felt little compunction about closing shop and returning to their comfortable Boston homes.

One of the most notable religious utopias was the Oneida community. Its founder, John Humphrey Noyes, believed that Christ's second coming had already occurred and that everyone alive was favored by divine grace, which Noyes saw as an imperative to live a better life. Perhaps surprisingly, the Oneidans embraced industry and commerce, achieving success in fruit packing, trap making, and silk thread winding. They owned everything communally, and this principle extended to each other. The Oneidans saw monogamy as a selfish act and asserted that the men and women of the community were united in one "complex" marriage; sex between any two consenting members was perfectly acceptable. The Oneidans maintained order solely through "criticism"—anyone acting out of line was made to stand before the other members and hear his or her faults recounted. Oneida remained viable for some thirty years, until the leadership devolved on Noyes' son, an agnostic. The old religious fervor died out, and the dream degenerated into a joint stock company.

Doubtless the most successful communalists were the Shakers, so called for the early propensity to tremble ecstatically during religious worship. Their guiding light, Mother Ann, espoused four key principles: Virgin Purity, Christian Communism, Confession, and Separation from the World. Though the Shakers were less adamant on the last point—maintaining social relations and some commerce with their neighbors—they insisted on the other three and renounced both personal property and sex. Men and women lived in a single large Unitary Dwelling and were considered complete equals, but they occupied separate wings and could speak together only if a third person were present. Despite their religious strictness, Shakers were known as simple, sincere, intelligent people, healthy and long-lived, producers of lovely books and hymns, and of furniture still prized for its quality and durability. In their heyday 6,000 Shakers lived in 58 separate "families" throughout the Northeast. Later their celibacy, combined with their strict discipline, led to a decline in numbers, but even today a small number of elderly Shakers in two communities in Maine and New Hampshire continue to keep the faith.

GO TO THE NEXT PAGE.

53. The passage implies that the end of the Brook Farm experiment was probably brought on by:

A. faltering commitment in the face of hardship.
B. a failure to attract members of sufficient intellect or ability.
C. the completion of the community's aims.
D. the incompetence of philosophers at field labor.

54. According to the passage, the Oneidans believed that:

A. men and women were equal in the eyes of God.
B. monogamy was wrong in principle.
C. rules and standards of behavior were unnecessary.
D. they were destined to witness Christ's second coming.

55. The passage implies that Brook Farm's economic system:

A. did not include the selling of produce outside the farm.
B. was based on the hiring of farm hands.
C. efficiently utilized time and labor.
D. was primarily intended to maximize collective profit.

56. According to the passage, all of the following were characteristic of the Oneida community EXCEPT:

A. complex marriage.
B. maintenance of order through social pressure.
C. belief in present grace.
D. shared living quarters.

57. The Shakers resembled the Oneidans in their attitude toward:

A. sexual practices.
B. equality of men and women.
C. personal property.
D. contact with the outside world.

58. It can be inferred from the passage that the cohesion of a secular workers' cooperative, based on the principles of collective ownership and the sharing of profits, would probably be weakened by:

I. diminished contact with the outside world.
II. increasing agnosticism.
III. considerable economic losses.

A. I only
B. II only
C. III only
D. I and II only

59. If the passage were to continue, the next topic the author would discuss would probably be:

A. a comparison between nineteenth- and twentieth-century communal living experiments.
B. a theory explaining why communal living might become popular again.
C. an analysis of why early communes attracted intellectuals and artists.
D. an investigation into why the three communes discussed were successful to varying degrees.

GO TO THE NEXT PAGE.

Due to ever-increasing paranoia about the transmission of hepatitis and AIDS via blood transfusions and the frequent difficulty of procuring matching blood donors for patients, researchers have been working at a feverish pace to produce disease-free and easy-to-use blood substitutes. The difficulty most synthetic blood researchers have had is in formulating a substance that combines qualities of sterility, high capacity for carrying oxygen to body tissues, and versatility within the human body. Three major substitute technologies have been developed to date; each has certain advantages and shortcomings.

"Red blood," the first of the blood substitute technologies, is derived from hemoglobin that has been recycled from old, dead, or worn-out red blood cells and modified so that it can carry oxygen outside the red blood cell. Hemoglobin, a complex protein, is the blood's natural oxygen carrier and is attractive to scientists for use in synthetic blood because of its oxygen-carrying capacity. However, hemoglobin can sometimes constitute a two-fold threat to humans when it is extracted from the red blood cell and introduced to the body in its naked form. First, hemoglobin molecules are rarely sterile and often remain contaminated by viruses to which they were exposed in the cell. Second, naked hemoglobin is extremely dangerous to the kidneys, causing blood flow at these organs to shut down and, ultimately, renal failure. Additional problems arise from the fact that hemoglobin is adapted to operate optimally within the intricate environment of the red blood cell. Stripped of the protection of the cell, the hemoglobin molecule tends to suffer breakdown within several hours. Although modification has produced more durable hemoglobin molecules that do not cause renal failure, undesired side effects continue to plague patients and hinder the development of hemoglobin-based blood substitutes.

Another synthetic blood alternative, "white blood," is dependent on laboratory-synthesized chemicals called perfluorocarbons (PFCs). Unlike blood, PFCs are clear, oil-like liquids, yet they are capable of absorbing quantities of oxygen up to 50 percent of their volume, enough of an oxygen-carrying potential for oxygen-dependent organisms to survive submerged in the liquid for hours by "breathing" it. Although PFCs imitate real blood by effectively absorbing oxygen, scientists are primarily interested in them as constituents of blood substitutes because they are inherently safer to use than hemoglobin-based substitutes. PFCs do not interact with any chemicals in the body and can be manufactured in near-perfect sterility. The primary pitfall of PFCs is in their tendency to form globules in plasma that can block circulation. Dissolving PFCs in solution can mitigate globulation; however this procedure also seriously curtails the PFCs' oxygen capacity.

The final and perhaps most ambitious attempt to form a blood substitute involves the synthesis of a modified version of human hemoglobin by genetically altered bacteria. Fortunately, this synthetic hemoglobin seems to closely mimic the qualities of sterility and durability outside the cellular environment, and oxygen-carrying efficiency of blood. Furthermore, researchers have found that if modified hemoglobin genes are added to bacterial DNA, the bacteria will produce the desired product in copious quantities. This procedure is extremely challenging, however, because it requires the isolation of the human gene for the production of hemoglobin, and the modification of the gene to express a molecule that works without support from a living cell.

While all the above technologies have serious drawbacks and difficulties, work to perfect an ideal blood substitute continues. Scientists hope that in the near future safe, synthetic blood transfusions may ease blood shortages and resolve the unavailability of various blood types.

60. The author mentions all of the following as weaknesses of synthetic bloods EXCEPT:

   A. naked hemoglobin can cause renal failure in humans.
   B. "red blood" can transmit viruses to a recipient.
   C. genetic engineering can be extremely difficult.
   D. "white blood" has a low oxygen-carrying potential.

GO TO THE NEXT PAGE.

61. According to the passage, PFCs are helpful in the synthesis of blood substitutes because they:

    I. mimic the oxygen-carrying capacity of blood.
    II. do not react with other body chemicals.
    III. break down in the blood within several hours.

    A. I only
    B. II only
    C. I and II only
    D. II and III only

62. According to the passage, all of the following are reasons for research into the development of synthetic bloods EXCEPT:

    A. Dangerous diseases can be transmitted by conventional blood transfusions.
    B. Synthetic bloods have greater oxygen-carrying capacities than naturally-produced human blood.
    C. Donor blood is sometimes in short supply.
    D. Certain blood types are not readily available.

63. We can infer that all of the synthetic blood technologies discussed in this passage:

    A. sustain submerged oxygen-dependent organisms.
    B. possess high oxygen-carrying capacities.
    C. maintain high standards of sterility.
    D. exhibit versatility in the human body.

64. Which of the following is mentioned in the passage as a problem specific to "red blood"?

    A. "Red blood" cannot be produced in large enough quantities.
    B. "Red blood" tends to form globules that block circulation.
    C. Hemoglobin does not carry oxygen effectively.
    D. "Red blood" exhibits poor durability in the bloodstream.

65. According to the passage, how much oxygen can be absorbed by a 300 cc sample of PFC?

    A. 50 cc
    B. 100 cc
    C. 150 cc
    D. 300 cc

66. It can be inferred from the passage that the difficulty of producing an ideal blood substitute is compounded by all of the following EXCEPT:

    A. There is no known way to isolate the DNA responsible for hemoglobin.
    B. Naked hemoglobin tends to break down in the bloodstream.
    C. Nonglobulating PFCs have significantly abbreviated oxygen-carrying capacities.
    D. The use of PFCs may lead to blood clotting.

GO TO THE NEXT PAGE.

Passage III (Questions 67–73)

The Russian wheat aphid, *Diuraphis noxia*, is a small, green insect discovered in southern Russia around the turn of the century. Agricultural researchers are not quite sure, but they believe the Russian aphid adapted itself to wheat about 10,000 years ago, when the crop was first domesticated by man. What is not in doubt is the insect's destructiveness. Spread by both wind and human transport, the Russian aphid has destroyed wheat fields throughout Asia, Africa, and Latin America.

Until a few years ago, the United States had been free of this pest. But in the spring of 1986, a swarm of Russian aphids crossed the Mexican border and settled a few hundred miles north, in central Texas. From there, it quickly spread to other Western states, destroying wheat fields all along its path. In fact, the level of destruction has been so great over the past five years that entomologists are calling the Russian aphid the greatest threat to American agriculture since the Hessian fly, *Phytophaga destructor*, was inadvertently brought to the colonies on ships by German mercenary troops during the Revolutionary War.

A combination of several factors have made it particularly difficult to deal with the threat posed by this aphid. First, Russian aphids reproduce asexually at a phenomenal rate. This process, known as parthenogenesis, often results in as many as 20 generations of insects in a single year. Although most generations remain in a limited geographic area because they have no wings, a few generations are born with wings, allowing the insect to spread to new areas. Second, because wheat is a crop with a very low profit margin, most American farmers do not spray it with pesticides; it simply is not economical to do so. And since the Russian aphid has only recently entered the United States, it has no natural enemies among North American insects or animals. As a result, there have been no man-made or natural obstacles to the spread of the Russian aphid in the United States.

Agricultural researchers seeking to control the Russian aphid have looked to its place of origin for answers. In Russia, the Russian aphid has been kept in check by predators which have evolved along-side it over many thousands of years. One species of wasp seems to be particularly efficient at destroying the aphid. The pregnant females of the species search the Russian aphid's home, the interior of a wheat stalk, sting the aphid into paralysis, and then inject an egg into its body. When the egg hatches the wasp larva feeds off the aphid, killing it in the process.

The introduction of predators like the wasp, coupled with the breeding of new strains of insect-resistant wheat, may substantially curb the destructiveness of the Russian aphid in the future. For the time being, however, American farmers are left to their own devices when it comes to protecting their wheat crops.

67. Which of the following statements would be most in agreement with the statements in the passage?

   A. It is no longer economical to grow crops with low profit margins.
   B. Humans are powerless against the forces of nature.
   C. Regional ecosystems are often severely damaged when new organisms are introduced.
   D. It is more difficult to stop the spread of an insect that reproduces asexually.

68. According to the passage, which of the following statements is/are true of Russian wheat aphids?

   I. Most are capable of flight.
   II. They are resistant to pesticides.
   III. They are capable of spreading rapidly.

   A. II only
   B. III only
   C. I and II only
   D. II and III only

GO TO THE NEXT PAGE.

69. It can reasonably be inferred that the author of the passage is:

   A. a botanist with an interest in wheat production.
   B. an agriculturist with an interest in pest control.
   C. a pest exterminator with an interest in agriculture.
   D. an entomologist with an interest in asexual reproduction.

70. The passage supplies information for answering all of the following questions EXCEPT:

   A. What measures were taken to combat the Hessian fly during the 18th century?
   B. Why does the Russian wheat aphid cause less damage in Russia than in other countries?
   C. Is it logical for American farmers to use pesticides in order to attempt to protect their wheat crops from the Russian aphid?
   D. What sorts of solutions have agricultural researchers investigated in their efforts to curb the destructiveness of the Russian wheat aphid?

71. The author suggests the best way to control the Russian aphid population in the United States is to:

   A. devote less acreage to the production of wheat.
   B. spray wheat fields with large quantities of pesticides.
   C. transplant its natural enemies from Russia.
   D. disrupt its reproductive process by sterilizing females.

72. According to the passage, the Russian wheat aphid and the Hessian fly are comparable with respect to:

   I. the amount of destruction they have caused.
   II. the means by which they reproduce.
   III. the ways in which they entered the United States.

   A. I only
   B. II only
   C. I and II only
   D. I and III only

73. The author most likely believes American farmers will:

   A. develop new types of aphid-resistant wheat.
   B. develop their own effective methods for dealing with the Russian aphid.
   C. stop producing wheat until the Russian aphid is brought under control.
   D. continue to lose a portion of their wheat crops for the foreseeable future.

GO TO THE NEXT PAGE.

Passage IV (Questions 74–79)

Our sense of smell is arguably the most powerful of our five senses, but it is also the most elusive. It plays a vital yet mysterious role in our lives. Olfaction is rooted in the same part of the brain that regulates such essential functions as body metabolism, reaction to stress, and appetite. But smell relates to more than physiological function: Its sensations are intimately tied to memory, emotion, and sexual desire. Smell seems to lie somewhere beyond the realm of conscious thought, where, intertwined with emotion and experience, it shapes both our conscious and unconscious lives.

The peculiar intimacy of this sense may be related to certain anatomical features. Smell reaches the brain more directly than do sensations of touch, sight, or sound. When we inhale a particular odor, air containing volatile odiferous molecules is warmed and humidified as it flows over specialized bones in the nose called turbinates. As odor molecules land on the olfactory nerves, these nerves fire a message to the brain. Thus olfactory neurons render a direct path between the stimulus provided by the outside environment and the brain, allowing us to rapidly perceive odors ranging from alluring fragrances to noisome fumes.

Certain scents, such as jasmine, are most universally perceived as appealing, while other, like hydrogen sulfide (which emits a stench reminiscent of rotten eggs), are usually considered repellent. But most odors evoke different reactions from person to person, sometimes triggering strong emotional states or resurrecting seemingly forgotten memories. Scientists surmise that the reason we have highly personal associations with smells is related to the proximity of the olfactory and emotional centers of our brain. Although the precise connection between emotion and olfaction remains a mystery, it is clear that emotion, memory, and smell are all sorted in a part of the brain called the limbic lobe.

Even though we are not always conscious of the presence of odors, and are often unable to either articulate or remember their unique characteristics, our brains always register their existence. In fact, such a large amount of human brain tissue is devoted to smell that scientists surmise the role of this sense must be profound. Moreover, neurobiological research suggests that smell must have an important function because olfactory neurons can regenerate themselves, unlike most other nerve cells. The importance of this sense is further supported by the fact that animals experimentally denied the olfactory sense do not develop full and normal brain function.

The significance of olfaction is much clearer in animals that in human beings. Animal behavior is strongly influenced by pheromones, which are odors that induce psychological or behavioral changes and often provide a means of communicating within a species. These chemical messages, often a complex blend of compounds, are of vital importance to the insect world. Honeybees, for example, organize their societies through odor: The queen bee exudes an odor that both inhibits worker bees from laying eggs and draws drones to her when she is ready to mate. Mammals are also guided by their sense of smell. Through odors emitted by urine and scent glands, many animals maintain their territories, identify one another, signal alarm, and attract mates.

Although our olfactory acuity can't rival that of other animal species, human beings are also guided by smell. Before the advent of sophisticated laboratory techniques, physicians depended on their noses to help diagnose illness. A century ago, it was common medical knowledge that certain bacterial infections carry the musty odor of wine, that typhoid smells like baking bread, and that yellow fever smells like meat. While medical science has moved away from such subjective diagnostic methods, in everyday life we continue to rely on our sense of smell, knowingly or not, to guide us.

GO TO THE NEXT PAGE.

74. According to the passage, the location of the olfactory and emotional centers of the brain helps explain all of the following EXCEPT:

A. why smells can evoke distant memories.
B. why odors elicit different reactions from person to person.
C. why a substantial part of the brain is devoted to smell.
D. which functions are rooted in the limbic lobe.

75. The passage implies that physicians no longer make diagnoses based on odors because:

A. the human sense of smell has considerably diminished over time.
B. the associations of odors with diseases proved largely fictitious.
C. such subjective diagnostic methods were shown to be useless.
D. the medical profession today favors more objective techniques.

76. The sense of smell in animals is different from olfaction in humans in that animals:

A. are unable to make associations between smells and past experience.
B. use smell only to communicate outside their own species.
C. rely on olfaction only for mating purposes.
D. more clearly exhibit behavior changes in response to odors.

77. The author describes the sense of smell as elusive because:

A. odiferous molecules are extremely volatile.
B. the functions of smell are emotional rather than physiological.
C. the function and effects of smell are not fully understood.
D. olfactory sensations are more fleeting than those of other senses.

78. It can be inferred from the passage that the emotional element of human olfaction would be better understood through investigation into:

A. the components and functions of the limbic lobe.
B. how pheromones regulate social behavior and organization.
C. the composition of certain highly evocative odors.
D. the pathway between outside environment and olfactory nerves.

79. Which of the following evidence does NOT support the author's statement that smell has an important physiological function?

A. Olfaction and metabolic function are located in the same area of the brain.
B. Animals with impaired olfaction frequently exhibit abnormal brain function.
C. A considerable amount of human brain tissue is devoted to olfaction.
D. Human beings with impaired olfaction are usually able to behave and function normally.

GO TO THE NEXT PAGE.

"Bebop lives!" cries the newest generation of jazz players. During the 1980s, musicians like Wynton Marsalis revived public interest in bebop, the speedy, angular music that first bubbled up out of Harlem in the early 1940s, changing the face of jazz. That Marsalis and others thought of themselves as celebrating and preserving a noble tradition is, in one sense, inevitable. After the excesses of experimental or free jazz in the 1960s and the electronic jazz-rock fusion of the 1970s, it is hardly surprising that people should hearken back to a time when jazz was purer, perhaps even at the apex of its development. But the recent enthusiasm for bebop is also ironic in light of the music's initial public reception.

In its infancy, during the first two decades of the 20th century, jazz was played by small groups of musicians improvising variations on blues tunes and popular songs. Most of the musicians were unable to read music, and their improvisations were fairly rudimentary. Nevertheless, jazz attained international recognition in the 1920s. Two of the people most responsible for its rise in popularity were Louis Armstrong, the first great jazz soloist, and Fletcher Henderson, leader of the first great jazz band. Armstrong, with his buoyant personality and virtuosic technical skills, greatly expanded the creative range and importance of the soloist in jazz. Henderson, a pianist with extensive training in music theory, foresaw the orchestral possibilities of jazz played by a larger band. He wrote out arrangements of songs for his band members that preserved the spirit of jazz, while at the same time giving soloists a more structured musical background upon which to shape their solo improvisations. In the 1930s, jazz moved further into the mainstream with the advent of the Swing Era. Big bands in the Henderson mold, led by musicians like Benny Goodman, Count Basie, and Duke Ellington, achieved unprecedented popularity with jazz-oriented swing music that was eminently danceable.

Against this musical backdrop, bebop arrived on the scene. Like other modernist movements in art and literature, bebop music represented a departure from tradition in both form and content and was met with initial hostility. Bebop tempos were unusually fast, with the soloist often playing at double time to the backing musicians. The rhythms were tricky and complex, the melodies intricate and frequently dissonant, involving chord changes and notes not previously heard in jazz. Before bebop, jazz players had improvised on popular songs such as those produced by Tin Pan Alley, but bebop tunes were often originals with which jazz audiences were unfamiliar.

Played mainly by small combos rather than big bands, bebop was not danceable; it demanded intellectual concentration. Soon, jazz began to lose its hold on the popular audience, which found the new music disconcerting. Compounding public alienation was the fact that bebop seemed to have arrived on the scene in a completely mature state of development, without that early phase of experimentation that typifies so many movements in the course of Western music. This was as much the result of an accident of history as anything else. The early development of bebop occurred during a three-year ban on recording in this country made necessary by the petrol and vinyl shortages of World War II. By the time the ban was lifted, and the first bebop records were made, the new music seemed to have sprung fully formed like Athena from the forehead of Zeus. And though a small core of enthusiasts would continue to worship bebop pioneers like Charlie Parker and Dizzy Gillespie, many bebop musicians were never able to gain acceptance with any audience and went on to lead lives of obscurity and deprivation.

80. According to the passage, which of the following is true about the bebop music of the 1940s?

   A. It followed the tradition of jazz from the 1920s.
   B. It differed markedly from the music of the Swing Era.
   C. It celebrated the songs of Tin Pan Alley.
   D. It did not require great improvisational skill.

GO TO THE NEXT PAGE.

81. According to the passage, which of the following is true about the jazz of the 1920s?

 A. It resembled the jazz played during the first two decades of the century.
 B. It placed greater demands on the improvisatory skills of its soloists.
 C. Its fast tempos foreshadowed those of bebop in the 1940s.
 D. It was primarily dance music.

82. Based on the information in the passage comparing bebop to other movements in the history of Western music, it is reasonable to conclude that:

 I. most movements in music history passed through a stage of experimentation before reaching mature expression.
 II. World War II prevented bebop from reaching a more appreciative audience.
 III. bebop did not go through a developmental stage before reaching mature expression.

 A. I only
 B. III only
 C. I and II only
 D. II and III only

83. It can be inferred from the passage that the innovations of Fletcher Henderson (lines 29–36) were inspired primarily by:

 A. his admiration for Louis Armstrong.
 B. a hunger for international recognition.
 C. the realization that the public favored large bands over small combos.
 D. a desire to go beyond the structural limitations of early jazz music.

84. The central thesis of the passage is that:

 A. the history of jazz is characterized by a constant search for new forms.
 B. the current revival of interest in bebop has damaged the careers of musicians who play jazz-rock fusion.
 C. bebop may represent the highest development of jazz, but it was largely unappreciated for many years.
 D. bebop would have been much more popular if it had been played by big bands instead of small combos.

85. According to the passage, all of the following are characteristic of bebop music EXCEPT:

 A. eminently danceable tunes.
 B. dissonant melodies.
 C. complex rhythms.
 D. intellectual complexity.

86. The author suggests that bebop seemed to represent a radical departure from earlier jazz in that it:

 A. grew to maturity before reaching a wide audience.
 B. attracted primarily a youthful audience.
 C. dispensed with written arrangements of songs.
 D. expressed the alienation of the musicians who played it.

87. The author mentions Wynton Marsalis and Charlie Parker as:

 A. pioneers of jazz-rock fusion.
 B. architects of the bebop movement.
 C. Swing Era musicians hostile to bebop.
 D. bebop musicians of different eras.

GO TO THE NEXT PAGE.

Passage VI (Questions 88–92)

Studies of photosynthesis began in the late 18th century. One scientist found that green plants produce a substance (later shown to be oxygen) that supports the flame of a candle in a closed container. Several years later it was discovered that a plant must be exposed to light in order to replenish this flame-sustaining "substance." Soon another discovery showed that the oxygen is formed at the expense of another gas, carbon dioxide.

In 1804, de Saussure conducted experiments revealing that equal volumes of carbon dioxide and oxygen are exchanged between a plant and the air surrounding it. De Saussure determined that the weight gained by a plant grown in a pot equals the sum of the weights of carbon derived from absorbed carbon dioxide and water absorbed through plant roots. Using this information, de Saussure was able to postulate that, in photosynthesis, carbon dioxide and water combine using energy in the form of light to produce carbohydrates, water, and free oxygen. Much later, in 1845, scientists' increased understanding of concepts of chemical energy led them to perceive that, through photosynthesis, light energy is transformed and stored as chemical energy.

In the 20th century, studies comparing photosynthesis in green plants and in certain sulfur bacteria yielded important information about the photosynthetic process. Because water is both a reactant and a product in the central reaction, it had long been assumed that the oxygen released by photosynthesis comes from splitting the carbon dioxide molecule. In the 1930s, however, this popular view was decisively altered by the stusdies of C. B. Van Niel. Van Niel studied sulfur bacteria, which use hydrogen sulfide for photosynthesis in the same way that green plants use water, and produce sulfur instead of oxygen. Van Niel saw that the use of carbon dioxide to form carbohydrates was similar in the two types of organisms. He reasoned that the oxygen produced by green plants must derive from water—rather than carbon dioxide, as previously assumed—in the same way that the sulfur produced by the bacteria derives from hydrogen sulfide. Van Niel's finding was important because the earlier belief had been that oxygen was split off from carbon dioxide and that carbon then combined with water to form carbohydrates. The new postulate was that, with green plants, hydrogen is removed from water and then combines with carbon dioxide to form the carbohydrates needed by the organism.

Later Van Niel's assertions were strongly backed by scientists who used water marked with a radioactive isotope of oxygen in order to follow photosynthetic reactions. When the photosynthetically produced free oxygen was analyzed, the isotope was found to be present.

88. Which of the following can be inferred about the scientists discussed in the passage?

   A. They relied on abstract reasoning in the absence of physical data.
   B. They never came to understand the role of light in photosynthesis.
   C. Each contributed to our understanding of the production of oxygen by plants.
   D. They tended to undervalue previous scientific findings.

89. According to the passage, C. B. Van Niel's experiments:

   A. provided the first model of photosynthesis.
   B. showed that the carbon dioxide molecule is split during photosynthesis.
   C. proved that some organisms combine hydrogen sulfide with carbon dioxide in photosynthesis.
   D. provided evidence that weakened the accepted model of photosynthesis.

90. According to the passage, the study of organisms that require hydrogen sulfide for photosynthesis:

   A. proved that oxygen is not produced in photosynthesis.
   B. contradicted the notion that oxygen is needed to support a candle's flame.
   C. disproved assumptions about the role of light energy in photosynthesis.
   D. clarified the role of water in photosynthesis among green plants.

GO TO THE NEXT PAGE.

91. Which of the following statements about photosynthesis would most probably NOT have been made by de Saussure?

A. It involves an exchange of equal quantities of gases.
B. It results in the conversion of light energy to chemical energy.
C. It produces oxygen.
D. It requires light.

92. The passage supplies information for answering all of the following questions EXCEPT:

A. Why is oxygen necessary for a candle to burn?
B. What was de Saussure's explanation of the function of water in photosynthesis?
C. What is the function of light in photosynthesis?
D. Is water required for all photosynthetic reactions?

STOP. IF YOU FINISH BEFORE TIME HAS EXPIRED, CHECK YOUR WORK. YOU MAY GO BACK TO ANY QUESTION IN THIS PART ONLY.

Writing Sample Test

Time—60 minutes

Two Prompts. Separately Timed:
30 Minutes Each

DIRECTIONS: This is a test of your writing skills. The test contains two parts. You will have 30 minutes to complete each part.

Your responses to the prompts given in this Writing Sample will be typed on the computer. You may work only on Part 1 during the first 30 minutes of the test and only on Part 2 during the second 30 minutes. If you finish writing on Part 1 before the time is up, you may review your work on that part, but do not begin writing on Part 2. If you finish writing on Part 2 before the time is up, you may review your work only on Part 2.

Use your time efficiently. Before you begin writing a response, read the assignment carefully and make sure you understand exactly what you are being asked to do. You may use scratch paper to make notes in planning your responses.

Because this is a test of your writing skills, your response to each part should be an essay composed of complete sentences and paragraphs, as well organized and clearly written as you can make it in the allotted time.

TURN TO THE NEXT PAGE TO BEGIN.

Part 1

Consider the following statement:

Voters should not be concerned about a political candidate's personal life.

Write a unified essay in which you perform the following tasks. Explain what you think the above statement means. Describe a specific situation in which voters should be concerned with a politician's personal life. Discuss what you think determines whether a politician's personal life is a public concern.

Part 2

Consider the following statement:

Great leaders are born, not made.

Write a unified essay in which you perform the following tasks. Explain what you think the above statement means. Describe a specific situation in which great leaders are made, not born. Discuss what you think determines whether great leaders are born or made.

GO TO THE NEXT PAGE.

Biological Sciences Test

Time—70 minutes

Questions 93–144

DIRECTIONS: Most of the questions in the following Biological Sciences test are organized into groups, with a descriptive passage preceding each group of questions. Study the passage, then select the single best answer to each question in the group. Some of the questions are not based on a descriptive passage; you must also select the best answer to these questions. If you are unsure of the best answer, eliminate the choices that you know are incorrect, then select an answer from the choices that remain. Indicate your selection by blackening the corresponding circle on your answer sheet. A periodic table is provided below for your use with the questions.

PERIODIC TABLE OF THE ELEMENTS

Hemoglobin (Hb) and myoglobin (Mb) are the O_2-carrying proteins in vertebrates. Hb, which is contained within red blood cells, serves as the O_2 carrier in blood and also plays a vital role in the transport of CO_2 and H^+. Vertebrate Hb consists of four polypeptides (subunits), each with a heme group. The four chains are held together by non-covalent attractions. The affinity of Hb for O_2 varies between species and within species depending on such factors as blood pH, stage of development, and body size. For example, small mammals give up O_2 more readily than large mammals because small mammals have a higher metabolic rate and require more O_2 per gram of tissue.

The binding of O_2 to Hb is also dependent on the cooperativeness of the Hb subunits. That is, binding at one heme facilitates the binding of O_2 at the other hemes within the Hb molecule by altering the conformation of the entire molecule. This conformational change makes subsequent binding of O_2 more energetically favorable. Conversely, the unloading of O_2 at one heme facilitates the unloading of O_2 at the others by a similar mechanism.

Figure 1 depicts the O_2-dissociation curves of Hb (Curves A, B, and C) and myoglobin (Curve D), where saturation, Y, is the fractional occupancy of the O_2-binding sites.

The fraction of O_2 that is transferred from Hb as the blood passes through the tissue capillaries is called the *utilization coefficient*. A normal value is approximately 0.25.

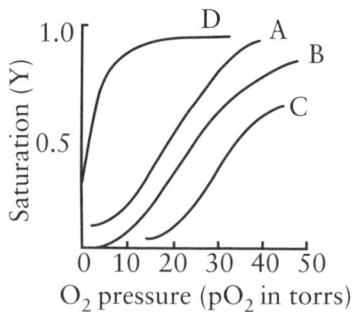

Figure 1

Myoglobin facilitates O_2 transport in muscle and serves as a reserve store of O_2. Mb is a single polypeptide chain containing a heme group, with a molecular weight of 18 kd. As can be seen in Figure 1, Mb (Curve D) has a greater affinity for O_2 than Hb.

93.   The llama is a warm-blooded mammal that lives in regions of unusually high altitudes, and has evolved a type of Hb that adapts it to such an existence. If Curve B represents the O_2-dissociation curve for horse Hb, which curve would most closely resemble the curve for llama Hb?

A.   Curve A
B.   Curve B
C.   Curve C
D.   Curve D

94.   If Curve B represents the O_2-dissociation curve for elephant Hb, which curve most closely resembles the curve for mouse Hb?

A.   Curve A
B.   Curve B
C.   Curve C
D.   Curve D

95.   If Curve B represents the O_2-dissociation curve for human adult Hb, which of the following best explains why Curve A most closely resembles the curve for fetal Hb?

A.   Fetal tissue has a higher metabolic rate than adult tissue.
B.   Fetal tissue has a lower metabolic rage than adult tissue.
C.   Fetal Hb has a higher affinity for O_2 than adult Hb.
D.   Fetal Hb has a lower affinity for O_2 than adult Hb.

GO TO THE NEXT PAGE.

96. The sigmoidal shape of the O_2-dissociation curve of Hb is due to:

   A. the effects of oxidation and reduction on the heme groups within the Hb molecule.
   B. the concentration of carbon dioxide in the blood.
   C. the fact that Hb has a lower affinity for O_2 than Mb.
   D. the cooperativity in binding among the subunits of the Hb molecule.

97. A sample of human adult Hb is placed in an 8 M urea solution, resulting in the disruption of noncovalent interactions. After this procedure, the α chains of Hb are isolated. Which of the four curves most closely resembles the O_2-dissociation curve for the isolated α chains? [Note: Assume that Curve B represents the O_2-dissociation curve for human adult Hb *in vivo*.]

   A. Curve A
   B. Curve B
   C. Curve C
   D. Curve D

98. The utilization coefficient is continually being adjusted in response to physiological changes. Which of the following values most likely represents the utilization coefficient for human adult Hb during strenuous exercise?

   A. 0.0
   B. 0.125
   C. 0.25
   D. 0.75

99. In sperm whales, the Mb content of muscle is about 0.004 moles/kg of muscle. If a sperm whale has 1,000 kg of muscle, approximately how much O_2 is bound to Mb, assuming that the Mb is saturated with O_2?

   A. 4 moles
   B. 8 moles
   C. 12 moles
   D. 16 moles

GO TO THE NEXT PAGE.

Just as the ingestion of nutrients is mandatory for human life, so is the excretion of metabolic waste products. One of these nutrients, protein, is used for building muscle, nucleic acids, and countless compounds integral to homeostasis. However, the catabolism of the amino acids generated from protein digestion produces ammonia, which if not further degraded, can become toxic. Similarly, if the same salts that provide energy and chemical balance to cells are in excess, fluid retention will occur, damaging the circulatory, cardiac, and pulmonary systems.

One of the most important homeostatic organs is the kidney, which closely regulates the excretion and reabsorption of many essential ions and molecules. One mechanism of renal function involves the secretion of antidiuretic hormone (ADH).

Diabetes insipidus (DI), is the condition that occurs when ADH is ineffective. As a result, the kidneys are unable to concentrate urine, leading to excessive water loss. There are two types of DI: central and nephrogenic. *Central DI* occurs when there is a deficiency in the quantity or quality of ADH produced. *Nephrogenic DI* occurs when the kidney tubules are unresponsive to ADH. To differentiate between these two conditions, a patient's urine osmolarity is measured both prior to therapy and after a 24-hour restriction on fluid intake. Exogenous ADH is then administered and urine osmolarity is measured again. The table below gives the results of testing on four patients. Assume that a urine osmolarity of 285 mosm/L of H_2O is normal.

Table 1

Urine Osmolarity (mosm/L of H_2O)

Patient	Before therapy	After fluid restriction	After ADH
A	285	765	765
B	180	765	765
C	180	180	400
D	180	180	180

100. An elevated and potentially toxic level of ammonia in the blood (*hyperammonemia*) would most likely result from a defect in an enzyme involved in:

　A. glycolysis.
　B. fatty acid catabolism.
　C. the urea cycle.
　D. nucleic acid degradation.

101. According to the passage, the catabolism of amino acids produces ammonia. Therefore, after a protein-rich meal, would you expect a build-up of ammonia in the lumen of the small intestine?

　A. Yes, because the ammonia will not be able to diffuse into the intestinal epithelium.
　B. Yes, because the rate at which digestive enzymes degrade ammonia is slower than the rate at which ammonia is produced.
　C. No, because the ammonia will diffuse into the intestinal epithelium and will be excreted by the kidneys.
　D. No, because the ammonia is produced inside individual cells, not within the lumen of the small intestine.

102. Which of the following substances would NOT be found in appreciable quantity in the urine of a healthy individual?

　A. Albumin
　B. Sodium
　C. Urea
　D. Potassium

GO TO THE NEXT PAGE.

103. Which of the following would you most likely expect to find in a patient with diabetes insipidus?

    A. Decreased plasma osmolarity
    B. Increased urine osmolarity
    C. Increased urine glucose
    D. Increased urine output

104. Based on the data in Table 1, which of the four patients most likely has central diabetes insipidus?

    A. Patient A
    B. Patient B
    C. Patient C
    D. Patient D

105. Based on the data in Table 1, which of the four patients most likely has nephrogenic diabetes insipidus?

    A. Patient A
    B. Patient B
    C. Patient C
    D. Patient D

106. What is the most likely cause of Patient B's dilute urine before therapy?

    A. Excessive water intake
    B. Dehydration
    C. Nephrogenic DI
    D. Central DI

GO TO THE NEXT PAGE.

Electromagnetic radiation from space constantly bombards the Earth. Most wavelengths are absorbed by the atmosphere; however, there are two windows of nonabsorption through which significant amounts of radiation reach the ground. The first transmits ultraviolet and visible light, as well as infrared light or heat; the second transmits radio waves. As a result, terrestrial organisms have evolved a number of pigments that interact with light in various ways: Some capture light energy, some provide protection from light-induced damage, and some serve camouflage or signaling purposes.

Among these compounds are many conjugated polyenes, which play important roles as photoreceptors. For every chemical compound, there are certain wavelengths of light whose quanta possess exactly the correct amount of energy to raise electrons from their ground state to higher-energy orbitals. For most organic compounds, these wavelengths are in the UV range. However, conjugated double bond systems stabilize the electrons, so that they can be excited by lower-frequency photons with wavelengths in the visible spectrum. Such a pigment, known as a chromophore, will then transmit the subtraction color, a color complementary to the one absorbed. For instance, carotene, a hydrocarbon compound with 11 conjugated double bonds, absorbs blue light and transmits orange. The wavelength that is absorbed generally increases with the number of conjugated bonds; rings and side-chains also effect wavelength.

Wavelength	Color	Subtraction Color
480 nm	blue	orange
580 nm	yellow	violet
680 nm	red	green

Among the many biological molecules that are affected by light is DNA, the genetic material of living organisms. DNA absorbs ultraviolet light, and may be damaged by UVC (< 280 nm) and UVB (280–315 nm). UVA (315–400 nm) and visible light can actually repair light-induced damage to DNA by a process called photorepair. For this reason UVA, which also stimulates tanning, was once considered beneficial. However there is now increasing evidence that UVA can damage skin.

107. The electrons that give color to a carotene molecule are found in:

   A. *s* orbitals.
   B. *p* orbitals.
   C. *d* orbitals.
   D. *f* orbitals.

108. Two pigments are identical except for the lengths of their conjugated polyene chains. The first transmits yellow light and the second red. What can be said about the sizes of the chromophores?

   A. The first is longer.
   B. The second is longer.
   C. One of the chromophores must be a dimer.
   D. The comparative lengths cannot be determined.

109. Why is benzene colorless?

   A. The absorption energy is of too high a frequency to be visible.
   B. The absorption energy is of too low a frequency to be visible.
   C. Benzene does not absorb light.
   D. Benzene is not conjugated.

110. Many crustaceans produce a blue or green carotene-protein complex. What is the most likely cause of the color change from green to orange when a lobster is boiled?

   A. Heat causes the prosthetic group to become partially hydrated.
   B. The increase in temperature permits the prosthetic group to absorb shorter wavelengths.
   C. The protein is separated from the carotenoid pigment.
   D. Heat causes the prosthetic group to become oxidized.

GO TO THE NEXT PAGE.

111. The four compounds represented by the electronic spectra below were evaluated as potential sunscreens. What is the correct sequence of sunscreen strength, from strongest to weakest, among these four?

I

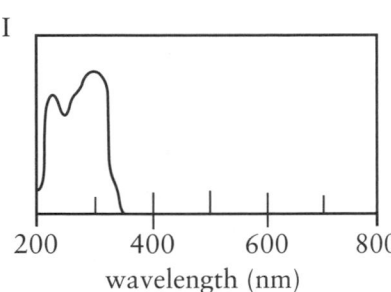

II

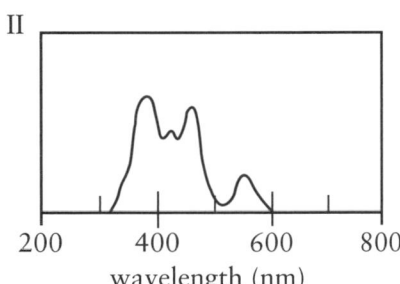

III

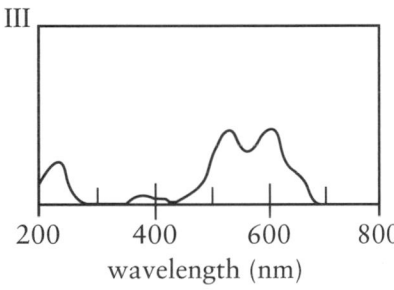

IV

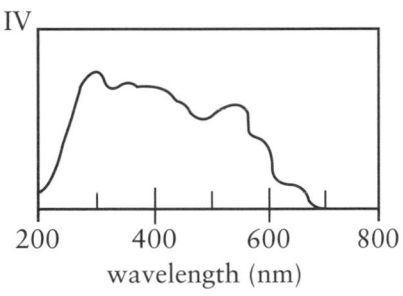

A. I, II, III, IV
B. IV, III, II, I
C. III, II, I, IV
D. IV, I, II, III

112. Which of the following compounds would be most likely to produce color?

A.

B.

C.

D.

113. The color-producing quality of conjugated polyenes is attributable to:

A. antibonding orbitals.
B. resonance.
C. polarity.
D. optical activity.

GO TO THE NEXT PAGE.

114. An increase in heart rate, blood pressure, and blood glucose concentration are all associated with stimulation of the:

    A. parasympathetic nervous system.
    B. sympathetic nervous system.
    C. somatic nervous system.
    D. digestive system.

115. Which of the following compounds share the same absolute configuration?

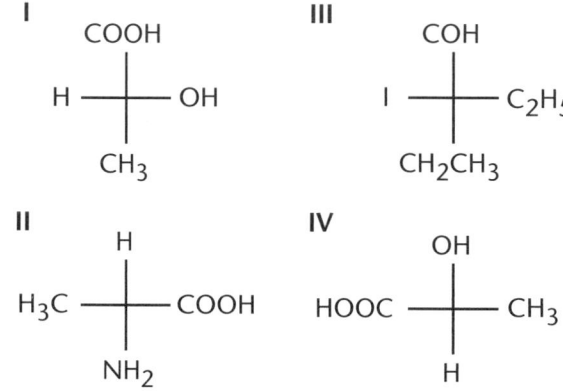

    A. I and III
    B. II and IV
    C. I and II
    D. II, III, and IV

116. Which of the following structures plays a role in both the male excretory and reproductive systems, but in the female excretory system only?

    A. Epididymis
    B. Prostate
    C. Urethra
    D. Ureter

117. The reaction $R-Br + Br^{*-} \rightarrow R-Br^* + Br^-$ is always accompanied by inversion. If this reaction is carried out on an optically pure sample of a chiral compound, which of the following statements will be true? [Note: Br* represents a radioactive isotope of bromine.]

    A. The rate of Br* incorporation is half the rate of racemization.
    B. The rate of Br* incorporation is equal to the rate of racemization.
    C. The rate of Br* incorporation is twice the rate of racemization.
    D. Cannot be determined.

118. Which of the following cell types does NOT contain the diploid number of chromosomes?

    A. Spermatogonium
    B. Spermatid
    C. Zygote
    D. Primary oocyte

GO TO THE NEXT PAGE.

Passage IV (Questions 119–124)

Aerobic respiration is the major process used by oxygen-requiring organisms to generate energy. During respiration, glucose is metabolized to generate chemical energy in the form of ATP:

$$C_6H_{12}O_6 + 6\ O_2 \rightarrow 6\ CO_2 + H_2O + 36\ ATP$$

The biochemical machinery necessary for cellular respiration is found in the mitochondria, small organelles scattered throughout the cytoplasm of most eukaryotic cells. The number of mitochondria per cell varies by tissue type and cell function.

Mitochondria are unusual in that they have their own genetic systems that are entirely separate from the cell's genetic material. However, mitochondrial replication is still dependent upon the cell's nuclear DNA to encode essential proteins required for replication. Despite this fact, mitochondria seem to replicate randomly, out of phase with both the cell cycle and other mitochondria.

The nature of the mitochondrial genome and protein-synthesizing machinery has led many researchers to postulate that mitochondria may have arisen as the result of the ingestion of a bacterium by a primitive cell millions of years ago. It is postulated that the two may have entered into a symbiotic relationship and eventually become dependent on one another; the cell sustained the bacterium, while the bacterium provided energy for the cell. Gradually, the two evolved into the present-day eukaryotic cell, with the mitochondrion retaining some of its own DNA. This is know as the *endosymbiotic hypothesis*. Because mitochondrial DNA is inherited in a non-Mendelian fashion (mitochondria are inherited from the maternal parent, who supplies most cytoplasm to the fertilized eggs), it has been used to look at evolutionary relationships among different organisms.

119. In which of the following phases of the cell cycle could mitochondrial DNA replicate?

    I. G_1
    II. S
    III. G_2
    IV. M

    A. IV only
    B. I and III only
    C. II and IV only
    D. I, II, III, and IV

120. Scientists have demonstrated that human mitochondrial DNA mutates at a fairly slow rate. Because mitochondria play such an important role in the cell, these mutations are most likely to be:

    A. point mutations.
    B. frameshift mutations.
    C. lethal mutations.
    D. nondisjunctions.

121. Which of the following mitochondrial genome characteristics differs most from the characteristics of the nuclear genome?

    A. Mitochondrial DNA is a double helix.
    B. Some mitochondrial genes code for tRNA.
    C. Specific mutations to mitochondrial DNA can be lethal to the organism.
    D. Almost every base in mitochondrial DNA codes for a product.

122. What is the net number of ATP molecules synthesized by an obligate anaerobe per molecule of glucose?

    A. 2 ATP
    B. 6 ATP
    C. 8 ATP
    D. 36 ATP

GO TO THE NEXT PAGE.

123. A mating type of wild-type strain of the algae *C. reinhardii* is crossed with the opposite mating type of a mutant strain of the algae, which has lost all mitochondrial functions due to deletions in its mitochondrial genome. All of the offspring from this cross also lack mitochondrial functions. Based on information in the passage, this can best be explained by the:

A. endosymbiotic hypothesis.
B. non-Mendelian inheritance of mitochondrial DNA.
C. recombination of mitochondrial DNA during organelle replication.
D. presence of genetic material in the mitochondria that is distinct from nuclear DNA.

124. Four different human cell cultures—erythrocytes, epidermal cells, skeletal muscle cells, and intestinal cells—were grown in a medium containing radioactive adenine. After 10 days, the mitochondria were isolated via centrifugation, and their level of radioactivity was measured using a liquid scintillation counter. Which of the following cells would be expected to have the greatest number of counts per minute of radioactive decay?

A. Erythrocytes
B. Epidermal cells
C. Skeletal muscle cells
D. Intestinal cells

GO TO THE NEXT PAGE.

Passage V (Questions 125–128)

A student was given a sample of an unknown liquid and asked to determine as much as possible about its structure. He was told that the compound contained only carbon, hydrogen, and oxygen, and had only one type of functional group. The student found its boiling point to be 206°C. Using mass spectroscopy, he determined its molecular weight to be 138 g/mol. Finally, he took the infrared spectrum of the compound, which is shown below.

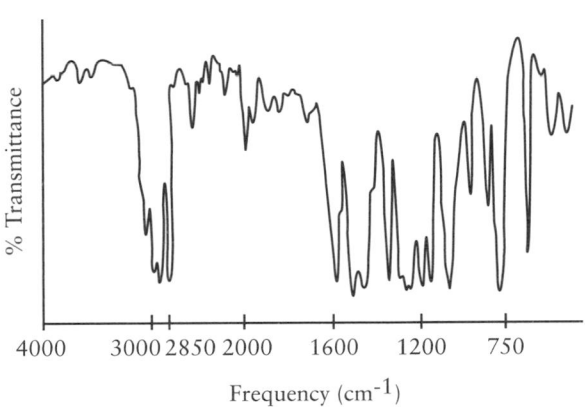

From this spectrum, the student quickly reached a conclusion about the functional group. He then turned his attention to the fingerprint region of the compound, which generally has a complicated pattern of peaks that are determined by the structure of the hydrocarbon portion of a molecule. The student decided that the large peak at 750 cm^{-1} must indicate that this was a disubstituted aromatic compound.

125. The correct formula for this compound could be:

A. $C_7H_{10}O_3$.
B. $C_8H_{10}O_2$.
C. $C_9H_{13}O$.
D. $C_7H_{21}O_2$.

126. The overlapping set of peaks near 3,000 cm^{-1} includes one peak at 2,850 cm^{-1}. What type of functional group could this indicate?

A. Methyl
B. Phenol
C. Carboxyl
D. Aldehyde carbonyl

127. Assuming that all of the student's deductions were correct, which of the following could be the structure of the unknown compound?

A.

COOH

CH$_2$CH$_3$

C.

CH$_2$OH

HOH$_2$C

B.

OCH$_3$

OCH$_3$

D.

COOH

128. The student decides to carry out some simple tests on the compound to confirm his identification. Which of the following statements is NOT true?

A. He could distinguish between a phenol and a benzoic acid by seeing if the unknown can be extracted with a weak base.
B. He could distinguish between a benzyl aldehyde and a benzyl ketone by seeing if the unknown will react with cold KMnO$_4$.
C. He could distinguish between a benzyl alcohol and a phenol by attempting to dissolve the unknown in an aqueous solution of HCl.
D. He could distinguish between a benzyl alcohol and a benzoic ester by attempting to dissolve the unknown in an aqueous solution of NaOH.

GO TO THE NEXT PAGE.

Although individual organisms have only two alleles for any given trait, it is possible for a trait to have more than two alleles coding for it. This phenomenon is know as multiple alleles. Multiple alleles are created when a single gene undergoes several distinct mutations. These alleles may have different dominance relationships with one another; for example, there are three alleles coding for the human blood groups, the IA, IB, and i alleles. Both the IA and IB alleles are dominant to the i allele, but IA and IB are codominant to each other.

A multiple-allele system has recently been discovered in the determination of hair coloring in a species of wild rat. The rats are found to have one of three colors: brown, red, or white. Let B = the gene for brown hair; b = the gene for red hair; and w = the gene for white hair. The results from nine experimental crosses are shown below. The males and females in Crosses 1, 2, and 3 are all homozygous for hair color.

Cross	Male	Female	Offspring
1	brown	red	all brown
2	brown	white	all brown
3	red	white	all red
4	brown	brown	3 brown : 1 red
5	brown	brown	all brown
6	red	red	all red
7	red	red	3 red : 1 white
8	brown	red	2 brown : 1 red : 1 white
9	brown	red	1 brown : 1 red

129. Based on the experimental results, what is the genotype of the male in Cross 6?

   A. bw
   B. bb
   C. bw or bb
   D. Bb or bw

130. If a large number of brown offspring from Cross 8 are mated with each other, what is the expected percentage of white offspring?

   A. 6.25%
   B. 8.33%
   C. 12.5%
   D. 25.0%

131. Based on the experimental results, what is the genotype of the female in Cross 5?

   A. Bb
   B. BB or Bb
   C. BB or Bw
   D. BB, Bb, or Bw

132. A white male is crossed with a heterozygous red female from Cross 9. What is the expected ratio of red to white offspring?

   A. 3:1
   B. 1:3
   C. 1:1
   D. 2:1

133. If it were discovered that the alleles for red and white hair were actually incompletely dominant and produced a pink hair color in rats with one copy of each allele, what would be the expected phenotypic ratio in a cross between a Bb male and a pink female?

   A. 2 brown : 1 red : 1 white
   B. 2 brown : 1 red : 1 pink
   C. 1 brown : 2 white : 1 pink
   D. 1 brown : 1 white

GO TO THE NEXT PAGE.

Passage VII (Questions 134–139)

Compounds containing a hydroxyl group attached to a benzene ring are called phenols (I). Derivatives of phenols, such as naphthols (II) and phenanthrols (III), have chemical properties similar to those of phenols, as do most of the many naturally occurring substituted phenols. Like other alcohols, phenols have higher boiling points than hydrocarbons of similar molecular weight. Like carboxylic acids, phenols are more acidic than their alcohol counterparts. Phenols undergo a number of different reactions; both their hydroxyl groups and their benzene rings are highly reactive. A number of chemical tests distinguish phenols from alcohols and carboxylic acids.

Thymol, a naturally occurring phenol, is an effective disinfectant that is obtained from thyme oil. Thymol can also be synthesized from *m*-cresol, as shown in Reaction A below. Thymol can then be converted to menthol, another naturally occurring organic compound; this conversion is shown in Reaction B.

134. Reaction A is an example of:

    A. a free radical substitution.
    B. an electrophilic aromatic substitution.
    C. an electrophilic addition.
    D. a nucleophilic aromatic substitution.

135. Comparing the K_a values for cyclohexanol ($K_a = 10^{-18}$) and phenol ($K_a = 1.3 \times 10^{-10}$) reveals that phenol is more acidic than cyclohexanol. Which of the following explain(s) the acidity of phenol?

    I. The exceptionally strong hydrogen bonding possible with phenol facilitates the loss of a proton, making it more acidic then cyclohexanol.
    II. Phenol's conjugate base, phenoxide, is stabilized by resonance to a greater extent than phenol itself.
    III. The negative charge of the oxygen atom on the phenoxide ion is delocalized over the benzene ring.

    A. I only
    B. II only
    C. II and III only
    D. I, II, and III

136. Which of the following shows the order of decreasing acidity among the four compounds below?

    A. I, III, IV, II
    B. IV, I, II, III
    C. IV, III, II, I
    D. IV, II, I, III

GO TO THE NEXT PAGE.

137. The reaction of phenol with dilute nitric acid produces which of the following compounds?

A.

$+$

B.

C.

D.

$+$

138. What simple chemical test could be used to distinguish between the following two compounds?

A.

B.

A. Compound B's solubility in $NaHCO_3$
B. Compound A's solubility in NaOH
C. Compound A's ability to decolorize a bromine solution
D. Compound A's solubility in $NaHCO_3$

139. Compound X ($C_{10}H_{14}O$) dissolves in aqueous sodium hydroxide but is insoluble in aqueous sodium bicarbonate. The proton NMR spectrum of compound X is as follows:

δ 1.3 (9H)	singlet
δ 4.8 (1H)	singlet
δ 7.1 (4H)	multiplet

Which of the following is the structure of Compound X?

A.

B.

C.

D.

GO TO THE NEXT PAGE.

Questions 140 through 144 are NOT based on a descriptive passage.

140. Which of the following compounds readily undergoes E1, S_N1, and E2 reactions, but not S_N2 reactions?

    A. $CH_3CH_2CH_2Cl$
    B. $(CH_3)_3COH$
    C. $CH_3CH_2CH_3$
    D. $(CH_3CH_2)_3CBr$

141. A certain drug inhibits ribosomal RNA synthesis. Which of the following eukaryotic organelles would be most affected by the administration of this drug?

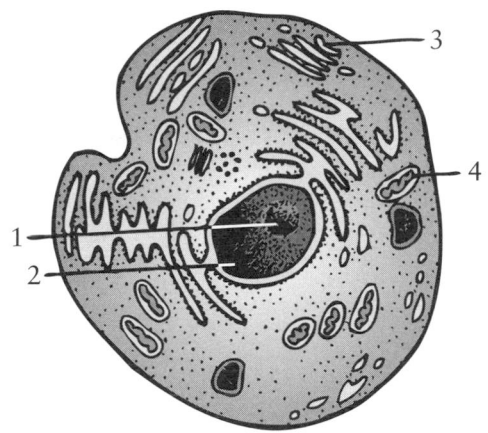

    A. 1
    B. 2
    C. 3
    D. 4

142. Exocrine secretions of the pancreas:

    A. raise blood glucose levels.
    B. lower blood glucose levels.
    C. regulate metabolic rate.
    D. aid in protein and fat digestion.

143. Destroying the cerebellum of a cat would cause significant impairment of normal:

    A. urine formation.
    B. sense of smell.
    C. coordinated movement.
    D. thermoregulation.

144. A cell with a high intracellular K^+ concentration, whose plasma membrane is impermeable to K^+, is placed in an ATP-rich medium with a low K^+ concentration. After several minutes, it is determined that the extracellular concentrations of both K^+ and ATP have decreased, while the intracellular K^+ concentration has increased. What is the most likely explanation for this phenomenon?

    A. The K^+ passively diffused from the medium into the cell.
    B. The K^+ entered the cell by way of facilitated transport.
    C. The ATP formed a temporary lipid-soluble complex with the K^+, thus enabling the potassium to enter the cell.
    D. The K^+ entered the cell by way of active transport.

STOP. IF YOU FINISH BEFORE TIME HAS EXPIRED, CHECK YOUR WORK. YOU MAY GO BACK TO ANY QUESTION IN THIS PART ONLY.

FULL-LENGTH PRACTICE MCAT
ANSWER KEY

1. D	31. D	61. C	91. B	121. D
2. A	32. B	62. B	92. A	122. A
3. D	33. D	63. B	93. A	123. B
4. C	34. A	64. D	94. C	124. C
5. B	35. C	65. C	95. C	125. B
6. A	36. C	66. A	96. D	126. A
7. A	37. C	67. C	97. D	127. B
8. D	38. B	68. B	98. D	128. C
9. D	39. C	69. B	99. A	129. C
10. C	40. A	70. A	100. C	130. A
11. A	41. D	71. C	101. D	131. D
12. B	42. C	72. A	102. A	132. C
13. C	43. D	73. D	103. D	133. B
14. D	44. D	74. C	104. C	134. B
15. B	45. C	75. D	105. D	135. C
16. C	46. B	76. D	106. A	136. D
17. B	47. B	77. C	107. B	137. A
18. D	48. C	78. A	108. B	138. B
19. C	49. B	79. D	109. A	139. B
20. B	50. A	80. B	110. C	140. D
21. D	51. D	81. B	111. D	141. A
22. A	52. D	82. A	112. C	142. D
23. B	53. A	83. D	113. B	143. C
24. B	54. B	84. C	114. B	144. D
25. C	55. C	85. A	115. B	
26. A	56. D	86. A	116. C	
27. C	57. C	87. D	117. A	
28. A	58. C	88. C	118. B	
29. D	59. D	89. D	119. D	
30. A	60. D	90. D	120. A	

FULL-LENGTH PRACTICE MCAT
SCORE CONVERSION CHART

PS Raw Score	PS Scaled Score	VR Raw Score	VR Scaled Score	BS Raw Score	BS Scaled Score
0 to 10	1	0 to 16	1	0 to 13	1
11 to 12	2	17 to 18	2	14 to 16	2
13 to 15	3	19 to 20	3	17 to 19	3
16 to 17	4	21 to 22	4	20 to 22	4
18 to 19	5	23 to 24	5	23 to 25	5
20 to 21	6	25 to 27	6	26 to 28	6
22 to 24	7	28 to 29	7	29 to 31	7
25 to 26	8	30 to 32	8	32 to 34	8
27 to 28	9	33 to 34	9	35 to 37	9
29 to 31	10	35	10	38 to 39	10
32 to 34	11	36	11	40 to 42	11
35 to 36	12	37	12	43 to 45	12
37 to 39	13	38	13	46 to 48	13
40 to 42	14	39	14	49 to 51	14
43 to 52	15	40	15	52	15

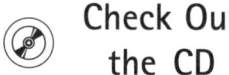 **Check Out the CD**

The tests on your CD-ROM offer a complete scoring analysis, including percentile ranks, essay scoring guidelines and more.

PHYSICAL SCIENCES: Answers and Explanations

ANSWER KEY

1. D	21. D	40. A
2. A	22. A	41. D
3. D	23. B	42. C
4. C	24. B	43. D
5. B	25. C	44. D
6. A	26. A	45. C
7. A	27. C	46. B
8. D	28. A	47. B
9. D	29. D	48. C
10. C	30. A	49. B
11. A	31. D	50. A
12. B	32. B	51. D
13. C	33. D	52. D
14. D	34. A	
15. B	35. C	
16. C	36. C	
17. B	37. C	
18. D	38. B	
19. C	39. C	
20. B		

EXPLANATIONS

Passage I (Questions 1–6)

This passage is about ideal gases and molecular motion. It requires you to know some basic facts about gases coming in, and also to gain a good conceptual understanding of the information presented in the passage. Gases are discussed in their own chapter in the General Chemistry section of this book.

1. D Standard temperature is usually expressed in either Celsius or Kelvin; for pressure, there are three different commonly used units. These are torr, atmospheres, and millimeters of mercury. If you know standard temperature and pressure in one set of units, you should be able to convert to other commonly used units. Conversion factors were not given in this problem, because you should know that 1 atmosphere of pressure is equal to 760 torr and 760 millimeters of mercury.

To convert from Celsius to Kelvin you simply add 273. If you recall that standard temperature is 0° Celsius, then it is a simple matter to convert to Kelvin. Since all of the choices are correct, (D) is the answer.

2. A According to Equation 5, the rate of effusion depends on the area of the pinhole, the pressures inside and outside the container, the molecular weight of the particles, the gas constant R, and the temperature. Since all four gases are in one container, subject to the same conditions, the only one of these factors that is different for the four gases is molecular weight. Since the rate of effusion is inversely proportional to the square root of the molecular weight, the rate of effusion increases as the molecular weight decreases. Thus, the lightest particle will effuse through the pinhole fastest. Molecular hydrogen is the lightest of the four species, with a molecular weight of two grams per mole, so it will effuse the fastest.

3. D The mean free path of a particle is the average distance the particle can travel before it collides with another gas particle or the wall of the container. The longer the distance that a gas particle travels between collisions, the farther apart the individual gas molecules must be. That means that the volume of the gas must increase to increase the distance between collisions. One way to increase the volume is to decrease the pressure of the gas, so (D) is correct. Choice (A) is incorrect because an increase in pressure leads to a decrease in the volume and thus mean free path. Thus the gas particles are closer together and more likely to collide, decreasing the average distance they travel between collisions. Choice (B) is incorrect because if the number of particles is increased while the volume remains constant, the likelihood of a collision will also increase. The pressure also increases as the number of particles per unit volume increases. Choice (C) is incorrect because the mean free path is analogous to the distance between collisions and if this is decreased, then the mean free path decreases as well. Basically, choices A, B, and C will all decrease the mean free path of a gas.

4. C If the ratio of the rates of effusion for the two gases is taken, and all factors that are the same for the two gases are canceled out, then one ends up with simply the inverse of the square root of the masses, as in choice (C). Since the gases A and B constitute a mixture, they are in the same container, at the same pressure and effusing through the same pinhole. Therefore, the pinhole area for A equals the pinhole area of B and the answer given in choice (B) can be condensed to the answer given in choice (C). Similarly, the pressure of the gas in the container is the same whether you are considering the gas A component or the gas B component, since they are in a mixture characterized by one pressure. Thus, the answer given in choice (D) also reduces to that in choice (C). Choice (A), which states that the ratio is 1, would be correct only if the two gases being considered had the same molecular weight. Although it is possible for this to be true, we have no indication of whether or not it is. Since the question states that they are two noble gases, it is a safer to assume that the two gases have different molecular weights.

5. B Equation 2 gives the formula for the average kinetic energy of an ideal gas. To answer this question, figure out which factor varies directly with the average kinetic energy. The rms speed, μ, has been canceled out of this equation, so choice (A) is wrong. The Boltzmann constant and universal gas constant, choices C and D, are the same for every value of the average kinetic energy, so they are also wrong. That leaves only temperature, choice (B). the correct answer. All you really needed to get this question was Equation 2 and an understanding of the various factors in it. However, you may have just made a beeline for choice (B) since you have probably had it drilled into your head in your study of gases that the temperature of a gas is a measure of the average kinetic energy of that gas.

6. A Equation 3 states that the root-mean-square speed, μ, is equal to $(3RT/M)^{1/2}$. Therefore, μ is proportional to $\sqrt{T}$ and $1/\sqrt{M}$. Since the temperature is held constant, we must look at the molar mass. If μ is proportional to $1/\sqrt{M}$, the molecule with the largest molar mass will have the smallest rms speed. Chlorine, choice (A), has the largest molar mass (71 g/mol) and is the correct response. Oxygen, carbon dioxide, and nitrogen have molar masses of 32 g/mol, 44 g/mol, and 28g/mol, respectively. When compared to chlorine, we can see that all of these molecules will have a larger rms speed.

Passage II (Questions 7–11)

7. A To do this question, you must remember the equation Q = CV, where Q is the charge stored, C is the capacitance, and V is the voltage across the plates. We are given that the capacitance is 10 micro farads, but we do not have a value for the voltage V, since the input voltage to the transformer is stepped up 50 times. From the diagram we can see that the input voltage is 160 volts. So the output voltage is 160 times 50, or 8,000 volts. Substituting the voltage and the capacitance into our equation gives a value for the charge of 8,000 times 10×10^{-6}, or 0.08 coulombs, which is choice (A).

8. D This question asks you to calculate the initial current through the patient, and this can be done by using Ohm's law, which states that the current is equal to the voltage divided by the resistance. We know that the resistance across the two electrodes is 1,000 ohms when a wetting gel is applied, but as in the previous question we do not have a value for the initial voltage. This may again be calculated. We know that the transformer increases the input voltage by a factor of 50, and since the input voltage is 160 volts, the output voltage will be 8,000 volts. This voltage charges the capacitor only, so the voltage across the capacitor when fully charged will be 8,000 volts. By substituting the values for the resistance and the voltage into Ohm's law, we find that the initial current flowing through the patient is 8,000 divided by 1,000, or 8 amps.

9. D The capacitance of a parallel-plate capacitor is given by $K \varepsilon_0 A/d$, where K is the dielectric constant, ε_0 is the permittivity of free space, A is the area of overlap of the two the plates, and d is the separation of the two plates. This implies that when a material with a dielectric constant K is introduced between the plates of a capacitor, the capacitance increases by a numerical factor K. In the question we are told that a dielectric with a value of K > 1 is introduced between the plates, which means that the capacitance will increase. So statement I is correct and choice (C) can be ruled out. It is important to note at this point that the voltage across the plates does not increase with the introduction of a dielectric. This is because the voltage across the plates of a fully charged capacitor is equal to the

voltage applied across the plates when it was initially charged. Since this is held constant at 8,000 volts, the voltage across the plates will remain at 8,000 volts. So statement II is false and choice (B) can be eliminated. To choose between choices (A) and (D), look at how the charge on the plates of a capacitor is affected by the introduction of a dielectric. The capacitance of a capacitor is related to the voltage across the plates and the charge stored by the equation C = Q over V, where C is the capacitance, Q is the charge stored, and V is the voltage. We have already said that the voltage across the capacitor remains constant when the dielectric is introduced. This implies that the capacitance of the capacitor is directly proportional to the charge stored. Since this is the case, as the capacitance increases, the charge stored on the plates must also increase. So statement III is true and choice (D) is the correct answer.

10. C When there is no ground connection, all the current is forced through the patient's heart, despite the relatively large resistance of the patient's body. However, if the patient is in contact with the ground, this provides a path of much less resistance than the patient's body, resulting in most of the current flowing through to the ground, rather than through the patient. This will render the defibrillator ineffective.

Choice (A) is incorrect because the resistance across the patient's body cannot change. Choice (B) is incorrect. If the defibrillator is not in contact with the patient when the doctor receives a shock, then the shock hazard has nothing to do with the patient being grounded or not. If, however, the electrodes are in contact with the patient when the doctor receives a shock, the ground will take most of the current, and thereby reduce the shock that the doctor experiences. So the doctor administering the treatment will be in less danger of receiving a shock when the patient is in contact with the ground. Choice (D) is incorrect since the burns received by the patient are due to the application of large currents over a small area of skin, and have nothing to do with the presence of a ground. Therefore, in order to reduce the burns that the patient receives, the area of the electrodes is increased to distribute the current and reduce the current density.

11. A   Since the capacitor is, in effect, connected to a constant voltage source, the potential difference doesn't change when a dielectric is inserted between the plates. Therefore, the charge on the plates must increase to compensate for the effect of the polarization of charge in the dielectric. The polarization of charge in the dielectric sets up an electric field opposite in direction and weaker in magnitude than the electric field due to the charge on the capacitor plates. This would decrease the net electric field between the plates if the capacitor were not connected to a constant voltage source. However, since it is connected to a constant voltage source when the dielectric is inserted, additional charge builds up on the plates to keep the potential difference constant. Therefore, the net electric field between the plates with the dielectric in place is equal to the net electric field between the plates with no dielectric and choices (C) and (D) are wrong. Since the charge on the plates increases, the energy stored will increase because the energy stored is given by (1/2)QV, where Q is the charge on the plates and V is the potential difference between the plates.

Discrete Questions

12 B   This question deals with the colligative properties of solutions. It brings up several critical points about solutions. One is that the presence of a solute in a solution *always* raises the boiling point and lowers the freezing point, compared to those of the pure solvent. The more concentrated the solution, the higher the boiling point and lower the freezing point will be. Thus it is clear that choice (A) is incorrect; since Solution Y's boiling point is higher than Solution X's, its freezing point must be lower as well. Actually, you don't have enough information to say that this answer is right or wrong since you don't know the original freezing point or freezing point depression constant for either solution. There must be a better answer. The second important concept is that of vapor pressure, which is the topic of both choices (B) and (D). A solution boils when its vapor pressure is equal to the atmospheric pressure. If a solution has a higher boiling point than another, it must have a lower vapor pressure. The vapor pressure of a solution increases as its temperature increases. Since it takes more heat to boil solution Y under the same atmospheric pressure, solution Y must have had a

lower vapor pressure to begin with. Choice (B) is therefore correct, and (D) incorrect. Choice (C) concerns the solubility of the two solutions in each other. Again, we don't have enough information to say that this answer is correct. After all, we know nothing about the two solvents of solutions X and Y, only that they have the same concentration of solute in them and what the resultant boiling points are. That leaves B as the correct answer.

13. C   In the question, we are told that the object is a distance of 10 centimeters to the left of the lens. To determine the position of the image, we simply plug the numbers into the equation: one over the focal length equals one over the object distance plus one over the image distance. This rearranges to give one over the image distance equals one over the focal length minus one over the object distance. Plugging in values for the focal length of 8 centimeters, and an object distance of 10 cm, we get an answer of 1 over 40 for the reciprocal of the image distance, which is equivalent to an image distance of 40 centimeters. Since we have a positive image distance, the image is on the real side of the lens, which is the right side of the lens. To calculate the magnification, we use the equation: Magnification equals minus the image distance divided by the object distance. Putting numbers into the equation, we get that the magnification is equal to –40 centimeters divided by 10 centimeters, or 4x. The minus sign indicates that the image is inverted. So the image is 40 centimeters to the right of the lens, with a magnification of 4x, which is answer choice (C).

14. D   This is a relatively simple concentration problem. Molality is defined as the number of moles of solute per kilogram of solvent. It is denoted by a lower case *m* instead of the upper case *M* that denotes molarity. Here, you must first calculate the molecular weight of maleic acid, or 116 grams per mole and determine the number of moles. Dividing actual grams by the grams per mole you get 0.25 moles. Since this is dissolved in 500 grams or 0.5 kilograms of ammonia you have a 0.5 molal solution, so choice (D) is the correct response.

15. B To answer this question, we simply apply the right-hand rule. Since the particle is an electron, the direction of qv is opposite to that of v or from right to left. When you point your thumb in this direction and your fingers into the page along the direction of the magnetic field, the palm of your right hand points in the direction of the force that is downwards.

16. C To solve this problem you need to remember the definition of *normality*, and know how acids and bases interact to neutralize each other. *Normality* is defined as the number of equivalents per liter of solution. Here nitric acid has one equivalent, that is, it has one proton to donate per mole. Thus, for this compound, normality equals molarity, and we have 2 moles in one liter, or 1.4 moles in 700 milliliters. Since acids and bases react in a 1 to 1 ratio of equivalents, in order to neutralize 1.4 moles of nitric acid, you must have an equal number of equivalents of the neutralizing substance present. Since sodium hydroxide also has 1 equivalent per mole, we need the same number of moles of each. Therefore, we need 1.4 moles of sodium hydroxide. Sodium hydroxide has a molar weight of 40 grams, 1.4 moles will have a mass of 56 grams.

17. B The main concept needed to answer this question is that the acceleration of gravity on the moon is one-sixth that on Earth. Since the object is dropped, its initial velocity is zero on both the Earth and the moon. Therefore, we use the kinematic formula: v squared equals 2ad, where a is the acceleration due to gravity and d is the distance. Dividing the equation for the velocity squared of the body on the moon by the equation for the velocity squared of the body on the Earth gives $v_m/v_e = \sqrt{a_m/g}$. The distance d cancels out since it equals 30 meters in each case. As given in the question stem, a_m/g is 1/6. Taking the square root, we get $\sqrt{1/6}$ which is choice (B). If you forget to take the square root, you get choice (A).

18. D To answer this question, you need to understand what it is that causes a molecular orbital to have high energy. In the first paragraph, we're told that when orbitals from different atoms with the same sign overlap to form bonds, they are called bonding orbitals. Also, we are told that bonding orbitals have lower energy than their component atomic orbitals. In the same way, we can say that when orbitals from different atoms with opposite signs overlap, they form antibonding orbitals. Antibonding orbitals are higher in energy than the original atomic orbitals.

Looking at the second paragraph, we are told that of the possible pi orbital structures for benzene, the one with the lowest energy has the plus region of all six p orbital functions on one side of the ring. From this we can conclude that another situation for the lowest energy would be for the negative region of all six p orbital functions on the other side of the ring. In choice (A), all the atomic orbitals have their negative sides facing the same direction, and this corresponds to the lowest energy molecular orbital—so we can rule out choice (A), because this gives the lowest energy state. Because you are told that the lowest pi energy orbitals are the ones with the plus region of all six p orbital functions on one side of the ring, you should be able to deduce that the energy level of a molecular orbital is determined not by whether the function signs are positive or negative, but by whether adjacent atomic orbitals are of the same or opposite sign. Examining choice (B), there is bonding from carbons one through three and four to six, but carbons three and four are antibonding. In choice (C), carbons one to two, three to four, and five to six are bonding but two to three and four to five are antibonding. Choice (D) is entirely antibonding, since there are no adjacent orbital functions of the same sign. Therefore the molecular orbital portrayed in choice (D) has the highest energy level.

19. C A photon of light can be absorbed only if its energy level is equal to the change in energy between two orbitals in the atom or molecule. Longer wavelengths of light have a lower frequency and thus lower energy level, so you can eliminate choice (D) immediately. The wavelength of light does not have to fit the length of the molecule, so choice (B) is wrong. This leaves you with choices A and C. To decide between these choices, think about what determines the energy of a quantum of light absorbed by an atom or molecule. The energy of the photon must be equal to the difference in energy between the ground state and the excited state. What is important is not the absolute energy level of the ground state, but the difference in energy level between the lower and higher orbital. Longer conjugated polyenes have a greater number of p electrons forming pi orbitals, and therefore a greater number of possible molecular orbitals. This produces smaller energy transitions, allowing for absorption of photons at a lower energy and longer wavelength.

20. B You are given the order of orbital filling in paragraph three and are told in the last paragraph what a triplet state is. Remember that when there are orbitals of equal energy, each one will be half-filled before any of the orbitals is completely filled, and all the half-filled orbitals will have electrons with the same spin. Looking at the answer choices for the question, you can see that they are all diatomic; thus, there will be 2 electrons in a hydrogen molecule, 14 in nitrogen, 16 in oxygen and 18 in fluorine. The passage does not describe how to fill the $n = 1$ shell, but from knowing that the $n = 2$ shell has the sigma 2s bonding orbitals and 1 sigma 2s antibonding orbital, there will be sigma bonding and antibonding orbitals in the $n = 1$ shell, and these will also hold 4 electrons. Therefore, molecular hydrogen will fill half the $n = 1$ shell with the total of 2 electrons that it has and there will be zero electrons in its second shell. Working in a similar way you will have 10 electrons in the second shell for molecular nitrogen, 12 for oxygen, and 14 for fluorine. When you fill in the molecular orbitals, you will find that nitrogen just fills the pi 2x and 2y bonding orbitals. Since there are no unpaired electrons, molecular nitrogen can't be a triplet. Molecular oxygen has 2 extra electrons, which go into the pi 2x and 2y antibonding orbitals. In other words it has unpaired electrons with the same spin.

21.   D In CH_4, methane, the single $2s$ orbital and the three $2p$ orbitals hybridize to form an sp^3 hybrid orbital. In C_2H_4, the 2s orbital hybridizes with only two of the p orbitals to form an sp^2 hybrid. The third p orbital remains separate and forms the second carbon-carbon bond. In C_6H_6, benzene, the six carbons also form sp^2 hybrid orbitals and the remaining p orbitals form the pi electron cloud above and below the plane of the ring. In C_2H_2, acetylene, only one p orbital hybridizes with the s orbital, and the two remaining p orbitals form the second and third carbon-carbon bonds. The C-H bonds of each of these molecules are formed by the hybrid sp, sp^2, or sp^3 orbitals. Since the s subshell is of lower energy than the p subshell, the greater the s character of an orbital, the lower will be its energy. Thus, the energy level transition from lowest to highest will go from sp to sp^2 to sp^3.

22.   A The molecular orbital you have been asked to choose is an antibonding sigma orbital. Examining the question, the star above the sigma sign indicates that the orbital is antibonding. You should know that sigma orbitals are formed in a straight line, choice (D) is a bonding sigma orbital and (A), the correct choice, is an antibonding sigma orbital. In pi orbitals, the lobes of the p orbitals are perpendicular to the line connecting the two atoms. When a pi orbital is bonding, the lobes above and below the plane of the molecule connect to form a shape such as that shown in choice (B). When a pi orbital is antibonding, the perpendicular p lobes cancel each other out where they overlap. This produces an electron cloud that looks as if the p orbitals were repelling each other, as in choice (C).

23.   B The first quantum number, n, is called the principal quantum number and this determines which principal energy level the electron is in, $n = 1$, $n = 2$, etc. This does not help specify between the p_x and p_y orbital, thus it is not the answer we are looking for. The second quantum number is the azimuthal number designated by l. This determines the subshell s, p, d, or f. Choice (A) is the azimuthal quantum number, and it does not help us in distinguishing the p_x orbital from the p_y orbital, so we can rule out choice (A). The third quantum number, the magnetic quantum number, specifies the particular orbitals within a subshell and is given by m_l. Each of these orbitals can hold two electrons. There's only one orbital in an s subshell, in a p orbital there are three, in a d subshell there are five, and in an f subshell there are seven. The three p orbitals are known as p_x, p_y, and p_z, so there we have our answer. The magnetic quantum number allows you to differentiate between the p_x and the p_y orbital, so choice (B) is the correct answer. Looking at the fourth quantum number, known as m_s, this tells us whether the electron has a plus or minus spin. Each orbital when filled contains two electrons of opposite spins, thus it is choice (B), the magnetic quantum number, m_l, that distinguishes the x, y, and z orbitals of the p subshell.

Passage IV (Questions 24–29)

24. B When the skier is at the top of the track, she is not moving, so all her energy is potential energy. So at the top of the track she has potential energy. When she leaves the jump ramp, she is moving. So she has kinetic energy equal to $1/2\, mv^2$. The difference in height between the top of the track and the point on the jump ramp where she jumps from is proportional to the amount of potential energy that gets converted to kinetic energy. Let h equal the height of the platform at the top of the track minus the height of the top of the jump ramp. In other words, let h be the vertical drop from the top of the track to the top of the jump ramp. The greater h is, the more potential energy gets converted to kinetic energy, and the greater will be the skier's speed when she jumps. Specifically, neglecting friction and air resistance, $mgh = 1/2\, mv^2$, and solving we find that $v = (2gh)^{1/2}$. In the question stem, we are told that the height of the ski jump ramp is increased; so h is decreased. Since $v = (2gh)^{1/2}$, we see that a decrease in h corresponds to a decrease in v. Therefore, answer choice (B) is correct.

25. C In this question, we are told that the ski jumper leaves the jump slope at a speed of 16 meters per second, and that she remains in flight for a time of 4 seconds. Using this information, we need to find the horizontal distance traveled. Now in the horizontal direction, there are no forces acting on the ski jumper; so the horizontal distance traveled is equal to the horizontal speed times the total time in flight. We know the total time in flight, but we don't have a value for the horizontal velocity. However, we do have the total velocity, and we know the angle at which she leaves the jump slope. We can use the equation $v_h = v_t \cos \phi$, where v_h is the horizontal component of velocity, v_t is the total velocity, and ϕ is the angle measured with respect to the horizontal. Substituting in, we get that the horizontal velocity $v_h = 16 \cos 30°$, which equals $16\sqrt{3}$ divided by 2, or $8\sqrt{3}$ meters per second. Using this we can calculate the hori-

zontal distance traveled, and we get that the horizontal distance traveled equals $8\sqrt{3}$ times 4, or $32\sqrt{3}$ meters, which is answer choice (C).

26. A Statement I says that increasing the vertical height h of the jump track would increase the jump distance. This is true. If we increase the vertical height h of the jump track, we give the ski jumper a greater initial potential energy, and therefore increase the overall chanae in potential energy. This means that the ski jumper's kinetic energy at the point that she takes off is greater, and thus her takeoff speed is greater. If her takeoff speed increases, then the jump distance must also increase. Since Statement I is true, we can eliminate choice (C). Statement II says that increasing the angle of incline of the jump increases the jump distance. This is untrue. By increasing the angle of incline, we do not increase the maximum potential energy of the ski jumper, and therefore the kinetic energy at the end of the ramp. Potential energy depends only on vertical height h, and not on how steep or how shallow the incline is. Therefore, the takeoff speed is not increased, and the jump distance is not increased. Since Statement II is false we can eliminate choice (B). Statement III states that increasing the total mass of the ski jumper increases the jump distance. As we saw in the answer to the previous question, the mass term cancels, which implies that all objects are accelerated at the same rate, irrespective of their mass. In other words, a ski jumper with a mass of 60 kilograms will have the same takeoff speed as a ski jumper with a mass of 100 kilograms. Therefore, statement III is false, and choice (A) is the correct answer.

27. C The work done by gravity equals W or mgh, where W is the object's weight, m is the object's mass, g is the acceleration due to gravity, and h is the vertical distance. The work depends only on the vertical distance and is independent of the actual path taken. When the work done by a force is independent of the actual path taken, the force is said to be a conservative force. Since gravity is a conservative force and the vertical distance is the same, the work done by gravity is the same.

28. **A** The track is just an incline, so this is an incline-plane problem. Neglecting friction and air resistance, the only force parallel to the track is the component of the skier's weight parallel to the track, which is W sin θ, or mg sin θ. This must be equal to ma, where m is the skier's mass, and a is the skier's acceleration down the track. So we have mg sin θ = ma. Note that the m terms cancel, so the result does not depend on the mass, and so is the same for all skiers, In the question stem, we are told that θ = 45°. Substituting into the equation a = g sin θ, we get that a = 9.8 $\sqrt{2}/2$, or 4.9$\sqrt{2}$. At this point we must approximate, as we don't know what the square root of 2 is. We know that it's going to be less than 2 but greater than 1, which tells us that a is between 4.9 and 9.8 meters per second squared. The only answer choice that is applicable here is answer choice (A), 6.9 meters per second squared.

29. **D** The only condition that changes in this question is the surface area of the skis. The normal force of the slope on the skier depends only on the mass of the skier, the acceleration due to gravity, and the angle of the slope. Therefore, changing the surface area of the skis would not affect the normal force, and choices (A) and (B) are incorrect. Therefore, the pressure exerted on the slope by the skis must depend on the surface area of the skis. The exact relationship is P = F/A, where P is the pressure on the slope due to the skis, F is the force exerted by the skis on the slope, and A is the surface area over which the force acts, which in this case is the surface area of the skis. The force exerted by the skis is just the component of the weight of the skier normal to the slope, or the normal force, which is constant. Therefore, the pressure is inversely proportional to the surface area of the skis. So the pressure decreases as the surface area increases, and choice (D) is the correct answer.

Discrete Questions

30. **A** The correct answer choice is (A), 1.6×10^{-12} joules. This question is a straightforward application of conservation of energy. The absolute value of the change in kinetic energy equals the absolute value of the change in potential energy. Since the particle starts from rest, the change in kinetic energy is just the final kinetic energy. An α-particle is a helium-4 nucleus consisting of 2 protons and 2 neutrons. The change in potential energy is equal to the charge times the potential difference. The charge of an α-particle is equal to two times the charge of a proton, or two times e. So the final kinetic energy is equal to the potential difference of 5×10^6 volts times the alpha particle charge of $2 \times 1.6 \times 10^{-19}$ coulombs. This is 1.6×10^{-12} joules, which is answer choice (A).

31. **D** The standard potential of a reaction is a measure of the driving force behind the reaction. When the potential is positive, as it is in this case, the reaction will take place spontaneously.

To answer this question, you first have to express the balanced equation given in terms of separate oxidation and reduction equations. When you do this, the equations you get are, for oxidation:

$$2Al \rightarrow 2Al^{3+} + 6e^-$$

and for reduction:

$$2Fe^{3+} + 6e^- \rightarrow 2Fe$$

The oxidation state of the oxide ions does not change, and therefore these are not taken into account when determining the voltage. Next, we determine and add up the standard potentials for these half reactions. You can see from the table that the standard potential for the reduction of aluminum is –1.66 volts. Since in this case the aluminum is being oxidized instead of reduced, we subtract the –1.66 volts, changing its sign from minus to plus. *We do not multiply the 1.66 by 2 for the 2 moles of aluminum in the balanced equation.* Next, we determine the reduction potential for iron from the +3 valence to 0. This is given in the table as –0.037 V. Finally, we add together the

−0.037 volts from the reduction of iron with the 1.66 volts from the oxidation of aluminum. This gives us a total of 1.62 volts for the total reaction.

32. **B** We need to calculate the kinetic energy of the particle, so we'll need to use the equation $K = (1/2)mv^2$, where K is the kinetic energy, m is the mass, and v is the velocity. In the question, we are told that the mass is m, but we're given nothing for the speed. Since the speed of the particle is uniform, it is related to the distance d, and the time t by the equation $v = d/t$. Now the distance that the particle moves through in one revolution is $2\pi r$, where r is the radius of the circular path, and since the particle goes through one revolution per second, its velocity equals $2\pi r$. Now we can substitute this expression for velocity into our equation for kinetic energy, and get that $K = (1/2)m(2\pi r)^2$. This gives us $K = 2\pi^2 mr^2$, which is answer choice (B).

33. **D** The points marked by the dotted lines in each graph are the equivalence points. These are the points at which the acid has been totally neutralized by the added base. To decide which of these graphs is accurate, there are two things you need to know. First, you need to decide how much of a weak base is required to neutralize a strong acid. Second, you must know what the pH will be after the acid has been completely neutralized. First, let's consider the amount of strong acid needed to neutralize a weak base. The question tells you that both the weak base and the strong acid are 0.1 normal. Since the weak base is only partly dissociated, the actual hydroxide ion concentration of the base will be considerably lower than the hydrogen ion concentration of the strong acid. For this reason, it may seem likely that the volume of acid that you would have to add to the base to bring about neutralization would be lower than the volume of the base you started with. In choices (A) and (B), only 15 milliliters of acid are added to bring 25 milliliters of base to the equivalence point. But the problem with this line of reasoning is that as soon as the small amount of free hydroxide in the basic solution has been neutralized, more of the base will dissociate and there will be more hydroxide. As you continue to add acid, eventually all of the base will dissociate. Thus, you'll end up having to add enough acid to neutralize all of the hydroxide in the base, just as if it

were a strong base. Since the number of equivalents are equal in this case due to the equal normalities, the neutralization of 25 milliliters of weak base will require a full 25 milliliters of strong acid and that means that you can eliminate choices (A) and (B). Next, you'll have to decide what the pH of the neutralized solution will be. When the base has been completely neutralized, a solution of salt water remains. But the cation, since it comes from a weak base, has a strong tendency to recombine with hydroxide ions from the water. The anion, because it comes from a strong acid, remains completely dissociated. This means that a process of hydrolysis takes place; the cation combines with the hydroxide from water molecules, while the resulting hydrogen ions remain free in solution. Thus, a neutralized solution formed from a weak base and a strong acid will be slightly acidic. Therefore, choice (D) is correct.

34. **A** The electric field has a magnitude given by kQ over r^2, where k is the electrostatic constant, Q is the magnitude of the charge, and r is the distance between the charge and the point in question. In the question we are told that the amount of charge of each particle on the corners of the square is the same. We also know that point P is the center of the square, which means point P is equally distant from each charge. So Q and r are the same for each charge and the magnitude of the electric field at point P created by each charge is the same. In other words, we have four electric field vectors of equal magnitude. To answer the question, we need to find the resultant vector. First, we need to figure out the directions of each of these fields. Hopefully, you remember that the electric field is directed along the line connecting the charge and the point in question, and that it points away from a positive charge and towards a negative charge.

Start with the positive charge in the upper left corner of the square. Here we want a vector along the diagonal of the square pointing away from the charge, and that's vector B. For the positive charge in the upper right corner, the electric field vector points along the other diagonal, still away from the charge, and that's vector D. Now for the two negative charges, remember, their electric fields will point towards them. The electric field vector for the charge in the lower right corner is vector B, and the direction of the electric field vector due to the negative charge in the lower left corner of the square is vector D. So, if you draw a vector diagram, you have two vectors pointing along the arrow of answer choice (B) and two vectors pointing along the arrow of answer choice (D). To find the resultant electric field vector, we can use simple reasoning. It certainly can't be answer choices (B) or (D), because if we chose one we would be neglecting the vectors in the other direction. Answer choice (C) doesn't fit the bill because it's pointing upward and none of the individual vectors have an upward component. The resultant vector should be in between the vectors being added.

Passage V (Questions 35–41)

35. C The enzyme participates in the reaction, but its concentration is so high that it can be treated as a constant and not included in the rate equation, so right away, choice (D) can be eliminated. To choose from the other three choices, we need to look at the graph and see whether the rate of the reaction is proportional to the concentration of A, or the concentration of B, or both. When we look at the graph, the results appear strange. A reaction usually slows down as time goes by, but this reaction starts slowly, and then speeds up. The length of the lag period increases as A increases and B decreases. This is just the opposite of what we would expect: Most reaction rates slow down as the product accumulates. What does this mean? Well, keep in mind that we don't see the ultimate rate of the reaction; we see a temporary lag period. The length of this lag period seems to be proportional to the ratio of A to B. The higher the concentration of product, the faster the reaction gets going. This suggests that the product is somehow participating in the reaction. The more B that is present, the faster A can react. Once the reaction gets started, more B is present and the rate then speeds up. At equal concentrations of B, the sample with a higher concentration of A takes longer to get started because a lower ratio of B is available. We don't know exactly how A and B interact, but we know that changing the concentration of either A or B affects the lag period and the rate, so both must factor into the rate equation. Thus, the best answer is choice (C). The reason x and y are used as exponents is that we do not know the actual effect the two species have on the rate, only that they do affect it, so the exponents are left unknown. That is also why this is a tentative rate equation, not an actual rate equation.

36. C We know that there is such an excess of reactant C that its concentration is virtually constant. So, as the passage says, we can treat this as a pseudo first-order reaction with respect to E. However, the rate predicted this way will be slightly larger than the true rate because the true concentration of C has been reduced slightly. In the question, we start with a concentration of E equal to 0.1 moles per liter and a concentration of C equal to 50 moles per liter. When the reaction has gone 50 percent toward completion, the concentration of E will be 0.05 moles per liter and the concentration of C will be 49.95 moles per liter. So the actual rate of the reaction will be k times 0.05 times 49.95, not times 50 as the pseudo first-order would predict. The percent difference between these two rates is just the amount of the difference divided by the true rate. So we find the difference between the two rates by subtracting the actual rate, (k x 0.05 x 49.95), from the calculated rate, (k x 0.05 x 50). This gives us a difference of k times 0.05 x 0.05. Then divide this amount by the actual rate, k x 0.05 x 49.95. We can cancel out the first two factors, and we are left with 0.05 divided by 49.95, or approximately 0.001. Now multiply this by 100 percent to convert to a percent, and we're left with 0.1 percent, choice (C).

37. C In this question, we are trying to find the rate of the second step of reaction 1. The rate of this step is equal to k_2 times the concentration of B times the concentration of D, where k, is the rate constant of step 2, as described in the passage. The problem is that we can't measure the concentration of B since it is an intermediate. But, according to the passage, we can figure out the concentration of B from the equilibrium constant of step 1. The equation for the equilibrium constant of step 1 is: $K_{eq} = [B] [C]/[A]$, or rearranging for [B], $[B] = K_{eq} \times [A]/[C]$. By combining this formula with the rate constant for step 2, we find that the rate of step 2 equals the K_{eq} of step 1, times k_2, times [A] times [D], all divided by [C]. But none of the choices is expressed in terms of the equilibrium constant; instead they're in terms of k_1 and k_{-1}, so to answer this question, you need to remember that the equilibrium constant for step one is equal to k_1, the rate constant for the forward reaction in step 1, divided by k_{-1}, the rate constant for the reverse reaction.

38. B The first statement says that k_1, the rate constant for the forward reaction, divided by k_{-1}, the rate constant for the reverse reaction, is equal to one. This might at first appear to be true, since, when a reaction is at equilibrium, the rates of the forward and reverse reactions are equal. But keep in mind that the reaction constant is only part of the reaction rate. In fact, statement I equals the equilibrium constant. So k_1/k_{-1} will not equal 1 at equilibrium, unless it happens that the concentrations of the reactants and products are exactly equal at equilibrium. Not all reactions meet this condition, so statement I is no good. Statement II says that the reaction potential, E, is equal to the standard potential for the reaction. There is a condition under which this is true, but that condition isn't equilibrium. The standard potential is defined as the reaction potential under standard conditions. Equation 2 says that the reaction potential is equal to the standard potential minus a pretty ugly expression. Under standard conditions, the concentrations of all the reactants and products are equal to one, so everything cancels out. The natural log of 1 is 0, so the ugly expression drops out, leaving the reaction potential equal to the standard potential. So statement II is true under standard conditions, but not true at equilibrium—unless equilibrium happens to occur under standard conditions. So statement II is not true either. Statement III, on the other hand, is true at equilibrium. At equilibrium, the voltage is zero, since the forward and reverse reactions are taking place at equal rates. We can rearrange the equation to find that the standard potential equals that ugly expression. And if we rearrange this equation, we're left with statement III.

39. C To answer this question, you need to understand the relationship between the concentration of reactants and the spontaneity and voltage of the reaction. First let's review what is meant by voltage. When a reaction takes place in a voltaic cell, the oxidation reaction at the anode produces excess electrons. Meanwhile, reduction at the cathode uses up electrons. For the reaction to continue, the cathode needs an additional supply of electrons. As a result of the two half-reactions, there is a movement of electrons through the wire from the anode to the cathode. The faster the reaction takes place, the greater the electrical force pushing electrons away from the anode and pulling them toward the cathode will be. This pressure on the electrons is called the electromotive force, or EMF. The electromotive force is measured in volts, and so is also known as the voltage. Don't confuse the voltage with the current—the voltage is the pressure on the electrons, while the current is the actual movement of electrons through the wire. The current depends not only on the pressure exerted by the EMF, but also on the amount of resistance of the wire. The voltage or electromotive force created by a redox reaction depends on the number of electrons exchanged in the reaction and the rate at which the reaction takes place. If the rate of the reaction changes, then the voltage or potential also changes. If the concentration of reactants is increased, then the reaction will move more quickly to the right, producing more electrons at the anode and using more at the cathode. This increases the voltage. So an increase in the concentration of reactants will increase the voltage. The spontaneity of a reaction is determined by Gibb's free energy, ΔG. If ΔG is negative, the reaction is spontaneous; if ΔG is positive, the reaction is not spontaneous. There is a direct relationship between the potential of a reaction and its free energy, given by the equation: $\Delta G = -nFE$, where n is the number of moles of electrons transferred in the reaction, F is Faraday's constant, and E is the cell voltage. So what will happen to the value of ΔG if we increase the concentration of the reactants? The reaction will proceed more quickly, increasing the flow of electrons, and therefore increasing the voltage, which in turn will make the value of ΔG more negative. As the value of ΔG becomes more negative, the reaction becomes more spontaneous.

40. A In order to answer this question, you have to manipulate equation 1, which states that the cell potential, E, is equal to the standard cell potential, $E°$, minus the product of RT/nF times the natural log of the concentration of products divided by reactants. The term $([C]^c[D]^d/[A]^a[B]^b)$ is often defined as Q, the mass action expression, where the reactants and products are raised to a power equal to their stoichiometric coefficients in the balanced reaction equation. The balanced reaction equation for the cell is as follows:

$$Cu^{2+}(aq) + Zn(s) \rightarrow Zn^{2+}(aq) + Cu(s)$$

How can we tell that copper is reduced and zinc is oxidized? The first clue is the standard cell potential: +1.10V. A positive cell potential means that the reaction is spontaneous and the cell must be galvanic. In galvanic cells, oxidation occurs at the anode and reduction occurs at the cathode. The species on the left-hand side of the cell diagram, i.e., zinc, is the anode, and the species on the right-hand side, i.e., copper, is the cathode. In other words, zinc is oxidized and copper is reduced. So, plugging our values into equation 1, we get $E = +1.10 - [(8.314 \times 298)/(2 \times 96,485)]$ ln $([Zn^{2+}]/[Cu^{2+}])$. Notice that $Zn(s)$ and $Cu(s)$ are not inserted into the equation because they are pure solids with a molar concentration of 1. Also notice that $n = 2$, since 2 electrons are exchanged in the reaction. The natural log of 0.2/0.02 is equal to 2.3, so the equation can be further simplified to $E = +1.10[(8.314 \times 298)/(2 \times 96,485)] \times 2.3$. The value of E works out to be +1.07V, choice (A).

Choice (B) is the cell potential under standard conditions of 1 atmosphere pressure and 1 molar concentration for each reacting species. Since the reaction takes place under nonstandard conditions, choice (B) is incorrect. If you incorrectly identified copper as the species being oxidized and zinc as the species being reduced, you would have ended up with choice (C).

41. D Activation energy is the minimum energy needed for a reaction to occur. Catalysts are effective because they lower the activation energy of the reaction; as a result, there are more reactant molecules with sufficient kinetic energy to collide and react with each other. An increase in the number of colliding molecules will result in a faster reaction, so choice (D) is correct. Choice (C) is incorrect because a catalyst ensures that the number of collisions between reactant molecules increases. In a chemical equilibrium, the rate of the forward reaction is equal to the rate of the reverse reaction. If a catalyst is added to increase the rate of the forward reaction, the system adjusts so that the reverse rate can rise to match the forward rate. A catalyst, therefore, does not affect the value of the equilibrium constant, but does affect the speed at which the equilibrium is reached. So, choice (B) is incorrect. Finally, choice (A) is incorrect because increasing the energy of the activated complex is the same as increasing the activation energy of the reaction. An activated complex forms when reactant molecules meet. These molecules can combine to form products or fall apart into their original reactants. Obviously, if the energy barrier to form this complex is higher, the reactant molecules will have more difficulty "climbing the energy hill." Therefore, an increase in the energy of the activated complex would decrease the rate of reaction, and choice (A) is incorrect.

Passage VI (Questions 42–47)

42. C Figure out the molecular weight of the compound being dissolved, which is Na$_2$EDTA • 2H$_2$O, or the dihydrate of the disodium salt of ethylene diamine tetraacetic acid. Right there is the trick in this question—you have to realize that we're not talking about exactly the same compound as the one in the table, but another, closely related species. This species is a salt consisting of one molecule of EDTA, plus two molecules of water, plus two atoms of sodium. The two sodium atoms will replace hydrogen atoms in two of the carboxyl groups of EDTA, so you have to subtract the weight of two hydrogen atoms from the weight of the EDTA molecule. You also have to add the weight of two sodiums and of two molecules of water. If we add these all up, we get a total of 372 as the molecular weight of the EDTA salt. To make one liter of a point five molal solution of EDTA, we need half a mole of this salt, which is 186 grams, choice (C).

43. D A buffer is a mixture of either a weak base and its conjugate acid, or a weak acid and its conjugate base. Tris, as it happens, is a base. Buffer solutions resist changes in pH when acid or base is added. If pH 8 is a good buffering region for Tris, the ratio of base (Tris) to its conjugate acid (protonated Tris) will be near to 1. The pH of this solution is equal to the pK_a + log [base]/[conjugate acid]. Therefore, if the ratio of base to its conjugate acid is near to 1, the pK_a must be near to the pH. Thus Roman numeral I is a true statement. To evaluate Roman numeral II, recall what a titration curve looks like. Titration is a procedure used for determining the normality of an acid or base. The procedure consists of adding an acid to a base, or a base to an acid, until the pH of the mixture reaches 7. The titration curve is a plot showing the pH of the solution as a function of the amount of acid or base added. Since the pH, as the dependent variable, is plotted on the y-axis, a steep part of a titration curve represents a rapid change in pH. But we just said that a buffer solution in its effective pH range, such as a pH 8 Tris solution, resists pH change, so the titration curve for Tris will actually be quite flat near pH 8, and so Roman numeral II is false. Adding sodium hydroxide, which is a base, to a pH 8 0 Tris solution also wouldn't change the pH

easily, so a large amount of the base would have to be added to affect the pH very much, and Roman numeral III is true. Since I and III are true, the correct choice is (D).

44. D To answer this, you have to know the definitions of two measures of solution concentration: percentage by mass and molality. The percentage by mass of a solution is the mass of the solute divided by the total mass of the solution, multiplied by 100. Thus, a 10% SDS solution has 10% of its mass in the form of sodium dodecyl sulfate and 90% of its mass in the form of water. The molality of a solution is the number of moles of solute per kilogram of solvent. Let's assume that this solution contains 1 kilogram of water. Remember that the water makes up only 90% of the total weight of the solution. We can find the total weight of the solution by using the formula 1,000 equals 0.9x. This tells us that the total weight of the solution is 1,111 grams, so the weight of the SDS must be 111 grams. Now we need to know how many moles of SDS there are in the 111 grams. The number of moles is equal to the mass of the SDS over its molecular weight: this comes to 0.385 moles. Since there are 0.385 moles of SDS for every thousand grams of water, the solution is 0.385 molal.

45. C The easiest way to do it is to figure out how much ethanol is in the solution at the end of the dilution, and work backward from that. Notice that the meaning of the percentage sign in this question and in the preceding question is different; there, it was percentage by mass, whereas in this question it's percentage by volume. Also, you're told in the passage that a 70% ethanol solution contains 70% ethanol and 30% water by volume. In practice, this is how researchers do usually measure solutions, just for convenience—it's easiest to measure liquids by their volume and measure solids by their mass. Five-hundred milliliters of a 70% ethanol solution will contain 350 milliliters of ethanol and 150 milliliters of water. So we need an amount of 95% ethanol that contains 350 milliliters of ethanol. If we call this amount X, then 0.95X equals 350 milliliters. So we want a choice that's just a little more than 350, and the only one that fits is C. If we solve the equation, we find that X equals 368 milliliters, choice (C).

46. B In the last step of the plasmid prep procedure, ethanol is added to the mixture, which is an aqueous solution, or a solution whose solvent is water. Then the test tube is incubated at low temperature for an hour, and finally the solution is centrifuged and a DNA precipitate forms. This happens because DNA, or deoxyribonucleic acid, is a highly polar substance, and is therefore more soluble in an aqueous solution than in a solvent composed mostly of ethanol. Thus choice (B) is correct. Remember the rule that like dissolves like; thus a highly polar substance will dissolve better in a more polar solvent—water—than in a less polar solvent—ethanol. Choice (C) is wrong because there's no evidence in the passage that DNA dissolves better in ethanol than in water; in fact, there's evidence against this conclusion, since the DNA is fully dissolved in the water solution but precipitates out of the water-ethanol solution. Choice (D) is wrong because centrifugation can't make a substance precipitate out of a solution; it can only make a precipitate that is suspended in the solution settle to the bottom. Finally, choice (A) is wrong because there's no evidence that DNA dissolves better at lower temperatures; on the contrary, the incubation at −20°C degrees apparently contributes to its precipitation.

47. B In an aqueous solution, sodium acetate is in equilibrium with its corresponding acid:

$$CH_3\,COOH + H_2O \qquad CH_3\,COO^- + H_3O^+$$

In this equilibrium, acetic acid acts as a weak acid and acetate acts as a conjugate base; this constitutes a buffer system. Buffer systems resist large changes in pH upon the addition of small amounts of acid or base. For example, when a base is added to the acetic acid/acetate buffer, the hydroxide ions are consumed by acetic acid to form acetate and water, so the pH doesn't rise too drastically. When an acid is added to the buffer, the hydrogen ions are consumed by acetate to form the undissociated acid, so the pH doesn't drop too drastically. In order to work out the change in pH, first calculate the initial concentrations of acetic acid and sodium acetate. We already know from Table I that the concentration of sodium acetate is $3M$. Plugging this into the Henderson-Hasselbalch equation, we can work out the concentration of

acetic acid. The Henderson-Hasselbalch equation is as follows: $pH = pK_a + \log [A^-]/[HA]$, where $[A^-]$ is the concentration of the conjugate base, and $[HA]$ is the concentration of the acid. Plugging our values into this equation, we get $5.2 = 4.74 + \log [3]/[HA]$. The concentration of acetic acid, therefore, works out to be $1M$. In a 100 mL solution, the number of moles of sodium acetate and acetic acid works out to be 0.3 and 0.1 moles, respectively.

What is the pH of the solution after 3.6 g of hydrochloric acid is added? The molar mass of hydrochloric acid is 36.5 g/mol, so the number of moles is 3.6/36.5 or 0.1. Remember, when an acid is added to the buffer, the hydrogen ions are consumed by acetate to form undissociated acetic acid. Therefore, if there are 0.3 moles of sodium acetate in the original solution, there will be 0.3–0.1 moles after the addition of hydrochloric acid. Similarly, if there are 0.1 moles of acetic acid in the original solution, there will be 0.1 + 0.1 moles after the addition of HCl. Therefore, the new concentration of acetic acid and acetate is $2\,M$. Plugging these new values into the Henderson-Hasselbach equation, we get $pH = 4.74 + \log [2]/[2]$. Since the log of 1 is 0, the pH is equal to the pK_a, 4.74. Choice (B) is, therefore, the correct response. Choices (C) and (D) can be discarded because we are adding an acid to the buffer system. The only way we can increase the pH of the stock solution is by the addition of base, since the equilibrium we talked about would then shift to the right to form acetate. Since a buffer resists drastic changes in pH, choice (A) is wrong.

Passage VII (Questions 48–53)

48. C The correct answer is choice (C), $k(L - L_0)/g$. When the mass is in equilibrium, the sum of the forces acting on it is equal to zero. There are two such forces in this case, which must therefore be equal in magnitude but opposite in direction. There is the downward pull of gravity on the mass, which is the weight of the mass, mg. Opposing this is the upward force exerted on the mass by the spring. This spring force is given by Hooke's law and is equal to the spring constant, k, times the amount the spring is stretched from its natural length by the hanging mass. If the mass were not present, the spring would be its natural length, L_0. When the mass is attached, it stretches to a length L. The difference between these two lengths, $L - L_0$, is the amount by which the spring is stretched when the hanging mass is in equilibrium. The corresponding spring force is then k times the quantity $L - L_0$. As we said before, when the hanging mass is in equilibrium the force of the spring equals the force of gravity. This implies that $k(L - L_0) = mg$. Solving for m we find that $m = k(L - L_0)/g$, which is answer choice (C).

49. B This question concerns energy conservation. If no energy were dissipated, the spring would oscillate forever. The total energy at any time is $1/2\,kx^2 + 1/2\,mv^2$, where x is the displacement of the mass from its equilibrium position and v is its speed. When the motion begins, the displacement is equal to A and the speed v is equal to zero. Therefore initially the total energy is equal $kA^2/2$. When all of this energy is dissipated, x and v will have to be zero and the mass will no longer oscillate.

50. A First, note that the motion of the spring-mass system is simple harmonic motion. When simple harmonic motion occurs, the speed is a maximum at the equilibrium position, so choice (A) is the correct answer. For a horizontal spring-mass system the equilibrium position of the mass corresponds to the spring being neither stretched nor compressed. But as the passage explains, with a vertical spring-mass system the situation is different. When the mass is in equilibrium, the spring is stretched—and that makes choice (B) incorrect. As for choices (C) and (D)—they represent the extreme positions in the motion of the mass. The mass is moving with simple harmonic motion, so in these positions the displacement from the equilibrium position is a maximum and the speed is zero. If you picked choice (C), the lowest point, you might have been thinking of something being dropped from a height h, but that is not what is happening here.

51. D Here you need to know the formula that relates period, T, to the spring constant k. It is $T = 2\pi\sqrt{m/k}$, where m is the mass. You should also know that the frequency, f, is one over the period. Therefore, the frequency of a spring-mass system is given by the $(1/2\pi)\sqrt{k/m}$. Squaring both sides and solving for the spring constant k, we find that k equals 4π squared times the frequency squared times the mass. We know the frequency is 2 Hertz and the mass is 5 kg. Working out the numbers gives us $80\pi r^2$ N/m.

52. D Keep in mind that all the springs, the two actual springs and the proposed single spring, are stretched by the same amount, x_e. For the system of two springs in the equilibrium position, the downward force due to gravity or the weight equals the sum of the two upward spring forces, or $W = F_1 + F_2$. For the proposed single spring in the equilibrium position, the weight equals the upward spring force, or $W = F'$. Since the mass stays the same, the weight W is the same in each case, so $F' = F_1 + F_2$. Applying Hooke's law to the single spring, we find $F' = k'x_e$. For the system of two identical springs, $F_1 = F_2 = kx_e$. Substituting into $F' = F_1 + F_2$, we find that $k'x_e = kx_e + kx_e$. Canceling the x_e's gives us that $k' = k + k = 2k$. Therefore the ratio of k' to k equals 2, which is answer choice (D).

VERBAL REASONING: Answers and Explanations

ANSWER KEY

53. A	68. B	83. D
54. B	69. B	84. C
55. C	70. A	85. A
56. D	71. C	86. A
57. C	72. A	87. D
58. C	73. D	88. C
59. D	74. C	89. D
60. D	75. D	90. D
61. C	76. D	91. B
62. B	77. C	92. A
63. B	78. A	
64. D	79. D	
65. C	80. B	
66. A	81. B	
67. C	82. A	

EXPLANATIONS

Passage I (Questions 53–59)

The first passage is a relatively straightforward, clearly structured historical passage about communal experiments in 19th century America. With little introduction, the author gets straight into detailed material, using each paragraph to describe a different commune in terms of its constitutional principles, economic system and historical track record. The first paragraph concerns the Brook Farm community, which the author tells us was founded for theoretical reasons by famous thinkers of the age. Paragraph two discusses the Oneida community, outlining the community's faith in the Second Coming, and how their belief in communal ownership extended to multiple marriage. In paragraph three the author describes the Shakers, another religious commune founded upon the four principles of Purity, Communism, Confession, and Separation.

53. A The last half of the first paragraph suggests that Brook Farm failed because the Farm's members, although interested in the theoretical aspects of their community, were not committed to maintaining the Farm in the face of hardship, choice (A). The first paragraph does suggest that Brook Farm was successful in meeting its aims, but it does not imply that such success led to the end of the experiment, as choice (C) suggests. You probably know that Margaret Fuller and Nathaniel Hawthorne were major American intellectuals of the 19th century; even if you don't, you are told that these two are among the Farm's more notable members. Thus, you can infer that Brook Farm was indeed able to attract members of sufficient intellect or ability, so (B) is wrong. Although the author notes that Brook Farm's members were thinkers, not workers, the fact that the members had more leisure than expected and outcompeted local farmers suggests that the Farm's philosopher-members were competent field hands; so (D) is incorrect.

54. B The Oneidans are discussed in paragraph 2. In the middle of that paragraph we learn that they felt monogamy was a selfish act, which implies (B). We're told that the Shakers held that men and women were equal, but the passage tells us nothing about what the Oneidans felt on that subject, so (A) is incorrect. John Humphrey Noyes, the founder of the Oneidans, believed Christ's second coming had already occurred, not that they were going to witness it, as choice (D) suggests. The Oneidans apparently did have certain rules and standards; otherwise they would not have needed to apply criticism to those who acted out of line, so (C) is wrong.

55. C   Brook Farm is discussed in the first paragraph of the passage. Brook Farm's system aimed to properly (hence efficiently) utilize time and labor, and we are told the system worked very well—choice (C). One measure of this success was their sales at the produce market, so (A) is wrong. The description of Brook Farm in the third sentence of paragraph one implies that the commune members did all the work; there is no mention of hired labor, suggested by choice (B). As for choice (D), if the Farmers had intended to maximize financial profit, whether individual or collective, their emphasis on properly utilizing time so as to pursue culture and leisure would not make sense. Their "free time" would have been put to generating greater profits.

56. D   In the middle of paragraph two, the author states that the Oneidans believed that all the men and women of the community were united in one complex marriage, choice (A). Order was maintained through criticism, a sort of social pressure, choice (B). You can infer that present grace, choice (C), refers to the Oneida founder's belief that the second coming of Christ had already occurred. But communal living, choice (D), is mentioned in relation to the Shakers, not the Oneidans. So (D) is correct.

57. C   The middle of the third paragraph states that the Shakers renounced personal property, while the second paragraph mentions that the Oneidans owned everything communally. These two statements reflect the same principle of community property. From this, we can infer that the two groups shared a similar view of personal property, choice (C). As for choice (A), the Shakers practiced celibacy while the Oneidans accepted sex between any two consenting adults. And, as discussed in question two, the Shakers believed in equality of men and women, but we are not told about the Oneidans' views on that matter, so there is no basis for choosing choice (B). As for choice (D), the Shakers rejected contact with the world in principle, though not in practice, while there is no indication that the Oneidans had any objection to such contact, so (D) is wrong.

58. C   Considering that the three communes discussed in the passage had varying degrees of contact with the outside world, and the author never mentions the amount of outside contact as a factor contributing to either the success or the failure of these communes, we cannot infer that diminished contact with the outside world (I) would weaken a secular workers' coop. Therefore, statement I will not be a part of the correct answer, eliminating choices (A) and (D). Because religious faith is not one of the bases of cohesion in a secular cooperative, it is unlikely that diminishing religious faith—increasing agnosticism (statement II)—would weaken the cooperative's cohesion, eliminating choice (B). The only remaining choice is (C), III only. Given that Brook Farm, a secular co-op, was drastically weakened by financial burdens (described in paragraph one), it is reasonable to infer that economic losses would weaken the secular workers' co-op described in this question stem.

59. D   This question asks about the next topic the author hypothetically might discuss. Consider the overall focus of the passage. This passage is primarily descriptive. Because of this descriptive tone and focus on the varying degrees of success achieved by several 19th century experiments in communal living, it would be logical to think the next topic the author might pursue would be a consideration of why these three communes were successful to varying degrees, choice (D). It is unlikely that the author would next compare 19th and 20th century communes, choice (A), since he had not previously made any mention of 20th century communes or suggestion of a comparison. A theory explaining why communal living might become popular again, choice (B). is an unlikely next topic because the passage is descriptive of the past, not predictive, in its focus. Although the first paragraph states that Brook Farm's members were artists and philosophers, this is just a detail of the passage; it is unlikely that the passage would later discuss the reasons such communes attracted artists and intellectuals, so (C) is wrong.

Passage II (Questions 60–66)

The passage starts by listing some of the reasons for research into synthetic blood—fear of disease and a shortage in matching donor blood. The passage continues to discuss the criteria for good blood-substitutes. It proceeds to discuss various synthetic blood technologies, pointing out their advantages and disadvantages. The second paragraph concerns "red blood"; the third is about "white blood"; and the fourth paragraph discusses genetically engineered hemoglobin. While accepting that each of these technologies has its drawbacks, the passage ends by reassuring us that scientists are continuing their efforts to perfect an ideal blood substitute. This clear and logical division of this passage's paragraphs is fortunate for the reader and helpful for the test taker trying to relocate details.

60. D Question 60 is a detail question that requires you to identify the answer choice which is not a weakness of synthetic bloods. Choices (A) and (B) mention that naked hemoglobin can cause renal failure in humans and that red blood can transmit viruses to a recipient. These facts are expressed in the second paragraph, which addresses red blood and the problems associated with it. The second half of that paragraph states that naked hemoglobin, the basis of red blood, can constitute a twofold threat to the human body as it can transmit viruses and is extremely dangerous to the kidneys, causing blood flow at these organs to shut down and results in renal failure. Choice (C) mentions that genetic engineering can be extremely difficult. Paragraph four is all about modified hemoglobin derived from genetically altered bacteria. Its last sentence emphasizes the challenges associated with the isolation and modification of the human hemoglobin gene. Although, in theory, genetic engineering can produce near-ideal synthetic blood, you can infer that a drawback of this process is the complexity of these procedures. So choice (C) is also a weakness, and therefore does not complete this question stem. Choice (D) mentions that white blood has a low oxygen-carrying potential. Were this true, it certainly would be a weakness, as one of the chief criteria of synthetic blood is that it mimic blood in

its high oxygen-carrying capacity. The third paragraph, regarding white blood, notes that PFCs, a primary component of white blood, have high oxygen-carrying capacities. The second and third sentences of this paragraph state that PFCs are capable of absorbing quantities of oxygen up to 50 percent of their volume and imitate real blood by effectively absorbing oxygen. From this we can infer that white blood is capable of transporting oxygen well. This contradicts choice (D). Since the passage never suggests that white blood has a low oxygen-carrying potential, choice (D) does not represent a weakness of synthetic blood and is the correct answer to question 60.

61. C In the third paragraph, where white blood and PFCs are discussed, the passage states that PFCs imitate real blood by effectively absorbing oxygen. It is true that PFCs mimic the oxygen-carrying capacity of blood, and option I will be part of the correct answer. The third and fourth sentences of the third paragraph establish that PFCs are inherently safer to use in synthetic bloods than hemoglobin is because PFCs do not interact with any chemicals in the body. Option II, therefore, also correctly completes the question stem. Finally, option III is a false statement. Nowhere does the passage suggest that PFCs breakdown in the blood within several hours. Rather, breakdown is mentioned as a problem associated with naked hemoglobin. Since option III is false, it cannot successfully complete the question stem. Only options I and II fit the question stem, so the correct answer is choice (C), I and II only.

62. B Choice (A) suggests that patients fear the transmission of dangerous diseases such as AIDS, via blood transfusions. This fear is mentioned in the opening sentence of the passage as one of the primary reasons for the desire to develop clean, sterile blood substitutes. Choice (A), therefore, is a reason for the development of synthetic bloods, and does not answer this question stem correctly. Choices (C) and (D) mention different aspects of the problem of procuring matching blood donors for patients, also described in the opening sentence as one of the reasons for the development of synthetic bloods. (C) and (D), then, do not correctly complete the question stem either. Choice (B) suggests that synthetic bloods have greater oxygen-carrying capacities than naturally produced human blood. This is not supported anywhere in the passage. The passage emphasizes that synthetic bloods should have high oxygen-carrying capacities, but there is no suggestion that synthetic bloods have higher oxygen-carrying capacities than blood.

63. B Choice (A) states that all of the synthetic bloods discussed in the passage sustain submerged oxygen-dependent organisms. The second sentence of the third paragraph notes that PFCs possess this ability, but there is no suggestion of this in reference to any of the other blood substitutes. Choice (C) is incorrect because, even though all synthetic bloods should have high levels of sterility, the passage explicitly states that the naked hemoglobin molecules of red blood are "rarely sterile and often remain contaminated by viruses to which they were exposed in the cell." Not all blood substitutes, then, maintain high standards of sterility. Finally, choice (D) is wrong in stating that all synthetic bloods exhibit versatility in the body. The passage makes clear that not all blood substitutes are particularly versatile. For one thing, the naked hemoglobin of red blood breaks down in the blood stream within several hours. Furthermore, PFCs tend to form globules, blocking blood circulation. Only choice (B) is mentioned in reference to all synthetic blood technologies. The second sentence of the second paragraph states that hemoglobin, the chief component of red blood, is "attractive to scientists . . . because of its oxygen-carrying capacity." The second sentence of the third paragraph implies that PFCs have high oxygen-carrying capacities as it mentions that PFCs can absorb oxygen up to quantities 50 percent its volume. The author goes on to note, in the following sentence, that PFCs imitate real blood by effectively absorbing oxygen. Finally, the passage explicitly states in the second sentence of the fourth paragraph that the synthetic hemoglobin produced by genetically altered bacteria "closely mimic(s) . . . (the) oxygen-carrying efficiency of blood."

64. D Since red blood is discussed in the second paragraph of the passage, refer there for details. Choice (A) is incorrect because the passage never says that "red blood cannot be produced in large quantities." In fact, the passage never at all mentions the extent to which red blood can be produced. The passage only mentions quantities of production of synthetic blood in the third sentence of the fourth paragraph, where it states, in reference to genetically altered hemoglobin, that "the bacteria will produce the desired product in copious quantities." Since the passage never mentions choice (A), it cannot be a problem specific to "red blood." Similarly, choice (B) distorts a detail of the passage which relates to another type of synthetic blood. The passage mentions in the fourth sentence of the third paragraph that the primary pitfall of PFCs is their tendency to form globules. The passage never says that red blood forms globules. Choice (C) also is not a true statement. The second sentence of the second paragraph states that hemoglobin is the blood's natural oxygen carrier and, in fact, is attractive to scientists precisely because of its oxygen-carrying capacity. You may safely conclude from this information, then, that hemoglobin does, indeed, carry oxygen effectively and (C) is not a problem at all. Only choice (D), which states that "red blood exhibits poor durability in the bloodstream," is mentioned in the passage as a problem specific to red blood. The passage states that "additional problems arise from the fact that hemoglobin is adapted to operate optimally within the . . . cell. Stripped of the protection of the cell, the hemoglobin molecule tends to suffer breakdown within several hours." One of the criteria for a successful blood substitute is that it be durable and versatile. The fact that red blood breaks down readily in the bloodstream shows that red blood is not durable in the bloodstream.

65. C   This application question requires you to apply information from the passage to solve a problem. The passage mentions that PFCs are capable of absorbing quantities of oxygen up to 50 percent of their volume. Applying this information, then, a 300 cc sample of PFC can absorb up to 150 cc, 50 percent of 300 cc. The correct answer, then, is choice (C), 150 cc, logically eliminating any of the other possibilities.

66. A   Which of the answer choices is not a factor that detracts from the production of an ideal blood substitute? Choices (C) and (D) present troublesome aspects of PFCs. The end of the second paragraph establishes that one of the drawbacks of PFCs is that they form globules, blocking blood circulation, choice (D). In order to bypass this problem, scientists have attempted to modify PFCs so that they do not form globules. These efforts have been thwarted, however, as such modified PFCs have curtailed oxygen-carrying capacities, choice (C). Choice (B) relates to problems with red blood. The third sentence of the second paragraph tells us that one of the problems of red blood is that its naked hemoglobin breaks down rapidly in the bloodstream. Choice (B), then, is a factor that has compounded the difficulty of producing an ideal blood substitute. Choice (A) presents a statement that, if supported by the passage, might very well compound the difficulties of producing an ideal synthetic blood. If there were no known way to isolate the DNA responsible for hemoglobin, then genetic engineering of modified hemoglobin would be hampered. But the passage never states that there is no known way to isolate the DNA responsible for hemoglobin. It does mention, in the last sentence of the fourth paragraph that genetic engineering is challenging because it requires the isolation of the human gene for the production of hemoglobin. But the passage does not say that there is no known way to do this. Choice (A) therefore, is not suggested as a complication in the production of synthetic blood and is the correct answer.

Passage III (Questions 67–73)

This short passage concerns the Russian wheat aphid, an insect that devours wheat. The first paragraph describes the Russian aphid's physical appearance, its adaptation to wheat ten thousand years ago, and its destructive spread throughout the wheat fields of Asia, Africa, and Latin America. The second paragraph concerns the pest's spread to the United States. Here we learn that the United States had been free of this insect until 1986 when a swarm of Russian aphids invaded Texas, spreading rapidly from there to other states. The third paragraph explains why it has so far been impossible to prevent or control the spread of the aphid in the United States. The fourth paragraph continues to consider the problem of controlling the aphid, this time by considering it in its place of origin—Russia. Finally, the fifth paragraph states that introducing the aphid's natural enemies into the United States, coupled with the breeding of new insect-resistant strains of wheat, may curb the aphid's destructiveness in the future. But this hopeful paragraph ends on a rather sour note—offering American farmers little hope by saying that for the time being American farmers will have to cope with this pest as best they can.

67. C One way to successfully approach this kind of question is to go through the options, considering the appropriateness of each and keeping an eye out for the one that really sounds consistent with the focus of the passage. Choice (A) indicates that it is no longer economical to grow crops with low profit margins. But the passage neither states nor suggests this. The only point in the passage regarding the economics of farming, made in the fifth sentence of the third paragraph, states that American farmers do not spray their wheat crops with pesticides because it is not economically logical to spray such low-profit margin crops with expensive pesticides. In other words, it is not economical to spray these crops—but that doesn't mean it is not economical to grow them at all. Further, this passage concerns just one type of crop—wheat crops. One cannot generalize this passage to make a statement regarding all low-profit-margin crops, so there's no basis for supporting choice (A). The sentiment expressed in

choice (B), that of human powerlessness in the face of nature, seems to be contradicted by the passage. The fourth and fifth paragraphs state that agricultural researchers are examining methods for controlling the Russian aphid in the United States, particularly by importing its natural enemies to the United States and breeding insect-resistant strains of wheat, and that these methods may curb the aphid's future destructiveness. In other words, the passage suggests that it probably is possible for humans to exercise some control over nature, so choice (B) is wrong. Choice (C) appears to accurately reflect one of the passage's principal ideas. The passage, particularly the first three paragraphs, strongly suggests that the Russian aphid has caused a great deal of destruction in areas outside of the Soviet Union because these areas had no natural defenses against this insect. Thus, a general statement to the effect that regional ecosystems are often severely damaged when new organisms are introduced into them, choice (C), accurately reflects a major idea conveyed in this passage and is the correct answer. Finally, the passage does indeed suggest, in the first two sentences of the third paragraph, that the aphid's rapid asexual reproduction is one reason for the difficulty in controlling this pest, but it would be wrong to read into this one detail of the passage that it is always more difficult to control asexual insects, so choice (D) is wrong. Notice that all of the incorrect choices in this question are strongly worded generalizations—sweeping conclusions that go way beyond the scope of this passage.

68. B The fourth sentence of the third paragraph tells us that most Russian aphids are born without wings (only a few generations have them), so most can't fly, making option I a false statement. Option II suggests that aphids are resistant to pesticides. We have no basis for concluding that this is true because the passage doesn't provide any information about whether or not Russian aphids are resistant to pesticides. In fact, the only piece of information the passage provides about pesticides is the fact, stated in the middle of the third paragraph, that American farmers haven't used pesticides against the Russian aphid for economic reasons.

So far, then, neither options I nor II are true statements. The third sentence of the second paragraph asserts that once Russian aphids invaded the United States, they spread rapidly to different areas. Option III, therefore, is a true statement. They are capable of spreading rapidly. Thus, option III is true, but options I and II are not, making choice (B), III only, the correct answer.

69. B   In order to answer a question about authorship, it is necessary to consider the passage as a whole, particularly its content and level of complexity. Two major themes are reflected in this passage: (1) Russian aphids have spread far and wide, causing serious damage to wheat fields in America and other countries, and (2) methods for controlling the aphid's destructiveness are currently being investigated by agricultural researchers. Given that the focus is on an agricultural crop being plagued by a destructive pest, an agriculturist with an interest in pest control, choice (B), is most likely to have written this passage. A botanist with an interest in wheat production, choice (A), is not likely to have written this passage because, although the passage deals with wheat and briefly mentions the possibility of producing insect-resistant strains of wheat (in the last paragraph), the passage certainly doesn't focus on the botany of wheat production. As for choice (C), if a pest exterminator with an interest in agriculture had written this passage we would expect a much more technical and detailed discussion about the ridding of this pest and the use of pesticides (and perhaps other chemicals) as possible means of controlling the aphid. And, this passage is unlikely to have been written by an entomologist with an interest in asexual reproduction, choice (D). Although an entomologist, or someone who studies insects, may be a likely author, the aphid's method of reproduction is a minor issue in this passage, confined to a couple of sentences in the first half of the third paragraph.

70. A   In the last sentence of the second paragraph, it is discussed that the Hessian fly was a major menace to American agriculture at the time of the Revolutionary War, but nowhere in the passage is it stated what, if anything, was done to combat this menace, so choice (A) is not answered in the passage and is the correct answer to this question. The second sentence of the fourth paragraph indicates that the Russian wheat aphid has done less damage in the Soviet Union than in other areas because natural predators which have evolved with it over the centuries have kept it in check, so choice (B) is addressed and is incorrect. In the fifth sentence of the third paragraph, we are told that it is not economical for American farmers to spray pesticides on their wheat in an attempt to protect their crops from the Russian aphid, so choice (C), too, is answered in the passage and is an incorrect choice. And, finally, the fourth and fifth paragraphs discuss possible means for controlling the aphid, particularly the introduction of the aphid's natural enemies, such as the female wasp, into new ecosystems and the breeding of insect-resistant strains of wheat, so choice (D), like (B) and (C), is answered and is wrong.

71. C   The last two paragraphs of the passage concern control of the aphid population. In the first sentence of the fifth paragraph, the author suggests that the introduction of the aphid's natural predators into the United States holds the possibility of controlling the aphid population in the future. In other words, the author thinks that transplanting the Russian aphid's natural enemies from the Soviet Union, choice (C), is a logical way of controlling the aphid population in the United States, so (C) is the correct answer to this question. Nowhere in the passage does the author state or suggest that reducing the acreage devoted to the production of wheat, choice (A), would control the aphid population in the United States, so A is wrong. Although some people might logically conclude that growing less wheat would lessen the aphid population in the long run, the author doesn't suggest this as a logical method of aphid control. The question stem asks for a suggestion of the author. As for spraying large quantities of pesticides on wheat fields, choice (B), the author indicates in the fifth sentence of the third paragraph that, for economic reasons, this is not a reasonable method of aphid control, so choice (B) is wrong. Finally, the author doesn't suggest that sterilizing female aphids is a logical way of controlling the aphid population in the United States, making choice (D) incorrect. In fact, in the first half of the third paragraph, the author makes a point of noting that aphids reproduce asexually at a phenomenal rate, so sterilizing females is not logical at all and certainly is not suggested by the author.

72. A   In the last sentence of the second paragraph, we are told that entomologists consider the Russian aphid so destructive that they have called it the greatest threat to American agriculture since the Hessian fly was brought over by German mercenaries during the Revolutionary War. Based on this, it is certainly reasonable to conclude that Russian aphids and Hessian flies are comparable with respect to the amount of damage they have caused to crops. Option I, therefore, does complete this question stem correctly, and will be part of the answer. The second sentence of the third paragraph states that Russian aphids reproduce asexually, but nowhere are we told by what means the Hessian fly reproduces, so we have no basis for concluding that Russian aphids and Hessian flies are comparable with respect to the means by which they reproduce, option II. The second sentence of the second paragraph states that a swarm of Russian aphids flew across the United States–Mexican border; i.e., they entered the United States on their own, with humans having nothing to do with their entry into this country. In contrast, the final sentence of the second paragraph clearly states that the Hessian fly was brought to the United States by humans, German mercenary troops, in boats. So, their methods of entry into the United States aren't comparable, making option III incorrect. Thus, since option I is a valid ending to the question, but options II and III are not valid, the correct answer is choice (A), I only.

73. D   The first sentence of the fifth paragraph asserts that new insect-resistant strains of wheat may be developed in the future and that these new strains may curb the destructiveness of the Russian aphid. But, the author neither states nor suggests that American farmers will be the individuals responsible for the development of these new strains of wheat, so choice (A) is wrong. Regarding choice (B), the last sentence of the fifth paragraph asserts that, until effective measures for controlling the Russian aphid are developed, American farmers are on their own when it comes to protecting their wheat crops. The tone of this sentence suggests that the author believes it is unlikely that American farmers can develop their own effective means of coping with this pest, the opposite of what is suggested by choice (B), so (B) is also wrong. The last sentence of the passage also suggests that the author believes American farmers will continue to produce wheat in the future, so choice (C) is wrong. Finally, the tone and content of the last paragraph—where the author states that American farmers will have to cope with the Russian aphid the best they can until methods are found for controlling its destructiveness—suggests that the author believes American farmers will lose a part of their wheat crops to the aphid for the foreseeable future, making choice (D) the answer.

Passage IV (Questions 74–79)

This next passage is about the physiological and emotional aspects of our sense of smell. The author mentions that while it's clear that smell is tied to such important physiological functions as metabolism and appetite, it's also related to memory and emotion in ways that aren't fully understood. In the first paragraph of the passage, smell, or olfaction, is called "vital yet mysterious," and throughout the passage the reader is given evidence of how smell is central to humans and other animals. But the passage also emphasizes that there are aspects and functions of this sense that are still unclear. One of these unknowns is how, and why, smell can evoke strong memories and emotions. The second paragraph says that smell differs from our other senses in that it reaches the brain almost directly. Then, the third paragraph mentions that scientists speculate that the reason smells evoke such personal reactions is that the olfactory and emotional centers are both rooted in the part of the brain called the limbic lobe. The fourth paragraph goes on to give three pieces of evidence that suggest that smell must have an important function. Next, in the fifth paragraph the author discusses olfaction in other animal species, and mentions the role of pheromones, which are chemical messages that influence important things like social order, communication, and reproduction in animals. Finally, the passage concludes in the sixth paragraph by saying that physicians used to use smell to detect illness, a practice that is no longer common. Then the author reiterates the fact that although smell doesn't always play an obvious role in our lives, it's clearly important in guiding us through life.

74. C   Choice (A) suggests that the location of the olfactory and emotional centers of the brain can not explain why smells can evoke distant memories. That is not the case at all—the third and fourth sentences of the third paragraph say that scientists surmise that the reason smells often evoke memories is because emotion, memory, and olfaction are all rooted in the brain's limbic lobe. Choice (B) mentions the fact that odors elicit different reactions from person to person. This is also explained by the location of the olfactory and emotional centers, and this point is detailed in the second and third sentences of paragraph three. Choice (C) questions whether the fact that a substantial part of the brain is devoted to smell can be explained by the location of olfaction and emotion. The second sentence of the fourth paragraph mentions that a large amount of brain tissue is in fact devoted to smell. But the author does not relate this to the location of the sense of smell and emotion. The author doesn't suggest that we can explain the large amount of brain tissue by its location, so (C) seems correct. Choice (D) says that the location of the olfactory and emotional centers of the brain helps explain which functions are rooted in the limbic lobe. The last sentence of the third paragraph says that the emotions and smell are indeed rooted in the limbic lobe, so (D) is true.

75. D   The fact that doctors used to use their noses to sniff out disease is discussed in the last paragraph of the passage. In the very last sentence of this paragraph, the author says that medical science has moved away from such subjective diagnostic methods. From this point, it can be inferred that contemporary medical science considers such diagnostic procedures too subjective, and prefer more objective methods, such as laboratory analyses. This is reflected in choice (D)—the medical profession today favors more objective techniques. As for the wrong answers, choice (A) says that physicians no longer make diagnoses based on odors because the human sense of smell has considerably diminished over time. There's nothing stated or implied in the passage about the sense of smell changing at all, and this answer choice is inapplicable. Choice (B) suggests that physicians no longer favor diagnoses based on odors because the association of odors with disease proved largely fictitious. This is not implied in the passage either. The author's tone in the last paragraph, where this issue is discussed, is not at all disparaging of these old subjective techniques. So (B) is wrong. Choice (C) says that such subjective diagnostic methods were shown to be useless. Again, the author never says anything disparaging about these subjective techniques. C then, is also wrong, and choice (D) is the answer.

76. D You're asked to identify how the sense of smell in animals is different from olfaction in humans. The author discusses olfaction in animals in the fifth paragraph, which begins with the statement that "the significance of olfaction is much clearer in animals than in human beings." Then, the author discusses the ways in which odors affect animals and bring about behavioral changes. Considering this information, the way smell in animals differs from that in humans is best expressed by answer choice (D)—animals more clearly exhibit behavioral changes in response to odors. Choice (A) says that animals are unable to make associations between smells and past experience. There is no instance in the passage that outright states or implies that. In actuality, the passage suggests that animals, with their clearly important sense of smell, probably are able to remember smells and what they signal or signify. So choice (A) is incorrect. Choice (B) states that animals only use smell to communicate outside their own species. This contradicts information in the second sentence of the fifth paragraph, which says that animals often rely on pheromones to communicate within their own species. Choice (C) suggests that animals rely on olfaction only for mating purposes. This is incorrect, as the fifth paragraph details the many functions of olfaction in animals—attracting mates is only one important aspect of smell in other animals species.

77. C Smell is described as being an elusive sense in the first sentence of the first paragraph. Although the author does not explicitly state why smell is an elusive sense, the author implies that smell is a mysterious process whose effects, means of functioning, and process of registering in the brain are not fully known. Considering this, then, choice (C) is the correct answer. One can infer that the author describes the sense of smell as elusive because "the function and effects of smell are not fully understood." Choice (A) suggests that the author deems smell elusive because odiferous molecules are extremely volatile. It is true that odiferous molecules are volatile, as this is stated in the third sentence of the second paragraph. The author, however, strongly implies that the mysterious functions of smell, not the actual makeup of odor molecules, is what is elusive about olfaction. Choice (B) says that the author characterizes smell as elusive because its functions are emotional rather than physical. This is not true. Throughout the first paragraph the author points out that smell has both physical and emotional functions. This is a central current of thought throughout the passage. Finally, choice (D) states that olfactory sensations are more fleeting than those of other senses. Even though the second sentence of the second paragraph says that smell reaches the brain more quickly than do sensations of other senses, and the third sentence of that paragraph says that odiferous molecules are volatile and dissipate quickly, we cannot confuse and combine these issues to conclude that olfactory sensations are more fleeting than those of touch, sight, or sound. The pace of olfactory sensations is an issue that simply is not addressed in the passage; choice (D) is wrong.

78. A Emotion and olfaction are discussed in the third paragraph. There it is stated that the "precise connection between emotion and olfaction remains a mystery" but that "it is clear that emotion, memory, and smell are all rooted in a part of the brain called the limbic lobe." From that it can be inferred that the role of olfaction in emotion would be better understood through investigation into the workings of the limbic lobe, or choice (A). Choice (C) suggests that investigation into the composition of highly evocative odors would shed light on human olfaction. But there's nothing in the passage that implies that the composition of smells effects our perception of them. Choice (B) states that the emotional element of human olfaction would be better understood through investigation into pheromones. However, the passage mentions pheromones in the fifth paragraph in considering animal, not human, olfaction. There's no connection made in the passage between pheromones and human olfaction, so that study of pheromones would not help scientists understand the emotional element of human olfaction. Choice (D) suggests that study of the pathway between outside environment and olfactory nerves would be helpful to our understanding of emotions and smell. The last sentence of the second paragraph states that olfactory neurons render a direct path between stimulus and brain. From this the author notes that smells reach the brain almost directly. But, the author does not say or imply that this anatomical fact has anything to do with the emotional aspect of olfaction. So, choice (D) is also wrong.

79. D The best approach to this type of question is to consider the answer choices in order. Choice (A) suggests that evidence that olfaction and metabolic function are located in the same area of the brain would support the author's contention that smell has an important physiologic function. The proximity of olfactory and metabolic centers in the brain is mentioned in the third sentence of the first paragraph—a fact that does indeed support the author's claim to the important physiological function of smell. So (A) is incorrect. Choice (B) presents the hypothesis that animals with impaired olfaction often exhibit abnormal brain function. The last sentence of the fourth paragraph gives this fact as evidence of the importance of smell, so it's certainly reasonable to apply this to the author's belief that smell plays an important physiological role. Choice (C) says that a considerable amount of human brain tissue is devoted to olfaction. This is true and is mentioned in the second sentence of the fourth paragraph as evidence that the role of smell must be profound. Choice (D) gives the evidence that human beings with impaired olfaction are usually able to behave and function normally. This completely contradicts the author's belief that smell has an important physiological function. If someone with an impaired sense of smell can function perfectly well, that is evidence against the author's theory of the importance of smell. Therefore, choice (D) does not support the author's statement and satisfies the question stem.

This passage is about bebop, a form of jazz music. The first paragraph offers three important points of information: that bebop was invented in the 1940s; that it has experienced a revival in the 1980s; and that this revival stands in ironic contrast to bebop's initial public reception—which implies that the initial public response to bebop was negative. The second paragraph provides historical background on jazz prior to bebop, proceeding chronologically. The author goes back to the infancy of jazz in the first two decades of this century, saying that, until the 1920s, jazz was rather simplistic. The music became more sophisticated in the 1920s—and gained its first international popularity. The 1930s are also covered in this second paragraph. This decade, the one immediately preceding the appearance of bebop, was known as the Swing Era, and featured big bands playing jazz-based dance music to large and enthusiastic audiences. In paragraphs three and four, the author describes bebop music and the radical departure it made from the jazz of previous decades. Paragraph three details the musical elements that made bebop so distinctive: its fast tempos, tricky rhythms and unusual chords and notes. Paragraph four describes the negative public response to the music, which ultimately resulted in jazz falling out of the mainstream of popular music.

80. B Choice (A), that bebop followed the tradition of jazz from the 1920s, is clearly wrong because the second sentence of paragraph three says that bebop "represented a departure from tradition in both form and content." Choice (B) is correct. Paragraph three, in its entirety, and the first sentence of paragraph four clearly show that bebop differed from music of the Swing Era. Bebop music was faster and harmonically more adventurous. Unlike swing music, it not danceable, and demanded intellectual concentration. Choice (C) contradicts the last sentence of paragraph three: bebop did not celebrate the songs of Tin Pan Alley. Bebop tunes were often originals, unfamiliar to audiences. And choice (D) is incorrect because, as the

second and seventh sentences of the second paragraph indicate, bebop sprang from improvisations. Its extremely fast tempos and ever-increasing musical sophistication clearly imply that playing bebop required extensive improvisational skill.

81. B The author says that Louis Armstrong, one of the two musicians "most responsible for" jazz's rise in popularity, "greatly expanded the creative range and importance of the soloist in jazz." In other words, Armstrong raised the stakes for jazz soloists. They had to improve, to rise above the "fairly rudimentary" improvisations that had been played during the first two decades of the century. So choice (B) is the correct answer. Regarding choice (A), it's clear from paragraph two that, in the 1920s, the innovations of people like Armstrong and Henderson really changed jazz, making it more sophisticated and expansive. Choice (A) says that 1920s' jazz resembled earlier jazz, and this goes against the grain of the author's argument; 1920s jazz was clearly different. Choice (C) is wrong because the author never specifies what kind of tempos were typical of 1920s jazz. The passage never indicates if they were fast or slow, so there's no support for choice (C). And choice (D) describes jazz music of the Swing Era in the 1930s, not the jazz of the 1920s.

82. A The phrase *Western music* appears only once in the passage. It's in the third sentence of the final paragraph, where the author compares bebop to "other movements in the course of Western music." The author says there that public alienation or estrangement toward bebop was intense because bebop seemed to have arrived "in a completely mature state of development, without that early phase of experimentation that typifies so many movements in the course of Western music."

This not only indicates something about bebop, it educates about most movements in the course of Western music—namely, that they go through at least two phases: an early, experimental phase, and a later, more mature, more fully developed phase. This is the substance of Roman numeral statement

I, which is a reasonable conclusion and therefore will be part of the correct answer. Notice that choices (B) and (D) do not include Roman numeral Statement I; thus, they can be eliminated. Since either choice (A), which offers statement I only, or choice (C), which offers statements I and II, must be the correct answer. One can review only statement II to determine the right answer. Statement II says that World War II prevented bebop from reaching a more appreciative audience. This is a distortion of the fifth sentence of the final paragraph, which says that a petrol shortage during World War II necessitated a three-year ban on the making of records. But, according to the author, it was not the recording ban that prevented bebop from reaching a more appreciative audience; it only compounded the problem (line 61). It was the radical elements of bebop itself that prevented the music from appealing to a wider audience. So statement II is false, and choice (A), statement I only, is the correct answer.

83. D Henderson's innovations are discussed in the sixth and seventh sentences of the second paragraph. Remember that the question stem seeks something that inspired Henderson. Sentence six says that Henderson, unlike many jazz musicians before him, had extensive training in music theory, and that he saw the creative possibilities in jazz played by a larger band. Sentence seven says that Henderson's song arrangements gave jazz soloists "a more structured musical background upon which to shape their solo improvisations." We know from the second sentence of that same paragraph that most jazz prior to the 1920s was played by musicians who couldn't read music, and who consequently had to keep their improvisations fairly simple. That is, the structure of early jazz was simple, but in Henderson's arrangements the structure was raised to a grander scale and more sophisticated levels of complexity and structure. It can therefore be inferred that Henderson was inspired by the desire to go beyond the simple structure of early jazz, to go beyond its structural limitations. Therefore, choice (D) is correct. Choice (A) is a strong distracter. Armstrong is mentioned in the passage as the other key figure in jazz of the 1920s. But whether Henderson admired Armstrong or not is never discussed, so you can't infer that

Henderson's innovations were inspired by his admiration for Armstrong. Choice (B) reflects the author's remark, in the third sentence of paragraph two, that jazz attained international recognition in the 1920s. This choice distorts that point in suggesting that Henderson hungered for international recognition. Choice (C) is correct in suggesting that one of Henderson's innovations was in the application of jazz to the big band setting. A problem with choice (C) is that the public's preference for big bands over small combos did not become apparent until a decade after Henderson's contribution—in the 1930s, during the Swing Era. Another problem with this choice is the implication that Henderson merely exploited the realization that the public liked the big band sound. The author gives only one reason Henderson was drawn to large bands—in the sixth sentence of paragraph two: Henderson was drawn to large bands because, with his training in music theory, he "foresaw the orchestral possibilities of jazz played by a larger band."

84. C According to the author, recently people have finally begun to appreciate bebop from the 1940s, an era when jazz music was perhaps "at the apex" or highest point of its development. But this newfound appreciation is ironic, argues the author, because when it was first introduced, bebop was not widely appreciated in its own time. This thesis is restated in choice (C): Bebop may represent the apex of jazz, but it was neglected for many years. Choice (A) may be an accurate statement about jazz history, but it's not the author's central thesis. The history of jazz is too broad to describe the author's interest. In fact, this choice doesn't even mention bebop, which is clearly of primary importance to the author. Choice (B) is fairly easy to eliminate, since the passage lacks any reference at all to those fusion musicians whose careers have supposedly been damaged by the revival of bebop. So (B) is only tangentially related and is also wrong. And choice (D) takes a detail from the passage, distorts it, and tries to raise it to the level of a central thesis. Although, the author does say that bebop was played by small combos rather than the big bands that had been so popular throughout the 1930s, but the author does not argue that bebop would have been much more popular if it had been played by big bands. In fact, he suggests that there were many other features of bebop that made it unpopular—its tricky rhythms, fast tempos that weren't danceable, and unfamiliar tunes. So, choice (D) is incorrect.

85. A The correct answer will be an item that the passage did not describe as a characteristic of bebop. Choices (B) and (C), complex rhythms and dissonant melodies, are mentioned in the fourth sentence of paragraph three as characteristics of bebop, so they can be eliminated. Choice (D), intellectual complexity, is referred to as a characteristic of bebop in the first sentence of paragraph four. Remaining is choice (A) as the correct answer. And indeed, the author never states that bebop "was eminently danceable." On the contrary, in the first sentence of the last paragraph the author states that bebop was not danceable. This choice confuses one of the author's comments regarding swing music. In the last sentence of the second paragraph, the author says that swing was eminently danceable.

86. A You're required to draw an inference about why bebop seemed to represent a radical departure from earlier jazz music. The key word here is *seemed*. In paragraph three, the author gives you several reasons why bebop actually was a departure from earlier jazz. But none of these reasons is among the answer choices. In fact, the reason why it seemed so radical a departure is stated in the middle of the final paragraph, and that reason is the recording ban that coincided with bebop's developmental or experimental phase. In its formative stage, bebop was not heard by a wide audience because there were no bebop records. By the time bebop was put on records, it had reached a mature stage of development, and must have seemed, to those hearing it for the first time, as if it had, in the author's words, "sprung fully formed like Athena from the forehead of Zeus." Choice (A), then, is correct in stating that bebop seemed a radical departure because it grew to maturity before reaching the public. Choice (B) is incorrect because the author never says that bebop attracted

primarily a youthful audience. The only issue mentioned about the audience for bebop in the 1940s is that it was small, representing only a fraction of the audience that had loved jazz in the Swing Era. Choice (C) is also unsubstantiated. The author says, in the final sentence of paragraph three, that bebop tunes were "often originals with which audiences were unfamiliar," but never that bebop composers dispensed with arrangements altogether.

Despite the author's reference to early bebop musicians leading lives of deprivation and obscurity in the final sentence of the passage, the fact remains that the passage contains no mention of the alienation of these musicians, and certainly does not suggest its expression as a reason bebop seemed radically different. Thus, Choice (D) is incorrect.

87. D Wynton Marsalis is mentioned in the second sentence of the passage as a musician who, in the 1980s, led the revival of interest in bebop. Charlie Parker, on the other hand, is mentioned in the final sentence of the passage as a "bebop pioneer." The only possible conclusion is that Marsalis and Parker are bebop musicians from different eras, which makes choice (D) correct. Choice (A) is irrelevant and unsubstantiated. The author does not identify any pioneers of jazz-rock fusion. Choice (B) is incorrect because only Parker was an architect of the bebop movement. Marsalis, playing forty years later, might be considered an architect of the bebop revival, but not the original movement. And choice (C) is patently false, since Parker and Marsalis were champions of bebop music, not of swing music.

Passage VI (Questions 88–92)

The first paragraph of this passage serves as an introduction to the importance of oxygen in the process of photosynthesis. The second paragraph notes that a scientist named de Saussure believed that in photosynthesis, carbon dioxide and oxygen combine, using energy in the form of light to produce oxygen and other substances. The third paragraph discusses the contributions of Van Niel, who revised de Saussure's hypothesis and postulated that the oxygen produced in photosynthesis was a byproduct of water, rather than carbon dioxide. The last paragraph serves as support for Van Niel's assertion stating that his hypothesis was supported and verified by subsequent experiments by other scientists.

88. C The unnamed 18th century scientists in paragraph one laid the groundwork for understanding the role of oxygen; de Saussure postulated the production of free oxygen during photosynthesis; Van Niel's conclusions revised our understanding of the actual source of oxygen in the photosynthetic reaction, and his findings were subsequently verified by other scientists. The generalization in choice (C) is thus accurate. Physical data are referred to throughout the passage, in all four paragraphs, so choice (A) is contradicted. Nothing suggests choice (B); the second paragraph makes it clear that de Saussure hypothesized that light energized the photosynthetic process, and then that scientists in 1845 added to our understanding by realizing that light energy is converted to chemical energy. Similarly, choice (D) is implicitly contradicted: All the scientists mentioned apparently benefited from and built on the work of previous scientists.

89. D The first three and final two sentences of paragraph three make it clear that Van Niel's studies "decisively altered" the traditional model of the photosynthetic reaction and supported a substitute conception. This idea is paraphrased in choice (D). De Saussure worked with a model of photosynthesis back in the early 19th century—a full century before Van Niel—so choice (A) is incorrect. Choice (B) summarizes an assumption that Van Niel disproved. As for choice (C), the passage never states that Van Niel discovered or proved that sulfur bacteria used hydrogen sulfide, merely that Van Niel studied these bacteria in order to make inferences about photosynthesis in green plants. In all likelihood it was another scientist who saw that these organisms used hydrogen sulfide to make their food.

90. D Paragraph three explains that Van Niel's investigation led to his conclusion that water plays a much different role in photosynthesis than had long been assumed—that water (rather than carbon dioxide) is split, into hydrogen and oxygen. The point is paraphrased in correct choice (D). Choice (A) is incorrect because, although oxygen isn't produced in the photosynthetic process occurring in the bacteria, it certainly is produced by green plant photosynthesis. Van Niel's study showed exactly where oxygen comes from in green plant photosynthesis. As for choice (B), Van Niel's study had nothing to do with a candle flame; that's an irrelevant detail from the eighteenth century, noted in paragraph one. Similarly, the role of light in photosynthesis as mentioned in choice (C) is never questioned.

91. B   De Saussure is discussed in the second paragraph. According to the last sentence of the paragraph, the conversion of light energy into chemical energy was not well understood until after de Saussure's work. According to the previous sentence, de Saussure was aware only that light supplied energy to plants. So it's unlikely that the statement made in choice (B) would have been made by de Saussure. Each of the other choices is mentioned earlier in this paragraph or in paragraph one as having been known to or discovered by de Saussure.

92. A   The question that's never answered in the passage is choice (A): It's never explained why (or how) oxygen supports a candle flame, or any other kind of combustion. Each of the other questions does get answered. Regarding choice (B), de Saussure claimed that water's function in photosynthesis is to combine with carbon dioxide as stated in the middle of paragraph two. For choice (C), light is described, in the last couple of sentences of paragraph two, as being the energy source for photosynthesis. Choice (D) can be found in paragraph three; water is not used by those bacteria that use hydrogen sulfide.

BIOLOGICAL SCIENCES: Answers and Explanations

ANSWER KEY

93. A	113. B	133. B
94. C	114. B	134. B
95. C	115. B	135. C
96. D	116. C	136. D
97. D	117. A	137. A
98. D	118. B	138. B
99. A	119. D	139. B
100. C	120. A	140. D
101. D	121. D	141. A
102. A	122. A	142. D
103. D	123. B	143. C
104. C	124. C	144. D
105. D	125. B	
106. A	126. A	
107. B	127. B	
108. B	128. C	
109. A	129. C	
110. C	130. A	
111. D	131. D	
112. C	132. C	

EXPLANATIONS

Passage I (Questions 93–99)

93. A The key to answering this question lies in knowing that at high altitudes, atmospheric pressure is low, meaning that there is less oxygen in the air than at sea level. We're told that the llama has adapted to life at high altitudes by evolving a different type of hemoglobin. Since the partial pressure of oxygen is lower up in the mountains, llama hemoglobin must be able to bind oxygen more readily at low partial pressures of oxygen. This means that for a given value of oxygen pressure on the x-axis of Figure 1, the llama's hemoglobin will be more saturated with oxygen than the horse's hemoglobin, since horses don't typically live in regions of unusually high altitude. In terms of Figure 1, this means that the llama oxygen-dissociation curve will be to the left of the horse's. So if Curve B is the horse curve, then the llama curve most closely resembles Curve A. Thus,

choices (B) and (C) are wrong. Curve D is also wrong: Remember, we're told in the passage that Curves A, B, and C are hemoglobin curves, while Curve D is the myoglobin curve.

94. C According to the passage, small mammals have higher metabolic rates and require a greater amount of oxygen per gram of tissue than larger mammals, and as a result, have hemoglobin that dissociates oxygen more readily than the hemoglobin of large mammals. A high metabolic rate implies that there's a lot of aerobic respiration going on. Metabolically active tissue needs lots of oxygen. The benefit of having Hb that easily dissociates oxygen is that when hemoglobin delivers oxygen to metabolically active tissue, it will readily give up its oxygen to the tissue. This means that for a given value of oxygen pressure, mouse hemoglobin will be less saturated with oxygen than elephant hemoglobin, since an elephant is much larger than a mouse and therefore has a much lower metabolic rate. In terms of Figure 1, the mouse Hb curve will be to the right of the elephant Hb curve. So if Curve B represents oxygen dissociation for elephant hemoglobin, then Curve C most closely resembles the curve for mouse Hb. Therefore, choices A and B are wrong. As for choice (D), we're twice told in the passage that Curve D represents oxygen dissociation for myoglobin. Since we're dealing with hemoglobin in this question, Curve D isn't even an option.

95. C Fetuses are 100 percent dependent on their mothers for all of their nutritional needs—oxygen being one of them. Oxygen is delivered to the fetus by way of diffusion across the placenta. According to the question stem, Curve A most closely resembles the oxygen-dissociation curve for fetal hemoglobin, assuming that Curve B is the curve for adult hemoglobin. This means that at a given oxygen pressure, fetal hemoglobin is more saturated with oxygen than is adult hemoglobin. This implies that fetal hemoglobin has a greater affinity for oxygen than adult hemoglobin has. In fact, at low partial pressures of oxygen, fetal hemoglobin has a 20–30 percent greater affinity for oxygen than adult hemoglobin. That is why oxygen binds preferentially to fetal hemoglobin in the capillaries of the placenta. In addition, fetal blood has a 50 percent higher concentration of hemoglobin than maternal blood, which increases the amount of oxygen that enters fetal circulation.

96. D The sigmoidal shape of the oxygen-dissociation curve for hemoglobin can be explained by the cooperativity among the subunits of the hemoglobin molecule. According to the passage, hemoglobin is composed of four subunits, each with its own heme group. Each heme unit is capable of binding to one molecule of oxygen, and so the entire molecule is capable of binding four molecules of oxygen. The binding of oxygen at the first heme group induces a conformational change in the hemoglobin molecule such that the second heme group's affinity for oxygen increases. Likewise, the binding of oxygen at the second heme group increases the third heme's affinity for oxygen, and the binding of oxygen at the third heme groups increases the fourth's affinity for oxygen. Therefore, the partial pressure of oxygen and the % oxygen-saturation of hemoglobin are not linearly proportional. As a consequence of these shifts in oxygen affinity with each binding, the line representing the oxygen-dissociation curve for hemoglobin is not straight, but rather a sigmoidal, or S-shaped, curve. Thus, choice (D) is the right answer. Choice (A) is wrong because when the iron molecule of the heme group binds to oxygen, it is reduced; when the iron releases the oxygen, it is oxidized. However, this neither results in the sigmoidal shape of the curve, nor does it affect it. The concentration of carbon dioxide in the blood, choice (B), is a factor that does affect hemoglobin's affinity for oxygen and therefore affects the positioning of the curve, but it is *not responsible* for the sigmoidal shape. A high concentration of carbon dioxide in the blood will decrease hemoglobin's affinity for oxygen, and will therefore shift the curve to the right. Choice (C) is also a true statement; myoglobin does have a higher affinity for oxygen than does hemoglobin, as shown in Figure 1. However, this does not affect the shape of the sigmoidal curve, so choice (C) is also incorrect.

97. D The four subunits in Hb are held together by noncovalent interactions. So placing a sample of human adult hemoglobin in an 8 *M* urea solution, which you're told disrupts noncovalent interactions, will cause the subunits to break apart. You're also told in the question stem that the alpha chains of this sample of hemoglobin were isolated. So you need to figure out what the oxygen dissociation curve of a single peptide chain would look like. From the passage you also know that myoglobin consists of a single polypeptide chain. Therefore, the oxygen-dissociation curve for one polypeptide chain of Hb would be expected to look similar to the curve for myoglobin. In fact, both the individual alpha chains and the beta chains of hemoglobin resemble the tertiary structure of myoglobin. Thus, the curve for the alpha chain will look like Curve D, so choice (D) is correct. The single chain of Hb will not look like Curves A, B, or C because these curves have a unique shape due to the cooperativity of the four hemoglobin subunits. Since you're now dealing with a single chain (because of that treatment with an 8 *M* urea solution), no cooperativity is possible.

98. D You're told that the utilization coefficient is the fraction of the blood that releases its oxygen to tissues under normal conditions, and that under these conditions, the value of the coefficient is approximately 0.25. During strenuous exercise, there is a greater demand for oxygen, especially in skeletal muscle, where oxygen supplies are rapidly depleted during cellular respiration. Under such conditions, one would expect that a greater fraction of the blood would give up its oxygen, and that the utilization coefficient would therefore be some value greater than 0.25. Also, during strenuous exercise, the utilization coefficient has been recorded at values ranging between 0.75 and 0.85, meaning that 75–85 percent of the blood gives up its oxygen in tissue capillaries. Since choice (D) is the only value greater than 0.25, it is the right answer.

99. A Figure out how much oxygen will be bound to myoglobin, if the myoglobin in this sperm whale is completely saturated with oxygen. All of the answer choice values are in moles. To equate the number of moles of oxygen that will bind to myoglobin, you need to figure out how many moles of myoglobin are present in the sperm whale's muscles. From the question stem you know that there are 0.004 moles of myoglobin per kg of muscle and the whale has 1,000 kg of muscle. Multiplying these two numbers together gives you 4 moles of myoglobin, implying that the whale has 4 moles of myoglobin in its muscles. Then, determine how many molecules of oxygen bind to a single molecule of myoglobin. The answer is one, because myoglobin consists of a single polypeptide chain, which contains a single heme group. Thus, myoglobin binds only one molecule of oxygen. If one molecule of oxygen binds to one molecule of myoglobin, then one mole of oxygen will bind to one mole of myoglobin. Since you know that the whale has 4 moles of myoglobin in its muscle, 4 moles of oxygen will be bound to myoglobin when myoglobin is completely saturated with oxygen.

100. C According to the passage, the catabolism of amino acids, which are the molecules that make up proteins, produces ammonia. Metabolism can be divided into catabolism and anabolism, and catabolism refers to pathways in which larger molecules are broken down into smaller parts. (If you have trouble remembering the difference between catabolism and anabolism, just associate anabolism with anabolic steroids. Anabolic steroids are used by weight lifters to build muscle, therefore anabolism must refer to the pathways in which smaller molecules are built into larger molecules). We know from the passage that if the ammonia that is produced as a byproduct of amino acid breakdown is not further degraded, it can become toxic, depending on its concentration in the blood. To answer the question, you need to recall that the end product of amino acid degradation is urea, which means that ammonia must feed into the urea cycle. The concentration of ammonia in the blood would become elevated and potentially toxic if one of the enzymes involved in the urea cycle was defective. Thus choice (C) is the correct answer. Choice (A), glycolysis, refers to the catabolism of glucose into pyruvate. Choice (B), fatty acid catabolism, refers to the breakdown of fatty acids into acetyl CoA. Choice (D), nucleic acid degradation, refers to the breakdown of DNA and RNA into nucleotides.

101. D To answer this question you need to recall the site of protein digestion, and the fate of the amino acids produced by this digestion. A brief review of the digestive system as it relates to proteins is in order. Food enters the stomach from the pharynx and esophagus. When protein-containing food reaches the stomach, its presence causes the release of the hormone gastrin, which stimulates the secretion of HCl, and pepsinogen, and muscular contractions of the stomach. HCl initiates the conversion of pepsinogen to its active form, pepsin. Pepsin breaks down proteins into peptides. The peptides then enter the small intestine. Three types of peptide-digesting enzymes are secreted into the small intestine: enterokinase, aminopeptidases, and dipeptidases. The combination of these three enzyme types breaks apart all peptide bonds, producing only single amino acids and dipeptides.

The single amino acids and dipeptides are then absorbed into the epithelial cells lining the small intestine by active transport. These molecules all enter the bloodstream by way of the capillaries of the villi. Villi are the fingerlike projections lining the small intestine that serve to increase the absorptive surface area of the intestine. From the bloodstream the amino acids enter individual cells. Inside these cells, the amino acids are used to either build new proteins or other biological molecules, or they are completely catabolized, in which case ammonia is produced. This ammonia then enters the urea cycle, and the urea produced in the process exits the cells and is excreted in the urine. So from this discussion of the digestion of protein, it is clear that ammonia is not produced inside the lumen of the small intestine, which makes choice (D) the correct answer.

102. A Albumin is a protein produced by the liver. It is very important in maintaining the plasma osmolarity of the blood. The glomerulus, which is the network of blood vessels enveloped by the part of the nephron known as Bowman's capsule, has small holes in its endothelial lining called fenestrations. When proteins travel through the glomerulus, they are prevented from entering the nephron due to the size of the fenestrations and the negative electrical charge of glycosylated proteins lining the fenestrations. Therefore, albumin is not normally found in urine because it is prevented from entering the nephron, so choice (A) is the right answer. The presence of protein in a urine sample is typically a sign of renal disease. Each of the other choices is normally found in appreciable quantity in the urine. Urea, choice (C), is the primary excretory byproduct of the urea cycle, while sodium and potassium homeostasis are kept in balance by the regulation of their excretion in urine.

103. D As explained in the passage, diabetes insipidus is a condition in which ADH is ineffective, and as a result, the kidneys reabsorb less water and are unable to concentrate urine. Very dilute urine is the result. So, urine output is increased in a patient with diabetes insipidus, which means that choice (D) is correct. Since water reabsorption is decreased, this means that plasma osmolarity will be increased, so choice (A) is wrong. Choice (C) is wrong because the presence of glucose in the urine is one of the symptoms and tell-tale signs of diabetes mellitus. Diabetes mellitus is the result of an insulin deficiency; without insulin, glucose is not converted into glycogen, and as a result, some of it gets excreted in the urine because the kidneys are overwhelmed by the excess glucose in the bloodstream. Choice (B) is incorrect because an increased urine osmolarity would mean that there was a greater concentration of dissolved solutes per liter of urine, which is not the case if there is an excess of water being excreted. It should be noted that a diabetes insipidus patient with an intact thirst mechanism and access to water will not become dehydrated. They will drink enough water to replace what is lost in the urine.

104. C You're told that a normal value for urine osmolarity is 285 milliosmoles per liter of H_2O. Since ADH increases water reabsorption in the kidneys, patients with diabetes insipidus are expected to have a decreased urine osmolarity. And if normal is 285 milliosmoles per liter of water, then, based on the information in Table 1, you should have concluded that Patient A does not have diabetes insipidus. Patients B, C, and D, have a very low urine osmolarity prior to therapy, indicating that there is something wrong. To answer this question you must have a good understanding of the mechanisms behind both central and nephrogenic diabetes insipidus. According to the passage, central diabetes insipidus is when ADH itself is either deficient in quantity or quality. Therefore, exogenous supplementation of ADH should alleviate the symptoms: that is, the kidneys should be able to concentrate urine, and therefore, urine osmolarity should greatly increase only after ADH is administered. It should not increase after the 24-hour restriction of fluid intake because water is not being reabsorbed. If you look at the results of the four patients, you'll see only Patient C's urine osmolarity increased after ADH was administered. So, choice (C) is the right answer. In the case of nephrogenic diabetes insipidus, it is the tubules themselves that are defective. Exogenous ADH would be ineffective as therapy since the patient's own ADH is sufficient in quality and quantity.

105. D Nephrogenic diabetes insipidus is when the kidney's collecting tubules are unresponsive to ADH. It's not that ADH is insufficiently produced or defective in any way, it's that the tubules do not concentrate urine by becoming more permeable to water when ADH is secreted by the posterior pituitary. Again, as in the previous question, you should have immediately ruled out Patient A because Patient A has a normal urine osmolarity prior to the therapy. A patient with nephrogenic diabetes insipidus would have a decreased urine osmolarity prior to therapy, which would remain low even after the restriction of fluid intake for 24 hours. This is because the tubules won't reabsorb water, regardless of the amount of fluid ingested. Likewise, the administration of ADH will not affect the urine osmolarity because, as said earlier, the patient's ADH is perfectly normal; it's the nephron tubules that are defective. If you look at Table 1, you'll see that only Patient D fits the bill. Patient D is most likely suffering from nephrogenic diabetes insipidus, which means that choice (D) is the right answer.

106. A Fluid restriction is the first step in the attempt to diagnose the pathology, if there is one, behind the inability to concentrate urine. Patient B had a low urine osmolarity prior to the onset of therapy. However, following the restriction of fluid intake, there was a substantial increase in urine osmolarity, indicating that Patient B's dilute urine is a function of the amount of fluid ingested. If a lot of fluid is drunk during the day, the urine formed will be dilute, assuming that the person's kidneys and ADH are both normal. Likewise, if there is very little fluid drunk during the day, the urine formed will be concentrated. Thus, the excessive intake of water seems to be the most likely explanation for the formation of dilute urine in Patient B. In fact, there are individuals who have a psychological condition in which they drink water excessively. This excessive intake causes the output of dilute urine. Simply restricting and observing fluid intake would enable the patient to concentrate urine. Fluid restriction had no effect on either Patient C or Patient D, indicating that they have a true pathology; choices (C) and (D) are wrong. If Patient B was dehydrated, then the body's response would be to produce concentrated urine from the start, which was clearly not the case here, since urine osmolarity was very low prior to therapy.

Passage III (Questions 107–113)

107. B Double bonds, like the ones in carotene, consist of one sigma bond, formed by the overlap of two sp^2 orbitals, and one pi bond, formed by the overlap of perpendicular p orbitals. It is the latter, the pi bond, that is stabilized by the conjugated polyene system. This conjugation enables the pi electrons to be excited by lower frequencies of light. Choice (A), s orbitals, is wrong because the pi electrons, which give conjugated bonds their stability, are not in s orbitals. (C) and (D) are wrong because carbon and hydrogen, which are the main or only components of organic molecules like carotene, don't have d and f orbitals.

108. B For each compound, the light that's transmitted is complementary in color to the light absorbed; thus, the first chromophore must absorb violet light and the second must absorb green light. Violet light has a shorter wavelength than green, meaning it has a higher energy. You're told that longer chromophores generally absorb longer-wavelength light than shorter ones, so the one that absorbs the green light, and therefore has a red color, must be the longer one. This makes (B) correct and (A) and (D) incorrect. Even though you know one pigment is longer, there's no basis for concluding that it is a dimer (meaning a compound made up of two identical subunits), so choice (C) is definitely wrong.

109. A The greater the number of conjugated bonds in a molecule, the more strongly electrons in excited states will be stabilized. Thus the more conjugated a molecule, the lower the frequency and the longer the wavelength that will excite it. Benzene, with only three double bonds, requires absorption of quite high energy light, higher than for the colored compounds discussed in the passage. In fact, the light required to excite benzene electrons is in the ultraviolet range, so no color is produced when benzene absorbs light, and benzene is colorless.

110. C The green color comes from absorption of light by the entire carotene-protein complex; as you know from the passage, the carotene by itself is orange. The fact that boiled lobsters are red and not orange is due to other pigments that are also present. When a lobster is cooked, the heat disrupts the intermolecular attractions that attach the carotene molecule, the protein's prosthetic group, to the protein itself. This change in the molecule causes the wavelength of light absorbed to change as well. As a matter of fact, it reduces the number of conjugated double bonds and therefore shortens the wavelength of light absorbed. The red color of the cooked lobster is the transmission color of the isolated carotenoid, with the conjugated bonds from the protein removed. Choices (A) and (D) are wrong because if carotene were hydrated or oxidized, it would break the chain of conjugation completely and produce a colorless compound. An increase in temperature, choice (B), is only a physical change and won't change the absorption wavelength.

111. D Substance IV would make the best sunscreen because it absorbs over a broad spectrum, including all three types of ultraviolet light. By the way, the absorption spectrum of melanin, the pigment which protects human skin from sunlight, is similar to this. The next best choice is I, which absorbs UVB and UVC, the most dangerous wavelengths of ultraviolet light. Choice II absorbs UVA, so it would prevent tanning but would let through the dangerous UVB and UVC, and therefore allow burning. Choice III would be of little value, since it absorbs almost exclusively in the visible range (greater than 400 nm).

112. C This molecule, which is called dopamine quinone, has four conjugated bonds and produces a brownish color. Choice (B) has a larger number of double bonds, but they are not conjugated, so its absorbance wavelength is below the visible range. Choice (A) has too few double bonds to produce color, and although choice (D) has six double bonds, they are conjugated in two sets of three, not one set of six, and it's also less likely to be colored.

113. B Resonance is responsible for reducing the frequency of light needed to excite an electron—that is, raise it to a higher-energy, antibonding orbital. Choice (A) is wrong because almost any molecule can absorb light and have an electron raised to an antibonding orbital. This process does not normally produce color because the frequency of light involved is usually outside the visible range. Resonance reduces the amount of energy needed, bringing the frequency into the visible spectrum. As for choices (D) and (C), optical activity, choice (D), is the property of being able to rotate plane-polarized light; this doesn't have anything to do with color. Polarity, choice (C), also has nothing to do with color.

Discrete Questions

114. B The vertebrate nervous system consists of two main parts: the central nervous system (the brain and the spinal cord), and the peripheral nervous system, which is divided into the sensory division and the motor division. The sensory division consists of those receptors and neurons that transmit signals to the central nervous system. The motor division transmits signals from the central nervous system to effectors and is divided into the somatic nervous system and the autonomic nervous system. The somatic system, choice (C), innervates skeletal muscle, and its nervous pathways are typically under voluntary control. The autonomic nervous system regulates the internal environment by way of involuntary nervous pathways. The autonomic nervous system innervates smooth muscle in blood vessels and the digestive tract, and innervates the heart, the respiratory system, the endocrine system, the excretory system, and the reproductive system. The autonomic system is further divided into the sympathetic division, choice (B), and the parasympathetic division, choice (A). The sympathetic division innervates those pathways that prepare the body for immediate action; this is known as the fight-or-flight response. Heart rate and blood pressure increase, blood vessels in the skin vasoconstrict and those in the heart vasodilate, pathways innervating the digestive tract are inhibited, and epinephrine, or adrenaline, is secreted by the adrenal medulla, thereby increasing the conversion of glycogen into glucose. This discussion makes it obvious that the correct answer is choice (B); activation of the sympathetic nervous system is associated with an increased heart rate, blood pressure, and blood glucose concentration. The parasympathetic system innervates nervous pathways that return the body to homeostatic conditions following exertion. Heart rate, blood pressure, and blood glucose concentration all decrease, blood vessels in the skin vasodilate and those in the heart vasoconstrict, and the digestive process is no longer inhibited.

115. B There are certain rules that you need to be familiar with in order to decipher the absolute configuration. First, the substituent with the lowest priority must be positioned vertically, that is, either up or down. Remember that in 3-D terms, vertical lines represent bonds going into the page. Second, to move your diagram around on the page you have to remember that interchanging any two pairs of substituents will give you the same compound—that is, it will preserve the absolute configuration. Interchanging just one pair of substituents will always reverse the absolute configuration. Also, you can hold one group steady while rotating the other three clockwise or counterclockwise. The third rule is that once you have the lowest-priority group positioned vertically, you should determine the order of priority among the other three substituents. If that order increases clockwise, that means the chiral carbon has an *R* configuration, while if it increases counterclockwise, the chiral carbon has an *S* configuration. If you look at compound I, you can see that the order of increasing priority is hydrogen, methyl, carboxyl, and hydroxyl. In order to get the hydrogen into a vertical position, you can hold the methyl group steady and rotate the others by 90°. The order of increasing priority is clockwise and so the configuration is *R*. For compound II, the hydrogen is already placed vertically, so you don't have to worry about moving the molecule around the page. The order of increasing priority is hydrogen, methyl, carboxyl, and amine, so when you draw arrows between the last three, the direction is counterclockwise and so the configuration is *S*. Therefore, you can discard choice (C) since these two molecules have opposite configurations.

Compound III may catch you off guard, because if you look at this molecule closely you can see that it is achiral. Although they are written differently, there are two ethyl substituents in this molecule; therefore, this molecule is neither *R* nor *S*, so choices (A) and (D) can be eliminated. In Compound IV, the hydrogen is positioned vertically and the order of priority is the same as in compound I. However, if you connect the arrows this time, you'll see that the direction is counterclockwise, so the configuration is *S*. This makes compounds II and IV the same, which means that choice (B) is correct.

116. C The epididymis, choice (A), is a group of coiled tubes sitting on top of the seminiferous tubules in the male reproductive tract. Sperm are produced in the seminiferous tubules and mature and acquire motility in the epididymis. Sperm are stored in the epididymis until ejaculation. Hence, the epididymis functions in the male reproductive system only; choice (A) is wrong. Choice (B), prostate, is one of the glands associated with the male reproductive tract; the prostate gland secretes an alkaline milky fluid that protects the sperm from the acidic conditions in the female reproductive tract. So, choice (B) also functions only in the male reproductive system. The urethra, choice (C), is a structure found in both men and women. During ejaculation, sperm travels from the epididymis, through the vas deferens, and through the urethra, which opens to the outside from the tip of the penis. The urethra is also directly connected to the bladder. Hence, in males, the urethra functions in both the reproductive and excretory systems. In females, however, the reproductive and excretory systems do not share a common pathway. Sperm enter the vagina and travel up through the cervix, uterus, and fallopian tubes, and urine leaves the body through the urethra; the vagina and the urethra never meet—they are separate openings. So, choice (C) is the right answer. Choice (D), ureter, is the duct connecting the kidney to the bladder. Urine is formed in the kidneys, travels down to the bladder by way of the ureters, and is stored there until it is excreted through the urethra. This process is the same in both sexes.

117. A Here you have to think about exactly what's happening as the stated reaction proceeds. Each time an alkyl halide molecule reacts, incorporating a radioactive bromine atom, it will be optically inverted; that is, it will go from *R* to *S* or vice versa. Each molecule thus inverted cancels out one of the molecules that still has the old configuration; thus each inversion event leads to the racemization of two molecules of alkyl halide. The rate of radioactive bromine incorporation is equal to half of the rate of racemization, and so the correct answer is (A).

118. B In gametogenesis in males, diploid cells called spermatogonia undergo mitosis to produce diploid cells called primary spermatocytes. The primary spermatocytes undergo the first round of meiosis to yield secondary spermatocytes, which are haploid. The secondary spermatocytes undergo the second round of meiosis, resulting in four haploid cells called spermatids. The spermatids then mature into sperm—the male gametes. So, choice (A) is incorrect because a spermatogonium is a diploid cell. We've already found the correct answer—choice (B), spermatid, is not a diploid cell, it's haploid. In female gametogenesis, a diploid cell called a primary oocyte undergoes the first meiotic division to yield two haploid cell—a polar body and a secondary oocyte. The secondary oocyte undergoes the second meiotic division to produce two more haploid cells—a mature oocyte, or ovum, and another polar body. So choice (D), primary oocyte, is also incorrect because these are diploid cells. During fertilization, an ovum and a sperm fuse; two haploid cells fuse to form a single diploid cell called a zygote. Thus, choice (C) is also incorrect.

Passage IV (Questions 119–124)

119. D During the G_1 phase, the cell undergoes intense biochemical activity. During the S phase, or synthesis phase, the nuclear DNA replicates. During the G_2 phase, the nuclear DNA condenses and the structures used during mitosis begin to assemble. During the M phase, or mitotic phase, mitosis occurs. Finally, the nuclear DNA segregates to opposite poles of the cell, the replicated organelles—mitochondria included—also segregate, along with the nuclear DNA, and the cell divides, forming two identical daughter cells. In the passage you're told that mitochondria replicate in a seemingly random pattern, out of phase with both other mitochondria and the cell itself. Remember that mitochondrial DNA must replicate in order for the mitochondrion itself to replicate. Basically, it can be inferred that mitochondrial DNA replicates throughout all of the phases of the cell cycle: G_1, S, G_2, and M. So, choice (D) is correct.

120. A Mitochondria are responsible for cellular energy production—they supply the cell with ATP. Mitochondrial DNA directs the synthesis of mitochondrial proteins, which ultimately play a major role in cell survival. Since mitochondria are so essential to eukaryotic cell life, one would therefore expect replication of its DNA to be highly accurate. Mutations that would cause a dramatic change in its DNA and its ability to produce proteins needed for ATP formation would be lethal to the cell. Since mutations do occur, the most likely type to occur would be one that causes the least damage. A point mutation fits the bill. Point mutations are defined as those in which only nitrogenous base is affected; for example, a cytosine is substituted for an adenine during replication. Point mutations are not usually lethal because of the redundancy of the genetic code; that is, each amino acid is typically coded for by more than one codon. Take the amino acid proline, for example. Proline is coded for by four codons: CCU, CCC, CCA, and CCG. Let's say that the codon is CCU; if there's a point mutation at the third base, no matter which of the remaining three bases is substituted for the uracil, the net product will still be proline. So a point mutation is the type of mutation least likely to affect their productivity. Thus, choice (A) is correct.

As to the other choices, Choice (B), frameshift mutation, is a mutation causing genetic material to be inserted or deleted during DNA replication or transcription. This produces a shift in the reading frame of the mRNA strand being translated, usually leading to the formation of nonsense polypeptides. Changes in protein synthesis would most likely be dangerous for the mitochondria and the cell itself. Lethal mutations, choice (C), are those that would cause the mitochondria to become nonfunctional. In choice (D), nondisjunction is the failure of homologous chromosomes to separate during meiosis. First of all, mitochondria have one circular chromosome—there aren't any homologous chromosomes. Second, mitochondria do not undergo meiosis—only specialized eukaryotic cells in sexually reproducing organisms undergo meiosis. So, choice (D) cannot even be a consideration.

121. D The nuclear genome is comprised of double-helical DNA that codes for mRNA, tRNA, and rRNA. Therefore, choices (A) and (B) are characteristics of the nuclear genome and are therefore incorrect. If a mutation occurred in the nuclear genome that rendered an essential gene nonfunctional, such as an enzyme involved in glycolysis, the organism would die. Thus, choice (C) is also a characteristic of the nuclear genome and an incorrect choice. Although the nuclear genome encodes many products, most of the bases of DNA are noncoding. That is, they are involved in the regulation of gene expression and do not themselves code for any product. So, choice (D) is not consistent with the nuclear genome, so choice (D) is the correct answer. The mitochondrial genome is so small, compared to that of the nucleus, that almost every nitrogen base has to code for a product; the mitochondrial genome doesn't have any DNA to waste!

122. A To answer this question, you must know how many ATP are formed from the catabolism of one molecule of glucose by an obligate anaerobe. An obligate anaerobe is an organism that must live without oxygen in order to survive. Obligate anaerobes produce ATP via fermentation, which includes both glycolysis and the reactions necessary to regenerate the NAD⁺ necessary for glycolysis to continue. Fermentation leads to a net production of 2 ATP; this ATP is generated during glycolysis. Therefore, an obligate anaerobe will produce 2 ATP per molecule of glucose. Aerobic organisms produce a net of 36 ATP, choice (D), per molecule of glucose, as shown in the equation provided in the passage. So, choice (D) is wrong, while choices (B) and (C) are just nonsense.

123. B From the question stem you know that the mating type of a wild-type strain, which has normal mitochondrial DNA, is crossed with the opposite mating type of a strain that lacks functional mitochondria due to deletions in the mitochondrial genome. "Mating types" is a way of referring to male and female in species that do not technically have opposite genders, such as algae and yeast. In addition, you're told that the offspring of this cross do not have functional mitochondria either. The offspring have the same deleted mitochondrial genome as the mutant strain. Now all you have to do is find the choice that best accounts for this occurrence. Choice (A) is incorrect because the endosymbiotic theory attempts to explain the derivation of mitochondria in eukaryotic cells, not the inheritance of mitochondria. Choice (B) is correct. Since you're told that the offspring lack mitochondrial functions, this implies that they inherited their mitochondria from the mutant strain mating type. In other words, the mutant strain was the organelle-donating parent—the female—in this cross. Therefore, the non-Mendelian inheritance pattern of mitochondria, as explained in the passage, best accounts for these experimental observations. If the mating type of the wild-type strain had been the organelle-donating parent, all of the offspring would have normal mitochondrial functions. Choice (C) is wrong because the word *recombination* implies the formation of new gene combinations due to crossing over events that occur during reproduction. If recombinations did occur, you would expect some of the offspring to regain mitochondrial functions, since wild-type mitochondrial DNA would replace the deleted segments of DNA in some offspring. Although choice (D) is a true statement, it does not explain the inheritance patterns observed in this cross.

124. C According to the question stem, four different human cell cultures were grown in a medium containing radioactive adenine. The first thing that you should be thinking about is DNA replication; while these cells are replicating they're going to incorporate this radioactive adenine into all of their DNA. This includes chromosomal DNA, as well as mitochondrial DNA. Mitochondria replicate independently of their cells. Since all autosomal human cells have the same amount of DNA in their nuclei, the only difference in radioactivity will be the amount that was incorporated into the mitochondrial DNA. This is why the cells' mitochondria were isolated via centrifugation, and the radiation from each sample was measure using a scintillation counter. The cells with the greatest number of mitochondria will have the highest radioactive count when their mitochondria are separated. So, you need to determine which of the four cell types would have the greatest number of mitochondria. This number is dependent on the energy needs of the tissue. Given the choices—erythrocytes, epidermal cells, skeletal muscle cells, and intestinal cells—you should know that the correct answer is choice (C), skeletal muscle cells. Muscle cells need a lot of energy in order to contract. ATP is required every time a molecule of myosin binds to actin in the sarcomeres. In general, muscle cells have a higher content of mitochondria than do any other type of autosomal cell. Erythrocytes, choice (A), do not even contain any mitochondria. Choice (B), epidermal cells, do not have any special energy requirements. The same thing applies to intestinal cells, choice (D).

Passage V (Questions 125–128)

125. B There's an easy trick to this question: to answer it, all you have to do is determine which of the answer choices has a molecular weight of 138 g/mol. The only compound which has a molecular weight of 138 g is choice (B): 8 carbons at approximately 12 g/mol is equal to 96 g, 10 hydrogens at approximately 1 g/mol is equal to 10 g, and 2 oxygens at approximately 16 g/mol is equal to 32 g. Adding these together gives a molecular weight of 138 g. The molecular weight of choice (A) is 142, and the molecular weights of choices (C) and (D) are both 137.

126. A The peak at 2850 cm^{-1} is characteristic of the C-H stretch of an alkyl group; in this case, it is attributed to the methyl group of the alkoxide. That's not a terribly exciting functional group, so you might not have known this right off the top of your head, but you could get it by a process of elimination. Choice (B), a phenol group, would produce a broad peak somewhere between 3,600 and 3,200 cm^{-1}, which represents the oxygen-hydrogen bond that is characteristic of all hydroxyl groups and pretty unmistakable. Since it's not present in this spectrum, choice (B) must be incorrect. Choice (C), a carboxyl group, would also produce a broad peak due to its hydroxyl group; this can be anywhere from 3,300 to 2,400 cm^{-1}, and tends to be even broader than a regular hydroxyl peak. The other peaks near the methoxy group peak are much too sharp to belong to a carbonyl group; they actually represent the carbon-hydrogen bonds of the aromatic ring. Whenever you look at the IR spectrum of an organic compound, remember that there will always be some kind of peak or peaks between 2,800 and 3,300 cm^{-1} that's simply due to the carbon backbone—alkane, alkene, alkyne, aromatic, or mixtures of all of these. A carboxyl group would also produce another peak associated with the carbon-oxygen double bond, around 1,700 cm^{-1}, and that's also lacking in this spectrum, so choice (C) is definitely wrong. Finally, choice (D), an aldehyde group, would have the same peak at about 1,700; it would also produce two characteristic peaks in the range of 2,720 and 2,820 cm^{-1}, called Fermi doublets, neither of which is present in the spectrum.

127. B This answer has two methoxy groups attached to an aromatic ring. The student theorized that the peak at 750 cm^{-1} indicates a disubstituted aromatic compound, and since we're told to assume that all of his deductions were correct, this allows us to eliminate choice (D), which has only one substituent on the ring. The passage also says that the compound contains only one type of functional group and so choice (A), which contains two different functional groups, is also clearly wrong. By the way, neither choice (A) nor choice (D) correspond to the correct molecular weight anyway. You are now left with choices (B) and (C), and to decide between these, you have to look back at the spectrum. If this were an alcohol, as in choice (C), the spectrum would contain a broad peak at about 3,350 cm^{-1} to 3,250 cm^{-1}, which is characteristic of a hydroxyl group. This is much like the peak we mentioned for a phenol and for the O-H group of a carboxyl group; like those, it's broadened by the fact that it can form hydrogen bonds. This is a very characteristic feature of any type of hydroxyl-bearing group, and since it's not here, choice (C) must be incorrect.

128. C Choice (C) is false because neither one will dissolve in aqueous hydrochloric acid. You could use base, not acid, to distinguish between these two; the slightly acidic phenol would dissolve, and the alcohol wouldn't. The other three choices are all true statements. For choice (A), the benzoic acid will become deprotonated, while the phenol won't. For choice (B), the aldehyde will be oxidized, yielding a carboxylic acid, while the ketone won't. Finally, for choice (D), sodium hydroxide will hydrolyze the ester, so it will dissolve, while benzyl alcohol will remain insoluble. Again, the only false statement is choice (C), the correct answer.

129. C The genotype of the red male in Cross 6 is either little b, w or little b, little b. Cross 6 is between a red male and a red female, and their offspring are 100% red. What we need to do is look at the offspring and work backwards to determine the genotypes of their parents. As we've just determined, there are two possible genotypes that correspond to a red phenotype—little b, little b and little b, w, since the b allele is dominant to the w allele. With these two genotypes, there are three possible types of crosses (you might want to write these down): little b, little b x little b, little b; little b, little b x little b, w; and little b, w x little b, w. Note that we're not taking into account the gender of the parents: We're not bothering with the fact that the little b, little b x little b, w cross can occur in two different ways—the male can be little b, little b and the female can be little b, w, and vice versa. All of the offspring of Cross 6 are red; therefore, we can eliminate the possibility of a little b, w x little b, w cross since 25% of their offspring would be white. We're left with the other two crosses, both of which produce 100% red offspring. If the male is little b, little b, then the female can be either little b, little b or little b, w; and if the male is little b, w then the female must be little b, little b. Hence the male can either be little b, little b or little b, w and the correct answer is choice (C).

130. A If a large number of the brown offspring from Cross 8 are mated with each other, 6.25% of the offspring are expected to be white. The first thing to do is to figure out the genotypes of the parents in Cross 8. Cross 8 is between a brown male and a red female. The fact that 25% of their offspring are white indicates that both parents are heterozygotes, since white fur is a recessive trait. This means that the genotype of the brown male must be big B, w, and the genotype of the red female must be little b, w. Now we need to figure out the genotypes of the brown offspring. A cross between this brown male and red female results in 25% ww offspring, which are white; 25% little b, w, which are red; 25% big B, w, which are brown; and 25% big B, little b, which are brown. So there are two different brown genotypes in the offspring—big B, little b and big B, w. If a large number of these brown offspring are mated with each other, there are four different crosses possible: (1) big B, little b x big B, little b; (2) big B, w x big B, w; (3) big B, little b x big B, w; and (4) big B, w x big B, little b (this is the second way that the third cross can occur). Now we need to figure out what percentage of the offspring produced in these crosses will have white fur. If we work out the Punnett squares, we find that neither the first, the third, nor the fourth crosses yield any white rats. On the other hand, the second cross, big B, w x big B, w, yields 25% white offspring. But 25% is not your answer. You have to take into account that only one-fourth of the total number of possible crosses between two brown rats yields 25% white offspring. One-fourth of 25% is 6.25%, which is the correct answer, choice (A).

131. D The genotype of the female in Cross 5 can either be big B, big B; big B, little b; or big B, w. In Cross 5, a brown male is mated with a brown female, and we're told that 100% of their offspring are brown. Since we know that the big B allele is dominant to the little b and w alleles, there are three types of genotypically distinct crosses between two brown parents that result in all brown progeny: (1) big B, big B x big B, big B; (2) big B, big B x big B, w; and (3) big B, big B x big B, little b. From this we see that at least one of the parents must be big B, big B. If the female is big B, big B, then the male can be big B, big B; big B, little b; or big B, w. Likewise, if the male is big B, big B, the female can be big B, big B; big B, little b; or big B, w. So, choice (D) is the correct answer.

132. C The ratio of red to white progeny in a cross between a white male and the heterozygous red female from Cross 9 is 1:1. This question is really quite simple because we're told that the red female has the heterozygous genotype, which we know is little b, w. We don't have to look at the progeny of Cross 9 and try to work backwards from there. Since white fur is recessive, the white male in the cross must have the genotype ww. So the cross is little b, w x w, w. Fifty percent of the offspring have the genotype b, w, which, phenotypically, is red fur; the other fifty percent of the offspring have the genotype w, w, which corresponds to white fur. Thus, the ratio of red offspring to white offspring is 50 percent to 50 percent, which is the same as 1: 1, choice (C).

133. B The ratio of progeny in a cross between a big B, little b male and a pink female would be 2 Brown:1 Red:1 Pink. What we need to do is figure out the genotype of the pink female. That's not so hard, since the question stem tells us that rats with pink hair have one copy of the red allele—little b, and one copy of the white allele—w. So, the genotype of the pink female would be little b, w. So if this pink female is crossed with a brown male, the cross is big B, little b x little b, w. If we work out the Punnett square, 25 percent of the progeny would be big B, little b, which is phenotypically brown; 25 percent would be big B, w, which is also brown; 25 percent would be little b, little b, which is red; and finally, 25 percent would be little b, w, which is pink if these two alleles are incompletely dominant. Thus, the phenotypic ratio of the offspring is 2 Brown:1 Red:1 Pink, choice (B).

Passage VII (Questions 134–139)

134. B Reaction A is an electrophilic aromatic substitution reaction, in which thymol is formed from *meta*-cresol. Both the methyl and hydroxyl substituents in *meta*-cresol are *ortho-para* directing activators. However, hydroxyl is the more powerful of the two and if you look at reaction A you can see that substitution occurs *ortho* to the hydroxyl group. However, we are not too concerned about substituent effects but rather the mechanism of the reaction, so let's briefly review what happens. Initially, phosphoric acid abstracts an electron from propene, creating a secondary carbocation. This carbocation then acts as an electrophile and adds to the electron rich benzene ring, *ortho* to the hydroxyl group. This results in the formation of an arenium ion and aromaticity is regained by loss of a proton, generating thymol. Therefore, this mechanism is electrophilic aromatic substitution, making choice (B) the correct answer. From this mechanism, it should be pretty easy to eliminate the other answer choices. Choice (C) is wrong, because although the carbocation adds to the ring, a proton is lost in order to regain aromaticity. Therefore, this is an example of substitution, not addition. Choice (D) is wrong because the carbocation which adds to the ring is acting as an electrophile, not a nucleophile. Remember that benzene is electron rich, and the substituents on *meta*-cresol enhance this, so there is no way that *meta*-cresol could be susceptible to nucleophilic attack. Finally, choice (A)—free radical substitution—is also wrong. There is nothing in reaction A to suggest that free radicals are formed and phosphoric acid will not induce radical formation.

135. C To answer this, you need to understand the resonance stabilization effect that makes phenols more acidic than aliphatic alcohols, such as cyclohexanol. In the phenoxide ion, the negative charge on the oxygen is dispersed throughout the benzene ring, which, in effect, acts like an electron sink, withdrawing electron density. This delocalizing charge effect, as it's called, stabilizes the phenoxide ion, and is described by statement III, which therefore must be included in the correct answer. So you can eliminate the choices that don't include III, which are choices (A) and (B). The phenoxide ion has more possible resonance structures than the undissociated phenol, which still has its proton; thus statement II is also correct. As for statement I, it's factually true—phenols can hydrogen-bond more strongly than aliphatic alcohols, as indicated by the higher boiling points mentioned in the passage—but this is really a consequence, not a cause, of phenol's greater stability. Even though statement I is true, it doesn't explain phenol's acidity, so choice (D), which includes statement I, is incorrect.

136. D In order to answer this question, you need to know what characteristics of a substituted phenol will tend to increase its acidity. The more electron-withdrawing groups a phenol has, the more any negative charge can be dispersed and stabilized by resonance. Since resonance stabilization stabilizes the phenoxide ion more than the phenol, increased resonance stabilization will make a phenol more acidic. Looking at the four phenols, three of them have varying numbers of nitro groups, which are strongly electron-withdrawing, and the fourth has a methyl group, which is electron-donating and should have the opposite effect from the nitro groups. Trinitrophenol (IV), which has the most nitro groups, is the most acidic, followed by dinitrophenol (II), then *para*-nitrophenol (I), and, finally, *para*-cresol (III) with the methyl group.

137. A To answer this question, you need to know that hydroxyl groups are electron-donating, so they activate aromatic rings towards electrophilic aromatic substitution. Like all electrondonating groups, hydroxyl groups are *ortho-para* directors. In this case, the nitro group will add to phenol to form two products, *ortho*-nitrophenol and para-nitrophenol. This means choice (A) is the correct answer. Choice (B) which has only para-nitrophenol, is incomplete and therefore wrong. Choices (C) and (D) can be eliminated because they both include *meta*-nitrophenol, which will not be formed. The only way to get *meta*-nitrophenol would be to start with nitrobenzene and turn it into a phenol—which would work because the nitro group is an electron-withdrawing, deactivating meta director. The reaction will produce only negligible amounts of *meta*-nitrophenol, if any.

138. B Compound A is *para*-cresol or *para*-methylphenol, and Compound B is benzyl alcohol, which behaves more like an aliphatic alcohol than a phenol. We can take advantage of this fact in order to distinguish between these two compounds. One of the easiest ways to do this is by their solubility behavior, which is also an easy way of separating them out of a mixture. Phenols are appreciably acidic, so they are quite soluble in aqueous sodium hydroxide. Alcohols, including benzyl alcohol, are not acidic and won't be soluble in aqueous sodium hydroxide. There is one exception: very small alcohols, with fewer than five carbons, are water-soluble, so they would dissolve in any aqueous solution. However, benzyl alcohol is too big a molecule to be water-soluble, so it won't be soluble in sodium hydroxide solution. So, the solubility of *para*-cresol, Compound A, in aqueous sodium hydroxide would provide an effective test to distinguish between the two compounds, and thus choice (B) is the correct answer. Notice that this means that you could separate a mixture of these two compounds by dissolving it in an organic solvent, and then extracting the solution in a separatory funnel with aqueous sodium hydroxide. The benzyl alcohol would stay in the organic layer, and the *para*-cresol would go into the aqueous layer. Choice (C) is wrong, because compound A won't react with a bromine solution and decolorize it. Both compounds will react under stronger conditions—namely the presence of a Lewis acid—but bromine in solution is too mild a reagent to react with the stable aromatic ring. Therefore, compound A—and compound B for that matter—won't decolorize bromine solution and choice (C) is incorrect. Choice (D) is incorrect because neither of the two compounds will be soluble in sodium bicarbonate. Sodium bicarbonate is a weak base, but since phenols are fairly weak acids, it takes a fairly strong base to make a phenol give up its acidic protons. Thus, *para*-cresol won't dissolve in sodium bicarbonate. As we've said, benzyl alcohol is an even weaker acid than *para*-cresol, so it certainly won't dissolve in sodium bicarbonate. And since neither compounds A nor B will be soluble in sodium bicarbonate, sodium bicarbonate can't be used to distinguish between them.

139. B All four answer choices are aromatic compounds, so Compound X must be aromatic. The chemical formula for this compound consists of carbons, hydrogens, and oxygens (which means you can eliminate choice (C) immediately, since that contains bromine atoms). The next piece of information in the question is that Compound X is soluble in aqueous sodium hydroxide, but not in aqueous sodium bicarbonate. This eliminates choice (A), which is a substituted benzoic acid which would certainly dissolve in sodium bicarbonate. From our discussion in the previous question, you should remember that the ability to dissolve in aqueous sodium hydroxide, but not in aqueous sodium bicarbonate, is characteristic of phenols. This suggests that Compound X is a phenol, which would make choice (B) correct and choice (D), which is a phenyl ether, incorrect.

Check other information in the passage to see if it supports your preliminary conclusion. The NMR spectrum has three separate peaks. The multiplet of area four has a chemical shift of 7.1, which is very far upfield; this represents the aromatic ring, and is due to the spin-spin coupling of four aromatic hydrogens. The singlet at a chemical shift of 1.3 has a peak area of 9 hydrogens; the chemical shift indicates carbon-hydrogen single bonds, and the fact that there are nine hydrogens that are all equivalent means that this represents a tert-butyl group. This would fit *either* choice (B) or choice (D). And finally, the second singlet peak, whose chemical shift is 4.8, has an area of one. If Compound X were choice (D), the single hydrogen peak that you'd get would be from the -CH group of the *tert*-butyl, next to the ether-group oxygen; this would be much further downfield, probably with a chemical shift of about 2.3 or 2.4, so choice (D) must be wrong. The fact that the signal from the single hydrogen is shifted much further upfield, to 4.8, indicates that the proton involved is deshielded, which in turn suggests that it's attached to a more electronegative element than carbon. This magnitude of shift is in fact characteristic of a phenolic hydrogen. This agrees with our previous conclusion, that Compound X is choice (B).

Discrete Questions

140. D E1 and S_N1 reactions are strongly favored by highly branched carbon chains and good leaving groups; E2 reactions are largely independent of the structure of carbon chains and are favored by good leaving groups which can easily be displaced, and by basic conditions. Finally, S_N2 reactions are strongly favored by unbranched carbon chains. Choice (A) is wrong because a primary alkyl halide will readily undergo S_N2 and E2, but not S_N1 and E1. Choice (B) also has a highly branched carbon chain, so it cannot undergo S_N2 In addition, OH⁻ is a very poor leaving group, so it will not readily undergo substitution. Choice (C) can be rejected because alkanes undergo neither elimination nor nucleophilic substitution. Finally, choice (D), a tertiary alkyl halide, has a highly branched carbon chain and an excellent leaving group—a bromide. It will not undergo S_N2, but can easily undergo E1, S_N1 and E2 reactions.

141. A You are presented with an unlabeled figure of a eukaryotic cell and asked to determine which of the four numbered structures would be most affected by a drug that inhibits ribosomal RNA synthesis. So basically, you have to know which structure is involved in the synthesis of ribosomal RNA. The nucleolus is the organelle responsible for ribosomal RNA synthesis, and in the figure, structure 1 is the nucleolus, and so choice (A) is correct. Structure 2 is the nucleus; structure 3 is the Golgi apparatus; and structure 4 is a mitochondrion. Therefore, choices (B), (C), and (D) are wrong, and choice (A) is the right answer.

142. D An exocrine gland is one that excretes its products into tubes or ducts that typically empty onto epithelial tissue, while an endocrine gland is one that releases hormones directly into the bloodstream. The pancreas functions both as an endocrine gland and an exocrine gland. As an endocrine gland, it produces and secretes three hormones: insulin, glucagon, and somatostatin. Insulin lowers blood glucose levels by stimulating the uptake of glucose into tissues, and its subsequent conversion into its storage form, glycogen. So, choice (B) is wrong. Choice (A) is incorrect because it is glucagon that raises blood glucose levels by stimulating the conversion of glycogen into glucose. Somatostatin suppresses both insulin and glucagon secretion. Choice (C) is incorrect because thyroid hormones are involved in the regulation of metabolic rate. As an exocrine gland, the pancreas secretes enzymes that are involved in protein, fat, and carbohydrate digestion; all of its exocrine products are secreted into the small intestine. Pancreatic amylase hydrolyzes starch to maltose; trypsin hydrolyzes peptide bonds and catalyzes that conversion of chymotrypsinogen to chymotrypsin; chymotrypsin and carboxypeptidase also hydrolyze peptide bonds; and finally, lipase hydrolyzes lipids. Thus, choice (D) is the correct answer.

143. C The cerebellum is part of the hindbrain, which is the posterior part of the brain and consists of the pons and the medulla oblongata, in addition to the cerebellum. The cerebellum receives sensory information from the visual and auditory systems, as well as information about the orientation of joints and muscles. In fact, one of the cerebellum's main functions is hand-eye coordination. It also receives information about the motor signals being initiated by the cerebrum. The cerebellum takes all of this information and integrates it to produce balance and unconscious coordinated movement. Damage to the cerebellum could damage any one of these functions. Total destruction of the cerebellum would eliminate all of them. Therefore, choice (C) is correct because destruction of a cat's cerebellum would seriously impair coordinated movement in the cat. Urine formation, choice (A), is the primary function of the kidneys, with a little bit of hormonal regulation to help things out. Choice (B), sense of smell, or olfaction, is a function of the cerebrum not the cerebellum, while thermoregulation, choice (D), is a function of the hypothalamus, which is a part of the cerebrum.

144. D A cell with a high intracellular potassium concentration is placed in a medium with a low potassium concentration and a high ATP concentration. The cell membrane is impermeable to potassium. If the cell were permeable to potassium, you would expect potassium to flow out of the cell, along its concentration gradient. This is clearly not the case: instead, the extracellular concentration of both the potassium and the ATP decreases, while the intracellular concentration of potassium increases. This implies that the potassium moved into the cell, across a membrane that is impermeable to it, and against its concentration gradient. What's the most likely explanation for this phenomenon? Choice (A) says that the potassium passively diffused into the cell, and choice (B) says that the potassium entered the cell by way of facilitated transport. Since both diffusion and facilitated transport occur along a substance's concentration gradient, not against it, both choices (A) and (B) must be incorrect. Furthermore, the potassium could not possibly diffuse across the membrane, because we know that the membrane is impermeable to it. And finally, neither of these choices accounts for the decrease in extracellular ATP concentration. Choice (C) sounds reasonable, except for two factors. First of all, we're told that the membrane is impermeable, yet ATP is not a very lipid-soluble complex with potassium; it enables the potassium to cross the lipid cell membrane and enter the cell. Second, there is no evidence to support the theory that ATP functions as a carrier molecule, shuttling potassium across cell membranes. ATP is the energy currency used by cells. Energy is stored in its high-energy phosphate bonds, and this energy is made available to cells when ATP is hydrolyzed to ADP and AMP. Thus, choice (C) is also incorrect. Choice (D), however, does make sense; it explains both the movement of potassium into the cell against its gradient, as well as the decreased extracellular ATP concentration. Active transport is the movement of a substance against its concentration gradient with the aid of carrier molecules and energy.

NOTES

NOTES

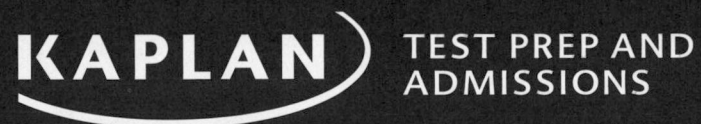

Tear-Out, Quick Reference Study Sheets for Biology, General Chemistry, Physics, and Organic Chemistry

The following MCAT Study Sheets are your one-stop resource for the key diagrams, charts, equations, and formulas that you are sure to see on the exam. This color-coded guide is separated into four MCAT subtopics: Biology, General Chemistry, Physics, and Organic Chemistry. Each topic features the most important highlights you will want to review in-between study sessions and before your test day. Carefully tear out the pages to create a light and portable on-the-go resource that you can use to study anytime, anywhere.

MCAT STUDY SHEET – BIOLOGY

THE CELL

FLUID MOSAIC MODEL AND MEMBRANE TRAFFIC

- Phospholipid bilayer with cholesterol and embedded proteins
- Exterior hydrophilic phosphoric acid region
- Interior hydrophobic fatty acid region

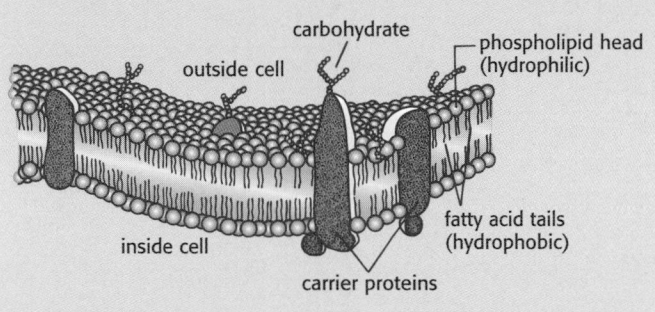

HOMEOSTASIS

HORMONAL REGULATION

Aldosterone

- stimulates Na^+ reabsorption and K^+ secretion, increasing water reabsorption, blood volume and blood pressure
- secreted from adrenal cortex
- is regulated by renin-angiotensin system

ADH

- increases collecting duct's permeability to water to increase water reabsorption
- is secreted from posterior pituitary with high [solute] in the blood

THE LIVER'S ROLES IN HOMEOSTASIS

1. gluconeogenesis
2. processing of nitrogenous wastes (urea)
3. detoxification of wastes/chemicals/drugs
4. storage of iron and vitamin B12
5. synthesis of bile and blood proteins
6. beta-oxidation of fatty acids to ketones
7. interconversion of carbs, fat, and amino acids

ENZYMES

REGULATION

- **Allosteric**: binding of an affector molecule at allosteric site.
- **Feedback inhibition**: end product inhibits an initial enzyme pathway
- **Reversible inhibition**: competitive inhibitors bind to active site; noncompetitive inhibitors to the allosteric site

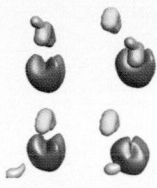

GLUCOSE CATABOLISM

Glycolysis occurs in the cell cytoplasm: $C_6H_{12}O_6 + 2ADP + 2P_i + 2NAD^+ \rightarrow 2Pyruvate + 2ATP + 2NADH + 2H^+ + 2H_2O$.

Fermentation occurs in anaerobic conditions. Pyruvate is converted into lactic acid (in muscle) or ethanol (in yeast).

Respiration occurs in aerobic conditions.

- **Pyruvate decarboxylation**: Pyruvate converted to acetyl CoA in the mitochondrial matrix.
- **Citric acid cycle**: Acetyl CoA enters, coenzymes exit.
- **Electron transport chain**: Coenzymes are oxidized, and energy is released as electrons are transferred from carrier to carrier.
- **Oxidative phosphorylation**: Electrochemical gradient caused by NADH and $FADH^2$ oxidation provides energy for ATP synthase to phosphorylate ADP into ATP.

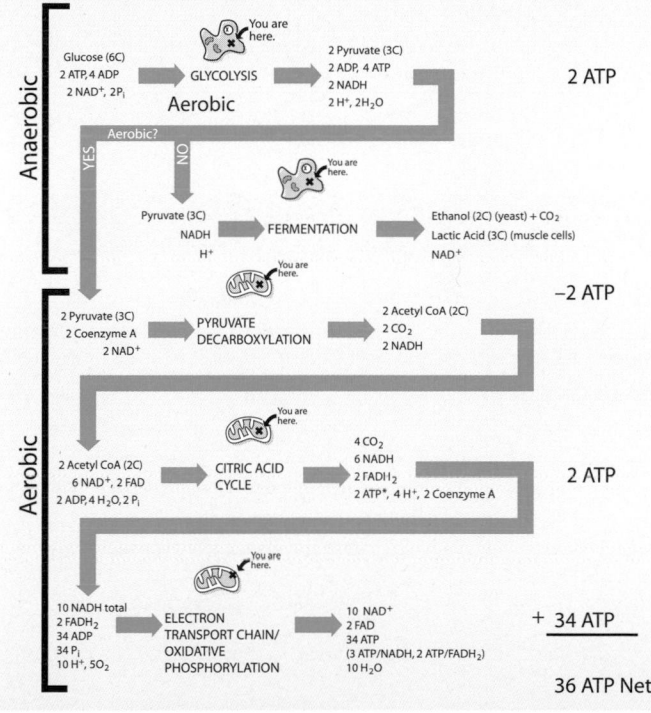

MUSCULOSKELETAL SYSTEM

Sarcomere

- contractile unit of the fibers in skeletal muscle
- contains thin actin and thick myosin filaments

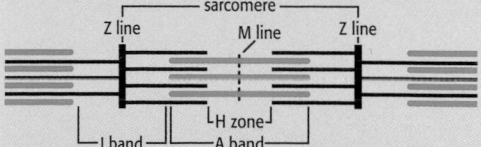

CONTRACTION

Initiation:

- Depolarization of a neuron leads to action potential.

BONE FORMATION AND REMODELLING

- Osteoblasts: builds bone
- Osteoclasts: breaks down bone
- Reformation: inorganic ions are absorbed from the blood for use in bone
- Degradation (Resorption): inorganic ions are released into the blood

ENDOCRINE SYSTEM

Direct hormones directly stimulate organs, tropic hormones stimulate other glands.
Mechanisms of hormone action: **Peptides** act via secondary messengers and **steroids** act via a hormone/receptor binding to DNA. Amino acid derivatives may do either.

Hormone	Source	Action
Follicle-stimulating (FSH)	Anterior pituitary	Stimulates follicle maturation; spermatogenesis
Luteinizing (LH)		Stimulates ovulation; testosterone synthesis
Adrenocorticotropic (ACTH)		Stimulates adrenal cortex to make and secrete glucocorticoids
Thyroid-stimulating (TSH)		Stimulates the thyroid to produce thyroid hormones
Prolactin		Stimulates milk production and secretion
Endorphins		Inhibit the perception of pain in the brain
Growth hormone		Stimulates bone and muscle growth/lipolysis
Oxytocin	Hypothalamus; stored in posterior pituitary	Stimulates uterine conteractions during labor, milk secretion during lactation
Vasopressin (ADH)		Stimulates water reabsorption in kidneys
Thyroid hormones (T_4, T_3)	Thyroid	Stimulate metabolic activity
Calcitonin		Decreases (tones down) blood calcium level
Parathyroid hormone	Parathyroid	Increases the blood calcium level
Glucocorticoids	Adrenal cortex	Increase blood glucose level and decrease protein synthesis
Mineralocorticoids		Increase water reabsorption in kidneys
Epinephrine, Norepinephrine	Adrenal medulla	Increases blood glucose level and heart rate
Glucagon	Pancreas	Stimulates conversion of glycogen to glucose in the liver, increases blood glucose
Insulin		Lowers blood glucose, increases glycogen stores
Somatostatin		Supresses secretion of glucagon and insulin
Testosterone	Testes	Maintains male secondary sexual characteristics
Estrogen	Ovary/Placenta	Maintains female secondary sexual characteristics
Progesterone		Promotes growth/maintenance of endometrium
Melatonin	Pineal	Unclear in humans
Atrial natriuretic peptide	Heart	Involved in osmoregulation and vasodilation
Thymosin	Thymus	Stimulates T lymphocyte development

REPRODUCTION

CELL DIVISION

- G_1: cell doubles its organelles and cytoplasm
- S: DNA replication
- G_2: same as G_1
- M: the cell divides in two
- Mitosis = PMAT
- Meiosis = PMAT × 2

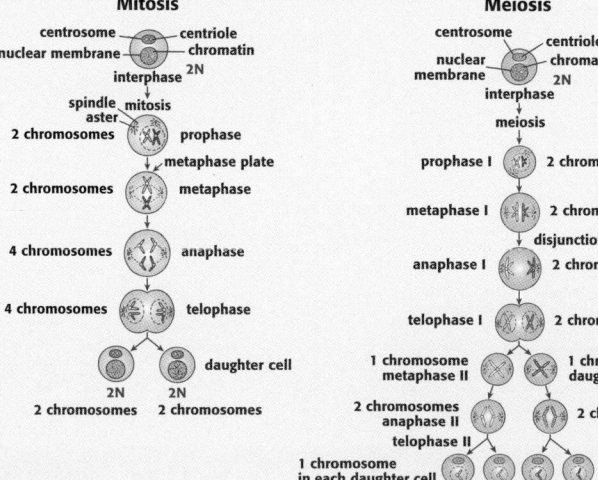

SEXUAL REPRODUCTION

Meiosis I:

- Two pairs of sister chromatids form tetrads during prophase I.
- Crossing over leads to genetic recombination in prophase I.

Meiosis II:

- Identical to mitosis, but no replication.
- Meiosis occurs in **spermatogenesis** (sperm formation) and **oogenesis** (egg formation).

FOUR STAGES OF EARLY DEVELOPMENT

cleavage: mitotic divisions
implantation: embryo implants during blastulation
gastrulation: ectoderm, endoderm, and mesoderm form
neurulation: germ layers develop a nervous system

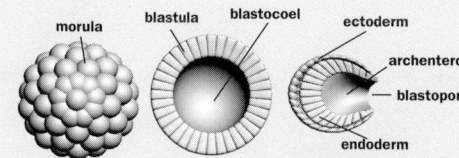

Ectoderm "Attract-o-derm"	Nervous system, epidermis, lens of eye, inner ear	Endoderm "Endernal" organs	Lining of digestive tract, lungs, liver and pancreas	Mesoderm "Means-o-derm"	Muscles, skeleton, circulatory system, gonads, kidney

DIGESTION

CARBOHYDRATE DIGESTION

Enzyme	Site of Production	Site of Function	Hydrolysis Reaction
Salivary amylase (ptyalin)	Salivary glands	Mouth	Starch → maltose
Pancreatic amylase	Pancreas	Small Intestine	Starch → maltose
Maltase	Intestinal glands	Small Intestine	Maltose → 2 glucoses
Sucrase	Intestinal glands	Small Intestine	Sucrose → glucose, fructose
Lactase	Intestinal glands	Small Intestine	Lactose → glucose, galactose

PROTEIN DIGESTION

Enzyme	Production Site	Function Site	Function
Pepsin	Gastric glands (chief cells)	Stomach	Hydrolyzes specific peptide bonds
Trypsin	Pancreas	Small Intestine	Hydrolyzes specific peptide bonds. Converts chymotrypsinogen to chymotrypsin
Chymotrypsin	Pancreas	Small Intestine	Hydrolyzes specific peptide bonds
Carboxypeptidase	Pancreas	Small Intestine	Hydrolyzes terminal peptide bond at carboxyl
Aminopeptidase	Intestinal glands	Small Intestine	Hydrolyzes terminal peptide bond at amino
Dipeptidases	Intestinal glands	Small Intestine	Hydrolyzes pairs of amino acids
Enterokinase	Intestinal glands	Small Intestine	Converts trypsinogen to trypsin

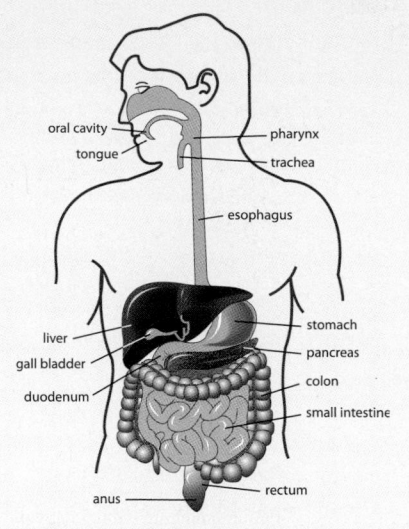

IMMUNE SYSTEM

- The body distinguishes between "self" and "nonself" (antigens)

HUMORAL IMMUNITY (specific defense)

B lymphocytes

memory cells
remember antigen,
speed up secondary
response

plasma cells
make and release antibodies
(**IgG, IgA, IgM, IgD, IgE**), which
induce antigen phagocytosis

- **Active immunity**: antibodies are produced during an immune response.
- **Passive immunity**: antibodies produced by one organism are transferred to another organism.

CELL-MEDIATED IMMUNITY

T lymphocytes

cytotoxic T cells
destroy cells directly

suppressor cells
regulate B and T cells to
decrease anti-antigen activity

helper T cells
activate B and T cells
and macrophages by
secreting lymphokines

memory cells

NONSPECIFIC IMMUNE RESPONSE

Includes skin, passages lined with cilia, macrophages, inflammatory response, and interferons (proteins that help prevent the spread of a virus).

LYMPHATIC SYSTEM

- lymph vessels meet at the thoracic duct in the upper chest and neck, draining into the veins of the cardiovascular system.
- vessels carry **lymph** (excess interstitial fluid), and capillaries (**lacteals**) collect fats by absorbing chylomicrons in the small intestine.
- **lymph nodes** are swellings along the vessels with phagocytic cells (leukocytes) that remove foreign particles from lymph.

CIRCULATION

BLOOD TYPING

Antigens are located on the surface of red blood cells

Blood type	RBC antigen	Antibodies	Donates to:	Receives From:
A	A	Anti-B	A, AB	A, O
B	B	Anti-A	B, AB	B, O
AB	A, B	None	AB only	All
O	None	Anti-A, B	All	O

Blood cells with Rh factor are Rh⁺ and produce no antibody. Rh⁻ lack antigen and produce an antibody.

MOLECULAR GENETICS

NUCLEIC ACID

- Basic unit: nucleotide (sugar, nitrogenous base, phosphate)
- DNA's sugar: deoxyribose. RNA's sugar: ribose.
- 2 types of bases: double-ringed purines (adenine, guanine) and single-ringed pyrimidines (cytosine, thymine, uracil).
- DNA double helix: antiparallel strands joined by base pairs (AT, GC).
- RNA is usually single-stranded: A pairs with U, not T.

TRANSCRIPTION REGULATION, PROKARYOTES

Regulated by the **operon**:

- structural genes: have DNA that codes for protein
- operator gene: repressor binding site
- promoter gene: RNA polyermase's 1st binding site
- Inducible systems need an inducer for transcription to occur. Repressible systems need a corepressor to inhibit transcription.

MUTATIONS

- **Point**: one nucleotide is substituted by another; they are silent if the sequence doesn't change.
- **Frameshift**: insertions or deletions shift reading frame. Protein doesn't form, or is nonfunctional.

VIRUSES

- acellular structures of double or single-stranded DNA or RNA in a protein coat.
- Lytic cycle: virus kills the host.
- Lysogenic cycle: virus enters host genome.

DNA REPLICATION

- **Semiconservative**: each new helix has an intact strand from the parent helix and a newly synthesized strand.

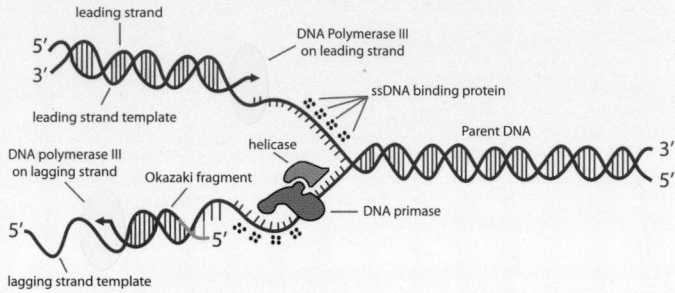

EUKARYOTIC PROTEIN SYNTHESIS

- **Transcription**: RNA polymerase synthesizes hnRNA using a DNA, "antisense strand" as a template.
- **Post-transcriptional processing**: introns are cut out of hnRNA, exons spliced to form mRNA.
- **Translation**: occurs on ribosomes in the cytoplasm.

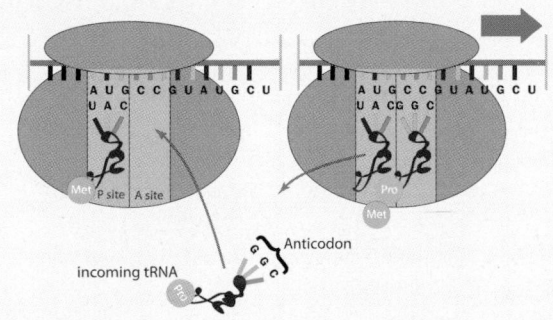

- **Post-translational modifications**: (i.e., disulfide bonds) made before the polypeptide becomes a functional protein.

EVOLUTION

- When frequencies are stable, the population is in Hardy-Weinberg equilibrium: no mutations, large population, random mating, no net migration, and equal reproductive success.

$$p + q = 1; p^2 + 2pq + q^2 = 1$$

p = freq. of dom. allele q = freq. of rec. allele

p^2 = freq of dom homozygotes

$2pq$ = freq of heterozygotes

q^2 = freq of recessive homozygotes

CLASSICAL GENETICS

- If both parents are Rr, the alleles separate to give a genotypic ratio of 1:2:1 and a phenotypic ratio of 3:1.

Law of independent assortment: Alleles of unlinked genes assort independently in meiosis.

- For two traits: AbBb parents will produce AB, Ab, aB, and ab gametes.
- The phenotypic ratio for this cross is 9:3:3:1.

STATISTICAL CALCULATIONS

- The probability of producing a genotype that requires multiple events to occur equals the *product* of the probability of each event.
- The probability of producing a genotype that can be the result of multiple events equals the *sum* of each probability.

GENETIC MAPPING

- Crossing over during meiosis I can unlink genes (Prophase I).
- Genes are most likely unlinked when far apart.
- One map unit is 1% recombinant frequency.

Given Recombination frequencies

X and Y: 8%

X and Z: 12%

Y and Z: 4%

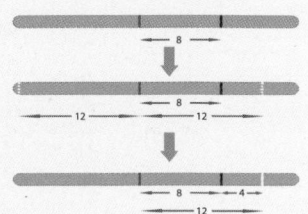

INHERITED DISORDERS in PEDIGREES

- Autosomal recessive: skips generations
- Autosomal dominant: appears in every generation
- X-linked (sex-linked): no male-to-male transmission, and more males are affected.

MCAT STUDY SHEET – GENERAL CHEMISTRY

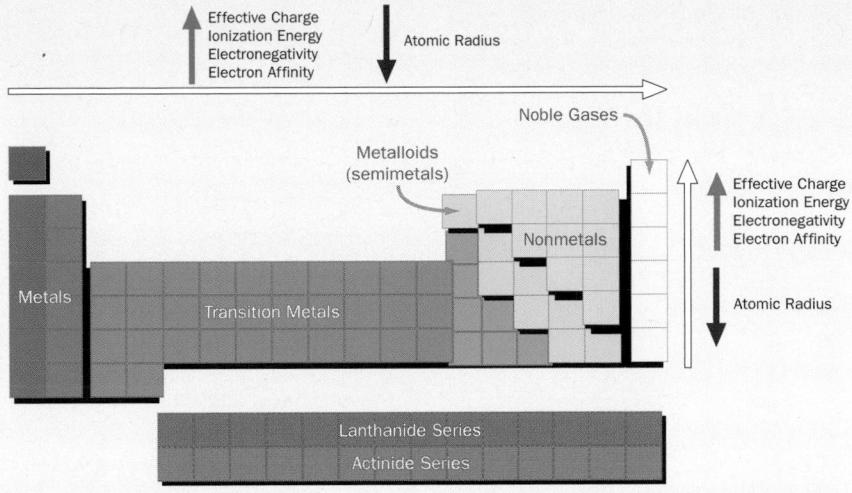

ATOMIC STRUCTURE

Atomic weight: the weight in grams of one mole (mol) of a given element and is expressed in terms of g/mol.

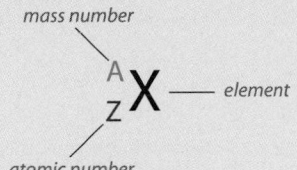

mass number

$$_{Z}^{A}X$$ — *element*

atomic number

A **mole** is a unit used to count particles and is represented by **Avogadro's number**, 6.022×10^{23} particles.

$$\text{Moles} = \frac{\text{grams}}{\text{atomic or molecular weight}}$$

Isotopes: For a given element, multiple species of atoms with the same number of protons (same atomic number) but different numbers of neutrons (different mass numbers).

Planck's quantum theory: Energy emitted as electromagnetic radiation from matter exists in discrete bundles called quanta.

Bohr's Model of the Hydrogen Atom

Angular momentum $= \dfrac{nh}{2\eta}$

Energy of electron $= E = \dfrac{-RH}{n^2}$

Electromagnetic energy of photons $= E = \dfrac{hc}{\lambda}$

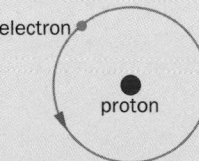

electron

proton

The group of hydrogen emission lines corresponding to transitions from upper levels $n > 2$ to $n = 2$ is known as the **Balmer series**, while the group corresponding to transitions between upper levels $n > 1$ to $n = 1$ is known as the **Lyman series.**

Absorption spectrum: Characteristic energy bands where electrons absorb energy.

Quantum Mechanical Model of Atoms

Heisenberg uncertainty principle: It is impossible to determine with perfect accuracy the momentum and the position of an electron simultaneously.

Quantum Numbers:

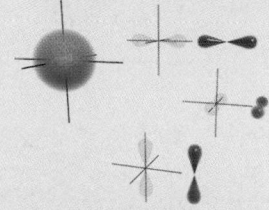

#	Character	Symbol	Value
1st	Shell	n	n
2nd	Subshell	l	From zero to n−1
3rd	Orbital	m_ℓ	Between l and −l
4th	Spin	m_s	½ or −½

Principal Quantum Number (n): The larger the integer value of n, the higher the energy level and radius of the electron's orbit. The maximum number of electrons in energy level n is $2n^2$.

Azimuthal Quantum Number (l): Refers to subshells, or sublevels. The four subshells corresponding to $l = 0$, 1, 2, and 3 are known as s, p, d and f, respectively. The maximum number of electrons that can exist within a subshell is given by the equation $4l+2$.

Magnetic Quantum Number (m_ℓ): This specifies the particular orbital within a subshell where an electron is highly likely to be found at a given point in time.

Spin Quantum Number (m_s): The spin of a particle is its intrinsic angular momentum and is a characteristic of a particle, like its charge.

Electron Configuration

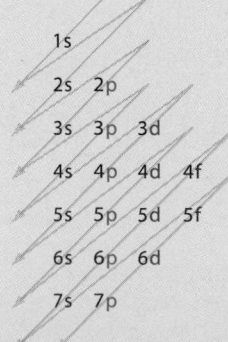

1s

2s 2p

3s 3p 3d

4s 4p 4d 4f

5s 5p 5d 5f

6s 6p 6d

7s 7p

Hund's rule: Within a given subshell, orbitals are filled such that there are a maximum number of half-filled orbitals with parallel spins.

Valence electrons: Electrons of an atom that are in its outer energy shell or that are available for bonding.

KINETICS & EQUILIBRIUM

Experimental Determination of Rate Law: The values of k, x, and y in the rate law equation (rate = k $[A]^x [B]^y$) must be determined experimentally for a given reaction at a given temperature. The rate is usually measured as a function of the initial concentrations of the reactants, A and B.

Efficiency of Reactions

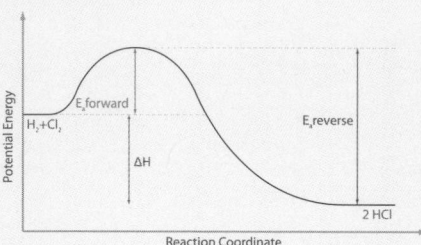

Factors affecting reaction rates: Reactant Concentrations, Temperature, Medium, Catalysts

Catalysts are unique substances that increase reaction rate without being consumed; they do this by lowering the activation energy.

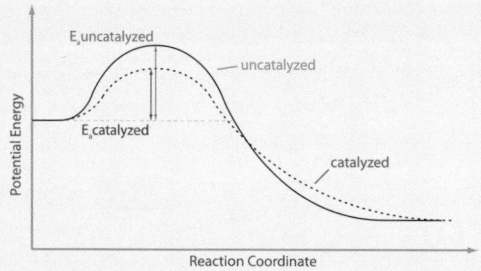

Law of Mass Action

$$a A + b B \rightleftharpoons c C + d D$$

$$K_c = \frac{[C]^c[D]^d}{[A]^a[B]^b}$$

K_c is the equilibrium constant. (c stands for concentration.)

Properties of The Equilibrium Constant

Pure solids/liquids don't appear in expression.

- K_{eq} is characteristic of a given system at a given temperature.
- If $K_{eq} \gg 1$, an equilibrium mixture of reactants and products will contain very little of the reactants compared to the products.
- If $K_{eq} \ll 1$, an equilibrium mixture of reactants and products will contain very little of the products compared to the reactants.
- If K_{eq} is close to 1, an equilibrium mixture of products and reactants will contain approximately equal amounts of the two.

A + B $\rightleftharpoons$ C + heat	
Will shift to **RIGHT**	Will shift to **LEFT**
1. if more A or B added	1. if more C added
2. if C taken away	2. if A or B taken away
3. if pressure applied or volume reduced (assuming A, B, and C are gases)	3 if pressure reduced or volume increased (assuming A, B, and C are gases)
4. if temperature reduced	4. if temperature increased

BONDING & CHEMICAL INTERACTIONS

Formal Charges

Formal charge = Valence electrons $- \frac{1}{2} N_{bonding} - N_{nonbonding}$

Intermolecular Forces

1. Dipole-Dipole Interactions: Polar molecules orient themselves such that the positive region of one molecule is close to the negative region of another molecule.

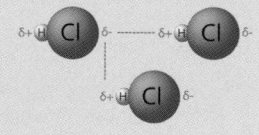

2. Hydrogen Bonding: The partial positive charge of the hydrogen atom interacts with the partial negative charge located on the electronegative atoms (F, O, N) of nearby molecules.

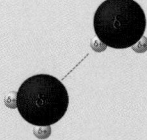

3. Dispersion Forces: The bonding electrons in covalent bonds may appear to be equally shared between two atoms, but at any particular point in time they will be located randomly throughout the orbital. This permits unequal sharing of electrons, causing rapid polarization and counter-polarization of the electron clouds of neighboring molecules, inducing the formation of more dipoles.

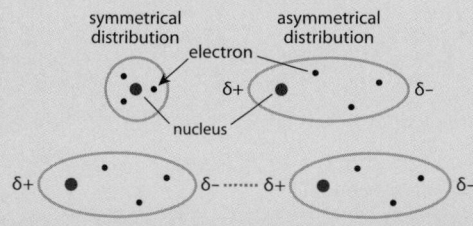

COMPOUNDS & STOICHIOMETRY

A **compound** is a pure substance that is composed of two or more elements in a fixed proportion.

A **mole** is the amount of a substance that contains the same number of particles that are found in a 12.000 g sample of carbon-12.

Combination Reactions: two or more reactants form one product.

$$S (s) + O_2 (g) \rightarrow SO_2 (g)$$

Decomposition Reactions: a compound breaks down into two or more substances, usually as a result of heating or electrolysis.

$$2HgO (s) \rightarrow 2Hg (l) + O_2 (g)$$

Single Displacement Reactions: an atom (or ion) of one compound is replaced by an atom of another element.

$$Zn (s) + CuSO_4 (aq) \rightarrow Cu (s) + ZnSO_4 (aq)$$

Double Displacement Reactions: also called metathesis reactions, elements from two different compounds displace each other to form two new compounds.

$$CaCl_2 (aq) + 2 AgNO_3 (aq) \rightarrow Ca(NO_3)_2 (aq) + 2 AgCl (s)$$

Net Ionic Equations: These types of equations are written showing only the species that actually participate in the reaction. So in the following equation,

$$Zn (s) + Cu^{2+} (aq) + SO_4^{2-} (aq) \rightarrow Cu (s) + Zn^{2+} (aq) + SO_4^{2-} (aq)$$

the spectator ion (SO_4^{2-}) does not take part in the overall reaction, but simply remains in solution throughout. The net ionic equation would be:

$$Zn (s) + Cu^{2+} (aq) \rightarrow Cu (s) + Zn^{2+} (aq)$$

Neutralization Reactions: These are a specific type of double displacements which occur when an acid reacts with a base to produce a solution of a salt and water:

$$HCl (aq) + NaOH (aq) \rightarrow NaCl (aq) + H_2O (l)$$

ACIDS AND BASES

Arrhenius Definition: An acid is a species that produces H+ (a proton) in an aqueous solution, and a base is a species that produces OH⁻ (a hydroxide ion).

Bronsted-Lowry Definition: An acid is a species that donates protons, while a base is a species that accepts protons.

Lewis Definition: An acid is an electron-pair acceptor, and a base is an electron-pair donor.

Properties of Acids and Bases

$$pH = -\log[H^+] = \log\left(\frac{1}{[H^+]}\right)$$

$$pH = -\log[OH^-] = \log\left(\frac{1}{[OH^-]}\right)$$

$$H_2O(l) \rightleftharpoons H^+(aq) + OH^-(aq)$$

$$K_w = [H^+][OH^-] = 10^{-14}$$

$$pH + pOH = 14$$

Weak Acids and Bases

$$HA(aq) + H_2O(l) \rightleftharpoons H_3O^+(aq) + A^-(aq)$$

$$K_a = \frac{[H_3O^+][A^-]}{[HA]}$$

$$K_b = \frac{[B^+][OH^-]}{[BOH]}$$

Salt Formation: Acids and bases may react with each other, forming a salt and (often, but not always) water in a neutralization reaction.

$$HA + BOH \rightarrow BA + H_2O$$

Titration and Buffers

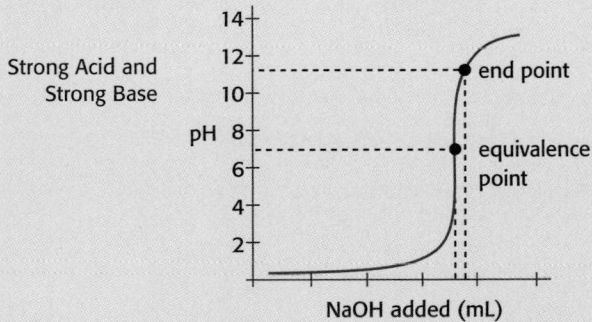

Strong Acid and Strong Base

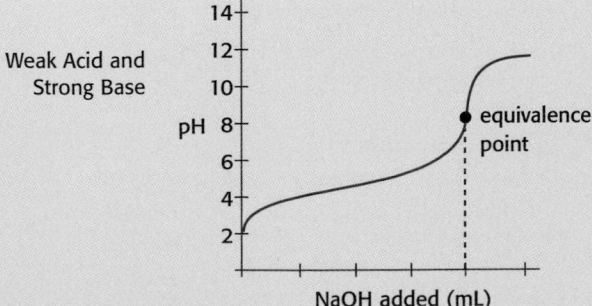

Weak Acid and Strong Base

Titration is a procedure used to determine the molarity of an acid or base by reacting a known volume of a solution of unknown concentration with a known volume of a solution of known concentration.

ACIDS AND BASES (cont.)

Henderson-Hasselbalch equation is used to estimate the pH of a solution in the buffer region where the concentrations of the species and its conjugate are present in approximately equal concentrations.

$$pH = pK_a + \log \frac{[\text{conjugate base}]}{[\text{weak acid}]}$$

$$pOH = pK_b + \log \frac{[\text{conjugate acid}]}{[\text{weak base}]}$$

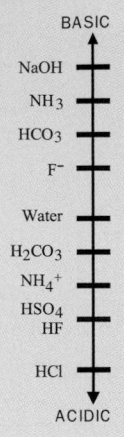

THE GAS PHASE

1 atm = 760 mm Hg = 760 torr

Do not confuse STP with standard conditions—the two standards involve different temperatures and are used for different purposes. STP (0°C or 273 K) is generally used for gas law calculations; standard conditions (25°C or 298 K) is used when measuring standard enthalpy, entropy, Gibbs free energy, and voltage.

Boyle's Law

$$PV = k \text{ or } P_1V_1 = P_2V_2$$

Law of Charles and Gay-Lussac

$$\frac{V}{T} = k \text{ or } \frac{V_1}{T_1} = \frac{V_2}{T_2}$$

Avagadro's Principle

$$\frac{n}{V} = k \text{ or } \frac{n_1}{V_1} = \frac{n_2}{V_2}$$

Ideal Gas Law

$$PV = nRT$$

Deviations due to Pressure: As the pressure of a gas increases, the particles are pushed closer and closer together. At moderately high pressure a gas' volume is less than would be predicted by the ideal gas law, due to intermolecular attraction.

Deviations due to Temperature: As the temperature of a gas decreases, the average velocity of the gas molecules decreases, and the attractive intermolecular forces become increasingly significant. As the temperature of a gas is reduced, intermolecular attraction causes the gas to have a smaller volume than would be predicted.

SOLUTIONS

Units of Concentration

Percent Composition by Mass: $= \frac{\text{Mass of solute}}{\text{Mass of solution}} \times 100 \, (\%)$

Mole Fraction: $\frac{\text{\# of mol of compound}}{\text{total \# of moles in system}}$

Molarity: $\frac{\text{\# of mol of solute}}{\text{liter of solution}}$

Molality: $\frac{\text{\# of mol of solute}}{\text{kg of solvent}}$

Normality: $\frac{\text{\# of gram equivalent weights of solute}}{\text{liter of solution}}$

PHASES & PHASE CHANGES

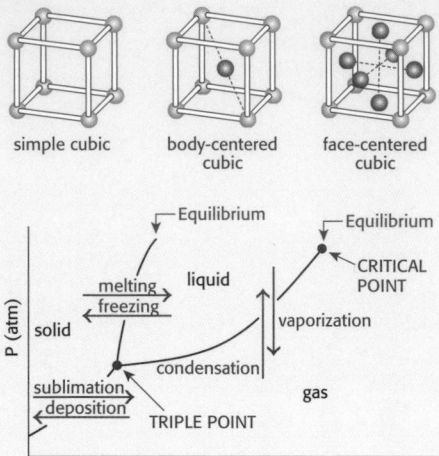

simple cubic   body-centered cubic   face-centered cubic

Colligative Properties: These are physical properties derived solely from the number of particles present, not the nature of those particles. These properties are usually associated with dilute solutions.

Freezing Point Depression

$$\Delta T_f = K_f m$$

Boiling Point Elevation

$$\Delta T_b = K_b m$$

Osmotic Pressure

$$\Pi = MRT$$

Vapor-pressure Lowering (Raoult's Law)

$$P_A = X_A P^\circ_A;\ P_B = X_B P^\circ_B$$

Solutions that obey Raoult's Law are called ideal solutions.

Graham's Law of Diffusion and Effusion

Diffusion: occurs when gas molecules diffuse through a mixture.

Effusion: is the flow of gas particles under pressure from one compartment to another through a small opening.

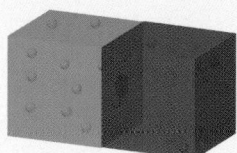

Effusion

Both diffusion and effusion have the same formula:

$$\frac{r_1}{r_2} = \left(\frac{MM_2}{MM_1}\right)^{\frac{1}{2}}$$

REDOX REACTIONS & ELECTROCHEMISTRY

Oxidation: loss of electrons

Reduction: gain of electrons

Oxidizing agent: causes another atom to undergo oxidation, and is itself reduced.

Reducing agent: causes another atom to be reduced, and is itself oxidized.

THERMOCHEMISTRY

Constant-volume and constant-pressure calorimetry: used to indicate conditions under which the heat changes are measured.

$q = mc\Delta T$, where q is the heat absorbed or released in a given process, m is the mass, c is the specific heat, and ΔT is the change in temperature.

States and State Functions: are described by the macroscopic properties of the system. These are properties whose magnitude depends only on the initial and final states of the system, and not on the path of the change.

Enthalpy (H): is used to express heat changes at constant pressure.

Standard Heat of Formation (ΔH°_f): the enthalpy change that would occur if one mole of a compound were formed directly from its elements in their standard states.

Standard Heat of Reaction (ΔH°_{rxn}): the hypothetical enthalpy change that would occur if the reaction were carried out under standard conditions.

$$\Delta H^\circ_{rxn} = \text{(sum of } \Delta H^\circ_{rxn} \text{ of products)} - \text{(sum of } \Delta H^\circ_{rxn} \text{ of reactants)}$$

Hess's Law: states that enthalpies of reactions are additive.

The reverse of any reaction has an enthalpy of the same magnitude as that of the forward reaction, but its sign is opposite.

Bond Dissociation Energy: an average of the energy required to break a particular type of bond in one mole of gaseous molecules:

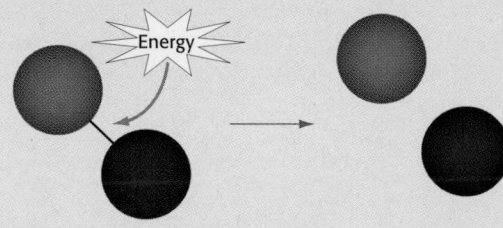

Entropy (S) the measure of the disorder, or randomness, of a system.

$$\Delta S_{universe} = \Delta S_{system} + \Delta S_{surroundings}$$

Gibbs Free Energy (G): combines the two factors which affect the spontaneity of a reaction—changes in enthalpy, ΔH, and changes in entropy, ΔS.

$$\Delta G = \Delta H - T\Delta S$$

if ΔG is negative, the rxn is spontaneous

if ΔG is positive, the rxn is not spontaneous

if ΔG is zero, the system is in a state of equilibrium; thus, $\Delta G = 0$ and $\Delta H = T\Delta S$

ΔH	ΔS	Outcome
−	+	Spontaneous at all temps.
+	−	Nonspontaneous at all temps.
+	+	Spontaneous only at high temps.
−	−	Spontaneous only at low temps.

Reaction Quotient (Q): Once a reaction commences, the standard state conditions no longer hold. For the reaction,

$$a\,A + b\,B \rightleftharpoons c\,C + d\,D$$

$$Q = \frac{[C]^c[D]^d}{[A]^a[B]^b}$$

MCAT STUDY SHEET – PHYSICS

KINEMATICS

Displacement (Δx): the change in position that goes in a straight-line path from the initial position to the final; it is independent of the path taken (SI unit: m)

Average velocity: $v = \dfrac{\Delta x}{\Delta t}$ (SI units: m/s)

Acceleration: the rate of change of an object's velocity; it is a vector quantity: $a = \dfrac{\Delta v}{\Delta t}$ (SI units: m/s^2)

Linear Motion

$v = v_0 + at$

$\Delta x = v_0 t + \frac{1}{2} at^2$

$v^2 = v_0^2 + 2a\Delta x$

$v_{avg} = \left(\dfrac{v_o + v}{2}\right)$

$\Delta x = vt = \left(\dfrac{v_o + v}{2}\right)t$

- When solving for time, there will be two values for t; when the projectile is initially launched and when it impacts the ground.
- To find max height, remember that the vertical velocity of the projectile is 0 at the highest point of the path.

Projectile Motion

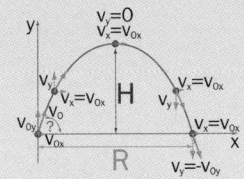

- vertical component of velocity $= v \sin \theta$
- horizontal component of velocity $= v \cos \theta$

Frictional Forces

Static Friction (f_s): is the force that must be overcome to set an object in motion. It has the formula: $0 \le f_s \le \mu_s N$

Kinetic Friction (f_k): opposes the motion of objects moving relative to each other. It has the formula: $f_k = \mu_k N$

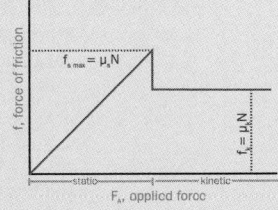

WORK, ENERGY & MOMENTUM

Work: For a constant force F acting on an object that moves through a distance d, the work is $W = Fd \cos\theta$. (For a force perpendicular to the displacement, $W = 0$.) [SI unit: Joule = N·m]

Power: the rate at which work is performed, and is given by:

$$P = \frac{w}{t} \text{ (SI unit: Watt = J/s)}$$

Mechanical Energy

Energy is a scalar quantity (SI unit: Joule).

Kinetic energy: the energy associated with moving objects. It is given by:

$$KE = \frac{1}{2}mv^2$$

Potential energy: the energy associated with a body's position. Gravitational potential energy of an object is due to the force of gravity acting on it, and it is expressed as: $U = mgh$

Total Mechanic Energy

$$E = U + K$$

Mechanical energy is conserved when the sum of kinetic and potential energies remains constant

Work–Energy Theorem

Relates the work performed by all forces acting on a body in a particular time interval to the change in kinetic energy at that time: The expression is:

$$W = \Delta KE$$

Conservation of Energy

When there are no nonconservative forces (e.g., friction) acting on a system, the total mechanical energy remains constant: $\Delta E = \Delta K + \Delta U = 0$

Momentum: a vector quantity. It is given by:

$$p = mv$$

	Before	After
Momentum:	$m_1 v_i$	$(m_1 + m_2)v_f$
Kinetic energy:	$\frac{1}{2}m_1 v_i^2$	$\frac{1}{2}(m_1 + m_2)v_f^2$
Conservation of momentum:	$m_1 v_i = (m_1 + m_2)v_f$	

NEWTON'S LAW

Newton's First Law (Law of Inertia): a body in a state of motion or at rest will remain in that state unless acted upon by a net force

Newton's Second Law: when a net force is applied to a body of mass m, the body will be accelerated in the same direction as the force applied to the mass. This is expressed by the formula $F = ma$ (SI unit: Newton (N) = kg·m/s^2).

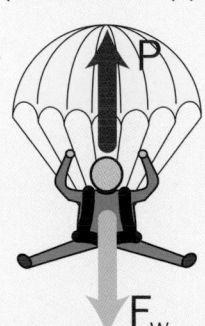

- $F_{gravity} > F_{parachute}$: person accelerates downward;
- $F_g = F_{parachute}$: terminal velocity is reached (person travels at constant velocity).

Newton's Third Law: if body A exerts a force on body B, then B will exert a force back onto A that is equal in magnitude, but opposite in direction. This can be expressed as, $F_b = -F_a$.

Newton's Law of Gravitation: All forms of matter experience an attractive force to other forms of matter in the universe.

The magnitude of the force is represented by: $F = \dfrac{Gm_1 m_2}{r^2}$.

- **Mass (m):** a scalar quantity that measures a body's inertia
- **Weight (W):** a vector quantity that measures a body's gravitational attraction to the earth ($W = mg$)

Uniform Circular Motion:

$a_c = \dfrac{v^2}{r}$

$F_c = \dfrac{mv^2}{r}$

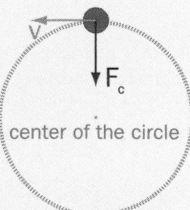

center of the circle

THERMODYNAMICS

Specific Heat

$Q = mc\Delta T$ (Mnemonic: looks like MCAT)

- can only be used to find Q when the object does not change phase
- $Q > 0$ means heat is gained, $Q < 0$ means heat is lost [SI Units: Joules or calories]

Heat of Transformation: the quantity of heat required to change the **phase** of 1 kg of a substance.

$Q = mL$ (phase changes are isothermal processes)

System Work

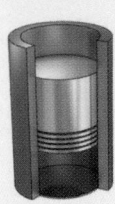 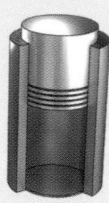

- When the piston expands, work is done by the system ($W > 0$).
- When the piston compresses the gas, work is done on the system ($W < 0$).
- The area under a P vs. V curve is the amount of work done in a system.

First Law of Thermodynamics: $\Delta U = Q - W$

Process	First Law Becomes
Adiabatic ($Q = 0$)	$\Delta U = -W$
Constant Volume ($W = 0$)	$\Delta U = Q$
Closed Cycle ($\Delta U = 0$)	$Q = W$

Second Law of Thermodynamics:
In any thermodynamic process that moves from one state of equilibrium to another, the entropy of the system and environment together will either increase or remain unchanged.

FLUIDS & SOLIDS

Density $(\rho) = \dfrac{m}{v}$ [SI units: kg/m³]

Specific gravity $= \dfrac{\rho_{substance}}{\rho_{water}}$ [no units]

$$\rho_{water} = 10^3 \text{ kg/m}^3$$

Weight (W) $= \rho g V$

Pressure: a scalar quantity defined as force per unit area:
$P = \dfrac{F}{A}$ [SI units: Pascal = N/m²]

- For static fluids of uniform density in a sealed vessel, pressure: $P = \rho g h$
- **Absolute pressure** in a fluid due to gravity somewhere below the surface is given by the equation $P = P_o + \rho g h$.
- **Gauge pressure:** $P_g = P_{abs} - P_{environment}$

Continuity Equation: $v_1 A_1 = v_2 A_2$

Bernoulli's Equation: $P + \dfrac{1}{2}\rho v^2 + \rho g h = \text{constant}$

Pascal's Principle

- A change in the pressure applied to an enclosed fluid is transmitted undiminished to every portion of the fluid and to the walls of the containing vessel.

$\Delta P = \dfrac{F_1}{A_1} = \dfrac{F_2}{A_2}$ and $W = F_1 d_1 = F_2 d_2$

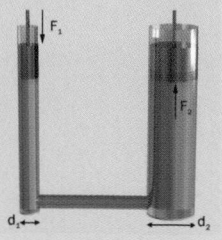

PERIODIC MOTION AND WAVES

Wave Formulas

$f = \dfrac{1}{T}$

$v = f\lambda$

	mass-spring	Simple pendulum
Force constant (k)	Spring constant (k)	mg/L
ang. freq. ω	$\sqrt{\dfrac{k}{m}}$	$\sqrt{\dfrac{g}{L}}$
frequency f	$\dfrac{1}{T}$ or $\dfrac{\omega}{2\pi}$	$\dfrac{1}{T}$ or $\dfrac{\omega}{2\pi}$
Kinetic energy K	$\dfrac{1}{2}mv^2$	$\dfrac{1}{2}mv^2$
K_{max} occurs at	$X = 0$	$\theta = 0$ (vertical position)
potential energy U	$\dfrac{1}{2}kx^2$	mgh
U_{max} occurs at	$x = \pm x$	Max value of θ
max acceleration	$x = \pm x$	Max value of θ

OPTICS

Spherical Mirrors

Mirror Equation: $\dfrac{1}{i} + \dfrac{1}{o} = \dfrac{1}{f} = \dfrac{2}{r}$

- Any of units of distance may be used, but all units used must be the same.

Concave Mirrors

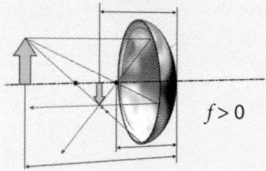

$f > 0$

- If an object is placed inside the focal length of a concave mirror, the image formed is behind the mirror, enlarged and virtual.

Convex Mirrors

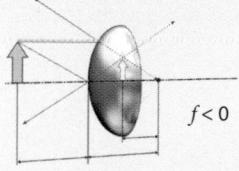

$f < 0$

- Regardless of the position of the object, a convex mirror forms only a virtual erect image.

Thin Spherical Lenses

Lens Equation: $\dfrac{1}{f} = \dfrac{1}{o} + \dfrac{1}{i}$

Converging Lenses

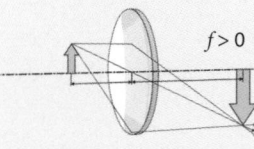

$f > 0$

- For an object beyond the focal point, the image formed is real and inverted.
- For an object inside the focal length, the image formed is virtual, erect and enlarged.
- No image at focal point.

Diverging Lenses

Magnification (m) $= \dfrac{-i}{o}$

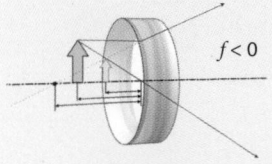

$f < 0$

- $|m| < 1$ image reduced; $|m| > 1$ image enlarged; $|m| = 1$ image same size
- Inverted image has a negative m, erect image has a positive m.

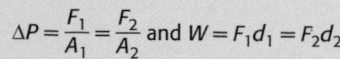

MAGNETISM

The Magnetic Field (B)

Magnetic fields are created by permanent magnets and moving charges.

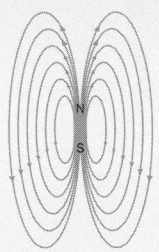

Magnetic field lines depict the direction a compass needle would point if placed in the field from the North Pole to the South Pole [SI Units = Tesla(T) = N·s/m·C]

Force on a Moving Charge

A charge moving in a magnetic field experiences a force exerted on it.

$F = qvB\sin\theta$

The magnetic force is zero when charges move parallel or antiparallel to the magnetic field.

Right-Hand Rule for Finding Direction of Force

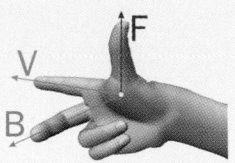

Note that the right-hand rule gives the direction of magnetic force exerted on a proton. The direction of force on an electron is simply in the opposite direction of the force on a proton.

Force on a Current-Carrying Wire

$F = iLB\sin\theta$

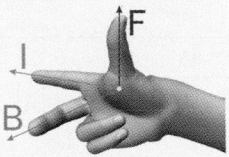

$X \rightarrow$ represents B fields pointing into the page, $\bullet \rightarrow$ represents B fields pointed out of the page.

Special Cases

Center of Wire Loop

$B = \dfrac{\mu_0 i}{2r}$

Around a Straight Wire

$B = \dfrac{\mu_0 i}{2\pi r}$

Right-Hand Rule for Direction of B Field produced by Current-Carrying Wires

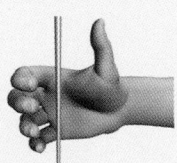

- Right thumb points in the direction of current flow
- Wrap your fingers around the wire as if you were grabbing it with your palm
- The direction that the fingers curl is the direction of the magnetic field

Wave Superposition
Constructive

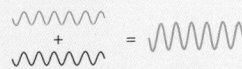

Waves can also be shifted with respect to one another by other fractions of a cycle, such as $\frac{1}{4}\lambda$, or 90° out of phase.

Destructive

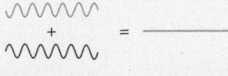

SOUND

Sound propagates through a deformable medium by the oscillation of particles along the direction of the wave's motion.

Intensity (I) $= P/A$ [SI units: W/m²]

Sound Level (β) $= 10 \log (I/I_0)$ [unit = decibel = dβ]

(Note that an increase in intensity by a factor of 100, for instance 40 W/m² to 4,000 W/m², corresponds to an increase in 20 dβ)

Beats occur when two waves that have slightly different frequencies are superimposed:

$f_{beat} = |f_1 - f_2|$

Refraction

$n = \dfrac{c}{v}$ (speed of light = 3×10^8 m/s)

Snell's Law: $n_1 \sin\theta_1 = n_2 \sin\theta_2$ when $n_2 > n_1$, light bends toward normal, when $n_2 < n_1$, light bends away from normal

Doppler Effect

- When a source and a detector move relative to one another, the perceived frequency of the sound received differs from the actual frequency emitted even though the source velocity and frequency is unchanged

$$f' = f \frac{(v \pm v_D)}{(v \pm v_S)}$$

ATOMIC AND NUCLEAR PHENOMENA

Blackbody Radiation

A **blackbody** is an object that absorbs all incident electromagnetic radiation upon it and emits energy that is characteristic to the system itself.

Wien's Displacement Law: $\lambda_{peak}T = $ constant

Stefan-Boltzmann Law: $E_{total} = \sigma T^4$

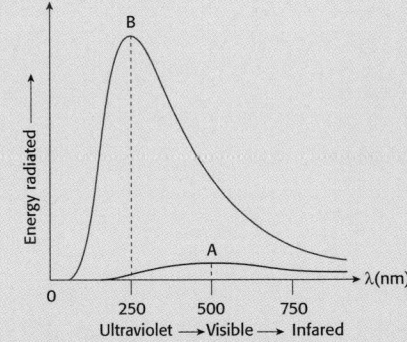

Photoelectric Effect

$E = hf = \dfrac{hc}{\lambda}$

$K = hf - W$

K is the maximum kinetic energy of ejected electron; W is the minimum energy required to eject an electron).

Nuclear Binding Energy

Mass defect: the difference between the sum of the masses of nucleons in the nucleus and the mass of the nucleus. The mass defect results from the conversion of matter to energy, embodied by: $E = mc^2$. This energy is the **binding energy** that holds nucleons within the nucleus.

Exponential Decay

Half Life

$n = n_0 e^{-\cdot t}$

Alpha Decay

$^{238}_{92}U \rightarrow {}^{234}_{90}Th + {}^4_2He$

Beta Minus Decay

$^{137}_{55}Cs \rightarrow {}^{137}_{56}Ba + {}^0_{-1}e^- + \overline{v}$

Beta Plus Decay

$^{22}_{11}Cs \rightarrow {}^{22}_{10}Ne + {}^0_{+1}e^+ + v$

DC AND AC CIRCUITS

Direct Current

Current: the flow of electric charge. Current is given by:

$I = \frac{\Delta q}{\Delta t}$ [SI units: Amp (A) = C/s]

(The direction of current is the direction positive charge would flow, or from high to low potential.)

Ohm's Law and Resistance

$V = IR$ (can be applied to entire circuit or individual resistors)

Resistance: opposition to the flow of charge. $R = \frac{\rho L}{A}$ (Resistance increases with increasing temperatures with most conductors)
[SI Units: Ohm (Ω)]

Circuit Laws

Kirchoff's Laws:

1. At any junction within a circuit, the sum of current flowing into that point must equal the current leaving.
2. The sum of voltage sources equals the sum of voltage drops around a closed circuit loop.

Alternating Current

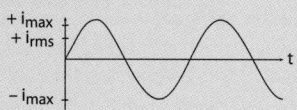

$V_{rms} = \frac{V_{max}}{\sqrt{2}}$

$I_{rms} = \frac{V_{max}}{\sqrt{2}}$

Series Circuits

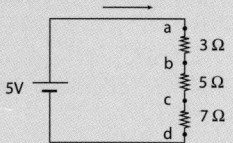

$R_{eff} = R_1 + R_2 + R_3 \ldots$
$V_{eff} = V_1 + V_2 + V_3 \ldots$
$I_{eff} = I_1 = I_2 = I_3 \ldots$

Parallel Circuits

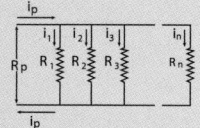

$1/R_{eff} = 1/R_1 + 1/R_2 + 1/R_3$
$V_{eff} = V_1 = V_2 = V_3 = \ldots$
$I_{eff} = I_1 + I_2 + I_3 + \ldots$

Power Dissipated by Resistors

$P = IV = \frac{V^2}{R} = I^2 R$

Capacitors

Capacitance: the ability to store charge per unit voltage.
It is given by: $C = \frac{Q}{V}$.

$C = \kappa \frac{\varepsilon_0 A}{d}$

Capacitors in parallel add
$C_{eq} = C_1 + C_2 + C_3$

Energy Stored by Capacitors:

$U = \frac{1}{2}QV = \frac{1}{2}CV^2 = \frac{1}{2}Q^2/C$

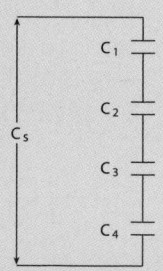

Capacitors in series add as reciprocals
$\frac{1}{C_{eq}} = \frac{1}{C_1} + \frac{1}{C_2} + \frac{1}{C_3} \ldots$

ELECTROSTATICS

Coulomb's Law

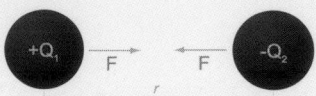

$F = \frac{kq_1q_2}{r^2}$ [SI units: Newtons]

Electric field

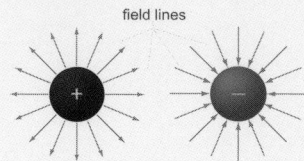

field lines

$E = \frac{F}{q} = \frac{kq}{r^2}$ [SI units: N/C or V/m]

- A positive point charge will move in the same direction as the electric field vector; a negative charge will move in the opposite direction.

Electric Potential Energy (U)

The electric potential energy of a charge q at a point in space is the amount of work required to move it from infinity to the point.

$U = q\Delta V = qEd = \frac{kq_1Q}{r}$ [SI units: V or J/C]

Electric Dipoles

- p is the dipole moment ($p = qd$).
- The dipole feels no translational force, but experiences a torque about the center causing it to rotate, so that the dipole moment aligns with the electric field.

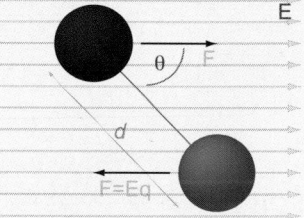

Electric Potential

The amount of work required to move a positive test charge q_0 from infinity to a particular point divided by the test charge:
$V = \frac{W}{q_0}$ [SI units: Volt = J/C]

Potential Difference (Voltage)

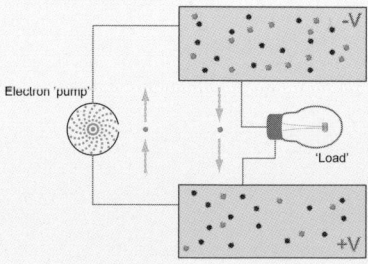

Voltage $(V) = \frac{w}{q} = \frac{kq}{r}$ [SI units: Volt = J/C]

- When two oppositely charged parallel plates are separated by a distance d, an electric field is created, and a potential difference exists between the plates, given by: $V = Ed$.

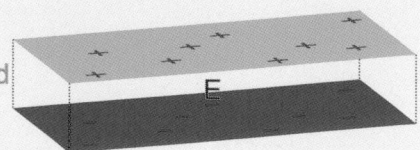

MCAT STUDY SHEET – ORGANIC CHEMISTRY

NOMENCLATURE

1. Find the longest carbon chain containing the principle functional group (highest priority groups are generally more oxidized).
2. Number the carbon chain so that the principle functional group gets lowest number (1).
3. Proceed to number the chain so that the lowest set of numbers is obtained for the substituents.
4. Name the substituents and assign each a number.
5. Complete the name by listing substituents in alphabetical order, place commas between numbers and dashes between numbers and words.

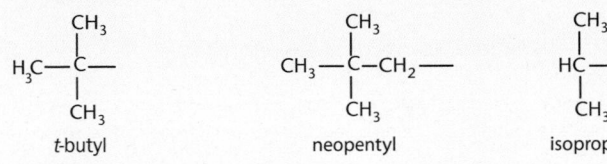

t-butyl   neopentyl   isopropyl

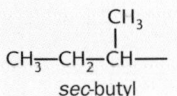

sec-butyl   isobutyl

Functional Group	Suffix	Functional Group	Suffix
Carboxylic Acid	-oic acid	Ketone	-one
Ester	-oate	Thiol	-thiol
Acyl halide	-oyl halide	Alcohol	-ol
Amide	-amide	Amine	-amine
Nitrile/Cyanide	-nitrile	Imine	-imine
Aldehyde	-al	Ether	-ether

ISOMERS

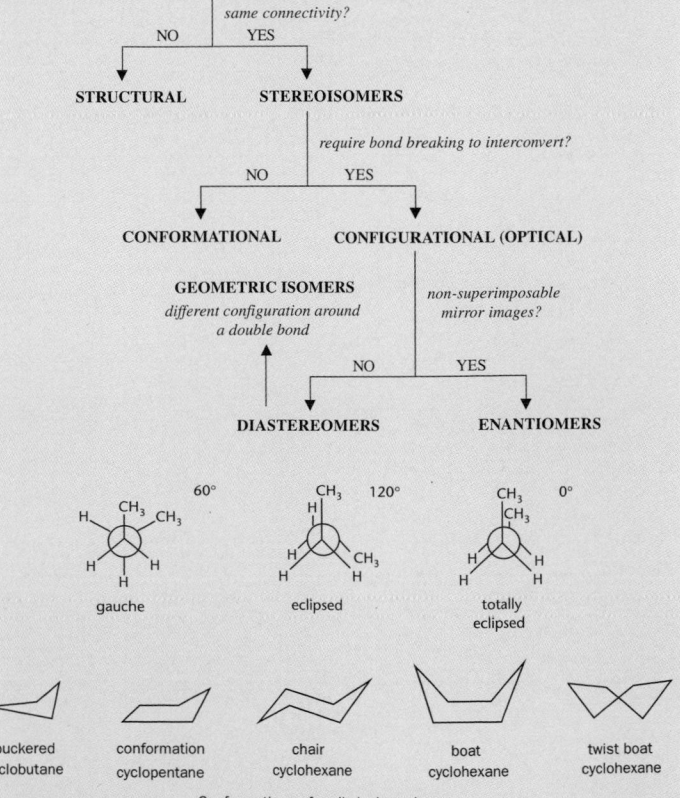

Conformations of cyclic hydrocarbons

BONDING

Bond order	single	double	triple
Bond type	sigma	sigma	sigma
		pi	2 pi
Hybridization	sp^3	sp^2	sp
Angles	109.5°	120°	180°
Example	C–C	C=C	C≡C

ALKANES

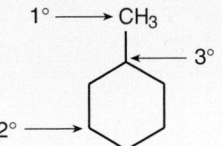

Free radical halogenation

- Initiation
- Propagation
- Termination

Combustion

$$C_3H_8 + 5O_2 \rightarrow 3CO_2 + 4H_2O + heat$$

Nucleophilicity and Basicity

$$RO^- > HO^- > RCO_2^- > ROH > H_2O$$

Nucleophilicity, size, and polarity

$$CN^- > I^- > RO^- > HO^- > Br^- > Cl^- > F^- > H_2O$$

Leaving groups (weak bases best)

$$I^- > Br^- > Cl^- > F^-$$

S_N1	S_N2
2 steps	1 step
Favored in polar protic solvents	Favored in polar aprotic solvents
3° > 2° > 1° > methyl	Methyl > 1° > 2° > 3°
Rate = k[RX]	Rate = k[Nu][RX]
Racemic products	Optically active and inverted products
Strong nucleophile not required	Favored with strong nucleophile

AMINO ACIDS, PEPTIDES, & PROTEINS

Amino acids have four substituents: amine group, carboxyl group, hydrogen, and R group. Amino acids are **amphoteric**—they can act as either acids or bases and often take the form of **zwitterions** (dipolar ions).

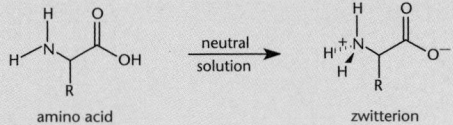

amino acid   neutral solution   zwitterion

Structure

Primary: sequence of amino acids
Secondary: α-helix, β-pleated sheet
Tertiary: disulfide bridges, hydrophobic/hydrophilic interactions
Quaternary: arrangement of polypeptides

Henderson–Hasselbalch Equation

$$pH = pK_a + \log [\text{conj. base}]/[\text{conj. acid}]$$

ALKYNES

Alkynes have a terminal hydrogen that is appreciably more acidic than hydrogens on alkanes and alkenes.

Synthesis via double elimination of geminal or vicinal dihalide

$$\xrightarrow[\text{Base}]{\text{Heat}} \quad CH_3C \equiv CCH_3 \quad + \quad 2HBr$$

Oxidation with $KMnO_4$, O_3

$$\xrightarrow[\text{2) } H^+]{\text{1) } KMnO_4, OH^-}$$

$$\xrightarrow[\text{2) } H_2O]{\text{1) } O_3, CCl_4}$$

Reduction with Lindlar's Catalyst or liquid ammonia

$CH_3C \equiv CCH_3 \xrightarrow[\substack{\text{Quinoline} \\ \text{(Lindlar's catalyst)}}]{H_2, \text{ Pd/BaSO}_4}$ cis-2-butene

2-butyne

$CH_3C \equiv CCH_3 \xrightarrow{\text{Na, NH}_3\text{(liq)}}$ trans-2-butene

2-butyne

Free radical addition

$$CH_3CH_2C \equiv CH + X \cdot \longrightarrow$$

Electrophilic addition (anti orientation)

$$CH_3C \equiv CH \xrightarrow{Br_2}$$

$$CH_3C \equiv CH \xrightarrow{2Br_2} CH_3CBr_2CBr_2H$$

Hydroboration (cis alkene formed)

$$3H_3CC \equiv CCH_3 + \tfrac{1}{2} B_2H_6 \longrightarrow$$

$$\xrightarrow{CH_3COOH} 3$$

ALKENES

Cis isomers have higher boiling points than trans isomers due to their net dipole moment. Trans isomers have higher melting points than cis isomers due to more effective arrangement, more efficient packing.

Catalytic Reduction

$$\xrightarrow[\text{Pd}]{H_2}$$

Electrophilic Addition of HX

$$\xrightarrow{+H^+} \xrightarrow{Br^-}$$

Electrophilic Addition of X_2

Anti-addition

Electrophilic Addition of H_2O

$$\xrightarrow[H_2O]{H^+} \xrightarrow{H_2O}$$

$$\xrightarrow[-H^+]{H_2O^+}$$

Free Radical Addition (anti-Markovnikov)

$$\xrightarrow{Br \cdot} \xrightarrow{HBr} + Br \cdot$$

most stable radical

Hydroboration (anti-Markovnikov, syn orientation)

$$R =$$

$$3 \xrightarrow{BH_3} \xrightarrow[OH^-]{H_2O_2} 3$$

Oxidation with $KMnO_4$

$$\xrightarrow[KMnO_4]{\text{cold, dilute}} + MnO_2(s)$$

Oxidation with O_3

$$\xrightarrow[\text{2) } Zn/H_2O]{\text{1) } O_3, CH_2Cl_2} 2$$

ALDEHYDES

The dipole moment of aldehydes causes an elevation of boiling point, but not as high as alcohols since there is no hydrogen bonding.

Synthesis

- Oxidation of primary alcohols
- Ozonolysis of alkenes
- Friedel–Crafts acylation

Reactions

Reactions of Enols (Michael additions)

$$\xrightarrow{\text{Base}} + \text{H:Base}$$

$$\longrightarrow + \text{Base}$$

Nucleophilic addition to a carbonyl

$$\xrightarrow{} \xrightarrow{H^+}$$

Aldol condensation

An aldehyde acts both as nucleophile (enol form) and target (keto form)

CARBOXYLIC ACIDS

Carboxylic acids have pKa's of around 4.5 due to resonance stabilization of the conjugate base. Electronegative atoms increase acidity with inductive effects. Boiling point is higher than alcohols because of the ability to form two hydrogen bonds.

Synthesis

Oxidation of primary alcohols with $KMnO_4$

Organometallic reagents with CO_2 (Grignard)

Hydrolysis of Nitriles

Reactions

Formation of soap by reacting carboxylic acids with NaOH; arrange in micelles

nonpolar tail   polar head

Nucleophilic acyl substitution

Ester formation

Acyl halide formation

Reduction to alcohols

ALCOHOLS

- Higher boiling points than alkanes
- Weakly acidic hydroxyl hydrogen

Synthesis

- Addition of water to double bonds
- S_N1 and S_N2 reactions
- Reduction of carboxylic acids, aldehydes, ketones and esters
  - aldehydes and ketones with $NaBH_4$
  - esters and carboxylic acids with $LiAlH_4$

Reactions

E1 dehydration reactions in strongly acidic solutions

Substitution reactions after protonation or leaving group conversion

Oxidation

- PCC takes a primary alcohol to an aldehyde

- Jones's reagent, $KMnO_4$, and alkali dichromate salts will convert secondary alcohols to ketones and primary alcohols to carboxylic acids

- Tertiary alcohols cannot be oxidized without breaking a carbon to carbon bond

Oxidation and reduction

Wittig Reaction

phosphonium salt   ylide

CARBOXLIC ACID DERIVATIVES

Acyl halides

Nucleophilic acyl substitution

Friedel–Crafts acylation

Reduction

Anhydrides

Synthesis via reaction of carboxylic acid with an acid chloride

Hydrolysis

Conversion into esters and carboxylic acids

Addition of ammonia to form amides

Friedel–Crafts acylation

Amines & Nitrogen Containing Compounds

Amide   Carbamate   Imine   Enamine

Azide   Nitrile   Isocyanate

Direct alkylation of ammonia

$$CH_3Br + NH_3 \longrightarrow CH_3\overset{+}{N}H_3Br^- \xrightarrow{NaOH} CH_3NH_2 + NaBr + H_2O$$

Reduction from nitro compounds, nitriles, imines, and amides

$$CH_3CH_2C\equiv N \xrightarrow{LAH} CH_3CH_2CH_2NH_2$$

Exhaustive methylation (Hoffman elimination)

Gabriel Synthesis

Amides

Synthesis via reaction of acid chlorides with amines or acid anhydrides with ammonia

Hydrolysis

Hoffman rearrangement converts amides to primary amines

nitrene   isocyanate

Reduction with LAH

Esters

Synthesis via condensation of carboxylic acids and alcohols

Hydrolysis in acid or base

Conversion to amides

Transesterification

Grignard addition

Claisen Condensation

Reduction